The Ultimate Medical School Rotation Guide

Stewart H. Lecker • Bliss J. Chang

Editors

The Ultimate Medical School Rotation Guide

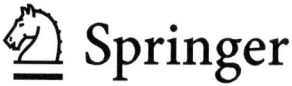 Springer

Editors
Stewart H. Lecker
Beth Israel Deaconness Medical Center
Boston, MA, USA

Bliss J. Chang
Harvard Medical School
Boston, MA, USA

ISBN 978-3-030-63559-6   ISBN 978-3-030-63560-2   (eBook)
https://doi.org/10.1007/978-3-030-63560-2

This Springer imprint is published by the registered company Springer Nature Switzerland AG
The registered company address is: Gewerbestrasse 11, 6330 Cham, Switzerland

To:
Ahn Hyee, Moon, and Bright

Preface

I remember the frustration of asking upperclassmen what resources they used to prepare for a rotation and being given a mélange of answers that all came back to one theme—existing board preparation resources such as First Aid, Step Up to Medicine, and Case Files. While these are great for standardized exams, they do not contain the depth or practical details necessary to be successful on a rotation. You cannot, for instance, merely know that the solution to heart failure exacerbation is "diuresis"; there is much more depth to providing great clinical care. What does it mean to "be helpful" when in the OR? What separates the superstars from the average student is all in the *details*.

This work was born to finally put to rest the age-old question of "How do I prepare for this rotation?" It is meant to be a concise, one-stop resource for you to use for your rotations. This work brings together twenty of the most talented medical students I know, utilizing their experience and expertise to distill down everything you need to know and do to ace your rotations. Without fluff, it covers the most common cases you will encounter as a medical student. We provide you with everything we knew at the end of a rotation that we wish we had known at the beginning. There is a true power and benefit to a work like this, written by medical students, for medical students.

With the upcoming Pass/Fail changes to USMLE Step 1 in 2022, clerkship performance will likely be by far the most important criteria for residency applications. In fact, the letter of recommendation from attendings you've worked with is already one of the most important factors—it is the best insight into your clinical skills and potential to be a stellar resident. Given the subjective nature of student evaluations, obtaining great evaluations is a daunting and uncertain prospect. However, our hope is that this book can help you convince even the most subjective of evaluators to provide you with the stellar evaluations you deserve so you can pursue your dream residency and career.

All the best in your studies. May medicine benefit from your successes on the wards.

Bliss J. Chang
Harvard Medical School
Class of 2020

Acknowledgments

Lead Editor
Bliss J. Chang
Harvard Medical School
Class of 2020

Co-Editor
Stewart H. Lecker, MD, PhD
Assistant Professor of Medicine, Harvard Medical School
Director, Nephrology Fellowship Training Program
Beth Israel Deaconess Medical Center
Boston, MA

Radiology Image Team
Sukjin Koh, MD
Department of Interventional Radiology
Brigham and Women's Hospital
Boston, MA

Colette M. Glaser, MD
Department of Radiology
Brigham and Women's Hospital
Boston, MA

Erika M. Chow, M.D., M.B.A.
Department of Radiology
Brigham and Women's Hospital
Boston, MA

Interpersonal Skills
Authored by:
Jeffrey Herrala
Harvard Medical School
Class of 2020

Faculty Reviewers:
Erik Alexander, MD
Professor of Medicine, Harvard Medical School
Director of Undergraduate Medical Education and the Principal Clerkship Experience
Executive Director of the Brigham Education Institute
Brigham and Women's Hospital
Boston, MA

William C. Taylor, MD
Associate Professor of Population Medicine, Harvard Medical School
Department of Population Medicine, Brigham and Women's Hospital
Director of Medical Education, Harvard Vanguard Medical Associates
Boston, MA

Student Reviewers:
Allison A. Merz
Harvard Medical School
Class of 2020

Pranayraj Kondapally
University of South Alabama Medical School
Class of 2022

Adam Beckman
Harvard Medical School
Class of 2022

Priya Shah
Harvard Medical School
Class of 2022

Lin Mu
Yale School of Medicine
Class of 2020

Wellness
Authored by:
Amira Song
Harvard College
Class of 2020

Student Reviewers:
Bliss J. Chang
Harvard Medical School
Class of 2020

What Attendings/Residents Look For
Authored by:
Bliss J. Chang
Harvard Medical School
Class of 2020

Stewart H. Lecker, MD, PhD
Assistant Professor of Medicine, Harvard Medical School
Director, Nephrology Fellowship Training Program
Beth Israel Deaconess Medical Center
Boston, MA

Faculty/Fellow/Resident Contributors:
Krishna Agarwal, MD
Melanie Hoenig, MD
Larissa Kruger, MD
Rahul Maheshwari, MD
Wilfredo R. Matias, MD
Edison K Miyawaki, MD
Subha Perni, MD
Celeste Royce, MD
Stephen Sozio, MD
Anonymous x3

Student Reviewers:
Curtis Bashore
University of Minnesota Medical School
Class of 2021

Jenna Fleming
University of Minnesota Medical School
Class of 2021

Amanda Zhou
Yale School of Medicine
Class of 2022

Clinical Tips and Pearls
Authored by:
  Bliss J. Chang
  Harvard Medical School
  Class of 2020

Student Reviewers:
  Cara Lachtrupp
  Harvard Medical School
  Class of 2021

  Lin Mu
  Yale School of Medicine
  Class of 2020

EMR Tips and Tricks
Authored by:
  Bliss J. Chang
  Harvard Medical School
  Class of 2020

Screenshots Courtesy of:
  Epic Systems Corporation
  1979 Milky Way
  Verona, WI 53593

Reviewed by:
  Epic Systems Corporation
  1979 Milky Way
  Verona, WI 53593

Student Reviewers:
  Daniel Michelson
  University of Minnesota Medical School
  Class of 2021

  Amrita Singh
  Yale School of Medicine
  Class of 2023

Internal Medicine
Authored by:
  Bliss J. Chang
  Harvard Medical School
  Class of 2020

Faculty Reviewers:
  Yamini Saravanan, MD
  Internal Medicine Clerkship Director, Cambridge Health Alliance Hospital
  Instructor in Medicine, Harvard Medical School
  Boston, MA

Student Reviewers:
  Simon Yang
  University of Minnesota Medical School
  Class of 2021

  Lucas Zellmer
  University of Minnesota Medical School
  Class of 2021

  Baraa Hijaz
  Harvard Medical School
  Class of 2024

General Surgery
Authored by:
  Selena Li
  Harvard Medical School
  Class of 2020

Faculty Reviewers:
  Roy Phitayakorn, MD MHPE (Med) FACS
  Associate Professor of Surgery, Harvard Medical School
  Director of Medical Student Education and Surgery Education
  Massachusetts General Hospital
  Boston, MA

  Elan Witkowski, MD
  Instructor in Surgery, Harvard Medical School
  Department of Surgery, Massachusetts General Hospital
  Boston, MA

Student Reviewers:
  Ameen Barghi
  Harvard Medical School
  Class of 2020

  Danny Wang
  WashU St. Louis School of Medicine
  Class of 2020

  Lena Trager
  University of Minnesota Medical School
  Class of 2022

  Huma Baig
  Harvard Medical School
  Class of 2021

OB-GYN
Authored by:
  Allison A. Merz
  Harvard Medical School
  Class of 2020

Faculty Reviewers:
  Celeste Royce, M.D.
  Assistant Professor of Obstetrics, Gynecology, and Reproductive Biology
  Beth Israel Deaconess Medical Center
  Harvard Medical School
  Boston, MA

Student Reviewers:
Jeffrey Herrala
Harvard Medical School
Class of 2020

Meagan Brockman
University of Minnesota Medical School
Class of 2021

Neurology
Authored by:
Iyas Daghlas
Harvard Medical School
Class of 2021

Faculty Reviewers:
Edison Miyawaki, MD
Assistant Professor of Neurology, Harvard Medical School
Department of Neurology, Brigham and Women's Hospital
Boston, MA

Student Reviewers:
Ellen Zhang
Harvard Medical School
Class of 2023

Apurv H. Shekhar
Yale School of Medicine
Class of 2023

Charlie W. Zhao
Yale School of Medicine
Class of 2021

Pediatrics
Authored by:
Aditya Achanta
Harvard Medical School
Class of 2021

Kelly Hallowell
University of Minnesota Medical School
Class of 2021

Faculty Reviewers:
Joanne Cox, MD
Associate Professor of Pediatrics, Harvard Medical School
Associate Chief, Division of General Pediatrics
Boston Children's Hospital
Boston, MA

Student Reviewers:
Margaret Irwin
Harvard Medical School
Class of 2021

Logan Beyer
Harvard Medical School
Class of 2023

Radiology
Authored by:
 Bliss J. Chang
 Harvard Medical School
 Class of 2020

Psychiatry
Authored by:
 Michael Dinh
 Harvard Medical School
 Class of 2020

Faculty Reviewers:
 Stuart Beck, MD
 Assistant Professor of Psychiatry, Harvard Medical School
 Department of Psychiatry, Massachusetts General Hospital
 Boston, MA

Student Reviewers:
 Catherine Bledsoe
 University of Minnesota Medical School
 Class of 2021

 David Johnson
 University of Minnesota Medical School
 Class of 2023

 Itamar Shapira
 UAB School of Medicine
 Class of 2023

Primary Care
Authored by:
 Bliss J. Chang
 Harvard Medical School
 Class of 2020

Faculty Reviewers:
 Yamini Saravanan, MD
 Internal Medicine Clerkship Director, Cambridge Health Alliance Hospital
 Instructor in Medicine, Harvard Medical School
 Boston, MA

Student Reviewers:
 Azan Virji
 Harvard Medical School
 Class of 2023

 Jack Inglis
 University of Minnesota Medical School
 Class of 2021

Emergency Medicine
Authored by:
 Alex Bonilla
 Harvard Medical School
 Class of 2020

Faculty Reviewers:

Susan E. Farrell, MD, EdM
Director, OSCE Program
Associate Professor, Emergency Medicine
Harvard Medical School
Boston, MA

Andy Jagoda, MD, FACEP
Professor and Chair Emeritus
Department of Emergency Medicine
Icahn School of Medicine at Mount Sinai
New York City, New York

Student Reviewers:

Lake Crawford
Yale School of Medicine
Class of 2023

John McGrory
University of Minnesota Medical School
Class of 2021

Critical Care

Authored by:

Balakrishnan Pillai
Medical University of South Carolina
Class of 2020

Ultrasound Images by:

J. Terrill Huggins, MD
Designated Education Officer
Ralph H. Johnson VA Medical Center
Professor of Medicine, Medical University of South Carolina
Division of Pulmonary, Critical Care, Allergy and Sleep Medicine
Charleston, SC

Faculty Reviewers:

Alice M. Boylan, MD
Professor of Medicine, Medical University of South Carolina
Chief, Acute, Critical, and Trauma Integrated Center of Clinical Excellence
Charleston, SC

Student Reviewers:

Amrita Singh
Yale School of Medicine
Class of 2023

Cardiology

Authored by:

Bliss J. Chang
Harvard Medical School
Class of 2020

Faculty Reviewer:
    Leonard S. Lilly, M.D.
    Professor of Medicine, Harvard Medical School
    Chief, Brigham/Faulkner Cardiology
    Brigham and Women's Hospital
    Boston, MA

Fellow Reviewer:
    Timothy J. Fernandez, M.D.
    Emory University
    Cardiology Fellow, Class of 2022

Student Reviewers:
    Ethan Katznelson
    Harvard Medical School
    Class of 2020

    Lena Trager
    University of Minnesota Medical School
    Class of 2022

Gastroenterology
Authored by:
    Emily Gutowski
    Harvard Medical School
    Class of 2020

Faculty Reviewers:
    Navin Kumar, MD
    Instructor in Medicine, Harvard Medical School
    Department of Gastroenterology, Brigham and Women's Hospital
    Boston, MA

Student Reviewers:
    Itamar Shapira
    UAB School of Medicine
    Class of 2023

    Hema Pingali
    Harvard Medical School
    Class of 2021

    Gaurav Suryawanshi
    University of Minnesota Medical School
    Class of 2020

Nephrology
Authored by:
    Bliss J. Chang
    Harvard Medical School
    Class of 2020

Faculty Reviewers:
    Stewart H. Lecker, MD, PhD
    Assistant Professor of Medicine, Harvard Medical School
    Director, Nephrology Fellowship Training Program
    Beth Israel Deaconess Medical Center
    Boston, MA

Infectious Diseases
Authored by:
  Bliss J. Chang
  Harvard Medical School
  Class of 2020

Faculty Reviewers:
  Simi Padival, MD
  Instructor in Medicine, Harvard Medical School
  Division of Infectious Diseases, Beth Israel Deaconess Medical Center
  Boston, MA

Student Reviewers:
  Azan Virji
  Harvard Medical School
  Class of 2023

  Bina Kassamali
  Harvard Medical School
  Class of 2022

Anesthesia
Authored by:
  Sarah Osmulski
  Harvard Medical School
  Class of 2020

Faculty Reviewers:
  Richard M. Pino, MD, PhD
  Division Chief, Critical Care
  Department of Anesthesia, Critical Care and Pain Medicine
  Massachusetts General Hospital
  Harvard Medical School
  Boston, MA

Student Reviewers:
  Michael Koller
  University of Minnesota Medical School
  Class of 2021

  Lovemore Peter Makusha
  Yale School of Medicine
  Class of 2020

Radiation Oncology
Authored by:
  Parsa Erfani
  Harvard Medical School
  Class of 2021

Faculty Reviewers:
  Matthew Abrams, MD
  Instructor in Radiation Oncology, Harvard Medical School
  Beth Israel Deaconess Medical Center
  Boston, MA

Resident Reviewers:
Subha Perni, MD
Resident, Harvard Radiation Oncology Program
Harvard Medical School
Boston, MA

Sharareh Koufigar, MS
Medical Physics Resident
Piedmont Cancer Institute
Atlanta, GA

Student Reviewers:
Grace Lee
Harvard Medical School
Class of 2020

Kerrie Greene
Yale School of Medicine
Class of 2023

Dermatology
Authored by:
Connie Zhong
Harvard Medical School
Class of 2020

Faculty Reviewers:
Jennifer Huang, MD
Dermatology Clerkship Director, Harvard Medical School
Boston Children's Hospital
Brigham and Women's Hospital
Boston, MA

Vinod Nambudiri, MD
Assistant Professor of Dermatology, Harvard Medical School
Department of Dermatology, Brigham and Women's Hospital
Boston, MA

Susan Burgin, MD
Associate Professor of Dermatology, Harvard Medical School
Department of Dermatology, Brigham and Women's Hospital
Boston, MA

Student Reviewers:
Amy Blum
Harvard Medical School
Class of 2021

Bina Kassamali
Harvard Medical School
Class of 2022

James Pathoulas
University of Minnesota Medical School
Class of 2021

Orthopedic Surgery

Authored by:
Ameen Barghi
Harvard Medical School
Class of 2020

Faculty Reviewers:
James Herndon, MD MBA
Chair Emeritus, Department of Orthopedics
Massachusetts General Hospital
Boston, MA

James D. Kang, MD
Chair, Department of Orthopedics
Brigham and Women's Hospital
Boston, MA

Edward K. Rodriguez, MD
Clerkship Director, Orthopedics
Associate Professor of Orthopedic Surgery
Beth Israel Deaconess Medical Center
Boston, MA

Collin May, MD, MPH
Clerkship Director, Pediatric Orthopedics
Instructor in Orthopedic Surgery, Boston Children's Hospital
Harvard Medical School
Boston, MA

Student Reviewers:
Lily Wood
University of Minnesota Medical School
Class of 2020

Neurosurgery

Authored by:
Malia McAvoy
Harvard Medical School
Class of 2020

Zack Abecaissis
Northwestern Feinberg School of Medicine
Class of 2020

Faculty Reviewers:
Richard Ellenbogen, MD
Chair, Department of Neurosurgery
University of Washington
Seattle, WA

G. Rees Cosgrove, MD
Lecturer on Neurosurgery, Harvard Medical School
Neurosurgery Program Director, Brigham and Women's Hospital
Boston, MA

Student Reviewers:

Tony Larson
University of Minnesota Medical School
Class of 2022

Julia Song
Harvard Medical School
Class of 2022

Charlie W. Zhao
Yale School of Medicine
Class of 2021

Ophthalmology
Authored by:
Theodore Bowe
Harvard Medical School
Class of 2020

Faculty Reviewers:

Yoshihiro Yonekawa, MD
Assistant Professor of Ophthalmology, Sidney Kimmel Medical College
Thomas Jefferson University
Wills Eye Hospital
Philadelphia, PA

Zeba A. Syed, MD
Assistant Professor of Ophthalmology, Sidney Kimmel Medical College
Thomas Jefferson University
Wills Eye Hospital
Philadelphia, PA

Student Reviewers:

Sameen Meshkin
Harvard Medical School
Class of 2022

Osama M. Ahmed
Yale School of Medicine
Class of 2021

Introduction

Welcome to *The Ultimate Medical School Rotation Guide*. We are thrilled to embark on a journey with you through the clinical years of medical school. Our mission is simple: to help you learn the most medicine while earning the best evaluations and maximizing your physical and mental well-being.

Clinical rotations are the highlight of medical school for many, if not most, medical students. It is a daunting period where you transition from the classroom onto the hospital wards and begin interacting with patients. Your actions take on consequences for your patient and your team. Despite all this, it is one of the most fun and rewarding periods of your life as you spend long days with your teams and hold intimate conversations with the ill. By the end of your rotations, you will be in awe at how much medicine you have learned and how you have matured as a clinician and person.

We encourage you to start by familiarizing yourself with the soft skills of medicine and general tips for success on the wards. These fundamental skills will form the foundation for any rotation, and are arguably as important if not more important than the content of a specific rotation. As you near the start of a rotation, you will ideally read through the respective chapter and then revisit it throughout your rotation.

We wish you all the best with your clinical endeavors and look forward to working with you in the future as our dear colleagues.

Contents

Contents

Contributors

Zack Abecaissis   Northwestern Feinberg School of Medicine, Class of 2020, Chicago, IL, USA

Aditya Achanta   Harvard Medical School, Class of 2021, Boston, MA, USA

Ameen Barghi   Harvard Medical School, Class of 2020, Boston, MA, USA

Alex Bonilla   Harvard Medical School, Class of 2020, Boston, MA, USA

Theodore Bowe   Harvard Medical School, Class of 2020, Boston, MA, USA

Bliss J. Chang   Harvard Medical School, Class of 2020, Boston, MA, USA

Iyas Daghlas   Harvard Medical School, Class of 2021, Boston, MA, USA

Michael Dinh   Harvard Medical School, Class of 2020, Boston, MA, USA

Parsa Erfani   Harvard Medical School, Class of 2021, Boston, MA, USA

Emily Gutowski   Harvard Medical School, Class of 2020, Boston, MA, USA

Kelly Hallowell   University of Minnesota Medical School, Class of 2021, Minneapolis, MN, USA

Jeffrey Herrala   Harvard Medical School, Class of 2020, Boston, MA, USA

Stewart H. Lecker   Assistant Professor of Medicine, Harvard Medical School, Boston, MA, USA
Director, Nephrology Fellowship Training Program, Beth Israel Deaconess Medical Center, Boston, MA, USA

Selena Li   Harvard Medical School, Class of 2020, Boston, MA, USA

Malia McAvoy   Harvard Medical School, Class of 2020, Boston, MA, USA

Allison A. Merz   Harvard Medical School, Class of 2020, Boston, MA, USA

Sarah Osmulski   Harvard Medical School, Class of 2020, Boston, MA, USA

Balakrishnan Pillai   Medical University of South Carolina, Class of 2020, Charleston, SC, USA

Amira Song   Harvard College, Class of 2022, Cambridge, MA, USA

Connie Zhong   Harvard Medical School, Class of 2020, Boston, MA, USA

Faculty Reviewers

Matthew Abrams, MD   Instructor in Radiation Oncology, Harvard Medical School, Boston, MA, USA
Beth Israel Deaconess Medical Center, Boston, MA, USA

Erik Alexander, MD Professor of Medicine, Harvard Medical School, Boston, MA, USA

Director of Undergraduate Medical Education and the Principal Clerkship Experience, Boston, MA, USA

Executive Director of the Brigham Education Institute, Boston, MA, USA

Stuart Beck Assistant Professor of Psychiatry, Harvard Medical School, Boston, MA, USA

Department of Psychiatry, Massachusetts General Hospital, Boston, MA, USA

Alice M. Boylan, MD Professor of Medicine, Medical University of South Carolina, Charleston, SC, USA

Chief, Acute, Critical, and Trauma Integrated Center of Clinical Excellence, Charleston, SC, USA

Susan Burgin Associate Professor of Dermatology, Harvard Medical School, Boston, MA, USA

Department of Dermatology, Brigham and Women's Hospital, Boston, MA, USA

Joanne Cox, MD Associate Professor of Pediatrics, Harvard Medical School, Boston, MA, USA

Associate Chief, Division of General Pediatrics, Boston Children's Hospital, Boston, MA, USA

Susan E. Farrell, MD, EdM Director, OSCE Program, Boston, MA, USA

Associate Professor, Emergency Medicine, Harvard Medical School, Boston, MA, USA

James Herndon, MD MBA Chair Emeritus, Department of Orthopedics, Massachusetts General Hospital, Boston, MA, USA

Jennifer Huang Dermatology Clerkship Director, Harvard Medical School, Boston, MA, USA

Boston Children's Hospital, Boston, MA, USA

Brigham and Women's Hospital, Boston, MA, USA

Andy Jagoda, MD, FACEP Professor and Chair Emeritus, Department of Emergency Medicine, Icahn School of Medicine at Mount Sinai, New York, NY, USA

James D. Kang, MD Chair, Department of Orthopedics, Brigham and Women's Hospital, Boston, MA, USA

Navin Kumar Instructor in Medicine, Harvard Medical School, Boston, MA, USA

Department of Gastroenterology, Brigham and Women's Hospital, Boston, MA, USA

Stewart H. Lecker, MD, PhD Assistant Professor of Medicine, Harvard Medical School, Boston, MA, USA

Director, Nephrology Fellowship Training Program, Beth Israel Deaconess Medical Center, Boston, MA, USA

Leonard S. Lilly, M.D. Professor of Medicine, Harvard Medical School, Boston, MA, USA

Chief, Brigham/Faulkner Cardiology, Brigham and Women's Hospital, Boston, MA, USA

Edison Miyawaki   Assistant Professor of Neurology, Harvard Medical School, Boston, MA, USA

Department of Neurology, Brigham and Women's Hospital, Boston, MA, USA

Vinod Nambudiri   Assistant Professor of Dermatology, Harvard Medical School, Boston, MA, USA

Department of Dermatology, Brigham and Women's Hospital, Boston, MA, USA

Simi Padival   Instructor in Medicine, Harvard Medical School, Boston, MA, USA

Division of Infectious Diseases, Beth Israel Deaconess Medical Center, Boston, MA, USA

Roy Phitayakorn, MD MHPE (Med) FACS   Associate Professor of Surgery, Harvard Medical School, Boston, MA, USA

Director of Medical Student Education and Surgery Education, Massachusetts General Hospital, Boston, MA, USA

Richard M. Pino, MD, PhD   Division Chief, Critical Care, Department of Anesthesia, Critical Care and Pain Medicine, Massachusetts General Hospital, Boston, MA, USA

Harvard Medical School, Boston, MA, USA

Edward K. Rodriguez, MD   Clerkship Director, Pediatric Orthopedics, Boston, MA, USA

Associate Professor of Orthopedic Surgery, Beth Israel Deaconess Medical Center, Boston, MA, USA

Yamini Saravanan   Internal Medicine Clerkship Director, Cambridge Health Alliance Hospital, Cambridge, MA, USA

Instructor in Medicine, Harvard Medical School, Boston, MA, USA

Zeba A. Syed, MD   Assistant Professor of Ophthalmology, Sidney Kimmel Medical College, Thomas Jefferson University, Wills Eye Hospital, Philadelphia, PA, USA

William C. Taylor, MD   Associate Professor of Population Medicine, Harvard Medical School, Boston, MA, USA

Department of Population Medicine, Brigham and Women's Hospital, Boston, MA, USA

Director of Medical Education, Harvard Vanguard Medical Associates, Boston, MA, USA

Elan Witkowski, MD   Instructor in Surgery, Harvard Medical School, Boston, MA, USA

Department of Surgery, Massachusetts General Hospital, Boston, MA, USA

Yoshihiro Yonekawa, MD   Assistant Professor of Ophthalmology, Sidney Kimmel Medical College, Philadelphia, PA, USA

Thomas Jefferson University, Wills Eye Hospital, Philadelphia, PA, USA

Student Reviewers

Osama M. Ahmed   Yale School of Medicine, New Haven, CT, USA

Huma Baig   Harvard Medical School, Boston, MA, USA

Contributors

Ameen Barghi   Harvard Medical School, Boston, MA, USA

Curtis Bashore   University of Minnesota Medical School, Minneapolis, MN, USA

Adam Beckman   Harvard Medical School, Boston, MA, USA

Logan Beyer   Harvard Medical School, Boston, MA, USA

Catherine Bledsoe   University of Minnesota Medical School, Minneapolis, MN, USA

Amy Blum   Harvard Medical School, Boston, MA, USA

Meagan Brockman   University of Minnesota Medical School, Minneapolis, MN, USA

Bliss J. Chang   Harvard Medical School, Boston, MA, USA

Lake Crawford   Yale School of Medicine, New Haven, CT, USA

Jenna Fleming   University of Minnesota Medical School, Minneapolis, MN, USA

Kerrie Greene   Yale School of Medicine, New Haven, CT, USA

Jeffrey Herrala   Harvard Medical School, Boston, MA, USA

Baraa Hijaz   Harvard Medical School, Boston, MA, USA

Jack Inglis   University of Minnesota Medical School, Minneapolis, MN, USA

Margaret Irwin   Harvard Medical School, Boston, MA, USA

David Johnson   University of Minnesota Medical School, Minneapolis, MN, USA

Ethan Katznelson   Harvard Medical School, Boston, MA, USA

Bina Kassamali   Harvard Medical School, Boston, MA, USA

Michael Koller   University of Minnesota Medical School, Minneapolis, MN, USA

Pranayraj Kondapally   University of South Alabama Medical School, Mobile, AL, USA

Cara Lachtrupp   Harvard Medical School, Boston, MA, USA

Tony Larson   University of Minnesota School of Medicine, Minneapolis, MN, USA

Grace Lee   Harvard Medical School, Boston, MA, USA

Lovemore Peter Makusha   Yale School of Medicine, New Haven, CT, USA

John McGrory   University of Minnesota Medical School, Minneapolis, MN, USA

Daniel Michelson   University of Minnesota Medical School, Minneapolis, MN, USA

Allison A. Merz   Harvard Medical School, Boston, MA, USA

Sameen Meshkin   Harvard Medical School, Boston, MA, USA

Lin Mu   Yale School of Medicine, New Haven, CT, USA

James Pathoulas   University of Minnesota Medical School, Minneapolis, MN, USA

Hema Pingali   Harvard Medical School, Boston, MA, USA

Priya Shah   Harvard Medical School, Boston, MA, USA

Itamar Shapira   UAB School of Medicine, Birmingham, AL, USA
UAB School of Medicine, Boston, MA, USA

Apurv H. Shekhar   Yale School of Medicine, New Haven, CT, USA

Amrita Singh   Yale School of Medicine, New Haven, CT, USA

Julia Song   Harvard Medical School, Boston, MA, USA

Gaurav Suryawanshi   University of Minnesota Medical School, Minneapolis, MN, USA

Lena Trager   University of Minnesota Medical School, Minneapolis, MN, USA

Azan Virji   Harvard Medical School, Boston, MA, USA

Danny Wang   WashU St. Louis School of Medicine, St. Louis, MO, USA

Lily Wood   University of Minnesota Medical School, Minneapolis, MN, USA

Simon Yang   University of Minnesota Medical School, Minneapolis, MN, USA

Lucas Zellmer   University of Minnesota Medical School, Minneapolis, MN, USA

Ellen Zhang   Harvard Medical School, Boston, MA, USA

Charlie W. Zhao   Yale School of Medicine, New Haven, CT, USA

Amanda Zhou   Yale School of Medicine, New Haven, CT, USA

Fellow Reviewer

Timothy J. Fernandez, M.D.   Emory University, Atlanta, GA, USA

Resident Reviewers

Sharareh Koufigar, MS   Piedmont Cancer Institute, Atlanta, GA, USA

Subha Perni, MD   Harvard Radiation Oncology Program, Harvard Medical School, Boston, MA, USA

Interpersonal Skills

Jeffrey Herrala

Contents

© The Author(s), under exclusive license to Springer Nature Switzerland AG 2021
S. H. Lecker, B. J. Chang (eds.), *The Ultimate Medical School Rotation Guide*,
https://doi.org/10.1007/978-3-030-63560-2_1

1

» The end of all knowledge should surely be service to others (César Chávez)

1.1 Introduction

From the start of a student's first clinical rotation, a shift in expectations occurs. In this new role, the value placed on an individual's performance (e.g., fund of knowledge, test scores) diminishes, and in its place rises the importance of a trainee's sincere motivation to serve their patients, families, and the medical team. The significance of a patient-centered and service-oriented medical student cannot be overemphasized. With this mindset, the student becomes a tremendous advocate, ally, and an irreplaceable teammate, vastly improving team interactions and patient care.

However, even with such intentions, the medical learning environment can be disorienting for trainees. In the absence of formal skills development, interpersonal habits (both desired and undesired) are left to be inherited from peers, from supervisors, or through trial and error. This process, commonly referred to as the "hidden curriculum," is a common source of stress for learners. Thus, this chapter seeks to accomplish the following: (1) describe the function of the medical learning environment, (2) provide an approach to forge interpersonal connections within the medical setting, and (3) improve patient care and alleviate student stress by outlining expectations and advice for common scenarios and relationships.

1.2 Sections

1. The Medical Learning Environment
2. The AMIGAS Framework
3. Suggestion Tables for Various Relationships and Scenarios Patients and Families
   (a) Attending and Fellows
   (b) Residents and Interns
   (c) Nurses and Staff
   (d) Peer Medical Students
   (e) Pre-rounds and Rounds
4. Special Topics Making Mistakes and Apologies
   (a) High-Stakes Conversations
   (b) The End of the Day
   (c) Feedback and Challenging Team Dynamics

1.2.1 The Medical Learning Environment

To be interpersonal experts, students must honor and equally value the contributions of each member of the medical learning environment, no matter their role: janitorial staff, clerks, attendings, and co-students alike. Each member of the team is uniquely skilled and mission essential for patient care and should be regarded as such. Outstanding medical students (as well as attendings, nurses, and residents for that matter) are patient-centered and ambitiously invest in interpersonal connection in all areas of the medical learning environment.

1.2.2 The AMIGAS Framework

While forging interpersonal relationships in the medical environment may come naturally for some, others may benefit from a formulaic approach for this skill. To this end, we offer the "AMIGAS" framework, one possible framework for relationship building. Each step—absorb, mirror, imagine, goal, ask, and serve—is described below. Once learned, these steps can be adapted to various situations and relationships.

▪▪ Absorb

This is the information gathering stage. As medical students, we are frequently placed in unfamiliar and complex situations before fully understanding their context. Asked to join a new team or meet a patient, we might speak or act in ways we regret once further information about the situation or individual becomes apparent. Classic examples of this are using technical jargon with someone who prefers another language or speaking in overly simplified terms to a patient we later learn is a physician. A student might joke only to realize that the tone was previously somber or speak too loudly when a team is using soft voices. We might walk slowly on rounds when others expect us to rush or move too quickly when a process demands meticulousness.

To avoid these situations, during the absorb stage, teach yourself to be maximally observant so you can keep learning and growing based on what you see. This is a habit of thought to be developed continually. Absorb everything about the scenario or an individual: what is the overall mood of the setting? What volume and cadence of speech is used in conversation? What is a patient's level of medical literacy? Where are ice chips and patient food located on the hospital floor? How long are patient presentations on this service? Interpersonal connections should be formed at a slow and steady rate, while each party learns from the other's cues. Remember the importance of this first step, even when pressured for time.

▪▪ Mirror

Mirror is a reflection stage and occurs simultaneously with the absorb stage. As we absorb information about an individual or a situation, we should subtly reflect the positive things we observe: a person's posture, head tilt, tone, voice, cadence, etc. People feel more comfortable and safe when they notice that others are willing to meet them where they are. We do this to communicate our desire to make others comfortable and show them that we are reliably there to take care of them. If an individual appears sad or overjoyed, adjust your mood and nonverbal communication to mirror them. Pay attention to how individuals respond to each of your gestures and adjust accordingly. When speaking, be sure to save space for others, especially patients, by pausing occasionally. Absorbing allows you to obtain as much information as possible about your surroundings before action is required, and mirroring appropriate gestures and affect sets others at ease while you identify next steps.*

*Only mirror *appropriate and professional behaviors* of patients and the medical team. As a human institution, the medical establishment is far from immune to the unacceptable behaviors and attitudes held by society at large (systematic discrimination, implicit bias, racism, sexism, classism, xenophobia) which significantly affect the health of the patients and communities we seek to uplift. As medical students, we are charged with the responsibility of intervening on any unjust practices within medicine which propagate disparity. If we recognize inappropriate behavior expressed by peers, senior clinicians, patients, or other team members (such as unequal treatment of a patient due to a given

Pearl: It is important to mention that "overasking" exists. By asking many questions, you may exhaust or distract others from patient care. If your teammate seems overwhelmed and distracted or meets your question with a brisk reply, allow them space to refocus and complete their immediate task before asking another question (unless your request is urgent or concerning important patient matters, in which case asking your attending/resident immediately is encouraged).

Pearl: Don't be limited by what you see in one patient's room, the whole hospital is your pantry! This is a great example of going the extra mile for your patient.

Pearl: You can learn a lot about the patient in indirect ways. Do they furrow their eyebrows when you use certain words, indicating confusion? Or, are they using highly medicalized terms which suggest prior healthcare experience?

Pearl: When asking a patient if they need an interpreter, consider normalizing with something like, "We're taught it's always better to ask, as some people with excellent English language skills prefer to have an interpreter present."

1

Pearl: Setting realistic expectations early avoids feelings of surprise or disappointment surrounding common issues within the clinic or hospital. If the issue does occur, the patient and family will react more acceptingly, as they anticipated that it may happen beforehand.

Pearl: Important caveats to taking ownership include sharing significant decisions or pieces of information without your team's permission. Examples include:

1. Informing patient of new cancer diagnosis
2. Informing patient of HIV result
3. Speaking with family about the death of a loved one under your care
4. Promising medications, discharge dates/times, or procedure timing
5. Telling a patient they can eat when they are NPO

Pearl: Anyone who has been hospitalized knows how difficult it can be to get privacy and sleep. Doors and curtains are often left open, and providers may speak audibly in the hallways and workstations, leading patients to spend days and night restless. Further, patients are often connected to I.V.s and monitors and cannot ambulate to the door or light switch themselves. Rest and privacy are crucial for healing. Always ask for patient preferences with lights, doors, and curtains before you depart

demographic factor or a microaggression or racist slur used against ourselves or a peer), we must intervene. For a framework on intervening in situations of this kind, reference the work *Disarming Racial Microaggressions: Microintervention Strategies for Targets, White Allies, and Bystanders* by Derald Wing Sue et al.

▪▪ Imagine

In the imagine step, try synthesizing what you observed in the absorb and mirror stages and empathize with the person with whom you are interacting. Empathy is defined as the "ability to understand and share the feelings of another." Practice this skill by exploring the possible priorities, concerns, desires, and plans of the other person. From what their actions and verbal and nonverbal communication suggest, how might they feel about this visit, procedure, or hospitalization? If you were them, how would you feel about a medical student overseeing your care? What is it like to go without food or fluids for a day? What words might you want to hear? These are only hypotheses, subject to continuous testing and reframing.

Practice the same with your medical teammates. Imagine you are the intern: how do you feel about your level of expertise? What might make your job easier? Imagine you are the chief resident: what is it like to orient multiple students? Imagine you are an attending: what matters to you while leading the team? After you absorb information and mirror, use empathy to imagine what an individual might be feeling about a situation and about you.

▪▪ Goal

Now that you have imagined the thoughts, priorities, and desires of your patient or teammate, anticipate what their immediate goal might be. How could you as a medical student bring them closer to achieving this goal? Does your patient need water? A tissue? Might their tired family member benefit from a cup of coffee or tea? Are they preoccupied by a question that is above your level of expertise? What does your attending need for the next step in a procedure? Does the intern have a long list of to-dos keeping them in the hospital? No task is too menial and often small actions have a large impact on patients. Furthermore, if you help out with small tasks, your team is more likely to have extra time to teach you. Go the extra mile and do what others will not do. Identify your patient or colleague's most important goal and make it your own.

▪▪ Ask

At this point, you have ideas on how to help your patient, classmate, resident, or attending achieve their goal. However, each step has been built upon assumptions regarding the person's goals and preferences. What if you are wrong? What if your plan to assist would offend a teammate or make a task more difficult? Thus, it is always best to ask for permission before helping out. For example: "Dr. [Attending], is now an appropriate time for a question about the surgical anatomy in our patient?" "[Patient], would you like to discuss your results right now with family, or at another time?" "[Intern], would it be helpful for me to work on obtaining your patient's medical records from an outside hospital?" Find their goal, plan a solution, and ask permission before proceeding.

▪▪ Serve

Now it is time to serve! Ask your timely and thoughtful question, assist with a step in the procedure, or complete a favor for a teammate. Do it carefully, efficiently, and when it's appropriate, use closed-loop feedback to inform the individual of their goal's completion. For example: "I received the records by fax, reviewed them, and placed them in our patient's binder." Closed-loop feedback ensures the other person is aware of the task's completion and, further, reminds them that your efforts helped move the team closer to its goal(s). It is crucial that you do not dwell on this success, though. Announcing loudly or repeatedly that a task is complete may cause patients, peers, staff, or superiors to question your intentions or find your actions self-serving. Solve the problem, use closed-loop feedback once, and then repeat the AMIGAS process from the beginning. Use of the AMIGAS method works best when applied within a situation or relationship repeatedly.

To ensure that you are communicating authentically and how you intend, try practicing with a friend or family member. Have them act as a clinic or preoperative patient, an attending, a nurse, or a clerk. If you have not done so before, film yourself in this practice environment to ensure that your body language, posture, and style matches what you hope to communicate.

Finally, though the AMIGAS framework might be helpful, making hypotheses about the feelings and needs of everyone around you can be exhausting! This style of interaction requires intense attention to detail, emotional energy, and persistence.

1.2.3 Suggestion Tables for Various Relationships and Scenarios

Using the AMIGAS method, it is possible to infer many ways to forge positive relationships on your medical team. However, specific examples may be useful, especially if you have never tried or seen them practiced before. In the tables below, we will provide recommendations as they apply to various relationships.

■ ■ Patients and Families

By default, the needs of the patient and their family must come first. If as a medical student you recognize a factor impeding a patient's care, you should bring it to the team's attention in a tactful and timely fashion. If done well, they should appreciate this intervention. See the table below for ideas for incorporating excellence into interactions with patients and families (◘ Table 1.1).

■ ■ Attendings, Fellows, and Advanced Practitioners

Leading the medical team, attendings (and in many clinical contexts, fellows and advanced practitioners) are tasked with crucial decisions for a large panel of patients: end-of-life discussions, surgical planning, ICU transfers, coordination with consulting services, etc. Similarly, though nuances exist between advanced practitioners (physician's assistants, nurse practitioners) and attendings, they should be treated similarly to attendings in most situations. Avoid the term "mid-level provider," as this can be seen as disrespectful. While attendings, fellows, and advanced practitioners may verify documentation, history and exam findings, and decisions, it is often difficult to be comprehensive due to competing demands. Therefore, closed-loop feedback and self-sufficiency in problem-solving while never appropriating decision-making beyond your level of responsibility are essential to earn their trust. Interactions with attendings should remain succinct, positive, triaged by your interns/residents/nurses, and reflect your decision-making ability and dedication to patients. Before asking a question, attempt to answer it yourself: if a patient's labs return abnormal, form your own differential, diagnostic plan, and initial treatment. If

Pearl: This is something you can ask for specific feedback on from your team and will demonstrate your thoughtfulness and dedication to patient-centered care.

Pearl: When a question is above your level, resist the temptation to provide inaccurate or incomplete answers. Elevate these to the team at the beginning or conclusion of your oral presentation.

Pearl: Unfortunately, this is surprisingly common by medical professionals. "I'll be back later" means that you will indeed visit them prior to leaving that day.

Pearl: Keep in mind that patients often nod "yes" to questions, even if they do not understand you, to be respectful.

Pearl: Attendings and residents cannot enter orders until you present to them, and this can be a significant source of delay for patient care. Aim for 30 minutes between being assigned a patient and presenting them to the team (though context dependent, e.g., shorter for ED patients, longer for new patient visits at PCP office).

1

□ Table 1.1 Patients and families

Encouraged	Avoid
• Knock and wait for a positive response prior to entering any room. • Awaken sleeping patients gracefully if you must interact with them. • Ask if now is a good time and if they would like family members in or out of the room. • Whenever possible, sit at the patient's bedside (if there is no chair, bring one in). • Speak slowly and gently. Pause often to allow for processing and questions. • Follow your patient's lead (smile if they are smiling, be serious if they are serious). • Introduce your role early and repeat your name several times (the hospital is a disorienting place—they will appreciate the reminder). • Ask how they prefer to be addressed and the proper pronunciation of their name. • Remember names for key family members. Jot them down if helpful. • Learn about them: what are they missing out on while in the hospital? Do they have any specific fears? What is their level of medical literacy? Do they have language preferences? • It's always okay to inquire respectfully with something like, "I wondered from your expression/pause/reaction if my comment might have upset/concerned/confused you." If appropriate, maybe add, "That certainly wasn't my intention" or some such clarifier. • Use layperson terms; avoid medical jargon. • Obtain an in-person or phone interpreter when needed. • To prepare for this, ask staff how to use the interpreter services on day #1, write down the phone number, and schedule this for the team whenever needed. • If an in-person interpreter is available, inform teammates of their scheduled arrival time before rounds. If using phone interpretation, call while walking to the patient's room to provide details they routinely request before entering the patient's room. This vastly improves patient care and team efficiency. • When using an interpreter, speak in 1–2 sentences at a time; this is better for patient comprehension and interpreter memory. • Ask permission before performing physical examinations, and inform patients of exactly what you are doing. • Set expectations early, for example: "Today will be a long day, Ms. G. Many patients in the Emergency Department find the wait exhausting. We will do our best to keep things moving quickly" or "Your procedure is scheduled for 2 PM, but changes and delays often occur. We will keep you up to date with any changes." • Communicate that your primary goal as medical student is to advocate for them, move care forward, answer questions, keep them comfortable, and ensure they are up to date with the plan. • Advocate: you often have more time for each patient than your teammates. Use this time to advocate for your patients. Was a medication dosage miscalculated? Has the patient been repeatedly awoken by labs or vitals that are now unnecessary for care? Your oral presentation on daily rounds provides you with a platform to advocate for any of these changes. • Take ownership: as permitted by the team, be the first to inform your patient of lab findings, changes in procedure timing, discharge plan, etc. As able, update family members at the patient's request. • In all of these situations, allow your attending/resident to determine who is the best person to inform the patient of particular information. • Provide patients (as allowed by the treatment plan) water, coffee, snacks, ice chips, and warm blankets. Whenever the opportunity presents itself, say the following: "My goal is to make you as comfortable as possible, what else can I do?" • If you find yourself without anything to do, check-in again with each of your patients. Do they have any new symptoms, questions, concerns, or requests? • Does the patient or family have any social concerns they are afraid to discuss (finances, legal issues, etc.)? Gently probe, and if present, offer a social work consultation. • When leaving any room, ask the patient if they prefer their door and curtain open or closed and if their lights should be on or off.	• Repeatedly mispronounce names, misgender a patient, or refer to them only by age and diagnosis—especially during patient-centered rounds, keep it personal. • Stand above a patient while talking. • Use overly technical or overly simplified language (too difficult = risk of misunderstanding; too simple = patronizing). • Examine a patient without their permission. • Leave a room without providing the patient time to ask questions. • Answer questions that are above your abilities or level of decision-making (regarding NPO status, admission, or discharge plan). • Break promises, such as forgetting to forward a request onto the team, fetch water, etc. This forces your patients to repeat requests to you or someone else (which can be embarrassing and difficult given vulnerable status of patients) and is deleterious to trust-building. • Rely on a suboptimal second language skill (on your part or a patient's part) to communicate information. Be humble; arrange a professional interpreter whenever necessary. • A history gathered without aid from a professional interpreter may yield inaccurate and potentially dangerous information. • Delay care by spending excessive time between gathering a patient's H&P and reporting your plan to the team. • Begin speaking to a patient or family member about clinical matters without first asking how they are doing. • Share medical matters in front of family members without gaining the patient's permission. Ideally, seek such permission before a family member is present

a patient has a rare condition, read as much as you can and share your plan with the team. If you are unsure of what to do next, suggest your own plan, and then ask for their input. Attendings (and all teammates for that matter) greatly appreciate the energy you invest in thinking through the details of your patient's care. In complicated cases, the time you spend thinking through a problem or reviewing the literature will refresh even your attendings memory and answer questions they may have otherwise needed to review.

Despite fewer interactions with your attending, their evaluations of your clinical care are most heavily weighted in your rotation performance. Furthermore, though students focus on oral presentations and responses to knowledge-probing questions, remember that attendings closely evaluate your interpersonal skills on rounds, in the work room, in clinic, and on the floor. Interpersonal skills are one of the core Entrustable Professional Activities (EPAs) which many schools are transitioning to for student evaluations (EPA 9: Collaborate as a Member of an Interprofessional Team, ▶ https://www.aamc.org/system/files/c/2/482214-epa13toolkit.pdf). Attendings often ask patients, nurses, and staff how you have been to work alongside. Respecting your patients, the medical team, and the janitorial staff is the right thing to do and is the way to learn to become the doctor you want to be. It's therefore not an accident that comments on these aspects of your behavior will find their way into your evaluations and medical school performance evaluation or dean's letter (◼ Table 1.2).

▪▪ Residents and Interns

Other than your peers, interns and residents are the closest to your stage in the medical training environment and can more easily relate to your current dilemmas and provide useful information for your success on the rotation, for example, attending style, daily workflow, and feedback on your proposed plans prior to rounds.

Generally, interns are on a steep learning curve and adjusting to the demands of clinical work. They will have less time to teach and will benefit significantly from your support. Most interns appreciate humble, speedy, and task-driven students, especially administrative work which prevents them from attending to more pressing clinical tasks. On the other hand, while senior residents appreciate a strong team player, like attendings, they focus more on a student's teachability, trustworthiness, critical thinking, fund of knowledge, and interpersonal skills. See below for general suggestions for interacting with interns and residents (◼ Table 1.3).

Pearl: It is always appreciated when students are self-motivated to learn details specific to a rotation.

If you have not been provided with necessary details for the rotation, in your first e-mail, demonstrate your background research: "I spoke with my classmate about the service who said to meet for rounds at 6:30 AM on floor 7A and prep for cases in OR 5. Please let me know if there have been any changes or if there is other material you would like me to prepare beforehand. Otherwise, I look forward to meeting you tomorrow!"

Pearl: Many trainees may provide ambiguous responses such as "I think it was X Y Z" when others ask clarifying questions about the history. Do not lie about anything, especially anything that could be relied upon as part of patient care. If you later learn you spoke in error, make sure you apologize and confirm that your correction has been received.

Pearl: Always keep track of all tasks (even the "smallest") on a task checklist.

Pearl: We are all human and have outside responsibilities; if you must direct attention elsewhere, be discrete or ask permission to step away.

Avoid being on your cell phone in front of your team unless they specifically requested you to research patient-related information.

Pearl: It may be difficult and anxiety-provoking to intervene on unprofessional attending behavior given the vulnerable status of students in the hospital. For more information on how to navigate these situations, see the section "Feedback and Challenging Team Dynamics" later in this chapter.

Table 1.2 Attending, fellows, and advanced practitioners*

Encouraged	Avoid
• Send an e-mail to your attending <3 days but >24 hours before your first day reminding them to expect you. Be brief and verify meeting time/location and any information helpful for preparation (patients' charts to review, content, etc.).	• Arrive late or in the wrong location.
• On the first day, introduce yourself in person using your name 2 or more times for memory's sake.	• Send a long e-mail with many questions or questions already answered within an introduction packet or e-mail.
• When able, ask for attending preferences regarding oral presentations, note writing, cosigning, timing for rounds, and other information they want their students to know.	• Leave without notifying the attending or team of your excusal.
• Some attendings have preferences for the professional attire of their team. If they are dressed especially conservatively, consider doing the same. If they wear their white coat, you might consider wearing yours.	• Lie about an exam finding or historical question you did not investigate.
• If you have conflicts that will take you away from the team, bring them to everyone's attention at the beginning of the week through e-mail or in person. On the evening morning of the conflict, remind your team again so that they are ready to cover for your clinical responsibilities.	• Forget to follow-up on requests (reading up on a concept, lead teaching on a clinical question, calling a consultant, etc.).
• If you disagree with a medical decision or action, clarify rationale by asking a question in a tone that comes across as open-minded rather than an accusatory or derogatory comment.	• Provide inefficient or disorganized presentations, as this will slow down rounds and force others to replicate your work.
• If an attending probes your knowledge in a weak area (we all have many), find a way to share related details you do know. Admit that you have not yet reviewed that concept, and follow briefly with concepts you do know (e.g., I am not familiar with treatment X, but have read about treatment Y and Z. How does treatment X differ?).	• Allow yourself to disengage during rounds, didactics, or impromptu teaching—be respectful of the time individuals dedicate to developing you.
• If you provide a suboptimal response to a knowledge-probing question, commit to reading on the topic at the end of the day. If appropriate, you may offer to share what you learned the following day.	• Ignore a mistake that is made by others out of fear of correcting—remember, the needs of the patient come first. Comment tactfully if something unsafe has occurred.
• After a few days of note writing and presenting, ask if your attending has any feedback on notes or areas they'd like you to expand or cut back.	• Pretend to understand a concept or procedure that you do not—medical school is about learning, after all. If an attending asks if you know something or if you have or have not attempted a procedure before, be honest.
• If a patient appears to be crashing (acute change of vitals or consciousness), immediately request help from your resident and/or attending.	• Make excuses for lack of knowledge in an area. Instead, say "I have not managed diabetic ketoacidosis before, but will read up on it tonight and share what I learned tomorrow."
• Attendings often have areas of expertise (airways, infectious diseases, geriatrics, etc.). If you know or identify this passion, it is wise to review these topics as permitted to best learn from your attending	• Ask for feedback on your first day or first presentation. This is often too early for others to grasp your specific abilities and weaknesses.
	• Ask for feedback during a time-pressured moment. If the team is busy, schedule feedback at a later time.
	• If you receive constructive feedback, avoid becoming defensive. Thank them for their honesty, and make a genuine effort to intervene on it immediately (assuming the feedback is reasonable)

□ Table 1.3 Residents and interns

Encouraged	Avoid
• On Saturday before a work week, it is helpful to e-mail the resident leading your team with your didactics schedule, conflicts, etc. so that they may be aware of them and include them if there is a weekly team e-mail on Sunday evening.	• Making comments to residents that you would not in front of a patient or attending. Although residents are more junior, your professional standards should be maintained when interacting with them.
• Early on, ask interns/residents how to best help the team: how are notes written? Are there computer functions you should know about? When are notes due? Who should cosign orders? What is the rounding style?	• Gossip about a teammate or patient. To provide feedback, refer to the subsection "Feedback and Challenging Team Dynamics." As much as possible, keep your comments positive and uplifting.
• If an attending asks a question clearly directed at another member of the team, allow the more senior trainees the opportunity to answer before answering. We are all learning.	• Compete with interns or residents during knowledge probing and teaching. Keep your contributions collaborative.
• Recognize that interns are adjusting to a substantial learning curve and might be overwhelmed. Just because they seem approachable does not mean they have the time or knowledge to answer all questions.	• Monopolize procedures (recognize that this is also their time to master content in the field). If they have done enough to become proficient, they may share the opportunity with you.
• If you join a busy team, acknowledge that it seems hectic and that you can wait until another time for an orientation, e.g., "Things seem busy today. Please feel no pressure to orient me. Maybe we can go over workflow and expectations at the end of the day or tomorrow?"	• Be distracting in the workroom. Use discretion when sharing about your personal life outside of the hospital.
• When a resident gets paged while preoccupied (in a procedure, presenting, or speaking), offer to take care of it if possible so they can continue with their immediate task.	• Eat the last doughnut (or the last of any communal food) or steal a person's workstation.
• When you grab food or water for yourself, offer to retrieve extra for your team. If they are busy and cannot attend "lunch conference," offer to bring back leftovers.	• Hover too closely behind your residents. It can be exhausting to be on display all day. Many will appreciate the space to grab a snack, use the restroom, or write a note alone. If unsure if you should join while they leave the room, ask "should I join you or stay here?"
• As permitted by administration and teammates, help write notes, update hospital courses, fax records, arrange interpreters, and prepare discharge paperwork ahead of time. There is often something to do which will benefit your patients.	
• If you have extra time and there is an abnormal delay in a patient's diagnostic results, therapeutic interventions, or procedure, consider offering to call the microbiology lab, the radiology technician, etc. to verify that the process is proceeding properly.	
• Remember, asking "How can I help?" requires the intern/resident to be creative to find ways for you to be useful. If overwhelmed, they may not have the bandwidth to consider how to use your skills/time. Always provide specific examples of how you might help, and request permission before proceeding. For example, "Would it be helpful if I start Patient X's discharge paperwork?"	
• Be flexible; every resident and attending has a different style, and every rotation creates new spaces to be useful. Sometimes, you will be essentially shadowing, others you will have full autonomy. Decide what is best for the patient and team, and remain flexible.	
• Learn the materials for common procedures, and have them ready at the bedside for your resident (lumbar puncture kits, suture kits, pelvic examination supplies, etc.).	
• Be enthusiastic. Say "Yes" to every educational opportunity offered to you, as long as you are comfortable with it	

■ ■ **Nurses and Staff**

Due to the ample experience, clinical know-how, and status as licensed providers, nurses should at all times be treated with equal respect and deference as attending physicians, no matter their stage or age! As described earlier, students must honor and equally value the contributions of each member of the medical learning environment, no matter their role. Each member of the team is uniquely skilled and mission-essential for patient care and should be regarded as such (□ Table 1.4).

1

Pearl: Staff and nurses will tire quickly when only approached for demands/requests. If you invest in them personally (chat briefly about family, sports, areas of shared interest, etc.), they will feel cared for as opposed to used and will have more energy to help you and your patient out!

Pearl: Asking before introducing yourself will quickly earn you a bad reputation among the nursing staff. Always warm up slowly and get to know your team by name.

Pearl: Remember, nurses spend the most time with your patients and are essential to enact any plan. If your nurse disagrees with a proposed plan (sees it as unfeasible; finds a procedure necessary/unnecessary, or dangerous; or is concerned with overly frequent labs, etc.), you want to know!

Pearl: Initiating open communication ahead of time is prophylaxis for more substantial disagreements in the future!

Pearl: Complements work wonders on team morale! Build up your teammates and positively reinforce excellent patient care whenever possible.
Moreover, when attendings and residents observe a student earnestly complement another, this signals maturity and personal security.

Pearl: Providing constructive feedback is a difficult but important skill. See the "Feedback and Challenging Team Dynamics" section for more on this

Table 1.4 Nurses and staff

Encouraged	Avoid
• Learn their names and use them (jot down if needed). If you are entering a room with a patient and a nurse, introduce yourself to *both* of them, not just the patient. • Before approaching a nurse or staff member with a question, greet them, ask how their day has been, and listen. • Probe their expertise: seek to learn as much as you can about their job, skills, and responsibilities. If they are willing to teach, learn how to change or remove I.V.s and adjust medication pumps, bandages, etc. • In the morning, ask the overnight nurse how things went for your patient and ask if they have concerns. • Respond to and follow through on nursing requests swiftly (e.g., fill medication orders, attend patient needs) with closed-loop communication (e.g., acknowledge receipt of request, provide interim update if necessary, communicate resolution of request). • When making a request of a nurse or staff member, ask if you can help with the process (reposition a patient for a dressing change, start a new I.V., etc.). • If possible, learn how to conduct a process on your own (if you ask a staff member to help fax something, ask them if they can teach you the steps so you can be self-sufficient the next time)	• Ignore pages, delay responding to pages, dismiss nursing concerns. • Interrupt nursing with nonessential requests when they are in a huddle or working on a procedure. • Ask a nurse to complete a task that you can complete safely on your own as a student (vitals recheck, patient ambulation, P.O. challenge, etc.). • Ignore nursing concerns about your proposed plan. • When provided an equal voice during plan formation, nurses will save you time and time again

■■ Other Medical Students

In most cases, you will be following other medical students when you begin a rotation and/or rotating with other medical students on your team. It is important to build a collaborative relationship with your medical student colleagues: your teamwork will both improve patient care and overall team function, and your evaluators will appreciate your ability to be a good team player (■ Table 1.5).

◻ Table 1.5 Other medical students

Encouraged	Avoid
• Before the first day, speak with peers who recently completed the rotation. Ask about best study materials, team workflow, patient lists to review, electronic health record tips, meeting areas and times, and team expectations. All of these steps will save you and your team's precious time, as you will be oriented before starting.	Withhold helpful information from peers: medicine is a team activity, and the rest of your career will be spent helping peers provide the best care they can.
• Pay it forward: at a rotation's conclusion, share lessons learned openly with peers. The more you share, the better their patients will be cared for.	Compete with each other—this will distract you, sap energy from patient care, and is deleterious to your team's function.
• If you are rotating alongside a peer, arrange a meeting beforehand to discuss expectations. It is helpful if you are on the same page for the entire rotation: agree on a time to arrive and depart the hospital, a plan for settling disagreements, and a mechanism to provide peer feedback as needed during the rotation.	Answer questions asked of your peer medical students before the question has been asked of you during didactics or teaching.
• Complement your peer's strengths with the team: if they give a strong presentation, give them a discrete high-five; if they discharge a patient efficiently or lead an excellent teaching session, give them the congratulations they deserve.	Try to arrive earlier or stay later than your co-student unless necessary for patient care—it is a marathon, not a sprint.
• If you feel the urge to compete with your peer, ask yourself: "how can I learn from their success and incorporate their strengths into my own routine?"	Undercut a peer's response during didactics. Instead, practice building on their response. For example, "I agree with Alex's response, and also thought we could add giant cell arteritis to our differential for headache."
• Be enthusiastic to work with your peer and support each other with your knowledge and skills; you will help fill each other's gaps.	Speak poorly of a co-medical student to interns, residents, nurses, attendings, or staff. If you have an issue with your peer, first discuss it directly with them in a nonthreatening setting. If you are still experiencing an issue, consider mentioning it to the clerkship director. However, if appropriate, try to address disagreements on the lowest level possible.
• When residents and attendings probe your knowledge during rounds, respond collaboratively. Always help the other person shine: if your peer was called on, give them ample time to think through an answer before attempting to answer. If you know the answer but they do not, share it humbly and give them credit for anything they shared. For example: "Just like Jerimiah was saying, I have read that postoperative fever is caused by many things, and recently learned the helpful mnemonic of the "5 Ws" to remember each of them."	
• If one of you intends to provide a "chalk talk" on rounds, encourage the other teammate to do the same so that you both learn from each other	

Pearl: Flexibility is key here. Maybe you conducted interesting research on a patient question and were so excited to share, but now, your team is far behind on rounds. Provide a brisk patient presentation, and find another time to share these learning points.

Pearl: Patient-first language honors patients as people first, not disease processes or habits.

Even if senior clinicians do not use patient-first language, lead by example, and they will learn from you!

Pearl: For example, while presenting your plan on patient-centered rounds, you might say: "Ms. Liu, given that you have both anti-phospholipid syndrome and a pulmonary embolism, I did some background research on which treatments are best for patients in your specific situation. I learned XYZ, and would suggest that we pursue XYZ option."

Pearl: Surgical teams move very quickly in the morning. If you are taking the stairs, try to move quickly enough to avoid others waiting on you.

Pearl: We are all human! Try your best to keep changing your gaze, laugh, and smile when appropriate to increase your engagement and retention.

■ ■ Pre-rounds and Rounds

Rounds are a critical time of each day during which major decisions about patient care are made and important teaching takes place. It is important to recognize the central position of rounding in the team's functioning and prioritize preparation for rounds (◻ Table 1.6).

1

■ **Table 1.6**   Pre-rounds and rounds

Encouraged	Avoid
• Elicit patient questions before rounds, answer those you are comfortable with, and write down those you will forward on to team.	• Surprise your patient with the rounding process. Imagine what it might be like to have 3–6 unexpected guests in your room while wearing a hospital gown.
• If conducting bedside rounding, inform your patient of how the process works, where you will sit, who will be in the room, and when to expect the visit. Rounds can feel intrusive, dehumanizing, or upsetting for patients who have never experienced them before.	• Be on phone (unless your team specifically asked you to use it to conduct work or research a question).
• Provide patients/family the option to have fewer people in their room if they prefer this or the option to have the team talk through the plan outside the room. Notify your attending of your patient's preferences.	• Trail behind the team or slow the team down.
• Arrive to rounds having thought about the crucial decisions for your patient (e.g., review literature for anticoagulation recommendations for a patient with unique/complicated history, surgical options for a patient with multiple past surgeries or unique anatomy).	• Sway back and forth while presenting or while listening to presentations. This may unintentionally communicate disinterest or inattention.
• Once your residents seem to have a handle on their own patients, ask to quickly run your management plan by them. Be quick; thank them for any feedback they offer.	• Zone out or focus on your own presentation when others are presenting or teaching.
• Arrive early to rounds. Though you may feel uncomfortable when presenting a plan, starting the morning off on the right foot by arriving early makes you feel more prepared and confident.	• Forget to close doors, turn off lights, or redrape patients before leaving the room.
• Before starting a presentation, gauge how rushed your team is; speed up or slow down your presentation based on this.	• Providing a lengthy or arrogant teaching. If you do plan to teach or hand out papers to fellow trainees, be sure to clear this with your peer medical student and resident beforehand to avoid seeming competitive; if possible, coordinate teaching sessions with your fellow student(s)
• Provide swift, organized, accurate, and thoughtful presentations in the style preferred by your team.	
• When rounding on your patient, try to be the one who introduces your patients to the team: "Hello, Mr. Z, this is the attending, Dr. F, and she will be leading your care." Introduce each teammate by name and position. This orients your patient to the care team and demonstrates initiative.	
• Sit beside your patient while presenting in their room.	
• Pay close attention to the verbal and nonverbal cues of your team: if they are not making eye contact with you, fidgeting with pens, staring off into the distance, and checking phones, this is feedback—focus on making your next presentation more succinct. If they are frequently interrupting you with questions like "Do they smoke?" or "Who takes care of them at home?," try to include answers to these questions in your future presentations.	
• Pay attention to verbal and nonverbal cues from patients and family: are they tearful? Provide a tissue. Hard of hearing? Move closer and speak slowly and slightly louder. Do they seem confused? Provide ample invitations for questions.	
• If appropriate, start presentations with a small personal factoid about the patient as a person (livelihood or hobbies for a patient, an interesting fact, favorite pet, etc.). This keeps the rounding process interesting and more person-oriented.	
• Use person-first language (e.g., "patient with diabetes" instead of "diabetic patient").	
• Provide a swift, non-assuming, and patient-focused teaching point for patients with a difficult medical decision.	
• This thoughtful and personalized approach will improve patient care, enhance your patient's understanding of the current thought process surrounding their medical decisions, and will encourage your team to think diligently about management decisions.	
• Finish presentations by forwarding on the list of questions you were unable to answer during pre-rounds. "Before I conclude, I know that Ms. J had questions about X, Y, and Z, and hopefully we have time to address those as a team now."	
• Invite the nurse to join for rounds if they wish to participate (if you know your team is headed to their patient next, consider walking ahead to find their nurse).	
• Organize interpreters for the team.	
• Replace dressings (when appropriate) and clear trash produced by team on rounds.	
• Even if not your patient, ask them about any preferences for the state of their room as you leave—would they like the lights on or off? The door open or closed?	

1.3 Special Topics

Making Mistakes and Apologies

If "practice makes perfect," it follows that trainee mistakes are a common and natural part of the learning process. However, while students are often forgiven by patients, overseeing providers, and staff for their errors, effective apologies build interpersonal resilience and prepare trainees for the demands of a career in medicine. Thus, it is crucial to master graceful apologies early on. That said, apologizing for mistakes is not always necessary. When deciding the threshold for an apology, ask: "Would I appreciate an apology in this situation?"

Below are common examples of medical student mistakes which may benefit from acknowledgment*:

- Arriving late or to the incorrect location for clinic, rounds, or didactics
- Misplacing a patient list with protected health information (PHI)
- Accidentally misinforming a patient or their family regarding results or plans
- Failing to review important patient information, anatomy, or medical knowledge expected before a clinic session or surgery
- Failing at a procedure after multiple attempts (e.g., suturing, I.V. placement, lumbar puncture, etc.)

**Remember, we are human! Most students will make most (if not all) of these mistakes while on the wards.*

After you conclude that an apology is indicated, provide one in a timely fashion. The length of an apology should, in general, correlate with the significance of the mistake (minor = brief apology; major = in-depth apology). If your apology demands time and attention, delay until after the current task is complete. The most effective apologies share the following traits ◘ Fig. 1.1.

1. State explicitly what error was made
2. Describe what happened
3. Acknowledge impact on others
4. Explain cause(s) for mistake
5. Provide a plan to prevent recurrence
6. Express sincere and genuine regret

You should think about this outline of your apology ahead of time, but avoid coming across as scripted; show an appropriate amount of true emotion, while keeping it professional (Gallagher, JAMA, 2003).

In summary, erring is an inevitable part of training, but significant mistakes left unacknowledged negatively impact our relationships. Though over apologizing is unnecessary, thoughtful and timely apologies demonstrate interpersonal expertise and reduce the deleterious effects of mistakes on crucial relationships. Outstanding apologies demonstrate professionalism, humility, respect for others, and naturally builds habits for continual interpersonal improvement. A proper apology can be a healing event, and by considering the items included in the list above, trainees are provided an opportunity to reflect and grow.

1

Anatomy of an Effective Apology

Explicit statement of error ➤ This morning, I made an error and left my patient list with protected health information in the cafeteria. The list was recovered by janitorial staff and the event was reported to our hospital's administration.

Impact on others ➤ My oversight not only put patient privacy at risk, but also left the hospital liable for a mistake I could have prevented.

Cause for mistake ➤ I believe I made the mistake because I do not have a dedicated place to put my patient list.

Plan to prevent recurrence ➤ To prevent this in the future, from here on out, I will place my patient list in the same white coat pocket each time and will verify the list's presence each time I leave a location.

Express sincere regret ➤ I am so sorry for the difficulty this mistake might cause, and am available if there is anything I can do to make it up.

Explicit statement of error ➤ Today I arrived ten minutes late to rounds after hitting traffic.

Impact on others ➤ My mistake delayed rounds and prevented me from pre-rounding and thinking through my patients' care. This will delay their results and hospital course.

Cause for mistake ➤ My lateness was caused by not allowing enough extra time for unexpected accidents on the road.

Plan to prevent recurrence ➤ From now on, I will arrive at the hospital an hour early, and use this additional time to prepare for patients and review for my end-of-course exam.

Express sincere regret ➤ I have apologized to each of my patients, but wanted to express my regret to the entire team as I know my mistake impacted each of you.

- ■ Explicit statement of error
- ■ Impact on others
- ▢ Cause for mistake
- ▢ Plan to prevent recurrence
- ■ Express sincere regret

▫ Fig. 1.1   Anatomy of an Effective Apology

▪▪ High-Stakes Conversations

Though interpersonal excellence is expected of all interactions, high-stakes conversations leave lasting impressions with patients and families and warrant special attention. Conversations that disclose significant clinical updates (affecting life or limb), probe personal content (sexual history, intimate partner violence), involve planning around life and death, or include multiple decision-makers may be high stakes. High-stakes interactions heavily shape an individuals' perception of the quality of care they have received, their healthcare providers, and comfort with a prognosis and plan. Further, students should remember that as health professionals, everything we say to patients may have a high emotional valence, and we must have astute attention to patients' verbal and nonverbal responses to detect these circumstances.

With this said, common high-stakes conversations include family meetings, sharing bad news, moments immediately surrounding traumatic accidents and loss of life, and goals of care discussions, to include discussion of code status. Excelling in these moments requires special attention to detail and is remembered by patients and families long after the event. Prior to leading these discussions as a trainee, be sure to first receive explicit permission and instruction from your attending/resident.

Begin the interaction by reflecting on your AMIGAS framework: *absorb* surrounding data, *mirror* the verbal and nonverbal cues from the group, *imagine* what their current mental and emotional state might be, consider their *goals*, *ask* permission to begin the conversation, and *serve*. To serve in high-stakes conversations, you should consider the widely practiced and highly effective SPIKES mnemonic. Though the details of this method can be found online, a paraphrased summary of the original paper (Baile et al. 2000) is provided below:

1. *Set-up.* Ensure privacy, invite significant others, and sit. Consider wearing your white coat and silencing electronic devices.
2. *Perception.* Assess the patient's perception and understanding of their medical prognosis and its severity.
3. *Invitation.* Obtain the patient's invitation to share results. Ask if this is a good time, who should be in the room, and how they would like you to deliver the information.
4. *Knowledge.* Provide the medical knowledge to the patient. Warn them ahead of time if it is bad news with a direct statement "I have some bad news." Speak in layperson terms, be honest and direct, but avoid unnecessary bluntness. Provide information in chunks and routinely check for patient understanding.
5. *Emotions.* Notice the emotions your patient expresses with open-mindedness (they may react with anger to news you would react with sadness or humor to news you'd respond to with anger). Provide time for silence, and then respond with empathetic statements. Common strategies include naming an emotion, "It seems that this news leaves you feeling lost." Avoid the urge to "fix them" with your words or share too much about yourself; these are self-soothing behaviors and are less effective in demonstrating genuine care for a patient's condition.

1

6. *Strategy and summary*. If the patient is emotionally ready (be sure to ask), provide them with a clear plan ahead: when is their next appointment? How long must they wait for their next results or for a procedure? Though it can be difficult to share prognosis information, some patients may ask for this immediately. Be prepared with your answer beforehand. The strategy and summary step relieves anxiety caused by medical uncertainty.

■■ The End of the Day

Unlike many jobs with clear "end times," one of the hardest parts about the clinical year is not knowing when you can go home. Some days, your team will run behind, asking you to remain long after you anticipated to help with admitting patients or to-dos; other times, a resident or attending might tell you to go home just after lunch. Unfortunately, the most awkward scenario is relatively common: a busy resident forgets to release their student at the end of the day, leading them to wander the hospital aimlessly while waiting for those magic words "go home." This uncertainty is a source of stress for students, as they do not want to appear unmotivated by asking to leave nor do they want to linger awkwardly without anything to be learned or done. Alternatively, while residents do not want to appear strict by making you stay, they might gladly accept the support of a willing and enthusiastic student who suggests completing helpful tasks.

Due to this ambiguity, the question "Is there anything else I can help with?" has become a mild alternative to the real question "Can I go home now?" when used by students with their overseeing residents. Asking a busy resident "What else [you] can help with?" puts the burden of identifying appropriate tasks on them and will often result in the reply, "I cannot think of anything else, you should just head home." Though tempting to ask this generic question when you want to go home or feel too exhausted to help, you will be surprised by how often residents will accept your help, even after hours, when you suggest a way to make yourself useful.

That said, while staying late will certainly catch the attention of your teammates, it will not always be good attention. It is not only about how long you stay in the hospital but your attitude and helpfulness while there. If you are planning to remain late, present yourself in a positive light. Stay off of your cell phone, and avoid studying for end-of-clerkship examinations while in the hospital without a resident suggesting this. It is better to leave the hospital on a positive note than linger. Just as the friend who overstays their welcome leaves you wanting alone time, residents spend many hours in the hospital and might enjoy some peace and quiet. If any resident gives you strong instructions to go home, do not resist this request more than once. They may be in need of space.

In summary, if you decide to remain late in the hospital, be sure to make this time high quality and productive. That said, all teammates appreciate honesty. If you would benefit from departing early on a particular day (you are celebrating a birthday, need to pick up a family member at the airport, etc.), bring this to the attention of your supervisor early in the day, and remind them when your tasks are complete.

Pearl: Your first interactions with a patient, staff member, or teammate heavily dictate the strength of future interactions. If you earn early trust (meet patients having thoughtfully reviewed their medical history, attend your first OR case with anatomy reviewed, deliver a practiced and conscientious patient presentation, etc.), you will earn trust which will aid future interactions. Similarly, you are also remembered by your final interactions with a person. Examples include providing thoughtful and clear discharge instructions for your patients, excellent sutures during your final surgery, or an exciting and helpful "chalk talk" on the last day of your rotation, as required. Avoid the temptation to relax your standards near the end of an interaction and finish strong.

■ ■ Feedback and Challenging Team Dynamics

With varied preferences, expectations, and leadership styles within each medical or surgical team, trainees will experience variable group chemistry throughout the ward experience. Eventually, students will encounter attendings, residents, peers, nurses, or staff with whom suboptimal interactions detract from patient care, team function, learning, and rotation performance. Though the culture of medicine prizes feedback and quality improvement, many trainees remain uncomfortable when resolving conflict with others. To make this process easier, consider the following steps on deciding how and when to intervene:

While you need not befriend everyone who teaches you, remember that you have something to learn from each person with whom you work!

1. *Ask*. Did your teammate's actions or words harm a patient, teammate, or staff member, or were they stylistic? If clear patient or teammate harm occurred as a result of an individual's actions, intervene swiftly and tactfully. Raise your concerns to the individual (if possible), and report the incident to your clerkship director as appropriate.
   - If the actions or words did not harm a patient or teammate but were merely stylistic, consider providing another opportunity for self-correction or apology before intervening or reaching a conclusion regarding an individual's performance and habits. What you witnessed may have been a behavioral outlier, miscommunication, or the result of an unusually difficult day.

2. *Introspect*. Before assigning blame, reflect on any tendencies or flaws that may have contributed to strained relations. Often, there is a contribution by both parties in a conflict. It is imperative for both individuals to own their component for the process of resolution to go well. How might internal changes prevent similar issues in the future?

3. *Invite*. Address the issue at the lowest level possible and invite the individual to choose a comfortable time and location for discussion. Before providing your thoughts, invite them to the conversation: "Are you OK to discuss some concerns at this time?"

4. *Provide balanced feedback*. When starting and ending feedback, consider positive traits that you noticed in the individual and wish to reinforce, and provide comment on these strengths before flanking the concerns you plan to raise.
   - When raising concerns, consider the following structure: "When [X] happened, I felt [emotion/impact]." Avoid the phrase "You are [adjective]." The former method differentiates a person's problematic actions from their worth and invites them to consider change in a nonthreatening way.

5. *Offer compromise*. As you request another individual to modify their behavior, you should offer to do the same. Suggest a solution that requires adaptation on both of your parts. For example, if a teammate is arriving earlier or later than you hope, offer to meet them at a midway point. If you disagree with a patient's management, offer an approach that utilizes strengths from your teammate's plan and your own.

6. *Wrapping up*. Conclude the interaction by thanking them for their willingness to work through disagreement together. Tell them that you are open to further discussion if they have thoughts later on.

7. *Follow-up*. If despite your intervention, you find the one-on-one interaction was ineffective in resolving an issue, determine the next best person to address it with (typically your clerkship director).

Note: This process can be uncomfortable. Consider role-playing your interaction with a trusted loved one before delivering it in person.

Pearl: When a supervisor provides you with constructive feedback, spend time reflecting on it. If you disagree, have a different perspective, or a different personality, still consider if their feedback is telling you something important. Often, those with whom we disagree will provide honest feedback on strengths/weaknesses, whereas others who like us often avoid constructive feedback to remain on favorable terms.

Wellness

Amira Song

2

"Medical school is a stressful time." This phrase is probably as familiar to you as the pages of your anatomy textbook or the hallways of your favorite library. Although you are no stranger to stress and dealing with its side effects, this chapter serves as a reminder to take care of yourself as you learn the ins and outs of caring for others and offers several tried-and-true tips on how to do so.

As obvious as it seems, it is incredibly easy to forget to take care of yourself, especially in between cramming for anatomy exams, caring for patients, and rushing to various meetings. During this time, you must remember that to take care of patients, you must consider your own well-being equally important if not more. This includes the basics: remembering to eat meals, exercise, and mentally check in with yourself occasionally to be in tune with your feelings and make sure everything is going alright. The following list of tips is not comprehensive, but it should serve as a general wellness checklist while on the wards.

1. *Prioritize sleep.*

   Sleep is essential to proper functioning, particularly intellectual function. You also don't want to be dozing off on rounds or in the operating room! Sleep is not only all about the length of time but also about quality. Ensure proper sleep hygiene, such as going to bed at around the same time each night and creating an environment (e.g., lights off, muting noises, comfortable bedding, avoiding caffeine at night) that facilitates good sleep.

2. *Stay hydrated.*

   It's all too easy to become dehydrated while caring for patients, putting in consults, and running errands. Bring a water bottle to keep hydrated throughout the day. Minimize your intake of sugary drinks—the sugar high and crash are real! You and your kidney will feel a lot better!

3. *Don't skip meals.*

   No matter how busy your rotations become, always eat! You may not have time to eat a full meal, but eat something. Keep some snacks in your backpack (personally, protein bars are great!). Thinking and walking throughout the hospital consume lots of energy, so it's important to keep your body fueled. Students have had vasovagal episodes after prolonged periods of fasting and standing; don't let that be you!

4. *Exercise.*

   You don't have to take an hour out of your day to complete a full training routine, but even 15 minutes of activity will make you feel energized and give your brain a break. Have an impromptu dance session, make up a bodyweight routine that can be completed anywhere, or go for a quick jog around the block if it's possible where you live. Here is a time-saving circuit that can be modified to your liking and will make you feel the burn in no time.

   50 jumping jacks
   40 butt kicks (both legs = 1 rep)
   30 squats
   20 sit-ups
   10 push-ups

5. *Take care of your relationships*

   Make sure to block out time for people that make you feel good. School is important, but so are people, and one cannot make meaningful conversation with textbooks or depend on them for emotional support and companionship. Maintaining a healthy support network and feeling the emotional support go a long way toward improving your mental state.

6. *Find a way of relaxation that works for you.*

   Meditation is a popular form of relaxation nowadays: many people speak about its benefits such as increasing self-awareness and helping develop concentration. However, meditation will not work for everyone, and it's up to you to find something that works for *you*. Examples include listening to music, playing music, writing/journaling, playing video games, cooking, practicing yoga, and watching movies. We all need to refresh and recharge, and medical students are no exception!

7. *Do something that has special meaning for you.*

   Whether it be volunteering, visiting a loved one, or otherwise, find something unrelated to classwork or medicine that makes you happy. If you had a hobby during high school or college that brought you a lot of joy, hold onto that hobby and make time for it during med school.

8. *Remember that in the grand scheme of things, nothing—not your grades, Step exams, nor residency—will make or break your life.*

   You got into med school, and now you just have to take it one step at a time. Don't fret over the little things and keep the big picture in mind.

Another key element of maintaining wellness is to avoid comparing yourself to others. It is all too easy to fall into the slippery spiral of self-doubt, self-loathing, and imposter syndrome. Remember, you earned your spot and you were chosen. We all have different strengths and weaknesses, and we should understand that we cannot always be the best at everything—but we make up for that with other attributes. Remember the following:

1. Life is not a competition of who has it worse. Sleeping fewer hours than your fellow classmate is an example of one-upping that benefits no one, especially yourself!
2. Remember that everyone is human and has faults and weaknesses.
3. Find friends who care about you for who you are rather than what you offer.
4. To borrow from the words of Marie Kondo, stop surrounding yourself with people who do not spark joy.
5. Use the mental health resources at your school! Medical school students have been shown to have a higher rate of psychological distress, including anxiety, depression, and suicidal ideation, relative to the general population [1]. If your school does not have a robust mental health service, or if the waitlist lasts many weeks, be sure you have a support network that you can count on. This could be your friends, family, mentors, or even strangers/pen pals over the internet with whom you can share your problems. Everyone knows that talking about your problems makes them better!

Lastly, medical school-induced stress can often cause burnout in many students, and it is not uncommon for individuals to lose sight of their vision. Regularly remind yourself of your goal. Write it in your journal, hang it on your wall, whatever will make you remember who or what you're doing this for.

Best of luck on your rotations, and remember—take care of yourself!

Reference

1. Quek TT, Tam WW, Tran BX, et al. The Global Prevalence of Anxiety Among Medical Students: A Meta-Analysis. International journal of environmental research and public health. 2019;16(15):2735. https://doi.org/10.3390/ijerph16152735.

What Attendings and Residents Look For

Bliss J. Chang and Stewart H. Lecker

Contents

© The Author(s), under exclusive license to Springer Nature Switzerland AG 2021
S. H. Lecker, B. J. Chang (eds.), *The Ultimate Medical School Rotation Guide*,
https://doi.org/10.1007/978-3-030-63560-2_3

3.1 Overview

As a medical student on clinical rotations, one of the most burning questions is, "what do my evaluators look for?" Evaluations are not the most important aspect of why students strive to do well on rotations but it is, for better or worse, a significant variable that shapes and determines our future careers. These evaluations (as part of the dean's letter or recommendation letters) are among the most important elements for residency applications, so students should work hard to achieve excellent evaluations.

The goal of this chapter is to provide a glimpse into what attendings and residents look for in medical students, beyond the generic answers we often hear such as "be yourself" and "help the team." How exactly do you best help the team? We will dissect these answers and provide specific recommendations about how one can tangibly improve performance on the wards.

3.2 The Unaltered Answers

We asked attendings, fellows, and residents, "What do you look for in medical students?" The unaltered, anonymized answers are below:

- As a clerkship director, I can say that, because there are so many different attending personalities and wants, evaluations are always somewhat subjective. The best students adapt to the personalities and demands of each team. I think the two most important traits are, in order of importance, being well liked and being clinically competent. Little can save a student who is clinically great but not well liked. However, being well liked alone won't get a student a good evaluation – we are evaluating clinical skills after all.
- The clinical years in medical school are unlike any other experience and truly mark the beginning of one's training as a physician. When I started my clinical year, I remember feeling the way I did when I moved to a new country for the first time, trying to learn despite not speaking the language or understanding the culture. In many ways, the qualities that allow medical students to excel, and thus the qualities that I look for as a resident in a medical student, are similar to the qualities that exemplify effective learners in new lands. The most important ones include humility, which allows for the space to integrate new information in a way that promotes growth, and kindness and commitment, which allow for the building of relationships between student, patient, and the care team that are essential for the delivery of compassionate and effective care. These qualities are necessary. Beyond this, the exceptional medical student is one who is present, who works hard, who sees every new scenario as a learning opportunity, and who seeks to understand. These qualities promote growth, which as a resident is my most important expectation of the medical students that I work with.
- Curiosity. Conscientiousness. Hustle.
- Sense of humor and ability to get along with everyone; clinical reasoning skills; sense of wonder, curiosity and inquiry; sincerity.
- Honesty, love for medicine and curiosity!
- They have to have read SOMETHING before starting the rotation. Then, it's all a matter of intellectual curiosity and commitment to work. Residents and staff know implicitly when a student doesn't care or is otherwise distracted.

- Enthusiasm and reliability – if you show up to work every day excited to learn, take care of patients and be a part of the process, and if you are dependable and have good follow-up, you make an excellent member of the care team and are also on your way to becoming an excellent career physician.
- Enthusiasm, Energy, Empathy, Curiosity, Teamwork. The best students exude those qualities and they are listed in rough order of importance.
- There are several key features: (1) the ability to work well with the team; (2) synthesizing information and coming up with a differential and plan; (3) desire to learn more; (4) desire to contribute to a patient's care and the work of the team; (5) interest in the area; and (6) just fun to have on the service.
- Self-motivation is critically important. Learning on their own, problem solving… these are the most important qualities in a trainee.
- Curiosity, proactivity, and empathy. Medical students that have great fund of knowledge and that are efficient and "get the job done" are appreciated, but the students that are truly remembered are the ones that are inquisitive, that ask when the formal explanation is not given, that try to connect physiology to the patient presentation and that push their preceptors past their first explanation. Students that stand out are the ones that also take on extra reading or bring articles that are important for their patients without prompting. Most importantly, empathy is a must. If you lack empathy and a "human sense" early in your career, this will be hard to develop later.
- The medical students I have most enjoyed working with possess an indefatigable intellectual curiosity. They genuinely want to learn the science in order to care for patients in the best way possible. This is very different from knowing all the answers, or even any of the answers. It's hard to quantify as it's different from volunteering for everything, staying the latest, or spending the most time with patients. It's just about showing that you care about the why. However, not everyone is going to be interested in everything and that's okay. But perhaps there is an element or angle of many things that could be interesting to one and that unique viewpoint could actually benefit residents and attendings.
- Curiosity and attitude are always number 1!

By now, it should be abundantly clear that there is no single attribute that ensures success on the wards. Rather, it is a combination of your characteristics, the depth of those qualities, and attending-specific preferences. Clinical evaluations are inherently subjective and this is a key reason to discuss expectations and engage in two-way feedback frequently throughout your rotations.

3.3 Dissecting the Answers

Despite the lack of a one-size-fits-all answer and plethora of attending philosophies and preferences, there are some medical students that repeatedly earn the best rotation grades and written evaluations. What is it that they do consistently so well?

In our experience, star students consistently do two things:

1. Always put in near-maximal effort regardless of whether it is a rotation that they enjoy or not.
2. Take their strongest qualities and use them to the max.

3

Let's be honest – most of you will not love every aspect of medicine and it is often apparent to others, whether that's leaving earlier, reading less, or simply not having the same spring in our steps. In order to perform consistently well, you must put in nearly the same amount of effort for rotations you dislike as for those you love.

Every student has a unique set of characteristics that they excel at, similar to how there are many different positions on a basketball team. For example, one could make it to the NBA as a point guard, a center, or a small forward. It's important to realize one's strengths and weaknesses and to utilize the strengths to make up for the weaknesses.

Take for example a student who has an extraordinary ability to deal with people. This person might not know the answer even half the time nor give great oral presentations, but their interpersonal skills are powerful – faculty and house staff want this person to succeed and so they may be quite liberal with how they give praise. Another example is the other extreme where a student isn't socially gifted (but also not terribly socially awkward) but has a remarkable knowledge base and drive to learn medicine. This student answers everything perfectly and gives the best oral presentations. Teams can depend on this student's work and it makes their lives easier.

Based on numerous student evaluations, the following are the main factors we believe that you should focus on.

3.3.1 Interpersonal Skills

The most important thing for any rotation is to have people you work with like you. They should want to spend more time having you on their team. Liking someone drastically changes, whether fair or not, how generous they are when writing evaluations. This doesn't mean that you should "suck up" or be artificially nice to people – this is easy to see through. If you're thinking of buying your team coffee each morning, forget it. Trying to hold the door open every time and before your fellow medical student? Forget it. But showing people that you are not only dependable, honest, curious, and diligent, but also fun to work with goes a long way! If you had two people with similar clinical ability, who would you want to work with? Refer to the ► Chap. 1 to learn how to grow your interpersonal skills!

3.3.2 Knowledge Base

This is undoubtedly the most debated characteristic, with staunch advocates (both students and attendings) on both extremes of the spectrum, believing that students should know nothing or everything. While knowledge base is not always explicitly mentioned, having a healthy knowledge base is critical to earning a great evaluation because it is the foundation for nearly every clinical skill. In order to string together a coherent oral presentation, or even to know what special exam maneuvers to perform, you need knowledge. While students without knowledge but with excellent interpersonal skills may initially thrive, there is a point at which even the most liberal of praise cannot cover up weak clinical skills. Furthermore, having a solid knowledge base is insurance against times when you work with an attending or resident who is particularly interested in assessing your clinical skills. As a student, it's very difficult to know how much to know. This book is unique in that it will provide you with essentially exactly what you need to know and do, as well as how to fill the remaining gaps for each rotation.

3.3.3 Clinical Reasoning

While a strong knowledge base is essential, your ability to reason through atypical cases without a clear-cut answer is important. Often, relying on fundamental concepts such as the presence or absence of a fever can be the deciding factor between two courses of action. Verbalize your reasoning rather only providing the answer. Whether right or wrong, you will demonstrate to your team where they can help clarify concepts and your willingness to think about what's going on. For example, instead of noting that you want to diurese with 40 mg IV lasix, note that you want to do so because the patient was not meeting diuresis goals and therefore you want to increase the dose.

3.3.4 Curiosity

Almost all medical students are curious – otherwise we wouldn't be where we are today. However, being curious and *appearing* curious are two very different things. This is one of those characteristics that can be interpreted very differently by different evaluators.

So how do you project the curiosity that you genuinely have? There are several ways, but try to think about how you express curiosity before looking below.

1. Questions: Perhaps the simplest yet among the most powerful tools, asking questions conveys interest, thoughtfulness, and curiosity. However, you will likely, at least over time, be judged on the quality and timing of your questions. You should ask genuine questions; never ask questions for the sake of asking them. You should display a certain level of thought in your questions – if you ask the most basic of questions too often, then people may think that you aren't making an effort to read/learn on your own. Furthermore, simple questions can usually be Googled – there is little point in asking easily searchable questions to members of a busy clinical team. Lastly, think about *when* it is appropriate to ask questions. If a patient is coding (cardiopulmonary arrest), you should save your question for later. Please refer to the Interpersonal Skills chapter for further details on how/when to ask questions.

2. Further reading: When we don't know the answer or want more information, we read something, whether in a book or online. However, this is an answer to our curiosity that is not always apparent to others. If you read a lot, it will naturally be apparent in your clinical performance and you need not make any further effort to explicitly demonstrate your curiosity. However, if you only read occasionally, one way to convey this is by teaching or printing out the journal article for your team, noting an interesting point(s). An easy rule of thumb is to try and learn one thing from every patient that you carry!

3. Staying involved: You don't always need to ask questions. Instead, you can learn through experience (remember shadowing?). For example, if you're on the cardiology rotation, you might ask your team to follow your patient to the cath lab for a few hours. Even if they say no, teams will notice and appreciate your enthusiasm.

Attendings appreciate when you ask questions about nuances of clinical thinking – as medical students we learn many hard and fast rules, and one hallmark of the clinical environment is that there is a large gray area. Seeking this out is a good way to find easy questions that many preceptors appreciate and to learn more about the practical nuances of medical decision-making.

There are many ways to express curiosity, and it is a trait best expressed through multiple methods. Try to cover all three points above regularly over the span of a rotation.

Note: one of the most common student, resident, and attending sins is telling patients that they will be back later. This means that the patient will indeed expect to see you later that same day. Make sure to report back to your residents with any changes or concerns.

3.3.5 Reliability

Always arrive a bit earlier than scheduled and do everything you say you will. If you're assigned a task or say that you're doing a task, make sure to circle back and let the team know your tasks were finished. This prevents misunderstandings and is overall better for patient care. Be prompt, honest, and unforgetting, and you will develop a reputation for reliability.

3.3.6 Honesty

This is absolutely critical in medicine. You should always be completely honest about everything. Asked if you heard a murmur but didn't? Then say you didn't (and follow up by asking for permission to listen again). You should never lie about anything, particularly physical exam findings. If you are caught lying, impressions can be irreparable and your future residency/career prospects can be bleak if such comments make it into your evaluations or letters. It is not worth lying to try and impress attendings – they are often looking for teaching opportunities! Lastly, honesty includes only reporting/noting findings that you actually checked for! It's quite easy to auto-pilot and regurgitate a normal exam when you haven't assessed for something like hepatomegaly. Attendings do take notice!

3.3.7 Enthusiasm

While enthusiasm is shown both through our body language and actions, we'll focus on our body language since the actions overlap with other characteristics (e.g., curiosity). Picture someone who you would describe as enthusiastic – they're likely smiling, appear interested, and perhaps even have a little spring in their step. When you're in the hospital, you should try your best to always be positive no matter how tough. You will have bad days in the hospital, but remember, each patient and your team deserve your best. Be humble and always be positive; never react negatively even if warranted. Refer to the Soft Skills chapter for more details.

3.3.8 Proactivity

Being proactive means doing things without explicit instruction and slowly (not on Day 1) doing more and more. You should remember that the name of the game is moving patient care along at all times. If you have time to do something that can help your team save time (e.g., obtaining patient records from an outside hospital), do it! Help your team and patient! However, make sure not to overdo things or overstep what you can do. We realize that as students, it can be hard to know what "be helpful in the OR" means – we've got you covered by providing you with checklists on exactly what you should do on each rotation.

3.3.9 Teamwork

Most students don't have trouble working with their interns, residents, and attendings, but may have more trouble working with fellow medical students or nurses. Simply put, treat everyone as family and as people more competent than yourself. Drop the exaggerated, unnecessary small things like competing with your fellow medical student on who can hold the door open more often. These petty things not only annoy your partner but are also obvious to your team. Help each other, whether it's reviewing a concept or offering to run a small errand – teams will notice! More details on teamwork in the Soft Skills chapter.

3.3.10 Professionalism

We've covered a lot of characteristics that contribute to professionalism. One thing to emphasize is to maintain good hygiene and dress conservatively. One of us remembers showing up to our first primary care clinic without a tie and being given a tie to wear! You should feel out what your team's preferences are and follow them.

As you work on teams, you'll notice the preferences of the attending and residents. On one rotation they may be funny and all about teaching medical students, whereas another might be more serious and old-school with significant expectations of your skills. It is extremely important to recognize this early so that you can tailor your strategy for the rotation. If you're constantly getting hammered with questions that you don't know the answer to, it's probably worth focusing more effort on expanding your knowledge base. If possible, talk with students who have completed the rotation for a heads up on what you can expect!

3.4 Example Evaluations

To wrap up this chapter, let's look at two real sample evaluations to get a sense for what things to do and what not to do.

First, let's look at this neurology clerkship evaluation since it offers a great look into the specifics that attendings consider when evaluating students. This attending focused a lot on my clinical skills, such as history-taking and communicating a treatment plan. Early in the rotation, the student could sense that this attending really cared about the student's clinical skills so that's what was focused on. You may notice that everything written here hinges upon a healthy knowledge base. Without the knowledge, you would not be able to do these clinical tasks well.

Without going through the evaluation in excruciating detail, let's consider the following:

1. Note what aspects of each clinical skill attendings analyze. For example, the oral presentation was described in terms of length/content (succinct, tailored to setting), organization, and eye contact (without using notes). We encourage you to go through the evaluation and pick out clinical skills that you want to work on and come up with tangible goals on how to improve them. For example, perhaps you want to take your oral presentation to the next level and decide to try using minimal notes this upcoming week. Want to improve your physical exam skills? Perhaps you can focus on the abdominal exam this week.

Pearl: Be specific with your goals and break down goals into manageable pieces.

Pearl: Share your goals with your team and seek feedback on those goals throughout the rotation.

3

2. Teams notice when students are easily taught, meaning that whenever you receive feedback or are taught how to do something (e.g., place orders), you shouldn't need to be shown/told again. To facilitate this, consider writing down every piece of feedback or instruction received and reflect on them intermittently.
    (a) Pearl: Develop a system to "learn" when taught once. This is best done by writing down key points for reference later.

███ did a superb job on his neurology rotation. His history-taking was completely entrustable by the middle of the rotation, able to gather a comprehensive history with only rare need for clarifying questions by his preceptor. His neurological examination improved steadily during the rotation and was also entrustable by the middle of the rotation, even for more complex patients. His preceptor was highly impressed by his ability to perform a complete examination of a Parkinson's patient and identify fairly subtle abnormal findings like mild rigidity and rest tremor. His oral presentations were succinct, organized, and effectively communicated without the use of notes. His preceptor found him to be quite flexible and able to tailor his oral presentations to the amount of time available, particularly helpful when the clinic was busy. He was promptly honest about information he didn't know or things he had not checked on exam, making him very reliable .

███ could generate a robust and appropriate differential diagnosis, raising several possible diagnostic considerations and spontaneously discussing their likelihood backed by clinical evidence. He researched and also committed to memory the diagnostic criteria of several clinical diagnoses (headaches, several dementias, CRPS), which demonstrated a fund of knowledge beyond his peers. He effectively recognized and could discuss pertinent clinical questions and was regularly able to plan a workup to answer these questions. His treatment plans were always appropriate and required little or no alteration by his preceptor. He was able to generate management plans at a level well above expected; for example, he was able to choose an appropriate headache preventative medication based on it's side effect profile. He was able to generate non-algorithmic solutions to problems; for example, suggesting overnight doses of Sinemet for a Parkinson's patient with a late-night schedule.

His preceptor felt ███ could independently communicate a treatment plan to his patients, including discussing the risks and benefits of proposed medications. He was able to enter orders for tests and medications into the electronic medical record, which few students at his level take on. His notes were completely entrustable and required little to no editing on the part of his preceptor. ███ preceptor noted that. ███ was one of the few students who actually improved the flow of his clinic on busy days, given his confidence in ███ abilities.

███ was highly professional and carried himself more like a resident than a medical student. He ensured that patients fully understood their plan at the end of the visit and accompanied them to the clinic front desk to ensure their care plan was accurately completed. He consistently developed a rapport with patients. His dedication to his patients was apparent and his preceptor witnessed numerous patients look to. as ███ their doctor with confidence throughout their visit.

███ often sought out feedback and responded to it exceptionally well, never needing to be reminded about something his preceptor suggested he change. He was extremely dedicated to learning, independently seeing 2-3 patients each clinic session and attending more than the required number of clinic sessions. He regularly searched the medical literature during and after patient visits, which often improved patient care (for example, in a patient with unexplained falls he found a case series showing that amiodarone increases fall risk in the elderly and realized that his patient's falls correlated with the initiation of amiodarone). In one patient with an unclear cause of symptoms he independently suggested a diagnosis of Raynaud's, which was very likely the correct diagnosis and not something his preceptor had considered.

His dedication to learning and teaching was best exemplified by the fact that he began writing a book to help his fellow students with board study in Neurology. His preceptor personally reviewed a chapter of this book (on dementia) and felt it was excellent. His preceptor witnessed ███ teaching several first year medical students and ███ was able to explain several clinical concepts in a manner appropriate for their level of training.

◻ **Fig. 3.1**   Neurology clerkship evaluation

Resident Comments:

1. It was a. ure working with ▮▮ He was an effective team member and contributing positively. ▮▮ had great presentation skills. Specifically, he went through a presentation on a patient with cirrhosis who presented with GI bleeding in an effective and logical manner. He also did the entire presentation by memory, showing that he knew this patient well. He acted professionally throughout the rotation and showed initiative. One example was asking to admit two patients during one of the evenings without prompting. He was an effective team member and willing to assist with work. He was very interested in learning and was willing to stay a little later for teaching. He also had great communication with our team and took effective histories. Additionally, his documentation was excellent. His as. ents were thorough and concise tying together the history, exam and labs.

2. ▮▮ was motivated. He knew his patients well and presented them with confidence. He was always asking how to assist in additional tasks. He referenced evidence based findings in his notes. He was thoughtful and took time with each of his patients

3. Excellent knowledge of primary literature and clinical trials. Great differential diagnosis but commits to what he thinks is going on and gives clinical evidence to support his reasoning.

Attending comments:

1. ▮▮ is one of the best subinterns that I have ever worked with in my twenty years at ▮▮ He is operating at the level of an intern. He excels at all of the subintern skills: his found knowledge, communication skills, presentation skills, and evaluation and management skills are all quite outstanding. He also quite skillfully ran a family meeting.

2. ▮▮ was very proactive in our discussions. He led a brief tutorial on CHF and did an outstanding clear job. He easily brought in the other students for a varied and interesting discussion. He was always punctual, well groomed, and a very good listener. He had good strong opinions on a variety of topics both w the cases as well as with career choices.

3. - Very impressive written documentation (H&P) for a patient with ESRD admitted with hypoxia and volume overload; demonstrated impressive fund of knowledge and ability to develop and communicate in written form a sophisticated care plan - Eager to learn and receptive to feedback

▣ **Fig. 3.2**   Medicine Sub-internship Evaluation

We encourage you to go back through ▣ Fig. 3.1 and dissect the various clinical skills yourself. This will be more memorable and useful rather than us dissecting it.

Now let's take a look at this medicine sub-internship evaluation to explore some other concepts (▣ Fig. 3.2).

A few notable points from this evaluation:

1. You might have noticed that students repeatedly focus on using my strengths. For example, both evaluations have noted how students do not use notes when presenting. Early on, if you find that your attending really prefers this, strive to do this for every patient. Many students summarize their history/physical with the patient at the end of each visit – wonderful for the patient and also a practice oral presentation. Consider also jotting down key discussion points to keep in mind. Refer to the Clinical Tips and Pearls chapter for more tips on how to improve your fundamental clinical skills.

2. There is a short mention of having" strong opinions" which can be perceived negatively, especially when reading in between the lines. This refers to when an attending had talked down upon a classmate's desire to pursue orthopedics: the student had interrupted and noted that it's actually one of the most intellectually challenging fields. Attendings may slip small comments like these into your evaluation, intentionally or not, so be careful of actions that deviate from the norm.

3

3.5   Dealing with Negative Evaluations

Receiving a negative (or even average) evaluation can be disheartening. However, it is important to realize that the process is inherently subjective and sometimes it is impossible for anyone to receive a stellar evaluation. Other times, the structure of a rotation is flawed and doesn't give students opportunities to shine. Regardless of the reason, it is rarely truly your fault. You will have many more opportunities throughout medical school to demonstrate your abilities and earn the evaluations you need for residency applications, so take a deep breath, try to learn as much as you can from the feedback, and carry forth.

3.6   Mid-Rotation Feedback

A key aspect to ensuring that you are on the right track is to check in frequently with your team. This is especially important at the mid-point of your rotation. While some clerkship directors will schedule mid-rotation feedback, you will need to take the initiative and seek feedback in other cases.

Seeking mid-rotation feedback accomplishes the following:

1. It demonstrates enthusiasm for learning, contributing, and improving. Be sure to be receptive to feedback without arguing – you do not want to be perceived as unreceptive to feedback. Regardless of whether you agree with the feedback or not, there is always something to learn. Furthermore, implementing feedback and actively demonstrating improvement really impress your team!
2. It provides you with a boost and fresh start since most teams change over during the middle of the rotation. Your new team will likely not be aware of how you performed in the first 2 weeks, and this can be a great advantage if you have been improving steadily throughout the rotation. By incorporating the feedback from your first team, you will be able to shine for your second team.
3. Some schools allow you to choose from among the people you have worked with for evaluations. If you seek feedback from each person that might evaluate you, you will get a sense of how enthusiastic they are about you and your performance.
4. You truly do learn a lot about your strengths and weaknesses. Knowing what these are allows you to maximize opportunities revolving around your strengths while being able to improve on weak points.

3.7   Concluding Remarks

Ultimately, the key to earning great evaluations is to identify the wants of your team, put in your best effort, take advantage of your strengths, and take small tangible steps toward improving your clinical skills. This is the best we can do as students in an inherently subjective process. Be sure to check out the details of your own school's evaluation system, and derive tangible goals for improvement from those rubrics, in addition to what we have covered in this chapter.

Clinical Tips and Pearls

Bliss J. Chang

Contents

© The Author(s), under exclusive license to Springer Nature Switzerland AG 2021
S. H. Lecker, B. J. Chang (eds.), *The Ultimate Medical School Rotation Guide*,
https://doi.org/10.1007/978-3-030-63560-2_4

This chapter is devoted to providing key tips related to the fundamental clinical skills that underlie almost all specialties. Specialty-specific differences are covered in their respective chapters.

Please refer to the following chapters for key topics not covered in this chapter:
- Interpersonal relationships & team work – ▶ Chap. 1
- Cultural competence and health disparities – ▶ Chap. 13
- Mental health – ▶ Chap. 2
- Dealing with negative evaluations – ▶ Chap. 3

4.1 General Rotation Considerations

Regardless of what specialty you rotate on, here are some principles for maximizing your intellectual, social, and emotional growth:
- *Prioritize the common.* Focus your studies on the bread and butter cases that will comprise 80–90% of what you will encounter. Avoid relying on board preparation books as they are too broad without enough relevant clinical depth.
- *Talk to past rotators.* Each rotation has nuances specific to its patients, teams, and services that won't be covered in any rotation guide. Past rotators are your best resource. Important nuances include team (attending, resident, nurse) preferences, what to keep in your pockets, where important supplies are located, room codes (bathroom, supply closet), and uncommon cases that are uniquely common at your institution (e.g., rotating at an institution linked to a cancer center dramatically increases the number of oncology-related cases you will see).
- *Develop a learning system.* You should have an idea of how to continue expanding your knowledge base throughout the rotation. Are you going to read nightly, solve a specified number of Anki flashcards, or watch concept videos on YouTube? While we believe this book is a great place to obtain a near-comprehensive overview of a rotation, we also provide links to excellent supplementary resources.
- *Create goals.* What do you want to improve over the rotation? Your goals may be completely different from rotation objectives. Knowing how you want to improve (whether improving your oral presentation or working on your ability to juggle time with friends on a tough rotation) will allow you to be more conscious of your actions, leading to faster improvements.
- *Self-reflect.* Think about your interactions with patients and team members. Consider what you do well clinically and what you can improve. Did a patient on your service pass despite the team's best efforts? Emotional, social, intellectual, and moral growth stem from recognizing and understanding past experiences. Thinking about recent experiences can be invaluable to your growth.
- *Keep in touch.* Did you hit it off with someone on your team? Thank them and keep in touch! They are an excellent resource for mentorship and recommendation letters.

4.2 Feedback and Learning

- *Jot everything down.* When you learn anything on the wards, you should always jot it down. Our memories are temporary but notes are forever. You can easily refer to what your attending thought you should work on, or the steps to preparing discharge paperwork. Learned a cool new fact? Jot it down! For example, some of the best surgical students I know use "attending preference" notecards (refer to the ▶ Chap. 24). Having notes and referring to this will allow you to improve yourself (and your evaluations) much more easily.

- *Set expectations.* At the start of a new rotation, set aside time with your resident and/or attending to discuss their expectations of you during the rotation. You can cover everything from what time they want you to arrive to whether they expect you to pend orders. Take note of these expectations and try to outperform them, but do not offer this verbally during this initial meeting.

- *Ask for specific feedback.* Try to ask for detailed feedback that identify exactly what you should work on to improve. Rather than asking "Do you have any feedback for me?," ask "What do you think about my oral presentation, and what specifically can I work on to take it to the next level?"

- *Be perceptive to various forms of feedback.* Feedback on a clinical rotation is not just narrative assessment in the end or a formal "feedback session" at the halfway point. It can take the form of minor suggestions at the end of your oral presentation, discussion about your differential diagnosis and clinical reasoning, or comments on how you position and drape the patient for surgery. Take feedback to heart and become a better doctor every day!

- *Accept feedback with humility and grace.* Feedback reflects perceptions by others, which may differ from intentions of your own. How you receive and process feedback is critical. Frowning, arguing, or making excuses will cast you in a negative light. Smile, be humble, and focus on opportunities for growth.

4.3 Pre-rounding

The goal of pre-rounding is to elicit information on how a patient's clinical status has changed since you last saw them yesterday. It is not meant to be a new patient evaluation.

- *The most complex for last.* If you have multiple patients, it can be helpful to round on your easier patients first and save the most complex patients for last so that they are fresh on your mind. This can also help you present with minimal use of notes.

- *Prioritize before seeing the patient.* Think about what you want to confirm with the patient prior to seeing them. Do you want to check for DVTs, a new murmur, or bleeding from a surgical site? What are your goals?

4.4 History-Taking

Despite access to powerful diagnostic tools, there are many conditions where a great history is more valuable than any test. Elements of the history are often the pivotal factor in differentiating between diseases. As such, you will be evaluated closely on your history-taking skills not only in person but also through your oral presentation as a reflection of what you've asked.

- *Obtain your own history.* It is so tempting (especially when crunched for time) to rely on the history obtained from others or the patient's chart. However, relying solely on others' information is a huge contributor to the propagation of incorrect and misleading information. Always obtain your information from the primary source (the patient) and compare it to what others have learned. Attendings will often ask you whether you have elicited X, Y, and Z history *from the patient.*

- *Develop trust.* You cannot and should not expect patients to trust you immediately. To elicit the best history, it is critical to earn the patient's trust. Patients have many reasons for holding distrust or failing to report accurate information. For example, a patient may not want to disappoint you and may not admit to being unable to adhere to a diabetic diet. Refer to the Interpersonal Skills chapter for more on building trust in a patient-physician relationship.

- *Ask what brings the patient in today.* Patients present with a chief complaint but your job is to discover why they're *really* coming to see you. Are they worried about their headache because they're concerned about a brain tumor or are they coming to see you for "pain" but unable to tell you that the pain is from physical (or emotional) abuse? These are, unfortunately, quite common scenarios that you will encounter. What made the patient decide to come see you today rather than yesterday or tomorrow? Did the pain get unbearable or did something else happen? What is the one question the patient wants to ask? What are they afraid of?

- *Details, details, details.* Medical education often teaches us to memorize, and that is no different for history-taking approaches. We learn the OPQRST mnemonic and memorize elements of a review of systems. However, there is so much richness to a patient's history that cannot be elicited by those memorized methods. The key to obtaining history is to think about what more you would want to know. Try to characterize each detail further – think, "what else could I know about this symptom?" We're very curious people – set your curiosity free and ask away (but also think about how each question can help your patient care)!

- *Think rather than recall.* We've all had those moments where we couldn't figure out the next question to ask. Practice *thinking* of what is relevant to ask next rather than trying to remember the next question you're "supposed" to ask based on a mnemonic. What do you really want to know?

- *Write notes.* Even the best memories are not as reliable as pen and paper. As a student, you have the luxury of time and you should strive to jot down key bits rather than rely solely on your memory. Writing also augments your memory so you can present better.

- *Elicit a story.* Unless pressed for time (as in during a heart attack), you should try to elicit a story from the patient. What happened first? How did the symptoms evolve? What made them decide to come in to see you today?

4.5 Physical Exam

As a medical student, the physical exam is the one thing that is almost completely within your control. You oversee what maneuvers to perform, and you have the freedom to perform most maneuvers, unlike ordering a diagnostic test. Given this great power and responsibility, it is one place where you can truly shine.

- *Describe what you find.* It's easy to get bogged down by fancy terms or findings named after someone. Don't worry about this – the terms will come with time. What's important is conveying exactly what you found, and there's no better way to state what you saw than in layman terms. For example, if you forgot what "clonus' means, you can always describe that the patient's foot flapped back and forth involuntarily three times when forcefully flexing the foot upward. If you don't know how to describe a heart murmur, try to mimic the noise! Not only will you likely make your team smile/laugh (in a good way), but also they'll really appreciate you trying to describe what you found whichever way you can.

- *Be detailed.* As with the history, try to be as specific as possible with your exam findings. How many beats of clonus were there? Was the murmur systolic or diastolic? Where on the back is the laceration located? The more details, the easier it is for others to follow along.

- *Take your time. Double and triple check.* As we learn exam techniques and new findings (e.g., a murmur you haven't heard), we are less confident in our findings. It is absolutely okay to take as long as you need to verify your findings. Don't feel pressured to take your stethoscope off to let others listen or because you feel you look incompetent if you take too long – everyone knows you are learning. In fact, people will rightly become suspicious if you can identify advanced exam findings with the speed of a seasoned veteran. This is the time to practice – the further you progress in your training, the more you will be expected to be facile with exam techniques and the less opportunity to learn in a judgment-free way.

- *Ask for demonstrations.* If you are unsure about a physical exam maneuver, ask your resident or attending to show you the appropriate technique. This really develops your examination skills as there are often limited resources particularly for advanced physical exam maneuvers.

4.6 Objective Data

This refers to anything that comes from a test, whether electrolyte values or radiographs.

- *Develop your own assessment.* Many data come back with interpretations by specialists. Always look at the primary data and develop your own thoughts, no matter your level of training. Not only will this help develop your own interpretation skills, but it can also catch mistakes (which aren't as uncommon as you'd think)!

- *Regularly check the EMR for new results:* New lab or imaging results will come in throughout the day – make sure you stay up-to-date with these, so you know the latest status of your patients. There are often EMR functions that alert you to new results and notes – refer to ▶ Chap. 5 for more details.

4.7 Oral Presentation

The oral presentation is the culmination of essentially everything you've done for a patient (history, physical, workup, analysis of data, coming up with a treatment plan, etc.). This is the most important way in which you demonstrate many of your clinical skills since your team is not always watching everything you do. You must learn to communicate your clinical skills effectively through the oral presentation.

4.7.1 General Tips

- *Fill in the gaps.* As you prepare the oral presentation, you may realize that you have forgotten to ask a question or perform an exam maneuver. It is completely acceptable, and encouraged, to go back and obtain the required information.

4

- *Make an argument.* Your presentation is a case for what you think is going on. You should reflect your thoughts on what's going on as early as the one-liner. What you choose to include and not include in your presentation reflect what you think is likely or not. The order in which you speak to one thing versus another and how you organize your thoughts all strengthen or weaken your argument. It is not necessary, and is in fact discouraged, to include every single piece of data in the presentation – incorporate the information that is absolutely necessary and/or depicts your argument.

- *Use cues.* Your friends weren't kidding when they say that attendings may only listen to your one-liner, only to zone out until you arrive at your assessment and plan. Humans naturally have a short attention span and need active cues to reel us back to what's going on. The burden is on you to keep your audience's attention. Explicitly outline what you're talking about as you go. Examples of directing people to where you are in the presentation include the following: "For past medical history…." and "In terms of radiology studies…".

- *Tell a story.* The best presentations are those that take the audience on a journey, starting from what initially happened to ending with what the future holds. As you present, try to think about whether what you're about to say fits with what you've been talking about.

- *Organize your thoughts.* Try to group things that make medical sense together. For example, the symptoms of fatigue, shortness of breath, and leg swelling could seem unrelated, but together they can be a classic presentation of heart failure. If you suspect heart failure, grouping those symptoms not only demonstrates your knowledge but also makes it much easier for your listeners to follow (and evaluate you fairly). Imagine burying those symptoms among 30 other review of symptoms – it would be easy for the listener to miss key information!

- *Present without notes.* To many attendings, presenting from memory demonstrates that you know your patient and his/her disease process well. When I was first told this, I was puzzled but now it's clear. Someone who knows exactly how heart failure exacerbation presents isn't really memorizing the encounter but rather checking off boxes in one's head and filling in the blanks. It's also impressive simply because most students don't even try – you'll be surprised at how much relevant information you remember and how much fluff you can cut out.

- *Practice presenting with your patient.* One great way to somewhat practice an oral presentation is to summarize everything you've talked about with a patient at the end of the encounter. This is not only awesome for patients but also is of great help for consolidating your memory prior to presenting to your team. Note: you should not actually present formally to your patient as you would to your team, but rather summarize the key history obtained from speaking with the patient.

- *Avoid editorializing.* The oral presentation can be divided into two parts: the facts and the analysis. The facts should be presented in their raw form – whatever the history, exam findings, or lab values. You should not interpret nor comment on the facts prior to your assessment and plan (A/P). For instance, students very commonly say "the temperature was afebrile to 98.4F" or "patient has hyponatremia to 131." You don't need to point these things out; everyone listening can interpret for themselves and come up with their own thoughts prior to hearing your A/P. However, it can be helpful to reference prior vales ("the sodium is down to 130").

- *Put your nickel down.* It is often appreciated when you state clearly what you think may be going on with a patient and what you want to do. It's okay to be wrong, but it's better to make a suggestion, show you've been thinking about the patient, and be wrong, than to shy away from "putting your nickel down!"

4.7.2 One-Liner

- *Be appropriately detailed.* Depending on what service you're on and who you're presenting to, your audience may be more interested in depth of details. On medicine clerkship, it may be fine to mention a history of CKD, but on the nephrology rotation, you should be more specific (a history of stage IIIb CKD with last Cr of 1.4 in Month/Year). Similarly, it may be fine to note a history of heart failure in the primary care clinic but on the cardiology service you should note the specific type of heart failure and most recent ejection fraction.
- *Frame your argument.* You should use your one-liner as if you were a lawyer about to argue to a case. If you think that heart failure exacerbation is most likely, you should include details relevant to that – very different from if you thought the patient had a pulmonary embolism.

4.7.3 History of Present Illness

- *Go in chronological order.* Start with what happened first, and unfold your story in chronological order, as if you are conveying a story about your day working in the hospital. This doesn't mean that everything must be strictly chronological, but strive to do this whenever possible.
- *Combine with the ROS.* Although ultimately up to the attending's preferences, you should try to weave in pertinent positives and negatives into the HPI. This often makes a lot more sense because listeners will begin thinking about a differential and are pulled one way or another with each of your words. It's much easier for the listener to consider pertinent negatives and positives while they're thinking about the conditions based on the history you just provided.

4.7.4 All Other History (Medical, Surgical, Medications, Social, etc.)

- *Stay relevant.* Focus on the key histories relevant to the case. For example, if a patient presents with abdominal pain, it is important to mention their history of abdominal surgery, but no need to mention a tonsillectomy.

4.7.5 Vitals

- *General order.* Unless specified by your attending, present in this order to maximize how many people you please: temperature, heart rate, blood pressure, respiratory rate, oxygen saturation.

4.7.6 Physical Exam

- *Head to toe.* Always go head to toe to ensure that you do not miss findings.

4

- *Only state what you actually examined.* It's easy to regurgitate a memorized script for the physical exam, especially early in your training. If you didn't check the first cranial nerve (smell), then you shouldn't report that all cranial nerves are intact! Furthermore, as painful it is to realize that you forgot to perform a basic exam maneuver such as checking the lower extremities for edema, you should own up to it and always state only what you checked.
- *Only present what is necessary.* Present the systems that you feel are relevant to the story you are painting – you may have done a neurological exam, but perhaps not super relevant for a patient with cellulitis. If your team wants to know more, they will ask!

4.7.7 Objective Data

- *Present the data.* As simple as it sounds, focus on presenting exactly what the data is, without interpreting it. You can, however, describe how they relate to a patient's previous/baseline data.
- *Pay attention to updates.* Some data may become available after you pre-rounded. Pay attention as you read through the data so you aren't caught off-guard when your team asks you about a new piece of data during your assessment and plan.
- *Stay relevant.* Focus on the key data that you will discuss in your assessment and plan. Unless your team has a strong preference, it is okay not to remark on everything. For example, you can present a BMP as notable for a sodium of 136 rather than reading out every value.

4.7.8 Assessment/Plan

This is the most important part of the presentation where you really shine.
- *Discuss with residents.* You will often have time to discuss with your resident prior to presenting. This time is often best spent discussing the assessment/plan as they often have many helpful pointers and know the common action items for various cases in accordance with your institution's guidelines.
- *Think rather than gather.* While gathering information is important, you should always try to interpret that information. At least try to interpret it using basic principles, even if you aren't sure.
- *Use a practical differential diagnosis.* Talk about the two to three most common competing differentials, and depending on the situation, include a do-not-miss diagnosis. Unlike the preclinical years, clinical teams will not want you to cover an exhaustive list of differentials, particularly of rare diseases such as pheochromocytoma that medical students love to remember.
- *Pay attention to what worked before.* Past diagnostic and treatment options that were successful are great clues to what might be a good course of action for patients with chronic medical problems. Of course, be sure to fully explore possibilities and avoid premature closure.
- *Does it change management?* For everything you want to do, ask yourself whether it would make a difference! Does the outcome change if you perform an action?
- *Incorporate literature.* Once you're comfortable with basic oral presentation, try to learn more about the patient's disease or its management by researching and incorporating primary literature (e.g., clinical trials) or secondary literature (e.g., society guidelines). You'll not only shine but also develop a habit of practicing evidence-based medicine.

4.8 Note-Writing

— *Use the appropriate template.* You don't need to spend time writing down all the various sections and formatting for a note. Find a template that your team approves of (such as borrowing from the resident). Focus your time on the content.

— *Explain your reasoning.* As a student, you should never just write down an abbreviated plan. You should spend ample time and words on explaining what you think is going on and why you think we should do what you're proposing. Yes, residents and attendings may take the shortcut, but you should not copy them.

— *It should not be a replica of your oral presentation.* Your note should reflect many differences from your oral presentation. First and foremost, it should reflect your learning from rounds – anything that wasn't quite right about the plan you presented should now be fixed along with an explanation to demonstrate your new understanding. Written notes also contain more detail, such as a complete past medical history.

— *Don't copy progress notes.* Always reassess the current state of your patient and write a new progress note. Don't fall into the habit of copy and pasting the same progress note each day. This is also a disservice to yourself later when you are preparing the discharge paperwork. Again, you may see residents and attendings may do this but you should not.

4.9 Calling a Consult

Refer to specialty chapters for further information on calling consults specific to each specialty.

— *Be prepared when calling a consult.* Consultants have a busy schedule and don't already know your patients, so you must help them help you. Call them early in the day when possible. Clearly identify yourself, your service, and reason for consult. Be ready to give them your patient MRN and name, your one-liner, and a brief summary of initial management and data relevant to the consultants.

— *Have a specific question.* It is critical to have a specific question, not only because people need to know why you're calling but also because it helps the consultant to respond positively and effectively. You may consider running the specific question by your resident prior to placing the consult.

4.10 Logistical Tips

— *Check on your patient throughout the day.* Patients in the hospital require close monitoring. Don't rely on the nurses to alert you, even though they often will. You should periodically check in with your patient, both to assess how they're doing and to build a stronger relationship with them. This may also include updating family members who are often anxious about everything happening.

— *Use a task sheet.* Always track every task, no matter how small, on paper. Not only does it feel great to check off a list of tasks, but it also ensures that you don't forget any tasks. With so many patients and the hospital bustle, you *will* forget tasks if you don't write them down.

4

- *Update your team frequently.* As you finish tasks or receive updates, you should let the appropriate person know, whether your resident, nurse, or attending. Nurses especially appreciate being kept in the loop.
- *Run the list frequently.* Running the list means going down through your checklist of tasks for each patient and the status of each task, as well as commenting on the general status of the patient. You should ask your resident (usually) or attending to "run the list" at least once in the afternoon to ensure that you communicate what you have been working on as well as provide an update to them about the patient.
- *Keep a separate place for learning/feedback.* It's very convenient for your learning to keep a separate notebook (or any other medium) full of all the clinical learning and feedback you receive. For example, if the attending just discussed the SPRINT Trial, you should jot some notes down! Trust me, you will forget a lot more than you think, so having notes to refer back to is a must!
- *Ask for help when needed.* If you don't understand a concept, a reason for doing something, or a task, don't hesitate to ask for clarification. It is very important to know your limits.

EMR Tips and Tricks

Bliss J. Chang

Contents

© The Author(s), under exclusive license to Springer Nature Switzerland AG 2021
S. H. Lecker, B. J. Chang (eds.), *The Ultimate Medical School Rotation Guide*,
https://doi.org/10.1007/978-3-030-63560-2_5

5

5.1   Overview

The EMR is an integral part of your clerkship experience. This chapter covers the must-knows of utilizing an electronic medical record (EMR) system to help speed up your workflow. Note that it is not meant to be a comprehensive manual on how to use an EMR. Since Epic is the most widely used EMR in the USA, we will use it in our examples; however, the underlying concepts should apply to most EMR systems. Remember, there are some stylistic differences between institutions and users, and these tips are not meant to be the only way EMRs can be used.

5.2   Prior to the Rotation

This section covers tips for setting up and customizing your EMR prior to seeing your first patient. Don't worry if your schedule doesn't allow this – setting it up at the end of your first day is fine too.

5.2.1   Create Patient Lists

At the beginning of each rotation, you should create your own patient list to track all the patients you see. This not only drastically reduces the time you spend locating your patient, but it also allows you to revisit the patient charts later for educational purposes after the patient's discharge. Many residents keep separate patient lists of interesting cases to review years later. These lists remain even if your account is deactivated during breaks, as long as you remain in the same hospital site.

To create a patient list, go to the Edit List button in the upper left corner and click Create My List from the dropdown.

You can customize what information your patient lists display. The best approach is to model this after your resident's patient lists as they have usually optimized this for slight institutional differences. Regardless of institution, you should at least have columns for location, patient demographics, MRN, attending, problem, new result or note flags, and admission date. These are among the most common information used around the clock on all rotations and will save you a lot of time. In particular, the new result and new note flags are one of my favorite features as they save me from manually opening charts to check for new data/notes constantly. For specific rotations, such as cardiology, specific information such as ins and outs (I/Os) can be great. These specific parameters are discussed in the respective specialty chapters. Here is one example (Fig. 5.1):

5.2.2   Smart Phrases

An excellent way to speed up your work flow is by using smart phrases (Fig. 5.2) which is a function that stores a template (such as for an admission note) which can be used with a short dot phrase (e.g., ".admissionnote"). You should create smart phrases for anything you use over and over. Some examples include various note types and your signature/pager signature.

You can also insert smart phrases using the green plus symbol in the notes (Fig. 5.3). If you need to view a list of all your smart phrases, this is easily done by clicking the button left of the plus symbol (Fig. 5.4).

While you can allow for easy access to your team's patients by ragging the premade team list to your own lists for easy tracking, you should keep a separate list only of patients you directly care for.

Many providers find the search box within patient lists to be very helpful, as it can search all currently admitted, recently discharged, or preadmitted patients.

Note that this screenshot shows what we call "column blocks" which make optimal use of space. MD Notifications, for example, shows new/panic results, new notes, orders needing cosign, and notes needing cosign.

EMR Tips and Tricks

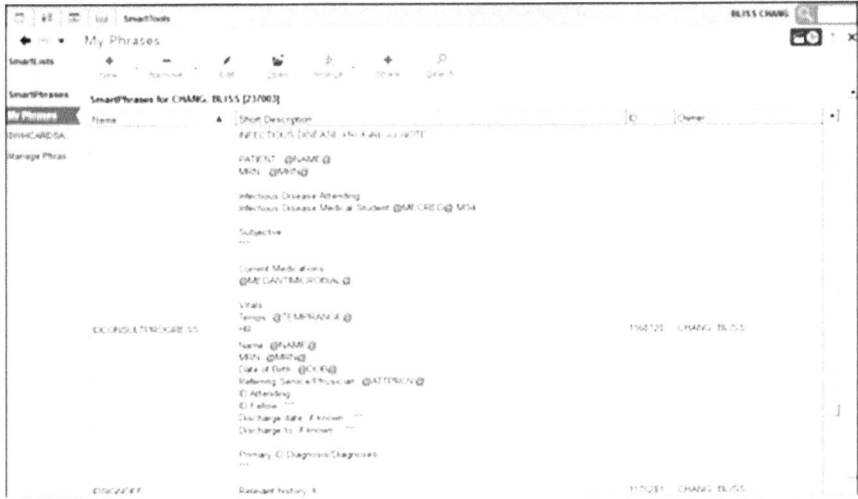

Fig. 5.1 Patient list fields. (© *2020 Epic Systems Corporation. Used with permission*)

Fig. 5.2 Smart phrases example. (© *2020 Epic Systems Corporation. Used with permission*)

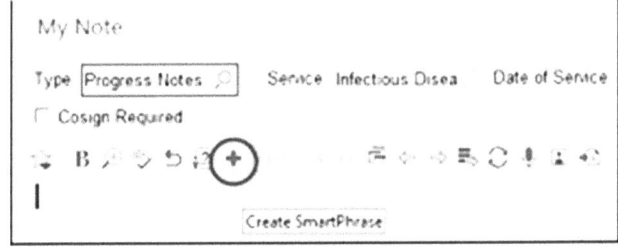

Fig. 5.3 Smart phrases example. (© *2020 Epic Systems Corporation. Used with permission*)

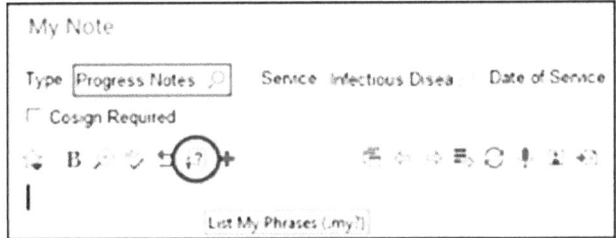

Fig. 5.4 Smart phrases example. (© *2020 Epic Systems Corporation. Used with permission*)

To edit to your smart phrases in Epic, you can click on the Smart Phrases button in the upper left corner. From there, your name will be auto-populated. Upon clicking Go, you will arrive at a list of all your phrases which are editable and shareable. One really helpful feature is the ability to look up smart phrases of anyone in the hospital system. This means you can borrow note templates and such from your residents, attendings, and even medical student friends. Even if you decide to create your own, it is often a good idea to browse your residents' note templates for an idea of what specifics they like to include. Of

5

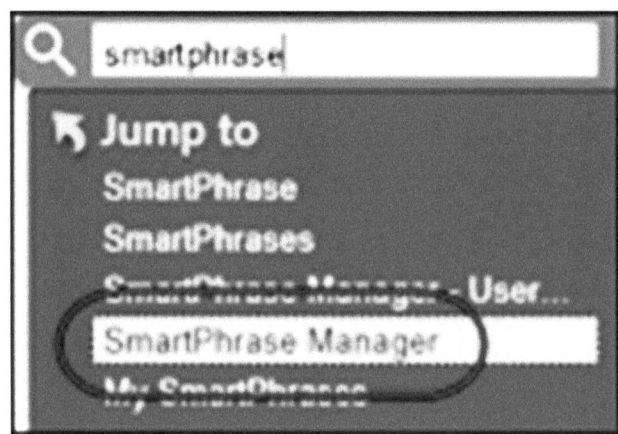

Fig. 5.5 Smart phrase lookup. (© *2020 Epic Systems Corporation. Used with permission*)

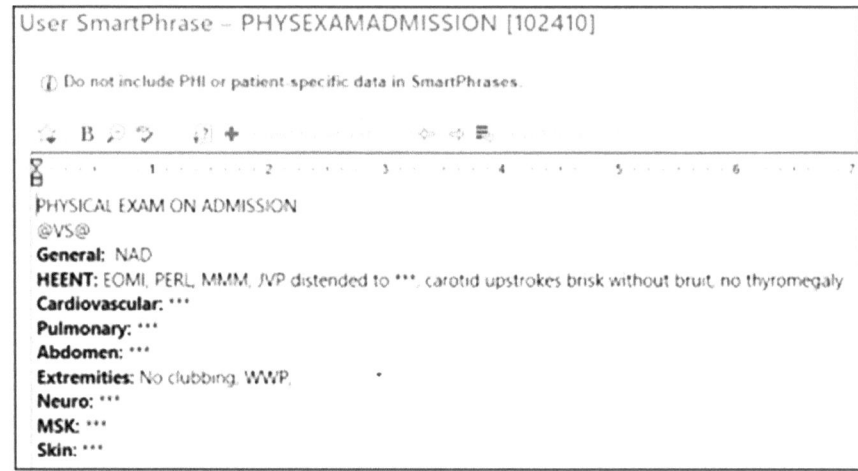

Fig. 5.6 Asterisk reminders. (© *2020 Epic Systems Corporation. Used with permission*)

course, you should ask people or at least let them know out of courtesy if you end up borrowing their phrases.

Note: You can also go to the Smart Phrase manager by searching "smartphrase" in the upper right corner of Epic (■ Fig. 5.5).

Remember to edit out the parts of the template that you did not check or do! This is best done by inserting a reminder in the form of three asterisks (■ Fig. 5.6) after each section when creating your smart phrase, as this will prevent you from submitting your note until these asterisks are removed.

5.2.3 Dot Phrases

These are similar to smart phrases, but rather than you creating them, they are already coded into the EMR. In Epic, you can bring up a list of dot phrases (such as for importing recent vitals or labs) by typing "." followed by any letters of interest (■ Fig. 5.7). You should take some time early on to explore what phrases are available as these are hospital-specific (there's a whole team that manages Epic for each hospital team!).

Lastly, some students create dot phrases of treatment plans for common conditions that they have managed, such as for heart failure exacerbation. This can be quite dangerous as an early medical trainee as it takes a lot of thinking

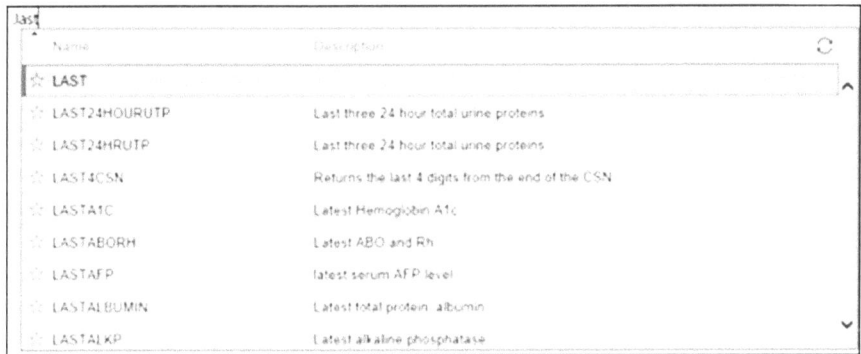

Fig. 5.7 Dot phrases. (© *2020 Epic Systems Corporation. Used with permission*)

out and may not benefit you educationally. This is an option for when you are very comfortable with a disease or when you're getting slammed with patients, but you should really try to avoid using automated methods for coming up with the majority of your plans. Whether you do this will not make a significant difference in how efficient you are, whereas it can greatly compromise your learning. I put this here mostly so you can stop this habit if you are doing it already.

A related but similar option is to look up the smart phrases of your consultants who will often save much of the routine plan recommendations. This is a great place to learn (again, try to not use these) what the management is for common conditions. It will also be very obvious if you just use these rather than crafting a medical student-style assessment and plan.

5.3 Daily Workflow

5.3.1 Creating Notifications

Have you ever wondered how your residents and attendings are always so on top of everything going on? Chances are that they're being notified when key results populate the EMR. You can set pager notifications that alert you to the availability of key results through the "Notify Me" bell (◘ Figs. 5.8 and 5.9). These notifications can trigger a push to Haiku (Epic's phone app), Canto (iPad), or Limerick (Apple Watch).

5.3.2 Chart Search

For patients with complicated medical histories, it's often very time-consuming and overwhelming to manually sort through their past notes and lab results. You should always utilize the search function in the upper right corner or on the left in patient charts in the storyboard area (◘ Fig. 5.10). Typing a snippet of what you're trying to find will pull up everything with that search term (◘ Fig. 5.11). The search function is built very well (if anything, more generous in its results), and you shouldn't need to worry about missing anything – in fact, you're more likely to miss something without the search function.

5

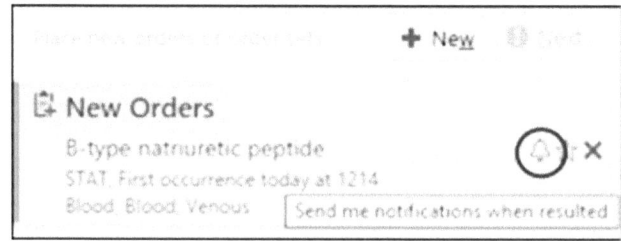

■ Fig. 5.8 Notify Me button (placing orders). (© *2020 Epic Systems Corporation. Used with permission*)

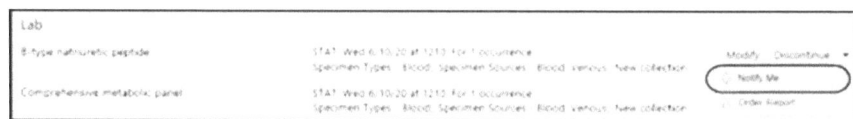

■ Fig. 5.9 Notify Me button (signed orders). (© *2020 Epic Systems Corporation. Used with permission*)

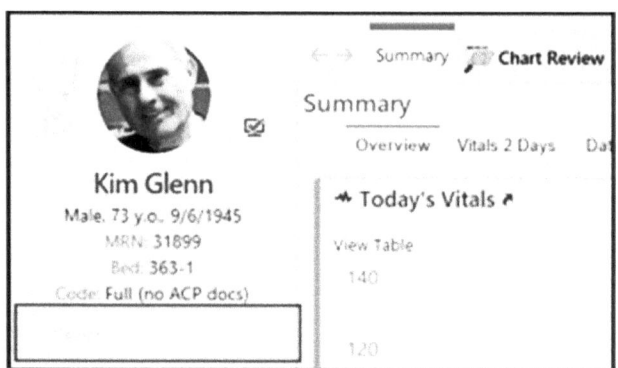

■ Fig. 5.10 The search function. (© *2020 Epic Systems Corporation. Used with permission*)

5.3.3 Chart Review Filters

When you want to find something (e.g., a prior clinic note) but don't have suitable search phrases to use in the search function, you can use filters on just about anything. Filters (■ Fig. 5.12) are a function built into many of the tabs (such as Notes) and allow you to target specific attributes such as specialty/department, physician, and date. A similar feature is to sort the notes, procedures, imaging, and such by attributes (■ Fig. 5.13).

Filters are great, but what many people really like about them is the ability to save them as QuickFilters, or checkboxes, that can be used to automatically filter things upon opening the activity (such as hiding nonclinical encounters or hiding nursing notes by default) or they can provide a single click to filter down to a common search (e.g., show me only my notes or quickly filter the imaging tab to MRIs only).

5.3.4 Time Mark Results

When you open up a patient's lab results, such as through Results Review, you may be spending a significant amount of time looking through the mess of results to find the new results. This is true even if you've already sorted the

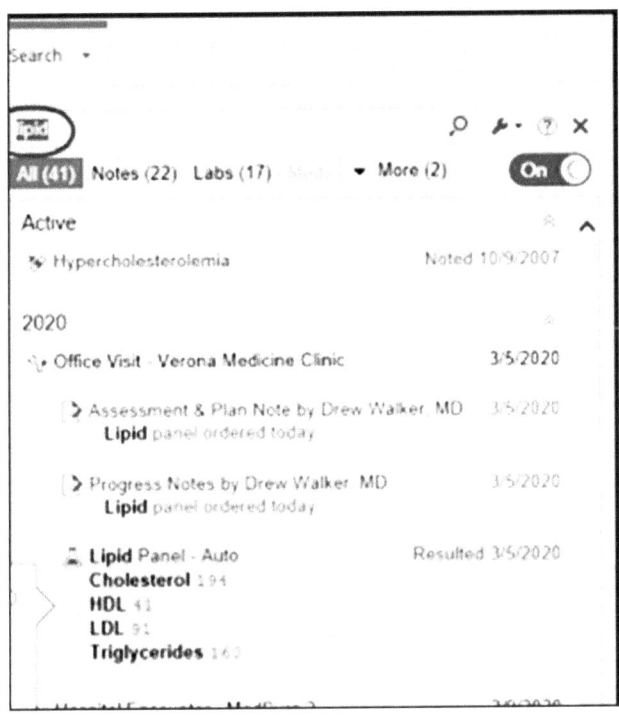

Fig. 5.11 Search results

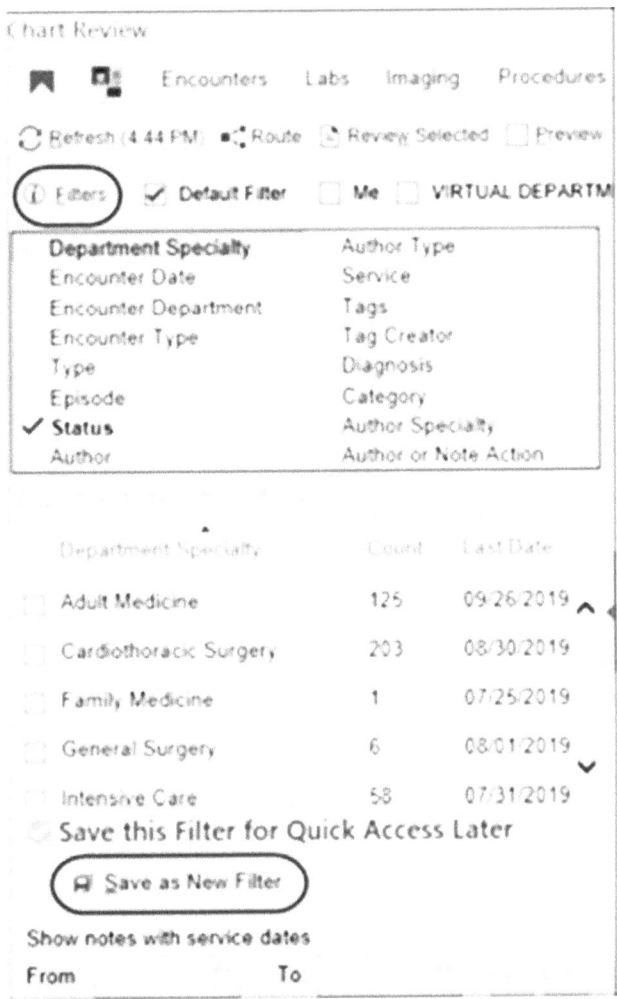

Fig. 5.12 Filter function. (© 2020 Epic Systems Corporation. Used with permission)

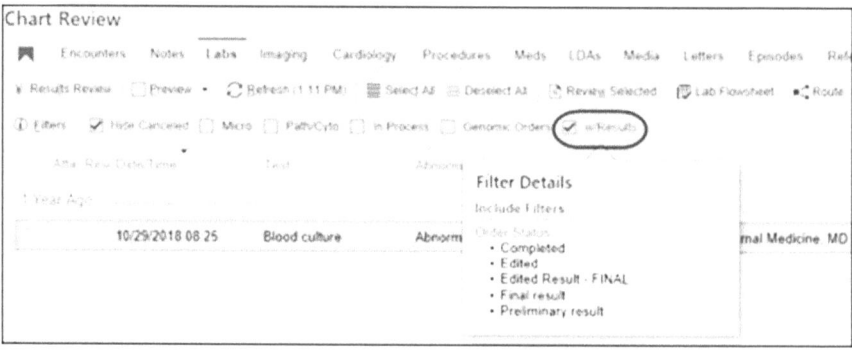

Fig. 5.13 Filter function. (© *2020 Epic Systems Corporation. Used with permission*)

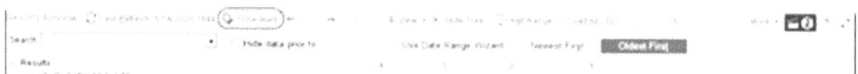

Fig. 5.14 Time Mark function. (© *2020 Epic Systems Corporation. Used with permission*)

	7	6	5	4	3
	10/4/2019 1121	10/10/2019 1413	10/16/2019 1725	10/17/2019 1351	10/17/2019 1352
LYTES/RENAL/GLUCOSE					
Sodium		139		138	137
Potassium		5.1		4.6	4.7
Chloride		96		97	97
Carbon Dioxide		31		26	26
BUN		56		44	45
Creatinine		2.15		1.98	2.01
GFR (estimated)		26		29	29
Glucose		98		118	119
Anion Gap		12		15	14

Fig. 5.15 Highlight row of values. (© *2020 Epic Systems Corporation. Used with permission*)

columns by date since there are often many results in 1 day. One way to only review the newest data that results is to use the Time Mark feature (Fig. 5.14). This will allow the system to remember to only show you data that results after the stamped time. Notably, to use the New Results Flag feature on your patient list, you must Time Mark. This feature is also found in many other sections such as Notes!

5.3.4.1 Compare Labs to Baseline/Prior Values

One of the most useful things to do for all key lab values is to compare current admission values to any priors. This is easily achieved through using the Show Selection in Flowsheet feature which allows you to avoid scrolling through years of results in horizontal fashion in Results Review. First, click the name of the lab result in question to highlight the row (Fig. 5.15). Next, right click to reveal an option to "Show Selection in Flowsheet" (Fig. 5.16). This should isolate the lab result in a vertical and chronological manner (Fig. 5.17), allowing you to see all the data for that lab in the EMR for that patient.

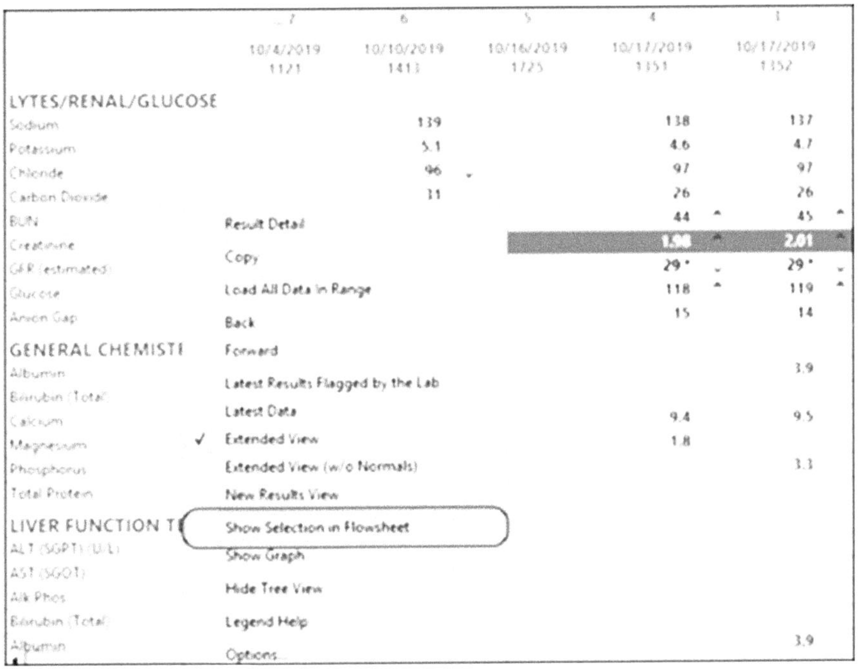

■ **Fig. 5.16** Select Show Selection in Flowsheet. (*© 2020 Epic Systems Corporation. Used with permission*)

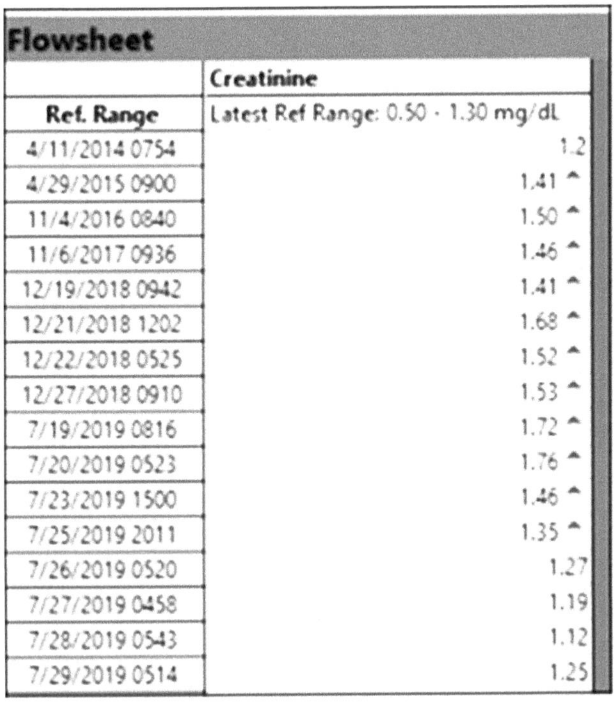

Flowsheet

	Creatinine
Ref. Range	Latest Ref Range: 0.50 - 1.30 mg/dL
4/11/2014 0754	1.2
4/29/2015 0900	1.41 ^
11/4/2016 0840	1.50 ^
11/6/2017 0936	1.46 ^
12/19/2018 0942	1.41 ^
12/21/2018 1202	1.68 ^
12/22/2018 0525	1.52 ^
12/27/2018 0910	1.53 ^
7/19/2019 0816	1.72 ^
7/20/2019 0523	1.76 ^
7/23/2019 1500	1.46 ^
7/25/2019 2011	1.35 ^
7/26/2019 0520	1.27
7/27/2019 0458	1.19
7/28/2019 0543	1.12
7/29/2019 0514	1.25

■ **Fig. 5.17** Flowsheet view of creatinine. (*© 2020 Epic Systems Corporation. Used with permission*)

5.3.5 Summary Tab

The Summary tab is a great tool for viewing key data in one place. It contains multiple tabs (■ Fig. 5.18), most notably Vitals, Comp, Fever, MAR, I/O, and 60-day Micro (also contained as part of the Fever tab).

5

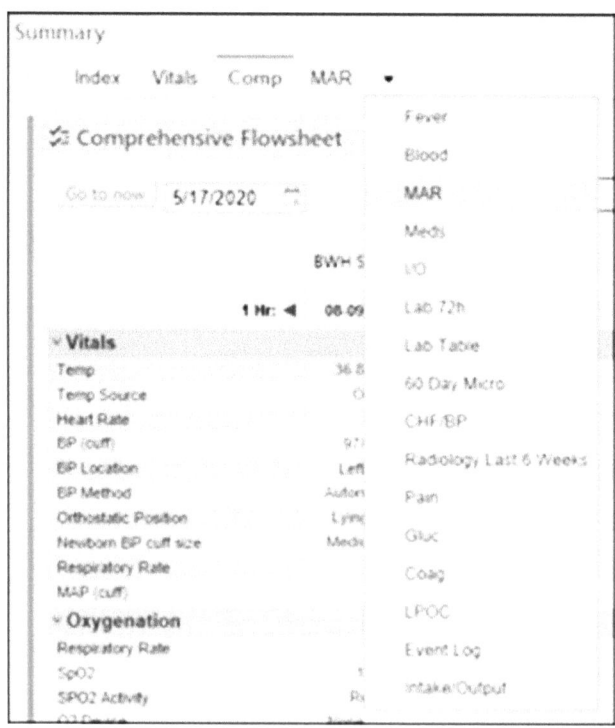

Fig. 5.18 Summary tabs. (*© 2020 Epic Systems Corporation. Used with permission*)

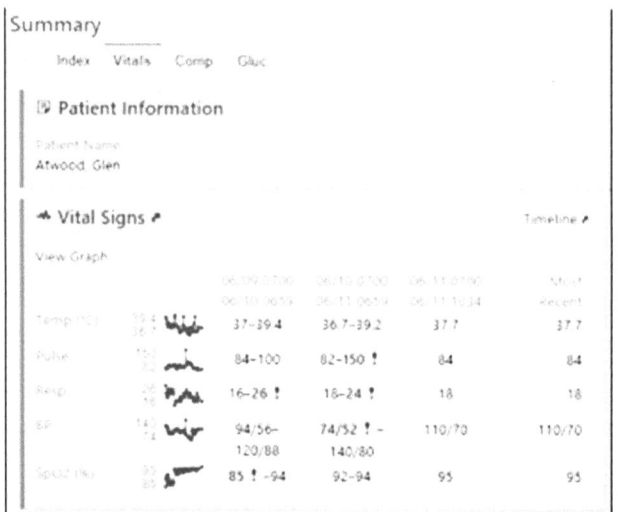

Fig. 5.19 Vitals tab. (*© 2020 Epic Systems Corporation. Used with permission*)

The Vitals tab (Fig. 5.19) conveniently puts all the vitals over the past 24–48 hours in one place, including the ranges. This is the best place to jot down vitals during pre-rounding. Do not read manually through all the data and try to find the ranges.

The Comprehensive Flowsheet (Comp) tab (Fig. 5.20) has great information that includes the vitals as well as other commonly used information such as ins and outs, SpO2, pain scores, and daily weights.

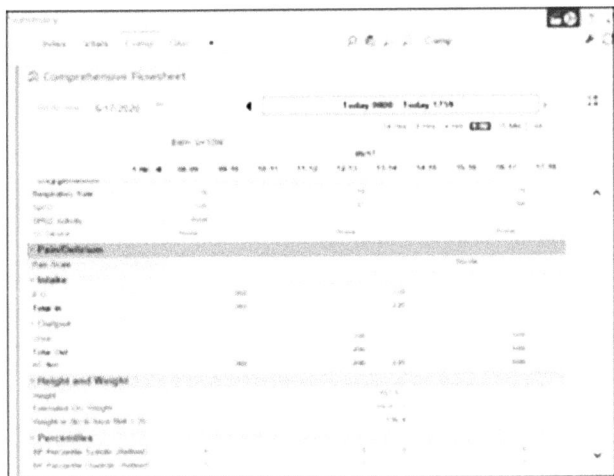

Fig. 5.20 Comprehensive tab. (© 2020 Epic Systems Corporation. Used with permission)

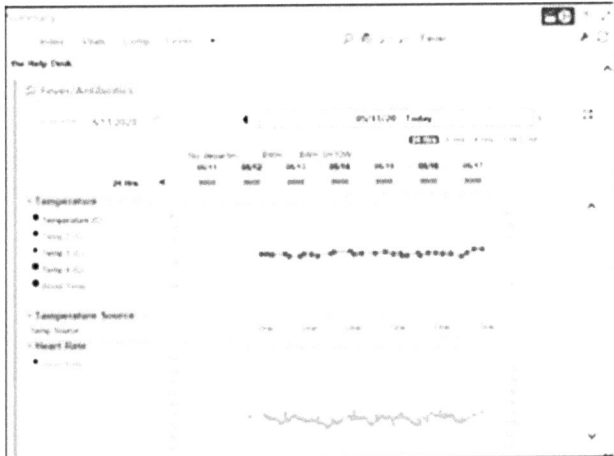

Fig. 5.21 Fever tab. (© 2020 Epic Systems Corporation. Used with permission)

⚫ Microbiology Results (last 60 days)

Collected	Updated	Procedure	Result Status	Component	Value
05/15/2020 1712	05/17/2020 0730	MRSA nasal screen (676/445324) Other from Nasal	Final result	Special Requests MRSA Nasal Culture	None NO METHICILLIN RESISTANT STAPHYLOCOCCUS AUREUS ISOLATED
05/16/2020 0740	05/16/2020 0749	Varicella zoster (VZV) antibody IgG (676998 740) Blood	In process	No component results	
05/16/2020 0740	05/16/2020 0749	Toxoplasma Gondii antibody IgG (676998 741)	In process	No component results	

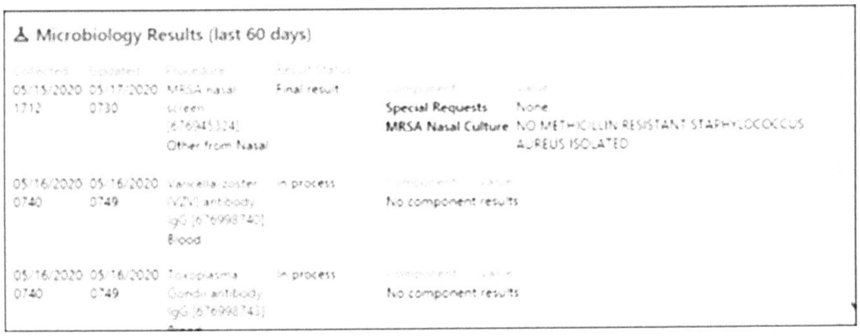

Fig. 5.22 60-day Micro tab. (© 2020 Epic Systems Corporation. Used with permission)

The Fever tab (□ Fig. 5.21) shows a graph of temperatures throughout the admission, allowing for easy identification of temperature spikes. If the patient is on antibiotics, all dose administrations are recorded in parallel with the fever curve, allowing you to examine whether the antibiotics had good effect.

The 60-day Micro tab (□ Fig. 5.22) is wonderful for looking at all the microdata. Many people do not use Results Review for this as it is much easier to visualize and compare all the results in this tab.

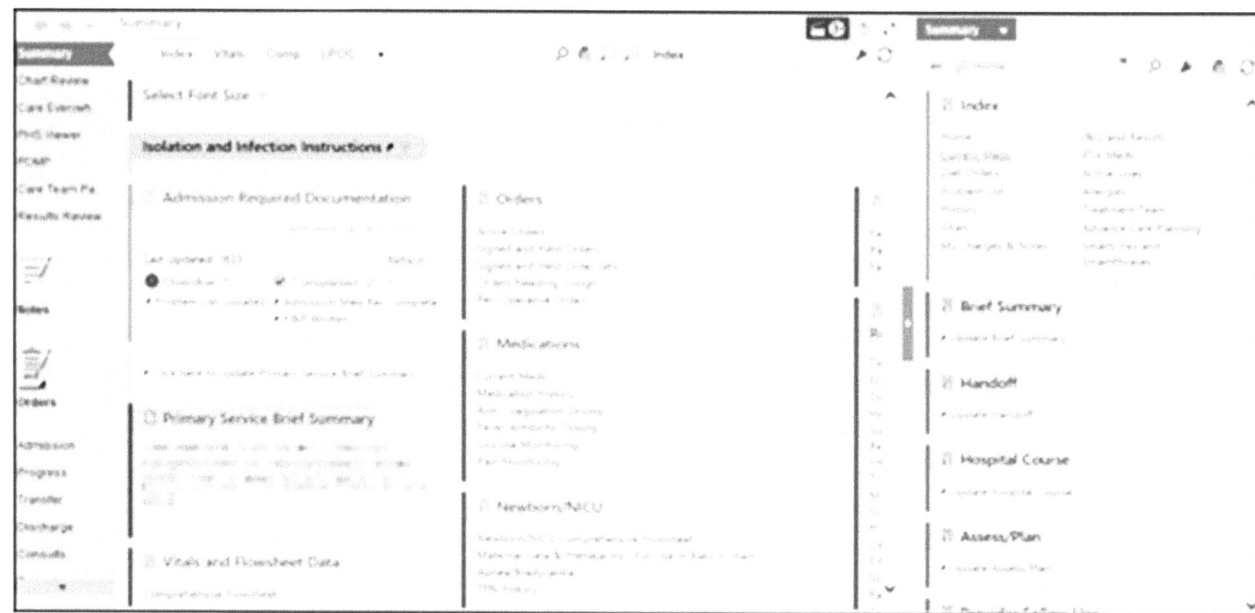

Fig. 5.23 Location of freehand fields in Summary tab. (© *2020 Epic Systems Corporation. Used with permission*)

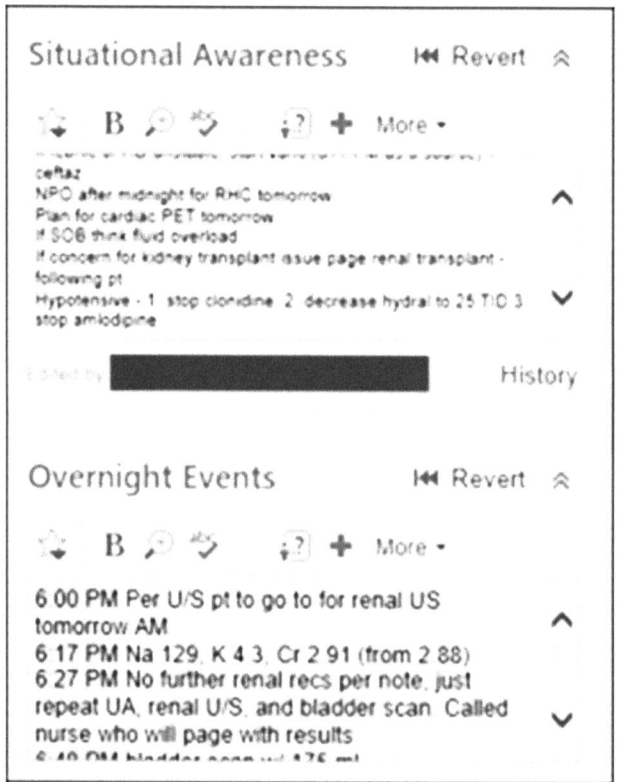

Fig. 5.24 Summary tab useful fields (foundation version). (© *2020 Epic Systems Corporation. Used with permission*)

On the far right side of the Summary tab (■ Fig. 5.23), there are a number of useful freehand fields such as Situational Awareness and Overnight Events (■ Figs. 5.24 and 5.25). This is a common place for members of the care team, usually residents, to keep important notes and reminders. This is a great place

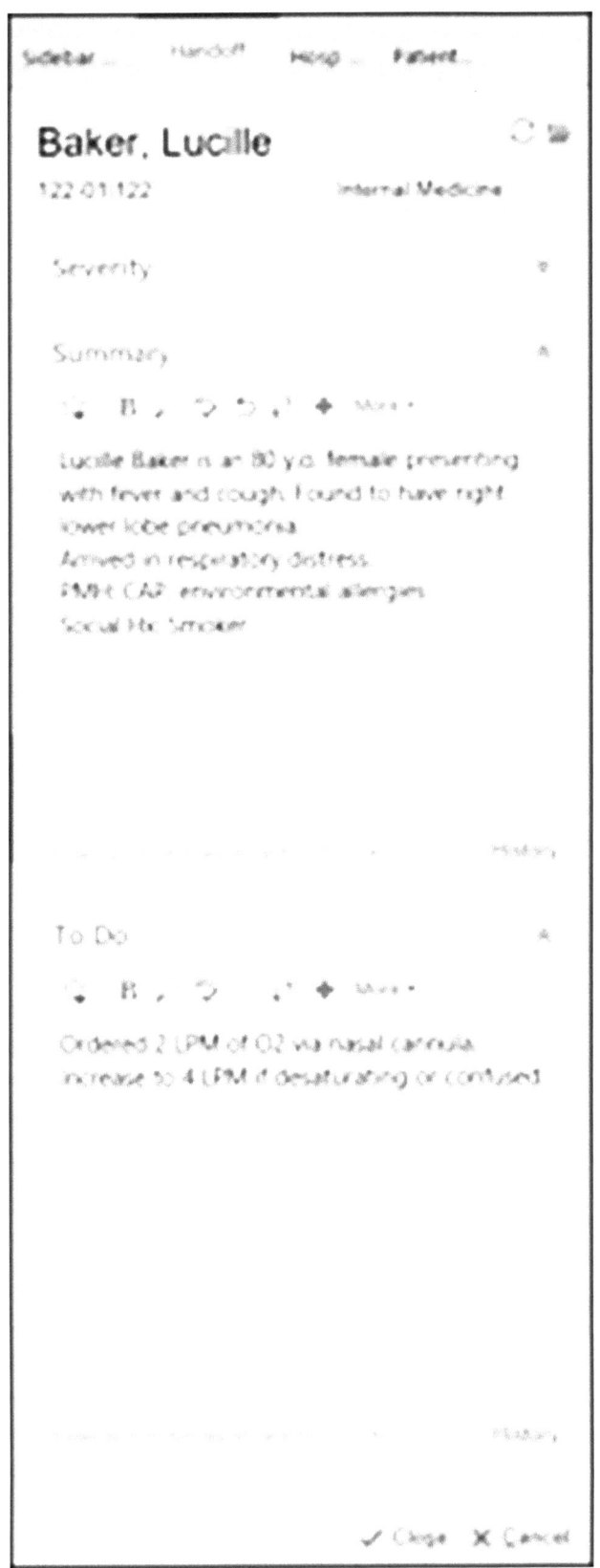

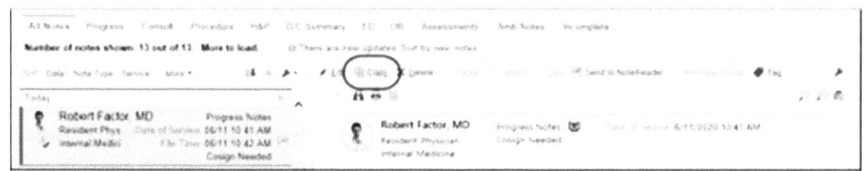

■ **Fig. 5.26**   Copy Note feature. (© *2020 Epic Systems Corporation. Used with permission*)

to check in the morning during your pre-rounding as well as prior to sign-out. While not foolproof, it does often contain a lot of the evolving management for your patient. Again, to facilitate your learning, you should not rely on these and come up with your own answers before checking.

5.3.6   Copy Note

For progress notes, a great feature is called Copy Note (■ Fig. 5.26) and literally copies the prior note you wrote for that patient but substitutes in relevant fields such as the date, updated labs, and so forth. You should always be writing an updated subjective, exam, and assessment for each progress note. However, this feature is very helpful in automating some of the more tedious things such as inserting objective data into a template and signing your pager info.

Internal Medicine

Bliss J. Chang

Contents

© The Author(s), under exclusive license to Springer Nature Switzerland AG 2021
S. H. Lecker, B. J. Chang (eds.), *The Ultimate Medical School Rotation Guide*,
https://doi.org/10.1007/978-3-030-63560-2_6

6.1   Overview

The Internal Medicine clerkship is a core requirement for all students regardless of their future specialty choice, and you will learn many principles that will serve as a foundation for the rest of your medical career. Excelling on your Medicine rotation is somewhat distinct from prior rotations in that you will need to blend many elements together, from compassion and effective communication to critical thinking, and the rotation will push you to integrate your knowledge across other disciplines. In particular, the breadth of presentations ranging from psychiatric to neurologic may be especially challenging for students.

Generally, medical schools and residencies (regardless of specialty) place a heavy emphasis on student performance in the Internal Medicine clerkship. This may lead to some level of anxiety and excitement prior to the rotation. Our goals in this chapter are to provide you with exactly what you need to know, and, arguably more importantly, *do*, to excel on your medicine rotation with less anxiety. More importantly, we wish to help you reach your maximum potential and be a treasured asset to your care teams and patients.

Don't worry about trying to distinguish your roles as a medical student versus a Sub-I in the Medicine wards. As a student, use the Sub-I role as your inner metric – over your clerkship and clinical year, you will need to grow your skills to become a Sub-I. Participate in as many aspects as you can, from contributing to the assessment/plan to calling consults.

This chapter begins with a framework to approach the clerkship through familiarization with clerkship components as well as personal goal setting. We then delve into fundamental clinical concepts, practical tips, and finally, the most common conditions you will encounter as a medical student on the rotation. Because the scope of the Internal Medicine clerkship often extends into conditions that are better described in subspecialty chapters, we may only briefly discuss some conditions in this chapter and refer to other chapters.

6.1.1   Setting Goals

The medicine clerkship is usually longer (3 months) and filled with more content than other rotations. Thus, it is especially important to set goals for your medicine clerkship to continue learning and building your foundational skills.

Throughout your rotation, set personal goals to improve daily. Students who do this stand out as independent and proactive learners. Attending and resident faculty will observe your growth over the clerkship and recognize your genuine and proactive desire to improve in your evaluations. It is often hard to know how to set achievable goals since we all have so much to learn. To identify and set achievable goals, I recommend using the Entrustable Professional Activities (EPAs), a list of clinical observable behaviors which more and more schools are using for clerkship evaluations (◘ Tables 6.1, 6.2, 6.3, and 6.4). Pay particular attention to the detailed descriptions underlying each EPA. These details can help you define specific goals and also ask for specific feedback around that behavior.

Actively striving towards goals is how you best improve. You should set aside a few minutes each day (or at least each week) to assess your own progress towards these goals. Identify what you've done well and what you want to work on the next day (or week). Keep these goals in mind by jotting them down in an easily visible place throughout your work day, such as in a corner of your task list for the day. This helps to constantly remind you and keep you from falling into a routine.

◻ **Table 6.1** Core EPAs, Part 1

EPA#	EPAText	Entrustable behavior	Emerging	Pre-entrustable
1A*	Gather a history:	Gathers complete and/or focused and accurate history (appropriate to patient presentation and setting), demonstrates relevant clinical reasoning useful in patient care. Communication is considerate, culturally sensitive, and patient/family centered	Gathers most relevant information, links most history/PE findings in a clinically relevant fashion. Communication is mostly patient focused, but still Somewhat unidirectional	Gathers too little/ too much information, and does not link information in a clinically relevant fashion. Communication is unidirectional and not patient focused. Does not tailor H&P to specific circumstances
1B*	Perform a physical examination:	Correctly performs basic and/or focused physical exam (appropriate to setting) and correctly identifies and interprets abnormal findings in the context of patient history	Correctly performs most of basic physical exam and identifies and interprets most abnormal findings. May have trouble tailoring exam to setting	Incorrectly performs or omits pertinent physical exam components. Does not tailor H&P to specific circumstances
2*	Prioritize a differential diagnosis following a clinical encounter:	Generates a thorough, appropriate, and reasoned list of possible Dx based on pathophysiology and epidemiology. Determines most likely based on H&P and initial labs. Outlines high value test strategy to confirm/exclude most likely and/or dangerous Dx	Generates a short list of possible Dx based on pattern recognition and reasoning about pathophysiology. Eliminates a few Dx based on H&P and initial labs. Outlines a simple evaluation using commonly available tests to confirm/exclude particular Dx	Generates 1–2 possible Dx, largely based on pattern recognition; has difficulty generating alternative hypotheses or explaining supporting mechanisms of disease. Unable to outline diagnostic evaluations to confirm/exclude particular Dx
3*	Recommend and interpret common diagnostic and screening tests:	Correctly interprets abnormal results for common labs/ imaging and impact on patient care. Identifies critical results with correct response/urgency. Recommends reliable, cost-effective patient-centered screening and evaluation of common conditions	Knows/finds normal common lab results. Gathers results and responds to critical ones w/ correct urgency; updates team. Identifies key tests for common conditions. Begins to interpret abnormal findings for common tests and impact on patient care	Misinterprets common results. Fails to recognize abnormal labs or responds to critical ones. Identifies order sets but cannot explain purpose. Identifies key tests for some common conditions. Repeats tests at incorrect intervals

◘ Table 6.2 Core EPAs, Part 2

EPA#	EPAText	Entrustable behavior	Emerging	Pre-entrustable
4	Enter and discuss orders and prescriptions:	Writes safe/indicated orders based on a clear ability to synthesize relevant information from a variety of relevant sources. Reliably incorporates pts' preferences. ID's potential safety concerns; demonstrates facility w/ paper and EMR orders	Demonstrates a developing sense of writing safe/reasoned orders/prescriptions. Assesses pt understanding of Rx instructions and contra-/indications for treatment, but unable to reliably apply to both straightforward and complex scenarios	Demonstrates familiarity with frequently ordered medications/tests/treatments. Neither writes safe and indicated orders nor takes into account patients' preferences in the context of an overall management plan
5*	Document a clinical encounter in the patient record:	Documents a timely, accurate, comprehensive but concisely captured patient story. Includes all relevant problems, DDx, testing and rationale in A&P. Provides accurate discussion germane to patient problem(s) and plan	Documents a timely and accurately captured patient story, but may have a few errors of omission/commission. Includes all relevant problems in A&P. Provides discussion of DDx, testing, rationale that is mostly pertinent to patient problems	Unable to accurately document or capture a cogent patient story. Includes errors of omission/commission and is primarily "cut and paste." Does not include relevant problems in A&P nor discussion of germane problems/testing
6*	Provide an oral presentation of a clinical encounter:	Provides a complete, accurate and logically sequenced oral presentation. Presents pertinent +/−'s w/out prompting. Requires <5 clarifying questions Spontaneously presents most H&P elements using notes only for reference	Provides a mostly complete, accurate presentation w/ general logical sequence. Distinguishes between important/unimportant H&P elements (pertinent+/−'s). Requires >5 clarifying questions. Spontaneously presents critical H&P elements without notes	Provides an incomplete, inaccurate presentation w/out logical sequence. Does not distinguish between important/unimportant details of H&P and labs (pertinent+/−'s). Requires multiple clarifying questions. Reads from notes when presenting

◘ Table 6.2 (continued)

EPA#	EPA Text	Entrustable behavior	Emerging	Pre-entrustable
7*	Form clinical questions and retrieve evidence to advance patient care:	Efficiently identifies, retrieves, assesses and prioritizes evidence directly related to patient's care. Forms questions that demonstrate understanding of the application of this evidence to contribute to patient's plan of care	Identifies, retrieves, assesses and prioritizes evidence and forms clinical questions related to patient care. Unable to use evidence to form complex questions to advance patient's plan of care	Identifies evidence and forms simple questions related to patient's clinical features. Unable to efficiently retrieve, assess, or prioritize information or apply it to form complex questions to advance patient care

Remember to create specific observable and achievable goals. For example, rather than "wanting to work on my oral presentation" which is a general skill which will take you more time to achieve, use the EPAs to further define your oral presentation goal as "I want to present physical exam findings in a more organized manner" or "I want to be more succinct and clear when presenting my clinical reasoning". Share your goals with the team so that they can pay better attention to what you want to work on, and help you with specific constructive feedback. Creating specific goals also helps to break down goals into manageable pieces. It's much easier to perfect your oral presentation if you work on each individual component and put them together as opposed to trying to fix everything at once.

On the first day of working with a new team, take the initiative and request 15 minutes with your team residents and/or attending to discuss your learning objectives and goals. At this time, also ask your team about their stylistic expectations for you – how would they want you to present, how many patients to follow, etc. Afterwards, check in with your team periodically (e.g., at the end of each week) to assess how you've been performing and what you can focus on for next week. These check-ins, especially when scheduled in advance, do not take much time and team members appreciate giving constructive feedback on specific goals. During these times, also ask your team what skills you should be focusing on.

Here are some larger clinical goals worth striving towards:

- [] Core: Pre-rounding, oral presentations, physical exam, note writing, etc.
- [] Logistical skills: Calling consults, obtaining collateral information, prioritizing tasks, etc.
- [] Workup and management: Disease-specific knowledge, clinical reasoning
- [] Procedural: IV lines, A-lines, lumbar puncture, wound care, etc.
- [] Communication: Tailoring language to patients, working with nursing/care coordination/pharmacy, etc.
- [] Empathy and patient-centered care

Throughout the rotation, you will be assigned tasks you perceive as "less clinical." An example is calling a pharmacy to reconcile medications. While

Table 6.3 Core EPAs, Part 3

EPA#	EPAText	Entrustable behavior	Emerging	Pre-entrustable
8	Give or receive a patient handover to transition care responsibility:	Organizes, prioritizes, and uses a handover communication template that is adapted based on patient, audience, setting, or context, without errors of omission/commission. Provides action plan demonstrating awareness of team and patient needs	Begins to use, organize, and prioritize handover communication based on patient, audience, setting, or context, with minimal errors of omission/commission. Provides action plan demonstrating awareness of team and patient needs	Unable to organize, prioritize, or adapt handover communication template based on patient, audience, setting, or context without making errors of omission/commission. Lacks awareness of team and patient needs
9*	Collaborate as a member of an interprofessional team:	Actively integrates into team to meet/exceed given role Understands role/responsibility of and effectively engages with all team members Develops/reiterates plans with input from patient/family Recognizes own role/limits; seeks help when needed	Takes initiative to integrate into team to meet given role; sometimes passive. May develop/reiterate plans w/out input from family or non-MD team members, but may seek their input at times. Recognizes own role/limits; seeks help when needed	Limits role in team discussion, passively follows others Develops/reiterates plans independent of patient, family, or other team members. Dismisses and does not seek non-MD input. Does not recognize personal role/limits
10	Recognize a patient requiring urgent or emergent care and initiate evaluation:	Recognizes abnormal VS/Sxs and need for higher level of care. Responds promptly to RN concerns Performs relevant H&P to begin evaluation of problem. Initiates stabilizing interventions, alerts superiors, and accurately communicates problem and plan	Sometimes recognizes abnormal VS/Sxs and need for higher care level. Mild delay in response to RN. Performs limited/non-relevant H&P. Formulates limited plan, alerts superiors w/ mild delay and communicates problem w/ little analysis of problem	Fails to recognize abnormal VS/Sxs or need for higher care level. Does not respond to RN. Unable to gather data to assess problem or formulate plan for initial stabilization and evaluation Does not alert superiors about patient in timely fashion

these are not the most direct patient-contact tasks, these are invaluable to your team's care of the patient and a way that medical students can especially help. When you are delegated such tasks, take pride in helping the overall care of the patient. That being said, there are ways to elicit more trust and hence tasks requiring more responsibility and usually more direct patient contact.

- *Knowledge*: Be diligent – use outside time to read and increase your medical content knowledge. As much as possible, tailor your readings based on the needs of your patients – this is not only a commendable motivator but you will also have to engage with the team around your patient's care. You should aim to reinforce and clarify concepts, striving to learn clinical pearls

Table 6.4 Core EPAs, Part 4

EPA#	EPAText	Entrustable behavior	Emerging	Pre-entrustable
11	Obtain Informed consent for tests and/or procedures:	Demonstrates understanding of informed consent. Engages pt/family in shared decision making w/ complete information; avoids jargon. Exhibits appropriate confidence yet seeks guidance as needed. Documents in a complete and timely fashion	Demonstrates understanding of informed consent. Begins to engage pt/family in shared decision making under direct supervision; avoids jargon Understands skill limit, confidence, and when to seek guidance. Prepare parts of documents in timely fashion	Lacks (full) understanding of informed consent Communication demonstrates errors of omission, personal bias, jargon or is unidirectional and lacks solicitation of pt/family preferences. Documents w/ errors of commission/ omission
12	Perform general procedures of a physician:	Demonstrates prep and reliable technique; applies knowledge of key issues (RIB/A, contra-/indications). Seeks appropriate help. Mitigates complications. Consistently uses universal precautions/aseptic technique. Provides complete/timely documentation	Demonstrates knowledge of prep and key issues (RIB/A, contra-/ indications). Begins to learn steps; use universal precautions/ aseptic technique Seeks appropriate help. Demonstrates knowledge of complication prevention. Provides documentation outline	Lacks knowledge of key issues (RIB/A, contra-/ indications) Unable to complete basic procedures. Lacks consistent skill and awareness of complications. Inconsistently uses universal precautions/ aseptic technique Provides incomplete documentation
13	Identify system failures and contribute to a culture of safety and improvement:	Demonstrates knowledge of systems of care and impact on safety. Participates in RCA and PDSA cycle for QI. Recognizes potential errors; reports errors/ near-misses. Adheres to pt safety protocols. Acknowledges personal knowledge/skills gaps	Demonstrates some knowledge of systems of care, impact on safety, and concepts of RCNPDSA. Recognizes potential errors at times; reports errors/ near-misses. Adheres to pt safety protocols w/ prompts. Often acknowledges personal knowledge/ skills gaps	Lacks knowledge of systems of care, impact on patient safety, and/or does not adhere to protocols. Unable to recognize potential errors or report errors/ near-misses. Unable to acknowledge personal knowledge/skills gaps

and nuances that are not obtainable from your readings. If you come to rounds without reading on your patient, an attending might discuss the basics which you could have gotten from a textbook. You would miss the rich discussion around the nuances of a presentation which is only based on experience.

- *Tasks:* There is no task that is below you. The team as a whole needs to complete a set of tasks, and your ability to complete even the smaller tasks contribute significantly to the team. As students, we study not only medicine but the system in which medicine is practiced. So, take the time to get a better history, call the pharmacy, grab the nurse when the team needs, understand the patient's insurance, and so forth, with enthusiasm. An excellent way to keep up with all these tasks for each patient is to pre-write these core tasks on your to-do list for each patient, without explicit instruction.

- *Taught once, learned forever:* You should ideally strive to learn and incorporate knowledge and feedback after being taught once. Not that your team doesn't want to help you, but due to the busy nature of clinical teams, you want to be professional and respectful of others' times. Every time you learn something again, it should be learned in a deeper manner. During my rotation, I kept a separate sheet in my notebook of feedback and things I learned, whether medical knowledge, social dynamics, logistics (e.g., consult numbers, how to call a transport), or otherwise to decrease the number of repetitious questions.

6.1.2 Rotation Structure

Your medicine rotation will likely be divided up into an inpatient portion (majority) and an outpatient primary care clinic. This chapter will focus specifically on the inpatient portion. You may refer to the "Primary Care" chapter for preparation for your outpatient rotation.

On the inpatient medicine rotation, you may be alone or paired with another medical student on a general medicine service. The general service cares for cases that do not typically require intense specialist management, but may be where overflow patients are admitted when other specialty services do not have bed space.

Refer to the "Interpersonal Skills" chapter for great advice on team dynamics such as introductions with team members, setting time for feedback, responding to feedback, and so forth.

6.1.3 Team Structure

You will generally have two interns on a team and one junior or senior resident. The interns primarily manage the patients, with oversight from the resident and attending. They are great for running your questions or plans by prior to presenting to the team. The resident usually takes on the primary teaching role for you and the interns. They are a great resource to turn to when the interns are busy or they (the interns) are unsure about your questions.

While residents often rotate for at least 2 weeks, your attending/hospitalist may change every week. Since every attending has some variation on expectations, asking what each attending is looking for early in the week would be beneficial. You can then demonstrate those qualities throughout the week.

Attendings and residents are your primary evaluators (often without differentiation of their rank); hence while you should make it a goal to learn as much as possible from them and ask intelligent questions, be aware that your interactions with them will, for better or worse, become a piece of your overall perceived performance. With questions, be inquisitive, but display thoughtfulness. For example, it's better to not ask the attending what diverticulitis is and rather ask them something confusing from your readings about diverticulitis. This demonstrates that you do your part in your learning and use your team to support and optimize your learning. If you do this, you will not only learn more and deeper, but your evaluations will reflect the depth of your medical knowledge and skills as a motivated student.

6.2 Practical Tips

In this section, we will cover the practical and logistical things you will encounter on your rotation. Overall, the logistics are similar to other nonsurgical rotations.

6.2.1 External Resources

While this chapter provides excellent practical tips, fundamentals, and a framework for approaching cases, you will need to refer to outside resources for conditions not covered in this book. We recommend using UpToDate as your go-to resource. It is not worth using other more board-oriented resources such as Online Med Ed, Case Files, etc. as they cover too many topics (which show up on the boards but not wards) without sufficient depth.

For expanding your knowledge base throughout the rotation, we recommend using UpToDate to gain deeper insight into common clinical cases and UWorld (the explanations are key) for more broad medical knowledge. UWorld has a surprising amount of depth (though less practical details such as dosing) for many of the topics it covers.

6.2.2 Shelf Prep

Whether you like standardized exams or not, medicine is filled with them. Many core rotations will culminate in a shelf exam consisting of 110 questions (100 scored). At most schools, you must score above a certain cutoff (approximately 70–80% of questions correct) to achieve honors. Thus, you should be studying regularly for the shelf exam throughout your rotation. It can be hard to do this on top of a busy clinical day, but studying for 30–60 minutes each day really adds up. The following cover two test-taking strategies you likely have not encountered.

Some students believe that preparation for the shelf exam is different than preparation required for daily patient care. A key secret is to apply one of the key skills from your wards experience to your shelf studies. Reading a set of answer choices is similar to listing your differential diagnosis or listing treatment options. For example, if a question stem presents a patient with memory impairment, the answer choices on the exam *most always* include mild cognitive impairment, Alzheimer's disease, and two other less prominent but potentially misleading answer choices such as delirium as diagnostic possibilities. From a test writer's perspective, they have to provide a set of answer choices that doesn't scream the right answer to the average test taker. This is done through building a common set of "differential" answer choices representing choices with some commonality, requiring a specific nuance to distinguish among them.

As an example, let's explore our example of memory loss further. A set of answer choices could be:
(a) Alzheimer's disease
(b) Delirium
(c) Mild cognitive impairment
(d) Depression

Each question has a learning (and testing) objective. Let's imagine that the goal of this question is to determine whether a student understands that memory loss is on a spectrum and what is required for a diagnosis of memory impairment. Let's explore behind the scenes with the above answer choices:

- We notice that choice A is Alzheimer's disease. This is the classic reflexive association students have when they think of "memory loss"; it is also not coincidentally positioned at the top of the answer list. Oftentimes, test writers position tempting but incorrect answer choices at the top of the list – many students see these, jump at it, and move on without considering the entire list. This is, in terms of clinical reasoning errors, premature closure.
- We notice that the two most similar answer choices are Alzheimer's disease and mild cognitive impairment. While these may not initially seem similar, as they represent opposite ends of the memory impairment spectrum, they are similar in that they both address the learning objective. This is another important point – think about what the tester is testing! Because these are the two key questions addressing the perceived learning objective, it's likely that one of them is the correct answer.
- The difference between A and C can be boiled down to the presence of functional impairment. Dementia is always associated with impairment in function. MCI is a normal part of aging, but patients can still carry on their activities of daily living (ADLs) independently. At this point, you scan the passage for functional status and unsurprisingly find that there is no impairment carrying out their ADLs.
- Choices B (delirium) and D (depression) represent transient states where memory can be impaired. For a diagnosis of true neurological memory impairment, you cannot have these alternative explanations.

This is how you should begin thinking about each question as you study. Over time, you will become more natural (and much faster) at reasoning through all this. Furthermore, this strategy perhaps ironically transfers over to your clinical differential diagnosis skills quite well.

One other key test-taking strategy to briefly touch on here is knowing how to read a question. Every word you read is an opportunity to come closer to the answer, but also an opportunity to be misled towards the incorrect answer. We've all experienced this where we think the answer is something and then one thing makes us feel uncomfortable and leads us to miss the question. Always start by reading the question and read backwards through the question stem. Usually, the most important details in shelf questions are located towards the end of the stem, whether in the lab results, physical exam findings, or otherwise. I can only guess that this is because most of the decisions you make need to be based on some objective information rather than simply symptoms. Lastly, I prefer not to read the answer choices first as they can bias you. Though we cannot delve into all the test-taking strategies here, try to spend some time each study session thinking about what the test writer thinks about as they develop these questions. You should be able to visualize what the two to three most similar answer choices will be and what "traps" they may set.

For resources, I recommend the UWorld question bank. Step Up to Medicine is not very high yield in my opinion and too long; you will obtain much more high yield information by studying the question explanations in UWorld. Be sure to take every NBME practice test available – sometimes the same questions appear on your real exam! Overall, there is a strong correlation between the number of questions you solve and your performance on these exams. Setting aside half an hour to do 20 questions each day is more than enough to get through all the practice questions in these resources.

6.2.3 **Pre-rounding**

While there is no "correct" way to pre-round, this section will cover some tips to optimize the process. The goal of pre-rounding is to understand your patient's status over the previous 24-hour period. Specifically, students will check in on a patient's symptoms and look at their response to any therapies. Additionally, it is important to identify any overnight events as well as consults done on your patient. Effective pre-rounding will give you the information to:

- Assess how the patient's status affects your differential and management. For example, if the SOB was thought to be CHF rather than COPD, did diuresis help? Or if the patient continued to spike a fever, what does that mean?
- Determine path to discharge. What does the patient need today to improve and be discharged?

Thus, we will focus on how you can best gather data, organize your thoughts, impress your team, and provide excellent patient care!

6.2.3.1 **Sign-Out**

You should begin by obtaining sign-out from the overnight team. They will tell you about any overnight events on your patient(s), as well as any interventions done or pending. This is also a great opportunity to get some insight to the overnight team's thoughts on course of action for the patient. If it is your first day, consider sitting and listening to the entire team's sign-out. It is a good way to learn how interns get information from the sign-out process.

6.2.3.2 **Pre-rounding**
Prior to Seeing Your Patients

Before seeing your patients, you should gather as much data as you can to maximize the value of your time with the patient. Begin with a quick chart review, using the following checklist to ensure you hit all the highlights.

Pre-rounding Chart Review Checklist
- [] Vital signs overnight
- [] Morning Labs, if back already (if not, try to check prior to rounds)
- [] Ins/outs
- [] New radiology studies
- [] Other new data (e.g., micro)
- [] New consult notes since yesterday
- [] MAR (Medication Administration Records) – check that the patient is taking the same medications as the day before, and if not, there should be a clear indication; identify any new medications given overnight

Remember to start tracking all of your tasks, including those above, in checklist format, as soon as you enter the hospital. You *will* forget tasks otherwise. Jot them down no matter how small a task. It's also quite satisfying to cross off completed tasks!

Next, obtain overnight events from the nurse. This is a great time to double check any of the objective data you obtained from chart review. One common thing worth double-checking is I/Os (they may not be most up to date in the EMR).

You are finally ready to see your patients. I recommend coming up with a systematic method for who to see first. My personal preference is to see patients I know well first, saving the newer patients for last. This helps to keep the new-

Pearl: Even though you are part of the general medicine team, you should still be up to date on what each specialty team's plans are for the patient.

est information freshest on your brain and is particularly helpful for presenting without notes. Similarly, among the familiar and new patients, sort them by complexity, saving the most complex for last. Rarely, you will have to see patients in another order, such as by acuity. Always think about whether you're arriving early enough to pre-round (e.g., give yourself more time the first week, more if you know of a complex new admit, etc.).

With the Patient

You should be entering the patient room with a good sense of what information you want to obtain. It's completely okay to gather your thoughts outside each room! Once you enter the room, be sure not to be completely engrossed in note-taking and give the patient the human connection they deserve.

Again, the goals behind your questions and exam maneuvers when pre-rounding are to (1) assess for common complications of hospitalization (e.g., DVT, infection) and (2) determine the progress towards recovery for your patient. Assessing for changes relative to the day before, as well as historic baselines, is very helpful.

Towards the end of your patient encounter, it can be quite helpful to summarize the information you gathered for the patient – this not only helps the patient understand what's going on but also helps you organize and synthesize the collected information. You'll be surprised at how effective this is. This, not a fabulous memory, was my secret for presenting without notes on rounds.

After Seeing the Patients

A great way to gather your thoughts for each patient is to run through the day's plan for them. This will tie together the key elements of history and objective data that guide your plan. Jot down bullet points for each key issue you intend to discuss in your plan. Regardless of your exact approach, you should always give yourself plenty of time to gather and organize your thoughts prior to rounds. If you're repeatedly rushing through this part, arrive earlier!

When time allows (for both you and your team members), you should run your plan by your intern or resident. Don't be afraid to ask questions! Furthermore, working on your progress note during pre-rounding is a good way to organize your thoughts and anticipate plans prior to presenting on rounds. This also allows you to quickly prep them after rounds so that it is ready for the resident to edit/co-sign.

6.2.4 Oral Presentation

Internists love to hear the entire story about the patient. Your presentations will thus be much longer, holistic, and detail-oriented than other services. However, this does not mean that you should include irrelevant details in your presentations. Always touch base with your team the first day on how they like your presentations – jot down their preferences so as to not forget.

While there are several ways to structure your presentation, the key is organization. If you've ever tried listening to another person present, you probably know how difficult it is to keep up when the presentation lacks structure and organization. Here are some tips for giving a clear and succinct oral presentation.

- Articulate transitions between each section ("For the physical exam,…").
- Grouping key information together in a logical fashion (e.g., if discussing COPD exacerbation, you should group discussion of the patient's cough, sputum, and SOB rather than spread them out in your history).

Pearl: Do not feel the urge to mimic the presentations of others on your team, whether a fellow student or intern/resident. There is often less formality in presenting for interns/residents, and you should always approach it seriously as described below unless specifically told otherwise.

– Avoid filler words such as "um" and "I think." It may feel awkward initially, but remaining silent is better than using tons of filler words! If you have read about your patient, you should have a hypothesis for the differential – state it and discuss it. Don't worry about being wrong – this is how you learn!

Let's explore the standard structure of a medicine oral presentation:

6.2.4.1 One-liner

This is among the most important parts to a presentation. You will be evaluated heavily based on your one-liner, and it is where you will either grab or lose your team's attention. Prior to reading on, refer to ▶ Chap. 4 for a primer.

The medicine one-liner is perhaps the most standard (◻ Fig. 6.1), with the following parts:
– Demographics: Always state the patient's age and gender; also state the race if relevant (e.g., sickle cell crisis).
– Relevant history: Only mention history relevant to the management of the *current* presentation
– Chief complaint: This should be detailed with the most important details (such as location or duration of pain) that you think will help in the workup and management of the patient.
– Current status (new admission, hospital day X, etc.).

Notice that the one-liner contains the three criteria used to determine a COPD exacerbation. Beginning with the one-liner, you're essentially making your case for what you think is most likely going on and why. Keeping this in mind can be very helpful when determining what to include or not in the one-liner.

6.2.4.2 History of Present Illness (HPI)

This is where you begin to make your case. It is a fine line between including everything the patient says and omitting important information. Include only relevant information which allows your team to sift through the differential or can otherwise affect the inpatient management of the patient. For example, A patient with COPD exacerbation who drinks heavily might need to be monitored for alcohol withdrawal and/or might want to be considered for an

> Pearl: Be as detailed as possible! Instead of saying diabetes, say "type 2 diabetes"; instead of saying CKD, say "stage III CKD with baseline Cr of 1.8."

> Preserving the patient's actual words can be really valuable. Avoid using too many medical terms when describing their symptoms.

Ms. A is a 63F with Grade III COPD (most recent hospitalization for COPD exacerbation six weeks ago) and type 2 diabetes presenting with three days of increasing shortness of breath, cough, and sputum production.

- Demographics
- Relevant History
- Chief complaint

◻ **Fig. 6.1** Anatomy of a one-liner

aspiration pneumonia. Similarly, a patient recently initiated on a biologic agent for psoriasis changes the potential differential of that patient's fever. The review of systems (ROS) should be integrated as part of the HPI rather than separating it out and going through each system exhaustingly. Lastly, remember that you're telling a story – stay organized and logical, and don't interpret.

6.2.4.3 Past History

There is no need to mention the exhaustive list of comorbidities many patients will have. Rather, mention any history not mentioned in the one-liner that is important to consider for this admission. These often include chronic problems managed by the primary team such as diabetes. It is also important to note unrelated yet significant comorbidities such as heart failure.

6.2.4.4 Medications

Run through the entire list of home medications, noting dosages for medications that are specifically relevant to the patient's hospitalization or used for inpatient management (e.g., units of basal Lantus). It can also be very helpful in newly admitted patients to compare what the patient is actually taking at home versus prescribed – this sometimes easily explains why the patient is hospitalized! At some institutions, a pharmacist with the team will be responsible for this section, but be sure not to zone out and pay attention!

6.2.4.5 Vital Signs

The vitals are typically reported in this order: temperature, heart rate, blood pressure, respiratory rate, and oxygen saturation. You should avoid editorializing, meaning translating the data into what it means. Everyone understands that a temperature of 98.8F is afebrile. While you may often hear residents do this, you should really be only providing the data here without interpreting it.

6.2.4.6 Physical Exam

Always be systematic and thorough here. We recommend a head-to-toe approach in order to ensure that you do not miss any systems. It is worth practicing saying the normal physical exam so that you can demonstrate that you have checked various things in a sophisticated manner. Use a resource such as Bates to understand physical exam maneuvers in more detail. If you have a patient with pneumonia, take the time to also percuss and practice egophony. You will never know how to do this or identify abnormalities if you only do the basic exam. It is always refreshing for the attending to have a medical student do a relevant and focused physical exam with other maneuvers. If you are unsure of a finding, inform your team and ask them to demonstrate the maneuver during rounds. If you are unsure of how to describe the finding using medical terms, it is completely acceptable to simply describe what you see or found. Here's a standard core physical exam upon which to build. Remember to only discuss parts of the exam you did.

- General: Alertness, overall appearance (well vs sick)
- Heart: Rate, rhythm, extra heard sounds
- Lungs: All sounds in all fields
- Abdomen: Soft, non-tender, non-distended; bowel sounds
- Extremities: Lower extremity edema or pain, dorsalis pedis pulses

6.2.4.7 Objective Data

Again, avoid editorializing – just read out the pertinent and most relevant lab values. Everyone can understand lab values, and if necessary, you can elaborate in your assessment/plan. You need not read all lab values, for example, from a BMP – note that significant findings ("BMP notable for a potassium of 5.2"). Note, for imaging data, you should present in a similar fashion ("opacities in the RUL") but also add your interpretation (and that of the radiologist's, if available).

6.2.4.8 Assessment/Plan

This is the most critical part of your presentation. You should always follow a systematic format as such:
1. Start by summarizing your patient briefly with a one-liner. This where you want to condense the patient's symptoms using medical terminology. For example, instead of saying "patient who had difficulty breathing that suddenly started," say "patient with acute dyspnea."
2. List out the top three problems (in order of importance) that you want to address so that you grab the attention of everyone. For example, "I'm going to address the patient's shortness of breath, hyponatremia, and diabetes."

Next, dive into the assessment by problem. For each problem, address the following, in order:
1. Differential Diagnosis
   1. State the most likely diagnosis and evidence (i.e., history, exam findings, medical content knowledge, and objective data) to support it.
   2. State two to three alternative diagnoses that you considered and why they are less likely:
      1. In new patients, include at least one do-not-miss diagnoses.
2. Diagnostic Approach
   1. Note any diagnostic tests you'd like to obtain and why.
3. Therapeutic Approach
   1. Suggest your treatment plan with why.
   2. Include evidence whenever possible.

■ Example A/P for #Shortness of Breath

"Ms. A's shortness of breath is most consistent with COPD exacerbation as evidenced by her meeting three of three criteria, specifically worsening dyspnea, cough, and sputum production. Moreover, she has a known history of COPD exacerbations which is the single best predictor of a future exacerbation per the ECLIPSE study. I considered lobar pneumonia but thought it less likely given the clear CXR and lack of infectious symptoms such as fever. Heart failure is also unlikely given no signs of volume overload on physical exam and no prior history of hypertension or coronary artery disease, the two most common causes of heart failure."

"Diagnostically, I would not currently favor obtaining further workup as this appears quite convincingly COPD exacerbation. If she worsens or does not improve over the next few days, we can consider obtaining a sputum culture."

"Therapeutically, we are admitting her for inpatient management given her persistent hypoxia to 84% despite supplemental oxygen. We will need to increase her oxygen saturation to at least 88% prior to discharge given her long-term COPD, and we should be cautious not to shut off oxygen drive by

Pearl: Try to avoid reading through lab values too rapidly – make sure you are also thinking about each as you read them! This will be important for the assessment/plan.

It is useful to provide an indicator of how a lab value changed compared to prior. For example, "The creatinine is up to 1.3" not only provides relevant data but also clues the listener into the trend.

promoting oxygen saturations higher than 92%. In terms of her acute exacerbation management, I'd like to treat with 60 mg prednisone for 5 days, which is supported over a 14-day course in the REDUCE trial which found no difference in clinical outcomes between 5- and 14-day steroid courses, and given the risk of adverse effects from steroids. I also recommend Duo-Nebs as needed. As for long-term management to prevent future hospitalization, this is a great opportunity to revisit smoking cessation as well as verifying proper inhaler technique. Her vaccinations for flu and pneumococcus are up to date."

A few aspects of the example that may have stood out follow:

- Rich details: For example, rather than mentioning "steroids," mention dose and agent (you will learn these over time, but until then, it's easy to look up and demonstrates your motivation to learn).
- Supported with evidence whenever possible (ECLIPSE, RESCUE studies).
- Clear organization and transitions to keep the listener engaged ("diagnostically", "therapeutically").
- Clear reasoning for everything that you suggest doing or not doing.
- Demonstrate a reasoning framework (acute versus long-term management).

Lastly, be sure to include chronic problems such as diabetes and hypertension that are to be managed. No problem is small enough for the primary team (you).

That's a wrap for oral presentations, but you should practice in the mirror or with a friend a few times prior to your rotation so you can get the structure of presentations down. This will allow you to fully focus on the medicine during your rotation!

6.2.5 Rounding

During rounds, you should aim to participate not only for your patients, but for all patients on the team. Rounds are filled with learning. You learn so much even from patients you are not taking care of. Be inquisitive and jot down all the pearls you learn in a section of your notebook. Here are some ways to actively participate for patients that aren't your own:

- Pay attention to labs when read (or if you have access to an EMR, review the labs yourself). There are many small lab abnormalities that may be passed over – feel free to point these out in an inquisitive manner. ("Do you think we should replete the magnesium? I've read that low levels may predispose to ventricular arrhythmias.") Not only does this demonstrate your knowledge but also provides the team with opportunities to teach you further. Practicing this for every patient also greatly enhances your ability to think quickly through key labs.
- Teams will frequently be unsure of a fact – you can volunteer to look this up and do bring back to the team, or if you're fresh from Step 1, your knowledge of mechanisms can really benefit teams!
- Contribute your experience from other rotations when teams are considering calling a consult on a case you managed on prior services (e.g., neurology).

6.2.6 EMR Setup

At the beginning of your rotation, you should ask your intern/resident whether they can help you customize an efficient EMR interface. Also, over the year, pay attention to the EMR interfaces of residents, interns, and attendings so you can always alter your own interface. Having the proper setup can greatly enhance your efficiency when collecting data on patients. An example of an efficient setup is below. Please refer to ▶ Chap. 5 for further information.

6.2.7 Calling Consults

Early on, I remember this was one of the things I would dread doing because I didn't quite know how to call a good consult, and it was intimidating to ask those more senior to come do something (see a patient). It also doesn't help that consult teams are typically busy particularly when medical students place them. In this section, we're going to cover the anatomy of an effective consult that will best enable consultants to help you.

6.2.7.1 Why Consult?

To better understand how to place superstar consults, let's think about why we place consults. We consult because we have a specific question which requires more in-depth expertise to help us answer our question. Our consult question should be so specific that there will also be a *specific* answer, be it further workup or management.

6.2.7.2 What Makes an Effective Consult?

Since we want a specific answer, we must ask a specific question. This really helps consultants know exactly what it is that we want of them, and how best they can help us. One of the most common mistakes is simply asking the consultant to come take a look at the patient. Why do we want them to come? What should they be looking for and helping us with?

Example of a specific question: "We would appreciate if you could assess for potential inotropic support and determine whether the patient merits CCU transfer." Note how not everything must be phrased in question format.

Context is key. You should provide a brief one-liner of the patient during the conversation with the consultant. You should also note a brief hospital course and what led to you place the consult. There are typically too few characters available to do so in the paging system.

Example of context: "She's an 81F with HFrEF (last EF of 30% a month ago) who we suspect may be acutely decompensating. She presented with increased shortness of breath yesterday and we began diuresing her with Lasix to which she responded well initially. This morning, however, her extremities appeared cold with MAP <65 and her mental status was markedly off from yesterday's."

Consultants receive many, many requests! Establish a sense of urgency for your consult to help them prioritize – is the patient stable, a watcher, or actively crashing? This can be done briefly either with a general descriptor such as "stable" or, preferably in unstable cases, through objective data such as "altered mental status with soft pressures."

The specific organization of these elements in a consult is largely stylistic, though certain institutions may have preferences. Personally, I think leading with the question is best as it frames everything nicely from the get-go.

In summary, here are the aspects to always consider for an effective consult in checklist format:

- [] Ask a specific question.
- [] Provide context.
- [] Establish urgency.

Other key elements to include are:
- [] Patient identifiers (name, MRN, room)
- [] Callback cell number +- pager number
- [] Your name

Putting it all together, here's an example consult to type into the paging system:

» Hi, we'd like to consult you for Doe 1234567890 in SH1010 regarding inotropic support and potential CCU transfer. Thanks, Bliss. p12345 123-456-7890.

This example includes key patient identifiers (name, MRN, room) as well as a sense of urgency (indicating potential need for a CCU transfer). It also asks a specific question – whether inotropic support and CCU transfer is merited. It wraps up by providing ample ways to reach you.

And here is an example conversation with the consultant:

Consultant: – Hi Bliss, you paged regarding Ms. Doe?

You: – Hi Sam, this is Bliss from the general medicine team. Thanks for getting back to me so quick. We wanted to consult you regarding Ms. Doe in room SH1010, MRN 1234567890. She's an 81F with HFrEF (last EF of 30% a month ago) who we suspect may be acutely decompensating. She presented with increased shortness of breath yesterday and we began diuresing her with Lasix to which she responded well initially. This morning, however, her extremities appeared cold with soft pressures and her mental status was markedly off from yesterday's. We wanted to consult you urgently regarding potential inotropic support and transfer to the CCU.

Consultant: – Sounds good – you're specifically interested in inotropic support and CCU management for acute decompensated heart failure, correct?

You: – That's right.

Consultant: – I'll go see her as soon as possible. Please go ahead and restrict fluid intake and start exploring any noncardiac etiologies.

You: – Got it, thanks!

Note the inclusion of all the important parts we discussed above. As you begin learning to place consults, use the checklist to help you ensure you're putting together a great consult.

6.2.8 Road to Discharge

Lastly, it's worth discussing how to know when to discharge patients. This is something that you should actively think about each day and discuss in your plans leading up to discharge. Specifically, you should ask yourself each day what is preventing your patient from discharge. Common issues to consider are listed in "Road to Discharge Checklist":

Road to Discharge Checklist
- [] Improvement in initial presenting symptoms
- [] Stable without need for intervention (no oxygen requirement, labile pressures, etc.)
- [] IV regimens converted to PO (antibiotics, fluids, electrolyte supplements, etc.)
- [] Short-term course of medications secured for patient
- [] Appropriate discharge destination (home, nursing home, rehab, etc.) & care coordination (PCP, barriers to care)

You can refer to this example as you make consults until you get the hang of it!

Transition to PO is typically done 1–2 days prior to discharge. Some attendings like to observe patients on a PO regimen (e.g., antibiotics) for at least a day prior to discharge, whereas some are okay with observing for a few hours.

6.3 Fundamentals

We will first examine some key clinical concepts from a general internist's viewpoint. It is helpful to know this perspective, because you can better identify how you can contribute meaningfully, particularly as you gather knowledge and skills from your other rotations where specialists may hold a significantly different view from internists even over common medical topics. We will also point out nuances and ways to stand out from these strong fundamentals.

6.3.1 Basic Metabolic Panel (BMP)

The BMP is part of the daily lab panels which are checked for inpatients. It is almost always obtained daily for hospitalized patients, usually without much thought. On admission, hospitalized patients need BMPs for general monitoring purposes given that their clinical status is less certain and many new interventions are being implemented.

You should familiarize you with the "fishbone" format of displaying lab values (■ Fig. 6.2):

There are three key ways to stand out when utilizing a BMP:

1. Be specific about what you want to check on the BMP and why. Every lab you recommend should have a rationale – this not only shows that you can think through things but also gives you a chance to learn about reasoning behind labs (■ Table 6.5). In your assessments, don't simply say that you want a BMP – say that you want a BMP to check the potassium because you just recommended initiating diuresis with furosemide which may cause hypokalemia.

2. Think critically about the need for obtaining a BMP for your patient. The reason should never be to "monitor for abnormalities." Rather, it should be specific – what abnormality are you concerned about, and how likely is it? What would be the significance of missing that abnormality? If you cannot answer those question, it is less likely that the patient needs a BMP. When the patient does not need a BMP, you should raise that point to your team – this shows that you think about even the "smallest" of actions you propose and that you are aware of the cost/benefit of tests.

3. Electrolyte rounds: This is a sort of mini-rounding on your own patients, led by you! In the morning while pre-rounding, take a few minutes to look at only the BMPs of your patients – are any of the values alarming? In need of repletion? Require close monitoring? Focusing only on the BMP can help expose action items that may easily miss the eye of others busier on your team.

Small but important actions like not ordering an unnecessary BMP can be set as daily goals! It only takes a few times of doing it to become quite good at it – but you need to remind yourself to do this until it becomes routine.

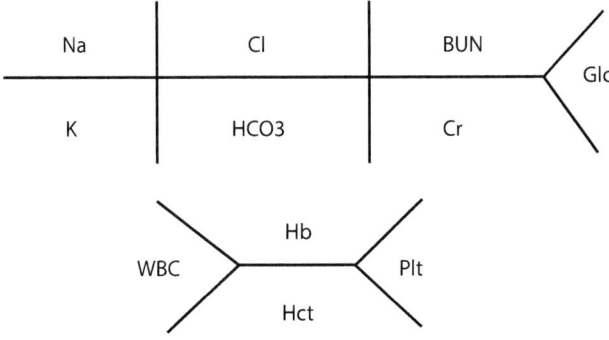

■ **Fig. 6.2** Fishbone labs

◻ Table 6.5 BMP components

Lab value	Common uses	Notes
Sodium	Sodium imbalance, cirrhosis (liver scores), heart failure (prognostic value), anion gap	High glucose levels may lead to pseudohyponatremia; use correction factor of 2.4 per 100 glucose above 100
Potassium	Potassium imbalance, diabetic ketoacidosis, anion gap	The majority of potassium is found intracellularly; thus blood potassium may not indicate overall body potassium balance
Chloride	Anion gap	
bicarbonate	Anion gap, acid-base status, volume depletion (contraction alkalosis)	
Blood urea nitrogen (BUN)	Kidney function, may speak to diet and GI bleed	
Creatinine	Kidney function, muscle mass	Important to always compare to baselines when available
Glucose	Diabetes	

6.3.2 Complete Blood Count (CBC)

This is another commonly obtained test, sometimes ordered routinely as part of the standard daily labs. Similar to the BMP, think about what value you're interested in and why you wish to obtain a CBC. You do not need to obtain this every day without reason.

A common change in the CBC is known as "hemodilution." This refers to a uniform decrease (sometimes may appear significant, e.g., change of hemoglobin by 1) in all three components (RBC, WBC, platelets) shortly after the patient receives fluids. This should not cause alarm, and you should simply note it as a change that you think is likely secondary to recent fluids rather than something like a GI bleed.

CBC with differential ("diff"): This is a special type of CBC in which the percentages of specific white blood cell types (e.g., monocytes, lymphocytes) are reported. This should be obtained when suspecting:

1. Infection: Primarily useful to check for lymphocytic (viral) or neutrophil (bacterial) predominance. One term you may hear often is "left shift" which simply refers to an increased production of immature WBCs, suggesting either infection or inflammation.
2. Hematologic malignancy: Increased proportions of certain lineages (lymphocytes, monocytes, basophils) may suggest a specific type of malignancy.
3. Allergic reactions: Increased presence of eosinophils signify allergic reactions to medications.

6.3.3 Physical Exam

As the primary team caring for the patient, you should always do a set of general exam maneuvers in addition to specifics relevant to your case. Always listen to the heart and lungs as they are among the most vital organs. It is also not

1 liter of IV fluids will typically cause a Hb drop of 1. This will correct within a few hours as fluids equilibrate among vascular compartments.

uncommon for patients to develop mild atelectasis (collapse of the lung) or pulmonary infections (e.g., pneumonia secondary to aspiration) while hospitalized due to limited mobility. Furthermore, patients can develop constipation or ileus frequently; thus, listen to bowel sounds and palpate the abdomen. Lastly, always check the lower extremities for signs of DVT (erythema, tenderness, swelling, asymmetry).

Let the following question guide your exam each day:
- What are the most important aspects of the physical exam to repeat daily?
  - E.g., for heart failure exacerbation, you would want to focus on markers of volume status such as leg edema, lung sounds, and jugular venous pressure.
  - E.g. for inpatient hospitalizations, you would want to assess for development of a leg DVT and thus check for calf tenderness, erythema, or edema.

If you would like a review of various physical exam maneuvers, a great resource is Stanford Medicine 25 (▶ stanfordmedicine25.stanford.edu).

6.3.4 Bowel Regimen

Almost all hospitalized patients receive a mild bowel regimen to help keep their bowels moving despite immobilization and various other factors such as change in diet. Some patients may not take these, but it is nice to offer it to them regardless. Common options are senna, docusate sodium (Colace), lactulose, and milk of magnesia. You should think of these options as a gradual stepwise escalation (◻ Fig. 6.3).

A few notes on common laxatives:
- Pearl: If suspecting severe constipation secondary to opioids, consider switching to tramadol or fentanyl which has weaker constipating effects.
- Avoid suppositories/enemas in patients with risk for GI/rectal bleed.
- Milk of magnesia can increase magnesium levels when in excess!

Pearl: All patients receiving any opioid analgesics should always receive a bowel regimen. This should become a reflex for you!

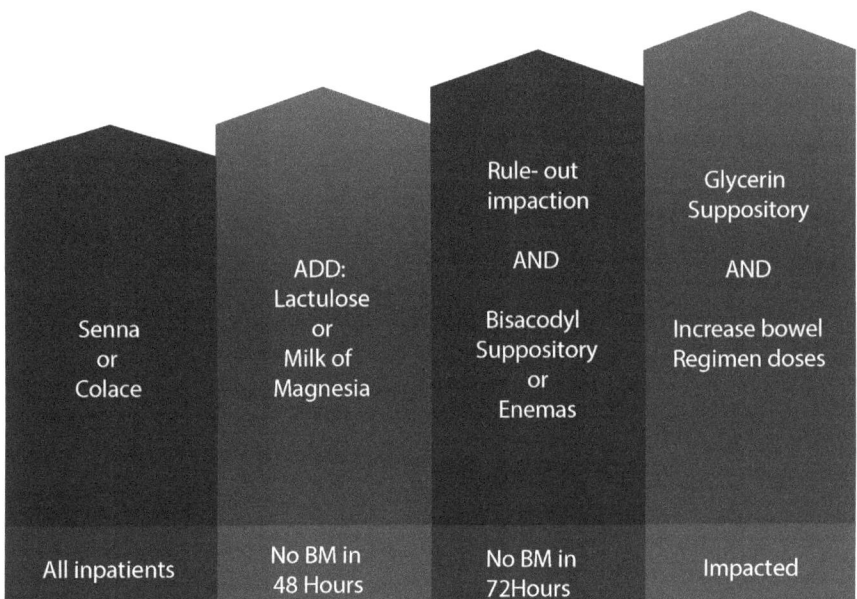

◻ **Fig. 6.3** Bowel regimen stepwise escalation

6.3.5 IV Fluids

Fluids are one of the most common interventions for patients. We won't go into all the reasons for giving fluids here but rather focus on some practical details.

6.3.5.1 Fluid Choice

There are three types of fluids that may be administered: crystalloids, colloids, and blood products.

- Crystalloids are those that contain small molecules, often electrolytes, which can easily cross cell membranes. Examples include normal (0.9%) saline, dextrose (D5W), and lactated ringers.
- Colloids contain large molecules such as albumin or gelatin that remain in and expand the intravascular space.
- Blood products may refer to any component(s) found in whole blood, such as packed RBCs, platelets, and fresh frozen plasma. Administration of blood products does increase intravascular volume.

In an inpatient general medicine ward, most of your patients will be classified as noncritically ill. In these patients, there is no difference between normal saline and lactated ringers, the two most common types of administered fluids, with regard to clinical outcomes per the SALT-ED Trial (NEJM 2018). A similar trial suggested a benefit for balanced crystalloids (lactated ringers) in critically ill patients (refer to ▶ Chap. 15).

Though there are other types of IV fluids, they are typically not administered on the inpatient general medicine floor. Fluids such as 0.45% NaCl and 3% NaCl are often used for sodium imbalance disorders which are typically ICU indications. Dextrose (D5W) may be administered in the improving (non-ICU) portion of management for diabetic ketoacidosis to aid in keeping blood glucose levels afloat in the setting of aggressive insulin administration.

It is important to note that while potassium chloride (KCl) may be repleted in IV form, oral tablets are preferred at most institutions since the IV form burns and is somewhat painful for the patient.

6.3.5.2 Volume

When suggesting how much fluids to give patients, there isn't a magical formula, and you do not need to calculate this using a formula as you might on your surgery rotation. Determining the volume to administer is quite easy once you do it a few times. There are two primary considerations:

- Degree of hypovolemia: Consider the blood pressure, heart rate, and urine output.
- Comorbidities that decrease ability to handle excess volume: Heart failure, CKD, and cirrhosis.

On the general medicine service, rarely will you need to provide a large amount of volume acutely. My personal approach is to provide 500 cc (1 L is fine, but no more than that at once) for most patients, and consider 250 cc in patients with cardiac or renal dysfunction. Using this approach, you can always administer more after reassessing.

6.3.5.3 Rate

This is largely stylistic and there is no correct answer though you should practice a systematic and consistent approach. The key variable in how fast to administer fluids is the urgency with which the patient requires this volume. If they aren't in the ICU, chances are that they don't need a bolus administered as fast as possible. The typical rate of fluid administration is anywhere from 100 to 250 ml/hr.

6.3.6 DVT Prophylaxis

Almost all patients who are hospitalized receive DVT prophylaxis which comes in two forms:
- Heparin: Typically low molecular weight heparin is injected subcutaneously although regular heparin may be used in cases such as renal impairment. The typical dose is 5000 U/day.
- Insufflation boots: These can have varying names but are essentially boots around the calve(s) that can inflate and deflate to gently squeeze the blood vessels of the lower legs. This is more commonly seen for post-op patients. The boots work by causing mechanically stimulated release of endogenous heparin. Thus, it is not mandatory for a patient to have both boots – one is acceptable.

Patients who are on DVT prophylaxis are unlikely to develop DVT/PE without significant risk factors for hypercoagulability. However, it is not impossible – you should continue to assess daily!

6.3.7 Insulin Management

Type 2 diabetes is among the most common secondary inpatient diagnoses. You will need to control these patients' blood sugars throughout the hospitalization. Due to the various interventions in-hospital, the blood glucose levels tend to fluctuate more. An insulin sliding scale is used to provide appropriate control, adjusted the next day if control was inadequate.

The total daily insulin (TDI) consists of a dosage that is split into basal (50%) and mealtime (50%). The mealtime insulin is divided further into thirds for a typical three-meal day. A finger-stick glucose should be checked prior to each insulin administration. The insulin sliding scale (ISS) means that if the patient is not meeting a sugar goal (typically 180) (■ Fig. 6.4), additional units of insulin are administered. At the end of the day, all the additional insulin administered is added to the total daily insulin dose.

Common scenarios that require an increase in the insulin sliding scale are steroid use and significant infections. Include insulin management as part of your plan and you will earn major bonus points!

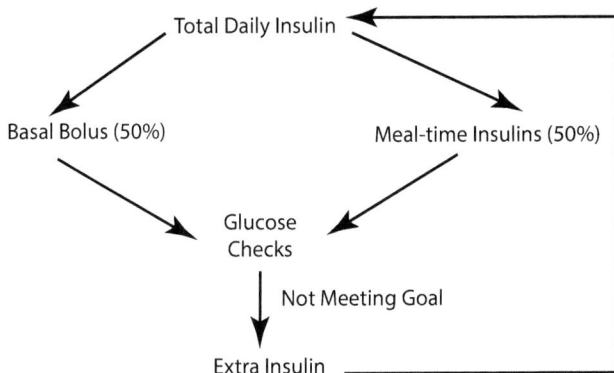

□ Fig. 6.4 Insulin sliding scale protocol

6.3.8 Approach to Supplemental Oxygen

Supplemental oxygen is a very common intervention for various inpatient hospitalizations. Let's explore when and how to provide oxygen below.

6.3.9 When to Provide Supplemental Oxygen

As trite as it may sound, supplemental oxygen is for when patients are saturating below 98% on room air. Tachypnea by itself is *not* an indication for supplemental oxygen. Also note that in patients with respiratory drive secondary to chronically elevated CO_2 levels (e.g., COPD), O_2 sat should be maintained lower than usual (goal 88–92%) to avoid respiratory failure.

Oxygen can be delivered in several methods (◘ Fig. 6.5), in escalating for persistent hypoxia:
- Nasal cannula
- Simple mask
- Non-rebreather (reservoir) mask
- Venturi mask

Note: Remember that the oxygen flow is less important than the FiO2 delivered!

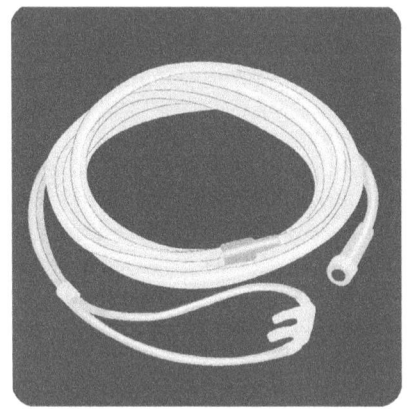

Nasal Cannula

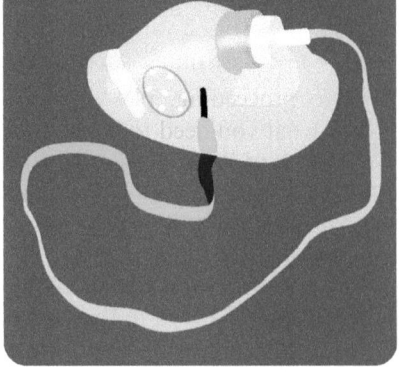

Simple Mask

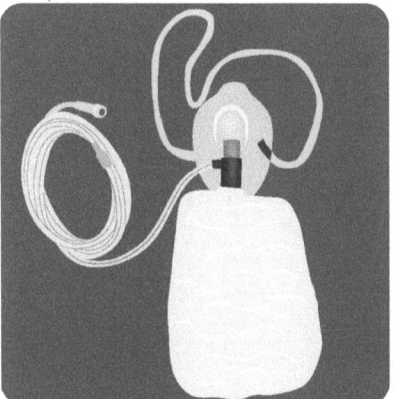

Nonrebreather Mask

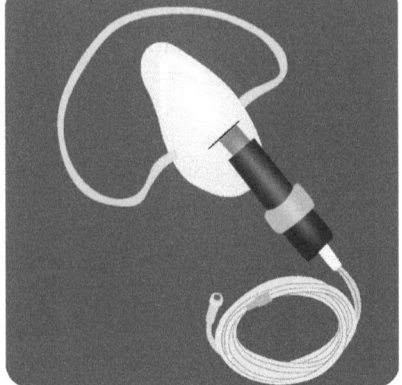

Venturi Mask

◘ **Fig. 6.5** Oxygen delivery methods

6.4 Common Cases

The following cases encompass the most common inpatient admissions that you will encounter. Certain conditions are referred to other chapters of this book as appropriate. Though patients will not present to the hospital with a nice label of their diagnosis on their foreheads, we defer to ▶ Chap. 14 for frameworks to approaching chief complaints since these common diagnoses are almost always made prior to admission to the general medicine service. Hence, it is better to delve into the specific diagnoses in this chapter.

The cases will be covered in the following format:

- Overview
- Framework – broad strokes for thinking about the disease
- Goals of admission – to help students think of why patients are admitted and what our goals are
- Presentation
- History
- Exam – details all major potential (not all possible) findings
- Workup
- Differentiating the differential – compares the most likely competing diagnoses; avoids the laundry list of possible diagnoses; focuses on key differentiating features that can be used in the A/P
- Management
- Contingencies – an advanced skill that students can begin to hone
- When to discharge – to help students think about the full course of management for the patient

Prior to proceeding, please note that although the following pages detail exactly what you need to know and do, you should strive to arrive at the content contained in these pages yourself through a multitude of study resources. This is the only way you will be able to extrapolate your success with cases beyond those here. As such, we will go through the first case in a question-based format that encourages this and shows you one method to effectively learning about a case.

6.4.1 Pneumonia (Question-Based Approach)

When learning about a disease for the first time, you should strive to understand what is the normal physiology versus what physiology becomes abnormal leading to the patient presentation. This is key to solidifying the disease entity in your memory and provides a firm foundation for all the "more clinical" learning that follows. A great resource for this is "Pathogenesis" section under a disease topic on UpToDate. An alternate resource includes Wikipedia (yes, it provides great starter information). Avoid resources such as First Aid – they do not delve into these details.

Task 1 Look up the pathophysiology of pneumonia. What aspect of physiology is altered? What would be the theoretical solution to fixing this abnormality?

Next, based on what you learned about the pathogenesis of the disease, try to understand the disease from different perspectives. In other words, categorize it in as many ways as possible as a thought exercise. The best way to do this is to search your classifications on UpToDate which will contain articles on all the major classifications you would desire knowing.

Pearl: While common diagnoses are often made prior to reaching the inpatient floor, you should always develop your own full admission H&P, differential, and treatment plan. Don't anchor to what the ED says!

Task 2 Look up common ways to classify pneumonia. What is the significance of these distinctions?

When the patient presents to the hospital, what is your goal as the provider? This is the time to think big picture prior to learning all the specific details such as symptoms, exam findings, and management. This part is a combination of reading, but also thinking about what's going on – you will not find such "Goals of Admission" in any resource other than this guide. Thinking through these goals is an excellent opportunity to assess whether you see the overall idea prior to painting the minute details. Don't worry – this part is hard, but for each disease, try to do this prior to reading our suggested goals of admission.

Task 3 Think about what you would want to do for the patient if they came in with a suspected diagnosis of pneumonia. Why is it important to do this?

Now we can delve into the specifics of the disease, from presentation to assessment and plan. While there are numerous places to learn this, UpToDate is my favorite. Be sure to use at least two resources to diversify the perspectives provided to you regarding a disease. Other great resources include MKSAP, AAFP, and many links on Google.

Task 4 Look up the disease specifics using your preferred resource. Try to stick to one resource when carrying out this task for any disease, so that you have familiarity and consistency.

Now is the time to refine the specifics you've just learned. After all, not everything that you read happens clinically on a routine basis. Try to get a sense for what the most common presentations and management strategies are – you will augment your understanding of this with clinical experience, but it's great to start thinking about this.

Task 5 Google what the most common symptoms and exam findings are for pneumonia. You should see many resources defining percentages. This gives you a sense for what is common (and thus more important to learn early on) and what is rare (something that you can add to your knowledge base later on).

Lastly, it is time to reflect on everything you've learned and connect the dots. This isn't to learn anything new per se but rather to solidify your own understanding of the disease. Practice active recall by talking through the disease from start to finish with a friend or simply aloud to yourself.

Now let's take a look at what information you may gather from studying a disease using the above method.

6.4.2 Pneumonia

Pneumonia is a very common cause of hospitalization and can also be a common iatrogenic problem which arises during a prolonged hospitalization. The run-of-the-mill pneumonia is not admitted; rather, pneumonia admissions are due to a significant abnormality in one of the vitals or high risk for decompensation (severity, age, comorbidities). The most common vital abnormality is a new oxygen requirement. There are several scoring systems such as the Pneumonia Severity Index (PSI) and CURB-65 that you may use on MDCalc that provides a sense of whether the patient is worthy of admission. Though you will not be responsible for making the decision to admit or not, these are worth briefly reviewing online so you can get a better sense for why patients are admitted for pneumonia.

Each time you suspect a pneumonia, think about it in these two distinct yet equally useful ways:

- Community-acquired pneumonia (CAP) vs hospital-acquired pneumonia (HAP)
- Bacterial vs viral

CAP is the most common type of pneumonia and is typically caused by bacteria, most commonly *Streptococcus pneumoniae* (gram-positive lancet-shaped diplococci), *Haemophilus influenzae* (gram-negative coccobacilli), and *Moraxella catarrhalis* (gram-negative diplococci). Atypical organisms such as *Legionella* and *Mycoplasma* are also not uncommon in the community. For HAP, the most common organisms are *S. aureus* and gram-negative rods (e.g., *Pseudomonas*). The principal value of considering HAP is for adding methicillin-resistant *Staphylococcus aureus* antibiotic coverage.

6.4.2.1 Goals of Admission

Practically speaking, most patients are admitted for pneumonia either for an oxygen requirement or for high risk (i.e., age, comorbidities) of complications. Your job will be to:

- [] Confirm the diagnosis of pneumonia.
- [] Rule out alternate do-not-miss and/or superimposed diagnoses.
- [] Treat the infection.
- [] Support oxygen requirement.
- [] Transition to outpatient management (e.g., antibiotics).

6.4.2.2 Presentation

The presentation of pneumonia is often a straightforward constellation of clinical symptoms that is largely consistent and readily visible in later stages. However, the symptoms during the initial phases of infection may be subtle, such as an isolated cough or fever. You're likely to notice more symptoms than not if the patient is being admitted.

History

- Chief complaint: variable – can range from cough, fever, dyspnea
- **O**: Acute (days; CAP) or subacute (weeks; viral, atypicals)
- **P**: Occasionally may involve chest pain with deep breaths (pleuritic pain)
- **Q**: Sharp
- **R**: Sometimes RUQ/LUQ, no radiation
- **S**: Mild to moderate severity
- **T**: Typically stable or worsening
- **A**: Fever, cough (productive, yellow/green), shortness of breath

Exam

- General: Possibly mild distress and ill-appearing, rarely altered mental status
- Cardiac: Potential physiologic tachycardia
- Lungs: Crackles, dullness to percussion, and egophony (E to A transition) in distribution of consolidation (if lobar)
- Extremities: Warm, well perfused without edema

6.4.2.3 Workup

By the time you are picking up a pneumonia patient, the core workup will likely have been done by the ED team or the overnight medicine team. However, here is a list of the key objective data you should use to guide your management (and suggest if not done yet):

- [] Lung exam – evidence of a new pulmonary process.
- [] CXR – evidence of (usually lobar) infiltrates.
- [] +-Sputum culture.
- [] Elevated WBC with left shift.
- [] MRSA Swab (98% NPV).
- [] Legionella and *S. pneumoniae* urine antigens.
- [] Flu swab (for deciding on single isolation room).
- [] If severe (e.g., blood pressures dropping, meeting SIRS criteria), consider blood cultures.

Differentiating the Differential

- COPD exacerbation: This will generally be in an older patient with a history of COPD. Though COPD exacerbation can be triggered by a pneumonia, typically there is no evidence of pneumonia such as lobar consolidation and improvement with duonebs.
- Heart failure exacerbation: Patients will usually have a history of heart failure or risk factors for new heart failure (e.g., CAD). Unlike pneumonia, there is typically prominent signs of volume overload and a lack of infectious signs, though infection can trigger HF exacerbation.
- PE: Usually much more acute than pneumonia, even that caused by *S. pneumoniae* which may be reported as an abrupt onset of SOB/chest pain. Patients with pneumonia are typically not tachycardic. Patients with PE may have risk factors for clotting such as recent immobilization or AFib.

6.4.2.4 Management

Goals

- [] Treat the infection.
  - [] Did I cover the most common organisms with empiric therapy?
  - [] Did I assess risk and cover, if applicable, for other microbes?
- [] Correct any oxygen requirements.

Treating the Infection

Initially, empiric coverage is used to cover the most common community pathogens (*H influenzae, Moraxella, S. pneumoniae* – remembered by the mnemonic *HMS*). Reasonable empiric regimens include CTX 1g QD or levofloxacin 750 mg PO QD. A few other coverage considerations to run through each time (including discussion in your assessment/plan) include:

- Atypicals: Typically included in empiric covered though varies by provider/institution
- Anaerobes: High risk or known aspiration; foul-smelling sputum
- MRSA: If HAP/HCAP or history of MRSA
- *Pseudomonas*: If HAP/HCAP, history of *Pseudomonas*, or severe chronic pulmonary comorbidities

> **Pearl:** Each hospital has its own antibiogram that displays antibiotic sensitivities for common bugs. These are excellent for deciding between multiple antibiotics that all cover the organism in question.

Reasonable coverage for atypicals is with levofloxacin or by adding azithromycin. Anaerobes may be covered with Zosyn and MRSA coverage is with vancomycin. *Pseudomonas* coverage may be obtained by using levofloxacin or cefepime instead of ceftriaxone. Please refer to ► Chap. 19 for further details on how to cover these organisms.

Contingencies

You should always have contingencies in mind, though not always necessary to present during rounds. Contingencies are more applicable when signing out your patients to the night team. These were always among the more difficult for me to think of independently, though it seems common sense after you get the hang of it. Remember, these should be in If-Then format.

- If labile pressures, then obtain blood cultures for potential sepsis.
- If new fever, then revert back to IV antibiotics (or switch IV antibiotics, depending on case).

The backbone inpatient empiric coverage for pneumonia is most commonly CTX 1g IV QD or levofloxacin 750 mg PO QD. MRSA coverage with vancomycin is added for all HCAP and patients with multidrug-resistant risk factors (e.g., recent hospitalization, prior MDR infection). If atypicals are suspected, levofloxacin may be chosen over CTX or azithromycin 500 mg PO QD added to the CTX. Rarer more severe infections with anaerobes or extended-spectrum beta-lactamases (ESBLs) may warrant Zosyn 4.5 mg IV q6h or meropenem 1 g IV q8hrs, respectively. Antibiotic regimens should be continued for 5 days if CAP is suspected, 8 days for HAP/HCAP, and 15 days for *Pseudomonas*. Refer to ▶ Chap. 19 for a great overview of the different antibiotic classes and their spectrum of coverage.

Pearl: Levofloxacin has greater side effects than CTX, including QT prolongation and increased risk of Achilles tendon rupture (in elderly).

Pearl: Meropenem covers *Pseudomonas*, whereas ertapenem does not.

6.4.2.5 When to Discharge?

Let's refer to our Road to Discharge checklist, modifying it to our case:

- [] No further SOB, cough, fever
- [] No oxygen requirement
- [] Ceftriaxone to PO levofloxacin
- [] Short-term course of medications secured for patient
- [] Patient able to go home and live independently

Now that we've covered all that you need to know for pneumonia, practice admission, and follow-up presentations for this case out aloud. You can also record yourself on video if you want to critique your oral presentation. Spending 5–10 minutes now will have tremendous returns later.

Again, prior to reading the COPD section, try to come up with your own illness scripts and then compare to what we provide here.

Pearl: The preference for IV antibiotics while hospitalized include:
- Better bioavailability (100%)
- Better penetration to certain tissues (e.g., bone)
- Faster onset of action

Pearl: You should suggest transitioning from IV to PO medication once the patient has been afebrile and improving for at least 24 hours.

6.4.3 COPD Exacerbation

COPD exacerbation is another staple case you should know well. The premise behind COPD exacerbation is that the patients are already teetering on the edge of their ability to efficiently use their lungs to deliver oxygen to the blood (alveolar ventilation defect). A slight disruption of that balance, such as with infection or forgetting maintenance medications, can lead to an "exacerbation" – a temporary worsening of already poor lung function.

6.4.3.1 Goals of Admission

- [] Stabilize lung function back to baseline (decrease lung inflammation).
- [] Support oxygen requirement.
- [] Rule out alternative causes of presentation.
- [] Identify triggers and counsel to prevent future episodes.
- [] Explore possibility of smoking cessation.
- [] Transition to outpatient management.

6.4.3.2 Presentation
History
The primary symptom for COPD exacerbation is shortness of breath but it may present without over SOB. Two out of three criteria below suggest the clinical diagnosis of COPD exacerbation, easily remembered by the mnemonic *SOB*:

- *S*putum (change in amount or color)
- *O*xygen (worsening SOB)
- *B*ark (new or increasing cough)

Notably, you should know that the most common risk factor for a COPD exacerbation is a prior COPD exacerbation. This is a consistent finding across multiple studies, such as the ECLIPSE Study (NEJM 2010). In cases where the patient is a poor historian and the diagnosis based on the presence of two or more criteria is less reliable, a history of prior COPD exacerbation and the lack of alternate diagnoses is a strong indicator that your patient is experiencing yet another COPD exacerbation.

Exam
- General: May have respiratory distress, accessory muscle usage, or altered mental status in severe cases
- Cardiac: Potential physiologic tachycardia
- Lungs: Coarse inspiratory crackles bilaterally with diminished and prolonged breath sounds throughout
- Extremities: Warm, well perfused without edema

Pearl: Always be as descriptive as possible, these details can really help support or refute a diagnosis!

6.4.3.3 Workup
- [] CXR – consistent with COPD changes (inc lung volume, decreased lung markings)
- [] Sputum culture
- [] If severe, consider ABG

Differentiating the Differential
- HF exacerbation: The best way to differentiate HF exacerbation is by eliciting a positive hepatojugular reflex which tests for the ability of the right heart to accommodate a transient increase in volume. You should not find a positive HJR with COPD exacerbation. There are also no signs of volume overload for COPD exacerbation.
- Pneumonia: Though pneumonia may trigger COPD exacerbation, this would usually manifest with obvious signs of infection on CXR, labs, and exam.
- Pulmonary embolism: This is a significant cause of mortality in patients with COPD admitted for presumed COPD exacerbation. PE usually presents with less of a cough/sputum picture and more SOB (including more tachypnea).

6.4.3.4 Management
Goals
- [] Treat the inflammation.
- [] Correct oxygen requirements.
- [] Reduce future exacerbations.
- [] Smoking cessation.

Treat the Inflammation

- Steroids (typically 40 mg prednisone) over 5 days is the core treatment to decrease inflammation in COPD exacerbation. You should be aware of the REDUCE Trial (JAMA 2013) which found no differences in clinical outcomes between a 5- and 14-day course of steroids, prompting a landmark shift to using 5 days given the potent side effects of steroids.
- Antibiotics are often administered for moderate to severe exacerbations (essentially, all inpatient admissions). This is backed by studies demonstrating decreased mortality and readmission rates when antibiotics are coupled to steroid therapy. An easy way to remember which antibiotics are administered is to recall the empiric inpatient options for pneumonia: ceftriaxone or levofloxacin. Pseudomonal coverage is added with cefepime or Zosyn when risk factors or prior history exists.

Pearl: Prednisolone may be used to bypass liver metabolism in patients with liver dysfunction.

Correct Oxygen Requirements

- Duonebs are administered typically q4h standing with Q2H PRN albuterol to help decrease the obstructive physiology.
- Supplemental oxygen should be delivered with a goal O2 sat of 88–92%. Since COPD patients live chronically with relative hypercarbia, a high O2 sat can cause decreased respiratory drive secondary to a decrease in CO_2 levels, leading to respiratory failure.
- Noninvasive positive pressure ventilation (NIPPV) may be considered in severe cases and has been shown to decrease mortality. However, if a patient requires NIPPV, they will be in the ICU rather than your general medicine service.

Reduce Future Exacerbations

One of the keys to managing a COPD exacerbation is to reduce the probability of future interventions. Though most exacerbations are caused by a viral or bacterial infection, there are several other common causes that may be targeted for reduction. These other causes include medication noncompliance, smoking, and exposure to heavy pollution. Explore these factors each admission with appropriate counseling.

Smoking Cessation

The possibility of smoking cessation should be explored each admission, as it both slows decline of pulmonary function (specifically decreases in FEV1) and decreases mortality. Speaking of mortality, a common topic that is tested by attendings and well worth knowing to round out your knowledge of COPD treatment are the three interventions that have been proven to improve mortality in COPD.

- Smoking cessation
- Chronic home oxygen therapy (>15 hours/day)
- Lung volume reduction

Contingencies

- If O2 sat >92%, then decrease supplementary O2.
- If new tachypnea (RR > 25) or accessory muscle use, consider ABG.

6.4.3.5 When to Discharge?

- [] Return to baseline oxygen requirements.
- [] Short-term course of medications secured for patient.
- [] Patient able to go home and live independently.

Actively assessing whether the patient is ready for discharge.

Common Knowledge Question: Females are more susceptible to UTIs because of their short urethra.

Pearl: Foleys should always be removed as soon as they are not needed, particularly in post-op patients. They should also be changed routinely if required long term.

Pearl: If *S. aureus* is found in the urine, always check for bloodstream infection. *S. aureus* is not a normal GU flora and 1/3 of patients with *S. aureus* in urine have *S. aureus* bacteremia.

Pearl: Symptoms are not always classical symptoms of bladder irritation such as dysuria, urgency, and frequency. UTIs may manifest in other ways such as altered mental status.

Pearl: AMS may present in many ways in elderly patients with comorbidities. Alternate presentations include falls and small changes in functional status.

6.4.4 Urinary Tract Infection (UTI)

UTI is a common diagnosis that you will encounter almost exclusively in females. Admission for UTI is usually in the elderly with many comorbidities and a low level of baseline function, often with an alternate chief complaint such as altered mental status. This is very important since UTI may go undiagnosed for longer than it should under the pretext of another problem such as AMS. It is also a common iatrogenic diagnosis often associated with prolonged hospitalization and indwelling Foleys.

The two most common bacteria that cause UTI are *E. coli* and *Klebsiella*, both gram-negative rods. Normally, the kidneys, ureter, and bladder are sterile. The presence of bacteria themselves in the KUB is less problematic; rather, it is the active inflammation that these microbes cause which leads to clinical consequences. This brings up an important point – typically, asymptomatic bacteriuria (bacteria in the urine without symptoms) does not require treatment.

UTIs are primarily classified as either uncomplicated or complicated. Complicated refers to the extension of the infection beyond the bladder, such as to the kidneys. Thus, any systemic symptoms (e.g., fever, chills) or symptoms outside the bladder (e.g., flank pain) indicate a complicated UTI. Pyelonephritis, infection of the kidney, is a subcategory of UTI. The utility of this binary classification lies in their distinct management.

6.4.4.1 Goals of Admission
- [] Categorize UTI as uncomplicated vs complicated vs asymptomatic bacteriuria.
- [] Treat UTI.
- [] Remedy modifiable risk factors for UTI.

6.4.4.2 Presentation
History

UTIs most often present with symptoms that indicate bladder irritation:
- Dysuria
- Frequency
- Urgency

Complicated UTIs may have additional signs and symptoms such as
- Fever
- Chills
- Flank pain
- Altered mental status

Exam
- General: usually no acute distress, though can have altered mental status
- Abdomen: suprapubic tenderness and/or fullness
- Back: costovertebral angle (CVA) tenderness
- GU: possibly an indwelling Foley

6.4.4.3 Workup
Is there an infection, and if so, with what bacteria?
- [] Urinalysis
- [] Urine culture

Urinalysis (UA)

A UA is always obtained for suspected UTI. Ensure that the sample is clean (ideally caught midstream) with few squamous epithelial cells (many squams suggest a dirty sample that is likely contaminated with bacteria from external genitalia). A UTI should have positive leukocytes (WBCs) and/or leukocyte esterase which is a protein found in leukocytes that is released into the urine when lysed by bacteria. Nitrites may also be in the urine, almost always indicating *E. coli*.

Pearl: In your oral presentation, you should always note the quality of the urine sample.

Urine Culture (UCx)

These are typically obtained along with the UA. While guidelines vary in terms of colony-forming unit (CFU) cutoffs that indicate a UTI, assuming that the urine was a clean sample, you shouldn't have much bacteria on culture. Furthermore, the culture is more important for speciating the bacteria and tailoring therapy. Officially, the CFU cutoffs vary between 10,000 (IDSA) and 50,000 (semi-traditional cutoff). There is likely a lot of influence practice patterns that dictate how CFUs are interpreted.

Pearl: Always check on the status of sensitivities and update the team both informally and in your oral presentations.

Differentiating the Differential

The diagnosis of a UTI is typically either established or not, and your goal is to differentiate between uncomplicated and complicated rather than considering a list of differentials. There is, of course, a differential, including some causes that may even facilitate recurrent UTIs (such as nephrolithiasis); however, they will not be discussed here.

6.4.4.4 Management
Goals
- [] Empiric antibiotics
- [] Reduce future UTIs

Empiric Antibiotics

Uncomplicated UTIs are managed with empiric antibiotics until urine culture results and/or sensitivities return at which time antibiotics may be narrowed. Symptoms typically begin resolving within 24–48 hours. First-line therapies are below:
- Nitrofurantoin (Macrobid) 100 mg BID x5 days
  - Present on Beer's list (avoid in elderly)
  - Avoid if GFR <60
  - Mechanism involves oxidative stress (avoid in patients with Mediterranean ancestry if their G6PD status is unknown)
- Bactrim DS BID:
  - IV Bactrim can artificially bump the Cr without affecting the GFR (avoid if concurrent AKI to avoid muddying the picture; Bactrim contains a sulfa moiety)
- CTX 1g QD x3–5 days
  - Requires IV access
- Ciprofloxacin 500 mg QD x3 days
  - Personally favor the other agents given increased side effect and resistance profiles
- Fosfomycin 3 g x1 dose
  - Convenient but expensive so usually not first line in practice

Complicated UTIs require better penetration to the kidneys, meaning that nitrofurantoin and fosfomycin are ineffective. Unsurprisingly, the regimens for complicated UTI are stronger and longer.

- CTX 1g QD x7–14d
  - Preferred
- Ciprofloxacin 400 mg BID x7–14d
  - Increasing resistance rates (be sure to check with your institution's nomograms)
- Gentamicin 5 mg/kg QD x7–14d
  - Typically avoided due to increased nephrotoxicity

Pseudomonal coverage is not routinely indicated and is added on in settings of increased risk for multidrug-resistant organisms or prior history of pseudomonal UTI. Repeat urinalysis is only indicated if suspecting treatment-refractory infection. It is not done to check for resolution of UTI.

Reduce Future UTIs
Risk factors for UTIs should be addressed when possible. The most common risk factor is inappropriate retention of a Foley long after its need has been exhausted. Always advocate to remove Foleys earlier rather than later, and challenge the patient to be self-sufficient. You can always put another Foley if needed, so just try! In patients with recurrent UTIs, some common underlying causes may be diabetes (control the blood glucose) and chronic nephrolithiasis.

Contingencies
- If UTI symptoms worsen or return, then switch to alternate empiric antibiotic and re-culture.

When to discharge? (if this is the primary reason for admission)
- [] Resolution of symptoms, most importantly systemic symptoms
- [] Appropriate supply of antibiotics to finish course as outpatient

6.4.5 Acute Kidney Injury

AKIs are a very common iatrogenic problem on the general medicine service, but may also be the cause of hospitalization. The vast majority of AKIs you will encounter on the general medicine service will be pre-renal (thus we will focus exclusively on that in this chapter), though you should be aware of the other types of AKI. Pre-renal AKI is caused by a lack of adequate perfusion to the kidneys due to decreased intravascular volume (think diarrhea, aggressive diuresis, poor PO intake). Please refer to the AKI section in ▶ Chap. 18 for a more detailed and complementary discussion, including the other AKI types.

Pre-renal AKI may range from mild to severe though most of the AKIs the general medicine service manages will be moderate. Severe AKI, defined as a Cr two to three times baseline, should result in nephrology consult for ICU transfer immediately. In mild to moderate AKI, it may be largely an invisible disease to you and the patient, only found incidentally on labs.

6.4.5.1 Goals of Admission
- [] Restore intravascular volume.
- [] Stabilize and improve renal function/urine output.
- [] Exclude secondary causes of AKI.
- [] Counsel on preventing future pre-renal AKIs, if applicable.

6.4.5.2 Presentation
History
Your goal is to obtain history that pinpoints the etiology of volume depletion. Common causes include:
- Absolute volume depletion
  - Diarrhea
  - Vomiting
  - Diuresis
- Effective volume depletion
  - HF exacerbation
  - Decompensated liver failure/hepatorenal syndrome
  - Sepsis
- Altered renal dynamics
  - NSAIDs
  - ACEi/ARB

You should also screen for use of medications that impair creatinine excretion without truly affecting the GFR, leading to a falsely elevated Cr:
- IV Bactrim (specifically, the trimethoprim)
- Famotidine/cimetidine

Exam
- General: No acute distress unless superimposed condition
- HENT: Dry mucous membranes, flat JVP
- Cardiac: Baseline, potential tachycardia
- Lungs: CTAB
- Extremities: DP 2+; no LE edema

6.4.5.3 Workup
The workup for AKI is primarily done to categorize the AKI into pre-renal, intrinsic, and post-renal to help narrow the etiology. There are occasionally secondary etiologies such as decompensated liver failure that leads to AKI which will be fairly obvious yet should be ruled out nonetheless. We will focus on the findings for pre-renal AKI.
- [] Creatinine
- [] BUN (increased from baseline, with BUN/Cr ratio >20)
- [] Urine electrolytes for FeNa (<1%) or FeUrea (<33%)
- [] Strict I/Os (decreased urinary output)
- [] Consider fluid challenge to support/refute pre-renal etiology
- [] Consider Foley to check for post-renal obstruction

6.4.5.4 Management
Goals
- [] Restore intravascular volume.
- [] Stabilize and improve renal function.

Restore Intravascular Volume
If the objective data supports a pre-renal AKI, you should administer either IV normal saline or lactated ringers. These are the best choices given that their volume remains in the intravascular space. If you used a non-isotonic fluid such as D5W or 1/2NS, it would be less effective in expanding the intravascular volume. The volume of fluid to administer is essentially trial and error; you typically begin with a liter and trend changes in Cr back towards baseline. Importantly, in patients with heart failure or baseline CKD, you should provide fluids in smaller boluses to avoid accidentally causing volume overload.

Pearl: A creatinine increase is always relative to baseline and a seemingly large (~0.5) increase at high creatinine levels (>2.0) does not reflect a large decrease in GFR. Refer to ▶ Chap. 18 for further details.

FeNa is not validated for use in CKD patients.

Use FeUrea rather than FeNa when a patient is currently (or recently) on diuretics.

Stabilize and Improve Renal Function

Regardless of the etiology of AKI, renal function should be prevented from worsening by avoiding nephrotoxins such as contrast, NSAIDs, and ACE inhibitors/ARBS. If there is a secondary cause such as decompensated liver failure, treat it!

Management Checklist

- [] Trend Cr daily.
- [] IV fluids (isotonic).
- [] Avoid nephrotoxins (contrast, NSAIDs, ACE inhibitors/ARBS).

Contingencies

- If Cr increases further with fluid administration, then consult nephrology immediately

6.4.5.5 When to Discharge?

Typically, AKI is not the principal problem but can still hold up a discharge.

- [] Cr trending back and in close proximity to baseline
- [] Adequate urine output
- [] Adequate PO fluid intake
- [] Patient restarted on home medications with nephrotoxic potential

6.4.5.6 Oral Presentation Pearls

- [] Include baseline Cr in one-liner.
- [] Include history of CKD with stage, if applicable, in one-liner.
- [] Always report I/Os broken down into specific components.

6.4.6 Chest Pain Rule-Out Myocardial Infarction (CPROMI)

One of the scariest and thus unsurprisingly frequent chief complaints is chest pain. In reality, most presentations of chest pain are noncardiac. Despite the wide differential for chest pain, due to the gravity of cardiac ischemia, each chest pain complaint is taken extremely seriously. If a patient is determined by the ED to have active ischemia, they are sent either straight to the cath lab or admitted to the cardiac service for observation. However, if there is no objective evidence for cardiac ischemia (negative troponins, non-ischemic EKG), but there is significant concern for early evolving cardiac ischemia, patients may be admitted to the general medicine wards. CPROMI is essentially a vigilance game that requires careful monitoring for new evidence of an ischemic process. Refer to "ACS" section of ► Chap. 16 for a complementary read.

6.4.6.1 Goals of Admission

- [] Rule in/out cardiac ischemia.
- [] Provide symptomatic relief of chest pain.
- [] Limited workup of noncardiac etiologies.

Presentation

Despite having had a thorough workup in the ED, you should be verifying all of their workup, including obtaining a completely new history and physical.

History

Chest pain is categorized as noncardiac, atypical (cardiac) chest pain, and typical chest pain based on how many of the following criteria are met (■ Fig. 6.6):

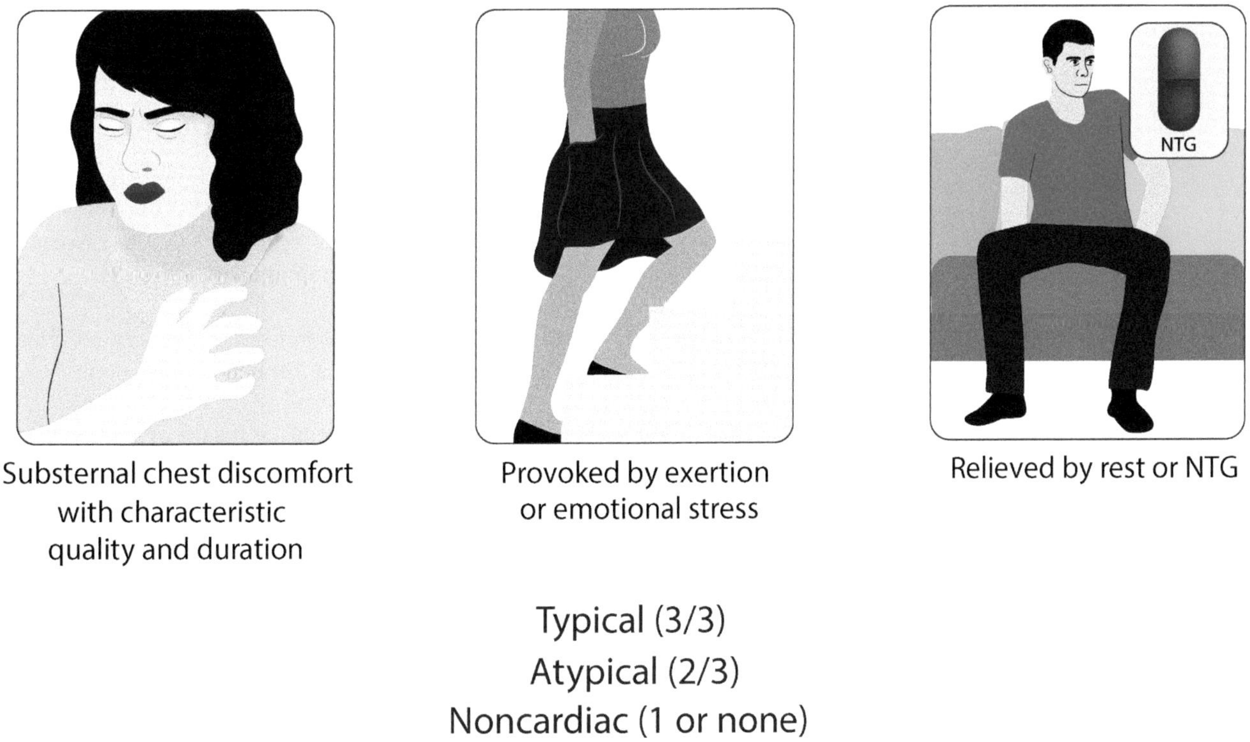
NTG
Substernal chest discomfort with characteristic quality and duration
Provoked by exertion or emotional stress
Relieved by rest or NTG
Typical (3/3)
Atypical (2/3)
Noncardiac (1 or none)

Fig. 6.6 Angina classifications

- Substernal chest pain/pressure lasting at least several minutes
- Worse with exertion or emotional stress
- Better with rest and/or nitroglycerin

Many ancillary features may associate with cardiac ischemia:
- Nausea/vomiting
- Diaphoresis
- SOB
- Musculoskeletal pain (arm, neck, jaw)
- Diabetes

Exam
The exam is largely benign in these cases, but you should pay close attention for any findings that may clue you into an evolving or active MI.

General: No Acute Distress
- HEENT: No JVD (JVD would hint either papillary muscle rupture or cardiogenic shock)
- Cardiac: RRR, no murmurs/rubs/gallops (mitral regurgitation most common new murmur from MI)
- Lungs: CTAB (diffuse crackles may suggest flash pulmonary edema)
- Extremities: No LE edema

Chest pain that is positional or reproducible with palpation is unlikely secondary to cardiac ischemia.

6.4.6.2 Workup
The extent to which you pursue a workup is largely attending and institution dependent. All providers must, however, continue observation for cardiac ischemia.
- [] Trend troponins q2h–q4h.
- [] Repeat EKG q4h.

- [] Telemetry.
- [] Reassess patient's symptoms and exams in-person frequently (e.g., q2h).
- [] BMP – to assess for electrolyte abnormalities that may be driving cardiac pain.

Differentiating the Differential

- Nonischemic cardiac
  - Aortic dissection: may have unequal arm blood pressures, associated with thoracic back pain, clear evidence on imaging
- Musculoskeletal
  - Costochondritis: reproducible pinpoint soreness or tenderness, worse with movement and does not improve with nitrates
- Gastrointestinal
  - GERD: pain typically comes on shortly after meals or recumbency; improves with TUMs/antacids; does not worsen with exercise and does not improve with rest
  - Esophageal spasms: difficult to ascertain during initial workup, but rare
- Pulmonary
  - Bacterial pneumonia: often has other infectious signs and symptoms; evidence of lower lobar consolidation on CXR
- Psychiatric
  - Stress-induced: recent events that would cause extreme stress
  - Panic attack: history of psychiatric diagnoses, including panic attacks

6.4.6.3 Management
Goals

- [] Rule Out MI

There are no specific treatments for this case. If a patient is found to have cardiac ischemia during observation, they are transferred either to the cath lab or cardiac unit for further management. Your only treatments here are for angina relief with nitrates.

Contingencies

- If recurrent chest pain, then obtain STAT EKG and repeat trops.
- If new murmur on heart exam, then obtain STAT TTE, EKG, and trops and consult cardiology.

6.4.6.4 When to Discharge?

- [] Negative troponins x2, spaced 4 hours apart
- [] No ischemic changes on EKG
- [] If applicable, outpatient provider referral for further workup of chest pain

6.4.7 Syncope

Syncope, distinct from the sensation of the room spinning known as vertigo, is another common reason for admission. The primary reason for these admissions is to rule out concerning etiologies and observe for repeated episodes. You should think about syncope by major etiology, presented here in descending order of how common they are:

- Vagal (neurocardiogenic)
- Orthostatic

- Cardiogenic
- Neurologic

For the first three, the ultimate mechanism of syncope is a lack of adequate perfusion to the head. When perfusion returns, consciousness follows. Let's examine how perfusion becomes transiently inadequate:

- Vagal: increase in vagal (inhibitory) tone (e.g., straining while urinating) leading to hypotension and/or decreased cardiac output
- Orthostatic: inadequate intravascular volume and/or baroreceptor dysfunction
- Cardiogenic: poor cardiac forward flow (e.g., arrhythmias, aortic stenosis)

Orthostatic hypotension is the most common cause of admitted syncope. Vasovagal syncope is typically observed in the ED but not admitted. Cardiogenic and neurologic syncope require more extensive management and hospitalization but are rarely discovered (difficult to capture the evidence, even if it is the cause) to be the cause of syncope.

On the other hand, neurologic syncope results from a true CNS deficit in the regions governing consciousness (e.g., reticular activating system) or diffuse cerebral dysfunction (e.g., seizure, large stroke).

6.4.7.1 Goals of Admission

- [] Observation.
- [] Rule out dangerous causes (cardiogenic, neurologic).
- [] Treat the underlying cause, if applicable.

6.4.7.2 Presentation

History

Upon presentation, patients will typically appear baseline and have no further symptoms. It is very useful to obtain first-hand accounts from any witnesses. Helpful elements of the history for distinguishing between syncopal etiologies include:

- Onset (immediate without warning vs gradual with prodromal symptoms)
- Other associated symptoms (tongue-biting, weakness, etc.)
- Post-syncopal symptoms

Exam

- General: Baseline; if seizures, may have evidence of tongue biting or incontinence
- Cardiac: Rarely abnormal upon inspection with murmurs or irregular rhythms or abnormal heart rates
- Lungs: Baseline
- Neuro: Baseline

Pearl: If the patient's new-onset symptoms, such as weakness or altered consciousness, continue to persist after syncope, seizure becomes high on the differential (Todd's paralysis, post-ictal state).

6.4.7.3 Differentiating the Differential

The differential for syncope exists but is usually irrelevant for a general medicine admission. The key thinking lies in differentiating between the various causes of syncope:

- Vagal: Some prodromal symptoms possible; long periods of standing
- Orthostatic: Most associated with prodromal symptoms (lightheadedness, sweating, heart racing); soon after standing/changing position
- Cardiogenic: Sudden onset without warning, history of arrhythmias
- Neurologic: May report prolonged symptoms after regaining consciousness

6.4.7.4 Workup

The inpatient workup of syncope is limited to ruling out the "very bad" causes; the rest can be done outpatient. The primary workup is in the form of tele overnight to check for arrhythmias. Further testing such as Tilt table testing and prolonged telemetry is done outpatient.

- [] Vital signs with orthostatics
- [] Full neuro exam
- [] Holter monitor

6.4.7.5 Management

Treatment is specific to the etiology of syncope. Typically, the most that is done in these admissions is administration of fluid.

- [] If orthostatic: IV fluids if orthostatic.
- [] If vasovagal/orthostatic: Patient education on preventing future syncopal episodes.
- [] If Cardiogenic or neurologic: Consult respective specialists inpatient.

Contingencies

- If patient syncopizes again during observation, then consider obtaining CT head.

6.4.7.6 When to Discharge?

- [] Patient stable without new signs or symptoms for several hours

6.4.8 Other Cases

There are a number of cases that may or may not be admitted to the general medicine floor based on the structure of your hospital. These cases typically are admitted to the specialty services when possible. Furthermore, some cases are simply better integrated into the specialty chapters. Please refer to those chapters for the following cases:

- Heart failure exacerbation (▶ Chap. 16)
- Decompensated liver failure (▶ Chap. 17)
- Constipation/bowel obstruction (▶ Chap. 7)
- Cellulitis (▶ Chap. 19)
- C diff colitis (▶ Chap. 19)

Remember to learn how to learn by going through the method we outlined prior to delving into these cases. Rather than going straight to the above chapters, try to learn about the topic yourself first. Good luck!

General Surgery

Selena Li

Contents

© The Author(s), under exclusive license to Springer Nature Switzerland AG 2021
S. H. Lecker, B. J. Chang (eds.), *The Ultimate Medical School Rotation Guide*,
https://doi.org/10.1007/978-3-030-63560-2_7

7.1   Introduction

Surgery is considered by many to be one of the more challenging rotations of your clinical year and can be a daunting start for many medical students. In this chapter, we aim to highlight the components that will help you both excel on and enjoy your surgery rotation. We consider the pillars of success for medical students on their general surgery rotation to be the following: clinical knowledge, practical and technical skills, and (arguably, most importantly) the proper mindset.

7.1.1   The Surgeon's Mindset

You are now a part of a team, and your primary job is to help that team accomplish its goals. Surgery can be compared to team-based sports, in which each athlete plays a specific role and, importantly, sets aside individual pride for the good of the team. As medical students, we are not the quarterbacks or the captains of the team. Some days, if we are lucky, we get to be a wide receiver. Other days, we might just be the water boy/girl, and in those cases, we should strive to be the best water boy/girl we can be. There is no such thing as a menial task, whether it is running to get supplies, positioning a patient, or printing out rounding reports for your team. Analogies aside, this is the mentality that you should have on your surgery rotation – be humble, work hard, and put the team and the patient first. Embody the following values, and not only will others appreciate working with you, you will be sure to enjoy your rotation and get the most out of it.

1. *Respect.* This should go without saying, but respect *every* person you encounter in the hospital – the patient, your attending and residents, the nurses, OR staff, and technicians. This goes for every person you meet, *regardless of how they treat you.* The hospital can be a demanding place to work, and most people are doing their best to get the job done. In the process, they may not appreciate a medical student interfering with their workflow, *and that is okay.*
   (a) ***Author's perspective.* In general, my mindset has been to regard others as higher than myself – not because I am a medical student and at the "bottom" of the hierarchy, but because I am a surgeon in training. And I plan to continue doing so even as a resident and an attending. I have found this to be very helpful in framing my mindset and earning respect rather than expecting it.
2. *Responsibility.* Your patients are now *your* patients, so step into the role of provider. Know every detail about your patients – their medical and surgical history, how many children they have, how many years since they quit smoking, and how many bowel movements they had yesterday. Be confident. Responsibility means knowing your abilities and knowing when to ask for help. Admit mistakes and never make up data. The patient always takes priority, not your desire to perform procedures. Ask your attending or resident to take you through a new procedure, and know your limits.
3. *Resiliency.* Surgical training is grueling. You will be challenged physically, mentally, and emotionally. There will be days when you feel like a superstar and days when you feel like a disappointment. When you make a mistake (and you will) or receive a reprimand, learn from it, and move on. In an environment of external validation and the desire to please others, find something within yourself that will anchor you and give you the drive to *keep going.*

7.1.2 Establishing Objectives

Throughout your education, you have received learning objectives for each of your classes and rotations, and your surgical rotation will be no different. These are the standards that your institution and the national board have established, but to truly get the most out of your rotation, start thinking about your personal objectives (◘ Table 7.1). This will help you to focus your energy on areas you are interested in or hope to improve and, at the end of the day, will help you to recognize small victories as well as points of weakness.

7.1.3 Learning in the OR

Before getting into the details of what you need to learn, first take some time to orient yourself on *how* to learn. This rotation will be inherently different than the others in that much of the learning is done by observing, practicing, or self-study rather than extended discussions. There will be opportunities to ask questions or to discuss differentials here and there, but much of your time will be spent in the OR, and learning during the case requires a different approach.

1. *Build a solid knowledge base before the case.* This means reading and reviewing to orient yourself to the indications, contraindications, general steps, and potential complications of the surgery. You should know why this patient is being operated on, why this specific approach to the operation, and what additional factors (comorbidities, preoperative risk, etc.) were taken into account. If you have time, try to look up the steps of the operation online so that you are familiar with operative flow.

    (a) This is where your clinical knowledge comes into play (discussed below).

2. *Watch for the steps of the operation.* The first time you see an operation, watch first for the general steps. Don't get too bogged down by the details of suture choice or needle angles yet.

3. *Watch the primary surgeon for technical skills.* Once you feel comfortable with the basics, watch how the surgeons handle their instruments, angle their bodies, and dissect the tissue (which layer are they focused on, etc.). Look at needle angles, forehand or backhand stitches, the size of the suture bites, and amount of travel. There is so much to learn just from watching, and this is something that every aspiring surgeon continues to do for the rest of their careers.

◘ **Table 7.1** Objectives sheet (with examples)

	Clinical knowledge	**Technical skills**
For the rotation	Understand first-line diagnostic tests and management for bowel obstructions	Subcuticular sutures (improving cosmetics of reapproximation)
For this block *(e.g., thoracic)*	Lung anatomy (lobes, segments, variants) and spatial relationship of airway, vein, and artery	Bronchoscopy
Daily	Chest tube output criteria	Chest tube sutures

4. *Watch the first assistant for how to assist.* This is the role that we will take most immediately, and being an excellent assistant is essential to being an excellent surgeon. This will teach you to anticipate the surgeon's next move and to train your instincts and good habits. Learn how to retract for optimal exposure, follow a suture line, and suction effectively.

5. *Watch the scrub nurse/tech to understand instrument choice and attending preference.* Different attendings will perform the same operation in different ways, and you should learn this as well. Knowing that one surgeon enters the abdomen with the Veress needle while another prefers Hassan technique (discussed in ▶ Sect. 7.7) will allow you to be more helpful and engaged in the operation. Often the best person to learn this from is the scrub nurse/technician.

6. *Ask questions selectively and thoughtfully.* Know when is a good time to ask questions (usually at the end of the case). If you have questions during the case, make a mental list. Then, separate that list into questions that you can look up easily after the case (fact-based answers) versus more nuanced questions (clinical decision-making).

7. *After the case, write down what you learned and look up what you still have questions about.*

7.2 Clinical Knowledge

Now that you have adopted the surgeon's mindset, the next step is to develop the knowledge base for your rotation. The following section will provide a framework for how to build your clinical knowledge, study for the shelf exam, and optimize your learning.

7.2.1 Resources

- *Pestana.* A good resource for common cases and scenarios, but lacking in detail. This book has great breadth but limited depth. Every piece of information is a must know for the shelf.
- *Surgical Recall.* Great resource for practical knowledge and for the wards. This book contains the answers for a lot of "pimp" and specialty-specific questions.
- *DeVirgilio.* Case-based textbook with corresponding questions at the end of each chapter to assess understanding.
- *NMS Surgery (National Medical Series).* A surgery textbook for content geared toward medical students, including USMLE-type questions.
- *Greenfield's Surgery.* A general surgery textbook focusing on the scientific foundations underlying different general surgery pathologies. This is a long read and more of a resident-level resource, but a useful reference to look up specific details the night before each case.
- *Cameron's Current Surgical Therapy.* This textbook is more advanced and addresses the most current surgical techniques and considerations. Usually higher-level residents will read this text, but it may be helpful for understanding the specifics of an operation.
- *Netter's Anatomy.* An anatomy atlas that you may have used during your preclinical years. Prior to each case, you should review the relevant anatomy, making sure to note important landmarks, potential variants, and the course of different structures in the region.

- *Zollinger's Atlas of Surgical Operations.* An amazing surgical atlas with helpful images and walks through most general surgery operations. It may be helpful to correlate *Netter's Anatomy* to a surgical atlas when preparing for a case.
- *UWorld question bank.* Limited in the number of surgery questions (~135 questions). For shelf review, many of the questions actually center on the diagnosis, workup, and management of each disease, and it may be useful to review the GI category of medicine questions as well.
- *Amboss question bank.* Good for both content review and questions. The learning cards provide a succinct way to review etiology, diagnostics, and management (including information on first-line and alternative treatment).
- *National Board of Medical Examiners (NBME) practice exams.* Past exams can be found online and serve as self-assessment tools prior to your shelf. Set aside time on the weekends leading up to your shelf exam to take a few practice exams and familiarize yourself with test questions.

7.2.2 Content Checklist

The following is a complete list of content areas to study, primarily focusing on topics that will be covered on the shelf exam. Subjects that are useful for the rotation but that may not be emphasized on the shelf exam are indicated with an asterisk*.

- Perioperative management
  - Preoperative assessment (cardiac, pulmonary, hepatic, renal, nutritional assessments)*
  - Discontinuation of medications*
  - Postoperative management (common complications, postoperative fever, perioperative hemorrhage, surgical site infection, urinary retention, ileus)
- Surgical intensive care unit (SICU) basics
  - Ventilatory support*
  - Hemodynamic monitoring
  - Fluids and electrolytes
  - Nutrition (parenteral vs enteral, routes of administration)*
  - Tubes/lines/drains*
- Skin/soft tissue
  - Burns (severity, rule of 9s, Parkland formula, complications)
  - Wounds (classification, types of repair)
    - Decubitus ulcers
    - Amputations
    - Bite wounds, stab wounds
  - Infection (impetigo, erysipelas, cellulitis, necrotizing fasciitis, folliculitis, skin abscess, ecthyma gangrenosum, paronychia, felon, dactylitis)
  - Suture selection (size, braided vs monofilament, absorbable vs nonabsorbable)
  - Skin cancer (melanoma, basal cell, squamous cell)
  - Sarcoma
- Ear, nose, and throat (ENT)
  - Congenital (thyroglossal duct cyst, branchial cleft cyst, cystic hygroma)
  - Orbital disorders (Graves' ophthalmopathy, orbital cellulitis, retinoblastoma)

- Ear (otitis media, mastoiditis, labyrinthitis, cholesteatoma, otosclerosis, ear barotrauma, decompression sickness, auricular hematoma)
- Nose (choanal atresia, deviated nasal septum, septal perforation, nasal papilloma, cleft lip and palate, juvenile nasopharyngeal angiofibroma)
- Throat (tonsillitis, peritonsillar abscess, parapharyngeal abscess, retropharyngeal abscess, temporomandibular joint dysfunction, laryngeal carcinoma)
- Salivary glands (sialadenosis, sialadenitis, sialolithiasis, parotid gland tumors)
- Oral and pharyngeal cancer
- Cardiac
  - Congenital (patent ductus arteriosus, aortic coarctation, atrial septal defects, ventricular septal defects, tetralogy of Fallot, transposition of great arteries, tricuspid valve atresia, hypoplastic left heart, total anomalous pulmonary venous return, Ebstein's anomaly, truncus arteriosus, aortic arch pathologies)
  - Coronary artery disease (angina, non-ST elevation myocardial infarction (NSTEMI), STEMI, indications for surgical treatment, complications after MI)
  - Valvular disease (aortic, mitral, tricuspid, and pulmonic stenosis/regurgitation)
  - Pericardial disease (acute and chronic pericarditis, pericardial effusion, tamponade)
  - Cardiomyopathies (dilated, restrictive, infiltrative)
  - Cardiac tumors (benign, malignant, metastatic)
- Thoracic
  - Infection (empyema)
  - Trauma (pneumothorax, hemothorax)
  - Pleural disease (effusions, pleuritis, mesothelioma)
  - Pulmonary embolism
  - Thoracic outlet syndrome
  - Hiatal hernias (sliding, paraesophageal, mixed, complex)
  - Lung cancer (small cell, adenocarcinoma, squamous cell, large cell)
    - Subtypes and variants (Pancoast tumor, bronchioloalveolar)
    - Workup of solitary pulmonary nodule
    - Screening recommendations
- Endocrine
  - Thyroid (Graves', Hashimoto's, hyper- and hypothyroidism, goiter, thyroid nodules, thyroid cancer)
  - Parathyroid (primary vs secondary vs tertiary hyperparathyroidism, hypoparathyroidism)
  - Pituitary (prolactinoma, pituitary adenoma, acromegaly)
  - Neuroendocrine (gastrinoma, insulinoma, VIPoma, neuroblastoma, Wilms tumor, multiple endocrine neoplasia types 1, 2A, and 2B)
  - Adrenal (Cushing's syndrome, Addison's, adrenal cancer, Conn syndrome, pheochromocytoma)
- Gastrointestinal (GI)
  - Esophagus (achalasia, Boerhaave syndrome, Mallory-Weiss tear, esophageal varices, diverticula, esophageal rings, Barrett's esophagus, esophageal cancer)
  - Stomach (gastroesophageal reflux, gastritis, peptic ulcer disease, gastric outlet obstruction, gastric cancer)
  - Gallbladder/bile ducts (cholelithiasis, choledocholithiasis, cholecystitis, gallstone pancreatitis, cholangitis, postcholecystectomy syndrome, cholangiocarcinoma)

- Liver (acute and chronic hepatitis, cirrhosis, benign liver tumors, hepatic cysts, pyogenic liver abscess, liver cancer)
- Pancreas (acute and chronic pancreatitis, cystic disease, pancreatic cancer)
- Spleen (splenic rupture, asplenia, postsplenectomy management)
- Small bowel (appendicitis, small bowel obstruction, ileus, small bowel neoplasms, carcinoid tumor)
- Bariatric surgery
- Other
  - Acute abdomen (differential based on location, specific signs)
  - GI bleeding (upper vs lower)
  - Hernias (ventral, umbilical, inguinal – direct and indirect, internal, femoral, obturator, flank hernias)
  - Peritonitis
- Breast surgery
  - Benign breast lesions
    - Screening in premenopausal and younger women vs postmenopausal women
  - Malignant breast lesions (ductal carcinoma in situ (DCIS), lobular carcinoma in situ (LCIS), inflammatory breast cancers, Paget's disease), DCIS, LCIS, Paget's disease
- Colorectal
  - Colon (diverticular disease, internal and external hemorrhoids, acute and chronic megacolon, large bowel obstruction)
    - Colorectal cancer (screening recommendations, classification, staging, treatment options)
    - Inflammatory bowel disease (Crohn's vs ulcerative colitis)
    - Intestinal ischemia (ischemic colitis, acute and chronic mesenteric ischemia)
  - Anal/rectal (pilonidal cyst, abscess and fistula, anal fissures, rectal prolapse, anal cancer)
- Renal
  - Congenital/pediatric (megaureter, polycystic kidney disease)
  - Cystic disease (solitary cystic lesions, polycystic kidney disease, medullary sponge kidney, obstructive cystic dysplasia, multicystic dysplastic kidneys)
  - Infection (lower UTI, upper UTI, and pyelonephritis)
  - Renal cell carcinoma (subtypes and classifications, paraneoplastic symptoms)
  - Retroperitoneal fibrosis
- Pediatric surgery
  - Bilious emesis (malrotation, duodenal atresia, jejunal/ileal atresia, Hirschsprung's, imperforate anus, necrotizing enterocolitis, meconium plug)
  - Non-bilious emesis (hypertrophic pyloric stenosis, gastroesophageal reflux disease (GERD))
  - Hyperbilirubinemia (biliary atresia, sepsis, Gilbert's, Crigler-Najjar)
  - Bloody diarrhea (necrotizing enterocolitis, intussusception, Meckel's diverticulum)
  - Newborn respiratory distress (congenital diaphragmatic hernia, choanal atresia, tracheoesophageal fistula, pneumothorax)
  - Abdominal masses (Wilms tumor, neuroblastoma)
  - Abdominal wall defects (omphalocele, gastroschisis, bladder exstrophy)
  - Hernias (epigastric, umbilical, direct, indirect)
  - Non-accidental trauma (child abuse, shaken baby syndrome, scalding burns, sexual abuse)

- Urology
  - Congenital malformations (bladder exstrophy, epispadias, hypospadias, posterior urethral valves, webbed penis)
  - Urinary tract (types of incontinence, retention, stricture, obstruction, vesicoureteral reflux, urolithiasis, urothelial cancer)
  - Prostate (benign prostatic hypertrophy, prostate cancer, prostatitis)
  - Testicle (testicular torsion, cryptorchidism, hydrocele, varicocele, spermatocele)
    - Testicular tumors (classification, staging, distinguishing features and associations)
  - Epididymis (acute and chronic epididymitis)
  - Penis (priapism, penile fracture, premature and delayed ejaculation, erectile dysfunction, penile carcinoma)
  - Genitourinary trauma (renal and ureteral, bladder, urethral trauma)
- Trauma
  - Primary and secondary survey*
  - Shock (hypovolemic, distributive, septic, obstructive, cardiogenic)
  - Blunt trauma (thoracic, abdominal, extremities)
  - Penetrating trauma (neck, thoracic, abdominal, extremities)
- Vascular
  - Aorta (thoracic vs abdominal aortic aneurysms and classification, aortic dissection, vascular ring)
  - Peripheral artery disease (ulcers, acute limb ischemia)
  - Venous disease (varicose veins, deep vein thrombosis)
  - Other
    - Aneurysms (cerebral, ventricular, popliteal, iliofemoral, carotid)
    - Renal artery stenosis
    - Carotid stenosis
- Orthopedic surgery (▶ Chap. 23)
- Neurosurgery (▶ Chap. 24)

7.2.3 Studying for Shelf

Learning material for the shelf exam differs in strategy and content from preparing for your clinical rotations. Both are necessary and should be pursued in parallel during the rotation. You will not be able to rotate through each of these electives while on your rotation, and it will be up to you to supplement your own learning for the shelf exam each evening. Essentially, you should have two study blocks each day – one for shelf content and one for your clinical rotation.

For each of the pathologies listed in the Content Checklist, make sure to review the following:
1. Epidemiology
2. Etiology
3. Pathophysiology
4. Presenting symptoms
5. Diagnostics*
6. Management*
7. Prognosis and complications

*Be explicit about first-line, second-line, and alternative tests and treatment plans. You will be expected to know not only the various options but also the order in which to proceed.

Recommended resources: Amboss learning cards and question bank, UWorld question bank, *First Aid for the USMLE Step 2 CS*

7.2.4 Studying for the Rotation

While your shelf studying will certainly help you on each of your rotations, you will be expected to go into deeper detail than what is necessary for the shelf exam. The timing of your electives also may not line up with your shelf schedule, and we would recommend treating these as separate entities.

For each patient case, you should know the following:

1. Anatomy
2. Differentials for common presenting symptoms (e.g., differential for RUQ pain when you are on your hepatopancreaticobiliary rotation)
3. Workup:
   (a) Diagnostic algorithms
   (b) Labs/imaging
4. Medical management
5. Indications for surgery
6. Contraindications to surgery
7. Treatment guidelines (e.g., National Comprehensive Cancer Network guidelines for esophageal cancer):
   (a) Relevant trials and novel treatments
8. Common operations:
   (a) Patient positioning
   (b) Approach (laparoscopic port sites, landmarks for incisions)
   (c) Steps of the procedure (may differ based on attending)
   (d) "Danger" areas and what to look out for
9. Complications (perioperative and long term):
   (a) Rates (e.g., ~16% of patients develop diabetes after a Whipple procedure)
   (b) Risk factors
   (c) Management

7.3 What to Expect

7.3.1 Before the Rotation

- Read through 1–2 textbooks of your choice (*Pestana, DeVirgilio,* etc.) to familiarize yourself with common cases. This can be a quick skim to orient yourself to the rotation and does not need to encompass specific details of each operation.
- Create a study schedule. Using the checklist above, set aside time every day to cover a portion of clinical content for shelf review. This should *be in addition to* your preparation for your cases the next day (e.g., if you finish your evening rounds around 6–7 pm, block out an hour at night to go over one section of shelf content. This could be unrelated to your current rotation, such as reviewing vascular, even when you are on a colorectal rotation. Then, having finished shelf review, proceed to prepare for your colorectal cases for the next day. This will ensure that you are both prepared for your clinical rotations and up to speed with your shelf exam knowledge.).
- Block out time to take at least 2 NBME practice tests in the weeks leading up to your shelf exam. You should aim to finish your content review prior to these tests, and the remaining time can be used to review areas of weakness.
- Practice basic suturing and knot-tying skills. You may be starting on a rotation in which you hit the ground running and might be asked to close a skin incision or tie in a tube or drain. If you are already comfortable with

this, you will likely be given more responsibility throughout your rotation and be able to participate more with each operation. See ▶ Sect. 7.7 for more information.

7.3.2 Team Roles

7.3.2.1 Attending Surgeon

Depending on your rotation, you will have one or more attending surgeons. A mentorship relationship with your attending is one of the most rewarding experiences of medical school and may define your future career trajectory. Establishing the proper framework for such a relationship is key early on and should be based on a foundation of professionalism and respect. An attending is your boss first and foremost and should be treated with a healthy level of reverence. While some attendings may decide to forgo the formalities, you should err on the side of caution unless explicitly told otherwise. After that, they may serve as a role model, educator, and mentor if you are lucky, but even then, a mantle of professionalism should be maintained.

Each attending has their own preferences in regard to team dynamics, surgical technique, and educational style. *Learn this!* (e.g., one attending may ask you to tie two-handed knots each time, while another will teach you one handed.) Adapt yourself to each attending, and if they teach you something different than what you previously learned, *then learn it again.* Your attending will be your primary evaluator on this rotation, but more importantly, you will learn so much from them!

7.3.2.2 Senior Resident

The role of a senior resident (often a chief resident) is to lead the team on a day-to-day basis (scheduling, assigning cases, communicating with the attending). They will be the ones to teach you surgical skills and procedures and may even take the time to go over different clinical topics. You will spend much more time with your residents than with the attending, and they are also involved in your evaluations. Like with the attending, your relationship with your resident should be professional. As you get to know each other better, this may change, but until then, think of your senior resident as your squadron leader. Be a good soldier, carry your weight, and do what you can to make their lives easier.

7.3.2.3 Junior Resident/Intern

Your job is to make your residents look good. The junior resident will likely bear the brunt of daily tasks, and the best thing you can do is help them relieve this. Ask them early on how you can be the most useful. Some interns may organize their to-do lists differently, and each has their own methods to ensure that no tasks fall through the cracks. As such, there are certain tasks that are not useful for you to do and may end up doubling their workload, so make sure to check and follow their lead. Your junior resident or intern will also be much closer to you in terms of perspective and experience. They can be helpful resources for the questions or concerns that you may feel uncertain asking your senior or attending.

7.3.2.4 Nurse Practitioner, Physician Assistants (Floor)

You may have additional help from nurse practitioners (NP) or floor physician assistants (PA). They are a major asset to the team, helping with floor work, discharge paperwork, pulling tubes and drains, and clinic work. The role of the

NP or PA will likely differ between institutions and departments, so make sure to clarify tasks and responsibilities early on. You can learn a lot from them (tips and tricks for floor procedures, attending preferences, institutional culture, etc.), and they should be treated with the same amount of respect as your residents and attendings.

7.3.2.5 OR Physician Assistants and Nurse Practitioners

An OR PA may serve as a first or second assistant in cases or may have a specific role (e.g., harvesting the saphenous vein in a coronary artery bypass graft or handing instruments through an assistant's port in a robotic case). They may be the ones to teach you how to position and prep the patient or even perform certain procedures. They will likely be a source of institutional knowledge and will help you navigate certain aspects like attending preferences.

7.3.2.6 Scrub Nurse/Tech

In the OR, the scrub nurse or surgical technologist is the glue that holds the surgical team together. A good scrub knows the steps of the procedures and the instrument the surgeons need before they even ask for it. Because of this, the best thing you can do is follow their lead. If they hand you an instrument (or importantly, if they do not hand you an instrument), this is for a reason. You can learn so much about the flow of the operation and anticipating next steps just from watching the scrub nurse. Remember your manners, say "please" and "thank you," and do not touch the Mayo tray.

7.3.2.7 Circulator

The circulator (nurse) remains unscrubbed during the case and serves as the point person for the surgical team. While it is important to introduce yourself to the entire team, it is especially important to meet the circulator when you enter the room. Follow their lead in terms of where to stand and how to be useful.

7.3.2.8 Anesthesia

Your anesthesia colleagues are an integral part of the surgical team. Remember that you are on your surgical rotation, but you can still learn from and help the anesthesia team as well. There will be times at which the surgical team is waiting for anesthesia and times at which anesthesia is waiting for you. Be kind and gracious at all times.

Sometimes anesthesia may not be aware that a medical student is closing skin. It may be helpful to let anesthesia know that you may need a couple more minutes so they can be prepared. Even if you feel the pressure to finish quickly, *never sacrifice quality for speed*. Take your time and do a good job.

7.3.3 Getting Started

Meet the team and discuss expectations on day one. Your resident will assign you 1–4 patients on the list (usually starting with one and working up from there).

1. Read up on your patients – all history and physical exams (H&Ps), clinic notes, prior op notes, and progress notes from the index hospitalization. Look at the imaging (not just the radiology reports) to begin training your eye.
2. Review the anatomy (broadly). You should know the details of the organ and its spatial relationship to adjacent structures, the blood supply (and

their course), and innervation. This is a broad overview to orient yourself before the rotation, but you will need to review in more detail the anatomy relevant to each operation the night before.

3. Start your content review early using Greenfield's or another more detailed textbook. You should know the basics and most common pathologies before starting the rotation. See checklist above in ▶ Sect. 7.2.2.

7.3.4 Schedule

Your weeks will consist of a mix of OR days and clinic days, in addition to floor work and rounding each day. During your acute care/trauma surgery block, you will likely spend the majority of your time in the ED. Expect to have call days and overnight shifts, which will differ based on your institution.

7.3.4.1 Sample OR Day

- Before 6 AM – Check on your patients. Check in with nurses for overnight events, vitals, I/Os, labs, and imaging. Print the lists for your team. Prep progress notes for the day (this may differ based on your institution's policy on pre-rounding).
- 6:00 AM – Receive handoff from night team.
- 6:30 AM – Team rounds (AM).
- 7:00 AM – Meet the patient in the postanesthesia care unit (PACU). Introduce yourself; help transport patient to the OR.
- 8:00 AM – Start first OR case. Depending on the rotation, cases can last anywhere from 20 minutes to >10 hours. Set your expectations depending on your rotation. At the end of the case, transport patient back to the PACU.
- As the day goes on, you may have 1–4 cases per day. In between each case, you may find the time to complete daily tasks, respond to pages, complete progress notes, and perform post-op checks.
- 5:00 PM – Pre-round again for PM rounds, gather info on vitals, labs, and day events.
- 6:00 PM – Team rounds (PM). Finish tasks, and hand off to night team.

7.3.4.2 Sample Clinic Day

- Before 6 AM – Pre-round on your patients. Check in with nurses for overnight events, vitals, I/Os, labs, and imaging. Print the lists for your team. Prep clinic notes (either in the morning or the night before), and look up relevant guidelines or management recommendations. See Examples section for sample clinic note.
- 6:00 AM – Receive handoff from night team.
- 6:30 AM – Team rounds (AM).
- 7:30 AM – Arrive at clinic. Set up your workspace and await instruction for patient assignments.
- 8:00 AM – Clinic start. You will see a mix of new patients for pre-op consultations, post-op visits, minor procedures, and long-term follow-up. You will go in first, conduct H&P, and prep your clinic note. When you are ready, you will present the patient to your attending (including your proposed plan) and go back in to see the patient together. Your attending will make adjustments to your plan and may give you some feedback. Return to your workspace, and finish the clinic note before moving on to the next patient.

- 5:00 PM – Clinic ends (will vary). Switch back to floor mode to pre-round; gather info on vitals, labs, and day events for your floor patients.
- 6:00 PM – Team rounds (PM). Finish tasks, and hand off to night team.

**The above sample schedules are hypothetical scenarios. You will likely run late on more than one occasion due to complicated cases during your OR days or delays in clinic, or you may end early if the OR schedule is light. Expect to stay however long it takes. Your mentality should be that you are in the trenches with the team at all times. You do not come and go as you please. You should be there helping, engaged, and focused until all of your team's goals are accomplished, *including* "scut work" and intern tasks at the end of the day.

7.4   A Practical Guide

7.4.1 The Floor

7.4.1.1 Preparing for Rounds

- Arrive early. Budget 15–30 minutes per patient, longer if you are just getting started or if this is a patient who is new to you.
- Start progress notes for each patient. Your team will likely provide templates for you at the start of the rotation, and some electronic medical records (EMRs) will allow you to carry over progress notes from previous days.
- Read the nursing progress reports (which will contain important information on overnight events) and any new notes that you have not yet seen from the previous day.
- Obtain info from the EMR (prior to seeing the patient).
  - Overnight events (from nursing note, later *confirm* with nurses and patient when you go see each patient)
  - Vitals
  - Tubes/lines/drains (type, location, output. Include info on what has been removed and how the insertion sites appear)
  - Intake/outputs (total and individual components) (◨ Table 7.2)
  - Labs and imaging (new)
  - Medications (any changes, PRN meds that were given)

Consult notes from the evening will contain recommendations that will guide the plan for the day.

◨ **Table 7.2**   Intake/output charting

	Volume	Route	Total
Intake	1.5 L	IV	2 L
	0.5 L	PO	
Output	2 L	Urine (Foley)	3 L
	0.75 L	Right chest tube	
	0.25 L	Mediastinal chest tube	
	3× (unrecorded amount)	Stool	
Net			-1 L

- Update the progress note with the data from above. Anticipate changes to the plan based on what has previously been discussed on rounds the previous day (e.g., plans to advance diet, remove drains, etc.) and any recommendations from consulting teams.
  - In many institutions, some cases have been moving toward enhanced recovery after surgery (ERAS) protocols. In this case, you can predict the plan for most patients unless there is a complication or reason to deviate.
- Print rounding lists for yourself and your team.
  - You may do this earlier and handwrite some of the key info obtained above, as you will need to have this data (vitals, labs, I/Os, imaging, etc.) when you present on rounds. Alternatively, some EMRs will allow you to call in these values with different commands, and you can incorporate that into your own rounding list.
- Go to the floor to see the patient.
  - Find the patient's nurse when you arrive. Ask about overnight events and any nursing concerns. Inform them that you will be going in to see the patient.
    - **The nurses are an *essential* part of the team, and no matter how much of a rush you are in to pre-round on your patients, take the time to acknowledge them. Remember too that depending on how early you are pre-rounding, you may be speaking with the overnight nurse at the end of a long shift! Kindness and respect goes a long way.
  - When you enter the room, look at the patient. Determine *sick or not sick?*
    - Look at the patient.
    - Look at the monitors (vitals, telemetry).
    - Look at drips (IV medications).
    - Look at ventilators and mechanical support.
      ***If there are *any* signs that the patient is unstable or their condition is worsening, ask for help immediately. Ask the nurse to page your resident and activate the appropriate codes or pathways for emergency response. See Critical Care and Emergency Medicine chapters for more information.
  - *Gently* wake the patient and introduce yourself and which team you are from. Remember that this will be very early in the morning!
    - *For patients at risk for delirium, it is worth asking your team whether their preference is to wake sleeping patients before rounds or to let them sleep.*
  - Ask the patient about the following:
    - Overnight events
    - Pain (including pain medications taken and subjective relief)
    - Symptoms (depending on operation – e.g., nausea or vomiting after gastrectomy)
    - Have they resumed normal bodily functions?
      - Ventilation (intubated? Type of ventilatory support, supplemental O2, etc.)
      - PO intake
      - Urine
      - Stool
      - Ambulation/activity
  - *Perform a focused physical based on the rotation and operation that were performed. You can obtain a good amount of information just observing the patient. Examine the color and quality of drain fluids. See Sample Progress Note [on page 149] for an example.*

– *Inform the patient that the team will be back later that morning to discuss the plan.*
– *Before leaving the room, ask the patient if there is anything you can help with (lights* on vs off, door opened vs closed, repositioning, etc.).
▬ Finish updating your progress note with the information obtained.

7.4.1.2 Presenting on Rounds

■ **General Guidelines**
▬ *Ask for team preferences* on your first day (how much information and order of presenting) as this will differ from team to team.
▬ *Be succinct but comprehensive.* Surgical rounds are much faster than medicine, as you will need to get to the OR or clinic to start your day. Now is not the time to bring up basic science journal articles or an exhaustive differential.
  – *Know everything but say the highlights.* While you are not bringing up every possible diagnosis for post-op fever, you still need to think through the full differential and workup *as you would on your medicine rotation.* However, you do not need to present all of this as you would on medicine rounds. Simply state the main bullet points, and be ready to go into detail if the team asks questions.
  – ***Potential pitfall. Understanding what to include or omit is a skill that many of us will continue to learn even into residency. You may feel the temptation to make your presentations shorter and shorter, but this should never be at the sacrifice of important information. As a medical student, you may not be entirely sure what is important or not, and in those cases, ask your intern prior to rounds, or just include the information.
▬ *Err on the side of formality.* Be ready to give the formal presentation for all patients at all times, but be able to adapt on the go. When you meet your team for PM rounds and your chief asks you how the patient is doing, you will not need to start with the one-liner and formal presentation order, but you will need to know the pertinent information.
▬ *Expect to be interrupted.* Whether this is for questions or your team asking you to speed up the presentation, expect that this will not be one fluid presentation, and don't let this fluster you. Answer the question or follow the request, and *make a mental note of this for the future.* If they are asking you for something, it is probably because you had left that detail out (or you had buried it within irrelevant data).
▬ As you present, *take notes on (1) changes to your plan and (2) tasks for the day.* Your rounding list will then become a to-do list for the rest of the day.

■ **Structure of the Surgical Presentation**
1. *One-liner*:
   ▬ Patient Name
   ▬ Age
   ▬ Need-to-know past medical history (PMH) (limit this to 1–2 diagnoses)
   ▬ Timing in relation to procedure (pre-op, POD ___)
   ▬ Procedure
     – Open vs lap
     – Index procedure and any major additional components. (Knowing what is pertinent to include here is a bit nuanced.)
       – *Example (cardiac): CABG x2, mechanical AVR, hemiarch replacement*
       – *Example (thoracic): VATS left upper lobectomy (do not include bronchoscopy, EBUS, etc.)*
   ▬ Current status/problems

Example #1: John Smith is a 65-year-old man recovering well on POD#3 from an open ventral hernia repair.

Example #2: Betty Boop is an 80-year-old woman with stage II pancreatic adenocarcinoma who underwent a Whipple procedure on 1/1/19, complicated by a bile duct leak that is being medically managed.

7

Example #1: No acute events overnight.

Example #2: Last night, Mrs. Boop developed a fever of 102 with RUQ abdominal pain. She underwent an abdominal CT, which demonstrated a large collection of subhepatic fluid concerning for an intra-abdominal abscess. She remained hemodynamically stable, was started on IV piperacillin/tazobactam, and is scheduled for IR drain placement this morning.

Example #1: The patient's pain is well-managed on IV Tylenol PRN. He is ambulating, tolerating a surgical soft diet, and urinating independently. He has not had a bowel movement in 2 days.

Example #2: This morning, the patient remains feverish and complains of RUQ abdominal pain, mildly improved since last night. She received oxycodone 5 mg once last night with good effect. She was up and out of bed to her chair yesterday. She remains NPO with an NG tube in place with minimal output. She has a Foley in place with clear yellow urine and had one episode of diarrhea last night.

Example #1: Total I/Os are net − 1 L with total intake of 2.5 liters, 800cc PO. Total output − 3.5 L urine. A M CBC and BMP are within normal limits. When I saw the patient, he was afebrile and hemodynamically stable, sitting comfortably in his bed. He was in normal sinus rhythm on tele; lungs were clear and abdomen soft and non-tender with dressing clean, dry, and intact. No peripheral edema. All tubes, lines, and drains have been removed.

2. *Overnight events*:

3. *Subjective data*:
   - New complaints
   - Pain:
     - **If the pain is new, treat this as a new complaint, and include all of the onset, position, quality, radiation, severity, and timing (OPQRST) information.
     - **If discussing normal postoperative pain, just focus on whether the pain is better/worse/unchanged and current management.
   - Activity (up and out of bed, ambulation)
   - Eating/drinking
   - Urine
   - Stool

4. *Objective data* (the order of this may differ based on team preference):
   - Intake/output (including tubes/lines/drains)
   - Labs (new)
   - Imaging (if applicable)
   - Micro (if applicable)
   - Vitals
     - **This varies significantly based on your team. "Afebrile and hemodynamically stable" may be sufficient for some attendings, while others prefer the actual numbers.
   - Physical exam (brief)

5. *Assessment/plan:*
  ▬ One-liner (abbreviated)
  ▬ Systems-based plans (include all in your note, but only say the pertinent changes during your presentation. Make sure to mention each of the systems, but you may not have any changes, in which case, it is acceptable to say, "nothing for ____."):
  – Neuro/pain
  – Cardiac
  – Respiratory
  – GI
  – GU
  – Heme
  – ID
  – Endocrine
  ▬ Discharge planning

7.4.1.3 Progress Notes

Progress notes will be team- and institution-dependent, and you will likely be given instructions with a template on your first day. The purpose of this section is to describe practically how to manage your time and efficiently complete your notes. See a Sample Progress Note on page 149 for more details.

Example #2: Tmax overnight was 99.9. Vitals this morning: BP 110/60, HR 86, RR 25, satting 100% on room air. Total I/Os are + 1.5 L. Total intake was 3 L IV. Total output was − 1.5 L: 500 cc through the NG tube and 1 L urine output through the Foley. Labs this morning are notable for K 5.5 and hemoglobin 7.5 down from 8 last night. Blood cultures from last night are growing 2/2 Klebsiella, sensitivities pending. When I saw the patient, she was alert and responsive lying in bed. No scleral icterus or jaundice. Cardiac exam was normal. Pulmonary exam notable for dullness to percussion in the RLL, no crackles or rhonchi. Abdomen was soft, tender to palpation in the RUQ without rebound or guarding and negative fluid wave. Dressings have been removed, staples intact, and incision is well-approximated without erythema or exudate. No peripheral edema.

Example #1: In conclusion, this is an otherwise healthy 65-year-old man recovering well on POD#3 from a ventral hernia repair. For neuro and pain management, we will transition him from IV to PO Tylenol. No cardiac or respiratory issues. GI, advance to a regular diet, and increase the bowel regimen. GU, Foley is out and he is urinating independently. No heme, ID, or endocrine issues. Plan for discharge tomorrow.

Example #2: In conclusion, Mrs. Boop is an 80-year-old woman, POD#7 from a Whipple, complicated by bile duct leak, now concerning for intra-abdominal abscess. For neuro, we will continue her on scheduled IV Tylenol and oxycodone PRN. No cardiac issues. Respiratory, incentive spirometry, up and out of bed. GI, NPO with NG tube in place; plan for IR drain placement this morning. GU, continue with Foley in place until after IR drain placement. ID, continue IV zosyn, and follow up sensitivities. Heme, Hgb drop likely dilutional, will recheck PM labs. Endocrine, continue sliding-scale insulin. Discharge planning pending resolution of abscess.

While different teams and attendings will have their own preferences for how aggressively to advance the diet, the general order of progression is as follows:

- *NPO (nil per os, or nothing by mouth)*
- *Sips of clears*
- *Clear liquids (juice, broth, etc.)*
- *Full liquids (includes dairy, protein shakes.)*
- *Surgical softs (includes mashed potatoes, pureed foods, etc.)*
- *Regular diet*

- *Pre-rounding.* Start your notes when you arrive in the morning. Carry over the template from your previous progress note, and update all of the objective data before going to the floor to see your patient. Your note should be 90% finished before you even round.
- *Subjective:*
  – Overnight events (based on nursing notes)
- Objective:
  – I/Os
  – Vitals
  – Labs
  – Imaging
- *Assessment/plan* (you can already anticipate what this will be based on consult note recommendations, previously established pathways, and team discussions the day prior):
  – Consult recommendations
  – Pain management (anticipated changes)
  – Diet (anticipated advances)
- Tubes/lines/drains (anticipated discontinuations based on output and objective data)
  – The general principle is that the longer these remain in the body, the higher risk of infection. Not only that, the patient usually has significant pain or discomfort with these in place that may be restricting mobility (e.g., large chest tubes causing pleuritic pain, so the patient takes smaller breaths, worsening atelectasis). However, if you take these out too early (i.e., there is still fluid accumulating), you may cause a fluid collection and need to replace the drain.
  – Most institutions and teams will have criteria for one to pull a drain (e.g., chest tube output <10 mL/hr).
- *After seeing the patient.* Complete your progress note tentatively by adding subjective data, physical exam, and adjustments to your anticipated plan.
  – Subjective:
    – Overnight events (confirm with patient)
    – New complaints
    – Pain
    – Activity
    – Eating/drinking
    – Urine
    – Stool
  – Objective:
    – Physical exam
  – *Assessment/plan.* Make adjustments to your plan as needed.

- *After rounds.* As you present on rounds, your residents will make adjustments to your plan, and once you meet with the attending to run the list, there will be additional changes. Make a note of this on your rounding list.
  – *Assessment/plan.* Make additional adjustments.
- *During the day.* Complete the tasks that have accumulated on your to-do list (calling consults, changing dressings, placing NG tubes, pulling drains, etc.). You will have random pockets of time in between cases that are optimal for completing these small tasks. This is also an opportunity to complete your progress note, which at this point should take only a few minutes since you have the bulk of the note already completed.
- *At the end of the day.* After sharing your note with your resident and finishing up for the day, make a point to *go back, and look at any changes/addendums* that your resident and attending make to your note. This is an important learning opportunity and will help you to refine this skill.

7.4.1.4 Handoffs/Sign-Outs

AM Sign-out   When you arrive in the morning, there will be a set sign-out time with the night team. They will update you on any overnight events and actions taken for your patients. Aim to have completed your pre-rounding prior to this, and it will make sign-out much smoother. You do not need to see all of your patients prior to sign-out, but try to have the objective data gathered and the list printed.

PM Sign-out   After your evening rounds, finish up your tasks for your patients and make sure that you complete any tasks that are remaining. This is where your daily checklist will come in handy. *Do not leave work for the night team to complete.* There are some cases in which this is inevitable (e.g., follow up on an evening lab), but everything else should be tidied up and ready to go.

- *Prior to sign-out*:
  – Complete all tasks.
    – AM labs ordered.
    – Tubes or drains pulled (if needed).
    – PRN orders in place.
  – Check in with nursing team.
    – Go over the plan and address any nursing concerns prior to sign-out. This will minimize the number of questions and pages the night resident receives.
- *What to include at sign-out*:
  – Abbreviated one-liner (if new patient or resident unfamiliar with this patient)
    – Name
    – Age

A common mistake that medical students make is prioritizing the progress note over tasks that need to be completed. The progress note can be signed at any time and instead should be completed during your free time (in between cases, etc.). Placing orders, calling consults, pulling drains, and bedside procedures are all time-sensitive and should take priority.

It may be tempting to copy notes forward, but remember that each daily progress note should reflect the findings of whether that's the subjective, vitals, physical exam, or the plan. Copying old notes that do not reflect the current plans is both detrimental to coordinating patient care and a potential for legal consequences.

    – Procedure

    – Time since procedure

    – Significant events

– Tasks with contingencies (contingencies should have clear thresholds and next steps. Instead of "if hypotensive, give fluids," try "if SBP<90, give 500cc bolus IV NS")

    – *Example: Please follow up on void trial at midnight. If patient has not voided, please ask for bladder scan. If > 400 cc, straight cath. If > 600 cc, replace Foley.*

– Potential pages

    – *Example: The nurses may page you for _____. PRN orders for __ are already in place.*

7.4.1.5 Consults

There are a few pathways by which your team will receive new patients: inpatient consults, ED admissions, and clinic. The latter two will be discussed in subsequent sections. While the overall structure is similar to H&Ps that you have conducted on other rotations, there are some nuances to the surgical approach that this section will focus on.

1. *Receiving the consult.* When your team is consulted, you will receive a page with patient identifiers, pertinent history, and the reason for the consult.
   - Look up the patient. Read the H&P for this hospitalization, most recent progress note, relevant clinic notes or op notes, and the discharge notes of any recent hospitalizations.
   - Start a consult note. See sample Consult Note at the end of the chapter for an example.
     - Fill in what you know from your chart review (one-liner, reason for consult, PMH, PSH, FH, SH, meds, allergies, vitals).
   - Review labs and imaging, and summarize in your admission note.
   - Call the consulting physician to receive handoff. Your goal should be to already have the objective data prepared and your note somewhat filled in before this phone call. You will be able to obtain most information from the chart and may even be able to read the note of the consulting physician. The phone call should really just be an opportunity to listen and confirm what you are reading. If you have any lingering questions (such as why the patient received a certain course of treatment), this is a good opportunity to ask. Your questions should really be to clarify the thought process and question of the primary team, not to obtain information that can be read in the chart.
     - Update your admission note with new information.
2. *Go see the patient.* When you arrive, check in with the nurse taking care of the patient. Take note of your surroundings, which will clue you in to the urgency of the consult.
3. *Sick or not sick?* This is the most important question to ask, before attempting to obtain the history or perform a physical. See "pre-rounding" for details. If the patient is unstable or may need an urgent procedure, let your resident know immediately.
4. *Conduct a targeted H&P.* The difference between an inpatient consult and an admission is that you are not the primary team. Think of yourself as a specialist who is tasked with answering a specific question.

Always confirm these elements with the patient if you are to include them in your note. It is easy to copy forward what other providers may have charted in previous encounters, but it is important that your note reflects accurate and current information that you have collected and confirmed with the patient.

- One-liner
- Reason for consult
- HPI:
  - Brief summary of why the patient is in the hospital*
  - Relevant details of hospital course*
  - Events leading to consult*
  - Current status
  - System-specific review of systems
- PMH, PSH, FH, SH, meds, allergies*

    *For these sections, you do not need to redo the H&P. "What brings you to the hospital?" is not an appropriate opener, given that they have likely been inhospital for several days and you are expected to have read the chart. You can explain to the patient that you have read about their history and discussed with the primary team, and to your understanding, this is what has been going on. Then, confirm whether this is accurate and whether they have anything to add.
- Targeted physical exam (relevant to your specific consult)
- Assessment/plan:
  - One-liner and reason for consult
  - 1–2 paragraphs explaining your evaluation of the patient and question
  - Bullet pointed recommendations
  - Ongoing involvement
    - "We will continue to follow" vs "Thank you for the interesting consult. We are signing off."

7.4.1.6 Discharge

Preparing for discharge requires a large amount of logistical work in which you can be useful. The more you anticipate and prepare ahead of time, the easier this will be for your team.

Every day (as early as day of admission or POD#1), evaluate the following:
- Anticipated discharge date
- Barriers to discharge
  - Patient condition (e.g., discharge pending resolution of _____)
  - Inhospital services (including plans to either transition to alternatives or to arrange home administration)
    - IV medications (transition to PO medication vs PICC placement for long-term IV medications)
    - Epidural (transition to PO medication)
    - Oxygen/ventilation requirements (wean O2 requirement vs arrange for home oxygen)
    - Parenteral nutrition (advance diet vs feeding tube placement vs PICC placement)
  - Logistics (rehab bed availability, transportation)

Prior to discharge:
- Update hospital course daily.
- Start and work on after visit summary (AVS).
- Work with case manager to organize destination after discharge (rehab vs home) and necessary home services.
- Contact PCP and outpatient providers (day before discharge).
  - Set up follow-up appointments.
- Confirm patient's preferred pharmacy.

Day of discharge:

- Finalize hospital course.
- Finish AVS and discharge instructions.
- Reconcile medications and send scripts to pharmacy.
- Confirm clinic follow-up (your team, relevant outpatient providers).
- Order follow-up labs and imaging.
- Print and go over follow-up instructions with the patient. Answer any last-minute questions.

7.4.2 The Operating Room

7.4.2.1 General Considerations

1. *Sterility.* At the start of your rotation, you will take a scrub class and learn about proper sterile technique. As you become more comfortable in the OR, this will become second nature, but you should always be conscious of this. Moreover, as a medical student, you will be heavily scrutinized for this and need to demonstrate that you understand how to conduct yourself in the operating room. It is better to do less than to contaminate yourself or others.
2. *Etiquette.* Introduce yourself to the team early. Ask the circulator where is the best place to stand and how you can be helpful (discussed below). During the operation, *never* grab an instrument without asking. The scrub nurse will hand you the appropriate tools.
3. *Awareness.* Be conscious of the people and equipment in the room and how you might be affecting the operation. Medical student mistakes are made more often because of lack of awareness rather than intentional misconduct.

    Be careful not to rest your weight on the patient's body beneath the drapes. Make sure you are not blocking the view of essential personnel. If your resident needs to step out or unscrub, you may step closer, but be aware of when they return and step back. You should never have to have somebody ask you to step back. Often times, residents or attendings will give you the opportunity to step closer, but on your end, it is better to wait for their lead.
4. *Focus.* Be engaged and focused during the operation. Start to anticipate the next step (regardless of whether or not you are involved in that step).

    During many cases, you will likely be doing very little during the critical portions of the case, but you can learn a lot from observing the choices that attendings make, anatomy, needle angles, and techniques. Learn the principles of surgery. Watch the resident and learn how to assist. Listen to the critiques that the attendings give the residents. The opportunities are endless!

7.4.2.2 Pre-op

The night before:

- Read textbook chapter (Greenfield or other) for the specific operation.
- Review anatomy.
    - In the past, you may have memorized structures and blood supply, but this time, think about the views that you expect to see these structures through. If it is a laparoscopic case, what are the camera views and where would you expect to see certain structures from different views.

A common mistake that trainees make is to only focus on what you get to do during an operation. Your training goes far beyond that, and you will get so much more out of your rotation if you learn how to learn.

 – Anticipate the steps of the procedure, and think about adjacent anatomy as well. What could be behind the structure that is being manipulated? What could be damaged in this area that you need to watch out for?
— Review surgeon-specific details. Read a prior op note to understand their particular approach and steps.

The day of the operation:
— For each patient, create an index card (or other pocket-sized note) with key details (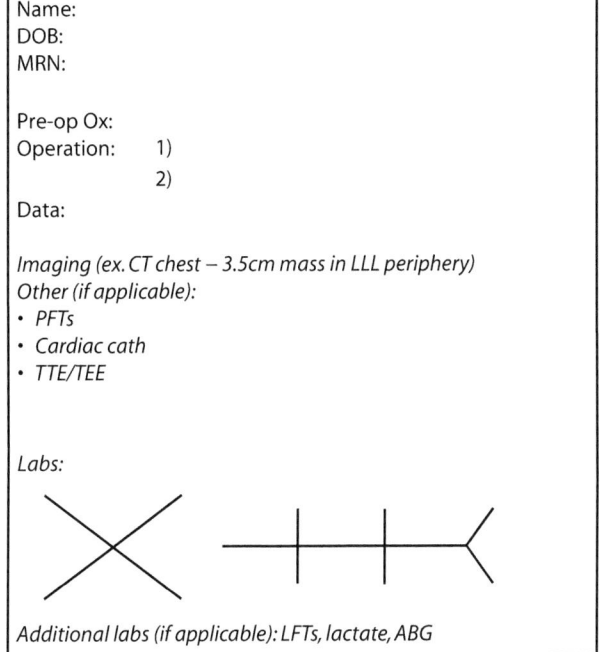 Fig. 7.1):
 – Patient ID, MRN, DOB
 – Pre-op diagnosis
 – Operation
 – PMH/PSH (pertinent to the operation or surgical risk factors)
  – *Thoracic example: insulin-dependent diabetes, L pneumonectomy in 2011*
 – Labs (with prior result if there is a change)
 – Imaging (brief)
  – *Surgical oncology example: CT – 3.5 cm mass in head of pancreas, no vascular involvement, +replaced R hepatic artery from SMA*
  – *Cardiac example: TTE – EF 25%, no AS, mild MR, no TR; left heart cath – 70% stenosis proximal LAD, 30% LCX, total occlusion of RCA*
 – Meds (pertinent to perioperative management)
  – Antibiotics
  – Antiplatelet/anticoagulation (held since ___)
  – Cardiovascular
  – Diabetes
 – Allergies
 – Additional considerations

☐ Fig. 7.1 Index card with key patient details

- Meet the patient in the PACU and introduce yourself.
- Go to the OR and introduce yourself to the OR team early.
- Pull your own gown and gloves, and open them for yourself if the circulator prefers.
- Help the anesthesiologists transport the patient to the OR.

7.4.3 In the OR

Preinduction (these tasks will be done by you, the circulator, and OR staff so follow their lead):
- Help the patient move onto the OR table.
- Move stretcher back into the hallway.
- Attach armrests to the OR table.
- Grab warm blankets for the patient.
- Attach safety belt.
- Connect sequential compression device.

After induction:
- Remove patient gown and blankets.
- Position the patient (according to each operation).
- Remove armrests from OR table.
- Place Foley catheter (if needed).
- Help anesthesia if needed (holding instruments, etc.).
- Open your gown and gloves (if they have not already been opened).
- Scrub in and gown up.
- Help the resident or scrub nurse drape the patient.
  - Blue drapes (sides, bottom, top handed to anesthesia)
  - Iodine band
  - Pockets (some drapes come with this, others will be folded and clamped to create pockets)
- Hand off suction tubing, Bovie wires, laparoscope wires, and/or wires for internal defibrillator paddles.
- For laparoscopic surgery, connect components of the scope; test the light and white balance.

During the operation:
  Your role in each operation will differ based on the rotation, your team, and your own personal skill and comfort level.
- Learning *goals*:
  - Steps of the operation
  - Surgical principles
  - Decision-making
  - Technical skills
- *Practical tips*:
  - Retracting
    - The goal is for the surgeon to see the area of focus. This may seem like a simple concept, but often times, you may find yourself retracting in a direction that optimizes your own view (subconsciously) rather than the view of the primary surgeon.
  - Suctioning
    - Again, a seemingly simple concept but actually a bit more nuanced and attending-specific. Some operations may have multiple suctions and suction tips. For example, in cardiac surgery, there will be a suc-

tion going into the bypass machine, a suction that separates out RBC from the fluid, and a waste suction. Make sure to know which suction to use and which tip to use before attempting to jump in there.

- *Suctioning fluid (large volume)*. The primary use of the suction is to improve visualization. When you are suctioning large volumes of fluid (blood, ascites, etc.), as long as the tip of your suction is submerged, you are fine. In those cases, aim your suction tip at the lowest point of the surgical field, out of the way of the surgical activity. Fluid runs down and will pool in that lowest point.
- *Suctioning fluid (spot suctioning)*. Additionally, you will use the suction to localize the source of bleeding. In these cases, you will see a small area of blood, and the technique is to suction that area and quickly move the tip away to be able to observe where the blood is coming from. Another technique may be to blot with a sponge or lap pad, which may be more effective.
- *Suctioning smoke*. The Bovie cautery generates quite a bit of smoke, and some surgeons prefer this to be suctioned. Use your judgment and remember that in the list of priorities of the operation, this is last. Keep the suction at a distance and do not obstruct the surgical field. If you feel that you cannot do this from a good angle, then it is better to just leave things alone.
- *Additional tips*. The suction is also a useful tool for retracting, and you may notice the residents use the suction to simultaneously clear the field and retract a bit of soft tissue. Observe how the residents and attendings are using the instrument, and learn from them! In the words of one my cardiac surgery attendings, at certain points of the operation, the suction is the most powerful tool you have.
- Suturing
  - During the operation, a lot can be learned by simply observing. At every level of your training, you will learn from watching before you get the chance to practice. Focus on how the attending and residents:
    - Select the suture (needle, size, material)
    - Handle the instrument
    - Choose the needle angle
    - Rotate their wrist or angle their body
    - Manipulate the tissue with their opposite hand
  - Protect the needle when you hand back the remainder of the suture. Practice safe sharps-handling, and notify the scrub nurse by saying "needle back." Remember that they need to count all of the needles at the end of the operation, so be cognizant of this, and keep track of your own needles.
  - A detailed how-to for skin suturing will be addressed in the Technical Skills section.
- Knot-tying
  - Two-handed vs one-handed. This may be attending-specific, so make sure to clarify with your intern before the operation. In general, start with two-handed and demonstrate that you understand the principles of tying tight, flat knots before attempting the one-handed knots.
  - Specific knot-tying instructions are included in the ▶ Sect. 7.7.
- Using the scalpel
  - You may be given the opportunity to make the skin incision. First and foremost, practice safe sharps-handling.
  - Use the belly of the blade to cut.

Be mindful of what setting the Bovie is on, as different settings will be used for different portions of the operation.

7

- The depth of the incision will depend on resident and attending preference. Some prefer to cut through the dermis, while others like you to stay superficial and complete the incision with the Bovie.
  - Hand the knife back handle-first and say "knife back."
- Using the Bovie
  - There are two settings (cut and coagulation) and varying levels of energy going through the cautery. Use cut for the skin and coagulation for dissection.
- The Bovie energy will travel through metal and stop at rubber. Keeping this in mind, you may use your gloved finger as a barrier to protect structures from the heat of the Bovie. On the other hand, you may use your forceps as a conduit for the Bovie energy. You may see your resident use the forceps to grab the end of a small vessel, and in that case, you can touch the tip of the Bovie to any portion of their forceps, effectively cauterizing the tissue that their forceps are touching.
- Use the tip of the Bovie, and be careful of what the rest of the metal tip may be touching. You may think that you are cauterizing one spot, but if the length of the Bovie tip is touching another structure, you could be unknowingly cutting into something else as well.
- Keep your finger off of the button while you are resting or doing blunt dissection. This will prevent you from unwittingly pressing down and cauterizing without meaning to.

After the operation:
- After the skin is closed, stay scrubbed in to help the scrub nurse dress the incisions.
- Unscrub and put on new (non-sterile) gloves. Help put the drapes in the trash.
  If planning to extubate in the OR:
  - Place arm boards back on the OR table.
  - Grab a new gown and warm blankets for the patient. When appropriate, place these back on the patient.
  - When anesthesia is ready to extubate, grab a towel or "Chux" underpad to place on the patient's chest. After extubation, this will be used to dispose of the used tube.
  - Bring the bed into the room (after asking anesthesia and nursing if it is a good time).
  - Help transfer patient from OR table to bed. Put side rails up.
  - Hang any chest tubes or Foley bags on the side of the bed.
  - Connect face mask to portable O2 chamber.
  - Transport patient back to the PACU. Make sure patient chart is travelling with the patient.
  If planning to remain intubated:
  - Grab a new gown and warm blankets for the patient. When appropriate, place these back on the patient.
  - Bring the bed into the room (after asking anesthesia and nursing if it is a good time).
    - The patient may also require a rack for IV medications, a travel monitor, and ventilator for transport. Bring these in with the bed and help transfer lines and plugs.

- Help transfer patient from OR table to bed. Put side rails up.
- Hang any chest tubes or Foley bags on the side of the bed.
- Transfer patient's vent to travel ventilator, and set vent settings according to anesthesia.
- Transport patient to ICU. Make sure patient chart is travelling with the patient.

7.4.4 Post-op

Sign-out to PACU/ICU nurses:
- One-liner:
  - Patient name
  - Age
  - PMH (pertinent to operation and post-op care)
  - Operation
- Significant events during the operation:
  - Complications
  - Intraoperative findings
    - *Example (surgical oncology – gastrectomy): We found a 4 cm mass in the antrum of the stomach without invasion into the adjacent structures and no gross metastatic disease. We resected the tumor in a distal gastrectomy. Preliminary path confirmed gastric adenocarcinoma with good margins.*

7.4.4.1 Post-op Check
Think of this as a brief progress note, conducted 2–4 hours after the operation:
1. Start the note and pull in objective data.
2. Check in with the nurse about:
   - Acute events
   - Pain management
   - Drain output (volume and appearance)
   - Urine output
   - Other concerns
3. Assess: sick or not sick?
4. Ask the patient:
   - New complaints
   - Pain
   - Brief ROS
5. Physical exam:
   - Let the following postoperative concerns guide your exam:
     - Postanesthesia. Mental status/delirium? Signs of drug reaction?
     - Cardiovascular. Hypotension? Volume status? Signs of hemorrhage (pallor, tachycardia)?
     - Airway/respiratory. Work of breathing? Oxygen requirement?
     - GI/abdominal. Soft vs rigid? Rebound or guarding?
     - Surgical sites. Check the dressings – clean/dry/intact?
     - Tubes/lines/drains. Hourly output? Appearance of fluid?
6. Complete your note. Depending on team preference, this may or may not include an assessment and plan (systems-based).

It may be difficult to remember all of these details during the operation, especially when you are scrubbed in and unable to take notes. In general, the main idea is (1) cancer or no cancer? and (2) margins clean? *When pathology calls in to the room, pay attention* and listen for these main points:
- Incisions/dressings:
  - *Example: The patient has four laparoscopic port sites (show the nurse where each of these are).*
- Tubes/lines/drains:
  - *Example: Patient's NG tube should remain in place overnight to low continuous wall suction.*
- Plan (systems-based):
  - Neuro/pain
  - Cardiovascular
  - Respiratory
  - GI
  - GU
  - Heme
  - ID
  - Endocrine

7.5 The Clinic

Your time in clinic is indispensable to learning clinical decision-making skills. As a surgeon, these skills are equally if not more important than your technical ones. Knowing when to operate (and when not to!), which operation, and how to advise your patient through the process is a skill that takes years to hone.

7.5.1 New Patients

Prior to clinic (either the night before or early in the morning):
1. Start the clinic note and fill out what you can from chart review:
   - One-liner:
     - Name
     - Age
     - PMH, PSH
     - Reason for visit (if known)
   - HPI:
     - Events leading up to referral to surgery (if known)
   - PMH
   - PSH:
     - Operation
     - Date
     - Surgeon/institution
   - FH (pertinent to presenting illness):
     - First-degree relatives
     - Additional relatives with familial syndromes (*example for gastric cancer patient – uncle with gastric adenocarcinoma diagnosed at age 54*)
     - Pertinent negatives (*e.g., otherwise negative for esophageal, gastric, or colorectal cancer*)
   - SH
   - Home medications
   - Allergies
   - Labs/imaging:
     - **Some patients may be referred with partial workup already completed. If so, make sure to look through the imaging and include the findings from the radiology report in the clinic note.
   - Assessment/plan:
     - **You will not be able to anticipate much here, but what you can do to prepare early is to look up treatment guidelines and institutional pathways or even references to trials that you can then include once you have assessed the patient.
       - *Resources*: NCCN guidelines (surgical oncology), AHA guidelines (cardiac surgery)

During clinic:
2. Introduce yourself to the clinic team (receptionist, medical assistants, nurse practitioners). Ask attending or resident how they like to structure clinic workflow, divide patients, etc.
3. Set up your workspace.
   ***Bring your laptop if you have remote access to electronic medical records. Clinic space is often cramped with limited computers, and you

will be last in line for computer use, so it will make the day smoother to be self-sufficient with your own laptop.

4. When the patient arrives, they will be brought to an exam room by the medical assistant who will see them first and take their vitals. When they are ready, the medical assistant will hand you the chart, which is your green light to go in and see the patient.

5. Introduce yourself, and inform the patient that you will be seeing them first, after which you and the attending will return to discuss the plan.

6. Perform an H&P as you would on other rotations.

7. Thank the patient and inform them that you will return with the attending.

8. Update your clinic note (as a way to organize your information before presenting to your attending).

9. New patient presentations should include the following:
   - One-liner:
     – Name
     – Age
     – PMH/PSH (pertinent)
     – Reason for visit
   - HPI
   - Relevant ROS
   - PMH/PSH
   - FH (pertinent)
   - SH
   - Home meds (abbreviated, since they will read your note which will include the full list)
   - Allergies
   - Vitals
   - Physical exam findings:
     – Pertinent findings to your evaluation. Do not go through all of the systems (HEENT, CV, resp, etc.). They will be able to read this in your note.
     – *Example of patient presenting with cholecystitis. On exam, the patient is well-appearing with no jaundice (peripheral or sublingual) or scleral icterus. The abdomen was non-distended, soft, and tender to palpation in the RUQ, without rebound or guarding. Murphy sign was positive. No abdominal masses were palpated.*
   - Labs/Imaging
   - Assessment and plan:
     – One-liner
     – Diagnosis
     – Recommended workup
     – Recommended treatment:
       – Surgical vs medical management
       – Type of surgery
       – Timing of surgery

10. Your attending will then give you some feedback, and you will see the patient together. Take note of his/her physical exam findings and how this may differ from your own. He will then communicate the plan with the patient.

11. Bring the patient back to the receptionist.

12. Complete your note with the corrections.

7.5.2 Follow-Up Visits

Prior to clinic (either the night before or early in the morning):

1. Start the clinic note and fill out what you can from chart review:
   - One-liner:
     - Name
     - Age
     - PMH/PSH
   - Procedure and date
   - Post-op diagnosis
   - HPI:
     - Brief summary of events leading to surgery and hospital course (1–2 sentences)
       - *Example: Briefly, Mr. Smith presented to the clinic 2 weeks ago with RUQ pain and was found to have acute cholecystitis. He underwent an uncomplicated laparoscopic cholecystectomy on 2/2/20 and was discharged on POD#0.*
     - The bulk of the HPI will focus on events since discharge, which you will fill out after seeing the patient.
   - PMH, PSH, FH, SH, allergies:
     - This will vary based on attending preference. Some post-op visit notes will not include this at all.
   - Home medications
   - Labs/imaging (new since discharge)
   - Assessment/plan:
     - **You will not be able to anticipate much here, and will fill this out on clinic day.

During clinic:

2. Introduce yourself to the clinic team.
3. Set up your workspace.
4. When the patient arrives, they will be brought to an exam room by the medical assistant who will see them first and take their vitals. When they are ready, the medical assistant will hand you the chart, which is your green light to go in and see the patient.
5. Introduce yourself and inform the patient that you will be seeing them first, after which you and the attending will return to discuss the plan.
6. Obtain the HPI information, focusing on events since the patient was last seen:
   - Acute events
   - Clinic visits, ED visits, hospital admissions
   - Pain:
     - Current pain medication regimen
   - Diet
   - Activity
   - Tubes/lines/drains:
     - They may be coming in to have the drain assessed and removed.
   - Surgical sites:
     - Sutures or staples that may need removal
7. Perform a physical exam (targeted):
   - System that was operated on
   - Surgical incisions (dressings intact or removed? Site clean and dry? Or is there erythema, exudate, dehiscence, etc.?)
   - Tubes/lines/drains (note both quantity and quality of the output):

- Insertion sites (similar to surgical incisions, is it clean and dry or weeping?)
    - **In some cases, the insertion site is significantly larger than the tube, which may saturate dressings. This is a common page that you or your intern may receive from the nurse taking care of your patient. A simple interrupted suture or U-stitch will solve this problem.
8. Thank the patient and inform them that you will return with the attending.
9. Update your clinic note (as a way to organize your information before presenting to your attending).
10. Post-op presentations should include the following:
    - One-liner:
        - Patient name
        - Age
        - Operation and date
        - Post-op diagnosis
    - Since the patient was last seen:
        - Acute events
        - Clinic visits, ED visits, hospital admissions
        - Pain:
            - Current pain medication regimen
        - Diet
        - Activity
        - Tubes/lines/drains remaining
    - Physical exam findings:
        - Pertinent findings to your evaluation
    - Assessment/plan:
        - One-liner
        - Medication changes
        - Plans for removal of any remaining tubes/lines/drains
        - Plans for follow-up
11. Your attending will then give you some feedback, and you will see the patient together. Take note of his/her physical exam findings and how this may differ from your own. He will then communicate the plan with the patient.
12. Bring the patient back to the receptionist.
13. Complete your note with the corrections.

7.6 The Emergency Department

7.6.1 Admissions

The initial process of ED admissions is similar to evaluating an inpatient consult. The main difference is the uncertainty of acuity and the "ownership" of the patient. As the consulting team, you are answering a specific question, whereas admitting a patient through the ED, you will be the primary team.

1. *Receiving the admission.* You will receive a page with patient identifiers, pertinent history, and presenting complaint:
    - Look up the patient. Read any notes from the ED providers or triage nurses for this hospitalization, any relevant clinic notes or op notes, and the discharge notes of any recent hospitalizations.
    - Start an admission note. See sample Admission Note at the end of the chapter for an example:
        - Fill in what you know from your chart review (one-liner, reason for consult, PMH, PSH, FH, SH, meds, allergies, vitals).

- Review labs and imaging, and summarize in your admission note.
- Review medicine administrative record (MAR) to see what the patient has received since arrival.

- Call the consulting physician to receive handoff. Your goal should be to already have the objective data prepared and your note somewhat filled in before this phone call:
  - Update your admission note with new information.

2. *Go see the patient.* When you arrive, check in with the nurse taking care of the patient. Take note of your surroundings, which will clue you in to the urgency of the consult.

3. *Sick or not sick?* This is the most important question to ask, before attempting to obtain the history or perform a physical:
   - *Look at the patient.*
   - *Look at the monitors (vitals, telemetry).*
   - *Look at drips (IV medications).*
   - *Look at ventilators and mechanical support.*
        ***If there are *any* signs that the patient is unstable or their condition is worsening, ask for help immediately. Ask the nurse to page your resident and activate the appropriate codes or pathways for emergency response. See Critical Care and Emergency Medicine chapter for more information.

4. *Conduct a full H&P:*
   - Chief complaint
   - HPI:
     - Events leading to presentation
     - ED course
     - Current status
     - System-specific review of systems
   - PMH, PSH, FH, SH, meds, allergies
   - Physical exam:
     - More extensive than your physical exam for consults or progress notes. This establishes the baseline for future exams.

5. Thank the patient, and inform them that you will return with the rest of the team in a few minutes.

6. Update your note and organize your presentation:
   - One-liner
   - HPI (as above)
   - PMH, PSH, FH, SH, meds, allergies
   - Physical exam:
     - Full physical documented since this is the initial note
   - Assessment/plan:
     - One-liner
     - Suspected diagnosis
     - Diagnostic workup:
       - Labs/imaging
     - Treatment
          **Some teams may prefer you to do systems-based A/P rather than this abbreviated format.

7. *Present to your resident.* In the ED, you will present and see the patient with your resident who will then staff the case with the attending. Treat this as you would an attending presentation unless your resident instructs you otherwise.

8. *See the patient together with your resident.*

9. *Adjust your note and A/P accordingly.*

7.6.2 Trauma

7.6.2.1 General Tips

- *Know the ED setting*. During a trauma, most likely you will be asked to fetch supplies or equipment, and this is where you can be the most useful. On the first day, find the supply room (and any access codes), and familiarize yourself with it. You should know the location of the following:
  - Warm blankets
  - Arterial line kit (and separate supplies– Fig. 7.2):
    - Disposable towel
    - Syringe
    - Scalpel
    - Gauze sponges
    - Silk suture
    - Arterial needle
    - Guidewire:
      - Be ready to use different wires with varying levels of stiffness.
    - PVC extension with stopcock
    - Catheter
  - Central line kit (and separate supplies– Fig. 7.3):
    - Sterile field drapes
    - Chloro-prep sticks or iodine
    - Syringe and needle for local anesthetic
    - 1% lidocaine vial
    - Syringe and introducer needle
    - Scalpel
    - Guidewire
    - Tissue dilator
    - Sterile dressing
    - Silk suture
    - Central line catheter (varies)
  - Chest tube kit (and separate supplies – Fig. 7.4):
    - Sterile field drapes
    - Chloro-prep sticks or iodine

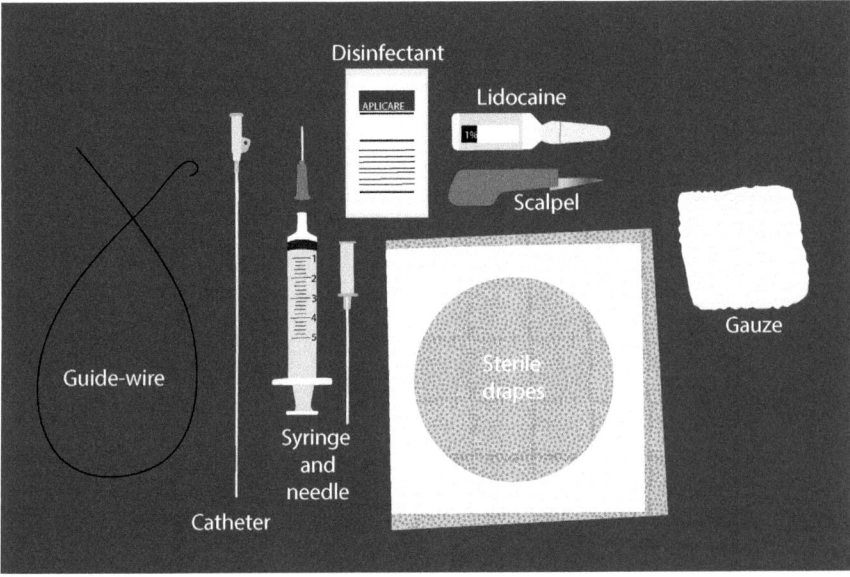

Fig. 7.2 Supplies within an arterial line kit

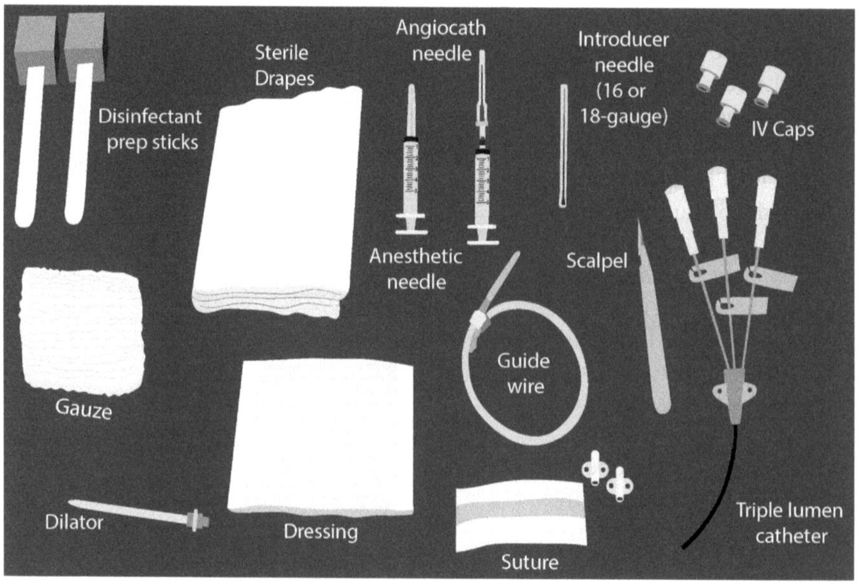

7

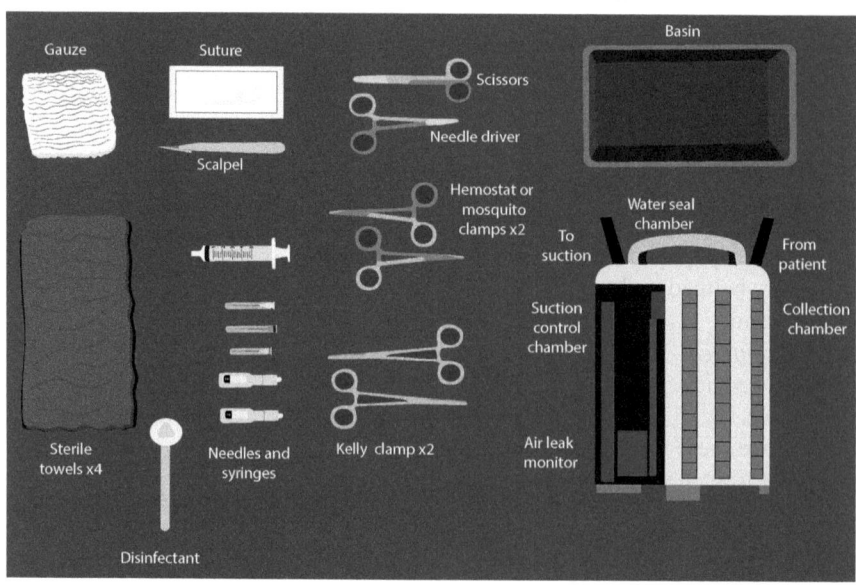

Fig. 7.3 Supplies within a central line kit

Fig. 7.4 Supplies within an chest tube kit

- Syringe and needle for local anesthetic
- 1% lidocaine vial
- Scalpel
- Forceps
- Curved Kelly forceps
- Argyle chest tube
- Silk suture
- Sterile dressing
- Tubing:
  - Connection to chest tube drainage system
  - Suction tubing
- Chest tube drainage system
- Sterile gauze

- Gown, personal protective equipment, sterile gloves
- Iodine or Chloro-prep sticks
- Lube
- Suction tubing
- Ultrasound
- Head lamps
- Mayo stand or table
- Tourniquet, c-collar, pelvic binder

- *Familiarize yourself with the equipment:*
  - Know what is in each kit (arterial, central, chest tube). Similarly, find out if there are important items missing from the kit that may be needed for procedures (e.g., sutures, ultrasound probe covers). If your institution does not use kits (or if your team prefers equipment that may be different), know what the necessary components are and how to obtain them.
  - Know how to operate the ultrasound. Turn it on; adjust gain and depth. Understand the different probes.
  - Know how to set up a chest tube. Placing the chest tube will be discussed below, but you should also know how to set up the water seal chamber and connect the chest tube to suction.
- *Memorize the ED radiology extension.* You will almost always be required to call for X-ray and CT. Know the extension and be ready to do this immediately.
- *Be attentive to your team.* During a trauma, there will be many personnel from different teams, and it can become quite chaotic. Look to your residents and listen to their instructions.
- *Be calm and focused.* You will be asked to do certain things (get supplies, hold pressure, etc.) and may feel lost at times. *Do what you need to do to get it done.* If you are asked to get something and you don't know where it is, ask for help (from somebody who is not otherwise occupied). If you feel overwhelmed or lost, take a deep breath, and focus on the immediate task at hand.
- *Be confident.* Your time in trauma is a great opportunity to learn and practice bedside procedures (peripheral IVs, central lines, arterial blood gas sticks, radial or femoral lines, chest tube placements, etc.) Don't be afraid to give these skills a try! This is how you will learn, and if you are not successful or if your resident feels that the patient is becoming unstable, you can hand this over. However, these skills improve with practice. Be confident and learn from your mistakes, so that the next time, you will be more likely to succeed.
- *Fill in the gaps.* There are many tasks and responsibilities *and many personnel to complete them.* If you are unsure of what you are doing, step aside, and let someone else take over. If you notice gaps, step in to help out. Because your role as a medical student is not clearly defined, the goal is to be available and helpful without getting in the way of others who do have clear roles.

7.6.2.2 What to Expect

1. Your team will receive a trauma alert page and head to the trauma bay to receive the patient. During this time, multiple teams will be gathering and setting up.
2. Grab trauma gowns and gloves for your team. Get the ultrasound which will be used for the focused assessment with sonography for trauma (FAST) exam.

3. The patient will arrive with paramedics and will be transferred over to the ED bed. If appropriate, help the team transfer the patient. At this time, the paramedics will begin giving handoff.

4. Your resident or the emergency medicine resident will begin the primary survey. At this time, you may help with exposure (removing clothing, positioning the patient) and grabbing supplies.

5. When indicated, call radiology to ask for portable X-ray, and alert the ED radiology department that you will be coming to the CT scanner.

6. A resident will perform the FAST exam with the ultrasound. Help plug in the ultrasound and adjust depth and gain if asked to.

7. Getting access – various personnel (ED nurses, anesthesia, your residents) will be obtaining peripheral IV access or central line access, getting an arterial blood gas or venous blood gas, and/or starting an arterial line (radial or femoral). If you feel comfortable, this may be a skill you are asked to perform. If not, step aside and allow someone else to do this.

8. When the team completes the primary survey, they will move on to a head-to-toe secondary survey. Help with logrolling the patient, and have gloves and lube on hand for the anal sphincter test.

9. At some point, X-ray will arrive. This will be a time to regroup with your team and await further instructions.

10. If the patient has stabilized, you may proceed to the CT scanner. Help transport the patient, and continue to be focused as the patient's status may change at any time, even in the scanner.

11. If the patient has not stabilized, you may proceed directly to the operating room (discussed below).

7.6.2.3 Primary Survey

A. Airway. Determine whether the patient can maintain an open airway or whether intervention (oral airway, laryngeal mask airway (LMA), intubation, or cricoid pressure) needs to be taken. You will not be the one to establish the airway but should understand when a patient needs intervention.
   - Is the airway patent and open *right now*?
     - *Tip: if the patient can talk, the airway is maintained.*
   - Will the airway *continue to be* maintained?
     - Neurologic compromise. If GCS score (see ▶ Chap. 24) is less than 8, the patient should be intubated. If the patient needs to be deeply sedated for any reason, they will also be intubated.
     - Upper airway compromise. If there is facial or neck trauma, intervention will need to be taken, and the type of intervention will depend on the location of injury.
     - Burns. If there is soot in the nose or mouth, consider intubation.
     - If a patient arrives with a prehospital airway, correct placement should be confirmed.
   - Cervical spine precautions: C-collar should be in place until the patient is cleared (clearance protocols vary by institution).

B. Breathing
   - Observe chest rise (equal and symmetric), respiratory rate, and O2 saturation.
   - Determine the need for rescue breathing (bag mask), mechanical ventilation, or veno-venous extracorporeal membrane oxygenation (ECMO).
   - Potential pathologies: penetrating chest trauma, hemo- or pneumothorax, flail chest, and pulmonary contusion.

C. Circulation
   - Perfusion. Look at the patient for signs of shock (warm vs cold, wet vs dry). Look at the monitors for blood pressure – arterial line if there is one – or cycle the BP cuff every few minutes. Feel for *bilateral* pulses:
     - *80-70-60 rule. If there is no reliable blood pressure monitoring, you can use this rule to get a rough sense of the systolic blood pressure.*
       - *Radial pulse ≥ 80 mmHg*
       - *Femoral pulse ≥ 70 mmHg*
       - *Carotid pulse ≥ 60 mmHg*
     - Mean arterial pressure (MAP) >60 mmHg is required for organ perfusion.
       - *MAP = 2/3*DBP + 1/3*SBP.*
   - Access. The patient should have at least two forms of access for large-volume transfusion and administration of IV medications:
     - Options for access:
       - Large-bore peripheral IV (16 gauge or higher)
       - Central line
       - Intraosseous
   - Temporizing interventions. If a patient is not maintaining tissue perfusion, the following interventions may be taken depending on the etiology:
     - Volume (IV normal saline or lactated Ringer's)
     - Transfusion
     - Medications (vasopressors, inotropes)
     - Chest compressions, cardiac massage, vascular clamping
     - Mechanical circulatory support (ECMO, intra-aortic balloon pump, percutaneous VAD)
   - Potential pathologies: hemorrhage, penetrating or blunt chest trauma, aortic dissection, cardiac tamponade, and pulmonary embolism
D. Disability
   - Baseline neurologic exam including pupils, signs of lateralization.
   - Glasgow coma scale (◘ Fig. 7.5):
     - Max score: 15
     - Min score: 3
E. Exposure
   - Remove all clothing.
F. FAST exam (with ultrasound)
   - Cardiac (most often subxiphoid):
     - Pericardium
     - Heart chambers
   - RUQ:
     - Hepatorenal recess (Morrison's pouch)
     - Right paracolic gutter
     - Lower right thorax
   - LUQ:
     - Subphrenic space
     - Splenorenal recess
     - Left paracolic gutter
     - Lower left thorax
   - Pelvic:
     - Rectovesical pouch
     - Rectouterine pouch (◘ Fig. 7.6)

Glasgow Coma Scale

BEHAVIOR	RESPONSE	SCORE
Eye opening response	Spontaneously	4
	To speech	3
	To pain	2
	No response	1
Best verbal response	Oriented to time, place and person	5
	Confused	4
	Inappropiate words	3
	Incomprehensible sounds	2
	No response	1
Best motor response	Obey commands	6
	Moves to localized pain	5
	Flexion withdrawal from pain	4
	Abnormal flexion (decorticate)	3
	Abnormal extension (decerebrate)	2
	No response	1
Total score:	Best response	15
	Comatose client	8 or less
	Totally unresponsive	3

◘ **Fig. 7.5** Glasgow coma scale

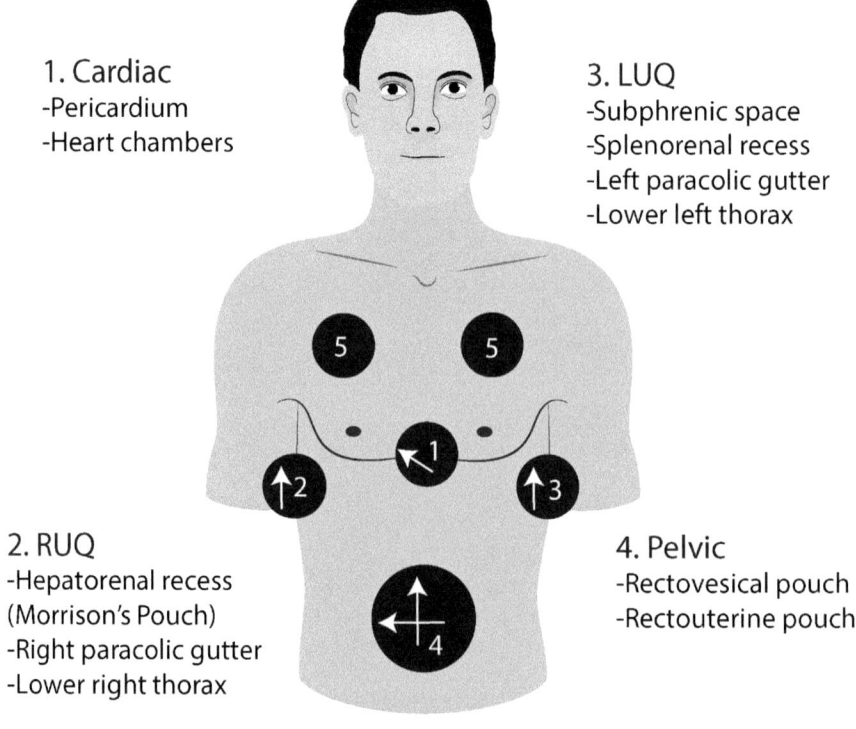

1. Cardiac
-Pericardium
-Heart chambers

3. LUQ
-Subphrenic space
-Splenorenal recess
-Left paracolic gutter
-Lower left thorax

2. RUQ
-Hepatorenal recess
(Morrison's Pouch)
-Right paracolic gutter
-Lower right thorax

4. Pelvic
-Rectovesical pouch
-Rectouterine pouch

5. Lung sliding (bilateral)

◘ **Fig. 7.6**   FAST exam sites

7.6.2.4 Secondary Survey

- Head and neck:
  - Signs of overt trauma
  - Eyes (pupil size and reactivity, EOM, bruising around eyes)
  - Ears (blood or fluid, foreign objects, Battle's sign – bruising over mastoid process)
  - Nose (blood or fluid, foreign objects, soot)
  - Mouth (lacerations, loose teeth or bony injuries, foreign objects, soot, etc.)
  - Neck (cervical spine trauma – c-collar should be on, bruising, asymmetry)
- Chest:
  - Signs of overt trauma:
    - Penetrating trauma
    - Blunt trauma (bruising, rib fracture, flail chest)
  - Chest rise:
    - Equal and bilateral?
    - Palpate chest bilaterally for focal tenderness
  - Cardiac auscultation
  - Lung auscultation
- Abdomen:
  - Signs of overt trauma:
    - Penetrating trauma
    - Blunt trauma (bruising, abdominal distension)
  - Tenderness
- Pelvis:
  - Signs of overt trauma:
    - Penetrating trauma
    - Blunt trauma (bruising, instability)
  - Urethral meatus:
    - **Blood at meatus is concerning for urethral injury, and retrograde urethrography needs to be performed prior to Foley placement.
- Extremities:
  - Signs of overt trauma:
    - Penetrating trauma
    - Blunt trauma (bruising, instability)
  - Fractures
  - Neurovascular status (pulses, capillary refill, mobility)
    - **Check for signs of compartment syndrome (5Ps – pain, pallor, pulseless, paresthesia, paralysis)
    - Gross sensory/motor exam
- Back:
  - Signs of overt trauma:
    - Penetrating trauma
    - Blunt trauma (bruising, instability, step-offs, asymmetry)
  - Anal sphincter tone:
    - **Performed during logroll. Have gloves and lube ready.

7.6.2.5 ED to OR

If the patient requires emergent surgery, you will proceed directly to the OR. This could be from the trauma bay, the CT scanner, or directly from the ambulance. These cases can be chaotic with several moving pieces that need to come together to prepare the OR.

Ways you can be helpful:
- Call the OR desk to alert them of the impending case.
- Help find and bring in equipment that may be missing (varies depending on the case):
  - Headlamps
  - Bronchoscope
  - Ultrasound
  - Step stools
- Grab masks and caps for the team. Open sterile gowns and gloves for the team.
- Transfer the patient to the OR table (as for any case).
- Hook up suction tubing if needed.
- Tie in surgical gowns for the teams scrubbing in.

Additional Tips:
- Remember to introduce yourself to the OR staff as you would for an elective case.
- Stay unscrubbed while the rest of the team is scrubbing in. At the start of the case (during prepping and draping), they will likely need extra hands to grab equipment or handle other tasks (calling or notifying additional people, taking care of other tasks that have been sidetracked). Wait and see where you can be the most helpful. There may also not be space for you to scrub in, and you should be flexible.
- Be prepared and follow instructions. The situation may change at a moment's notice, and you need to be ready to respond (chest compressions, holding pressure, etc.).
- Be proactive! This is a great opportunity to get involved, learn new skills, and help your team out.

7.7   Technical Skills

7.7.1   References/Resources

- Introduction to the operating room: ▶ https://www.youtube.com/watch?v=wNi-q8XSTbw
- Instrument guide: ▶ https://www.facs.org/-/media/files/education/medicalstudents/common_surgical_instruments_module.ashx
- Surgical technique videos:
  - Animated knots: ▶ www.animatedknots.com
  - Medical University of South Caroline (MUSC) technique videos: ▶ https://medicine.musc.edu/departments/surgery/education/medical-student-information/3rd-year-info/suture-techniques-video
  - Chest tube insertion: ▶ https://www.youtube.com/watch?v=kEc5fn6ownc
  - Chest tube maintenance: ▶ https://www.youtube.com/watch?v=Ui0eKmEk38M

7.7.2   Bedside Procedures

Prior to performing any of these procedures, make sure you have read about and gone over the steps with your resident. Often times, you will observe the first and perform the next one, or you may be able to practice in simulation first. Make sure you are comfortable and realistic about your own skills to ensure that you are prioritizing patient safety.

7.7.2.1 Chest Tube Placement
Equipment Required (See ▶ Sect. 7.6)

- Sterile field drapes
- Chloro-prep sticks or iodine
- Syringe and needle for local anesthetic
- 1% lidocaine vial
- Scalpel
- Forceps
- 2 curved Kelly forceps
- Chest tube (28 to 40 Fr)
- Silk suture
- Sterile dressing
- Tubing:
  - Connection to chest tube drainage system
  - Suction tubing
- Chest tube drainage system

Positioning

There are several ways to position a patient for chest tube placement depending on the urgency of the procedure, setting, and type of chest tube. The best way to achieve a feel for the various positions is to watch some videos on YouTube.

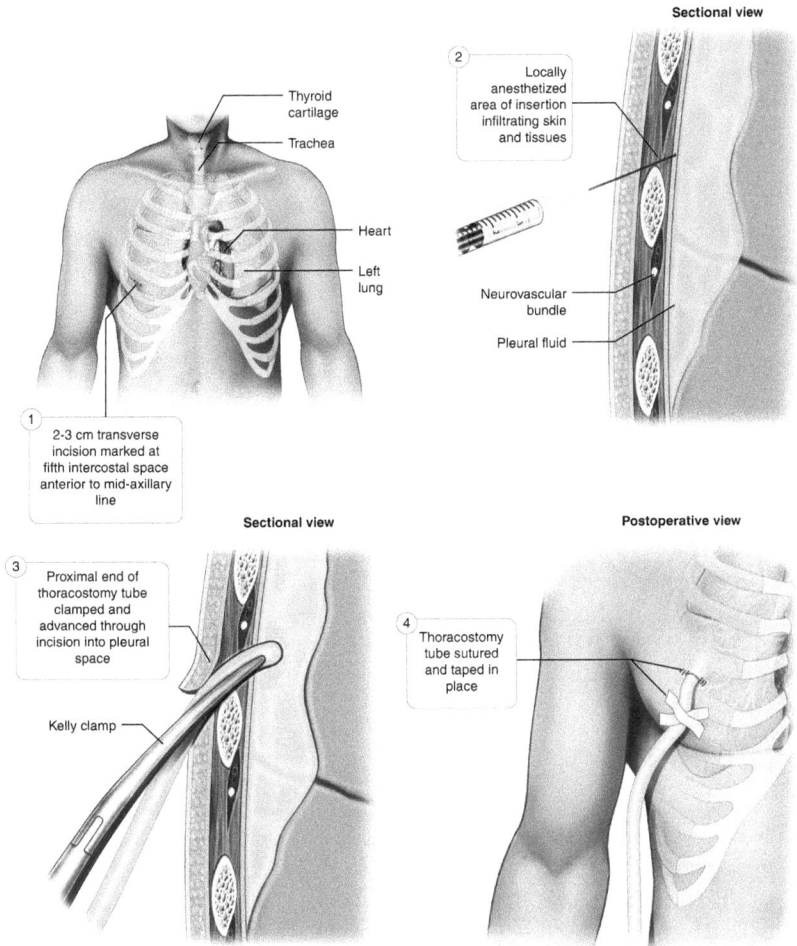

**During emergent situations, the patient is NOT placed in lateral decubitus position (position C) due to risk of bleeding compromising the "good lung," which is down. Furthermore, some patients may not be able to handle the hemodynamic changes. In these patients, position A is the safest method to gain access and will be discussed below.

1. Ask the patient to place the ipsilateral arm over their head.
2. Place a shoulder bump (typically a rolled up blanket or IV saline bag) under the ipsilateral side to provide elevation.

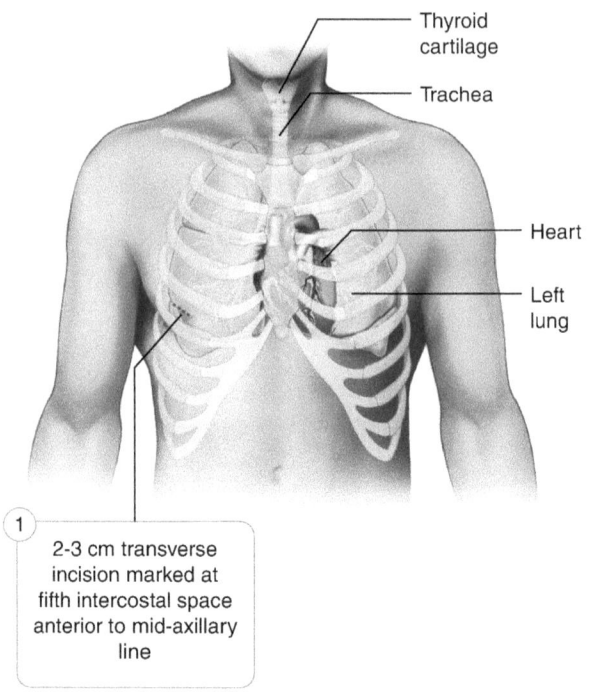

3. Identify and mark landmarks:
   The "triangle of safety"
   (a) Anterior axillary line (pectoralis major muscle)
   (b) Posterior axillary line (latissimus dorsi muscle)
   (c) Nipple or inframammary/pectoral crease
4. Palpate and count ribs. Plan for insertion in the 4th–5th intercostal space.
   **Be aware of the liver in a right-sided chest tube insertion and the spleen on the left side, which may be elevated or enlarged. Know the patient history, and if there is a CXR, take the time to look at this and estimate the level of the diaphragm.
5. Plan your incision site. You will be angling the chest tube cranially, so plan for your skin incision to be a few inches lower than the intercostal space you plan to enter.

Placing the Tube

1. Sterilely prep and drape the patient. Put on your sterile gown and gloves.
2. Draw up your local anesthetic (typically lidocaine). Anesthetize the skin where you plan to make your incision, then angle your needle deeper along your planned track, and continue to inject anesthetic into the deeper muscle layers.
3. When you reach the bone, carefully march the needle along the superior edge of the rib, and continue to inject the anesthetic. At some point, you will feel a "pop" as you enter the pleural space. You may confirm this with drawing back fluid, and then continue to inject the remainder of the anesthetic.

**Remember your anatomy: the neurovascular bundles run along a groove at the inferior border of each rib. By hugging the superior border, you are lessening your chances of injuring these structures.

4. Make a 1–2″ horizontal skin incision with the scalpel where you had previously marked.

5. Using a curved Kelly clamp, bluntly dissect through the subcutaneous fat and muscle layers. The curve of the clamp should face down toward the patient, and as you press down, open the clamp to spread the muscle fibers. You may alternate using the Kelly and your finger to complete the dissection.

   **The Kelly clamp is sharp and can injure structures, so make sure you know where the tip of the clamp is to avoid injury to the liver, spleen, lung, or even the heart.

6. When you reach the bone, again march along the superior border of the rib, and pop into the pleural space.

7. Once you are in the pleural space, replace the Kelly with your finger, and bluntly sweep 360 degrees along the pleural space. This ensures that there are no lung adhesions and will reduce your risk of causing lung injury with the tube.

8. Using one Kelly clamp (or other large clamp), clamp the blunt end of the chest tube to avoid spilling any fluid onto the floor before the suction is connected.

9. With another Kelly clamp, clasp the tip of the chest tube. Guide the chest tube with the clamp and your finger along the track that you have just created.

   **Make sure the tip of the chest tube does not surpass the tip of the clamp. Feel with your finger that you are correctly in the pleural space. Both of these actions will reduce the chance of tunneling the tube into the wrong location.

10. Unclasp and remove the Kelly clamp. Guide the chest tube while rotating the tube clockwise, aiming for the tube to sit along the posterior chest wall. Stop at resistance to avoid kinking the tube.

11. Place a silk suture in the skin and tie the chest tube in. Clean the incision site and place sterile dressing.

12. Connect the chest tube to the drainage system, which should be connected to continuous wall suction (never connect a chest tube directly to wall suction!). Note the time of placement.

13. Monitor chest tube output (quality, volume, and rate) to guide further management.

14. Dispose of sharps, clean the field, and help to reposition the patient before leaving the room.

15. Order a portable chest X-ray to confirm location of the chest tube.

7.7.2.2 Nasogastric Tube Placement

Types and Indications
- Levin: small bore, used for delivering nutrition or medication
- Salem Sump: large bore, used for aspiration and decompression
- Dobhoff: weighted small bore, used for delivering nutrition or medication

Equipment Required
- Disposable underpads (Chux)
- Nasogastric tube
- Lube or lidocaine jelly
- Cold water in a cup with a straw
- Suction tubing and canister
- Bucket or basin
- Tape and safety pin

Positioning the Patient

1. Adjust the angle of the bed so that the patient is sitting as upright as possible.
2. Place the disposable pad on the patient's chest, and hand them the basin (as a precaution in case of nausea and vomiting) and the cup of water with the straw.
3. Explain the procedure to the patient as they will need to participate in the placement of the tube. Instruct them that you will insert the tube until it reaches the back of the throat. At that point, they will need to tuck their chin to their chest and begin drinking through the straw. Have them practice this a few times before you attempt to place the tube.
4. Set up your supplies. Open the tube and stretch out the end to create a slight curve. Lubricate the tip with lube or lidocaine jelly. Open the suction tubing and connect this to the canister preemptively.

Placing the Tube

5. When you and the patient are ready, take the tube, and begin to insert the tip into the nare. This should enter *parallel to the nasal floor (along the inferior nasal concha)*.

    **Remember your anatomy. Do not be tempted to angle this upward into the nose, as the tube will need to make a sharper turn to enter the nasopharynx.
6. When the tip reaches the angle of the mandible (you should be able to estimate this), pause. At this point, instruct the patient to tuck their chin down and begin drinking the water as practiced.

    **This move will open the epiglottis and help you to insert the tube into the esophagus rather than slipping into the airway.
7. Continue pushing the tube in at a smooth, quick pace. If you hit resistance, do not keep pushing. Make sure to talk the patient through this and encourage them, as this part of the procedure is *extremely* uncomfortable. Be ready with the basin in case of emesis.
8. When you reach 50–60 cm, you should be in the stomach. Stop and ask the patient to speak to you (say their name, etc.). If they can speak, you know that the tube is not in the trachea.
9. Secure the tube with tape at the nose, and safety pin the tube to their gown.
10. For Salem Sumps, connect the tube to suction tubing and the canister at continuous wall suction. Take note of the quality and volume of output.
11. Clean the field, and help to reposition the patient before leaving the room.
12. Order a KUB to confirm location of the nasogastric tube. **The side port of the tube should be past the diaphragm on X-ray.

7.7.2.3 Additional Procedures

There are a number of other bedside procedures that you may want to include in your personal objectives to learn and practice. For detailed descriptions, see other chapters (Chaps. ▶ 14, 15, and 20).

- Central line placement:
  - With PA catheter
- Subclavian line placement
- Arterial line placement:
  - Radial
  - Femoral
- Ultrasound-guided IV
- Bronchoscopy

General Surgery

7.7.3 Operating Room Skills

There are many resources (videos and textbooks) available that explain the basics of technical skills, but nothing beats hands-on practice and learning in person during your clerkship. Because of this, the focus of this section will be tips and tricks that may not be mentioned in other resources.

7.7.3.1 Knot-Tying

Two-Handed

The principle of the two-handed knot is learning how to lay knots down flat and in alternating directions. This improves the strength of the knot and allows for a tighter hold (▶ www.animatedknots.com).

Tips:
- Observe your knot as it is coming down – there will be a direction in which it lays down flat. This may require you to cross your arms as you pull the knot tight.
- Even though you are tying two-handed, you can still push the knot. Maintain tension with one hand, and push *next to* your knot (not directly on top) in the opposite direction.

Resources:
- Animated knots: ▶ www.animatedknots.com

One-Handed

During a one-handed knot, one hand is your "post," which maintains tension, while the other hand does the work of tying. This is useful when tying in deep cavities and can be faster than the two-handed. Note that most attendings will want to see you master the two-handed knot before allowing you to tie one-handed (▶ www.animatedknots.com).

Tips:
- Practice one-handed knots with both hands. You may have one that you prefer, but you should be ready to tie with either hand.
- Slip knots:
  - There are cases in which you may tie two knots in the same direction. This is useful for getting a tighter seal and being able to push both knots down further. For example, as you tie the first knot, this may loosen as you pull back, and the second knot (in the same direction) allows you to push both knots down even tighter. You can do this a few times in a row, and your next knot (in the opposite direction) will "lock" this in place.
- Depending on the tissue and location of the stitch, the tightness of the knot may be achieved either by pulling up with your non-tying hand or by pushing down on the knot as described above:
  - In general, if you are tying soft tissue such as bowel or abdominal structures, you want to avoid from pulling up on the suture, as this can tear the tissue.
  - If you are tying in a chest tube, your knot needs to really secure this structure in place, and in this case, you would simultaneously pull up with one hand, while pushing the knot down with the other.
  - Observe your residents (and importantly, your attendings' feedback to your residents) to learn the nuances of when to pull up vs push down. Similarly, observe during the case which types of knots really need to be pulled tight vs purposeful airknots, etc.

Resources:
- Animated knots: ▶ www.animatedknots.com

7.7.3.2 Suturing

The goal of this section is to review the basic principles of suturing in general surgery (types of sutures, basic stitches, tips for technique). As you progress in your training, you will learn alternative needle angles and techniques to accommodate different tissues, suture types, and purposes of the stitch that are beyond the scope of this chapter.

Types of Sutures

There are three basic classifications of sutures (◻ Table 7.3), each with their own advantages and disadvantages:

— Braided vs monofilament
— Absorbable vs nonabsorbable
— Synthetic vs natural

Suture and Needle Size

Sutures are numbered based on size of the diameter. Thick sutures number from 0–10, with larger numbers signifying larger diameters. Thin sutures are numbered 1–0 ("one-oh") to 12–0 ("twelve-oh"), with larger numbers signifying smaller diameters. The strength of a suture depends both on material and size.

Needles can be straight or curved, with the curve of the needle at different lengths. The curve comes in ¼, ½, 3/8, or 1/3 of a circle (and if you forget, you can look at the packaging which has a life-size image of the needle). The size and shape combination will have a specific name like CT-2, SH, and UR-6. The

◻ **Table 7.3** Suture characteristics

	Advantages	Disadvantages	Notes
Braided	Greater shear strength More flexible Needs fewer knots	More abrasive to the tissue Can be a nidus for infection	Multifilament Should be tied with knots lying flat (rather than slip knots) Min: 2–3 knots
Mono-filament	Smooth tissue passage Less tissue reaction	Breaks more easily Needs more knots to secure	Single strand Can slide knots by tying slip knots (2 in the same direction) Min: 4–5 knots, up to 10 for smaller sutures
Absorb-able	Decreased risk of infection Less likely to cause foreign body reaction	Possible increased risk of wound dehiscence	Degrades over time (half-life varies depending on suture) Good for biliary or GU tracts
Nonab-sorbable	Permanent Preferred when healing may be slow or when consequences of suture failure are high	Nidus for infection	Good for heart valves, vascular anastomosis
Synthetic	Less tissue reaction Less inflammation	Cost	
Natural	Economical Easy handling and knotting	Causes stronger tissue reaction and suture antigenicity	Less frequently used

tip of the needle can be either cutting or tapering (which is also shown on the packaging). Cutting needles have three sharp edges and look like a triangle en face, whereas tapering needles have smooth edges.

**Be aware of what type of needle you are using, as a cutting tip can sometimes cut your own suture without you meaning it to.

Basic Stitches

While this chapter will not go through a step-by-step of each type of suture (as we feel this is something better learned and practiced in person), there are a number of basic stitches that you should know and master by the end of your rotation, listed here (◻ Fig. 7.7):

Interrupted:

━ Simple interrupted
━ Vertical mattress
━ Horizontal mattress
━ Figure of 8

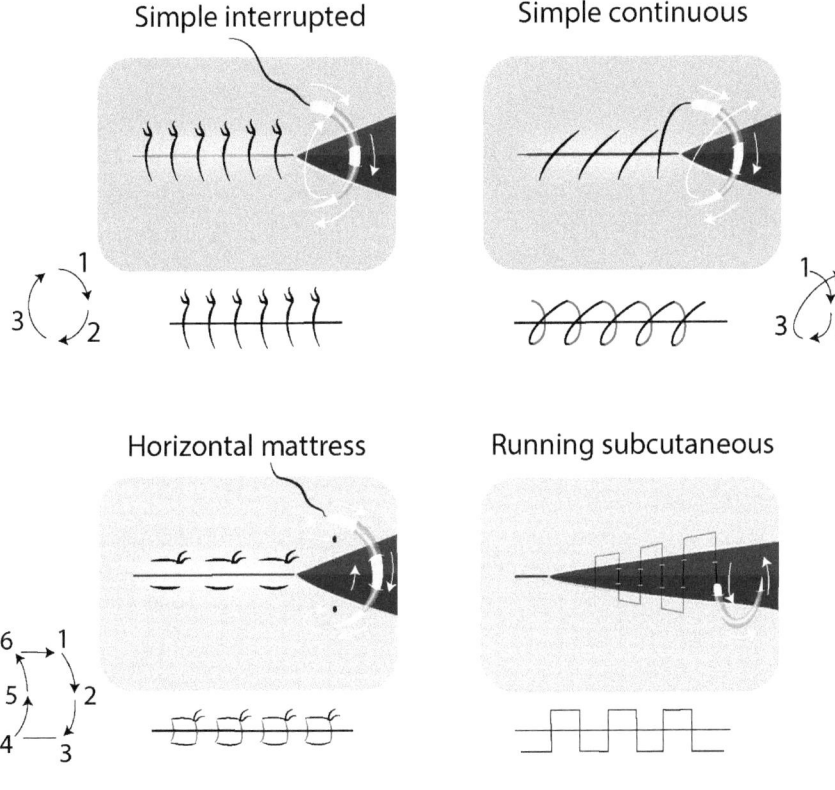

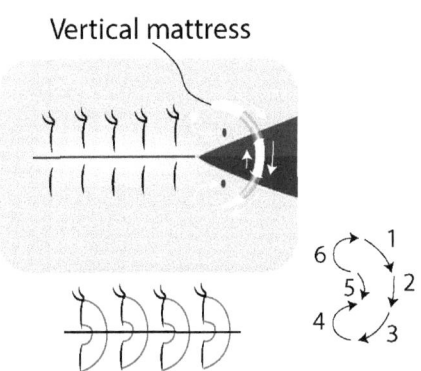

◻ **Fig. 7.7** Basic suture types

Continuous:
- Simple running
- Running subcutaneous/subcuticular
- Locked

Resources:
- MUSC (Medical University of South Caroline) suture technique videos:
  - ▶ https://medicine.musc.edu/departments/surgery/education/medical-student-information/3rd-year-info/suture-techniques-video

General tips (for general surgery, as these may no longer apply in subspecialties such as cardiothoracic that requires different maneuvers and needle angles):
- Holding the needle driver:
  - Tip: you can gauge a lot about technical skill based on the way that a person handles the instrument, even before any stitches are placed! Watch how your attendings and residents use each of the instruments, and emulate them. If something feels awkward or unnatural, practice it the correct way – it is better to build good habits now, even if it temporarily slows you down, than to get the job done but reinforce bad habits.
  - Put your thumb in one hole and your ring finger in the other. Your index holder should be braced on the side of the driver for additional control.
    - **Keep your hand relaxed and your fingertips just inside the holes of the driver. The driver should not go further than your DIP joint. This makes the handling of the instrument easier.
- Load your needle either:
  - In the center, at a 90 degree angle
  - 2/3 away from the tip, at a slightly obtuse angle
- *Your needle should enter the tissue at a perpendicular angle*. This angle is between the tip of the needle and the tissue (rather than the angle of your needle driver, hand, etc.). This is accomplished by pronating your wrist and adjusting your body or your hold of the instrument.
- *Follow the curve of the needle*. After you have pushed the needle into the tissue at a 90 degree angle, rotate your wrist to follow the natural curve of the needle (this is why choice of needle size is important). If you deviate, you may be putting tension or torque on the tissue which can lead to injury.
- When your needle emerges, let go of the needle with the needle driver. With a forceps in your opposite hand, grasp the needle, and rotate your wrist to pull the needle out (still along the curve of the needle).
- *Do not touch the tip of the needle* with your instruments. This will blunt the tip and make it more difficult to push through tissue on your next bite.
- *Think of the needle driver as an extension of your body*. Placing the stitch depends not only on the use of the driver but also your wrist and arm, the way that your body is facing, etc. This is less obvious now but will come into play when you are throwing stitches either deep in the body or at difficult angles. Try to stand up straight and not hunch down toward your hands.

7.7.3.3 Basics of Laparoscopy

Laparoscopic surgery is the minimally invasive technique of performing operations through port sites in an insufflated abdomen. First adopted by gynecologic surgeons, laparoscopy became widely adopted by general surgeons in the 1990s eventually becoming standard of care for cholecystectomies, appendectomies, and many foregut operations.

All general surgery residents are expected to reach competency in core laparoscopic operations. There is a widely adopted national curriculum – the

Fundamentals of Laparoscopic Surgery – which consists of five didactic modules, manual skills training, and a two part written and practical exam. Most academic centers will have laparoscopic trainers available to residents and medical students for practicing laparoscopic skills.

The components of the manual skills examined are:

- Peg transfer
- Precision (pattern) cutting
- Ligating loop (endoloop)
- Extracorporeal knot-tying
- Intracorporeal knot-tying

Camera Driving

As a medical student, you often play the integral role of driving the camera during a laparoscopic operation.

1. *Setting up.* There are a few crucial components to a laparoscopy setup. You should familiarize yourself with these different components and recognize how they come together as you may be asked to help assemble the system.
   - Laparoscope (variety of sizes and degrees – which refer to the angle of view compared to the shaft):
     - Size refers to the outer diameter. Most commonly 5 mm or 10 mm but sometimes 3 mm or 8 mm scopes are used.
     - Some scopes have a bevel at the tip (0–90 degrees):
       - 0° scope: sometimes used upon entry of the abdomen to check for bleeding or injury
       - 30° scope: used for most operation, allows views around corners
     - Camera head (attached to laparoscope, sends image to monitor).
   - Fiber-optic cord (connected to light source)
     - **The light cord can reach very high temperatures and set the sterile drapes on fire, so it should never be set directly on the drapes.
   - Monitor

It is important to remember that the laparoscope and all its components are very expensive and sterile during the operation, so you should remain vigilant about taking the appropriate precautions. In addition to the light cord and camera cord, lines for CO_2, suction and irrigation, and energy devices will also be secured on the sterile field and passed off. Some newer platforms integrate several of these functions.

2. *White balancing.* After setting up the laparoscope, the camera should be white balanced with the light and magnification already adjusted to the anticipated settings using a white object such as a gauze sponge or lap pad. If available, the laparoscope may be put in warm antifogging solution before use.

3. *Driving the camera.* The cardinal rule of laparoscopic camera driving is that the camera controls are oriented upward toward the ceiling.
   - Most camera heads will have three dials – a coupler, optical zoom, and focus. These are usually not adjusted after initial setup. Some devices will have automatic or digital/integrated function.
   - When adjusting the camera angle, *only the light post should be moved.* The camera head should stay level, ensuring a stable horizon so that "up" on the screen also refers to "up" in the patient whether that's the diaphragm or abdominal wall.
   - The light post and cord are also always oriented opposite to the bevel of the scope angle (e.g., when the light cord is at 12 o'clock on an imaginary clock, the scope is angled 30° downward toward 6 o'clock. It follows that control of the light cord is inverted; turning the cord right will look left in the abdomen and turning left will look right).

- Generally, the camera should center the active instrument on the middle of the screen and avoid any unnecessary movements or sudden movements as much as possible. As one can imagine, it is also easier to maneuver an instrument looking at it from an angle rather than down its shaft. If blood or fluid gets on the scope, remove the scope, clean, and dehumidify before reinserting. **Alternatively, you may try to carefully wipe the scope off on the bowels or liver; however this is a more advanced maneuver and should be done carefully and with the permission of your attending/residents.
  - **Similar to knowing when to suction, understanding when to clean the scope is a bit more nuanced. If the lens is completely soiled, do this immediately. However, if it is only a bit fogged or smudged but nonobstructive, look at the surgical field, and gauge whether this is a good time. Most times, they will ask you to clean the scope, or if you are unsure, you can ask if it's a good time.

Entry/Port Sites

The beginning of every laparoscopic operation involves insufflating or filling the abdomen with carbon dioxide.

Types of entry:

- *Veress needle.* A beveled sharp needle with a blunt spring-loaded tip is used to penetrate the layers of the abdominal wall. You will be taught to feel 3 "pops" through the fascial layers. As you can imagine, this method of entry can cause injury to abdominal contents (bowel, liver, stomach, etc.). Different attendings/residents may teach you different techniques, but classically, the safest area is the LUQ ("Palmer's point").
- *Hassan technique.* Using direct visualization, a small incision is made, dissection is taken down to the fascia, and the peritoneal cavity is entered. A blunt port is then inserted and secured. Many variations exist.

Insufflation:

1. After gaining entry, purge the CO_2 line of room air, and then *connect the CO_2 line.* If you are in the right location, the abdomen will begin to insufflate.
2. *Look at the three monitors:*
   - Flow. This can be set to low, medium, or high settings. Starting flow should be low (<0.5 L/min). Once placement is confirmed, this can be turned up to high (>10 L/min). Watch for bradycardia during rapid insulation and stop if needed.
   - Pressure. Initial pressure should be 0–7 mmHg and ultimately reach 12–15 mmHg. If initial pressures are high (with low flow), this is a sign that you may not be in free peritoneal space.
   - Volume. Varies depending on body habitus.

7.8   Conclusion

A final word of encouragement: every student is different, and there is no one right way to go about this rotation. At the end of the day, if you show up and are genuinely engaged, focused, and excited to learn, this is what matters! Nobody expects you to be perfect or to know all of the right answers, so take a breath, be yourself, and enjoy the rotation.

7.9 Examples

Admission Note Template

*** **Surgery Service Consult Note**

Name:
MRN:
Date:

Attending: **Senior:**   **Intern:**

Consulting Physician:

Reason for Consultation:

History of Present Illness:

PMH	PSH
	**Include year, hospital, surgeon
Social History	**Family History**

Prior to Admission Medications

Allergies

Review of Systems:

Physical Exam:
Vitals:

Gen:	Lying in bed comfortably, well nourished, well kept
Psych:	Alert, oriented, appropriate mood and affect, good insight to condition
Neuro:	Sensation intact to light touch, no noted asymmetry of CNVII
Head:	NC/AT, no evidence of trauma
Neck:	Supple, symmetrical, trachea midline, no lymphadenopathy
Lungs:	Clear to auscultation bilaterally, respirations unlabored

Heart:	Regular rate and rhythm, S1 and S2 normal, no murmur, rub, or gallop
Abdomen:	Soft, non-tender, non-distended***
Musculoskeletal:	Extremities normal, atraumatic, no cyanosis or edema
Skin:	No rashes or signs of trauma noted
Pulses:	2+ and symmetric

Labs:
CBC
BMP
LFT
PT/PTT/INR

Imaging:

Assessment and Plan:
One-liner.

N: *PRN narcotics*
CV: *Hemodynamically stable within normal limits*
P: *Maximum pulmonary toilet, IS, OOB*
GI: *NPO/IVF*
GU: *Monitor UOP, Strict I/O*
- *Trend Creatinine*
Heme: *Heparin SC TID, SCDs*
ID: *Trend fever curve, no indication for abx at this time*
Endo: *No active issues*
Dispo:

The patient was seen and discussed with Dr. ***, who agrees with the above assessment and plan.

_____

This patient was seen and evaluated by the ED Surgery Team; for further management please page responding inpatient clinician and team noted above.

Progress Note Template

*** Surgery Service Progress Note

Name:
MRN:
Date:
Time:

Hospital Day:
POD:

Procedure:

Brief Summary: One-liner
24 hour events:

Current Diet:

Vitals:

Fluid Balance:

Exam:

Gen:	Lying in bed comfortably, well nourished, well kept
Psych:	Alert, oriented, appropriate mood and affect, good insight to condition
Neuro:	Sensation intact to light touch, no noted asymmetry of CNVII
Head:	NC/AT, no evidence of trauma
Neck:	Supple, symmetrical, trachea midline, no adenopathy
Lungs:	Clear to auscultation bilaterally, respirations unlabored
Heart:	Regular rate and rhythm, S1 and S2 normal, no murmur, rub, or gallop
Abdomen:	Soft, non-tender, non-distended***
Musculoskeletal:	Extremities normal, atraumatic, no cyanosis or edema
Skin:	No rashes or signs of trauma noted
Pulses:	2+ and symmetric

<table>
<tr><td>Medications:
IVF:
SCHEDULED:
PRN:</td></tr>
<tr><td>Labs:
CBC
BMP
LFTs
Coags (PT/PTT/INR)

Other if applicable</td></tr>
</table>

Tubes, Lines and Drains:

Assessment and Plan:
One-liner.

N:
CV:
R:
GI:
GU:
Heme:
ID:
Endo:
Ppx:

Dispo:

Code Status:

<u>Clinic Note Template</u>
(Post-Op Visit)

Patient:
MRN:
DOB:
Date:

Date of Procedure:
Procedure:

*** <u>Surgery Clinic Note</u>

History of Present Illness:
_____ is a _____ who presents for follow-up after ***.

Since his operation, the patient has been recovering well. He was weaned off opioids and pain is well-controlled with Tylenol PRN. He has resumed his daily activities. He is tolerating a ____ diet without nausea, vomiting, abdominal pain or discomfort.

He complains of _____. Denies fever, chills, ____

Review of Systems: As mentioned in HPI.

Physical Exam:

Pathology:

Imaging:

Labs:
CBC
BMP

Other (if applicable): tumor markers, LFTs

Impression/Plan:

The patient continues to recover from his operation. Pain is well-controlled without opioids. All tubes, drains, and staples have been removed. He may resume _____, with the exception of _____. We will see him back for follow-up in _____.

Post-Op Check

POST-OP CHECK

Patient:
MRN:
Date:
Time:

Procedure:
Complications:
EBL:

Subjective: Pain well controlled with ***. No nausea/vomiting. ***Irritation from NGT. No flatus. UOP adequate. SCDs. No fevers/chills/CP/SOB/calf pain.

Current Diet:

Vitals:

Fluid Balance:

Physical examination:
General: NAD, AAOx3, laying in hospital bed, NGT with minimal bilious output ***
CV: RRR ***
Pulm: Breathing comfortably ***
Abdomen: Soft, appropriate incisional tenderness, non-distended. Dressings C/D/I. JP SS. ***
GU: foley in place draining clear yellow urine ***
Ext: WWP

Assessment/Plan:
One-liner

N: Continue dilaudid PCEA
CV: D5LR@85
Pulm: IS/PT
GI: NPO, continue NGT to LWS
GU: continue foley, monitor UOP
ID: cefoxitin x 2
Heme: SQH
Endocrine: NTD
Disposition: to floor

► Author's Disclaimer

This chapter is based on our collective experiences in general surgery at our institutions but by no means encompasses the entirety of rotations, experiences, or culture of general surgery across the board. These are the tips and tricks that have helped us succeed during our rotations, but it is up to you to determine what fits you and your institution.◄

Obstetrics and Gynecology

Allison A. Merz

Contents

© The Author(s), under exclusive license to Springer Nature Switzerland AG 2021
S. H. Lecker, B. J. Chang (eds.), *The Ultimate Medical School Rotation Guide*,
https://doi.org/10.1007/978-3-030-63560-2_8

8.1   Introduction

8.1.1   Overview

There are many aspects of obstetrics and gynecology (OB-GYN) that differ from other medical specialties. These differences make the rotation simultaneously exciting and meaningful but also challenging and potentially overwhelming. OB-GYN uniquely blends surgery, medicine, and patient advocacy, which is what draws many medical trainees to it. Your days and weeks can vary considerably: one day you're in the OR, the next you're on the Labor and Delivery (L&D) floor, and the next you're in clinic. At most medical schools, you will spend time in all of these settings – most commonly you'll have an OB block (the L&D floor ± antepartum service), a GYN block (benign GYN, GYN oncology, and sometimes more subspecialized services), and a clinic block or clinic time interspersed throughout the rotation. During any one of these blocks, you will also likely see GYN and sometimes OB consults from the ED and other parts of the hospital. It is a challenging rotation, with early mornings, pathologies you may not have previously learned about, procedures and acronyms not encountered in other medical specialties, and sometimes hectic and stressful clinical situations. Despite these challenges, most students find it to be very enjoyable and meaningful.

OB-GYN residents and faculty tend to understand that most students are not going to pursue careers in their field. However, all doctors will take care of patients with female reproductive organs at some stage of training and/or practice. As a result, there are some fundamental concepts, diagnoses, procedural skills, and treatment plans related to OB-GYN that all physicians should know. Furthermore, 100% of the population has been or will be affected by a pregnancy and delivery experience that went smoothly or could have gone better! Your instructors will want you to recognize this and will be looking for you to be enthusiastic about learning the important and fundamental principles and skills of the field.

Regardless of your specialty ambitions, recognize that what you learn during your OB-GYN clerkship will inform your practice as a physician. If you do know which specialty you're interested in, consider how the knowledge and skills you acquire during your OB-GYN rotation will impact your practice. Identify specific learning goals related to the intersections between OB-GYN and your field of interest, and bring these up with your preceptor.

If you think you might be interested in pursuing a career in OB-GYN, let your clerkship director, residents, and attendings know so that they can help you think about how to optimize your rotation. Regardless of your specialty ambitions, the guidelines outlined in this chapter will help you make the most of your rotation, earn the best possible evaluations, and have fun in the process!

8.1.2   An Introduction to the Specialty

Approximately 90% of OB/GYNs are generalists and begin practice after completing a 4-year residency in OB/GYN. There are also subspecialties within OB-GYN that you may or may not gain exposure to, depending on your hospital. These include:

- Obstetrics-related (i.e., related to pregnancy)
  - Maternal-Fetal Medicine (MFM) – high-risk pregnancy and prenatal diagnosis
  - Genetics

- Gynecology-related (i.e., everything except pregnancy)
  - Gynecologic Oncology (a.k.a. "GYN ONC") – cancers of the female reproductive tract and associated organs
  - Reproductive Endocrinology and Infertility (REI) – infertility and gynecologic endocrine disease
  - Female Pelvic Medicine and Reconstructive Surgery (FPMRS, a.k.a. "Urogynecology") – advanced pelvic surgery and urologic problems involving the female urogenital system
  - Minimally Invasive (Gynecologic) Surgery (MIS or MIGS) – advanced laparoscopic and robotic benign GYN surgery
  - Family Planning (FP) – complex contraception and abortion
  - Pediatric and Adolescent Gynecology (PAGS) – GYN-care for children and adolescents

8.1.3 Before Your Rotation: Resources to Download or Subscribe to

Disclaimer   These resources are current as of March 2020 but may change over time.

- **Textbooks**
- *Obstetrics & Gynecology* (Beckmann & Ling)
- Blueprints (Callahan & Caughey)
- *Case Files* (Toy, Baker, Ross & Jennings)

Be aware that these exist. It may be unrealistic to expect that you could read an entire textbook while completing a time-intensive rotation and studying for a shelf exam. Instead, use these books to dive into specific topics as they come up during your rotation. Beckmann and Ling's *Obstetrics and Gynecology* and *Blueprints* are both good comprehensive resources – if you're able to obtain these through your school's library, see which one "speaks to you," and use that to build your knowledge base about specific (patho)physiologic and management concepts as you encounter them clinically and during didactics. *Case Files* is useful for shelf preparation.

- **Anatomy**

YouTube videos: Playlist "Pimped – Welcome to Ob/Gyn Recommended Videos" ▶ https://www.youtube.com/playlist?list=PLXjtJli4WDYrxVHHD-pzmSdG8OU6vsoeb and this video with pelvic anatomy labeled from a laparoscopic view: ▶ https://www.youtube.com/watch?v=WFS-IUxVQL0
- Watch one of the "anatomy review" videos before the rotation begins.
- Watch videos for individual procedures you know you'll be attending.

- **Podcasts**
- Pimped app ($) & podcast (free)
  - Directed at medical students and with 16 episodes only, this is by no means a comprehensive review tool, but the episodes are quick and include some very high-yield pointers for specific situations (e.g., "before your first hysteroscopy," etc.). You can listen to them on your way to the hospital in the mornings when you know you'll be in a specific setting that day.

8

- CREOGs over Coffee (free)
  - This is a podcast created by two OB-GYN residents at Brown that can be exceptionally helpful on OB-GYN specialty electives and sub-I's. The content is aimed at review for the CREOGs (the OB-GYN residency in-service exams) so it's technically above medical student level, BUT it's a very efficient way to review specific topics if you know you'll be encountering them and/or if you have extra time while commuting or exercising.

- **Apps and Websites**
- APGO Educational Objectives and Videos (free)
  - The Association of Professors of Gynecology and Obstetrics (APGO) is the national organization that governs medical student education in OB/GYN. Their educational objectives and accompanying videos, compiled by clerkship and residency program directors, residency selection committee members, and National Board of Medical Examiners (NBME) question-writers, are generally very high-yield. Most medical schools pay for student access to the materials associated with the free objectives and YouTube videos.
  - Objectives: ▶ www.apgo.org/educational-resources/apgo-medical-student-educational-objectives
  - Videos: ▶ https://www.youtube.com/channel/UCB67eiHQzqqLUB-HrDJzYdtQ
- Pregnancy wheel (many free apps)
  - Use these to estimate pregnancy dating in clinic, when seeing ED consults, and in OB triage.
- CDC Medical Eligibility Criteria ("CDC MEC") for Contraceptive methods (free app)
  - This app and a PDF available online contain guidelines for contraindications to contraceptive methods; it will be useful for contraceptive counseling.
- ▶ Bedsider.org (website for patient-facing infographics and articles)
  - You can refer patients to this website for information about sexual health and contraception. It also has some useful charts and graphs that you can print and share with patients or use in contraceptive counseling.
- CDC STI Treatment guidelines (free app)
  - This app contains guidelines for STI treatment. Use it to make your treatment plans when you encounter any patient with any suspected or confirmed STI in any setting (e.g., new diagnosis vs. recurrence of genital herpes in pregnancy, seeing a patient in the ED with pelvic inflammatory disease, etc.).
- ASCCP (app for $, or ASCCP PDFs (▶ https://www.asccp.org/management-guidelines) for free)
  - Guidelines for Pap testing and management of cervical pathology. Every time you see a patient in gyn clinic, you should be aware of her Pap history and have a plan for her related follow-up testing and/or treatment using these guidelines.
- LactMed (website (▶ https://www.ncbi.nlm.nih.gov/books/NBK501922/), free)
  - Database with information on drugs and other chemicals' levels in breast milk and infant blood and possible adverse effects in nursing infants. Use this for treatment planning for pregnant and nursing patients and for answering patients' questions.

- Online Med Ed (OME) (website, free videos)
  - OME's videos are useful for providing overviews of specific concepts, frameworks through which to approach certain clinical scenarios, and tips for test-taking.
- UpToDate (website and app)
  - ('nuff said) – Useful for developing diagnosis and treatment plans for specific presentations or conditions.
- ACOG app (you can join ACOG for free as a med student!)
  - First, if you tell your resident that you joined ACOG, they will be *thrilled*.
  - The app contains easy access to ACOG Practice Bulletins and Committee Opinions (incredibly useful resources that OB-GYNs rely on for providing evidence-based care), an estimated due date calculator, an "Indicated Delivery" interface in which you can input a patient's gestational age and conditions and see when they should be delivered, vaccination guidelines, and more. Useful in all clinical settings during your rotation.
- AHRQ ePSS (primary care guidelines) (free app)
  - This app allows you to enter the age, sex, and smoking status of your patient, and then it tells you which screening tests they should be undergoing. It is useful in GYN clinic given the sometimes-primary care-ish role of OB-GYNs – as you'll see below, a comprehensive OB-GYN H&P includes "Healthcare maintenance." All this being said, you should do everything you can to plug your OB-GYN patients into primary care if they don't have a PCP – this will both improve their care and win you brownie points!
- OBG Project (website, can buy monthly subscription to "OBG First" if interested in OB-GYN)
  - Easily searchable, practical, and evidence-based professional standards and guidelines for women's healthcare. Useful for learning about a specific topic and for developing diagnosis and treatment plans for specific presentations or conditions, similar to UpToDate, but with more varied resources such as lit reviews, timely topic reviews, an ultrasound atlas, and more.

Standout Tip: If you are tasked with presenting on a specific topic during your clerkship, start with the relevant (1) ACOG Practice Bulletin and (2) UpToDate page. These two resources will cover 99% of what you should know and pack into a quick presentation and are full of references to primary literature that you could dive into if needed.

8.1.4 OB-GYN Fundamentals

OB-GYN has its own language and acronyms. Here are some of the most important concepts:

1. *Gs & Ps* (or GTPAL):
   - G = # of pregnancies.
     - Each pregnancy didn't have to result in a birth – it could end in a miscarriage or a termination, it could have been ectopic, or it could have resulted in a birth, either vaginal or cesarean.
     - For every patient, ask "have you ever been pregnant? How about any miscarriages, losses or abortions? How many deliveries? Any ectopic pregnancies?"
     - Multiple gestations (i.e., twins, triplets) count as one pregnancy.
   - P = Parity.
     - The four spaces behind "P" are for T, P, A, and L.
       - Term = pregnancies ending with deliveries at 37 weeks or later
       - Preterm = pregnancies ending with delivery between 20 weeks and 36 weeks 6 days

– Abortion = pregnancies ending before 20 weeks, for any reason (i.e., miscarriage, ectopic pregnancy, elective termination)
– Living children
– Multiple gestations (i.e., twins, triplets) count as one delivery, no matter how many fetuses are delivered.
– Pay attention to the L! If it's more than the "T/P," they could have had a twin pregnancy; if it's less, they have lost a child.
– Be prepared to expand on all of the "TPAL" numbers – e.g., if someone had an ectopic pregnancy, you'll want to know about how it was managed (more below).
– If TPAL is straightforward (e.g., G1P0000 or G2P2002), you can shorthand to: G_ P_ (e.g., G1P0, G2P2).

2. *The LMP.* You ALWAYS want to know when the last menstrual period (LMP) was!
   ▬ If they've never had a period (e.g., prepubertal or primary amenorrhea), that's important to know.
   ▬ If they are of reproductive age, you want to know whether periods are regular, whether they could be pregnant, etc.
   ▬ If menopausal, you want to know age of menopause.

3. *The management ladder.* A general principle of all management options, outlined in ◼ Fig. 8.1, is: *expectant* (i.e., observe and do nothing) → *medical* (i.e., use medication) → *surgical.* This is a good way to frame your decision-making when talking to a resident or attending about many OB-GYN conditions. For example:
   ▬ 19-year-old G0 with dysmenorrhea and cyclic dyschezia concerning for endometriosis. Expectant management would be inappropriate given significant symptom burden. Recommend medical management (e.g., trial of NSAIDs and birth control pills) for now, and be aware of potential to escalate to surgical management (e.g., laparoscopy for definitive diagnosis and potential excision).
   ▬ 29-year-old G1P1 s/p normal spontaneous vaginal delivery 30 minutes ago, now with persistent vaginal bleeding, total estimated blood loss 1.5 L, on pitocin and s/p rectal misoprostol. Expectant management (i.e., observation) would be inappropriate given significant blood loss (>1 L meets threshold for postpartum hemorrhage). Recommend trial of medical management (e.g., carboprost, methergine, TXA), and be aware of potential to escalate to surgical management (e.g., balloon tamponade (most often with a Bakri balloon) → uterine artery embolization → hysterectomy).
   ▬ 32-year-old G2P0 presenting after spontaneous rupture of membranes, q3 minute contractions, cervical exam is 5 cm / 80% / -1, progressed from 2 cm / 40% / -2 2 hours ago. Plan to manage expectantly given satisfactory natural labor progression.

4. *The pelvic exam.* This is an invasive and uncomfortable experience and should be discussed with the patient before it is done. This way, they know what to expect and have the opportunity to provide fully informed consent, even if they've had a pelvic exam in the past. Never do a pelvic exam alone – an instructor and/or chaperone should be present with you, serving as both a teacher/observer and second pair of hands. All maneuvers should be done gently, but try not to be overly timid – the longer the exam takes, the more uncomfortable it is for the patient. As much as you can, explain what you are doing at all times and what the patient should expect.

8

Pearl: Expectant management can also include surveillance, for example, h/o cervical intraepithelial neoplasia (CIN) 3 needing annual Pap tests.

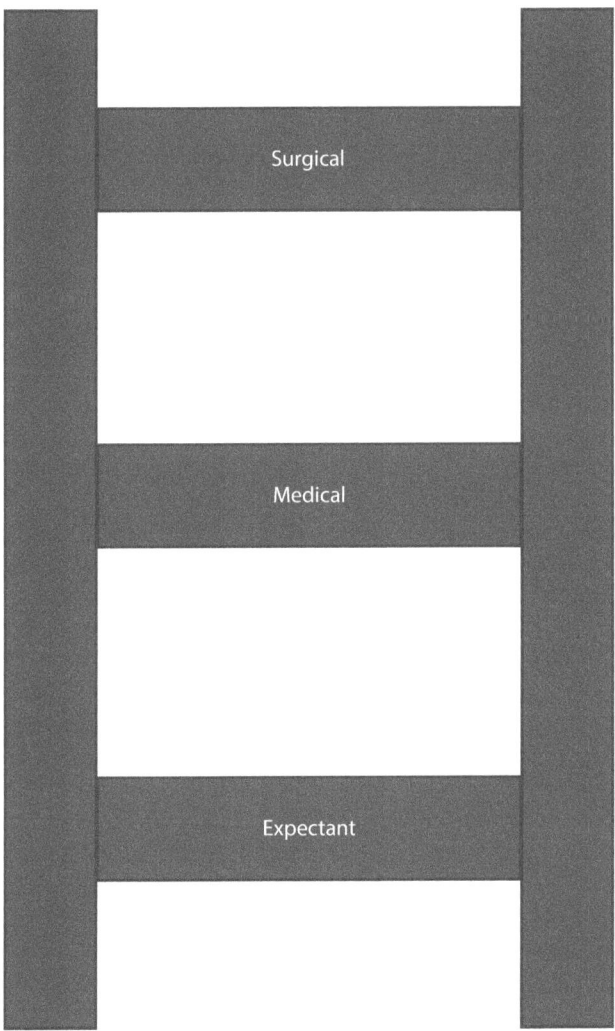

◻ Fig. 8.1 The OB-GYN management ladder. Treatment options for nearly all conditions in OB-GYN can be thought of in a stepwise framework, beginning with observation (a.k.a. "expectant management," i.e., doing nothing or observing), then stepping up to medical management, and then finally to surgical management

1. Setting up:
   (a) Provide the patient with privacy so that they can put on a gown and remove any undergarments (only from the waist down, unless you are also conducting a breast exam).
   (b) Allow them the opportunity to urinate prior to starting as a full bladder can make the exam uncomfortable.
   (c) Ensure that you have:
      - A speculum
      - Gel/lubricant
      - A light source
      - Gloves
      - Any specimen collection tools you need (e.g., swabs for a wet mount, Pap test kit, Gonorrhea/Chlamydia (GC/CT) swabs)
      - Tissues for the patient to wipe off excess lubricant after the exam
      - A pad for the patient to use if desired (Paps and swabs can sometimes cause spotting)

! Common Error: Avoid using the term "stirrups," as this term connotes riding horses and can be dehumanizing for patients.

For example: "I imagine it's very hard to do right now, but as much as you can, try to let your legs fall out to the side, and relax your bottom into the exam table."

Historical fun fact: Pap tests were formerly called Pap "smears" because they involved smearing a sample of cells onto a glass slide. Back then, performing the bimanual exam with non-water-soluble lubricant before collecting the Pap sample increased the "uninterpretable" rate on Paps, so it was important to do the bimanual exam after the speculum exam. Now with modern technology and water-soluble lubricants, it doesn't matter which is first, and in fact, conducting the bimanual exam first enables acquisition of haptic information as to where the cervix is, so you know where to place the speculum.

2. Positioning:
   (a) The patient should be in the dorsal lithotomy position (supine). Elevate the head of the table to 30 degrees (this usually makes the exam more comfortable – check with the patient).
   (b) Extend the footrests and ask the patient to place their feet in them.
   (c) Ask the patient to move toward the end of the table so that their bottom reaches the edge (you can put your hand at the side of the table's end so that they have a target to reach).
   (d) Arrange the sheet so that that it covers up to their knees.
   (e) Use verbal cues to assist them in positioning their legs, such that they relax them out to the sides. DO NOT push them open with your hands.
3. External inspection:
   (a) Inspect the vulva, urethra, and perineum. Make note of the general appearance, whether there are skin changes or excoriations and whether there is any appreciable discharge or blood.
4. The bimanual exam (see ◘ Fig. 8.2a):
   (a) Place the first two fingers of your dominant hand inside of the vaginal introitus, and place your nondominant hand just above the pubic symphysis, at the level of the uterus.
   (b) Palpate the cervix, uterus, and adnexae. Note the size of the uterus in centimeters (estimate the distance between your fingertips); any tenderness of the cervix, uterus, or adnexae; and whether you note any masses. Move the cervix gently to check for cervical motion tenderness.
5. Inserting the speculum (see ◘ Fig. 8.2b and c):
   (a) Place two fingers just inside or at the introitus to separate the labia, and gently press down on the perineal body.
   (b) With your other hand, hold the closed speculum with the blades between your index and middle finger. Introduce the closed speculum past your fingers at a 45° angle downward – push the speculum POSTERIORLY (i.e., toward the patient's bottom) as much as possible, avoiding the more sensitive anterior wall and urethra.
   (c) After the speculum has entered the vagina, remove your fingers from the introitus.
   (d) Open the speculum after full insertion, and maneuver the speculum gently so that the cervix comes into full view.

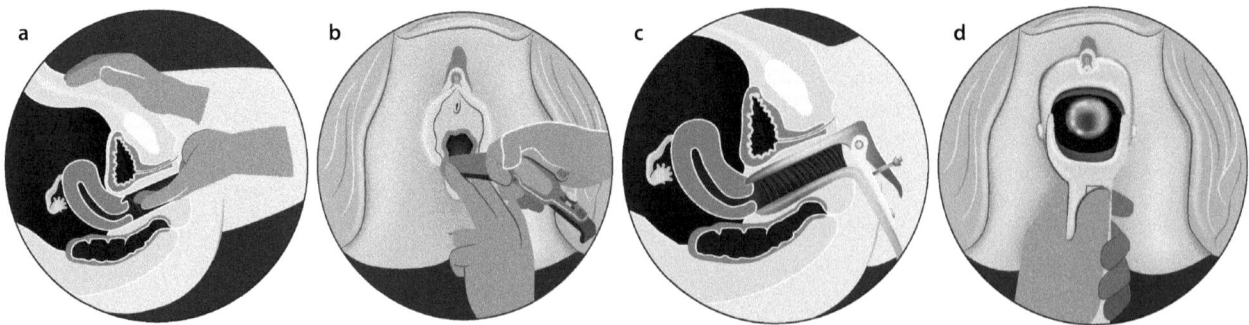

◘ **Fig. 8.2** The pelvic exam. Steps of the pelvic exam. **a** The bimanual exam. Note how the left thumb is folded over the palm of the hand to avoid touching the more sensitive anterior vulvovaginal structures. **b** Speculum insertion. Note how the nondominant hand separates the labia, keeping them away from the speculum machinery. **c–d** Speculum position. Note how the posteriorly angled orientation enables visualization of the cervix

6. Internal inspection (see ◘ Fig. 8.2d):
   (a) Note the position and color of the cervix, including the appearance and location of the os and whether there is any discharge or bleeding.
   (b) Note the appearance of the vaginal mucosa.
7. Remove the speculum: Undo the screw or plastic lever to allow the speculum to close, but leave open slightly to avoid pinching the vaginal walls. Retract slowly and gently.
8. Rectovaginal exam:
   (a) Change gloves (to avoid cross-contamination from the vagina to the anus), and coat the first two fingers of your dominant hand with gel.
   (b) Let the patient know what to expect: "You will now feel me placing a finger in your vagina and a finger in your rectum to better assess your uterus and ovaries."
   (c) Ask the patient to bear down ("as if having a bowel movement") and as they do, insert your index finger into the vagina and your middle finger into the rectum to the first knuckle of your middle finger, and then pause. Wait for the internal sphincter to relax, and then insert the rest of the way as the patient continues to bear down.
   (d) Assess the rectovaginal septum with the two inserted fingers by scissoring them. Expect to feel stool, but no fixed masses.
   (e) Retract both fingers slowly and gently.
9. Conclusion:
   (a) Redrape the patient and remove your gloves out of the patient's sight (as there may be visible discharge or stool). Throw the gloves into the trash unless they are needed for a stool sample.
   (b) Tell the patient to push back to sit up and offer them a wipe.
   (c) If there were no pathological findings, tell the patient that everything appears "healthy and normal" and that you are going to send the samples to the lab.

Indications for a pelvic exam:
1. Cervical cancer screening (i.e., Pap tests)
2. STI screening
3. Lower abdominal or vaginal symptoms (e.g., vaginal bleeding or discharge, lower abdominal/pelvic pain, vaginal masses/ulcers)
4. Pregnancy (during initial prenatal visit, and for certain complications during pregnancy)
5. GYN procedure or surgery, to characterize the size and shape of the uterus (e.g., prior to IUD placement)
   Note that pelvic exams are NOT indicated for an *asymptomatic* patient undergoing an "annual physical" unless the patient is due for cervical cancer or STI screening.

5. *Relationships with team members.* In OB-GYN, it is essential to be as friendly and deferent as possible to every member of the team, especially nurses. OB nurses in particular are often motivated by a fierce sense of patient advocacy and a desire to protect patients and their families during a particularly vulnerable time.
6. *Trauma-informed care.* Many patients have experienced physical or sexual trauma that they may or may not disclose. Survivors of trauma report that speculum and pelvic exams can be both painful and anxiety-inducing. A trauma-informed approach can help providers create a safer space for patients: with all sensitive exams and procedures, allow the patients to have

Pearl: The rectovaginal exam is not necessary in many patients but is important in patients with pelvic pain, rectal symptoms, or a pelvic mass. It can also provide a sample for fecal occult blood testing.

Pearl: As an alternative to collecting samples for STI screening during a pelvic exam, you can screen with NAAT (nucleic acid amplification testing) of urine. However, this has decreased sensitivity compared to vaginal swab (~78% vs. 98%).

Pearl: In a patient with vaginal discharge, pelvic exam should also include wet prep and STI testing.

Common Error: If a patient opts out of a pelvic exam, efforts should be made to sensitively ascertain why, as this may impact their care in important ways.

For example: "Do you have a difficult time with pelvic exams? Is there anything I should know to make it less difficult for you?"

For example: "What can I do to help you be more comfortable?"

For example: "Is it okay to begin the exam now?"

For example: "Would you like the door open or closed while you wait for the doctor?"

For example: "Is it okay if I examine your neck to feel your thyroid gland?"

For example, instead of "bed," say "exam table;" instead of "stirrups," say "footrests;" instead of "spread," say "separate;" and instead of "everything looks good", say "everything looks healthy and normal."

For example: "Is it okay if I ask you a few questions?"

For example, bring a chair or kneel so you can speak to patients at their eye level. Do not sit on their hospital bed, stand above them, or get unnecessarily close to them while speaking, as these gestures suggest a power differential.

as much control over their care as possible, and move slowly. Patients can opt out of pelvic exams. Several specific actions you should take to provide more trauma-informed care include:

- Ask if there is anything the provider needs to know about patient's previous experiences that may make an exam more difficult, or if they have ever had a painful experience with pelvic exams before.
- Ask the patient about their preferences and honor those preferences.
- Ask for permission to begin an exam or procedure.
- Allow the patient to maintain as much control as possible: have them move/remove their clothes instead of doing it for them, keep them as covered as possible, and avoid overly personal questions when they aren't relevant to the patient's care. When conducting a pelvic exam, offer to elevate the head of the table past 30 degrees so that the patient can more easily see what is happening during the exam; this can make the experience less uncomfortable for some patients.
- Offer patients choice.
- Explain what you will do, how you will do it, and why it is necessary.
- Use more medical/scientific words to make your language as neutral as possible.

7. *A note for male medical students*: It can be challenging to be a male learner in a field with mostly female patients receiving care for often-intimate concerns, from mostly female providers. Patients may prefer to have you not participate in their care or perform pelvic exams on them. The extent to which you respect your patients' autonomy and preferences will factor into how you are evaluated – the tenets of professionalism in medicine include respecting patient autonomy, prioritizing patient welfare, and demonstrating compassion and respect for others.

That said, it would be a disservice to your education to complete an OB-GYN rotation without effectively learning to conduct a pelvic exam or other important principles of the field. With this balance in mind, you can optimize your OB-GYN learning as a male medical student by:

- Asking for permission early and often
- Speaking slowly and doing your best to maintain a calm presence
- Using unassuming body language

– Always deferring to your patient's preferences
8. *Sex and gender*. This chapter sometimes uses the terms "female," "woman/women," and she/her pronouns when referring to patients with pelvic anatomy that may include a vagina, uterus, ovaries, and/or fallopian tubes. However, this should not be prescriptive, and OB-GYN can often involve care for patients with nonbinary genders. Sex typically refers to a patient's sex assigned at birth (female, male), while gender refers to a patient's gender identity, which can fall anywhere on a spectrum and may or may not align with biological sex. As the medical community works to be more inclusive and welcoming, we sometimes make mistakes; feedback helps us to grow toward a healthier learning environment together.
9. *The OB-GYN H&P*. Since OB-GYN has many conditions and questions that are not encountered in other parts of medicine, the H&P has additional aspects that are different from a typical medical or surgical H&P. Here is a *full* OB-GYN H&P template:

■■ ID and Chief Complaint

Include age, Gs & Ps, LMP (if not pregnant) or gestational age (if pregnant), and CC.

■■ HPI

Conventional format – OPQRSTAA (onset, provoking factors, quality, radiation, severity, timing and duration, alleviating factors, associated symptoms)

■■ ROS

Conventional format, with particular attention to …
– GYN-related:
  – Abdominal/pelvic pain
  – Vaginal: abnormal discharge, abnormal bleeding, dyspareunia (pain with vaginal intercourse)
  – Urinary: dysuria, hesitancy, urgency, incontinence
  – Bowel: change in bowel habits, rectal bleeding, dyschezia (pain with bowel movements)
  – For post-/perimenopausal woman – hot flashes/night sweats, vaginal dryness, abnormal bleeding, irritability, depression, mood changes
– OB-related ("the 5 questions")
  – Vaginal bleeding?
  – Leaking fluid or discharge?
  – (only if >20 weeks) Do you feel the baby moving? If so, how often?
  – (only if >20 weeks) Are you having contractions? If so, how often and how strong?
  – (only if >20 weeks) Any headaches, vision changes, or right upper abdominal pain?

■ Past Gyn History
  – Menses:
  – Age at menarche and/or menopause
  – LMP
  – Frequency, duration, and quality of periods
    – If heavy, attempt to quantify pad or tampon use, and ask about passage of clots
  – Pain with periods (dysmenorrhea)?

For example, say: "it's important to me that patients' preferences for their type of provider are honored, so please let me know if you'd prefer for someone else to conduct this exam. As a student doctor, I feel comfortable performing the exam with the assistance of a chaperone, who may provide feedback. What is your preference?"
If the patient is comfortable with you conducting the exam, say "If at any time you feel uncomfortable, please let us know and we will pause or switch places – whatever you prefer."

Standout Tip: Practice taking a full OB-GYN H&P with a classmate before doing so with a patient. There are many elements that do not appear elsewhere in medicine, and asking some questions can be awkward. If you're able to collect and present a comprehensive OB-GYN H&P early in your rotation, you will take more from the rotation, and your preceptors will be impressed.

Question Box: Can you think of why each of these questions is important during pregnancy? We'll dive into this in detail in "OB" Section 8.2.3.3.

Question Box: Can you think of why this is important? Answer: Early menarche and late menopause are associated with some breast and ovarian cancers.

Common Error: Remember that these are intimate questions, so stick to what is clinically relevant; if a patient has a new sexual partner, it may be important to complete STI testing. Though some clinicians ask patients how many lifetime sexual partners they have had, this information is often not relevant if they haven't had new partners recently.

Pearl: To aid nonjudgmental contraceptive counseling for patients at risk for unplanned pregnancy, ask: "Could you get pregnant with any of your sexual partners?"

Standout Tip: Questions to ask to assess for complications: "Did they give you any medicines for bleeding?" "Did you need a transfusion or other procedures or surgeries?"

Pearl: It can be uncomfortable to ask patients about abortion given the stigma associated with it. However, one in four women in the United States has at least one abortion, and this aspect of the history can be important in some circumstances. All patients should be screened alone for IPV, sexual partners, and prior pregnancies or STIs. The presence of partners, family members, and even children may lead patients not to disclose their entire history.

- Sexual History:
  - Sexually active? Partner(s) of same sex, opposite, or both? New partners in the last 6 months?
  - Pain with sex? (dyspareunia)
  - Hx of STIs? (Gonorrhea, Chlamydia, Trichomonas, HSV, HPV, syphilis, HIV, Hep B)
- Contraception (if heterosexually active):
  - Current past/methods? STI prevention (i.e., condoms?)
- Pap History:
  - Last Pap?
  - Prior abnormals?
- Other GYN problems? (e.g., fibroids)
- If menopausal:
  - Hot flashes, night sweats?
  - Vaginal dryness?
  - History of hormone/estrogen replacement therapy?

- **Past OB History**
- G _ P _ _ _ _ (TPAL)
  For each pregnancy beyond the first trimester...
- Date and type of delivery (vaginal, operative vaginal, C/S – if C/S, indication?)
- Gestational age, sex, birth weight
- Complications?
  To fill in "TPAL," ask specifically about other pregnancies, including...
- Spontaneous abortions (a.k.a. miscarriage). If yes,
  - Did they pass spontaneously, or require a procedure?
  - Any complications?
- Induced abortions (a.k.a. therapeutic or elective interruption of a pregnancy). If yes,
  - Medical or surgical?
  - First or second trimester?
  - Any complications?
- Ectopics. If yes,
  - Treated medically or surgically?
  - If surgery was performed, was the tube conserved or removed?
  - Did they require blood transfusion?

- **Past Medical and Surgical History**
- Ask about any chronic/ongoing medical problems including diabetes, cardiovascular disease, pulmonary disease, neurologic problems, GI issues, etc.
- Ask whether they've had surgeries. If they've had abdominal surgery, ask:
  - Which surgery
  - If it was open vs. laparoscopic
  - Whether there were complications

- **Non-OB-GYN Health Maintenance**
- Risk assessment for cardiovascular disease and diabetes
- Mammograms (if >40 or elevated risk)
- Colonoscopies (if >50 or elevated risk)
- Osteoporosis screening (if menopausal or elevated risk)
- *Medications*
- *Allergies*

- **Family History**
- History of bleeding disorders? (e.g., significant bleeding with dental procedures, after childbirth, after surgery)
- Cervical, endometrial, ovarian, breast, or colon cancers?

- **Social History**
- Ask who they live with and who else lives there
    - Relationship status and screen for intimate partner violence (IPV)
- Work
- Tobacco/alcohol/substance use

Pearl: Use the AHRQ ePSS app in clinic to check which primary care screenings your patient is due for. OB-GYNs are sometimes the only healthcare provider their patient sees and often manage breast cancer screening. That said, OB-GYNs are not primary care providers – if you can, you should do everything you can to plug your OB-GYN patients into primary care if they don't have a PCP.

Question Box: Why do we ask about these cancers specifically? Answer: A significant family history of some/all of these malignancies could suggest Lynch syndrome (a.k.a. HNPCC) or other familial cancer syndromes.

Pearl: IPV screening has an "A" evidence rating from the USPSTF. The more often these difficult questions are asked, the less stigmatizing they become for patients, and the more likely disclosure is, enabling intervention if safe and desired.
One example of a screening protocol (the STAT tool) includes the questions:
Have you ever been in a relationship where your partner has pushed or slapped you?
Have you ever been in a relationship where your partner threatened you with violence?
Have you ever been in a relationship where your partner has thrown, broken, or punched things?

Question Box: What do these questions indicate?
Answer: These signs indicate a state of hyperandrogenism, often seen in anovulatory conditions, such as polycystic ovarian syndrome, or in congenital adrenal hyperplasia.

Question Box: Why is evaluating for distention or ascites important in the OB-GYN physical?
Answer: These are often the only physical exam findings present in early ovarian malignancy.

Pearl: Use a systems-based approach to develop your differential.

Standout Tip: Always include (1) the most dangerous and (2) the most likely diagnoses in your differential.

Pearl: Specify that you're interested in the first day of the LMP when talking to patients; many people think of when their period ended when asked "when was your last period?", but it's the first day that matters for pregnancy dating.

- **Physical Exam**
  - Vitals
  - General appearance (Hirsutism? Acne? Virilization?)
  - Examine thyroid, lymph nodes, heart, lungs, (± breasts), abdomen, extremities
  - Look for surgical scars on the abdomen and evidence of distension or ascites, and palpate for masses, organomegaly, or herniation.
  - Pelvic exam (only if a resident/attending present explicitly told you to, and never without a chaperone/assistant):
    - Inspect the vulva, urethra, and perineum.
    - Bimanual exam (palpation of the cervix, uterus, and adnexa).
    - Speculum exam >inspect cervix and vaginal walls; take Pap and STI samples if needed.
    - Rectovaginal exam can be performed for patients with known/suspected GYN malignancy, endometriosis, pelvic pain, or adnexal masses and in patients over 50 to check for anal/rectal masses or malignancy.

Not every point above is relevant for all encounters. For example, for a patient with a ruptured ectopic in the ED, her family history is largely irrelevant, and for a menopausal patient presenting for routine gynecologic care, the details of her pregnancy history are not necessarily important. For a patient coming in for a new OB visit, on the other hand, a comprehensive history should be taken.

Broadly speaking, your notes should be complete and include all of the important information, but as brief and to the point as possible. OB-GYNs are surgeons and do not often write out the long differentials, reasoning, etc. that is sometimes seen in medicine notes. That said, especially as a student, the more you explain about your reasoning, the better. Explain why a reasonable diagnosis isn't on your differential.

8.2   Obstetrics

8.2.1   OB Fundamentals

"OB" (short for "Obstetrics") indicates everything related to pregnancy, including both general obstetrics (low-to-moderate-risk pregnancies) and maternal-fetal medicine (high-risk pregnancy and prenatal diagnosis). A few important principles for OB:

1. *Pregnancy dating*
   - Estimated Due Date (EDD/EDC) = 40 weeks from first day of the LMP (because this is easier to track than date of conception, which we don't always know)
   - Preterm <37 weeks
   - Term = 37 weeks to 40 weeks 6 days
   - Late term = 41 weeks to 41 weeks 6 days
   - Post-term ≥42 weeks
2. A history of something (e.g., preeclampsia, preterm delivery) in a prior pregnancy is almost always a risk factor for the same (something) in subsequent pregnancies.

Obstetrics and Gynecology

3. *The OB one-liner*. For every single OB patient you present, include:
   - Age
   - Gs & Ps
   - Gestational age and method of dating (ultrasound vs. LMP vs. in vitro fertilization (IVF) embryo transfer date)
   - CC

   For example: "This is a 31-year-old G3P1011 at 32 weeks 4 days by 9-week ultrasound consistent with LMP, here for a routine prenatal visit."
4. *Nulliparity/primiparity/multiparity*
   - "nullip" = no prior deliveries (used if this is their first delivery)
   - "primip" = one prior delivery (used if this is their second delivery)
   - "multip" = >1 prior delivery (used if this is their third pregnancy or higher)
5. *The five questions*
   - For pregnancies <20 weeks, no matter the setting, ALWAYS ask patients about:
     1. *Vaginal bleeding* ("Have you noticed any vaginal bleeding?")
     2. *Leaking fluid or discharge* ("Have you noticed any leaking fluid or discharge?")

Question Box: Why is each of these points important for providers to know?
Answer: Age is almost always relevant, for both medical and social reasons.
Gs & Ps put the patient into the OB context; is this a first pregnancy, or have they had many before? What were the outcomes of prior pregnancies? All of these factors impact clinical decision-making.
Gestational age is important for all pregnancy-related care.
CC – the reason you are evaluating and presenting the patient – is critical for obvious reasons.

Pearl: These are the technical definitions. In real life, patients having their first baby (i.e., nulliparous patients) are sometimes referred to as "primips," or "primiparous," and patients who have had at least one baby (i.e., primiparous and multiparous patients) are all often referred to as "multips."
To make sure you are being clear and it doesn't seem like you misunderstand these often misused terms,
If it's their first delivery, say they're nulliparous.
If they've had more than one prior delivery, say they're multiparous.
If you ever feel uncertain, just say how many prior deliveries they've had.

Pearl: Think of these five questions as the "ROS" of pregnancy. ALWAYS include the answers to them in your notes and presentations. We'll get into why they are so important in ► Sect. 8.2.3.2.

8

Question Box: Why is right upper abdominal pain important in screening for preeclampsia?
Answer: In the preeclamptic state, liver swelling causes stretching of "Glisson's capsule," which in turn activates pain receptors localizing to the RUQ.

Common Error: Not emailing a preceptor before a clinic session with them is a missed opportunity to demonstrate your initiative and preparation. This email is an opportunity to clarify questions you have about clinic location and timing, access to medical records, and expectations. For example, "My understanding is that your clinic is located in the Green Zone of Building C, 3rd floor. Is this correct for Thursday?", or "I am able to view your schedule in the online medical record; are there any specific patients you recommend I prepare to see?"

For pregnancies >20 weeks, no matter the setting, ask (1) and (2) and add:

3. *Fetal movement* ("Have you been feeling the baby move? If so, how often?")
4. *Contractions* ("Have you been feeling any contractions? If so, how often and how strong are they?")
5. *Preeclampsia symptoms* ("Any headaches, vision changes, or right upper abdominal pain?")
6. There are MANY abbreviations in OB care. Consider printing an online chart of the most common, and have it handy as you encounter unfamiliar terms.

This section contains content on *prenatal care* (i.e., everything leading up to delivery), *intrapartum care* (i.e., management of labor and delivery), *postpartum care* (i.e., management after delivery), and certain high-risk conditions. You will find the following checklists and note templates:

Checklists:
- New OB clinic visit
- Return OB clinic visit
- OB triage
- Postpartum visit

Templates:
- OB triage note
- OB triage patient presentation (includes example)
- Laboring patient presentation (includes example)

8.2.2 Prenatal Care

Refer to ◘ Fig. 8.3 for an overview of key points related to pregnancy dating, maternal and fetal physiology, and the clinical care schedule throughout pregnancy.

8.2.2.1 Preparing for OB Clinic
Introduce Yourself (1–3 Days Before Clinic)

To prepare for OB clinic, email your preceptor ahead of time to introduce yourself, and ask what you can do to prepare. If possible, send this email

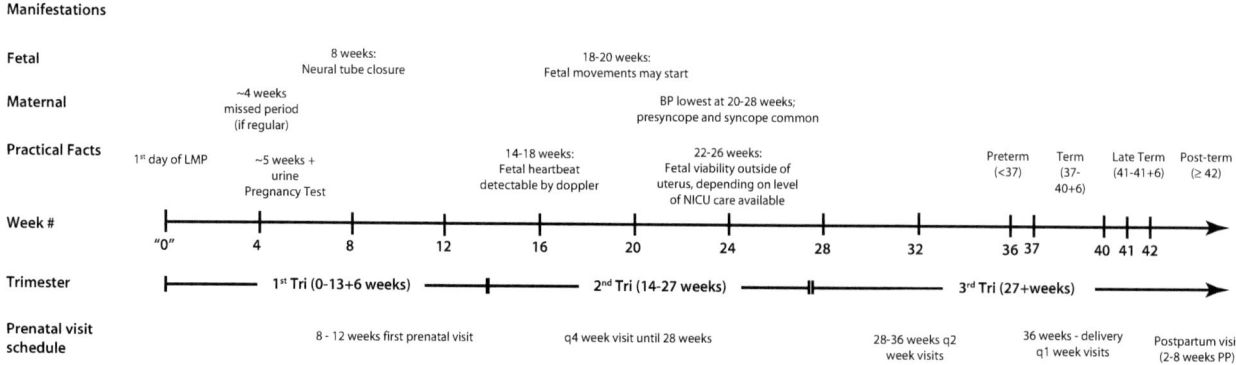

◘ **Fig. 8.3** Maternal and fetal physiology, pregnancy dating, and prenatal care schedule

24–72 hours beforehand so that you have time to complete any preparatory tasks they recommend.

If they respond with specific instructions, e.g., "read this chapter" or "prepare to see patients x, y and z," do those things! If they name specific patients you should prepare to see, follow the "prep your list" instructions below. If they don't respond or if they respond but say "nothing to prepare," this doesn't mean you're off the hook. If you have access to the medical record, prepare to see all patients by prepping a patient list per the "prep your list" instructions below. If you don't have access to the medical record, prepare blank templates for at least four patients on a sheet of paper or notecards per the instructions below. Regardless of medical records access, you should have at least one learning objective for each clinic session. This way, you'll be ready for anything.

Prep Your List (0–24 Hours Before Clinic)

Prepare a sheet of paper divided into sections for each patient, or make a notecard for each patient. For each patient, organize a notecard/section of paper into nine sections (◘ Table 8.1):

For each patient:

- Populate sections 1a–6 and 8 on your paper/notecard by:
  - Reading their most recent OB clinic note
  - Skimming through their other OB clinic notes for this pregnancy
  - Supplementing with other (non-OB) notes or info in their patient profile
- Leave space 1b–c (the HPI and ROS) and 7 (the exam) blank so that you can fill them in during the clinic visit.
- For 9 (A&P), fill in the predictable routine prenatal to-dos based on the checklists below, and leave space for any other to-dos for issues that come up during the visit.

Here is an example of what one completed pre-clinic template could look like (◘ Table 8.2):

If you're thinking about prepping a full clinic session's worth of patients, you may be thinking: "this is crazy! There are 20 patients on this list for a half day of clinic, there's no way I'm going to see all of them. Why should I prepare all of them?" You're right – OB clinic lists are crazy! But if you want to get the

Standout Tip: If there is social space, tell your preceptor about your learning objectives, and ask if they can help you achieve them and provide feedback. For example, for your first clinic, this might be "taking an OB-GYN history," or "performing a pelvic exam"; by the end of your clerkship, this might include "take a complete history in 10 minutes, perform a pelvic exam, and discuss a plan of care with the patient." They will be impressed by your initiative!

! Common Error: Recognize that this paper or note card contains confidential information! Be very careful about its storage and disposal to protect patient privacy.

! Common Error: Though it is important to prepare, avoid getting bogged down in the details and spending hours preparing for clinic. The histories don't need to be perfectly detailed unless they're pertinent to the pregnancy. Aim to spend about 1.5–2 hours TOTAL preparing for clinic. This means that you'll skim many patients' notes instead of reading them all thoroughly. If you've skimmed over them all, though, you'll encounter conditions, complaints, treatments, etc. that you haven't heard of before, and you should ask your preceptor questions about those things if/when you don't understand them.

◘ Table 8.1 OB clinic prep

1. Header/one-liner
   (a) CC
   (b) HPI
   (c) ROS (*the five questions if >20 weeks; the two questions if <20 weeks*)

2. OB Hx
   (a) This pregnancy
   (b) Prior pregnancies

3. Gyn Hx
   (Pap hx, STI hx, pertinent sexual hx, contraception)

4. Med/Surg Hx

5. Fam/Soc Hx

6. Meds/all

7. Exam
   BP ___ Weight ____
   Fetal heart rate ____
   Fundal height ____

8. Labs/imaging
   Urine dip ____

9. A/P

■ Table 8.2 Example of complete OB clinic template

8:00 AM Marisol H. 29ys G2P1001 　CC: New OB visit 　HPI: 　ROS: 　　Vaginal bleeding ____ Leading fluid/Discharge _____	
OB Hx 　G2: Current 　G1: Uncomplicated spontaneous vaginal 　delivery at 39 weeks, 19 months ago	**Med/Surg Hx** 　Iron deficiency anemia, Hgb 10.1 　Appendectomy (lsc, age 18)
Gyn Hx 　Last Pap 3 years ago, no hx of abnormal 　Paps 　Chlamydia at age 19, treated w/o 　complications 　Sexually active with male partner, 　previously used birth control pills	**Fam/Soc Hx** 　Fam: Mother s/p hysterectomy for 　endometrial cancer at age 58 　Soc: Lives with partner, denied IPV 　previously; Works full-time as chemical 　engineer; No hx of smoking, 4 drinks/week 　outside of pregnancy; no other substance use
	Meds/All 　Prenatal vitamin, Fe tablets 　Allergy to penicillin (anaphylaxis)
Exam 　BP ___ Weight ____ 　Fetal heart rate ____ 　Fundal height ____	**Labs/Imaging** 　Urine dip _____
A/P 　-　1st tri labs (Blood type & Ab status, CBC, Hep B, Hep C, HIV, Syphilis, Rubella, Varicella) 　-　Pelvic exam ☐ Pap (due bc 29 ys and last 3 yrs ago), GC/CT 　-　Urine culture 　-　1st tri screenings (aneuploidy and/or genetics) 　-　+/- ultrasound depending on LMP (not needed if pt is asymptomatic and certain of LMP 　　with regular periods)	

8

most out of clinic and show your preceptor that you're an engaged learner, then yes, you should prepare – at least briefly – to see every single patient. As Louis Pasteur said, "chance favors the prepared mind" – if you're ready for everything, you're setting yourself up for success. When your preceptor sees that you read about every patient and had questions about their care, they will be impressed with your diligence. Further, when you do see patients, you'll know exactly what to think about and present in your "plan" if/when you present the patient because OB clinic is so formulaic.

Learn and Shine (in Clinic)

Your templates are prepped, you've read about pregnancy and prenatal care (in the section below this one), and you're ready to go! Your role in OB clinic will depend on the clinic and its structure, staffing, and volume. There will likely be non-physician providers who conduct the initial OB visit counseling and check vitals and fetal heart tones, run the urine dipstick, and ask "the five questions" at each visit. Some of these routine tasks are great opportunities for you to make yourself useful and to get the hang of some concrete skills. Do not be disappointed if you prepared the entire list only to find that your resident or attending prefers that you shadow – you should creatively weave in the questions you prepared the night before to demonstrate that you closely reviewed their histories (e.g., I noticed that Ms. L received RhoGAM after vaginal bleeding early in her pregnancy due to her Rh- blood type, do we typically provide RhoGAM a second time during the same pregnancy?)

8.2.2.2 Prenatal Care: Important Content and Checklists

The New OB Visit

- Is this pregnancy planned? Desired?
- Full OB-GYN history and physical (per template in Introduction).

Pearl: Wards' life is busy – if you absolutely cannot prep the full list in detail, it is better to get the name, patient age, gestational age, and chief complaint, and jot down a list of "to-dos" for all of the patients than be overly thorough and miss these basic details for patients at the end of your list. Triage as necessary.

Standout Tip: Befriend the medical assistant(s), nurse(s), and advanced practitioner(s) who work at the clinic, and ask them how you can help. If it feels appropriate, ask if you can (1) observe a "new OB" intake/counseling visit, and (2) spend a visit or clinic session working with them to learn how to check for fetal heart tones, measure the fundal height, and interpret a urine dipstick. Once they've shown you these things, if it feels appropriate, ask if you can try. All of these actions will help you learn about prenatal care and demonstrate that you are engaged learner.

This is a long one! All subsequent OB visits are much shorter.

Common Error: Never assume that a pregnancy is a good thing – pay attention to the patient's emotions and ask this question as it seems appropriate. By stating whether the pregnancy is desired/undesired in your oral presentation, you demonstrate to your resident/attending that you have situational and social awareness and make their job easier!

Pearl: Uncontrolled DM in early pregnancy increases risk for miscarriage and congenital malformations.

Pearl: The 1-hour GTT screening test is only validated in the third trimester of pregnancy, so it isn't always clear exactly what should be done with its results during the first trimester. On the other hand, the pregnancy increases RBC turnover, artificially decreasing the Hgb A1c compared to that in nonpregnant individuals. Remember these physiologic principles as you consider diabetes screening during the first trimester.

Question Box: Do you know why asthma history is important during pregnancy?
Answer:
(1) Patients may experience exacerbations during pregnancy, and (2) it is a contraindication to the medication carboprost (a prostaglandin analog that can cause bronchospasm), which can otherwise be used to decrease blood loss in postpartum hemorrhage.

Standout Tip: All patients should be screened for IPV at least once during pregnancy. This is often done by an intake nurse at the first prenatal visit, but the more often these questions are asked, the less stigmatizing they are for patients, and the more likely disclosure is, enabling intervention if safe and desired. Each time you present a patient, report the result of your IPV screen.

- In your medical history, ask specifically about:
  - Hypertension (outside of or within pregnancy)
    - If yes, get baseline preeclampsia labs and urinalysis
  - Diabetes
    - If they have obesity or a history of gestational diabetes, screen for pre-gestational diabetes with a 1-hour glucose tolerance test (GTT) or Hgb A1c.
  - Asthma
    - If yes, how severe?
    - Meds? Hospitalizations? History of intubation?
- Depression/psychiatric screen (PHQ-2 or other validated screening tools).
- Screen for IPV and human trafficking.
- Pregnancy dating:
  - By LMP: if the patient has a certain LMP and had regular periods, they had a positive urine pregnancy test, and they have no symptoms concerning for abnormal pregnancy (i.e., pain, vaginal bleeding, fever), they don't need an ultrasound! That said, <50% of women know the first day of their LMP.
  - By ultrasound: the earlier, the more accurate for dating (ideally within first trimester, or before 13w6d).
  - If IVF, date by embryo transfer date.
- Labs: Blood type and Ab status, CBC, Hep B, Hep C, HIV, syphilis, rubella, varicella.
- Pap: if >21 and no Pap in the last 3 years, refer to ASCCP guidelines.

▣ Table 8.3 Risk of aneuploidy by age

Age	Risk of Trisomy 21	Risk of any aneuploidy
30	1/1000	1/400
35	1/350	1/175
40	1/100	1/60

- GC/CT if age <26 or history of STIs.
- Urine culture (screening for asymptomatic bacteriuria).
  - Asymptomatic bacteriuria = high levels of bacteria in urine without symptoms
  - Dx criteria: single bacteria strain (>10^5 CFU CFU/mL in two consecutive voided samples or >10^2 in one catheterized sample)
  - Trt: Abx tailored to culture results, and f/u to ensure clearance
- Offer genetic screening (cystic fibrosis, Hgb electrophoresis, Tay-Sachs, spinal muscular atrophy).
- Offer screening for aneuploidies.
  - Risk of aneuploidy goes up 3× for every 5 years over age 30 (▣ Table 8.3).

Question Box: Unlike everywhere else in medicine, asymptomatic bacteriuria should be treated during pregnancy! Can you think of why?
Answer: In the setting of pregnancy, asymptomatic bacteriuria increases risk for UTI due to urinary tract stasis and changes in immune system function, and UTIs can lead to adverse pregnancy outcomes. Thus, all patients should be screened at least once in early pregnancy (12–16 weeks) and treated if bacteriuria is present.

Pearl: In patients with sickle cell trait, check culture each trimester due to increased risk for pyelonephritis.

Question Box: Why is trimethoprim-sulfamethoxazole, a first-line treatment for UTI outside of pregnancy, contraindicated in the first trimester?
Answer: Because it interferes with folic acid metabolism, affecting neural tube development.

Common Error: It is important to recognize that these screening tests are not diagnostic – they help with risk stratification, but do not give definitive answers.
Patients should thus recognize the implications of testing. For example, for aneuploidy risk, if the test came back as "elevated risk" and they subsequently were diagnosed with an aneuploid pregnancy, what would they do about it? Further, in screening for CF and hemoglobinopathies, results have implications for the patient's families.

8

Pearl: The quad and sequential screens are older and now less common, but still useful and accurate, especially if patients can't or don't present for care early in pregnancy or their insurance doesn't cover newer screening tests (as many don't). The sequential screen in particular is used less frequently these days.

! • Common Error: Prenatal screening tests help with risk stratification, but do not provide diagnoses. To definitively diagnose any condition prenatally, the chorionic villi or amniotic fluid must be sampled.
Remember: "testing involves tissue"!

Pearl: BP decreases during first to second trimesters, is lowest at 20–28 weeks, and then returns to normal during the third trimester. High BP in third tri should raise concern for hypertensive disorders of pregnancy.

Pearl: Fundal height should be within ± 2 cm of weeks after 20 weeks; 2 readings outside of this should prompt ultrasound to assess fetal growth.

– Quad screen (12 weeks).
  – AFP, ß-hCG, estriol, inhibin A
– Sequential screen (Part 1 @ 11–14 weeks, Part 2 @ 15–18 weeks).
  – 11–14 weeks: Nuchal translucency & PAPP-A
  – 15–18 weeks: AFP, ß-hCG, estriol, inhibin A
– Cell-free DNA (MATERNAL serum, looking at fetal DNA) (after 10 weeks).
  – T13, 18, 21, X&Y chromosomes, but doesn't tell you about other anomalies
– F/u with definitive testing.
  – Chorionic villus sampling (CVS) (10–13 weeks) (0.2% miscarriage)
  – Amniocentesis (15–20 weeks) (0.1–0.3% miscarriage) (IAI, alloimmunization in Rh-negative mothers)
= Plans for breastfeeding. There are higher rates of starting breastfeeding when providers discuss at a first or early visit.
= If patient has had a prior cesarean, discuss their plans for route of delivery. Some patients will want to have a trial of labor after cesarean (TOLAC). Check delivery note from prior birth for contraindications to TOLAC (surgery involving the contractile, or top, portion of the uterus – most often a classical cesarean section or myomectomy).

The Return OB Visit
= BP (compare to priors).
= Weight.
= Review pre-pregnancy BMI to see how much they should be gaining.
= Track weight along curve (often available in office or in online record, or can search for one online; see recommendations below).
= Fetal heart rate (FHR) (after 10–14 weeks; auscultate for 30–60 seconds).
= Normal findings:
  – In early pregnancy, FHR is typically in the 160 s.
  – After 28 weeks, FHR increases with fetal movement (evidence of maturing autonomic nervous system).
  – Near term, FHR ranges from 110 to 160.
= Potentially abnormal findings:
  – Absence of fetal heart sounds, which may indicate early pregnancy, improper technique, faulty equipment, or fetal death
  – Any decrease in FHR that doesn't return to baseline immediately
= Fundal height (cm ≈ weeks).
= Urine dipstick.
  – Proteinuria could be evidence of preeclampsia.
  – Glucose could be evidence of gestational diabetes.
  – Blood and leukocyte esterase could be evidence of asymptomatic bacteriuria (which you treat, unlike everywhere else in medicine!)
= Review labs.
  – Second visit: Blood type and Ab status, CBC, Hep B, Hep C, HIV, syphilis, rubella, varicella
  – Subsequent visits: per ◻ Fig. 8.3
= Review any new US results.
= The five questions:
  – <20 weeks: (1) VB, (2) leaking fluid/discharge?
  – >20 weeks: Add (3) fetal movements (start at 18–20 weeks), (4) contractions, and (5) preeclampsia symptoms?

— Additional tasks based on gestational age:
  – 11–14 weeks: Offer first trimester screening.
  – 15–20 weeks: Offer second trimester screening if first trimester screening was not done.
  – 18–20 weeks: Fetal survey (ultrasound).
  – 24–28 weeks:
    – CBC
    – tDAP
    – 1-hour glucose tolerance test (GTT) → if >140, f/u with diagnostic 3-hour GTT
    – Antibody screen if RH negative > RhoGAM if Rh neg and ABS is negative @28 weeks
  – 26–30 weeks: Depression screen and re-screen for IPV.
  – 32 weeks:
    – Contraception plan
    – Birth plan (TOLAC, or "trial of labor after cesarean," discussion if needed)
  – 36 weeks:
    – Group B Strep (GBS) screening (not needed if patient has/had GBS-bacteriuria)
    – Ultrasound for position and EFW
  – 38–40 weeks: Cervical exams.
  – 41 weeks: Recommend induction of labor; if expectant management; twice weekly antenatal testing

To write up new and return OB clinic notes, ask your preceptors if they have a template they prefer, as they are the ones following up on your documentation. If they don't, construct a note following the format of the checklists above and the "OB-GYN H&P" template in the introduction to this chapter.

Key Points for Pregnancy Counseling

— Weight gain: "eating for two" is a MYTH! In reality, they'll be eating for ~1.15
  – Weight gain recommendations depend on pre-pregnancy BMI.
  – Normal weight before pregnancy → gain 25–35 pounds
  – Underweight before pregnancy → gain 28–40 pounds
  – Overweight before pregnancy → gain 15–25 pounds
  – Twin pregnancy, normal weight before pregnancy → gain 35–45 pounds
  – Too little weight gain → risk for small for gestational age infants and associated difficulty with breastfeeding, risk for illness, and developmental delay.
  – Too much weight gain → risk for large for gestational age (macrosomia), cesarean delivery, gestational diabetes mellitus, preeclampsia, postpartum weight retention, and offspring obesity.
— Foods and substances to avoid:
  – Unpasteurized dairy or juices (listeria)
  – Large fish (swordfish, tuna, king mackerel) (excess mercury)
  – Un/undercooked meat or fish (salmonella)
  – Preserved deli meats (nitrites, which are teratogenic)
  – Alcohol, tobacco, marijuana

Pearl: The flu shot can and should be given anytime during pregnancy. Pregnant patients are more likely to develop severe disease with influenza infection; vaccination reduces risk by ~40% and protects their newborn.

Standout Tip: The Edinburgh Postpartum Depression Scale (EPDS) is a validated, frequently used tool for depression screening in the perinatal period and is free online.

Standout Tip: Planning for postpartum contraception should be done well before delivery and, in fact, can be discussed throughout pregnancy. Always document postpartum contraception plans (or if the patient hasn't decided on a method, document what they're considering). This is especially important if they're interested in a postplacental IUD (i.e., an IUD placed immediately after delivery of the placenta), as this needs to be made obvious to the inpatient team when they're admitted to the L&D floor.

Question Box: Why do you think postpartum contraception is important?
In addition to facilitating reproductive autonomy, contraception enables more effective pregnancy planning. As we'll discuss below, up to 40% of patients do not attend their postpartum visit, which often means that they do not obtain a reliable contraceptive method in the postpartum period. Optimal pregnancy spacing for maternal and child health includes waiting at least 18 months to become pregnant again after a delivery, and shorter interpregnancy intervals have been associated with increased risk of preterm birth, low birth weight, and preeclampsia.

8

Pearl: Prenatal vitamins should be taken daily and should contain 800–1000 mcg of folic acid. If a patient can't tolerate prenatal vitamin, they can try folic acid by itself.

Question Box: Why should NSAIDs be avoided during pregnancy?
Answer: NSAID use in early pregnancy increases likelihood of miscarriage and malformations, whereas use after 30-week gestation is associated with premature closure of the fetal ductus arteriosus.

Common Error: Be careful to avoid anchoring in on pregnancy-related diagnoses in pregnant patients. Anytime you see pregnant patients and they have a complaint, treat their complaint as if it were occurring in a nonpregnant patient. If they are stable, though, see if their complaint could be related to the normal physiology of pregnancy or is a common pregnancy-related problem.
Though pregnancy is often the cause of many somatic complaints, other causes should still be ruled out as in a nonpregnant patient, but with attention to potential effects of imaging and diagnostic tests on the fetus.

Pearl: Pregnant people develop a respiratory alkalosis (increased TV decreases the expiratory reserve volume, and with a constant respiratory rate, minute ventilation increases > increased alveolar (PAO2) and arterial (PaO2) PO2, decreased PACO2 and PaCO2).

- Medications:
  - Prenatal vitamin for all
    - Tylenol (acetaminophen) OK
    - Colace (docusate sodium) OK
    - NO NSAIDS (Advil, Aleve, Motrin, Dayquil, NyQuil, etc.)
- Exercise:
  - Generally, continue whatever regimen the patient participated in before pregnancy; however, avoid any activity that could leave a belly bruise or involves significant pressure changes – no SCUBA diving or skydiving!
- Sex:
  - No restrictions unless the patient has placenta previa or vasa previa

Common Complaints and Diagnoses During Pregnancy

- *Lower quadrant pain* could be round ligament pain.
  - The round ligaments attach the uterus to the pelvic side wall and descend down through the inguinal canal; they stretch with the growing uterus, and this hurts!
- Common complaints that tie into physiology of pregnancy.
  - Syncope/presyncope during second trimester often related to low BP from vasodilation.
  - Anemia (dilutional) related to relatively greater increase in plasma volume compared to RBC volume (>rarely, this can cause the symptom "pica," which is the consumption of non-nutritional substances such as dirt or paper).
  - Dyspnea without other signs/symptoms could be related to elevated diaphragm >decreased total lung capacity (TLC) (tidal volume (TV) actually increases during pregnancy, but the compressed diaphragm means that TLC decreases).
  - *Dyspnea with tachycardia, hypoxia, chest pain, and/or associated lower extremity edema* could be a sign of pulmonary embolism (given elevated thrombotic risk during pregnancy) or peripartum cardiomyopathy.
  - *Lower extremity swelling* related to compression of veins returning to the IVC by gravid uterus; OR, during third trimester, can be a sign of preeclampsia > check the BP and urine dipstick!
- *Urinary symptoms* (burning, frequency, urgency).
  - The gravid uterus pushes down on the bladder, causing urinary frequency (polyuria), but this could also be due to a UTI.
  - UTI (lower) = acute cystitis (infection in bladder)
    - Dx criteria: symptoms + leukocyte esterase, WBC count, nitrites; culture 10^5 CFUs/mL of a single organism
    - Trt: OK to treat presumptively with symptoms
  - UTI (upper) = pyelonephritis (infection in urinary system above bladder); + fever, chills, N/V, back/flank pain, CVA tenderness on exam. Pregnant women with pyelo can become VERY sick – 20% develop severe complications like septic shock and can even progress to ARDS.
    - Dx criteria: UA and UCx; CBC with leukocytosis, anemia; typically not imaging, but can use imaging in patients with risk factors for severe complications (e.g., to look for stone). Without radiation, bedside ultrasound can offer clinically useful information on both pyelonephritis (fat stranding) and nephrolithiasis (obstructed ureter → hydronephrosis).
    - Trt: Parenteral abx (admit! This is a complicated UTI based on pregnancy and its ascent in the urinary tract); convert to oral when afebrile for 24–48 hours.

- *Carpal tunnel syndrome* (numbness/tingling in the thumb and first to third fingers).
  - Dx: Phalen's sign, Tinel's sign
  - Trt: Expectant (observe) ➜ wrist splints and physical therapy ➜ surgery if severe

In Summary, to Prepare for and Shine in OB Clinic

- Email your preceptor 1–3 days in advance.
- Complete any advised preparatory reading.
- Prep your list (per instructions above).
- Be nice to/befriend clinic staff.
- For each patient you see, make note of and, if abnormal, incorporate into your A&P:
  - Blood pressure
  - Weight
  - Fetal heart rate and estimated fetal weight at 37+ weeks
  - Fundal height
  - Urine dipstick results
  - Answers to the five questions
- Thank everyone at the end of the clinic session.
- Complete any clinic notes you write from the clinic session that same day/evening

Antenatal Testing: Indications and Interpretations

1. *OB Ultrasound*

There are many indications for ultrasound throughout pregnancy and many findings you should be able to identify.

In the *first trimester*…

- Indications (when to do it?)
- Dating – if LMP is uncertain and/or if periods were not regular
- If any symptoms of potentially abnormal pregnancy – pain, vaginal bleeding, fever
- Screening for aneuploidy (nuchal translucency) – can be done before 14 weeks

- Interpretations (what to look for?)
- Location (intrauterine?).
- Sac (and how many).
- Fetal heart activity?
- Crown-rump length (CRL) – most accurate way to date pregnancy before 14 weeks.
- There are criteria for diagnosing a failed pregnancy (e.g., certain sac size w/o embryo, certain CRL without fetal heart tones, lack of tones after sac has been present for 2 weeks, etc.) – do not memorize them, but know that they exist.

In the *second trimester*…

- Indications
  - Anatomy scan (18–22 weeks)
  - Growth (biometry – biparietal diameter, head circumference, Abd circumference, femur length) (see ◼ Fig. 8.4)
  - Cervical length screening (transvaginal)

! Common Error: Don't duplicate work! Communicate directly with your preceptor regarding which note(s) you are writing.

Pearl: In the first trimester, quality of transvaginal scans is usually better than that of transabdominal scans.

Pearl: Pregnancies without an US before 22 weeks should be considered "sub-optimally dated."

Standout Tip: If you see a patient with a specific anomaly, read about that anomaly – e.g., How sensitive/specific is US for it? What implications does it have for the health of the fetus, both short and long-term?

8

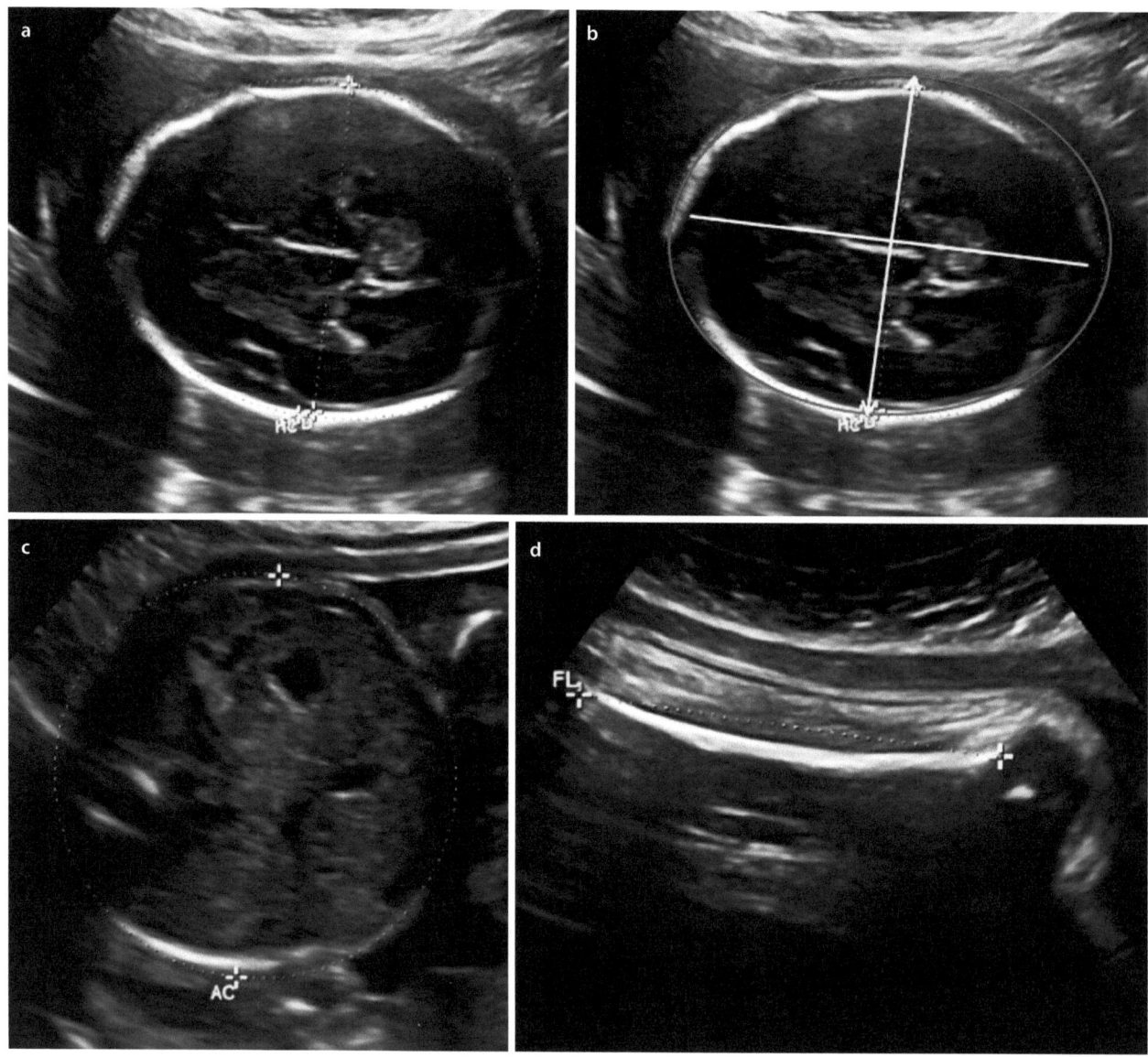

☐ **Fig. 8.4** Biometry. **a** Biparietal diameter. **b** Head circumference. **c** Abdominal circumference. **d** Femur length

- ■ Interpretations
- ═ Placenta
- ═ Fetal anatomy
- ═ Biometry
- ═ Cervix

In the *third trimester…*

- ■ Indications
- ═ Scanning for position and fluid volume.
- ═ Growth (e.g., multifetal gestation, IUGR, gHTN, GDM), q3–4 weeks – in the third tri, this is least accurate (can be off by 20%).
  - – EFW by Hadlock (biometry measurements)
- ═ Decreased fetal movement ➜ biophysical profile (BPP).

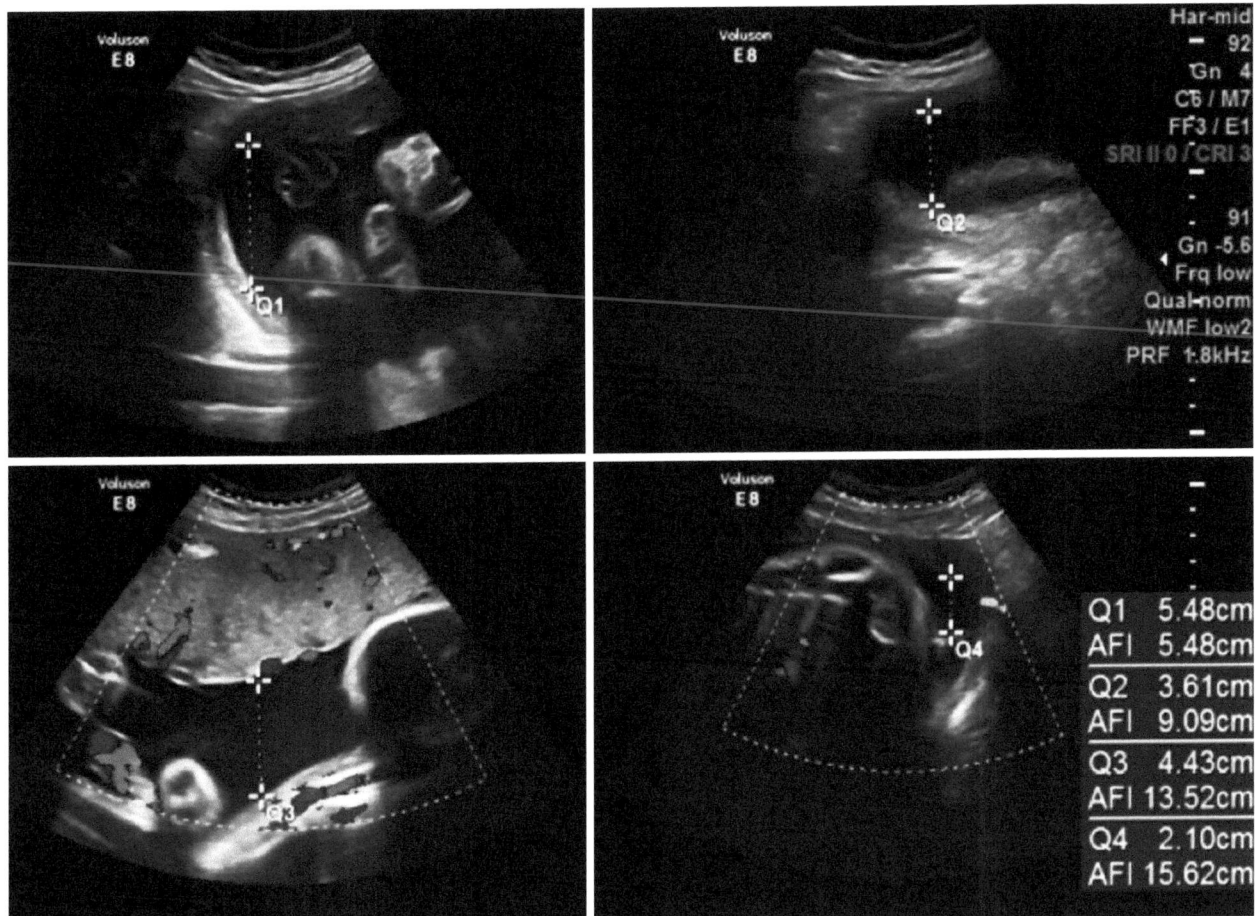

Fig. 8.5 Amniotic fluid index. The deepest pocket devoid of umbilical cord and fetal parts is measured vertically in each of four quadrants of the uterus. The amniotic fluid index, or AFI, is the sum of the four measurements, with normal ranging from 5 to 25 cm. The MVP is obtained by measuring the depth of the single greatest pocket devoid of cord and fetal parts, and normal is 2–8 cm

▪ Interpretations

═ Scanning for position

═ Fluid: AFI (amniotic fluid index; see ▪ Fig. 8.5) or MVP (maximum vertical pocket)
  – Probe along mother's cephalocaudal axis, perpendicular to floor.
  – Make sure there are no fetal parts or cord where you're measuring.
  – Studies have shown less interventions for oligohydramnios when MVP is used (compared to AFI) without negatively impacting perinatal outcomes.
  – Oligo = too little fluid; poly = too much.

═ Growth: Fetal growth restriction ≤ 10%ile
  – Consider umbilical artery Doppler measurements.

═ Biophysical profile (BPP): Five components, score of either 0 or 2 for each (a BPP of 8 to 10 is reassuring):
  – Amniotic fluid volume
  – Fetal tone (>2 flexions/extensions of extremities)
  – Fetal activity (movement of extremities)
  – Fetal breathing movements (>30 seconds continuous effort)
  – Nonstress test (NST) (a test of the fetal heart rate – see below)

Standout Tip: Ask your instructors when they use AFI vs. MVP to assess fluid volume in pregnancy.

Pearl: Normal blood flow through the umbilical artery involves higher-pressure flow during systole and lower-pressure flow during diastole. If there is placental resistance (e.g., due to placental calcification in the setting of preeclampsia), flow during diastole can decrease or become absent or even become reversed.

2. *NST (Non-stress Test)* – commonly used in high-risk pregnancies beginning at 32–34 weeks, or in low-risk pregnancies who have not yet delivered at 40–41 weeks
   - The NST is considered formally reactive (a reassuring sign) if there are two accelerations of the fetal heart rate (FHR) in 20 minutes that are at least 15 beats above the baseline heart rate and last for at least 15 seconds (see ◘ Fig. 8.9a).
   - If non-reactive, assess the fetus with ultrasound.
3. *CST* (contraction stress test, a.k.a. oxytocin challenge test, or OCT) – can be used to determine if a fetus will tolerate labor for patients undergoing induction
   - Obtained by administering oxytocin or nipple stimulation to trigger at least three contractions in 10 minutes and analyzing the FHR tracing during that time
   - Positive (i.e., suggestive of fetal intolerance of labor) if greater than 50% of contractions are associated with late decelerations

8.2.3 Labor and Delivery

The Labor and Delivery (L&D) floor can be highly variable experience depending on the hospital, and within a single L&D floor, days can range from being "slow" with a lot of downtime to "crazy" with no chance to sit down for an entire 12-hour shift. Because of this craziness, a lot of learning happens through observation and participation as you're directed in the moment. There may not be time for formal teaching, but there is often space for questions "on the go," and residents and attendings tend to want to get you as involved as possible if you demonstrate that you are engaged and prepared. To this end, it may be wise to bring your own lunch and/or snacks. Since L&D can be so unpredictable, if you leave the labor floor for lunch, you may miss an opportunity to deliver a baby (among other tasks and learning opportunities!). In general, the more time you spend out on the floor, the more you'll see and do. No active patient issues or deliveries occur in the resident workroom or breakroom!

Things to DO:
- Do your best to be "following" one laboring patient at all times.
  - Introduce yourself to them with a provider.
  - If it feels appropriate, stay in the room with them while they are pushing; be their cheerleader! Help coach them by cheering them on, counting to 10 during pushes if they want counting, get them water, etc.
- When you are not following a patient who is actively pushing, try to work with/follow a resident.
  - The more you are with someone, the less you will miss; that said, give them space (both physical and mental) to do their job.
- When you aren't with a resident, stay near the nursing station so you don't miss updates – things happen in an instant, and you are less likely to miss them if you're working on notes or reading at the nursing station as opposed to a secluded workroom.
- Say "Yes" to all opportunities offered, as long as you feel comfortable with them – e.g., "Do you want to come with me to examine the patient in 3?", "Do you want to try scanning for position?" (YES!)

Pearl: This is a very important time for patients, family members, and friends. L&D nurses are usually the ones managing the second stage. Follow their lead on coaching – they have a TREMENDOUS amount of knowledge and are an underutilized resource in learning about labor! Be sure only to assert yourself and assist in ways that the patient and family deem helpful. Ask, "Is my coaching helpful, or would you prefer something different or quiet?" If other members would like to be more involved in coaching, do not steal the limelight.

- Seize as many opportunities as you can to evaluate patients on your own in triage, write notes, and present patients at signout. The more you do these things, the more you will learn, and the more your evaluators will be able to give you feedback.
- Identify at least one specific, reasonable learning/development goal for yourself each day (e.g., take <5 minutes to present a patient you saw in triage, signing out two patients, etc.) and tell your resident about it at the start of the shift. That way, they can provide feedback on that specific goal.
- If you ever feel uncertain about where you should be (a common experience on the L&D floor), ask for help!

Things to NOT do:
- Be overly close to residents or assume familiarity/friendliness – as stated above, give them space (both physical and mental) to do their job.
- Retreat to the workroom when you feel uncertain of where you should be or when you don't have an actively laboring patient to follow – instead, ask someone if there are things you can help with, or better yet, suggest a topic you could read about and then present to your team when there is downtime.

8.2.3.1 Signout

Five minutes before signout begins at the beginning of a shift, obtain a blank sheet of paper and fold it into eight sections. During signout, do your best to listen closely and take down notes about the laboring patients, filling in each section of your paper with one patient. Try to write down everything that is said as illustrated below with three sections: (1) maternal, (2) fetal, and (3) to-dos. Leave space so that you can update their course throughout your shift.

8.2.3.2 OB Triage

- OB Triage Checklist
- Chart prep (5–10 minutes).
  - Vitals.
  - Start a note (either in the computer or jot down on a piece of paper, using the same framework as the "OB clinic" box) containing the sections in the template below.
  - Populate:
    - History of the current pregnancy
    - Medical and surgical history
    - Past OB history
    - Meds and allergies

> Standout Tip: Don't passively wait to be asked to see a patient in triage. Actively keep an eye on the triage board, and ask your resident/attending if you can quickly go see a new patient as soon as you notice one.

> Standout Tip: By taking notes this way, you'll be aware of what is going on with all of the laboring patients on the floor and will be able to reference your notes for their history in case an opportunity to participate in their care arises, or if a resident or nurse has a question about a patient.

> Common Error: If your patient is hemodynamically unstable or looks "sick" (e.g., seems abnormally fatigued or "out of it," or is in excruciating pain), tell your resident right away. Patient safety is always the #1 priority.

```
Rm 2 - Velasquez                                              To do:
                                                              ☐  Epidural
30 ys G1P0 @ 39 w 6 d (9 wk US), spont labor.    EFW 3496 g   ☐  Re-check @ 9AM
11 PM SROM, 4/60/-3 ☐ 2AM Pit started            Cephalic
☐ 5AM 5/80/-2. Pit now @ 6.                      Cat I
                                                 GBS –
                                                 Rh +
```

▣ Box 8.1 L&D signout template

- See patient (10 mins).
  - History (new and verify info from chart – see below)
    - Ask the five questions!
  - Physical
    - Pay attention to the BP.
    - Estimated fetal weight by Leopold's.
    - Speculum and cervical exam only with resident/midwife/attending.
- Make your plan and prepare to present (5–10 minutes).

If your plan includes a bedside US (most of the time it will), get the ultrasound machine, including gel and a towel, on your way to seeing the patient with your resident.

If your plan includes a cervical exam, get a sterile glove and lubricant jelly ready for your resident.

If your plan includes a speculum exam, get a speculum, lubricant jelly, a few cotton swabs, and nitrazine paper ready (ask a triage nurse to help with this), and leave it in the patient's triage area/room

- Jot down an outline of your presentation using the template below.

- **History**
- CC.
- Confirm the LMP/EDD/gestational age.
- HPI (including "history of the present pregnancy"; see "common OB triage complaints" below for specific questions to ask).
- ROS (ALWAYS ask THE FIVE QUESTIONS).
- Med Hx:
  - "Do you have Diabetes or any problems with blood sugar that you know of?"
  - "Have you ever had Preeclampsia or problems with your blood pressure that you know of?"
  - "Do you have Asthma?" (if yes, how bad? Meds? Hospitalizations? Ever been intubated?) (if YES to ANY of these questions, no carboprost)
  - "Anything else that your doctor was watching or worried about during your pregnancy?"
- OB Hx:
  - Confirm Gs & Ps.
  - For any prior deliveries:
    - Mode of each delivery? (spontaneous vaginal, operative vaginal, i.e., forceps or vacuum, cesarean delivery; if cesarean, why?)
    - Complications?
  - Hx blood transfusions?
- GYN Hx:
  - STI Hx (any active STIs?)
- Surg Hx:
  - Any abdominal surgery?
- Meds, allergies.
- Social Hx: alcohol/tobacco/substance use/IPV screen, "anyone here with you today?"
- Family Hx: typically noncontributory.

Standout Tip: Prepare for your preceptor to be able to efficiently see the patient and carry out a full evaluation.

Reminder! THE FIVE QUESTIONS: Contractions? Leaking fluid? Bleeding? Do you feel the baby moving? Preeclampsia symptoms? (headache, vision changes, RUQ, or epigastric pain?)

Pearl: Triage is the third time/place to ask about IPV and trafficking, since patient can be isolated from attendants easily.

- **Physical**
  - Vital signs!
  - General appearance
  - Cardiopulmonary exam (Always have your stethoscope, because OB-GYNs often don't carry them and sometimes need them!)
  - Abdominal exam (Do they have scars? Can you feel contractions?)
  - Estimated fetal weight (EFW). Determined by Leopold's maneuvers:
    - Palpate the abdomen for the size of the uterus.
    - General estimates:
      - Football sized = 5 lbs or 2500 g
      - Soccer ball sized = 7 lbs or 3300 g
      - Basketball sized = 9 lbs or 4000 g
    - Also used to check position of fetus (breech, transverse, or cephalic)
  - Lower extremity exam
  - If elevated BP, neuro exam (CNs, sensory, motor, reflexes, coordination; at minimum, reflexes, and check for clonus)
  - With a resident/midwife/attending:
    - Sterile speculum exam (Never do a spec or vaginal exam on your own, unless you have been explicitly told to do so by a resident/attending who has seen you do them before!)
    - Cervical exam (see ☐ Fig. 8.6) (You will likely not be doing cervical exams on patients, since they are very invasive and painful and require a

> **Question Box:** Why do we care about reflexes and clonus in an OB patient with elevated BP?
> Answer: Hyperreflexia and clonus are common findings in preeclampsia and can be a warning sign of potential for seizure.

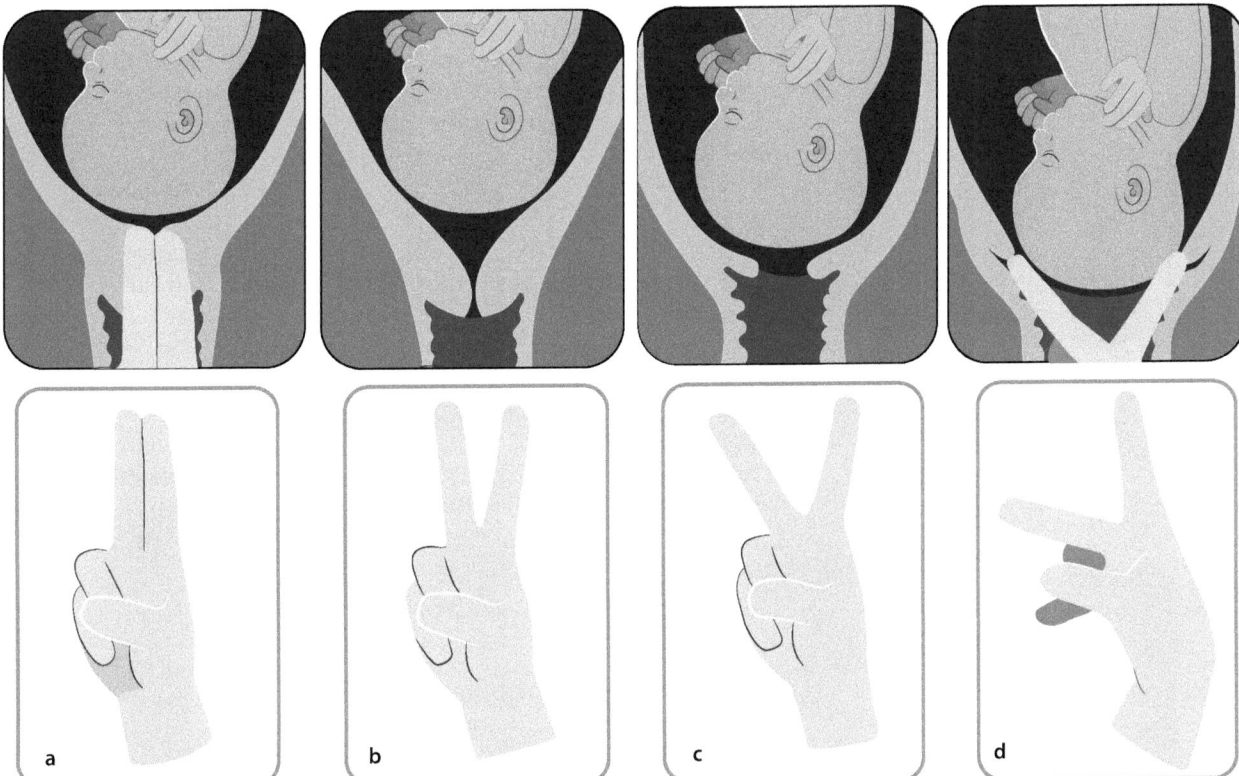

☐ **Fig. 8.6** The cervical exam. A cervical exam during labor involves measuring the dilation and effacement of the cervix and the position of the fetal head relative to the maternal ischial spines. The dilation measures the amount of horizontal space between the edges of the internal os. In **a**, the cervix is 2 cm dilated (wide enough for two fingers to fit through) and 0% effaced. In **b** the cervix is 3 cm dilated and 50% effaced. In **c**, the cervix is 4 cm dilated and 80% effaced. In **d**, the cervix is 8 cm dilated and 100% effaced

lot of practice to do accurately; that said, here is a description of what they're assessing…)

– Dilation: 0–10 cm.
– Effacement (cervical thinning) – the normal cervix is 3–4 cm long; during labor it shortens to just a few mm; the % of this "thinning" is called "effacement," and it's reported as a percentage (0 being a cervix that has not started thinning at all, 100% being a completely thinned-out cervix that's ready for a baby's head to go through it).
– Station: where the fetal head is relative to the mother's ischial spines (IS) (these can be felt in the vagina) – above the IS = negative, at IS = 0, below IS = positive.
– Example: 2 / 50% / -3 means cervix is 2 cm dilated and 50% effaced, and fetal head is 3 cm above IS.
– Once a cervical exam has been done, calculate their Bishop score (calculators available online); >8 means favorable for labor.

8.2.3.3 Common CCs in OB Triage

Here we will cover "the big 5," which are the reasons you ask THE FIVE QUESTIONS.

1. "I'm having contractions"
   ▬ Put them "on the monitor" (i.e., tocometer; note that this does NOT tell you strength of contractions; only frequency).
   ▬ Labor = regular, painful contractions + cervical change
     – Braxton hicks (a.k.a. "practice contractions") are intermittent and not so painful that the patient cannot talk during them.
     – Labor contractions are regular and more painful – "Breathing through contractions" (i.e., taking long, slow breaths to tolerate pain of a contraction) can be a sign that they're the real deal.
   ▬ When to admit?
     – If nothing else is going on, generally admit when >4 cm dilated, and/or making fast change (e.g., two exams over 2 hours in triage 2 cm → 6 cm), and/or multiparous with a history of speedy deliveries.
2. "I think my water broke"
   ▬ What we care about: rupture of membranes (ROM)
     – Preterm ROM: prior to term (i.e., <37 weeks)
     – Premature ROM: no contractions or cervical change yet
     – Spontaneous ROM (SROM): after labor has started
   ▬ Common non-ROM phenomena: urine (fetus is compressing bladder; hard to distinguish between urine and amniotic fluid), normal vaginal secretions/discharge, semen from recent intercourse.
   ▬ How to distinguish: you're looking for THREE things – pooling, nitrazine blue, ferning
     – Speculum exam
       – Pooling → +ROM
       – Sample of fluid:
         - pH: use nitrazine indicator paper (yellow → dark blue/green means the pH is consistent with amniotic fluid).
           - Important causes of false-positive pH: blood, semen (i.e., this is useless if there is any blood, and/or if they've had sex recently)
         - Look at fluid under the microscope → ferning.
           - Important causes of false positive: cervical mucus (→ very important to only collect the clear fluid; avoid mucus)
     – Tricks for getting the right fluid/distinguishing what's going on:
       - Valsalva ("cough").

- If they cough and you see urine come out of the urethra, it's not amniotic fluid. If they cough and fluid comes out of the vagina, it's more likely to be amniotic fluid.
    - Have the patient walk around with a pad.
    - Ultrasound → do they still have enough fluid? (compare to prior if possible)
        - DVP or AFI.
- When to admit?
    - If they're ruptured
3. "I'm bleeding"
    - Do they have a known placental issue?
        - Placenta previa *mother's blood*.
        - Vasa previa *baby's blood*; this is BAD (emergency if bleeds) as a fetus has a very small blood volume.
        - Placental abruption *mom's blood*, but this is a potentially BAD one because the bleeding can be concealed, and the fetus can have inadequate blood supply.
        - Risk factors: smoking, cocaine, trauma ("classic" = car accident)
    - Ultrasound to look for placenta (position and is there an abruption?)
        - If any of these things are present, it can indicate urgent/emergent delivery.
4. "My baby stopped moving"
    - HPI (for how long? Are you doing kick counts? etc.).
    - Get an NST and/or BPP.
    - If everything is normal (i.e., their NST is reactive), send them home and teach about kick counts:
        - Lie down/sit quietly for 1 hour; if you feel ten movements, that's good.
        - If patients ever feel worried or like something has changed, they can always come in and be put on the monitor.
5. *Headache, visual change, shortness of breath, nausea/vomiting, or upper abdominal pain*
    - Check BP, urine protein/Cr, CBC, uric acid, AST/ALT,
        - If BP >160/110 sustained for 15 minutes, lower blood pressure with medication.
    - Get an NST and/or BPP.
    - For further work-up and management guidelines, see "Preeclampsia" section (8.4.2.1).

! Common Error: Though sometimes visualizable, placental abruption cannot reliably be seen on ultrasound. Lack of sonographic evidence of abruption does not mean there is no abruption.

8.2.3.4 Key Terms/Definitions for the Labor Floor

- "Spontaneous labor" = regular contractions with cervical change
- "Augmentation of labor" = intervention to increase contractions that are already happening
    - Options (2): oxytocic agents, artificial ROM (amniotomy – done with cervical hook)
- "Induction of labor" = starting labor with interventions
    - Options:
        - Prostaglandins (misoprostol, dinoprostone)
            - Contraindications: maternal asthma or glaucoma, prior c-section, non-reassuring fetal testing
        - Oxytocic agents (Pitocin)
        - Mechanical dilation of the cervix
        - Artificial ROM
    - Bishop score of 5 or less may lead to a failed induction as often as 50% of the time.

8.2.3.5 Normal Labor

- *Stage 1*: onset of labor → complete dilation and effacement
  - Latent: 0–6 cm
  - Active: 6–10 cm (expect >1 cm/hour in nulliparous patient; 1.2 cm/hour in multiparous patient)
- For each patient you are following on the labor floor, you should check on them and write a progress note at least every 4 hours if they're in stage 1 latent phase (<6 cm) and every 1–2 hours if they're in stage 1 active phase (>6 cm).
- *Stage 2*: complete dilation and effacement → delivery of infant

  Allowed 3 hours (4 if epidural) in nulliparous pt; 2 hours (3 if epidural) in multiparous pt
- During stages 1–2, progression depends on the 4 P's:
  1. Power – how strong are contractions? (measured by Montevideo units (MVUs), >200 MVUs considered "adequate"; measurement requires a device called an intrauterine pressure catheter); how well is the patient pushing? (nulliparous patients or patients with an epidural may not push effectively and may need time and practice during the second stage)
  2. Passenger – how large is the baby? In what position?
  3. Pelvis – how large is the pelvis?
  4. Placenta – is the fetus tolerating labor? Measured by fetal heart tracings.
- *Stage 3*: delivery of infant → delivery of placenta
  - *Group B Strep (GBS) prophylaxis*

8.2.3.6 Fetal Monitoring

External fetal monitoring is the most commonly used method for fetal monitoring in the United States: it is used in >85% of labors. It involves simultaneous and continuous fetal heart rate (FHR) and contraction detection.
- FHR detected by ultrasound (→ visual pattern reflects auditory signals).
- Contractions detected by tocography (detects changes in tension of abdomen).
- It's a screening test, not a diagnostic tool.
- Normal fetal heart tracing (FHT) virtually precludes fetal hypoxia, i.e., has HIGH negative predictive value for normal fetal acid-base status.
- Abnormal FHT is not necessarily predictive of adverse fetal outcomes.
- Tocometer (contraction pattern) interpretation:
  - Can only estimate frequency and duration; to quantify strength of contractions requires an intrauterine pressure catheter.
  - Normal CTX frequency is <= 5 within 10-minute period, averaged over 30 minutes.
  - Tachysystole = >5 CTX within 10 minutes averaged over 30 minutes.
- FHT interpretation (see ◘ Fig. 8.8)
  - Baseline (>2 minutes within a 10-minute segment)
    - Normal 110–160
    - Bradycardia <110
    - Tachycardia >160
  - Variability (fluctuation of HR around the baseline; see ◘ Fig. 8.8)
    - Absent = no variation in FH
    - Minimal = variation ≤ 5 bpm
      - Transient loss of variability can be due to fetal sleep cycle or maternal meds such as magnesium and opioids.
      - Persistent absent or minimal variability is concerning for fetal acidemia.

Pearl: Variability is the best indicator of fetal acid-base status! Moderate variability effectively rules out fetal acidemia.

- Moderate (normal) = variation 6–25 bpm
- Marked ≥25 bpm
- Accelerations
  - Abrupt increase in FHR.
  - Gestational age of fetus is important: at ≥ 32 weeks, accels should be 15 bpm range × 15 seconds; before 32 weeks, 10×10.
  - Accel lasting >10 minutes is a change in baseline.
- Decelerations
  - Abrupt decrease in FHR.
  - There are multiple types:
    - *Early*: symmetrical, directly mirroring a contraction, usually 30 seconds or more; nadir of decel coincides with peak of contraction intensity.
      - Associated with fetal head compression
      - Clinically benign; not associated with fetal acidemia
      - Only decel that falls into Cat I
    - *Variable*: abrupt and deep (<30 seconds) (>15 seconds below baseline); random, with no apparent relationship to contraction.
      - Associated with cord compression.
      - Assess for frequency; recurrent (>50% of the time in a 20-minute period) is associated with acidemia.
    - *Late*: gradual decrease in FHR with return to baseline, associated with contraction; nadir occurs after peak of contractions and resolution after end of contraction.
      - Associated with uteroplacental insufficiency.
      - Recurrent late decels require intervention.
    - *Prolonged*: decrease ×15 bpm or more × more than 2 minutes, but <10 minutes.
  - Decel lasting >10 minutes is a change in baseline.
- Sinusoidal pattern (extremely rare) = fetal acidemia
  - ×20 or more minutes.
- Fetal sleep cycles are typically 20 minutes but can last up to 60 minutes and can lead to loss of variability.
  - To elicit variability, vibroacoustic stim or fetal scalp stimulation

> Pearl: Use the VEAL CHOP acronym to remember important causes of EFM findings:
> - V – C: Variable decels are often due to cord compression.
> - E – H: Early decels are often due to head compression.
> - A – O: Accels are OKAY!
> - L – P: Late decels are due to placental insufficiency.

NICHD Categories:
- Cat I: Normal; indicates normal fetal acid-base status
  - Normal baseline with moderate variability
  - Accels OK but not necessary
  - Early decels OK
  - No variable or late decels
  - Review q30 minutes during stage 1 labor; q5–15 minutes during stage 2 labor
- Cat II: Indeterminate; requires more evaluation – everything that isn't I or III
  - Majority (~80%) of tracings
- Cat III: Bad; indicates fetal acidemia, though predictive value for fetal encephalopathy is poor
  - Absent variability AND any of…
    - Recurrent late decels (>50% of contractions in 20-minute window)
    - Recurrent variable decels (>50% of the time in 20-minute window)
    - Bradycardia
    - Sinusoidal

Management of Cat II and III tracings:
- Note that EFM is not a great test; it is a screening test (high sensitivity, low specificity for fetal distress) and is not diagnostic!
- Cat I: do nothing
- Cat II or III:
  - Cat III: fetal acidemia ~25% of the time (best predictor of abnormal acid-base status at time of delivery).
  - For both II and III, often initiate multiple measures at once…
    1. Reposition mother.
    2. IV fluid bolus (increase maternal blood volume → increased blood flow to fetus).
    3. Closely observe the contraction pattern; if there is tachysystole, this could be the culprit! Turn down/off pit (if on), or use terbutaline if no pit is on.
    4. Supplemental oxygen (though controversial, this is often pursued).
    5. Intrauterine resuscitation – amnioinfusion – only if membranes are ruptured (goal is to reduce cord compression; typically, only done in case of recurrent variable decels, since they're associated with cord compression).
  - If non-reassuring Cat II or Cat III persists despite resuscitative measures, proceed to delivery.

8.2.3.7 Presenting the OB Triage Patient: Template

This is a ___ year-old G _ P_ _ _ _ patient at __ weeks by ___ presenting with ____.

(HPI). She has (not) had vaginal bleeding, leaking fluid, or contractions, and she endorses normal fetal movement.

This pregnancy has been complicated by ___.

She has a medical history notable for ___. She has a surgical history notable for ___.

She takes ___ for ___.

She (has no allergies) or (is allergic to ___).

Her exam is notable for ___.

Her toco tracing is notable for ___.

Fetal heart monitoring is notable for ___.

Recent labs are notable for ____.

Her most recent ultrasound on __ showed __.

In summary, this is a ___ year-old G _ P_ _ _ _ patient at __ weeks presenting with ____ concerning for ___. (Outline pertinent points of H&P and reasoning leading up to your proposed plan). I think we should ____ **disposition** (admit her/observe her in triage/discharge her to home with follow-up in __ days).

Standout Tip: Mention up to three abnormal things if they are pertinent to the presentation). If her vitals are all normal and she had no abnormal exam findings, say "her exam was unremarkable including normal vitals. She hasn't had a vaginal or cervical exam yet."

8.2.3.8 Presenting the OB Triage Patient: Example

This is a 32-year-old G1P0 patient at 39 weeks 6 days by 12 week ultrasound presenting with after a gush of fluid 1 hour ago and painful contractions every 4 minutes.

She has been feeling intermittent contractions for the last 24 hours or so, now every 3–5 minutes and increasingly painful, such that she is now unable to talk during them. About 1 hour ago, after a contraction, she stood up from the couch and felt a gush of clear fluid, so she decided to come to the hospital. Review of systems was unremarkable otherwise. She has not had vaginal bleeding, and she notes normal fetal movement.

This pregnancy has been uncomplicated. She has a medical history notable for hypothyroidism, for which she takes levothyroxine 100 mcg daily, and no surgical history. She has no allergies.

On exam, she had normal vitals and is generally well-appearing but was unable to speak during a contraction she had while I was in the room. Her fetus is cephalic by Leopold's with EFW 7 lbs or 3300 g. She hasn't had a vaginal or cervical exam yet.

Her toco tracing is consistent with contractions every 3–5 minutes. Fetal heart monitoring is notable for a baseline of 150 with moderate variability, occasional accels, and no decels. Recent labs are notable for her being Rh negative s/p RhoGAM at 28 weeks and GBS positive 2 weeks ago. Her most recent ultrasound at 37 weeks showed a fetus in cephalic presentation with anterior placenta with estimated fetal weight 3196 g.

In summary, this is a 32-year-old G1P0 patient at 39 weeks 6 days presenting with painful contractions every 4 minutes and leaking fluid concerning for spontaneous rupture of membranes, overall potentially consistent with labor. Her tocometer shows contractions every 3–5 minutes, and her fetal heart tracing is Category I. I think we should perform a sterile speculum exam to assess for rupture of membranes, a cervical exam to assess for cervical change, and a bedside ultrasound to confirm cephalic presentation. If we confirm rupture of membranes, I think we should admit her to L&D for labor management and start penicillin for intrapartum GBS prophylaxis.

8.2.3.9 Intrapartum Fever: Differentiating the Differential

- Fever can simply happen from labor itself! One isolated intrapartum temp 38–39 without an obvious source is unlikely to be due to infection.
- If a patient has any additional infectious symptoms or >1 elevated temp, this merits work-up and treatment.
- Intra-amniotic infection (IAI) or chorioamnionitis.
- Transient reaction to epidural – symptoms can include fever, hypotension, and tachycardia.
- Non-genital region infection (e.g., upper respiratory infection or pneumonia – cough, shortness of breath).
- DVT/PE – lower extremity swelling (DVT), tachycardia, and/or pleuritic chest pain (PE).
- UTI – urinary symptoms, flank pain, hx of UTIs (especially in pregnancy).

8.2.3.10 Intra-amniotic Infection (IAI)

Background
- IAI is an umbrella term for:
  - Chorioamnionitis = infection of chorion, amnion, or both (i.e., anything in the uterus while fetus, placenta, etc. are present)
  - Endometritis = infection of endometrium (i.e., in the uterus after delivery)
- Risk factors:
  - Longer ROM; longer labor; multiple digital cervical exams; cervical insufficiency; nulliparity; meconium; internal fetal monitoring; other genital tract pathogens (STI, GBS, BV, etc.); hx of IAI; EtOH and/or smoking
- Why do we care?
  - Chorioamnionitis: Associated with acute neonatal morbidity (PNA, meningitis, sepsis, death)
  - Either chorioamnionitis or endometritis → dysfunctional labor leading to C/S, postpartum hemorrhage d/t atony, peritonitis, sepsis, death

Diagnosis

— One temp >39° C OR one temp between 38° C and 38.9° C + one or more risk factors (maternal or fetal tachy), WBC >10K, OR two temps >38 within 30 minutes.
  - No time for culture or gram stain intrapartum → ends up being a clinical dx
  - Postpartum endometritis = fever, tachy, uterine tenderness, foul smelling lochia, leukocytosis

Treatment

— See OB-GYN Antibiotics Guide.
— IV fluid bolus; cooling blankets, ice. (Bring tachycardia down!)
— Treat until afebrile for 24 hours regardless of route of delivery.

8.2.3.11 The Vaginal Delivery

Meet the patient before you attend her delivery. Review the following beforehand:

— Hemoglobin or hematocrit
— Number of prior deliveries (both vaginal and cesarean) and any complications
— Whether the patient has asthma and/or high blood pressure
— Fetal presentation

Here's what will typically happen during a normal vaginal delivery:

— After a patient is "fully dilated" to 10 cm, they can start pushing.
— Stay in the room with the patient while they push. They should work to have three pushes lasting 10 seconds during each contraction. If it feels appropriate, help with counting and coaching.
— For example, ask the patient if they would like hearing a ten-count during each push, what kind of encouragement they want, etc. You can be a great labor coach, and the nurses, residents, and attendings will notice if you are engaged, invested, and doing a good job helping your patient through labor.
— You may be able to gown and glove with the resident, ± deliver the baby "hands over hands." If you're offered the chance to do the delivery or do hands over hands, put three fingers on the top of the baby's head, and support the perineum with your other hand → head restitutes (turns to one side or the other) → put your hands on either side of the head, parallel to the floor and fingers toward the face → anterior shoulder → posterior shoulder → "catch!" (i.e., slide your hand under the bum), and then bring it straight to the mother's chest for skin to skin if this is what the patient prefers.
— As soon as the newborn is delivered:
  1. The providers will start Pitocin (starting "Pit" immediately after delivery has been shown to decrease blood loss and doesn't affect placental delivery).
  2. They will clamp the cord after 60 seconds ("delayed cord clamping," which has been shown to improve neonatal outcomes, thought to be related to increased placental blood transfusion). If the neonate is in distress, however, the cord may be clamped earlier to facilitate resuscitation.
  3. Be ready to collect cord gases! Insert the needle into the umbilical vein slowly at a 45° angle; avoid going completely through the vein. Allow the (self-filling) syringe to fill with blood. Obtain 0.5–1 mL and then remove the needle from the cord.
  4. Someone (potentially you!) will deliver the placenta.

Question Box: Remember why we care so much about asthma and high blood pressure on the L&D floor?
They are contraindications to the postpartum hemorrhage medications carboprost (Hemabate) and methylergonovine (Methergine), respectively.

Standout Tip: There is often limited time for questions during a delivery, but there often IS time for questions after, so watch what happens carefully and have questions ready. During the delivery, there is typically neither time nor "social space" for questions or extensive teaching. If your attending/resident wants you to do something, they will hand it to you, or gesture with their hands, guide your hands, etc.

Pearl: Remember that the umbilical vein carries the mother's oxygenated blood to the fetus from the placenta and then that the two umbilical arteries carry deoxygenated fetal blood back to the placenta.

Pearl: The three signs of placental release are:
1. Gush of blood.
2. Cord lengthening.
3. The uterus gets smaller and firms up.

= Once the placenta is delivered, someone (potentially you!) will massage the uterus to (1) assess its tone and (2) help it "clamp down." Someone (potentially you!) will examine the placenta, including seeing how many vessels are in the cord (there should be three).

= Lacerations Grading Scale
  – Vaginal mucosa only → first degree.
  – Muscle → second degree.
  – External anal sphincter → third degree.
  – All the way through and through to rectal mucosa → fourth degree.
  – The resident/midwife/attending will repair any lacerations with sutures.

8.2.3.12 The Cesarean Delivery

There are several important concepts you should know related to the medical, social, and surgical aspects of a cesarean delivery. Always meet the patient in the preop area before they are taken to the OR. Here are the important things to know about your patient beforehand and select important facts about cesarean deliveries.

■ Important things to know about a patient before a cesarean delivery

= Why is it happening?
= Preop hemoglobin or hematocrit
= Placental location
= Presentation of the fetus
= Whether the patient has asthma and/or high blood pressure
= Whether they've had prior cesarean deliveries (if yes, how many? any complications?)
= Any other abdominal surgeries

■ Medical knowledge

= Reasons for planned CS (plan for 39 weeks to avoid them going into labor):
  – Repeat
  – Breech/transverse (malpresentation)
  – Hx uterine surgery (myomectomy – only if the uterine cavity was entered)
  – Abnormal placentation (previa, accreta, increta, percreta)
  – Multiple gestation with at least one babe not cephalic
  – Elective
= Indications during labor
  – Arrest of dilation – must be in active labor (i.e. at least 6 cm) for this to happen (this is when we expect consistent change)
    – Zhang curve – the patient should make 1 cm of change every 4–6 hours with adequate contractions (based on IUPC).
      - If you have an IUPC in, they get up to 4 hours with adequate (>250 MVUs/10 minutes) or 6 hours with inadequate CTX.
      - If you don't have an IUPC in place, they get up to 6 hours.
  – Arrest of descent (have reached complete dilation, but pushing isn't bringing the baby down).
    - Nullip with epidural gets 4 hours with NO change.
    - Nullip without epidural gets 3 hours with NO change.
    - Multip with epidural gets 3 hours with NO change.
    - Multip without epidural gets 2 hours with NO change.
  – Non-reassuring fetal heart tracing/fetal intolerance to labor.
    - Cat II, non-reassuring (wide variability)
    - Cat III → emergent (stat) C/S
    - Sinusoidal

Pearl: Atony (i.e., the uterus not clamping down) is the most common cause of postpartum hemorrhage.

Pearl: Search online for "vaginal delivery laceration degrees" images or illustrations, and this will become clearer. If you're asked what degree it is and you have no idea, guess second, as it's the most common.

Pearl: The vast majority of the time, the patient is awake, so be conscious of your words during the surgery!

Standout Tip: If your institution has a system/board to monitor every patient's tracing on the floor, keep an eye on it. If you think you recognized a prolonged decel or a Cat III tracing, (1) alert someone (they likely noticed before you) and (2) rush to the bedside (you can get accidentally left behind since this is an emergency).

Pearl: Cord prolapse is an EMERGENCY with "all hands on-deck" to get the patient into an OR for a cesarean delivery as quickly as possible.

Standout Tip: Make sure you know how to gown and glove yourself properly without help. It comes in handy in these situations! You can ask a scrub tech to practice with you during down time, or find YouTube video and ask for supplies to practice on your own.

Standout Tip: Familiarize yourself with the PPH treatment ladder! This is great question fodder because (1) it's common and deadly, and (2) the PPH meds aren't really used anywhere else and have specific indications and contraindications.

Pearl: PPH was previously defined as >500 mL for vaginal delivery.

Question Box: Risk factors include a prolonged second stage and infection (IAI). Can you think of why these would increase risk for poor tone after delivery?
Think of the active phase of labor as a workout – the uterus is a muscle working very hard to expel a fetus! If that workout is very long, or if the muscle is inflamed because of infection, it will be harder for the muscle to contract at the end of the workout.

  - Absent variability with recurrent late/variable decels
  - Absent variability with bradycardia
– Cord prolapse – slips between presenting part and maternal pelvis → restricts blood supply.
– Malpresentation.
– Abruption (if bad, will cause non-reassuring fetal heart tones).

- **Social knowledge**
  - Help transfer patient to table.
  - Put on compression boots.
  - Write your name on the board.

- **Surgical knowledge**
  - Prep: chlorhexidine needs to dry for 3 minutes because it's alcohol based → flammable.
  - Abdominal layers, outside → inside: Campers → Scarpa's → Rectus sheath (external, internal, oblique) → preperitoneal fat → peritoneum.
  - The surgeon may or may not dissect a bladder flap; if there is social space, ask about their practice.
  - They will ask you to retract a bladder blade toward the patients' feet. *Hold it with all of your might!*
  - Hysterotomy – note location of uterine vessels.
  - If you're given the opportunity to tie a knot or suture fascia or skin, this is your time to shine! Your preceptors will be watching, and it's usually obvious if you have been practicing.

8.2.3.13 Postpartum Hemorrhage (PPH)

Everyone bleeds with a delivery. Hemorrhage is >1 L for both vaginal and cesarean delivery.

- **The 4 T's of PPH**
  - TONE (Atony) – THE MOST COMMON CAUSE (~70%)!
    – TRT: ladder; see ◘ Fig. 8.10.
  - TRAUMA (laceration) (~20%)
    – TRT: repair (suture)
  - TISSUE (retained products – membranes or placenta) (~10%)
    – TRT: sweep → D&C
  - THROMBIN (coagulopathy – DIC, low platelets, etc.) (~1%)
    – Diluting coagulation factors; hypothermia can further inhibit coagulation cascade.
    – TRT: FFP, platelets, pRBCs → cryoprecipitate

8.2.3.14 The L&D Handoff/Signout: Checklist and Example

- Age, Gs & Ps
- Gestational age, by ___ (dating mechanism)
- Reason for admission (e.g., labor, PPROM)
- Most recent cervical exam @ __ time, & labor progress
- Augmentation
- Estimated fetal weight (EFW)
- Fetal status and position
- ± presence of epidural
- GBS/rubella/Rh status

- **For example**

"Ms. Z is a 30-year-old G1P0 at 39 weeks 6 days by 9-week ultrasound admitted in labor. She arrived at 11 PM after SROM at home and was having q4 minute contractions at that time. She was started on Pit at 2 AM and most recently she was 5 / 80 / -2 at 5 AM. Her fetus has an EFW of 2496 g and is cephalic with a category I tracing. She would like an epidural but has not yet gotten one. She is GBS negative, Rubella immune and Rh positive."

8.2.4 MFM (High-Risk Pregnancy): Select Conditions

There is a 3-year-long fellowship devoted to mastering high-risk pregnancy conditions. Thus, we will not attempt to cover this subspecialty in great detail. We will, however, provide frameworks with which to think about several common and important conditions that you will almost certainly encounter during your rotation.

8.2.4.1 Hypertensive Disorders of Pregnancy

- **Background**
- These are a spectrum of diseases involving elevated blood pressure, all of which are thought to be related to placental dysfunction.
- Complicate up to 10% of pregnancies.
- Spectrum includes chronic hypertension, gestational hypertension, preeclampsia, eclampsia, and HELLP syndrome.

- **Diagnosis**
- Any BP > 140/90 during pregnancy is considered elevated (a.k.a. "mild range").
  - 160/110 is classified as "severe range."
  - A patient needs two or more elevated BPs greater than 4 hours apart to earn any of these diagnoses.
- Chronic HTN (cHTN): predates pregnancy, or elevated BPs < 20 weeks
- Gestational HTN (gHTN): HTN > 20 weeks, no other body system involvement
- Preeclampsia (PEC) ("superimposed PEC" if cHTN; plain old PEC if gHTN)
  - Proteinuria (protein/creatinine ratio > 0.3 vs. 24 h urine >300 mg)
- Severe features of PEC:
  - BP > 160/110
  - Headache/visual disturbance/neurologic symptoms
  - Hepatic dysfunction (AST or ALT >2x upper limit of normal)
  - Renal dysfunction (Cr >1.1 mg/dL or doubling compared to baseline)
  - Low platelets (<$100 \cdot 10^9$/L)
  - Pulmonary edema
- HELLP: Hemolysis, Elevated Liver enzymes, Low Platelets
  - LDH > 600 U/L
  - AST ≥ 70 U/L
  - Platelets <$100 \cdot 10^9$/L

- **Treatment**
- The only treatment is removal of the placenta, i.e., delivery!
- Blood pressure can be managed with medications, most often labetalol and/or nifedipine.

Standout Tip: Consults to MFM and neonatology (the NICU) are often needed for patients presenting with high-risk conditions, if these services are available at your institution. These are important tasks that you can help with and follow up on.

Pearl: Since placental dysfunction is the driving force behind all of these disorders, the only way to "cure" them is by removing the placenta – i.e., delivering the fetus. Elevated blood pressures can be managed with medications, but these disorders tend to worsen as pregnancy progresses, and a dysfunctional placenta can mean that the fetus isn't getting enough nutrients. Making decisions about when to deliver these patients can be challenging and involves weighing risks of adverse effects on maternal vs. fetal health.

Standout Tip: Calculate this ratio yourself! The lab may "round up," so a ratio of 0.27 would be falsely rounded up to 0.3. That said, if it's reported at <0.2 or >0.4, it doesn't matter, as the patient clearly rules in or out with those numbers.

Pearl: Remember that Cr normally decreases during pregnancy, to a normal range of 0.4–0.8 mg/dL. Can you think of why?

Pearl: Different hospitals and anesthesiologists have different thresholds, but thrombocytopenia is often a contraindication to epidural analgesia for pain control during labor. Remember to address pain control in your plans for patients.

8

◻ **Table 8.4** Recommended delivery timing for hypertensive disorders of pregnancy

Diagnosis	Delivery timing[a]	Comments
cHTN	39	
gHTN	37 – 37 + 6	d/t higher risk of IUFD >38 weeks
PEC w/o SF	37 – 37 + 6	d/t higher risk of IUFD >38 weeks
PEC w/ SF	34	Earlier if maternal or fetal status is unstable

[a]For gHTN and PEC diagnosed after 37 weeks, deliver expediently once diagnosed

- Seizure prophylaxis: IV magnesium sulfate is often administered intrapartum to prevent eclamptic seizures.
- If eclamptic seizure, break with IM or IV Mg; can use Ativan (like outside of pregnancy), but this is not first line.
- Delivery timing (◻ Table 8.4):

8.2.4.2 Gestational Diabetes (GDM)

■ Background
- Progesterone and human placental lactogen (HPL) make the body more insulin-resistant during pregnancy > elevated blood sugars.
- Complicates 6–9% of pregnancies.

■ Diagnosis
- All pregnant patients should be screened 24–28 weeks.
- 1-hour GTT screen (non-fasting): 50 g glucose load, screen is positive if glucose >140 1 hour later.

- 3-hour GTT diagnostic test (fasting): 100 g glucose load, test is positive if fasting blood glucose >95, 1 hour 180, 2 hours 155, 3 hours 140 (thresholds may differ depending on your institution).

- **Treatment**
- Antenatal
  1. What are mom's sugars? Typically check four times daily: fasting and after each meal:
     (a) Fasting goal: <95 g/dL
     (b) Postprandial goals: 1 hour <140 or 2 hours <120
  2. Diet and exercise (though there aren't great data for efficacy of diet/exercise modification).
  3. Medications
     (a) Insulin injection – mainstay of GDM treatment; doesn't cross the placenta
     (b) Oral meds – controversial and not FDA-approved for GDM
        - Metformin – crosses the placenta, and some studies have shown accumulation in fetus; long-term outcomes unknown.
        - Glyburide (SFU) – increased risk for hypoglycemia, and macrosomia rates may be increased compared to insulin.
- Delivery timing
  - If well-controlled, can deliver at 39 weeks or later
  - If poorly controlled, weigh risk of prematurity with risk for stillbirth; generally, 37 – 38 + 6, but sometimes earlier can make sense if inpatient attempts at blood glucose control are failing.
- Intrapartum
  - Closely monitor blood glucose to avoid both hypo- and hyperglycemia
  - In active phase, check blood glucose q 2–4 hours if diet-controlled, q hour if med-controlled.
- Postpartum (◘ Table 8.5)
  - Increased risk for persistent impaired glucose tolerance postpartum

> Common Error: Remember the difference between a screening test and a diagnostic test! The 1-hour GTT is a screening test; the only way to earn a diagnosis of GDM is through a positive 3-hour GTT, which is a diagnostic test.

> Common Error: Not all patients with GDM need medications! Consider medication if >50% of blood glucose values are above goal.

> Pearl: Intrapartum blood glucose >140–180 is associated with increased risk for neonatal hypoglycemia and maternal ketoacidosis.

> Standout Tip: R/o occult T2DM with 2 h GTT postpartum (potentially even in hospital).

◘ **Table 8.5** Abnormal placentation and related conditions

	Description
Placental abruption	Separation of placenta from uterine wall
Placenta previa	Placenta develops over the cervical internal os; can be complete or partial
Low-lying placenta	Placenta develops near but not overlying the cervical internal os (previously "marginal placenta previa")
Placenta accreta spectrum	Accreta: abnormal adherence of part or all of placenta to uterine wall Increta: placental invasion of uterine myometrium Percreta: placental invasion through myometrium to uterine serosa
Vasa previa	Fetal vessels pass over cervical internal os (seen with velamentous cord insertion, velamentous placenta, or succenturiate placenta)

Pearl: When evaluating a patient presenting with symptoms concerning for PTL, conduct the speculum exam BEFORE the digital cervical exam so that you can collect specimens (GC/CT, GBS, wet prep) and evaluate for ROM (i.e., look for pooling and collect a sample to test pH and look for ferning under the microscope).

Note that these PTL treatment guidelines are relevant for viable fetuses, typically defined as >24 weeks. Pre-viable PTL may be managed differently and depends on the patient and institution.

Question Box: Contraindications to tocolysis include IUFD, non-reassuring fetal status (i.e., baby sick), anything that makes mom unstable (i.e., mom sick), and PPROM. Can you think of why these conditions would make tocolysis dangerous?

Question Box: Do you know why Indomethacin should not be administered for more than 48 hours, and not after 32 weeks? Answer: It is an NSAID and can cause premature ductus arteriosus closure.

Pearl: There is now evidence that antenatal steroids also decrease risk for intraventricular hemorrhage and necrotizing enterocolitis in premature infants, and some data suggest benefit up to 37 weeks.

8.2.4.3 Preterm Labor (PTL)

- **Background**
- 12% of births are preterm, ~50% of which are preceded by PTL.
- ~30% of PTL spontaneously resolves, but it's nearly impossible to predict who this will be.

- **Diagnosis**
- This is a clinical diagnosis! PTL is defined as the onset of painful contractions leading to cervical change (i.e., labor) after 20 weeks but prior to 37 weeks.
- To make this diagnosis, you need evidence of regular, painful contractions (typically with a tocometer) and evidence of cervical change (by conducting a digital cervical exam).

- **Treatment**
- A patient presenting in preterm labor will be admitted for at least 48 hours while within the "beta window." Once they are beta complete and off of fluids/tocolytics (medications to stop contractions), you'll re-evaluate their status.
- In true PTL, tocolytics (medications to stop contractions) are usually only administered until the patient is "steroid-complete" (i.e., 48 hours), because all available evidence suggests that true PTL does not stop once it has started, and risks of facilitating continued pregnancy with tocolysis typically outweigh benefits.
  - <32 weeks, indomethacin, no more than 48 hours
  - ≥32 weeks, nifedipine (*pay attention to BP*)
- IV magnesium sulfate (fetal neuroprotection to prevent cerebral palsy), 24–32 weeks.
- IM steroids (facilitate fetal lung maturity), 24–34 weeks.
- Antibiotics.
  - GBS ppx if GBS status unknown, because PT delivery is associated with elevated risk for neonatal GBS disease (see ❑ Fig. 8.7)
- Bed rest, pelvic rest, sedation, and hydration do NOT HELP.
  - Hydration WILL sometimes stop contractions that don't have associated cervical change (i.e., pre-labor contractions) but has NOT been shown to stop true PTL.

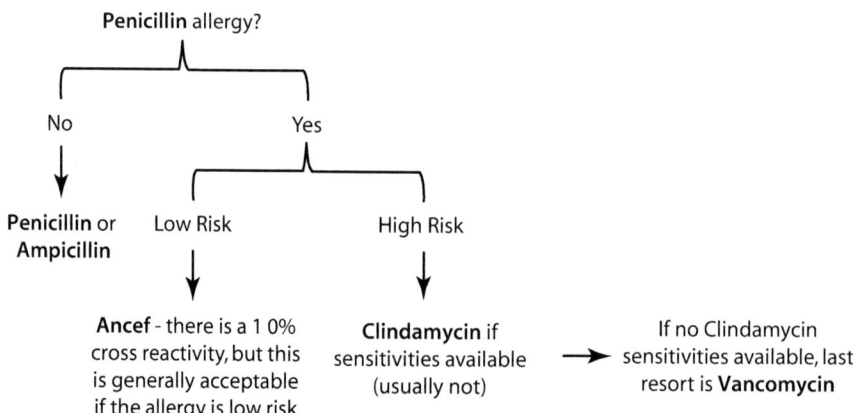

❑ **Fig. 8.7**   Intrapartum GBS prophylaxis flowchart

8.2.4.4 PPROM (Preterm Pre-labor ROM)

- **Background**
- Birth occurs within 1 week in 50% of patients diagnosed with PPROM.
- 15–25% have intra-amniotic infection (IAI), 15–20% get postpartum endometritis, and 2–5% are complicated by placental abruption.
- PPROM is often thought to be caused by a subclinical infection; having abx on board prevents infection from worsening.

- **Diagnosis**
- Clinical diagnosis defined as evidence of ROM prior to labor without contractions or cervical change after 20 weeks but prior to 37 weeks

- **Treatment**
- These patients will typically remain admitted to the hospital for the duration of their pregnancy.
- IV magnesium sulfate (fetal neuroprotection to prevent cerebral palsy), 24–32 weeks.
- IM steroids (facilitate fetal lung maturity), 24–34 weeks.

Note that similar to PTL, these PPROM treatment guidelines are relevant for viable fetuses, which is typically defined as >24 weeks. Pre-viable PPROM may be managed differently and depends on the patient and institution.

Pearl: There is now evidence that antenatal steroids also decrease risk for intraventricular hemorrhage and necrotizing enterocolitis in premature infants, and some data suggest benefit up to 37 weeks.

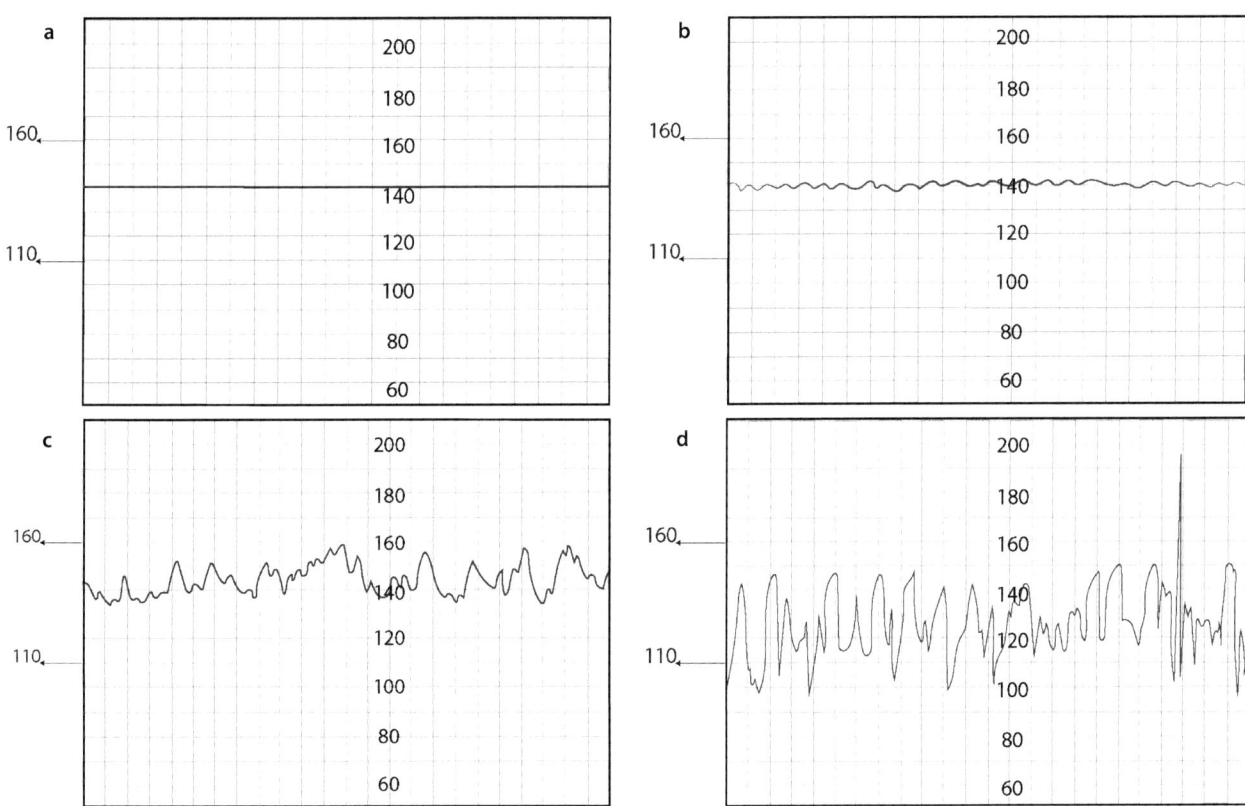

☐ **Fig. 8.8** Fetal heart tracing variability. Baseline variability is the fluctuation in the fetal heart rate from beat to beat. Variability is characterized as absent **a**, minimal (<5 bpm, **b**), moderate (6–25 bpm, **c**), or marked (>25 bpm, **d**)

8

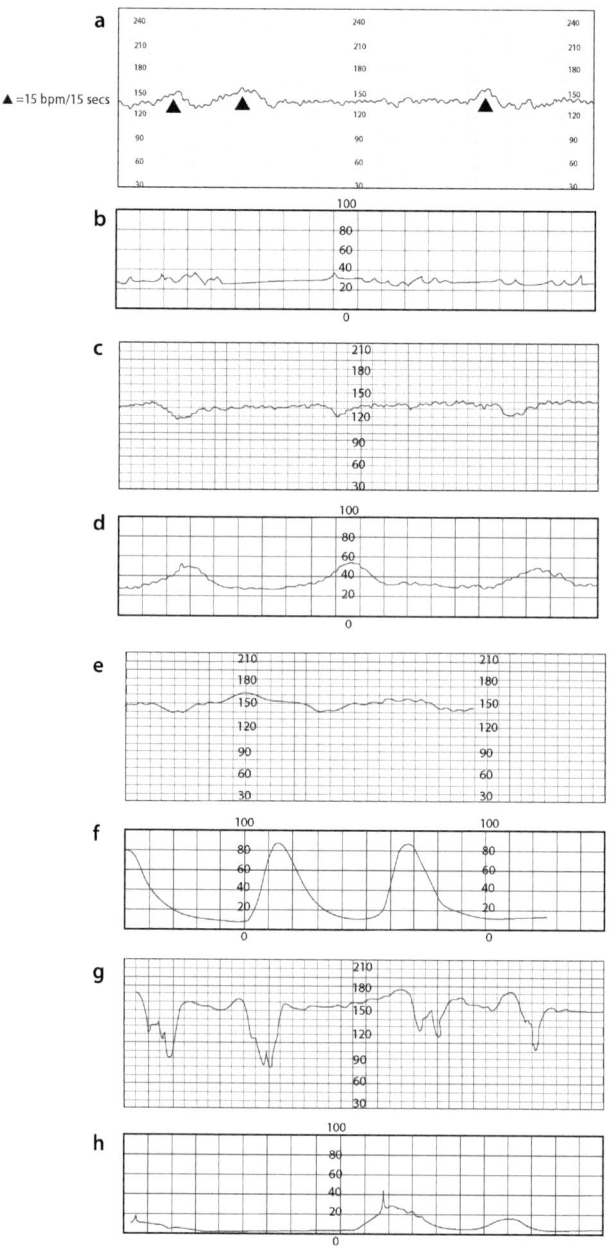

Fig. 8.9 Fetal heart tracing accelerations and decelerations. Panels **a, c, e,** and **g** represent fetal heart tracing, while panels **b, d, f,** and **h** represent maternal tocometry. **a** Accelerations are defined as an abrupt increase in heart rate (at least 15 bpm) and return to baseline in a short time frame (15 seconds or more). **b** No evidence of maternal contractions. **c, d** Early decelerations are symmetrical, directly mirroring a contraction, usually 30 seconds or more, and the nadir of the decelerations coincides with peak of contraction intensity. They are often due to head compression. **e, f** Late decelerations are a gradual decrease in fetal heart rate in which the nadir occurs after peak of contraction, and the heart rate returns to baseline after the end of the contraction. They are often due to placental insufficiency. **g, h** Variable decelerations are abrupt, deep, and random and have no apparent relationship to contractions. They are often due to cord compression

?Question Box: Can you think of why "latency antibiotics" may be helpful in PPROM?

PPROM is typically thought to be caused by some kind of subclinical infection, and/or having antibiotics on board prevents infection from brewing and worsening the clinical situation. Antibiotics have been shown to prolong pregnancy (and therefore decrease gestational age-dependent mortality) and decrease rates of both maternal and neonatal infection.

− Antibiotics.
  – GBS ppx if GBS status unknown, because PT delivery is associated with elevated risk for neonatal GBS disease (see ◻ Fig. 8.7)
  – Latency abx
− Bed rest, pelvic rest, sedation, and hydration do NOT HELP.

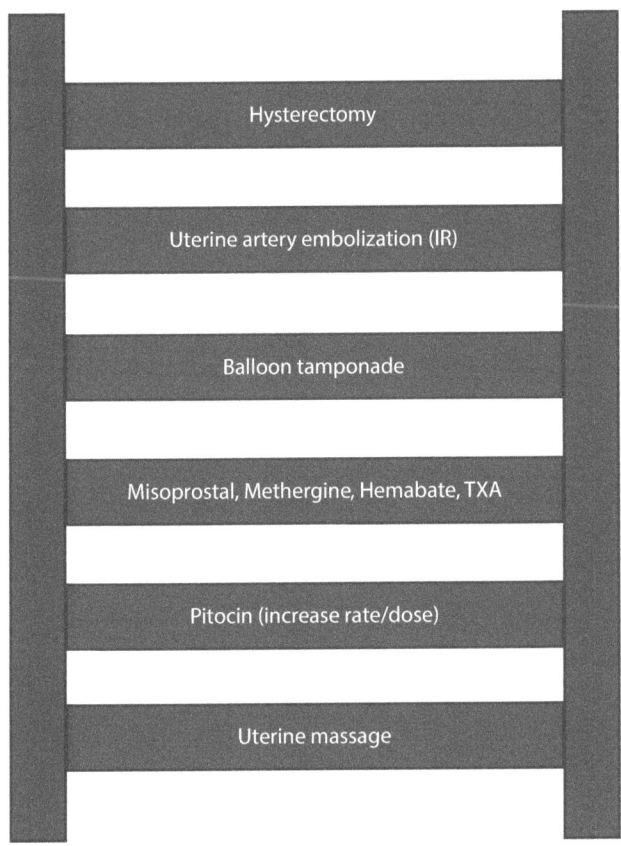

Fig. 8.10 Postpartum hemorrhage management ladder. Treatment options for postpartum hemorrhage. All patients should receive uterine massage and Pitocin (IV or IM), as studies have shown that administering Pitocin after anterior shoulder delivery decreases blood loss without affecting placental delivery. Notable contraindications to the PPH medications include avoiding methylergonovine (Methergine) in hypertensive patients (given its vasoconstrictive action) and avoiding carboprost (Hemabate) in patients with asthma (given its beta-adrenergic properties). If all medication options have been given and the patient is still bleeding, mechanical intervention options include balloon tamponade (inside of uterus), which can be placed after both vaginal and cesarean deliveries, uterine artery embolization (typically done by interventional radiology), and, as a last resort, hysterectomy.

— Tocolytics?
– NO! Often, ROM is provoked by pathology – worse than a preterm baby is an infected preterm baby!
— Deliver at 34 weeks (earlier if maternal or fetal instability, IAI, placental abruption).

8.2.5 Postpartum Care

Patients typically stay in the hospital for 24–48 hours after a vaginal delivery, or 2–4 days after a cesarean delivery, depending on their clinical status.

8.2.5.1 Postpartum Fever: Differentiating the Differential
— Wind (atelectasis, upper respiratory infection, pneumonia – cough, shortness of breath)
— Water (UTI – polyuria, dysuria, hematuria)
— Womb (uterus – go through risk factors – e.g., retained products of conception, manual placental extraction, operative VD, CD?)

Pearl: There is some evidence that expectant management until 37 weeks may be associated with improved fetal outcomes in patients with PPROM – guidelines may change soon, and this is a good question to ask your preceptors about!

Pearl: If the fever is persistent, yet no clear source has emerged, treat presumptively for endomyometritis, and this is a good topic to ask your resident about.

! Common Error: There is typically no need to obtain cultures for patients presenting with signs/symptoms concerning for postpartum endomyometritis. This is a clinical diagnosis (fundal tenderness + fever = postpartum endomyometritis), and cultures don't tend to help. Treat with Gent + Clinda.

- Wound – CD? Infected lacerations?
- Walking (DVT/PE) – calf tenderness, pleuritic chest pain, dyspnea, tachycardia?
- Weaning breastfeeding – engorgement (transient low-grade temp, 2–3 days PP) and mastitis (red-shaped indurated area of pain). Trt if concerned for mastitis: dicloxacillin. If mastitis, rule out abscess with ultrasound.
- Wonder drugs (misoprostol! or any other drugs they received on L&D)

8.2.5.2 The Postpartum Visit

After leaving the hospital, the next contact with a healthcare provider is typically at the postpartum visit. Postpartum care planning should be individualized, but generally speaking, patients with cesarean deliveries should be seen 2 weeks postpartum, while patients with vaginal deliveries should be seen 6 weeks postpartum. A nurse, midwife, or physician may make phone contact with the patient at 2–6 weeks. Importantly, the postpartum visit is underattended, with up to 40% of patients missing it, and there is a significant effort under way in the field to prioritize continued care during this medically and socially vulnerable time in patients' lives.

8.2.5.3 Postpartum Visit Checklist

If you see a patient for a postpartum visit, think about the patient's physical, psychological, and social well-being using the 9 B's.
  9 "B's":
- Breast – If breastfeeding, any issues or complications?
- Belly – Abdominal exam (if cesarean delivery, examine incision).
- Bottom – Perform pelvic exam (bimanual and speculum), with specific attention to lacerations; can do Pap, GC/CT if needed; can insert IUD.
- Bleeding – Lochia is red/brown (2 weeks) > pink/watery > yellow/white (up to 8 more weeks).
- Bladder – Assess for urinary incontinence; refer for pelvic floor PT and/or Urogyn evaluation PRN.
- Bowels – Assess for fecal incontinence; encourage stool softeners PRN for constipation (common).
- Birth control – Contraceptive counseling, if not yet done; combined hormonal methods can be started 6 weeks postpartum (not earlier due to estrogen increasing already-elevated thromboembolic risk related to pregnancy); OK to resume sexual intercourse if pelvic exam is normal.
- Blues – Edinburgh Postpartum Depression Scale or other validated screening tools.
  - This is also the time to screen again for IPV or family violence. The stress of a newborn can lead to new or exacerbate existing interpersonal conflict.
- Baby – How is the newborn? Are they connected to pediatric care?

8.3 Gynecology

8.3.1 GYN Fundamentals

Gynecology includes care for all female reproductive organs outside of pregnancy: outpatient preventive healthcare, pregnancy prevention/termination, assisted reproductive technology, surgery for benign indications such as fibroids and incontinence, and surgery/chemotherapy for gynecologic malignancies. You will likely spend time in GYN clinics and be assigned to at least one GYN inpatient team. On your inpatient team(s), you will go to OR cases and see consults in the ED and/or other parts of the hospital. Some points that are specific to GYN are:

1. *Vulva vs. vagina* (Fig. 8.11). Mixing up the vulva and the vagina is common! Being able to describe vulvar anatomy will distinguish you as a well-prepared learner. In brief:
   - Vulva = labia majora, labia minora, vestibule, and perineum
   - Vagina = internal
2. *Imaging in the GYN patient.* After the H&P, imaging is a very important tool in gynecology, and ultrasound is almost always the first step. CT scans are generally not useful in gynecology as the pelvic organs are poorly visualized – except for patients with acute pelvic pain in whom you need to rule out non-GYN etiologies (e.g., appendicitis, diverticulitis), oncologic patients, or concern for immediate postop complications such as bleeding or abscess, you should almost never order a CT as the first pelvic imaging test for a GYN patient.
3. *Rule out pregnancy and do pelvic exams.* It is (almost) always a good idea to get a pregnancy test and conduct a pelvic exam.
4. *Consider malignancy.* Always think of malignancy in constructing your differentials. There are many GYN malignancies, some of which present in younger patients – though rare, these are "can't miss" diagnoses.
5. *Surgical nomenclature.*
   - "Hyster-" = uterus
   - "Salping-" = fallopian tube
   - "Oopher-" = ovary

For example, a "bilateral salpingo-oophorectomy" is removal of the tubes and ovaries. A "hysteroscopy" is looking into the uterus with a camera.

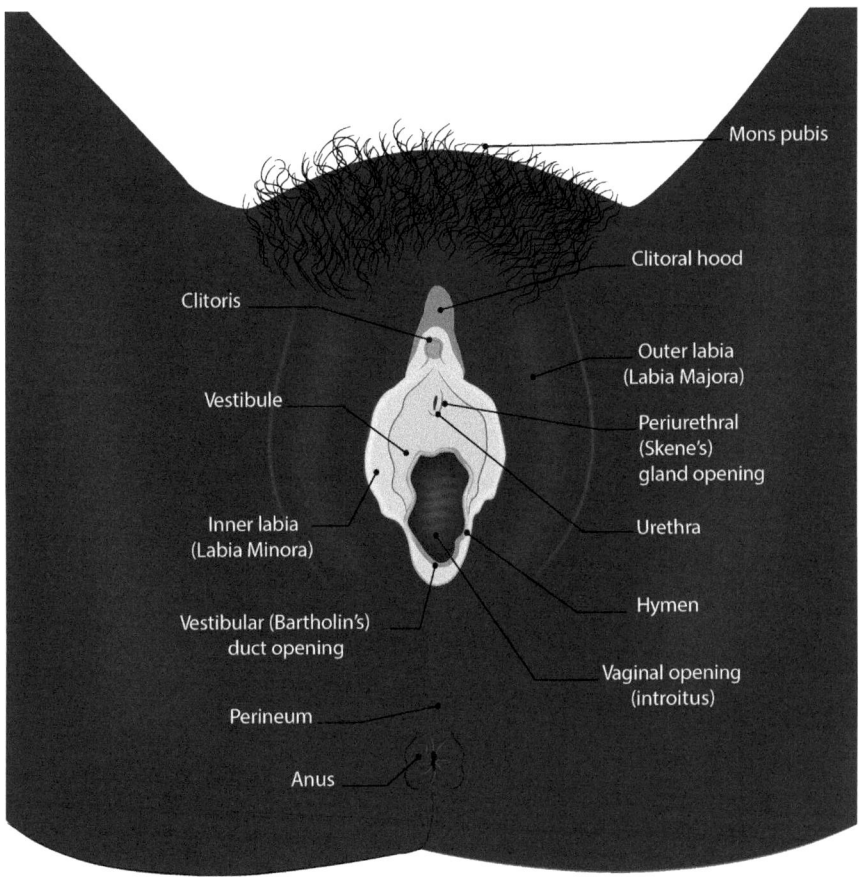

 Fig. 8.11 Vulvar anatomy

Pearl: Practice with real suture material rather than string or yarn, and practice tying knots with sterile gloves on. Instead of tying endless knot-chains on your water bottle handle, practice with one end of the suture attached to a surgical tool (e.g., a clamp); this way, you are simulating the conditions in which knots are often tied in the OR and can practice the often-clumsy task of starting the knot from the proper orientation.

- "-ectomy" = removal
- "-otomy" = opening or incision
- "-oscopy" = view with scope

6. *Suturing and knot-tying.* Practice, practice, practice! You will have the opportunity to showcase your suturing and knot-tying skills in the GYN OR. Be sure to have your two-handed knots and subcuticular stitches mastered. When you are handed a tool in the OR, you have a few minutes to shine, and you want your practice to show. With this said, do not be discouraged if your first few stitches in a series are a bit slow. It takes a while to warm up after watching for so long. Stay confident, even if your hands are shaking.

This section of the chapter contains content on *Outpatient GYN* (i.e., GYN clinic), *Inpatient GYN* (i.e., GYN consults and surgery), and select *Subspecialty* content related to Family Planning, Reproductive Endocrinology and Infertility, Pediatric and Adolescent Gynecology, Urogynecology, and GYN Oncology. You will find the following checklists and examples:

- GYN clinic checklist
- GYN consult checklist
- Anatomy checklist
- OR checklists: "OR Prep" and "Entering the OR and setting up"
- Pre-rounding checklist
- Postop milestones (discharge checklist)
- Postop patient presentation example

8.3.2 Outpatient GYN

8.3.2.1 GYN Clinic Checklist

Essentially the same as for OB clinic (refer to Section 8.2.2.1), but without the OB-specific points. In summary:

- Email your preceptor 1–3 days in advance.
- Complete any advised preparatory reading.
- Prep your list (1.5–2 hours TOTAL, per instructions in "OB Clinic" Section 8.2.2.1, review patients' charts, and populate the clinic template in the "OB" section, but without the OB-specific points).
- Be nice to/befriend clinic staff.
- Take a complete OB-GYN history for all patients per the "OB-GYN H&P" template in this chapter's Introduction (Section 8.1.4, Item 9).
- Never conduct a pelvic exam without a preceptor present.
- When conducting pelvic exams, ask for permission, use a trauma-informed approach including neutral language, and point the speculum DOWNWARD to avoid irritating the more sensitive anterior vaginal structures (see ◻ Fig. 8.2).
- Use the *expectant → medical → surgical* management ladder framework in constructing and presenting your plans.
- Thank everyone at the end of the clinic session.
- Complete any clinic notes you write on the day of the clinic session, and communicate explicitly with your preceptor about which notes you're writing.

8.3.2.2 Common Outpatient GYN Conditions
Well-Person Care

ACOG recommends that patients see an OB-GYN once annually for routine health maintenance and screenings, that is, to undergo routine testing (e.g., blood pressure check, breast cancer screening), mental health screening and counseling, lifestyle (diet and exercise) screening and counseling, and when applicable, STI screening, cervical cancer screening, family planning counseling, and menopause-related care.

- STI Screening
  - Annual GC/CT if <25 years old and/or if increased risk for infection
  - HIV at least once in patients aged 15–65, more frequent screening if increased risk for infection
  - Syphilis, hepatitis B and C if increased risk for infection

- Cervical Cancer Screening (the Pap Test)
  - For an average risk patient, start at age 21, and repeat every 3 years if the findings are normal.
  - Beginning at age 30, add testing for HPV > interval may be extended to every 5 years (assuming everything is normal).
  - Some abnormal Paps will necessitate additional testing (e.g., colposcopy, biopsy) and treatments (see ASCCP guidelines for specifics).

- Family Planning
  - "Are you interested in becoming pregnant in the next year?"
    - If YES, preconception counseling and prenatal vitamins
    - If NO and they could become pregnant in the next year, contraceptive counseling

- Non-GYN Health Maintenance
  - Follow USPSTF guidelines (in AHRQ ePSS app).
  - Highlights:
    - Weight management – diet and exercise counseling
    - Blood pressure
    - Cholesterol
    - Colorectal cancer screening and rectovaginal exams if >50
    - Breast cancer screening
    - Osteoporosis if at elevated risk (post-menopause)
    - Living and work conditions
    - Intimate partner violence screening
    - Mental health screening: PHQ-2
    - Seat belt use, helmet use for bikes

Vulvovaginitis

Vaginal itching/burning/discharge/odor is common. The history, exam, and wet mount often give you an answer; labs (other than GC/CT swab) and biopsies are often not useful initially. That said, biopsy is the only way to

---

Pearl: Historically, the pelvic exam (i.e., inspection of external genitalia, speculum exam, bimanual exam, and rectovaginal exam) was done routinely as a screening tool in asymptomatic patients for GYN cancer or infection; however, there is very limited evidence that pelvic exams in asymptomatic patients are actually useful screening tools. Cervical cancer screening (via Pap and/or HPV testing) and STI screening may require a pelvic exam, but if the patient is not due for these screening tests and is asymptomatic, there is technically no need for a pelvic exam. This is NOT the case for patients with pelvic or vaginal symptoms of any kind (e.g., abnormal bleeding, pain, discharge, etc.), in whom a pelvic exam is almost always indicated.

Pearl: According to the USPSTF, all patients who could potentially become pregnant should take daily folic acid supplementation (e.g., with a prenatal vitamin).

Nearly half of pregnancies are unintended. Outside of relatively rare conditions, anyone having heterosexual intercourse – however rare – could become pregnant. To inquire sensitively, ask "is there any chance you could become pregnant with any of your partners?"

! Common Error: Not all vulvo-vaginitis is yeast! In one study of 200 patients presenting to a specialty vulvar clinic with vaginitis who thought they had yeast infections, diagnoses included:
- Contact dermatitis (20%)
- Recurrent yeast (20%)
- Atrophic vaginitis (13%)
- Vulvar vestibulitis (13%)
- Lichen sclerosis or lichen simplex chronicus (11%)
- Bacterial vaginosis (7%)

8

Pearl: All "lichens" are treated with topical steroids.

Rare, but can't miss!

definitively diagnose lichen planus and sclerosis, which increase risk for vulvar cancer.

- **History**
- Typical OSPQRSTAA history.
- Where specifically is the itching? (e.g., inside the introitus vs. outside on the vulva)
- Vulvar hygiene history: What menstrual products do you use? Do you douche or wash inside the vagina? Do you use any "feminine hygiene" soaps or washes? Do you use lubrication for penetrative sexual activity? Shaving or waxing? What kind of underwear?
- Menstrual and/or menopausal history.

- **Physical**
- Quick skin exam – other eczematous rashes? Psoriasis?
- Pelvic exam:
  - Inspect vulva: Rash? Global vs. localized? Size of introitus? Discharge?
  - Speculum exam: Vaginal walls? Discharge? Cervicitis?

- **The Wet Mount (Sample of Vaginal Discharge on a Glass Slide)**
- pH (normal 3.8–4.5)
  - <4.5 normal or yeast
  - >4.5 BV or Trichomonas
- Whiff test (KOH ➜ fishy odor = BV)
- Microscopy
  - Pseudohyphae ➜ Candida
  - Clue cells ➜ BV
  - Trichomonads ➜ Trichomonas

- **Differentiating the Differential: Vulvovaginitis**
- Candida vaginitis – *Thick*, white discharge + *itching;* pseudo-hyphae on wet mount.
- Bacterial vaginosis – *Thin*, white discharge + *fishy* odor.
- Trichomoniasis – *Yellow, frothy* discharge + odor.
- Chlamydia and/or Gonorrhea – Cervicitis; can be asymptomatic.
- Contact dermatitis – Changes in hygiene practice, non-cotton underwear.
- Atrophic vaginitis – Menopausal patient, thin, friable vulvar and vaginal tissue.
- Lichen planus – Vulva AND vagina; look for affected oral cavity or other skin involvement.
- Lichen simplex chronicus – "Eczema of the vulva"; vulva only.
- Lichen sclerosis – "Cigarette paper" thin skin; a/w neoplasia and painful narrowing of introitus.
- Extramammary Paget's disease (rare malignancy).
- VIN (vulvar intraepithelial neoplasia)/vulvar cancer (usually squamous cell carcinoma) – Dx by biopsy.

Treatment is condition dependent. Refer to the CDC STI app for all antimicrobial options. Since contact dermatitis is so common, know about common vulvar irritants:
- Shampoos and body washes with scents (clean with water only)
- Non-cotton underwear (100% cotton underwear are least irritating!)
- Panty liners

If itching is not improving with topical steroids and hygiene measures (cotton underwear, etc.), biopsy!

Chronic Pelvic Pain

Chronic pelvic pain is common and burdensome. It is defined as a pain syndrome perceived to originate from pelvic organs or structures, typically lasting >6 months. It is often multifactorial, has a long differential, and is often associated with negative cognitive, behavioral, sexual, and emotional consequences. It is important to approach pelvic pain systematically.

Pearl: Central sensitization is a key concept in understanding chronic pelvic pain. The reactivity, or sensitization, of the nervous system is "turned up" such that it is constantly reactive. It lowers the threshold for a stimulus to cause pain and then makes it more likely for pain to stick around after the stimulus is removed.

- Differentiating the Differential: PPUBS
- P: Pain – Chronic or cyclic?
  - Cyclic > endometriosis, adenomyosis
  - Chronic > pelvic mass(es), chronic PID, non-GYN causes
  - Related to mood/stress > consider psychosocial element of pain
- P: Periods – thorough menstrual history
  - Key question: when did your painful periods start? (distinguish primary vs. secondary dysmenorrhea)
- U: Urinary symptoms (urgency, frequency, dysuria, and timeline)
  - Interstitial cystitis (painful but improves after urination)
- B: Bowels (constipation, diarrhea, both?)
  - Bowel irregularity > IBS, IBD, other functional GI disorders
  - Pain with defecation > endo or dyssynchronous pelvic muscle firing
- S: Sexual function (dyspareunia (superficial vs. deep), timing (before vs. during vs. after penetration?), and is pain preventing them from having sex?)
  - Superficial/before penetration > vulvodynia, vulvovestibulitis, vaginismus
  - Deep/during penetration > endometriosis
  - After penetration/during orgasm > musculoskeletal spasm

PPUBS acronym courtesy of Dr. Mark Dassel, Center of Pelvic Pain Director of the Center of Endometriosis OB/Gyn & Women's Health Institute, Cleveland Clinic; via CREOGS over Coffee.

- Treatment
- Multimodal! If you don't target every aspect of the patient's pain, it is unlikely to get better.
- Treat the underlying condition.
  - For example, if cyclic, block ovulation with OCPs.
  - For example, if interstitial cystitis, consider trialing NSAIDs, TCAs, antihistamines, PT, and biofeedback.
- Anxiety and depression can be very reasonable responses to pelvic pain; pain is often improved with improved management of comorbid mental health conditions.
- Pelvic floor PT – can be very helpful, but address other pelvic pain generators before going to PT.

Abnormal Uterine Bleeding (AUB)

"AUB" is an umbrella term that replaced the old terminology of "menorrhagia," "metrorrhagia," and "menometrorrhagia." AUB can include prolonged menstrual bleeding, heavy menstrual bleeding (formerly menorrhagia), irregular bleeding (formerly metrorrhagia), oligomenorrhea (bleeding cycles >35 days apart), and polymenorrhea (cycles <21 days apart), among others. Specifics of the bleeding history in AUB are essential to pointing toward a diagnosis; if further work-up beyond an H&P is needed, this will often include ultrasound, labs, and endometrial biopsy (either in the office or in the operating room with hysteroscopic guidance).

8

■ **The Bleeding History**
— Regular or irregular?
— Heavy or light? (quantify – how many pads or tampons per day?)
— Pain? If so, is it associated with the bleeding, or does it come during other times in the menstrual cycle?
— Family history – other family members with abnormal bleeding?
— Medications

■ **Exam**
— Evidence of P COS? (hirsutism, virilization, acanthosis nigricans) (>ovulatory dysfunction)
— Weight gain or loss, sweating (>endocrine dysfunction > ovulatory dysfunction)
— Petechiae, ecchymoses, skin pallor, swollen joints (>coagulopathy)
— Pelvic exam (polyps sometimes protrude through cervix; uterine size and consistency >adenomyosis, leiomyoma; cervical cancer sometimes visible at external os, if advanced)

! ● Common Error: Not every patient will require all of these options; use your history and exam and the pointers in "differentiating the AUB differential" to select appropriate testing options.

■ **Comprehensive Testing Options for a Patient with AUB**
— Labs:
 – β-hCG
 – CBC with platelets
  – Make sure Hgb hasn't dropped to a level at which you'd need to transfuse.
  – Platelet quantity and function can significantly impact clotting.
 – TSH (both hyper- and hypothyroidism can be associated with AUB)
 – As indicated: Free T (if hirsutism), prolactin (if oligomenorrhea), PTT/PT/fibrinogen OR thrombin time OR vWD diagnostic panel (if heavy menses since menarche and family history of heavy bleeding)
— STI screen, Pap
— Office endometrial sampling
— Transvaginal ultrasound and/or saline infusion sonography
— Hysteroscopy (in office or in OR, depending on provider and institution)

Pearl: Cervicitis and cervical cancer can cause heavy bleeding.

Pearl: Everyone over age 45 and those under age 45 with risk factors for endometrial hyperplasia (e.g., unopposed estrogen, obesity) should undergo endometrial sampling.

The differential for AUB can be worked through using the acronym PALM-COEIN (see ▣ Fig. 8.12).

! ● Common Error: No matter what, make sure that your differential includes pregnancy and malignancy!

■ **Differentiating the Differential: PALM COEIN**
PALM = structural causes
— P: Polyps (epithelial proliferation of endometrial stroma and glands)
 – Dx: Ultrasound suggestive; technically must biopsy for diagnosis
 – Trt: hysteroscopic polypectomy
— A: Adenomyosis (endometrial tissue in myometrium)
 – Boggy, tender, enlarged uterus on pelvic exam
 – Dx: Ultrasound and/or MRI suggestive (start with US; MR typically only used for surgical planning); technically must biopsy for diagnosis
 – Trt: ladder (same as fibroids; see below)
— L: Leiomyoma (a.k.a. fibroids) (benign proliferation of smooth muscle cells and fibroblasts of the myometrium)
 – Irregular, enlarged uterus on pelvic exam.
 – Dx: Ultrasound and/or MRI suggestive (start with US; MR typically only used for surgical planning); technically must biopsy for diagnosis.
 – Trt: ladder (see below).

ABNORMAL UTERINE BLEEDING: PALM COEIN

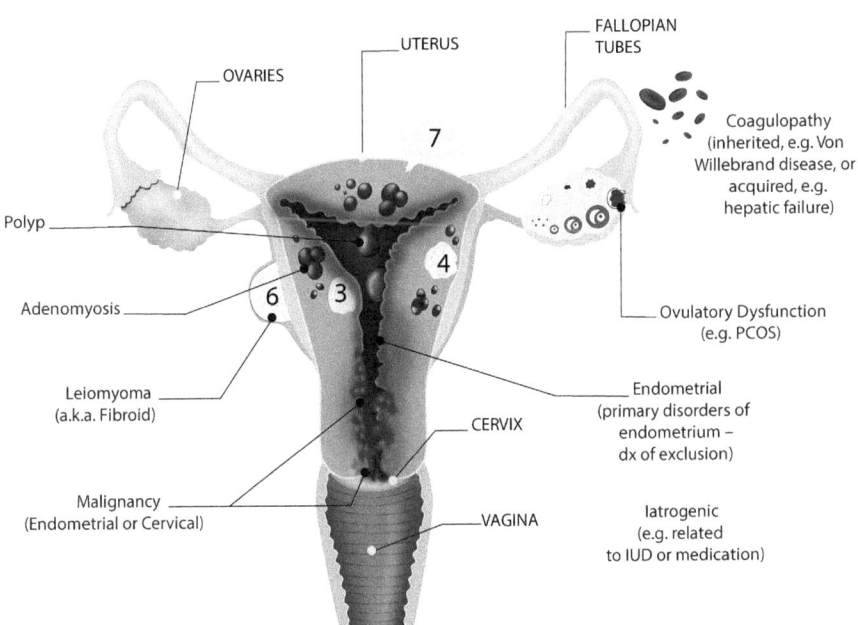

☑ Fig. 8.12 PALM COEIN. Fibroids (leiomyoma) are numbered according to FIGO classification

- M: Malignancy and hyperplasia (most often endometrial hyperplasia or cancer; sometimes cervical)
  - Endometrial cancer is the most common GYN malignancy and often presents with AUB.
    - Endometrial thickness >4 mm in post-menopausal patient with AUB is concerning for malignancy (see ☑ Fig. 8.13).
  - Cervical cancer can cause intermenstrual bleeding.
  - Ovarian cancer typically does not cause vaginal bleeding.
  - Dx: Biopsy.
  - Trt: Per ONC; typically, combination of surgery and chemotherapy, depending on grade and stage.

  COEIN = nonstructural causes
- C: Coagulopathy
  - Up to 20% of patients presenting with heavy bleeding have an underlying bleeding disorder. Start work-up for hemostatic disorders if:
    - Heavy menstrual bleeding since menarche AND
    - Hx of PPH, heavy bleeding with surgery, bleeding with dental work OR > 1 of frequent bruising, nose bleeds, gum bleeding, or family history of bleeding symptoms
  - Consider acquired bleeding disorders from:
    - Medications (e.g., anticoagulants, NSAIDs, contraception, supplements, and herbs (which may impact other medications' efficacy or directly affect the coagulation cascade))
    - Medical conditions (e.g., hepatic failure)
  - Dx: Labs (CBC, PT/PTT, smear, specific functional assays)
  - Trt: Condition-specific

Pearl: Endometrial lining thickness is really only useful in post-menopausal patients and can be used to rule out malignancy. In a menstruating patient, the endometrial lining may range from 1 mm to 30 mm, and any value in that range is normal.
In a post-menopausal patient with vaginal bleeding, thickness >4 mm is concerning for malignancy and should prompt further work-up.
In a post-menopausal patient with no symptoms who has an ultrasound for another indication, >11 mm is concerning for malignancy and should prompt further work-up.

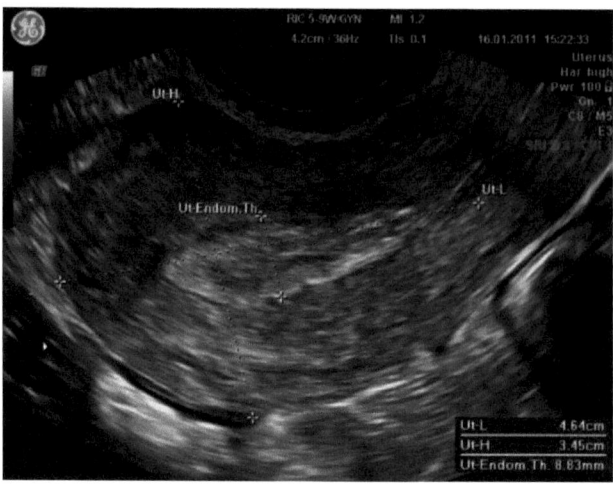

◻ Fig. 8.13 Ultrasound with thickened endometrium. Longitudinal view (transabdominal) of the uterus demonstrating thickened endometrium. (From "Ectopic Pregnancy" by Togas Tulandia, Springer 2015)

- O: Ovulatory dysfunction
  - Anovulatory cycles >irregular menses and endometrial proliferation and thickening (due to unopposed estrogen).
  - Etiologies:
    - Extremes of reproductive age
    - Endocrine disorders that disrupt the hypothalamic-pituitary-ovarian axis (PCOS, hypothyroidism, hyperprolactinemia)
    - Metabolic dysregulation and stress: obesity, anorexia, weight loss, mental stress, and extreme exercise
  - Dx & Trt depend on etiology (treat the underlying condition).
- E: Endometrial (i.e., primary disorder of endometrium)
  - Diagnosis of exclusion; no clinically available specific tests or biomarkers and no specific therapies available.
- I: Iatrogenic
  - IUD
  - Meds: e.g., GnRH agonists, aromatase inhibitors, SERMs
- N: Not otherwise specified/not yet classified

Courtesy of CREOGs over Coffee.

Really, don't let anyone leave your care without a pregnancy test.

DDX by Age

Teenagers/adolescents (13–18) – Most commonly, this is persistent anovulation due to immaturity or dysregulation of the HPO axis, which can represent normal physiology. Otherwise, it could be hormonal contraception use, pregnancy, infection, coagulopathies, or occasionally, tumors.

Reproductive-age (19–39) – Mostly, think about pregnancy! Don't miss early pregnancy bleeding. Once pregnancy is ruled out, consider structural causes (P, A, L). Anovulatory cycles are also common (e.g., in PCOS). Consider meds (e.g., contraception). Lastly, consider hyperplasia, esp. in patients with risk factors (e.g., unopposed estrogen, obesity, PCOS).

40–Menopause – Most often anovulatory bleeding, which can be normal and related to declining ovarian function. This group is more likely to have structural causes such as fibroids and polyps and more likely to have endometrial hyperplasia or cancer. Always check HCG!

Uterine Fibroids

- Background
= Most common pelvic tumor in women.
= They are noncancerous and arise in reproductive-age women from the smooth muscle cells and fibroblasts of the myometrium.
= Depending on population studied, they are present in 20–80% of people with a uterus.
= 50% are asymptomatic; when symptomatic, they often present with AUB and/or pelvic pain/pressure.
= No reason to intervene unless they're causing problems (e.g., heavy bleeding, "bulk symptoms" (pelvic pain, pressure, bowel and bladder dysfunction), necrosis, infertility, and adverse pregnancy outcomes).
= Extremely rarely, can be malignant (leiomyosarcoma), which is diagnosed by biopsy.

- Diagnosis
= Ultrasound and/or endometrial cavity evaluation (biopsy and/or hysteroscopy/D&C)
= Location – pedunculated intrauterine, submucosal, intramural, subserosal (including pedunculated subserosal)

Standout Tip: Read about the FIGO classification, and know the classification of fibroids in patients you see/go to the OR for.

- Treatment
= Expectant often not the answer if they're symptomatic
= Medical options:
  - Combined oral contraceptive pills (suppressing ovulation >halt growth)
  - Levonorgestrel IUD, though distortion of uterine cavity due to fibroids is a relative contraindication to IUD placement
  - GnRH agonists (Depo Lupron, leuprolide) – most effective medical therapy for fibroids, but only available as injection (constant GnRH activity >downregulates HPG axis)
    - Often used in anticipation of surgery to shrink fibroids preoperatively.
    - Decrease bone mineral density >don't use for more than 6 months without some kind of estrogen + progestin add-back therapy.
  - GnRH antagonists (Orlissa, elagolix) (lack of GnRH activity >downregulates HPG axis) – available orally (unlike the GnRH agonists)
    - Decrease bone mineral density >don't use for more than 6 months without some kind of estrogen + progestin add-back therapy.
  - Progesterone-only options – arm implant, injection, pills – second line, but can help with bleeding
  - NSAIDs associated with decreased menstrual bleeding, decreased pain
= Surgical/procedural options:
  - Uterine-conserving procedures and surgeries
    - Uterine artery embolization (cut off blood supply) – interventional radiology. This is contraindicated if future pregnancy is desired.
    - Endometrial ablation (not an option if cavity-distorting fibroids, and bad idea if there is any concern for malignancy because scarring precludes future endometrial sampling). This is contraindicated if future pregnancy is desired.
    - Myomectomy (abdominal, hysteroscopic or laparoscopic).
  - Hysterectomy (definitive)
    - Minimally invasive (vaginal and/or laparoscopic) preferred, if possible. Obviously, this is contraindicated if future pregnancy is desired.

! Common Error: If you are ever uncertain, err on the side of rounding/spending more time with your team, rather than less.

✓ Standout Tip: Ask your team if you can present on a specific topic relevant to a patient you care for. These typically last 5–10 minutes and can be great opportunities to strengthen your knowledge base and show your team how much you know and how hard you're working. Keep it BRIEF and high-yield!

? Question Box: Why is each of these tests important?

ⓘ For example, "I suspect missed abortion based on the ultrasound showing an embryo with crown-rump length consistent with an 8-week pregnancy but no fetal heart activity."

ⓘ For example, "I am not concerned about a septic abortion given her lack of fever and normal white blood cell count."

ⓘ For example, "This was a highly desired pregnancy and the patient prefers to let the pregnancy pass in the most natural way possible, so I suggest we give her misoprostol to induce uterine contraction and evacuation of the pregnancy."

8.3.3 Inpatient GYN

Your role on your inpatient GYN team is similar to that on other surgical teams. In general, your team should tell you where to go and what to do. Although most days you will wear scrubs, if you aren't sure, err on the side of wearing "professional" attire and changing into scrubs if you go to the OR. If you have an off-site clinic for part of the day, you may or may not join your inpatient team to round before and/or after clinic, but discuss this with your chief. Before you leave each day, ask your residents where and when you should meet them the next day and what you should do to prepare. Specific potential tasks include:

- Pre-rounding on patients whose surgeries you were in
- Presenting patients on rounds
- Writing daily progress notes for patients
- Preparing for and attending assigned OR cases
- Seeing consults from the ED or other parts of the hospital
- Preparing signouts
- Preparing discharge paperwork
- Giving "chalk talks"

8.3.3.1 GYN Consults
GYN Consult Checklist

- Spend 5 minutes reviewing the patient's chart before going to see them, and fill in as much of their templated OB-GYN H&P as possible from that information.
- Spend 10 minutes with the patient gathering their H&P and confirming their history.
- If they are of reproductive age, your plan should probably include:
  - Pregnancy test (often already done before you see them).
  - Pelvic exam including speculum exam; collect STI swabs if any concern for PID.
  - Ultrasound.
  - CBC.
- In your plan, make sure you address:
  - The diagnosis you suspect most
  - The most serious/life-threatening diagnoses you want to rule out
  - Patient stability
  - Patient preferences, if applicable
  - Contraception, if appropriate and desired
  - Follow-up plan

8.3.3.2 Common Conditions
Acute Pelvic Pain (◨ Fig. 8.14)

Differentiating the Differential: Acute Pelvic Pain in the Reproductive-Age Patient

- Ovarian torsion – SUDDEN onset ➜ waxing and waning pain, nausea and vomiting; "worst pain of my life."
- Ovarian cyst complications (e.g., hemorrhagic corpus luteum cyst, ruptured follicular cyst) – tender to palpation, rebound tenderness.

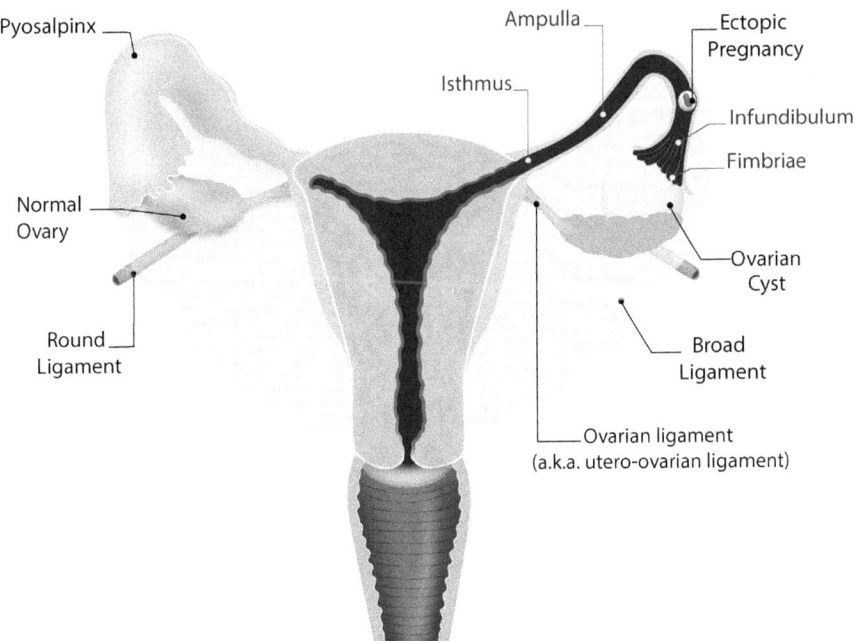

Fig. 8.14 Common causes of acute pelvic pain in the reproductive-age patient

- Pelvic inflammatory disease – fever and pelvic pain with uterine, adnexal, or cervical motion tenderness.
- Ectopic pregnancy – positive pregnancy test, pain, watch out for hemodynamic instability.
- Nephrolithiasis – presents very similar to ovarian torsion with colicky "worst pain of life" pain. Key to differentiation is an abnormal urine analysis (blood, crystals) and ultrasound findings consistent with hydronephrosis.
- Appendicitis – fever, nausea and vomiting; pain migrates from umbilicus to RLQ.
- Diverticulitis – fever, LLQ pain/tenderness, abdominal distention, ± constipation or diarrhea.
- Functional GI pain – absence of "organic" cause; often + diarrhea or constipation.

Ovarian Torsion

- Background
- Complete or partial rotation of the adnexa ➜ ischemia.
  - More commonly involves both ovary and tube
- Early dx and treatment are essential to keep the ovary alive.
- More common in reproductive-age patients (less common surrounding and after menopause).
- Risk factors:
  - Large ovarian mass (>80% have ovarian mass 5 cm or larger; size of mass is proportional to torsion risk).
  - Ovulation induction.
  - Benign masses (e.g., teratoma) torse more often than malignant masses, because malignant masses become fixed to surrounding structures.
  - Patients presenting with torsion under age 15 are more likely to have normal ovaries.

Question Box: What is cervical motion tenderness (CMT) anyway? During the bimanual exam, if there is a marked increase in pain with motion of the cervix, this may be a sign of inflammation; if in doubt, ask your resident or attending to verify your findings.

Question Box: Think of the conditions that increase risk for large cystic masses during pregnancy – are there further studies you want to consider?

Pearl: Ovarian torsion without infection can also cause fever, probably due to edema and inflammation of the ovarian tissue.

Pearl: Though decreased/absent Doppler flow has high specificity for torsion, presence of Doppler flow does NOT rule out torsion.

Pearl: Once diagnosed with PID, patient should undergo testing for HIV and GC/CT, and all sexual partners should be treated presumptively for GC/CT.

Additional suggestive criteria (not necessary for dx, but help narrow down)
Oral temp >101F
Abnormal cervical mucopurulent discharge
Cervical friability
White cells on saline microscopy of vaginal fluid
High ESR/CRP
GC/CT documented
Biopsy (endometrial bx showing organisms)
Imaging (US → pyosalpinx, TOA)
Laparoscopy showing Fitz-Hugh-Curtis syndrome – filmy adhesions going up to liver.

- Can happen during pregnancy (10%), typically between 10 and 17 weeks.
- Presentation: acute onset lower abdominal pain, nausea, vomiting.

- **Diagnosis**
- Ultrasound (first-line diagnostic tool).
- Torsed ovary will be enlarged and edematous compared to contralateral ovary
- Can be decreased or absent Doppler flow in torsed ovary – high specificity
- MR (expensive, but can be used for diagnosis if US is non-diagnostic).
- CT generally not useful except for ruling out non-GYN etiologies for acute pelvic pain such as diverticulitis or nephrolithiasis not captured on ultrasound.
- Direct visualization (i.e., surgery, typically laparoscopy) is needed for definitive diagnosis and is also the only option for treatment.

- **Treatment**
- Surgery! (this is also the only way to confirm diagnosis)
  - Assess ovarian viability (by inspection) and preserve the ovary if possible.
  - Even black or blue-ish ovaries can maintain function following detorsion; the earlier the detorsion, the more likely the tissue will retain function.
  - Cystectomy often done for benign ovarian mass to reduce risk for re-torsion.
  - Management in pregnant patients same as nonpregnant patients: laparoscopy.
  - If c/f malignancy, salpingo-oophorectomy.
- Risk for recurrence (unknown)
  - Reduce risk with oral contraceptive pills and ovarian fixation (to pelvic sidewall) (though both of these approaches lack long-term, systematic study).

Pelvic Inflammatory Disease (PID)
- **Background**
- Infection of the upper female genital tract, i.e., endometritis, salpingitis, tubo-ovarian abscess (TOA), pelvic peritonitis.
- PID can be caused by many infectious diseases; we think of GC/CT most commonly, but <50% of PID patients test positive for these organisms! Other organisms are vaginal flora bacteria and Gram-negative organisms.
- Presentation: Pelvic pain, fever.

- **Diagnosis**
- "Minimum criteria"
- Pelvic pain with no other identifiable cause for illness
- One or more of the following: cervical motion tenderness, uterine tenderness, adnexal tenderness

- **Treatment**
- Hospitalize? This is a complicated decision which generally considers the following:
  - Are they pregnant?
  - Do they have a high fever or signs of septic shock?
  - Do they have nausea and vomiting requiring IV antiemetics?

- Would they be able to follow an outpatient antibiotics regimen and follow up in 24–72 hours?
  - Is there an abscess?
- Empiric, broad-spectrum antibiotics (see CDC STI app and OB-GYN Antibiotics Guide).
- Complicating factors:
  - TOA (consider if no improvement with 24–48 hours of IV antibiotics)
  - IUD in place?
    - Consider removal if no clinical improvement in 48–72 hours.
- Follow-up: 72 hours of treatment should lead to improvement (so for patients being treated as outpatient, schedule a f/u clinic visit in 72 hours); if no improvement, admit for IV antibiotics, additional w/u, etc.

8.3.3.3 Early Pregnancy Complications

Acute complaints during the first trimester of pregnancy are generally considered GYN territory. If a patient comes in for vaginal bleeding, pain, or fever and has a positive pregnancy test, ultrasound is ALWAYS an important step in the work-up. Note how nearly all of the diagnoses in the differential below are differentiated based entirely on ultrasound. Quantitative β-hCGs are also often important in these patients. A key principle of early pregnancy physiology is that the serum β-hCG should increase by at least 53% every 48 hours in a normal intrauterine pregnancy; if it is not increasing at that rate, this raises concern for an ectopic or failing pregnancy. Further "normal pregnancy" milestones to be aware of are (1) an intrauterine pregnancy should be seen on transabdominal ultrasonography with β-hCG levels greater than 6000 mIU/mL and (2) a fetal heartbeat should be seen with β-hCG level greater than 5000 mIU/mL.

Differentiating the Differential: Vaginal Bleeding in a Patient with a Positive Pregnancy Test

- Ectopic pregnancy – pain, ultrasound without intrauterine pregnancy, ± hemodynamic instability.
- Spontaneous abortion (SAB) – ultrasound with evidence of non-viable intrauterine pregnancy.
- Subchorionic hematoma – ultrasound with evidence of blood between the uterine lining and the chorion (the outer fetal membrane, next to the uterus) or under the placenta.
- Postcoital bleeding – patient reports recent intercourse; ultrasound without evidence of abnormality.
- Vaginal or cervical lesions or lacerations – seen on pelvic exam.
- Extrusion of molar pregnancy – ultrasound with molar pregnancy.

Ectopic Pregnancy

- Background
- A pregnancy that implants outside of the uterine cavity – this happens in <1% of pregnancies. 95–99% of ectopics are in the fallopian tube (see ◘ Fig. 8.15), mostly within the ampulla.
- Any female patient of reproductive age presenting with vaginal bleeding and/or abdominal pain should always be evaluated for ectopic pregnancy! A ruptured ectopic pregnancy is a true emergency – it can result in rapid hemorrhage, leading to shock and death.
- Risk factors: prior ectopic, prior tubal surgery, PID (tubal scarring from prior infection can block fertilized egg passage to the uterus, and chronic

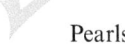 Pearl: Because many patients with ectopic pregnancies are young and otherwise healthy, such signs of intra-abdominal hemorrhage may not occur until the patient has lost a LOT of blood.

Pearls:
Monitor for signs and symptoms of rupture – increased abdominal pain, bleeding, or signs of shock. If treating with methotrexate, advise the patient to come to the ED immediately in case of such symptoms. Remember contraception, if patient desires it – patients may resume sexual activity before the come back to see a clinician in follow-up, and it may not yet be safe to become pregnant if they are recovering from treatment/surgery.
If a patient is treated surgically for ectopic pregnancy, they can continue prenatal vitamins. If treating with MTX, they should stop taking any folic acid. MTX is a folic acid antagonist, so giving concurrent folic acid is counterproductive. Patients who desire pregnancy can resume taking prenatal vitamins when the HCG level drops to zero.

Pearl: Before administering MTX, collect baseline CBC, transaminases and creatinine.

infected state may cause intrauterine scarring in a condition known as "Asherman's syndrome," which is highly associated with ectopic pregnancy), assisted reproductive technology, endometriosis, prior abdominal surgery (adhesions), smoking, pregnancy i/s/o in-place IUD (IUDs prevent pregnancy, but in the <1% who become pregnant with an IUD in place, those pregnancies are much more likely to be ectopic because the IUD prevents normal implantation in the uterus).

- **Diagnosis**
- History: unilateral pelvic or lower abdominal pain and vaginal bleeding
- Physical: ± tender adnexal mass, SGA (small for gestational age) uterus, and bleeding from the cervix
  - If ruptured, may be hypotensive, tachycardic, or unresponsive or show signs of peritoneal irritation secondary to hemoperitoneum
- Labs:
  - Quantitative β-hCG, CBC, blood type, and antibody screen
- Ultrasound:
  - Looking for adnexal mass or extrauterine pregnancy (see ■ Fig. 8.12); a hemorrhaging, ruptured ectopic pregnancy may reveal intra-abdominal fluid throughout the pelvis and abdomen.
  - Gestational sac with a yolk sac seen in the uterus on ultrasound indicates an IUP.
  - At early gestations, neither an IUP nor an adnexal mass can be seen on ultrasound.

- **Treatment**
- Unstable → surgery
- Stable (i.e., uncomplicated, nonthreatening) → surgery or methotrexate (MTX)
  - Can treat with MTX only if small ectopic pregnancies (as a general rule, <4 cm, serum β-hCG level < 5000, and without a fetal heartbeat), if there are no contraindications to MTX, and for those patients who will be reliable with follow-up (to verify declining β-hCG)

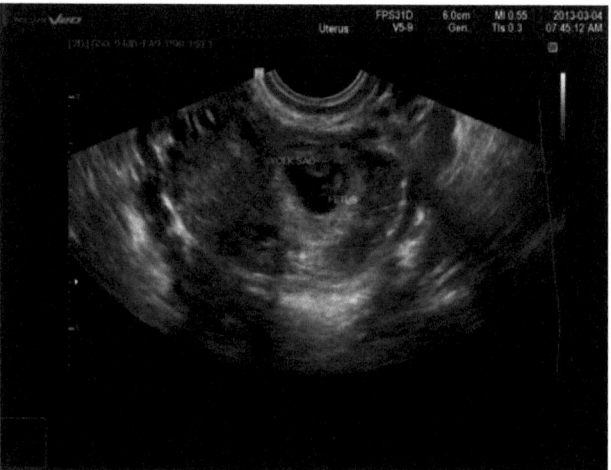

■ **Fig. 8.15**   Tubal ectopic pregnancy. Ultrasonographic image of tubal ectopic pregnancy with both embryonic pole and yolk sac visible within the gestational sac. (From "Ectopic Pregnancy" by Togas Tulandia, Springer 2015)

Spontaneous Abortion (SAB)

- Background
- 15–20% of all pregnancies
- Type of SAB depends on the amount of products of conception (POC) that have passed and whether the cervix is dilated:
    - Complete – complete expulsion of all POC before 20 weeks
    - Incomplete – partial expulsion of all POC before 20 weeks
    - Inevitable – no expulsion, but cervix is dilated and viable pregnancy is unlikely
    - Threatened – any VB before 20 weeks (no cervical dilation or POC expulsion; pregnancy is still viable)
    - Missed – death of embryo/fetus before 20 weeks; no bleeding or symptoms (i.e., POC still all in uterus)

- Diagnosis
- History: VB, cramping, abdominal pain, and decreased symptoms of pregnancy
- Physical (VS, abdominal exam, bimanual exam, speculum exam): BP (hypotensive?), Temp (fever?), sources of bleeding other than uterine, changes in the cervix suggestive of an inevitable abortion
- Labs: Quantitative β- hCG, CBC, blood type, and antibody screen
- Ultrasound: assess fetal viability, placentation, r/o ectopic

- Treatment
- Depends on (1) viability of pregnancy and (2) patient preferences.
    - If pregnancy is not viable (i.e., missed ab, incomplete ab), can manage expectantly, medically (mifepristone, misoprostol), or surgically (D&C) – depends on clinical stability and patient preferences
    - If pregnancy is potentially viable and desired, can manage expectantly with close f/u; if not desired, may proceed with medical or surgical ab

8.3.3.4 The OR

When you go to the OR, the more you know about the patient and the case, the more you will get out of being there and the more opportunities you will have to participate. Introduce yourself to any patient whose procedure you will observe. Ask your resident if you can help with documentation including op notes, postop orders, prescriptions, and postop instructions. Things you should definitely do, if possible, include a postop check and note and (pre)rounding on the patients for as long as they're in the hospital, including writing their daily progress notes.

Anatomy Checklists

Be able to recognize the following structures when looking down into the pelvis from a laparoscope:
- Uterus
- Cervix
- Uterine support structures:
    - Uterosacral and cardinal ligament complex
    - Round ligaments
    - Broad ligament
- Ovaries
- Fallopian tubes
- Ureters
- Sigmoid colon

Pearls:
If there is uncertainty about viability of the pregnancy, serially follow the quant β-hCG every 48 hours to see if it is increasing appropriately (it should rise by 67% – double every 48 hours).
Rh-negative patients get RhoGAM if they bleed during pregnancy, regardless of pregnancy viability (to prevent isoimmunization and risk for fetal anemia in future pregnancies). Remember contraception, if patient desires it – patients may resume sexual activity before the come back to see a clinician in follow-up, and they may not desire pregnancy right away/ it may not yet be safe to become pregnant if they are recovering from a treatment regimen or surgery. Advise patient to continue prenatal vitamins, as all patients with potential for pregnancy should take a daily folic acid supplement.

Pearl: Imagine that you are the attending surgeon and the buck stops with you in terms of the patient's care – if a complication arises intraoperatively, if they have an adverse reaction to a drug, etc., you want to know as much as possible about the patient to keep them safe and inform your decision-making.

Pearl: It is common for attendings/residents to prefer writing their own notes and for them to ask you to just focus on learning. This is OK! As long as you offered each person, you are off the hook and enjoy the rare opportunity to just learn without administrative responsibilities.

Pearl: The APGO videos are an excellent resource for anatomy review!

- Anterior cul-de-sac
- Posterior cul-de-sac ("pouch of Douglas")
- Vesicovaginal space

Be able to draw out the course of the following blood vessels:
- Common iliac artery >external and internal iliacs (internal a.k.a. hypogastric)
- Internal iliac artery (a.k.a. hypogastric artery) >anterior and posterior branches
- Anterior branch of internal iliac >obliterated umbilical, uterine, superior vesical, obturator, vaginal, and inferior gluteal and internal pudendal arteries
- Blood supply to the uterus, tubes, and ovaries (derives from the uterine arteries and the ovarian arteries)

Checklist: Preparing for the OR
- Who is the patient and why are they having surgery? Know:
  - The indication for the procedure
  - Their OB-GYN and medical history
  - Their surgical history
  - Their medications and allergies
  - What procedure are they having done? If it's a planned procedure, look it up the night before – find a YouTube video of the surgery, and memorize:
    - The anatomy relevant to the procedure
    - The steps and/or stages of the procedure
    - The common complications
- Self-care:
  - Eat breakfast.
  - Use the bathroom before heading into the OR.
  - If you are getting queasy, step away from the table and sit down (the last thing you want is to faint and land in the surgical field). It's okay to ask for a cold compress for the back of your neck.
- Before the surgery, go to the pre-op area ~30 minutes ahead of time (and/or with your resident – will depend on your team), and introduce yourself to the patient.
- If it's an urgent or emergent procedure, it may or may not be worthwhile to go to the bathroom or step out of the OR for a moment, and it won't be obvious that you're gone to read on your phone about the procedure. If your resident tells you to go to the bathroom before the procedure, or if you're waiting outside of the patient's pre-op bay, spend 3 minutes reviewing the patient's record and/or the procedure (whichever you know less about). If there is no time for that, though, don't worry about preparation – your being present with your team is more important than your patient-specific knowledge in an urgent/emergent setting.

Checklist: Entering the OR and Setting Up
- Before entering the OR, make sure you're wearing personal protective equipment (PPE):
- Scrubs
- Hair cover
- Mask
- Eye protection
- Shoe covers

Standout Tip: If it's a planned procedure and you can prepare the night before, write all of this down on a notecard, and keep that notecard in your scrub pocket.

For example, say "Hi, I'm ___, and I'm the medical student member of your surgical team. If it's okay with you, I'll be watching and assisting with your surgery today."

Common Error: If a hospital computer or tablet is available, use one of those rather than reading on your phone. One of the most common complaints residents have about students is that they are on their phones and no one knows if they are studying, looking at social media, or texting. This is one of the biggest reasons students get negative comments and is especially common in the downtime around surgeries. If you can use a hospital computer or tablet where the screen is visible, everyone can see what you're up to, and you'll be more likely to get kudos.

8

- Introduce yourself by name to *everyone* in the OR, and ask for their name and remember them – the scrub nurse, the circulating nurse, the anesthesia team, and, of course, your surgical team (the attending and resident(s) or assistant(s))
  - You want to connect with every member of the OR team (see the "Soft Skills" chapter for more tips on this). This is *key*. Repeat your name a few times so they can remember it.
- Write your name on the board, including your full name (first and last), and what year of medical school you are in.
- Help transfer the patient to and from the PACU. Ask your resident to show you how to set up the leg rests so that you can help; do your best to learn this so that you can be trusted to do it on your own after one to two rounds with help.
- Ask if it would be helpful to place the Foley. Be careful to practice working with the materials beforehand, and review the anatomy of the clitoris, urethra, and vagina. A common mistake in catheterizing is placing the catheter in the vagina, or attempting to insert it into the clitoris (painful). You will be watched like a hawk by the scrub nurse and residents for general sterility and proficiency of this procedure if you ask to do it. If done well, this demonstrates competence.
- Find out if you are scrubbing in: Ask your resident politely, "Do you know if I should scrub?" If they say yes, ask the resident and/or scrub nurse if you can get the resident's and your own gown and gloves. If they say yes, get them, and then ask if you can hand them to the scrub nurse.
- Before scrubbing, make sure you have:
  - Checked with the attendings/residents that it's time to scrub
  - Pulled your gloves (and those of your resident(s), if not already pulled) for the scrub nurse
  - Removed watches/rings/bracelets, etc. from your hands and wrists
  - Silenced your phone
  - Donned PPE

Pearl: Because the vagina isn't sterile, you CANNOT use the same gloves in the vaginal and abdominal surgical fields; if you move from the vagina to the abdomen, you must change gloves.

Common Questions and Pearls for the OR

Use antibiotics if entering (i.e., cutting tissue of) (1) the uterus, or (2) the vagina.

- Prep: Clean the Skin
- ChloraPrep (alcohol based). This evaporates/dries; it's flammable (common question), so it has to dry before drapes are placed on top of them!
- Prep the vagina – it will never be sterile, but we make it "surgically clean"
- Betadine (iodine-based).
- Chlorhexidine (alcohol based). This has a lower concentration (<4%) to avoid burning the vaginal mucosa; more common in more bloody procedures (e.g., Urogyn).

Draping is usually not a medical student job due to risk for contamination. Most procedures start in the vagina, with an exam under anesthesia (to facilitate surgical planning), urinary catheter insertion, and speculum exam to facilitate placement of a uterine manipulator.

Standout Tip: Manipulators are varied and complex, but if you can get good at manipulating the uterus, you will be loved! Focus on this.

- Laparoscopy: Abdominal Entry, Insufflation, and Port Placement
- Entry location: often through umbilicus
  - Exceptions to umbilical entry: multiple prior laparoscopic surgeries, umbilical hernia, distorted anatomy for other reasons; in these cases, can go in through Palmer's point (RUQ)

Standout Tip: *Review your anatomy!* Laparoscopy is a great opportunity for teachers to probe your knowledge and teach because everyone can see everything.

Question Box: Why enter at the umbilicus?
It has the minimum depth between skin and peritoneum and is avascular.

Question Box: Why CO2?
O2 is flammable; NO2 will give the bends; CO is toxic.
CO2 is inert – not all of the gas will come out, and it's OK for it to be absorbed by the abdominal wall/tissue. That said, know that CO2 can cause minor irritation (shoulder pain related to peritoneal irritation is a classic post-op complaint to be aware of).

- Insufflation: fill the belly with CO2, 12–15 mmHg.
- Before placing ports:
  - Transilluminate to make sure you aren't hitting vessels, and look for the abdominal wall folds to make sure you're avoiding the inferior epigastric vessels.
  - Inside (closer to peritoneum) = inferior epigastric.
  - Outside (closer to skin) = superficial perforating veins and/or arteries.

When closing, incisions and port sites >5 mm require closure of the fascia to decrease risk of hernia; smaller port sites (<5 mm) are less likely to have herniation. All port sites require skin closure, which can be by subcuticular suture (your time to shine!) or skin glue.

Most laparoscopic cases can go home the same day or the next day.

Procedure-Specific Tips and Pearls

- **D&C ("Dilation and Curettage")**
- Dilate the cervix and "scrape" off endometrium with curette.
- Dilators are numbered by the circumference, whereas we care about the cervix diameter → if you want to dilate to 8 cm, use a (8 × 3 + round up = 25) (common question).
- Relatively short procedure; "gritty" texture means the procedure is complete.

- **Hysteroscopy**
- Camera looking into the uterus through the cervix.
- Speculum → dilate cervix as needed for scope → insert camera → insert fluid → look at uterine cavity ± intervention.
- Fluid choices – two categories:
  - Electrolyte-containing (normal saline, lactated Ringers)
  - Non-lyte-containing (sorbitol (3%), mannitol (5%), glycine (1.5%), dextrose (5%))
- "The deficit": fluid used to distend the uterine cavity is absorbed systemically, so be aware of your patient's fluid and electrolyte status.
- You want to SEE the ostia (opening of the tubes) – this is how you know you were truly in the uterine cavity and it was completely visualized.

- **Hysterectomy**
- Three approaches – know the basics of each:
  - Abdominal
  - Laparoscopic (lsc) – physician manipulated (straight stick), robot assisted, lsc-assisted vaginal (use of ports, but ultimately removing uterus through vagina as opposed to port sites)
  - Vaginal
- Indications:
  - AUB – fibroids, polyps, endometrial hyperplasia (hysterectomy is last resort for these, but is definitive treatment)
  - Prolapse
  - Cancers – ovarian, uterine, endometrial, cervical
- The tubes and ovaries – take them or leave them?
  - Tubes are needed for natural passage and union of eggs and sperm. Outside of this function for fertility, they only increase risk for ovarian cancer. Therefore, in patients having their uterus removed, the tubes are also often removed for cancer risk reduction unless doing so cannot be done safely.

Pearl: Common question! A significant body of evidence suggests that many ovarian cancers originate in the fallopian tubes.

- Ovaries provide estrogen and progestin, which have many health benefits.
  - If the patient is premenopausal, leave the ovaries if possible. There are significant negative effects of oophorectomy and resultant surgical menopause: increased risk for cardiovascular disease, osteoporosis, and all-cause mortality.
  - If the patient is post-menopausal, the ovaries may still be providing some benefit…
    - Around age 55, it can be reasonable to remove the ovaries.
    - After 65, ovary removal is strongly encouraged.
- Important steps, regardless of approach:
  - Cutting the round ligament
  - Ligation of the ovarian blood supply
  - Avoiding the ureters and inspecting for ureteral injury
    - Can occur at the pelvic brim, medial to the infundibulopelvic ligament, at the level of the internal os, where it passes under the uterine artery ("water under the bridge"), or just lateral to vaginal cuff closure (right before it implants into the dome of the bladder)
  - Ligation of the uterine arteries (uterus should start to blanch (turn white) at this point)
  - Vaginal cuff closure

8.3.4 Postoperative Care

8.3.4.1 Post-op Check and SOAP Note

This is quite similar to the general surgery rotation, so refer to ▶ Chaps. 1 and 7 for guidance on post-operative milestones and rounding. Offer to write these notes and plan to (pre)round the next day(s) for patients who stay in the hospital.

8.3.4.2 Pre-rounding Checklist

- Open a note in the chart and fill it in as you gather information.
- Chart review:
  - Overnight events?
    - Read ALL notes (nursing, Physical Therapy, etc.) since the last time you reviewed the chart.
  - Vitals
  - UOP
  - Morning labs, if any
- Check in with nursing.
  - As with other rotations, get overnight events directly from the overnight nurse – sometimes there will be events that have not yet been entered into the chart.
- See the patient.
  - Examine the patient's belly.
  - Do NOT perform a pelvic exam, but ask if they have had vaginal bleeding.
  - Look at their pad to assess the volume of any blood.
- Write your progress (SOAP) note (this also serves as prep for your presentation).

8.3.4.3 Presentation Example

"Ms. Z is a 38-year-old, G4P2 who is postop day #1 s/p laparoscopic total abdominal hysterectomy for symptomatic uterine fibroids. Her past medical history is non-significant, and she has had no prior surgeries. Intraoperatively

Question Box: What artery runs inside the round ligament? Answer: Sampson's!

Question Box: What structure contains/conceals the blood supply to the ovary? The IP (infundibulo-pelvic) ligament (a.k.a. suspensory ligament of the ovary).
Note that this can hemorrhage and build up in the posterior peritoneum before bleeding into the peritoneal cavity and becoming recognized – it is a direct branch off of the aorta and can BLEED.

Pearl: Pay attention to location of ureter relative to the IP ligament! Thermal energy can spread and cause delayed thermal injury to surrounding structures including ureters.

Pearl: Be aware that vaginal cuff dehiscence is a complication of hysterectomy. What's sitting behind the cuff? Bowel – patients can come into the ED with bowel hanging out of their vagina after a cuff dehiscence. This is why it's important for patients to avoid insertion of anything into their vagina for at least 6 weeks after hysterectomy.

Pearl: The Enhanced Recovery After Surgery (ERAS) Protocol is an evidence-based guideline for postoperative care. If your hospital uses it, follow the guidelines closely. If your hospital doesn't use it, ask your resident about it by saying "I read about the Enhanced Recovery After Surgery protocol online – does our hospital use that?"

8

Standout Tip: Ask your team for explicit details and examples of how they present ins and outs (e.g., do you report UOP in cc/kg/hour, or cc/24 hour?).

Common Error: If there is gauze covering incisions, do not remove it, but comment on how saturated it is and the color (e.g., 20% saturated with serosanguinous fluid).

Pearl: GYN patients typically don't actually need to eat before leaving the hospital, but you want to be sure they won't immediately vomit when they eat at home – this will prevent a bounce back.

Pearl: A "trial of void," typically done by nursing, means either back filling the bladder with normal saline ("active trial") or encouraging the patients to drink ("passive trial"), letting them pee on their own, and seeing how much comes out; if they're unable to void on their own, they need to have a catheter replaced.

she was found to have a large fibroid uterus which was morcellated in a bag prior to removal through a mini-laparotomy. EBL was 500 cc.

Subjectively, she is doing well with Tylenol and gabapentin for pain control, had mild nausea last night, but feels thirsty this morning.

Objectively, her vitals are ___. She is receiving IV LR at 125 cc/hour and made 0.8 cc/kg of urine per hour overnight. On exam, she is alert and oriented. Heart and lungs are clear. Her abdomen is soft, appropriately tender, and non-distended, with normoactive bowel sounds. Her incisions are clean, dry, and intact with Steri strips in place. She has a Foley in place draining clear, yellow urine, and she has no bleeding on her pad. Her calves are nontender and she is wearing SCDs.

In summary she is progressing appropriately postoperatively. The plan for today is to D/C her Foley for a trial of void, start clear liquids as tolerated, and check a CBC today, with likely discharge to home this afternoon."

8.3.4.4 Post-op Milestones (Discharge Checklist)

The key question for postoperative patients is "when can they be discharged?" Below are the milestones you'll be monitoring closely to determine the appropriate timing.

- Nausea/vomiting is controlled.
- Able to eat and drink.
- Foley is out; can void on their own (otherwise, can go home with a catheter).
- Passing gas (gas is important, but patients don't need a bowel movement before going home – the bowels are often slow to return to normal function after surgery in the peritoneum, even if they weren't touched).
- Ambulating (at or near whatever their baseline ambulatory status was preoperatively).
- Check for acceptable:
  - Vitals
  - UOP
  - CBC if done

8.3.5 Select Subspecialty Topics in Gynecology

8.3.5.1 Family Planning

Contraception

A full list of contraceptive methods can be found in the CDC MEC app, along with absolute and relative contraindications. We will not discuss details of individual methods here; instead, we will address several important concepts to understand and think about as you discuss contraception with your teachers and patients.

1. Typical-use vs. perfect-use failure rates. "Typical use" describes the failure rate of a method averaged among patients using this method in the real world (e.g., the average patient taking birth control pills may miss several pills each month, or take the pills at a slightly different time each day). "Perfect use" describes the failure rate of a method averaged among patients using this method in the real world (i.e., a user taking the birth control pill at the exact same time every single day, without ever missing a day). A major advantage of long-acting reversible contraceptions (LARCs) (IUDs and the arm implant) is that their typical use and perfect use failure rates are equal because they do not require user action to work, unlike short-acting methods such as the pill, patch, ring, or shot.

2. Mechanism of action – pregnancy can be prevented by:
   - Preventing ovulation (arm implant, pill, patch, ring, injection)
   - Making the uterus inhospitable to a pregnancy (IUDs)
   - Blocking entry of sperm into the uterus, mechanically (barrier methods) or by thickening the cervical mucus (hormonal contraception)
3. Postpartum contraception. Combined hormonal methods (pill, patch, ring) should not be used in the first 6 weeks postpartum due to elevated thromboembolic risk from pregnancy. All other methods are safe to use while breastfeeding and can be initiated immediately postpartum.
4. Hormonal vs. non-hormonal. The only highly effective non-hormonal option is the copper IUD. Less effective non-hormonal options include barrier methods and fertility awareness.
5. Return of fertility. Among reversible methods, the Depo-Provera injection is the only method for which fertility may not return immediately after stopping (it can take up to 6 months for ovulation to return, and up to 18 months to achieve a pregnancy). For all other reversible methods, fertility returns rapidly after stopping the method.
6. Emergency contraception (EC). These methods can be used after unprotected intercourse (UPI), imperfect contraceptive use or barrier failure, or forced sex without contraception. The copper IUD is the most effective form of EC and can be inserted up to 5 days after UPI. Oral EC options include ulipristal acetate (an antiprogestin which can be used up to 5 days after UPI) or the norethindrone pill ("Plan B" which can be used up to 3 days after UPI). The earlier EC is administered, the more effective it is.

Contraceptive Counseling
- Ask the patients about their goals/priorities (e.g., privacy, decrease bleeding, future fertility, etc.).
- Ask if they'd like to hear about all vs. some vs. none of the options.

Standout Tip: Contraceptive decision-making is often influenced by prior experiences and the experiences and opinions of an individual's social network. For each method you discuss, start with "what do you know about X method?"

Pregnancy Options Counseling
- Typically, there are three options for a pregnancy:
  - Continued pregnancy
  - Abortion
  - Adoption
- Unexpected pregnancy can be stressful, scary and isolating, or exciting and joyous for patients. Either way, it's a common experience – nearly half of all women in the United States have an unintended pregnancy at some point in their lives. If you see patients who did not expect to be pregnant and have a positive pregnancy test, share information with them objectively and non-judgmentally so that they can make their own informed decisions.

Pearl: If you are telling a patient about a positive pregnancy test result, say: "The pregnancy test was positive" in a clear, neutral voice, and then leave space for them to respond.

Abortion
- Approximately one in five of pregnancies ends in abortion.
- At 2014 rates, about one in four (24%) women will have an abortion by age 45.
- Abortion-related morbidity and mortality increase with gestational age; however, the average mortality rate associated with abortion is approximately 14 times lower than that associated with continued pregnancy.
- Abortions can be done medically or surgically.
  - Medication abortion is an option until 10 weeks.
    - Mifepristone (progesterone antagonist; halts growth of pregnancy) + misoprostol (prostaglandin analog; induces uterine contractions)

– Surgical abortion
  – Dilation and curettage (D&C) (<14 weeks)
  – Dilation and evacuation (D&E) (>14 weeks)

A note on abortion regulation:
- Abortion is the most regulated medical procedure in the United States, with more than half of states having imposed specific restrictions on abortion provision (a.k.a. "Targeted Regulation of Abortion Provision," or "TRAP" laws) that increase barriers to accessing safe abortion care. As a result, availability of abortion varies widely between institutions and regions.
- ACOG upholds that abortion is part of comprehensive reproductive healthcare and opposes legislation that increases barriers to accessing abortion services.

8.3.5.2 Pediatric and Adolescent Gynecology (PAGS)

Approach to the adolescent patient:

ACOG recommends that female patients should be introduced to the gynecologist between ages 13 and 15. This visit may not involve a pelvic exam; rather, it's an opportunity to introduce a confidential space to discuss reproductive health, menstruation, sexual orientation, gender identity, contraception, etc. At this stage, patients may be in early, mid, or late adolescence, and discussion should be tailored to their emotional and intellectual development. Don't rush! Give them TIME.

Key issues in this population:
- Confidentiality and consent.
  - In most states, healthcare surrounding contraception and STI diagnosis and treatment is confidential for patients under age 18, though most STI diagnoses must be reported to departments of public health.
  - Pregnancy: In most states, patients under 18 who are pregnant can consent to their own healthcare, as well as that for their child. Notably, however, most states require parental or guardian consent to obtain an abortion.
  - Abuse: State laws mandate reporting of physical or sexual abuse that is disclosed to a healthcare provider.
- Sexuality and sexual activity.
  - Nonjudgmental counseling surrounding safer sex (contraception and STI prevention) is essential.
  - 47% of girls aged 15–19 years have already engaged in sexual intercourse, yet a minority of these individuals use contraception.
  - Adolescents aged 15–19 account for 50% of new STI diagnoses.
- Pelvic exam, STI screening, and Pap testing recommendations are the same in adolescents as in adult patients. That is to say,
  - Pelvic exams should only be done if a patient has symptoms (though an external pelvic exam can be done for staging Tanner stages of development if this is pertinent to the patient's care).
  - STI screening: if patient has had sexual intercourse, annual screening for GC/CT is recommended. This can be urine sample or vaginal swab (more sensitive). HIV screening should be done at least once.
  - Pap testing: does not start until age 21, regardless of HPV vaccination status or sexual activity.
- Vaccination against Human Papillomavirus (HPV) is recommended by the FDA for all patients, female and male. It is a two-shot regimen for patients under age 14 and a three-shot regimen for patients aged 15 and older. Its use has been extended up to age 45.

PAGS subspecialists care for patients with both medical reproductive endocrine issues (e.g., PCOS, ovarian insufficiency) and surgical issues (e.g., cysts, congenital anomalies of the reproductive tract).

Pearl: In visits with adolescents, start with patient and parent together, then parent only, then patient only, and then all together again.

Standout Tip: Many patients and families are unaware of the difference between a pelvic exam and a Pap test; this is a great opportunity for education!

Pearl: Immune compromise is an exception to the "Paps start at 21" rule.

8.3.5.3 Reproductive Endocrinology and Infertility (REI)

Infertility is the most common condition encountered in REI. It is defined as lack of conception despite regular intercourse for 1 year (or 6 months if female is >35 years old). Overall incidence is 12–18%, and incidence increases with age (30% in women aged 40–44). Many couples have multiple reasons for infertility, and treatment is often multimodal. The approach to infertility involves (1) identifying the underlying cause(s) and (2) correcting reversible cause(s) and overcoming irreversible cause(s) in order to conceive a pregnancy.

Evaluation of infertility always starts with a thorough OB-GYN history. Additionally, it most often involves looking for the following conditions with the following tests:
- Male factor: Semen analysis/male work-up
- Ovulatory dysfunction: "Day 3 labs" (day 3 FSH and estradiol) ± AMH, antral follicle count (normal is 3–8 follicles per ovary), TSH
- Tubal damage: Hysterosalpingogram
- Uterine cavity distortion: Sonohysterogram
- Endometriosis: History and physical, pelvic ultrasound, laparoscopy
- Coital problems

Treatment options include (1) lifestyle modification and (2) condition-specific treatments.
1. Lifestyle:
   - Stop smoking.
   - Reduce excessive alcohol and caffeine (>250 mg/day) consumption.
   - Work toward a normal BMI (20–25) (both under and overweight can contribute to infertility).
   - Appropriately timing intercourse (just before and around the time of ovulation – you want sperm waiting for the egg; can use ovulatory predictor kits).
2. Condition-specific:
   - Ovulatory dysfunction.
     - Induce ovulation with a selective estrogen receptor modulator (SERM) (works at the level of the brain) or aromatase inhibitor (works at the level of the ovary).
   - Tubal factor (blocked tubes) – both tubes are blocked, sperm and egg cannot meet >need IVF.
   - Male factor.
     - Low sperm count
       - Intrauterine insemination
       - Inject each egg with a single sperm
     - Obstructive → Surgically obtain sperm from the testes directly
   - Cavity (mechanical issues).
     - Remove any fibroid(s) and/or polyp(s).
     - Uterine septum should be corrected – can be hysteroscopically resected.
     - Intracavitary adhesions (e.g., Asherman's syndrome) can be hysteroscopically removed.
   - Same sex couples and single patients.
     - Donor sperm insemination.
     - Female-to-male transgender patients can freeze eggs prior to hormone-assisted transition.

Pearl: Male factor infertility is the most common identifiable cause of infertility. A semen analysis is easy to do and should always be the first step!

Question Box: Can you think of why each of these tests is useful in the work-up of suspected ovulatory dysfunction?

Question Box: Can you describe the physiology underlying how these medications induce ovulation? Answer: Both aromatase inhibitors and SERMs trick the brain into thinking estrogen is low → FSH goes up → triggers follicle development

8.3.5.4 Urogynecology

Urinary Incontinence

- **Background**
- Affects 1/3 of women, but many don't talk about it. There are two types (stress and urge), though patients often have a mix of them.
- SUI (stress urinary incontinence) is leaking with some kind of physical activity (cough, jump, sneeze) and is typically a small volume of urine.
- Urge incontinence (a.k.a. overactive bladder or OAB) is due to muscle spasm of the detrusor muscle (think of this as "Afib" of the detrusor) and can produce a larger volume of urine.
- Risk factors: Pregnancies; heavy lifting; obesity

- **Diagnosis**
- Hx: What happens, how often, how much urine, how much does it bother you?
- Physical: Cough stress test (in lithotomy position); POP-Q exam
- Testing: Cystometry (fill bladder with catheter, look at detrusor contraction); urodynamic studies

- **Treatment**
- The first step is always a diary including beverage intake and episodes of incontinence; lifestyle modification can go a long way.
- Physical therapy & Kegels (10 reps 3× daily) → 50% improvement
- SUI
  - Vaginal inserts (pessary)
  - Surgical treatments: slings, Burch procedure (neck of the bladder is suspended from nearby ligaments)
- OAB
  - Avoid bladder irritants (caffeine, artificial sweeteners, ocean spray, crystal light).
  - Pharmacotherapy (anticholinergics and/or beta agonists – take ~4 weeks to work).
  - Bladder retraining (timed voiding and pelvic floor PT → retrain the bladder so that the capacity increases).

Pelvic Organ Prolapse (POP)

- **Background**
- Affects 11% of women, but many don't talk about it. There are three main types.
- Anterior wall prolapse ("cystocele"): prolapse of the bladder into the vagina.
- Posterior wall prolapse ("rectocele"): prolapse of the rectum into the vagina.
- Uterine or cuff prolapse: prolapse of the uterus or vaginal cuff (after hysterectomy).
- Risk factors: pregnancies; heavy lifting; obesity.

Pearl: Pelvic organ prolapse (POP) (see below) is another common condition often treated by urogynecologists and can often contribute to urinary incontinence. The POP-Q exam is a systematic method for classifying POP.

Question Box: Can you describe how SUI treatments work?
To conceptualize them, imagine the urethra as a hose; stepping on that hose blocks flow through it. Pessaries, slings, and the Burch procedure all put pressure on the urethra to prevent urine leakage.

8

- ■ Diagnosis
- ▬ Hx: do you have a vaginal bulge or lump? how much does it bother you?
- ▬ Physical: cough stress test (in lithotomy position); POP-Q exam; stage of prolapse.

- ■ Treatment
- ▬ Physical therapy and Kegels (10 reps 3× daily)
  - – Vaginal inserts (pessary)
  - – Surgical treatments: anterior or posterior colporrhaphy (bringing the pelvic floor tissues together to support the prolapsing wall); cervical or cuff suspension from sacrum or sacrospinous ligament; hysterectomy

8.3.5.5 Menopause

Menopause is defined as the permanent cessation of menstruation after 1 year without menses. In North America, median age at menopause is 51, which means that on average, women spend >1/3 of their life in menopause. The cardinal signs and symptoms are generally all caused by declining and then absent estrogen.

Symptoms include:
- ▬ Vasomotor symptoms (i.e., "hot flashes") – up to 80% of perimenopausal patients
  - – Sudden flushes of heat, typically starting in the face/chest and spreading through the body; typically 1–5-minute long
  - – Can last up to 8 years
- ▬ Genitourinary syndrome of menopause (a.k.a. vulvovaginal atrophy and concomitant urinary symptoms) – 10–40% of menopausal patients
  - – Vaginal dryness, itching, irritation, dyspareunia, urinary symptoms, and frequent UTIs
- ▬ Sleep disturbance
- ▬ Mood changes

Treatment options:
- ▬ Lifestyle modifications: control surrounding environment and avoid vasomotor triggers; avoid alcohol and caffeine; use air conditioning if possible, dress in layers, drink cool drinks; weight loss can be helpful.
- ▬ Nonhormonal medications:
  - – SSRI
  - – Gabapentin
  - – Clonidine
- ▬ Hormonal therapy:
  - – Low-dose vaginal estrogen is a first-line treatment for vulvovaginal atrophy in the genitourinary syndrome of menopause.
  - – Systemic estrogen + progestin is a highly effective treatment option but is associated with increased risk for cardiovascular disease in older patients.
  - – Generally, in younger patients, initiating estrogen + progestin for vasomotor symptoms within 36 months of their final menstrual period is thought to be safe.

> Pearl: How these medications help with menopausal symptoms is not well-understood.

> Pearl: Unopposed estrogen is associated with increased risk for endometrial cancer. Systemic estrogen should always be administered with a progestin to people with a uterus.

8.3.5.6 Gynecologic Oncology (GYN ONC)

GYN ONC training includes a 3-year-long fellowship devoted to mastering the medical and surgical management of gynecologic malignancies. Thus, we will not attempt to cover this subspecialty in great detail. We will, however, share some important concepts and frameworks with which to think about the most common conditions you'll encounter during a GYN ONC rotation.

Broadly, when it comes to all oncologic disease, the importance of the basics cannot be underscored enough! Some important concepts:

- Cancer screening attempts to identify early-stage malignancy. Pap testing (screening for cervical cancer) is a major cancer screening success story and one of the great public health victories of modern medicine.
- Definitive diagnosis of all malignancy requires biopsy, which can be done in the clinic setting in the case of easy-to-access organs (e.g., a vulvar or cervical lesion), or can require surgery (e.g., suspected ovarian malignancy).
- Carcinoma in situ vs. invasive cancer: "in situ" means that the cancerous cells have not invaded the epithelial basement membrane; in invasive cancer, they have broken through this barrier.
- Grade = what do cells look like under the microscope?
- Stage = how extensive is the cancer in the body?

Approach to GYN malignancy, regardless of the site, includes:

- Staging: this is the process of determining the degree of spread in the body, based on magnitude of primary tumor and extent of metastatic spread.
  - Stage 1: limited to the organ
  - Stage 2: local spread
  - Stage 3: regional spread
  - Stage 4: distant metastasis
- Biopsy is needed to establishing tumor grade; depending on the malignancy, this can be done pre- or intraoperatively.
- Surgery: often, hysterectomy + bilateral salpingo-oophorectomy (hyst + BSO) with lymph node evaluation.
- Chemotherapy: neoadjuvant (before surgery) vs. adjuvant (after surgery).
- Radiation: Brachytherapy and/or whole-pelvis radiation.
- Consideration of fertility preservation options in younger patients who may be interested in childbearing.

Some key facts and concepts related to the three major GYN malignancies are listed below.

Cervical Cancer

- The incidence and mortality of cervical cancer in the United States have each decreased by >50% since the introduction of Pap testing.
- The vast majority of cervical cancer is caused by HPV, >70% by strains 16 and 18 > HPV testing is part of routine screening.
  - Individuals with competent immune systems tend to clear HPV on their own, typically between 8 and 24 months after exposure; thus, HPV co-testing with Paps is not typically recommended until ≥30 years of age.
- Colposcopy can be used to obtain cervical biopsies in patients with abnormal Paps.

- Cervical intraepithelial neoplasia (CIN) is a precancerous condition which can be excised with cryotherapy or loop electrosurgical excision procedure (LEEP).
- Invasive cervical cancer is treated surgically or by chemo/radiation therapy, depending on stage.

Endometrial Cancer

- Cancer of the lining ("endometrium") of the uterus makes up >90% of uterine cancers and is increasing in incidence.
- Two major types:
  - I (80%; bread and butter – estrogen-driven, typically low-grade, endometrioid histology, favorable prognosis)
  - II (10–20%; higher-grade, more aggressive, worse prognosis)
- Often presents with AUB, and amount of bleeding is NOT related to risk for cancer. ANY bleeding in a post-menopausal patient is abnormal.
- Can also present via Pap (atypical glandular cells).
- Incidental finding on imaging.
- Diagnosis: endometrial biopsy or hysteroscopy/D&C.
- Treatment: Surgery!
  - Typically, Hyst + BSO with some kind of lymph node evaluation (often sentinel node biopsy).
  - Minimally invasive approaches are preferred due to lower perioperative morbidity and are not associated with worse cancer outcomes.
- Most stage 1 patients are cured after surgery.
- Most stage 2–4 patients require some kind of adjunctive chemotherapy, ± brachytherapy or whole-pelvic radiation.

Ovarian Cancer

- Most deadly of all the GYN malignancies. There is no identified/established screening tool, and most present at stage 3 or later because of its varied presentation and symptomatology.
- Often presents with abdominal discomfort, fullness, and/or early satiety due to ascites and abdominopelvic tumor burden.
- Though family history is always important and there are cancer syndromes that increase risk for ovarian cancer (e.g., HNPCC, BRCA), the vast majority of ovarian cancer cases have no genetic tie.
- Three main types:
  - Epithelial (85–90%)
  - Germ cell
  - Sex chord stromal
- Diagnosis and treatment: Surgery!
  - Typically, Hyst + BSO with some kind of lymph node evaluation (often sentinel node biopsy)
- Tumor markers (CA-125, CEA, and sometimes CA 19-9) which are not indicated for primary screening; rather, they are used in follow-up for surgical patients to assess for treatment response and recurrence.
- Most patients require some kind of adjunctive chemotherapy, ± radiation.

Pearl: Risk factors for type I include:
- Estrogen (exogenous, e.g., menopausal hormone therapy, tamoxifen; and endogenous, e.g., elevated circulating estrogen levels related to obesity, or an estrogen-secreting tumor)
- Diabetes
- Nulliparity
- Genetics (Lynch syndrome, Cowden syndrome)

Protective factors include:
- Progestin-containing contraception
- Breastfeeding
- Increasing gravidity and parity

Pearl: Carboplatin + paclitaxel is often the endometrial cancer chemotherapeutic regimen of choice.

Pearl: Brachytherapy is local radiation (cylinder in the vagina) after a hysterectomy to decrease risk of recurrence at the vaginal cuff (most likely site of recurrence) – often used in "high-intermediate"-risk patients.

Appendix (◻ Table 8.6)

◻ **Table 8.6** OB-GYN antibiotics

Condition	Regimen	Covering	Comments
Asymptomatic bacteriuria and lower UTI in pregnancy	Per culture results Typically beta-lactam (Cephs, 'penems), nitrofurantoin (usually 3–7-day course), or fosfomycin (single dose)	*E. coli* (~70%), *Klebsiella, Enterobacter*, GBS	Bactrim contraindicated in first trimester due to interference with folate metabolism Patients with sickle cell trait or disease should be tested every trimester during pregnancy (higher risk of pyelo)
Upper UTI during pregnancy	Start with ceftriaxone (or other broad-spectrum beta-lactam) If second trimester, Bactrim OK; If extended spectrum beta-lactamases (EBSLs), consider meropenem or ertapenem Avoid nitrofurantoin and fosfomycin because these don't achieve adequate concentrations in the kidneys	*E. coli* (~70%), *Klebsiella, Enterobacter*, GBS	Consider continuing prophylactic antibiotic therapy if recurrent UTI
PPROM, latency antibiotics	Ampicillin + erythromycin (or Azithro) × 48 hours (IV) followed by amoxicillin + erythromycin (or Azithro) × 5 days (PO)	GBS, GU flora	PPROM is typically thought to be caused by some kind of subclinical infection, and/or having abx on board prevents infection from brewing and worsening things Abx have been shown to prolong pregnancy (and therefore decrease gestational age-dependent mortality) and decrease rates of both maternal and neonatal infection
Intrapartum GBS prophylaxis	Penicillin (PCN) or ampicillin if not allergic If PCN allergy, may use Ancef, clindamycin, or vancomycin depending on clinical scenario (see ◻ Fig. 8.7)	GBS, GU flora	If GBS status is unknown, antibiotic prophylaxis should be given If PCN allergic and GBS +, obtain sensitivities as resistance to clindamycin is common
Intra-amniotic infection (IAI)	Mostly polymicrobial, but cover GBS with AMP, GU flora with Gent + Clinda If postpartum and/or if PCN allergy, only Gent + Clinda	GBS, GU flora	Why does ampicillin become less important after delivery? Because it primarily covers GBS, which we treat only to reduce risk for neonatal GBS infection

◻ **Table 8.6**   (continued)

Condition	Regimen	Covering	Comments
Pelvic inflammatory disease (PID)	Multiple options in CDC STI app If admitted, start with parenteral abx with transition to PO in 24–48 hours if clinically improved If outpatient (mild-moderate acute PID), treat with PO abx with close f/u for 72 h; if no improvement or worsening, admit for IV abx	GC/CT	If tubo-ovarian abscess, surgery is often needed to contain the source of infection

OB Triage Note Template

Referring Provider: _
   Primary OB Provider: _
   ID/CC: _ year old G_ P_ _ _ _ at _ weeks _ days gestational age by LMP consistent with _week ultrasound (EDD _) presenting with _.
   Pregnancy Dating
   EDD _ by (US on _ at _ weeks gestation) vs. (sure LMP)
   Problem List
   1. _ (list any active problems)
   2. Postpartum contraception plan
   3. Plans for birth
   4. Plans for breastfeeding
   5. Plans for pediatric care
   Hx of Current Pregnancy: Complicated by the above problem list. She presents to L&D with _.
   ROS: Pertinent findings noted in the above history of present illness and triage intake form, all other systems are negative. *List THE FIVE QUESTIONS*
   Physical Exam
   VS: _
   GENERAL: No acute distress.
   CARDIOVASCULAR: RRR, _murmurs. 2+ peripheral pulses
   RESPIRATORY: Effort normal, lungs clear to auscultation bilaterally posteriorly
   ABDOMEN: Nontender, gravid. No palpable masses, or hernias. Fundal height _. EFW _ by Leopold's.
   EXTREMITIES: _ edema, symmetrical strength and movement. No calf tenderness. Patellar DTRs normal and symmetric.
   SKIN: No rashes, lesions.
   NEURO: Alert and oriented. No gross deficits.
   PSYCH: Mood/affect appropriate.

PELVIC: Normal external genitalia, _ lesions.
SSE: _ pool, nitrazine _, fern _
SVE: _ / _ / _
LEOPOLD's: _ cephalic, EFW _#
FHT: baseline _, _ variability, _ accels, _ decels.
TOCO: _
Labs: _
Bedside US: cephalic _, placenta _, fetal cardiac motion _, AFI/DVP _
ASSESSMENT & PLAN: _ year old G_ P_ at _ WGA by _ with _.
_.
_.
Fetal well-being: _reactive on monitor
Follow up in _ weeks with _ (provider)
Note cc'd to provider/clinic: _

8

Neurology

Iyas Daghlas

Contents

© The Author(s), under exclusive license to Springer Nature Switzerland AG 2021
S. H. Lecker, B. J. Chang (eds.), *The Ultimate Medical School Rotation Guide*,
https://doi.org/10.1007/978-3-030-63560-2_9

9

9.1   Overview

Neurology can sometimes feel like a black box. It is my hope that this chapter will open that black box and help you confidently enter and enjoy your neurology rotation. Neurology is quite similar to internal medicine, sharing the fundamental principles of history-taking, differential diagnosis, and the oral presentation. I would thus advise you to review the internal medicine chapter (▶ Chap. 3) prior to reading this chapter. However, there are several features unique to neurology including:

1. The neurological examination
2. Lesion localization in the assessment
3. Consideration of neurology-specific diagnostics and treatments in your plan

In this chapter, we will focus on these elements that are specific to neurology. We begin by discussing the physical examination, where we introduce a hub-and-spoke model to help organize your approach to the neurological patient. We then discuss the oral presentation, review the approach to brain imaging in neurology, the assessment and plan, and four commonly encountered neurological conditions (delirium, headache, first seizure, and bacterial meningitis). We end the chapter with a review of five landmark clinical trials that inform clinical practice in neurology and may be used in your oral presentations to support treatment decisions.

9.2   The Neurological Examination

9.2.1   Overview

We have all been there – seeing a consult and then later realizing that you forgot a key physical examination maneuver. The trick to overcome this problem is to build a "muscle memory" for the neurological examination by performing the maneuvers in the same order each time. However, we know that some patients will require special physical examination maneuvers - how does this fit into the principle of doing the examination in the same order each time?

The answer is the "hub-and-spoke" model of the neurological examination. In essence, there is a "hub" for the neurological examination that represents the core maneuvers that you will perform nearly every time when evaluating patients on your rotation. When required, you can add one of the spokes – for example, detailed strength testing in the setting of weakness – to accommodate a specific patient presentation. In this section we will discuss the core physical examination and then talk about some high-yield spokes to consider in special scenarios. What follows is a list of the core neurological examination maneuvers, which you may use as reference on your rotation, with additional details to follow (▶ Box 9.1).

Act out the examination a few times before proceeding in the chapter and practice the examination for the few days preceding your rotation with the aim of having the examination memorized by the day you start your rotation. We will now go into more detail for each part of the core neurological examination.

Box 9.1   The Steps to Performing the Core Neurological Examination

Mental Status

Alert and oriented to person, place, and time. Able to say the days of the week backward. Speech fluent with intact repetition and without aphasia or word-finding difficulties. Followed one- and two-step commands without difficulty. 3/3 memory at 5 minutes

CN II-XII

- II – Visual fields full to confrontation in each eye individually. Pupils equally round and reactive to light
- III, IV, VI – No ptosis. Extraocular movements intact without nystagmus
- V – Sensation to light touch intact on face bilaterally
- VII – Face symmetric with normal forehead wrinkle, blink, smile, and cheek puff
- VIII – Able to hear finger rub bilaterally
- IX, X – Palate midline with elevation. No uvular deviation
- XI – 5/5 shoulder shrugs bilaterally
- XII – Tongue midline with protrusion

Motor Examination

Normal bulk and tone with no fasciculations or bradykinesia. No myoclonus, asterixis, or tremor. No pronator drift. 5/5 strength bilaterally in upper and lower extremities

Sensory Examination

Diffusely intact to light touch in upper and lower extremities. No extinction to bilateral simultaneous stimulation

Reflexes

Deep tendon reflexes normal and symmetric bilaterally at the triceps, biceps, brachioradialis, quadriceps, and soleus. Toes down-going bilaterally

Cerebellar Examination

Normal finger to nose and heel to shin. No dysarthria

Gait

Normal gait with intact toe, heel, and tandem gait

9.2.2   The Mental Status Examination

9.2.2.1   Arousal

- The mental status examination begins *as soon as you step into the room*. By simply looking at the patient, you can immediately assess their level of consciousness – are they awake or are they sleeping? If asleep, what kind of stimulation does it take to wake up the patient? There is a substantial difference between the patient being arousable to name vs. arousable only to sternal rub.
- Incomplete reporting: *"The patient was stuporous."*
- Good reporting: *"The patient fell asleep multiple times during the examination and was unable to arouse to voice but could be woken up by light touch."*

The idea that the mental status examination begins the moment you step into the room is also relevant to the practice of psychiatry!

This highlights a general principle that *more detail is better* when it comes to relaying the physical examination. The same principle can be applied to the assessment of orientation. If the patient was unable to answer a question, then relate the answer they gave:

- Incomplete reporting: *"The patient was oriented to person, place, but not time."*
- Good reporting: *"The patient was oriented to person, place, but not time, as they thought the year was 1950."*

the patient saying "1950" is quite different from the patient being able to state the year, but missing the month.

9.2.2.2 Attention

We began with an assessment of arousal because the mental status examination may be unreliable if the patient is sleepy. The same principle holds for *attention*, which reflects the ability of the patient to concentrate on a task. If a patient is inattentive, they would not be expected to perform well on a memory test. I like to test attention by asking the patient to state the days of the week backward, but others prefer tests like "serial 7s" (starting at 100 and sequentially subtracting 7). While there may be small variation in sensitivity and specificity for these tests, the specific test used often ends up being a matter of style.

9.2.2.3 Memory

When testing memory, it is helpful to use the same three words each time. That way, you will not forget the words when the patient is repeating them to you. A commonly used trio of words is "purple," "ball," and "chair." Ensure that the words are unrelated so that the patient must rely on their short-term memory to get them right.

I sometimes (ironically) forget to ask the patient to repeat the three words. It can thus be helpful as a backup to thus ask the patient to remind you to ask them about the words in a few minutes. In a way, this serves as an additional test of memory.

9.2.2.4 Language

- Asking the patient to repeat a phrase, such as "today is a sunny day in Boston," tests two basic language modalities at the same time: fluency and repetition (and dysarthria, although that is not considered a domain of language per se – more on this later). To test for the ability to start with a one-step command (e.g., point to the ceiling), then a two-step command (e.g., point to the ceiling after pointing to the door).

9.2.2.5 Spokes

The mental status examination has several "spokes" that can be deployed in patients with suspected cognitive deficits.

1. The Montreal Cognitive Assessment, more commonly referred to as the MoCA, features one page of questions (readily accessible via the Internet) that assess different domains of cognition. Some of these overlap with domains that you routinely test – such as attention and memory – while other domains are not typically tested in the 'hub' examination (e.g., visuo-spatial function). I recommend conducting a MoCA any time you admit a patient who is being worked up for cognitive decline or dementia. This does not necessarily have to be on the same day you admit the patient – in fact, it is preferable to wait until the daytime or when a delirious patient has improved (despite these precautions, an in-hospital MoCA may still not be representative of a patient's function at home). Once the MoCA is com-

Patients with a Broca's/expressive aphasia can have an intact ability to sing, which can be elicited on the physical examination.

Difficulty following commands can be seen with a Wernicke's/fluent aphasia.

□ Table 9.1 Steps for eliciting several frontal release signs

Reflex	Steps
Grasp reflex	Place a finger at the base of the palm of the patient's hand. Sweep your finger toward the patient's fingers. If the patient reflexively grasps your finger, they are considered to have a positive grasp reflex
Myerson's sign	Tap the patient's forehead between their eyes. Patients typically blink with the first few taps then stop blinking. If the patient continues to blink they are considered to have the Myerson's sign, which is a frontal release sign
Palmomental reflex	Drag your finger from the patient's thenar eminence up to the base of the thumb. Watch the ipsilateral corner of the patient's mouth for a twitch

plete, take some time to analyze the results on the page and synthesize the deficits into domains of mental status (e.g., visuospatial vs. memory).

You can also have the patient draw a clock in isolation if you do not feel the need to do the full MoCA. If you do this, then make sure you bring a picture of the clock to rounds and upload the picture to the patient's medical record.

2. Frontal release signs are reflexes that are typically found in infants and disappear in adulthood. These reflexes can re-emerge in the setting of frontal lobe pathology (e.g., in frontotemporal dementia). Although these signs tend to not have a high sensitivity or specificity, they can provide helpful evidence for a diagnosis of dementia. Choosing between the reflexes is oftentimes a matter of style. Here are some examples (□ Table 9.1).

9.2.3 The Cranial Nerve Examination

Always examine the cranial nerves in numerical order (with the exception of V, which is typically examined after III, IV, and VI). I have never tested the first cranial nerve in the hospital setting. This test may be indicated if you suspect an early presentation of a neurodegenerative disease (e.g., Parkinson's or Alzheimer's disease), but these cases are more typical in the outpatient setting. Do ensure that you only report what you test (e.g., CN II-XII intact). Prior to your rotation, I recommend practicing the cranial nerve examination until you perform do it smoothly from memory. Here we will go into more depth for most of the cranial nerves, with the exception of CN VIII and CN XI (as those will not generally be assessed at a "spoke: level on your inpatient rotation).

9.2.3.1 Visual Fields (CN II)

Everybody has a different approach to testing the visual fields. Here is my approach:

1. Sit or stand a few feet away from the patient at the same eye level.
2. Cover your eye, and have the patient mirror the action so that they are covering the opposite eye (e.g., you cover your right while they cover their left).
3. Now, take your free hand and extend it out far into one of the corners of the four quadrants until you can no longer see the hand. Ensure that your hand is equidistant from you and the patient (see □ Fig. 9.1).
4. Now start wiggling1 the fingers and bring the hand closer until the patient reports seeing the hand. Note whether this happens at the same time that

Don't forget that visual field testing, pupillary light reflex, and visual acuity all test the second cranial nerve!

---

1 An alternative approach is to flash 1 or 2 fingers and ask the patient to name how many fingers they see.

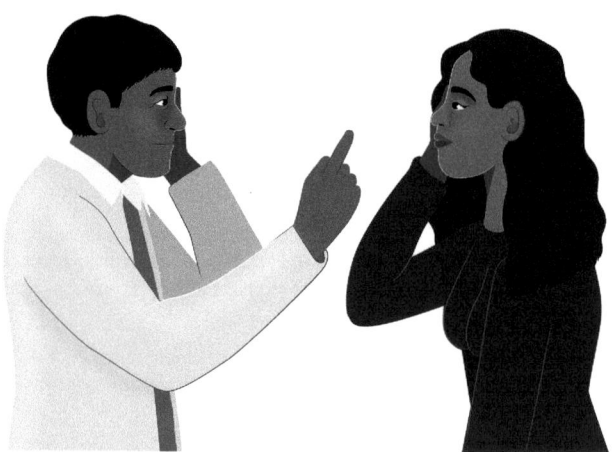

☐ **Fig. 9.1** Visual field testing

the hand enters your field of view – this would be a normal finding. If the hand needs to come in closer, then the patient may have a compromised visual field. Repeat this for all four quadrants, then for the other eye.

9.2.3.2 Extraocular Movements (CN III, IV, VI)

A common error when testing extraocular movements (III, IV, VI) is to not move your fingers far out enough in the visual field. This may cause you to miss subtle ocular weakness or nystagmus. Once you reach the "limit" of the extraocular movement, hold your finger in position for a moment and look closely for nystagmus. In patients reporting diplopia, this part of the examination may clarify which eye movements elicit the diplopia.

9.2.3.3 Nystagmus

On the subject of nystagmus, it is important to remember the principle of describing the examination in as much detail as possible. A limited presentation may simply relate that there was nystagmus associated with extraocular movements. An advanced presentation would, at the very least, include:
1. What direction of eye movements elicited the nystagmus? When was the nystagmus most pronounced?
2. A description of how the eyes moved during the nystagmus – was it vertical, horizontal, or torsional nystagmus?
3. The direction of the fast and slow phase of nystagmus
4. Roughly how many beats of nystagmus did you see? A few beats or sustained nystagmus?

9.2.3.4 Facial Nerve (CN V)

When performing the maneuvers that test CN V (normal forehead wrinkle, blink, smile, and cheek puff), keep in mind the difference between upper and lower motor neuron patterns of facial weakness.
- *Upper motor neuron injury*: contralateral, lower face weakness that spares the forehead
- *Lower motor neuron injury*: ipsilateral weakness involving the whole face

It is not accurate to say that strokes always cause an upper motor neuron pattern of facial weakness. This is because a brainstem stroke injuring the facial nerve nucleus or facial nerve tract can cause a lower motor neuron (whole face) pattern of weakness.

Another pearl concerns the pattern of facial weakness in Bell's palsy. As a reminder, Bell's palsy is an idiopathic facial nerve palsy that is thought, in many cases, to be caused by a viral infection. You may therefore expect this syndrome to be characterized by weakness of the whole face. Unfortunately for the diagnostician, patients do not always present with a "complete" Bell's palsy and may thus initially present with weakness of the lower face. Stroke may be on the differential in these cases.

The House-Brackmann scale is a standardized way to grade facial paralysis in Bell's Palsy. It is worth looking up if you happen to see a patient with a Bell's!

9.2.3.5 Glossopharyngeal (CN IX) and Vagus Nerves (CN X)

There is overlap in the function of these two nerves and it is therefore generally difficult to tease them apart one from another. Keep in mind that in the setting of weakness of these nerves, the uvula will deviate toward the *intact* side. To remember this, think of two vectors pulling the uvula upward and to the side. When strength is equal, these vectors cancel out. When one side is weak, the other side will dominate and pull the uvula toward that side.

9.2.3.6 Hypoglossal Nerve (CN XII)

One approach to test for subtle tongue weakness (CN XII) is to place your index finger on the outside of the patient's cheek and have them push their tongue against you from the inside of their cheek. Compare on each side. If you try it on yourself, you will find that the tongue is actually quite strong at baseline!

The approach to thinking about tongue weakness is flipped relative to the uvula. This is because the vectors from the muscles are pushing the tongue out, rather than pulling the tongue in. Therefore, if the muscles on the right side are weak, then the vectors from the left side will dominate in pushing the tongue out toward the right side. Keep in mind that this description is in reference to the location of *muscle* weakness. The location of the lesion will differ depending upon whether the lesion is an upper or lower motor neuron lesion. In lower motor neuron lesions (e.g., brainstem stroke), the muscle weakness will be ipsilateral to the lesion in the nervous system. In upper motor neuron lesions (e.g., cortical stroke), the muscle weakness will be contralateral to the lesion in the nervous system.

In addition to testing for weakness, don't forget that tongue fasciculations can be a sign of amyotrophic lateral sclerosis.

9.2.4 The Motor Examination

The motor examination also begins with observation. This point was emphasized to me by a case I will never forget. I was on the neurology consult team seeing a patient with suspected amyotrophic lateral sclerosis. I knew it was important to look for fasciculations, so I briefly looked at the patient's muscles during my strength examination. I reported back to the team that there were no fasciculations. If you've spent any time in a hospital as a medical student, you can probably see where this is going. Indeed, when the attending came in to see the patient, she identified fasciculations on her physical examination. What was the difference? She took her time carefully looking at each of the limbs and used a penlight to illuminate the muscle from the side, casting a shadow that helped highlight the fasciculations. The specific lesson here certainly pertains to fasciculations, but the broader point is to be slow and mindful in your examination when you can afford the time. This will help you pick up subtle examination findings that can make or break a diagnosis.

9

9.2.4.1 Hyperkinetic Motor Findings

The nomenclature of the hyperkinetic motor examination findings – tremor, asterixis, and myoclonus – can be confusing. Think of a tremor as a *continuous, predictable* oscillation. Below are several commonly encountered tremors (☐ Table 9.2).

In contrast to a tremor, myoclonus is a *discontinuous, unpredictable* paroxysmal contraction of a muscle; you can think of it as a twitch. Asterixis, most classically seen in hepatic encephalopathy, is a *negative myoclonus*. In other words, it is a *discontinuous, unpredictable* paroxysmal *loss* of muscle tone. Think of the outstretched, upright hands that flap in asterixis. The reason the hands flap down is because the muscle tone that is extending the hands is being lost. It is not unheard of to see all three of these in sick, encephalopathic patients. These are reviewed in the table below (☐ Table 9.3).

9.2.4.2 Strength Testing

Now for the meat of the motor examination – strength testing – first, make sure you know the patient's handedness, as they are expected to be stronger on that side. Specifically, if patients are right-handed and their right hand is subtly weaker relative to their left hand, then you would be suspicious of right-hand weakness (especially with other supporting history and examination findings).

Neurologists have a semi-standardized way to grade strength. For beginners, the most difficult task is to distinguish a 4/5 from a 5/5. You may notice

☐ **Table 9.2** Commonly encountered tremors on the wards

Tremor name	Disease association	Description
Resting tremor	Parkinson's disease	Moderate-low-frequency resting tremor, sometimes transiently alleviated by movement
Physi-ologic tremor	This is present in all individuals regardless of disease state	High-frequency tremor that is present when hands are outstretched ("postural" tremor) or when trying to use the limb ("action" tremor). Not present at rest. Exacerbated by certain settings including anxiety, caffeine intake, and hyperthyroidism
Essential tremor	Essential tremor	Similar to physiologic tremor but lower frequency and therefore more visible and disruptive. Similar triggers but can be alleviated by alcohol. Typically accompanied by a strong family history
Intention tremor	Lesions to a cerebellar hemisphere	Moderate frequency tremor that emerges and increases in amplitude as the individual reaches out to a target (e.g., in the finger-to-nose test)

Note: Although the hands are used for the description of the tremor, these movements can occur in other body parts

☐ **Table 9.3** Review of the three core hyperkinetic movements

Movement	Description
Tremor	Continuous, predictable oscillation
Myoclonus	Discontinuous, unpredictable paroxysmal contraction
Asterixis (negative myoclonus)	Discontinuous, unpredictable paroxysmal *loss* of muscle tone

■ **Table 9.4** Guide for grading strength in the neurological examination

Score	Finding
0/5	Motionless
1/5	Flicker of a movement
2/5	Can move within the horizontal plane, but cannot lift limb
3/5	Can lift limb against gravity, but cannot bear any resistance
4/5	Can move limb against some resistance
5/5	Can move limb against full resistance

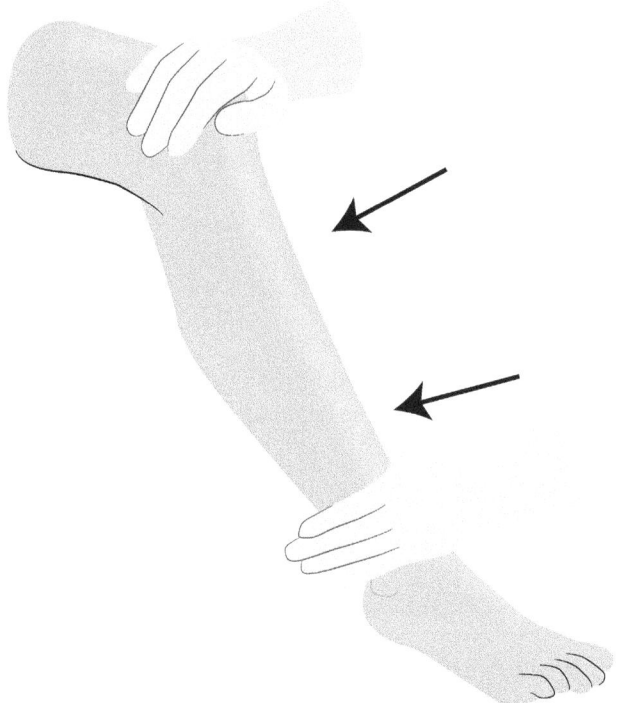

■ **Fig. 9.2** Demonstration of joint isolation. The hand on the knee is stabilizing the joint. The arrows demonstrate the direction of force that is being applied to the leg

that residents and attendings sometimes add +/− to their score – I would recommend against this for the start of your rotation and would instead focus on first mastering the 0–5 scale (■ Table 9.4).

Although there is a component to strength testing that simply requires experience, there are some principles to maximize accuracy of your examination that can be remembered as the three *S*s:

1. *S*ame: when testing finger strength, oppose the patient with the same finger that you're testing. For example, if testing index finger strength, then use one of your index fingers, not your whole hand!
2. *S*tabilize: use one of your hands to test strength and the other hand to stabilize the most proximal joint (■ Fig. 9.2). For example, when testing bicep strength, use one hand to oppose the bicep and the other to hold the elbow. Neglecting to stabilize the limb in this manner may result in an inaccurate examination.

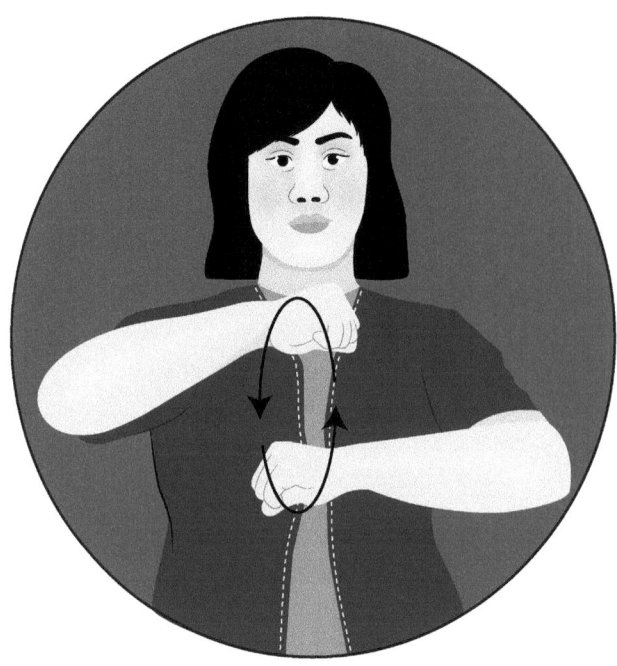

☐ **Fig. 9.3** Demonstration of how to perform the orbiting maneuver

3. *Symmetry*: assess whether the patient's strength is symmetric. Asymmetry can be a helpful clue in cases of subtle weakness.

It can be difficult to confidently identify subtle muscle weakness. Here, one can make use of the "orbiting" examination maneuver (☐ Fig. 9.3). In effect, you ask the patient to rotate their arms around each other. If one of the arms doesn't move as much, the other (more mobile) arm will look like it is orbiting this arm.

9.2.5 Sensory Examination

Detection of a distinct border on the back below which there is sensation loss is concerning for a spinal injury.

You may have noticed that sensation to light touch included in the core examination. By and large, this will be sufficient in the hospital as an initial, sensitive screen for sensory loss. It is when you detect sensation loss through this initial check that you should deploy some "spoke" tests for sensation. As a minimum, you should check for sensation loss in more specific modalities (proprioception/vibration for the dorsal tract/large fibers and pain/temperature for the spinothalamic tract/small fibers), and you must delineate the boundary of sensory loss (e.g., where does it start and where does it end).

A "spoke" test to consider in the sensory examination is a test for "extinction" to double simultaneous stimulation. What we mean by extinction is that the patient is able to sense touch on each side when tested independently, but when both sides are tested simultaneously, they are no longer able to perceive the sensation. Patients who are unable to perceive simultaneous bilateral touch may have neglect, which is most commonly caused by a lesion in the nondominant (primarily right) parietal lobe. This maneuver is therefore frequently performed when examining a patient with a confirmed or suspected stroke.

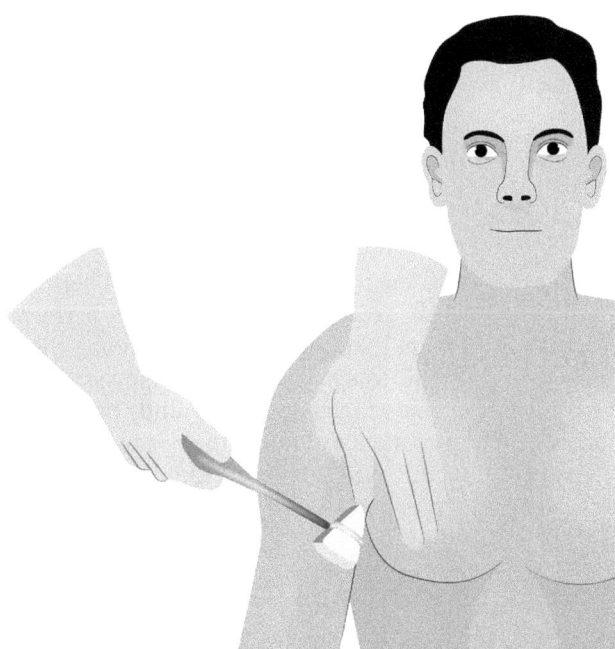

■ **Fig. 9.4** Demonstration of pectoral reflex

9.2.6 Reflexes

9.2.6.1 Tips for Getting It Right

Using a proper tool is the first step to set yourself up for success with reflexes. The shape of the tool – whether it looks like a ray gun or a classic hammer – doesn't matter as much as whether the tool is properly weighted. You should avoid using evenly weighted hammers, as these do not fall effectively enough to reliably elicit a reflex. I said "fall" because you want to loosely grip the hammer and primarily allow gravity and the instrument's weight do the work (in contrast to tightly gripping and swinging the hammer). Think of gently guiding a falling pendulum to its target.

9.2.6.2 The Pectoral Jerk

One of the highest-yield "spoke" reflexes is the pectoral jerk. To elicit this reflex, you place your index finger on the pectoral tendon and tap the hammer (■ Fig. 9.4). Any contraction of the pectoral muscle is an abnormal finding. This is useful to confirm an upper motor neuron (UMN) lesion (localizing to C2/C3 or C3/C4), especially in the setting of ALS where a single UMN finding may confirm the diagnosis. It has come in handy many times on my rotations.

9.2.7 Cerebellar (Coordination) Examination

9.2.7.1 Overview

The "cerebellar" examination is a bit of a misnomer. Many of the maneuvers, such as the finger-to-nose test, actually test multiple neurological domains at the same time – for example, you may imagine that muscle weakness and spasticity may influence one's ability to properly do a finger-to-nose test. Keep this in mind while interpreting the data you gather in this portion of the examination.

It is worth noting that examination findings supporting a cerebellar lesion may be found in other portions of the examination:

- As you observe the patient sitting upright, you may see them swaying with truncal ataxia.
- While listening to the patient speak, you may note dysarthria.
- The cranial nerve examination may reveal nystagmus.
- The gait and strength examination may reveal limb ataxia.

After observing, there are a few things to consider when performing specific maneuvers for the cerebellar examination. The key to performing a good finger-to-nose test is to ensure that the patient is extending their arm out as far as possible when trying to touch your finger. Many students place their finger too close to the patient, which can miss a subtle intention tremor that would only be seen with the patient extending their arms completely outward. This maneuver can also reveal "past pointing," which is seen when the patient extends their finger past yours as a consequence of cerebellar pathology.

9.2.7.2 Spoke Movements

Additional spoke movements to consider for patients in whom the history or "core" examination yield evidence concerning for cerebellar pathology include:

- Testing rapid alternating movements. This can be done by having the patient place one hand in the palm of another, then rapidly flipping the placed hand back and forth. Inability to perform this maneuver is known as "dysdiadochokinesia."
- Testing for limb hypotonia. There are a variety of ways to test this, each depending upon the limb. For the upper extremity, you can have the patient lay their arm onto a table with the wrist hanging off the edge. You can then lift and set down the arm and look to see whether the wrist looks "floppy" and whether the wrist swings back and forth like a pendulum – this would indicate decreased tone.
- Test for ability to tap a rhythm. Tap out a rhythm on a table and ask the patient to do the same. Inability to tap out a rhythm may be consistent with an ipsilateral cerebellar lesion.

9.2.8 Gait Examination

From a neurological perspective, the assessment of gait offers two streams of information. First, a deficit in gait can support a problem in one of the other components of the neurological examination – sensation (e.g., proprioception of the feet), motor (e.g., strength and tone), and cerebellar function (coordination). Second, a characteristic gait can be an independent piece of evidence for a diagnosis. An example of this would be a shuffling gait in Parkinson's disease. Although the gait examination is most commonly performed in the neurological setting, it remains informative in most medical settings. For example, in the emergency department, it can help you determine whether a patient with acute back pain is stable enough to walk around safely. It is very impressive to the team if, in your clinical assessment, you report a patient's ability to ambulate independently as evidence for discharge safety.

9.2.9 Non-neurological Examination

It is important to perform a screening general examination (HEENT, heart, lungs, abdomen, extremities), particularly when the patient is first admitted to the hospital. After all, patients on neurology floors have medical problems too, and many neurological problems can be triggered or exacerbated by medical conditions. For example, patients with a history of stroke can have their stroke deficits re-emerge in the setting of an acute illness. This is called "recrudescence" and can mimic a new stroke!

There are a few neurological perspectives on the general examination that are worth highlighting:

1. Vitals:
    1. Very high blood pressure may acutely precipitate intracerebral hemorrhage, hypertensive encephalopathy, or posterior reversible encephalopathy syndrome.
    2. Chronic hypertension is a risk factor for cerebrovascular disease and vascular dementia.
    3. Cushing's triad, a sign of increased intracranial pressure, can manifest with irregular, decreased respirations, bradycardia, and systolic hypertension.
2. Skin:
    1. Bacterial meningitis may cause a petechial rash.
    2. Stigmata of cirrhosis (jaundice, spider angioma) places hepatic encephalopathy on your differential for altered mental status.
3. HEENT:
    1. Tongue biting can be an indication that a patient has experienced a seizure.
    2. Nuchal rigidity may be a sign of meningitis.
    3. Signs of head trauma: ecchymoses around the eyes ("raccoon eyes") or at the mastoid process ("Battle's sign") are consistent with a basilar skull fracture.
    4. Scalp tenderness may be consistent with giant cell arteritis.
4. Cardiovascular examination:
    1. An irregularly irregular heartbeat can raise suspicion for atrial fibrillation (AF), which is a stroke risk factor (although most admitted patients get an EKG, which is a better test for AF).
    2. A new murmur in the setting of infectious symptoms may be a sign of bacterial endocarditis, which places the patient at high risk for stroke.
5. Abdominal examination:
    1. A rectal examination can assess for impaired reflexes in the setting of spinal injury.
6. Extremities:
    1. A straight-leg test can assess for radiculopathy as a cause of back pain.

This is why it's relevant to know the location and clinical presentation of prior strokes when admitting a patient!

9.3 The Oral Presentation

As mentioned at the beginning of the chapter, the neurological oral presentation will be similar to that in the internal medicine rotation. The same best practices of presenting the history chronologically, presenting pertinent positives and pertinent negatives, and providing an organized assessment and plan still apply here. If you need a refresher, please revisit that section of the book. There are several nuances to consider when giving an oral presentation on your neurology rotation, which we will discuss here. When put together, the oral presentation for a new patient admission will look like this (► Box 9.2).

9

1. One-liner (*including handedness*)
2. History of present illness (HPI)
3. Emergency department course
4. Events since arrival to floor
5. Past History with focus on aspects that are relevant to neurologic conditions
6. Medications (with focus on medications with relevance to neurology such as AEDs, antiplatelets, anticoagulants)
7. Vitals/exam (brief description of general examination, with most of the focus on the neurological examination)
8. Objective data (with focus on neurological diagnostic studies; here is where you typically go over the imaging with the team)
9. Repeat one-liner
10. Assessment with localization
11. Point-by-point plan with diagnostics and therapeutics, *with a discussion of whether neurology-specific diagnostics are indicated.*

9.3.1 One-Liner

Classically, the neurological oral presentation includes the patient's handedness (e.g., a 65-year-old right-handed man). If the patient has a history of neurological disease, it is important to place their baseline in context. For example, rather than state "a 65-year-old right-handed man with a history of R (right) MCA (middle cerebral artery) stroke," it would be preferred to state "a 65-year-old right-handed man with a history of R MCA stroke with residual mild left hemiparesis."

9.3.2 History

The same internal medicine principles of presenting the history *chronologically, concisely, and with pertinent positives and negatives* apply to neurology.

Many patients you present will have chronic neurological illnesses with intermittent flares (e.g., multiple sclerosis). These patients often have long-term relationships with outpatient physicians. In these cases, make sure that you know the following information, much of which can be obtained by review of the medical record:

1. Physician name
2. When the patient last saw their physician
3. History and trajectory of the patient's illness, including last hospitalization
4. What the management strategy has been (e.g., what medications the patient is currently taking, what has been tried in the past, etc.)

Knowing the medications that have been tried by a patient can be a useful shortcut for you and the team to understand the severity of the patient's disease.

Do not underestimate the value of a call or email to the patient's provider in providing invaluable information. This also signals to the team that you're taking initiative in caring for the patient.

9.3.3 Examination

It is generally permissible to be concise when presenting the general medical examination – something to the effect of "the heart, lung, abdominal, and extremity examinations were unremarkable." Do not forget that some neurological diseases have non-neurological examination findings. For example, a patient with meningitis may have nuchal rigidity, which does not necessarily fit into a subsection of the neurological examination. Listing these pertinent positives or negatives demonstrates your knowledge, critical thinking skills, and signals the diagnoses on the differential that you are considering in your assessment.

The presentation of the neurological examination follows the same "hub-and-spoke" model used to guide the conduct of the examination. For a patient with isolated acute right arm weakness, the "spokes" may be additional details regarding the strength and reflex examinations, over and beyond the hub examination. Your team will expect to hear a detailed strength examination covering all parts of the arms, all the upper extremity reflexes, a pronator drift, and a test for orbiting. The team will not be as interested to hear about the mental status spoke examination, such as results from the MoCA.

For a patient with altered mental status, the key "spoke" would be the mental status examination. In this case, a MoCA would be helpful, but the team would not necessarily want to hear about spokes from the reflex examination (e.g., pectoral reflex).

9.3.4 Objective Data

As with the examination, I conceptualize the presentation of objective data on the neurology wards as "non-neurological" and "neurological." For the former, I use the system of "Labs" (e.g., basic metabolic panel, complete blood count, liver function tests), "micro" (e.g., urinalysis, blood cultures), and "imaging" (e.g., chest X-ray, echocardiogram, EKGs).

It is essential to be very familiar with the patient's objective neurological data. These include EEGs, lumbar punctures (make sure you know the characteristic CSF findings associated with various meningitis syndromes!), electromyograms (EMG) and nerve conduction studies (NCS), and, most importantly, brain imaging studies. For the tests that you report, make sure you know the following facts:
1. Date of study.
2. Indication for study (i.e., what were the presenting symptoms?)
3. Details of how study was conducted (e.g., with or without contrast?)
4. Major findings of the study. Always look at brain imaging yourself – this is helpful from a learning perspective, but also because you can sometimes (even as a medical student) catch things that may have been missed in the radiology report.

Everyone has a different approach to working though imaging studies. The following are the steps I like to take (▸ Box 9.3).

If you are having difficulty understanding an image, check to see whether a neuroradiologist is available to go over the image with you. I also found ▸ radiopaedia.org to be the best resource for finding examples and explanations of MRI and CT findings. Knowing your imaging is essential, as you will often be asked to present the imaging to the team on rounds. Here are multiple CT and MRI scans demonstrating various pathologies that you may encounter on your rotation (◻ Figs. 9.5, 9.6, 9.7, 9.8, 9.9, 9.10, and 9.11).

Maneuvering through these radiology programs can be tricky. Make sure to carefully watch how your resident does it on rounds and don't be afraid to ask for a tutorial if there's free time in the afternoons!

9

Box 9.3   The Approach to Interpreting Neuroimaging

1. Mentally review the clinical scenario and ask yourself where you think the lesion is located. This ensures that you pay extra close attention to this part of the scan.
2. If there is an older scan available, pull that scan up alongside the scan you're looking at for comparison.
3. Start with axial images from the T2 FLAIR sequence – this is generally the best imaging sequence to start with for identifying pathology. Start at the most caudal (bottom) part of the scan and slowly scroll up. Make sure you know where you are in the brainstem (i.e., medulla, pons, pons) – see below for tips and representative imaging. For abnormal findings, describe the location, shape, size, and how it compares to prior images. Findings that are bright relative to the surrounding tissue are called hyperintensities, and findings that are darker than the surrounding tissue are described as hypointense. In addition to the parenchyma (another word for brain tissue), I assess the following:
   1. Do the carotids appear normal?
   2. How do the ventricles look – do they appear "squished" or too big? What is the position of the midline of the brain – is it shifted?
   3. Can I see the distinction between the gray and white matter, or are there parts of the scan with "loss of this gray-white differentiation"?
   4. Is the superior sagittal sinus open (to assess for a thrombosis)?
4. It can then be helpful to pull up the sagittal and coronal planes to further characterize any observed pathology.
5. Proceed to the T1 with contrast (if available). Note, that on T1 images, gray matter appears gray and white matter appears white. This is in contrast to T2, where gray matter appears white and white matter appears gray. Ask yourself the following questions:
   1. Do any lesions enhance with contrast? This suggests loss of patency of the blood-brain barrier, consistent with inflammation.
   2. If there is enhancement, is it uniform or is there a ring-enhancing pattern?
6. Proceed to diffusion-weighted imaging to assess for acute ischemic injury. For any abnormal findings on DWI, pull up the "ADC" image and check whether that spot is dark (called an "ADC correlate"). Sometimes you get a lesion that is bright on DWI but with no ADC correlate – this false-positive DWI lesion can actually be driven by T2 signal, a scenario called "T2 shine through." Going through this exercise of comparing DWI to ADC and identifying T2 shine through is an impressive skill to demonstrate on rounds.
7. Proceed to susceptibility-weighted imaging (SWI). This is the best sequence to identify blood, particularly cerebral microbleeds, which appears black. A microbleed is defined as small, chronic, brain hemorrhages that are typically individually asymptomatic but in aggregate may cause cognitive dysfunction. They are also helpful for diagnosis – a substantial burden of lobar microbleeds may be consistent with cerebral amyloid angiopathy (CAA)

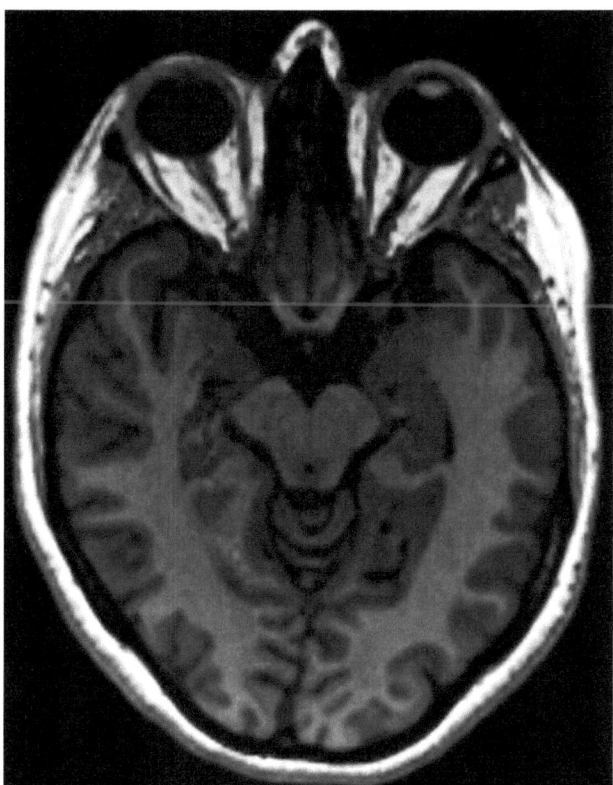

Fig. 9.5 Representative T1 MRI axial imaging of the midbrain. A helpful way to remember the appearance of the midbrain is to look for the brainstem section that looks like "mickey mouse"

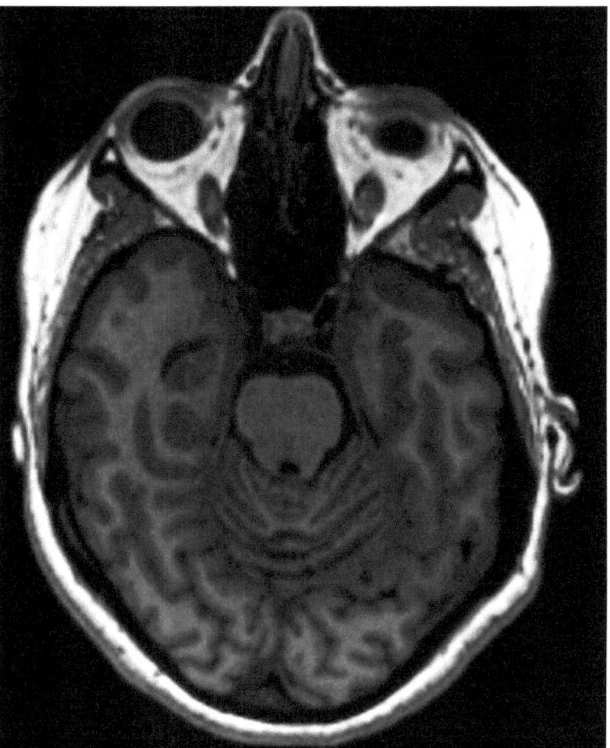

Fig. 9.6 Representative T1 MRI axial imaging of the pons. The mickey mouse appearance to the brainstem disappears at the pons. Instead, the pons has a bulbous appearance

9

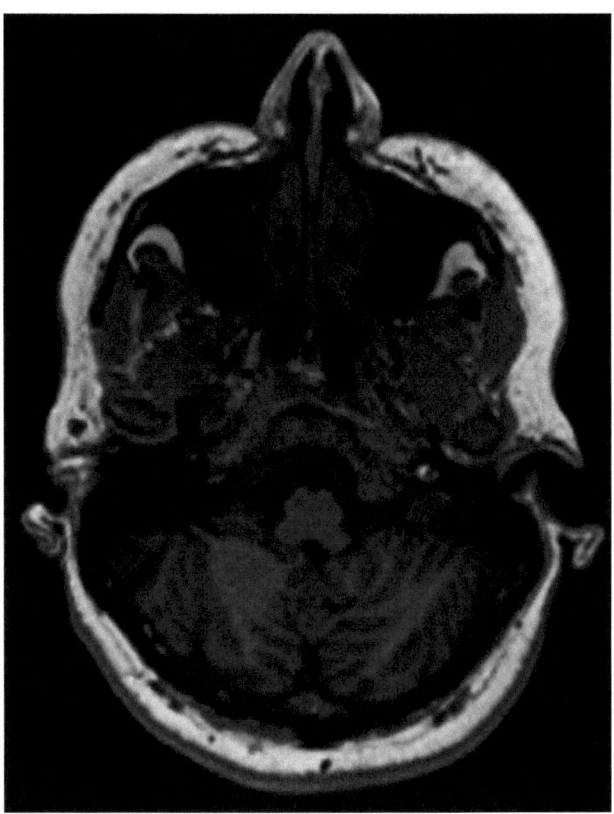

■ **Fig. 9.7** Representative T1 MRI axial imaging of the medulla. Notice how, in contrast to the pons, the medulla has two little "feet" sticking out posteriorly

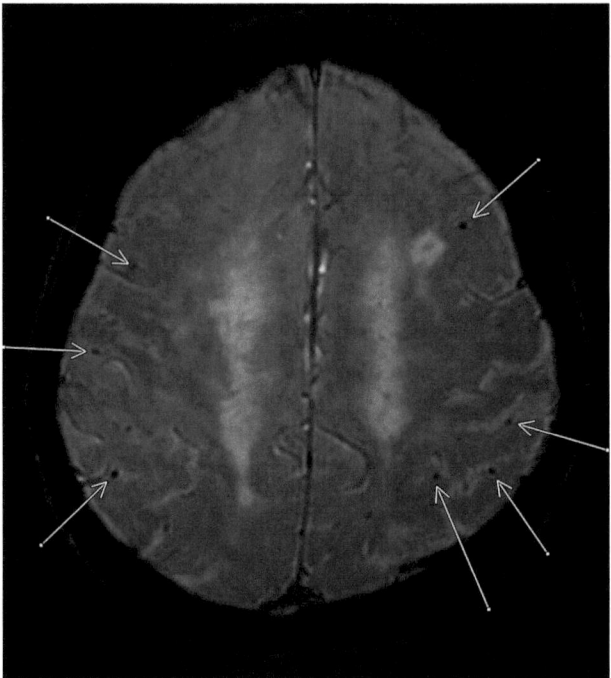

■ **Fig. 9.8** Cerebral amyloid angiopathy (CAA). The arrows point to cerebral microbleeds, which show up as black dots on susceptibility-weighted MRI. Remember to include CAA on your differential for patients with a lobar intracerebral hemorrhage

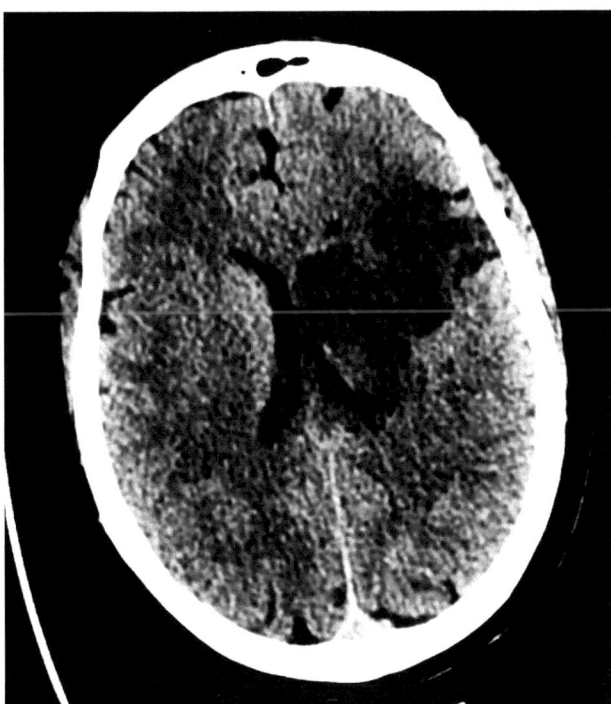

Fig. 9.9 Appearance of acute ischemic stroke on CT scan without contrast. The infarction is demonstrated by the white arrow pointing to the hypodensity. Although diffusion-weighted MRI is the best scan for diagnosing ischemic stroke, large strokes can sometimes be seen on CT scan (which are typically obtained when trying to rule out a hemorrhage)

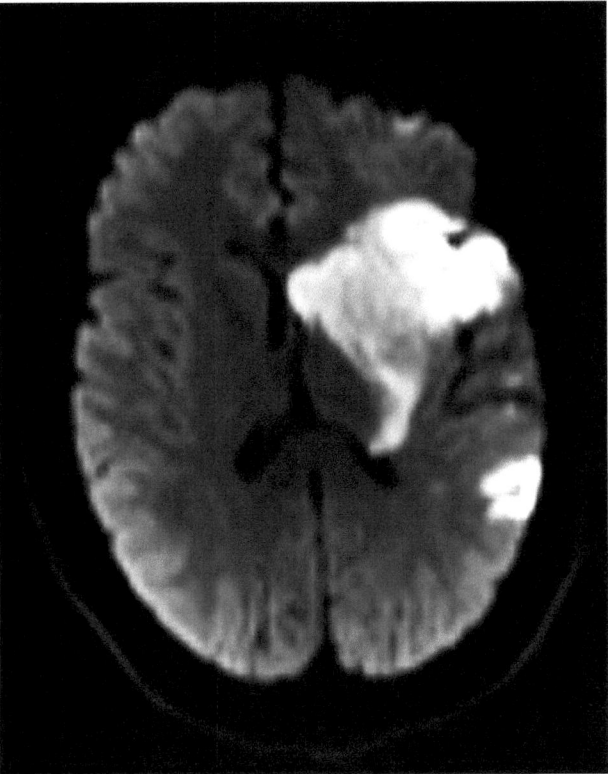

Fig. 9.10 Appearance of acute ischemic stroke on diffusion-weighted MRI scan. The bright white areas mark the infarcted regions

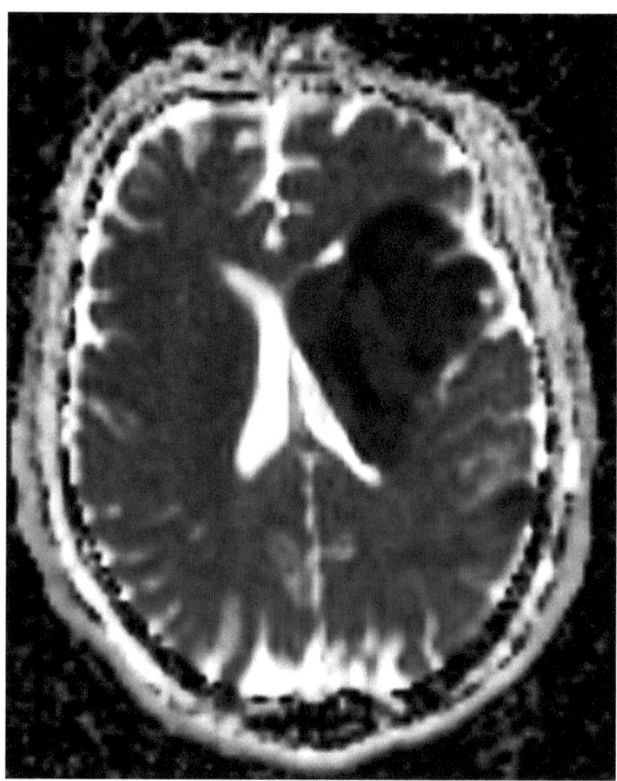

Fig. 9.11 ADC correlate of diffusion-weighted lesion. ◻ Figure 9.8 demonstrates a finding on diffusion-weighted imaging that is very concerning for stroke. As stated in the text, such a finding must be confirmed with the ADC imaging series. Here we see that the bright areas on the DWI are black on the ADC series, which is consistent with ischemic infarct

9.3.5 Assessment

The following are the steps I recommend for the neurological assessment component of the oral presentation:

1. Restate the patient's one-liner ("A 65-year-old right-handed man with a history of R MCA stroke with residual mild left hemiparesis who presents with R-sided arm weakness.")

2. Relate your thought process about localization. Here is where you list the pertinent elements of the history and physical examination followed by your hypothesis about possible neurological localizations. This could sound like: "the patient's history is notable for acute-onset right upper extremity weakness (RUE), and the examination was notable for 4/5 strength throughout the RUE with pronator drift and hyperreflexia. I am most suspicious for a left-sided stroke in the region of the motor cortex supplied by the left middle cerebral artery. An internal capsule localization is less likely given the full strength in the ipsilateral face and legs, and a brain stem localization is less likely given the absence of cranial nerve deficits."

3. You then give your differential diagnosis. As stated in the medicine chapter, you generally want to put your nickel down on what you think is most likely: "I think an ischemic stroke is most likely given the patient's history of untreated atrial fibrillation, the acute onset of symptoms, and examination findings of upper motor neuron weakness in the right upper extremity." You then list other diagnoses that are possible but less likely: "I also considered migraine with aura; however the patient's symptoms were not associ-

ated with a headache, there were no other aura symptoms, and the diffusion-weighted imaging was consistent with an ischemic lesion." It is generally appropriate to include 2–3 other diagnoses on the differential. Avoid providing a long laundry list.

9.3.6 Plan

Just like the internal medicine presentation, you should divide your plan into different problems and then divide each problem by proposed diagnostics and therapeutics. This makes it easy for others to follow your line of thinking.

Broadly speaking, you want to consider a set of "special" diagnostic tests on your neurology rotation (◘ Table 9.5). I recommend saving this checklist somewhere on your phone and always referring to it when considering your treatment plan (◘ Table 9.6). These include the following.

◘ **Table 9.5** The various neurology-specific tests to consider for your clinical plan

Test	Settings to order	Considerations
EEG	1. Concern for seizure 2. Unexplained change in mental status or prolonged delirium (e.g., in nonconvulsive status epilepticus)	Hospitals typically provide the option of either a "routine EEG," which lasts about half an hour, or "EEG with long-term monitoring (LTM)," which can monitor the patient for a much longer period of time (hours to days) Consider which is more appropriate for your clinical scenario and when sharing your plan specify the type of EEG that you would like to order
LP	1. Neuroinfections (meningoencephalitis) 2. Neuroinflammatory disease 3. Subarachnoid hemorrhage with a negative CT scan 4. Pseudotumor cerebri	Make sure you specify what additional studies you would like to obtain on the LP (e.g., cell counts, gram stain, protein/glucose, cultures, etc.) There is generally no reason not to obtain an opening pressure when doing an LP, so make sure you are prepared to measure this during the LP
EMG/NCS	1. Concern for neuropathy or myopathy 2. Concern for motor neuron disease	These tests are useful in evaluating suspected neuropathy, myopathy, or amyotrophic lateral sclerosis Sometimes these tests are not readily available in the inpatient setting. In these cases you must ask yourself the question of whether they are urgent enough to delay a patient's discharge or whether they could instead be obtained as an outpatient
Brain imaging	(Too many to list!) 1. CNS malignancy 2. Stroke 3. Seizure work-up 4. Dementia work-up 5. Neuroinflammatory diseases Head trauma	CT vs. MRI? Contrast or no contrast? Vessel imaging?

EEG electroencephalogram, *LP* lumbar puncture, *EMG* electromyogram, *NCS* nerve conduction study

◘ Table 9.6 Indications for imaging in the setting of stroke

Imaging study	Clinical scenario
CT scan without contrast	This is the best test to rule out an intracranial hemorrhage (ICH), which must be ruled out prior to administering intravenous thrombolysis Ischemic strokes are not typically acutely visible on CT scans but eventually become visible as hypodensities
MRI with diffusion-weighted imaging sequences (DWI) [1]	This is the most sensitive test for an acute ischemic stroke – ischemia can be visible within a few minutes of onset. Strokes appear hyperintense
MRI with T2 FLAIR sequence [1] (this does not require contrast)	Ischemic strokes are visible on FLAIR after ~4.5 hours. You can thus date a stroke by assessing for a FLAIR hyperintensity in the same location as the DWI lesion. *Make sure you include an assessment of stroke timing in your analysis of the radiologic findings!*
CT angiography (CTA; requires contrast)	This test visualizes the patient's blood vessels, which permits identification of blood clots and stenosis. These can guide important treatment decisions and inform the stroke mechanism
MRA – can either be with or without contrast	Just like the CTA, this test assesses the cerebral blood vessels. A potential advantage of vessel imaging with MRI is that you can avoid the administration of contrast. This may be done by ordering an "MRA time-of-flight"

9.4　Common Cases

Armed with the tools to examine patients and conduct effective oral presentations, we will now review four common clinical scenarios that neurologists encounter in the hospital. We have elected to not include ischemic stroke in this chapter, as the approach to its diagnosis and management is rapidly evolving and may be obsolete by the time you read this.

9.4.1　Delirium

» My dad spiked a fever and started coughing up green phlegm. Since last night he hasn't been himself – he can't hold a conversation with us, and his words sometimes stop making sense.

In organizing your approach to the history and physical in a patient with suspected delirium, you need to gather data that answers the following questions:
1. Does the patient actually have delirium?
2. Is there an identifiable cause for delirium?
3. Is this patient at risk for delirium?

9.4.1.1　Does This Patient Actually Have Delirium?

A useful tool to assess whether a patient has delirium is the "Confusion Assessment Method" [1] (CAM) which has high sensitivity and specificity for the diagnosis of delirium. The following are the CAM criteria for delirium, which I recommend committing to memory:
1. Acute onset of symptoms with fluctuation throughout the day
2. Inattention
3. One of either (i) disorganized thinking or (ii) alterations in level of consciousness

Much of this information can be gathered by interacting with and observing the patient. It is helpful to speak with family members and/or care providers who can characterize how distant the patient is from their baseline state.

9.4.1.2 Is There an Identifiable Cause for Delirium?

There are a substantial number of possible etiologies for delirium. Preclinical students are often surprised that some of the below causes – such as urinary tract infections and dehydration – can trigger delirium. In reality, any shock to a vulnerable patient's system, including pain, can precipitate delirium. One therefore needs to approach the history and examination with a broad differential. I like to use the following mnemonic each time I encounter delirium (▶ Box 9.4). Keep in mind that this list is not exhaustive and should only be used as a starting point for formulating your approach.

Your history will typically be anchored on a particular symptom or complaint, such as a focal neurological deficit. You will conduct an HPI on this "anchoring" problem. You will then conduct a broad review of systems, touching on each of the elements of the mnemonic. For example, to assess risk for an infection, you could ask about fever/chills/night sweats (general infectious symptoms), cough/dyspnea/chest pain (respiratory infection), headache/neck stiffness/photophobia (meningitis), skin rashes (cellulitis), abdominal pain/vomiting/diarrhea (intra-abdominal infection), and dysuria/lower back pain (urinary tract infection).

Box 9.4   Mnemonic for Causes of Delirium

I WATCH DEATH

- *I*nfection – meningoencephalitis, urinary tract infections, pneumonia, sepsis
- Withdrawal – alcohol, benzodiazepine withdrawal
- Acute metabolic change – electrolyte derangement, hypercalcemia, liver injury, kidney injury
- Trauma – head trauma, pain
- CNS disease – seizure
- Hypoxia/hypercarbia
- Deficiencies – vitamin B12 deficiency
- Endocrine – hypo-/hyperthyroidism
- Acute vascular event – myocardial infarction, hypertensive emergency, ischemic stroke, hemorrhagic stroke
- Toxins (including iatrogenic injury) – review the patient's medication list (be on the lookout for medications with CNS activity including opiates, benzodiazepines, anticholinergics, etc.)
- Hypovolemia – dehydration, over-diuresis

Old patients with baseline cognitive impairment can take a very long time to fully recover to their cognitive baseline after a seizure.

9.4.1.3 Is This Patient Generally at Risk for Delirium?

Delirium is no exception to the rule that the greatest risk factor for diseases in medicine is a history of the disease – be sure to look through the medical record for prior hospitalizations for delirium. Another important risk factor is baseline cognitive impairment or dementia – if a patient has a lower baseline level of cognition (e.g., "cognitive reserve"), then it takes less of a systemic insult to trigger delirium. Risk for delirium also increases linearly with older age and number of comorbidities.

9.4.1.4 Examination

Your examination will follow the theme of "does this patient have delirium" and "what could be a trigger for this patient's delirium?" The former is assessed with a thorough neurological examination with an emphasis on the mental status examination and an assessment for inattention. These data will be useful for your CAM assessment.

Triggers are assessed by conducting a thorough general medical examination. For example, assessing infectious causes of delirium would involve testing for nuchal rigidity, listening to the lungs, looking for rashes, conducting an abdominal examination, and testing for suprapubic or costovertebral angle tenderness.

9.4.1.5 Work-Up and Treatment

Your work-up of delirium will vary depending upon what you find in your history and examination. Again, it is helpful to group potential diagnostics by the I WATCH DEATH mnemonic.

1. Infection: urinalysis, blood cultures, chest X-ray, CBC
2. Withdrawal: urine toxicology screen, assessment for symptoms via "Clinical Institute Withdrawal Assessment of Alcohol Scale" (CIWA-Ar)
3. Acute metabolic change: CHEM-7, liver function tests, kidney function tests, ammonia (although controversial as to whether this test adds value)
4. CNS disease (seizure): EEG
5. Hypoxia/hypercarbia: arterial blood gas/venous blood gas
6. Deficiencies: vitamin B12 levels
7. Endocrine: TSH
8. Acute vascular accident: EKG, troponins, MRI, chest X-ray
9. Dehydration: lactate, serum creatinine, serum sodium, serum chloride, FeNa

9.4.1.6 Treatment

Your approach to treatment depends on what you find in your work-up. For example, infections will be treated with appropriate antibiotic coverage, and volume depletion will be treated with an infusion of normal saline. If it is necessary, agitation can be treated with an antipsychotic (e.g., haloperidol, quetiapine), however these are not believed to impact the duration or clinical course of delirium.

In addition to addressing the underlying cause of delirium, the following interventions may be helpful for stabilizing a delirious patient:

- Ensure good sleep hygiene and consistent sleep timing. Turn off the lights to permit the normal nightly rise of melatonin, and open the blinds in the morning to allow sunlight into the room. Minimize disruptions to sleep through strategic timing of medication administration and vital sign checks. Consider a small dose of melatonin as low as 0.30 mg (commonly used doses like 3 mg are supraphysiological and may have a net deleterious effect on sleep).
- Ensure the patient has access to their eyeglasses and hearing aids.
- Orient the patient each day to person, place, and time. If possible, have a clock visible to them in the room so they can keep track of the time.
- Ensure adequate pain management (preferably non-opioid medications).
- Minimize deliriogenic medications (anticholinergics and benzos in particular).
- If the patient is able to ambulate at baseline, arrange for them to be seen by the physical therapy team for ambulation.

9.4.2 Headache

Headache is a commonly encountered neurological problem on both the inpatient and the outpatient settings. The most important determination you must make as a neurologist is whether the patient has a primary or secondary headache disorder.

The most common primary headache disorders to consider are migraine, tension headache, and cluster headache. In reality, the vast majority of primary headache cases you see will either be migraine or tension headaches, as cluster headaches are rare. The following are some pearls that you may find helpful in differentiating the two:

- The POUND [2] mnemonic is a clinical tool that helps to (i) rule in migraine and (ii) keep track of some relevant headache features. Patients meeting 4 or more features have a likelihood ratio of 24 for the diagnosis of migraine, those with 3 features a likelihood ratio of 3.5, and those with 2 or fewer features a likelihood ratio of 0.41 (i.e., lower risk). The mnemonic stands for:
  - *P*ulsatile in quality
  - Duration of 4–72 hours
  - *U*nilateral location
  - *N*ausea or vomiting
  - *D*isabling nature of the headache
- You can take these features and flip them for tension headache:
  - Squeezing
  - Lasts 30 minutes to 7 days
  - Bilateral location
  - Generally no nausea/vomiting
  - Generally not disabling
- Migraine auras can happen before, during, or after the headache and may present as basically any neurological symptom. "Hemiplegic migraine" is an aura subtype that involves acute weakness that can mimic a stroke. One pearl to know is that weakness is never the only aura during a hemiplegic migraine episode [3].
- In my experience, the disabling nature of a migraine headache is quite helpful in differentiating migraine from tension headache. "Disabling" means that the patient cannot continue on with the activities they were doing prior to the headache onset. In contrast, patients with a tension headache are typically able to continue on with their daily activities. Ask the patient "are you able to continue on with what you were doing before the headache started or do you have to stop?"

In addition to the primary causes of headache, you must consider "secondary" etiologies. This is my preferred mnemonic (▶ Box 9.5).

Box 9.5   Mnemonic for Causes of Secondary Headache

VOMIT
- *V*ascular – intracranial hemorrhage (especially subarachnoid hemorrhage), venous sinus thrombosis, cervical artery dissection, hypertensive emergency, reversible cerebral vasoconstriction syndrome, eclampsia
- *O*verflow/underflow – high intracranial pressure (e.g., mass lesion, hydrocephalus, idiopathic intracranial hypertension), low intracranial pressure (post-LP headache)

- *M*edication side effects – nitrates, medication rebound headache, caffeine withdrawal
- *I*nfection/inflammation – meningoencephalitis, intracranial abscess, systemic infections, sinus infections, giant cell arteritis
- *T*rauma/tumor – concussion, primary CNS malignancy, metastasis

As with delirium, your line of questioning and examination will assess evidence for each of these etiologies in turn. It is particularly essential to ask questions about headache "red flags" that include (☐ Table 9.7).

☐ **Table 9.7**   Red flags for dangerous causes of secondary headaches

Symptom or risk factor	Potential etiology
Older age (>50)[a]	Most of the secondary causes (e.g., giant cell arteritis, malignancy, vascular)
Thunderclap onset – maximal pain very soon after onset "Worst headache of my life"	Vascular: Intracranial hemorrhage (particularly subarachnoid hemorrhage), hypertensive emergency, venous sinus thrombosis, reversible cerebral vasoconstriction syndrome (RCVS) *Note that although cervical artery dissection is a vascular cause of headache, it does not typically have a "thunderclap" onset*
Any neurological signs or symptoms	Vascular causes of headache, increased ICP, CNS infection, malignancy
Infectious symptoms: fever, chills, night sweats, meningismus	Meningoencephalitis Cerebral abscess (don't forget that systemic infections like influenza can cause headaches!)
Immunocompromised state (HIV, iatrogenic)	CNS infection
History of malignancy, weight loss	Secondary CNS malignancy
Symptoms of increased intracranial pressure: Worse when flat and improves when standing Worse with increased abdominal pressure (sneezing, coughing, Valsalva) Worse in the morning Vision changes (blurring or diplopia)	Intracranial mass lesion, idiopathic intracranial hypertension
Systemic symptoms, proximal muscle weakness, jaw claudication, loss of vision, scalp tenderness	Giant cell arteritis

[a]The most memorable patient I saw in the emergency department was an older man with a history of hypertension who presented with a new headache. Apart from his age, he had no red flags, nor did he have neurological signs or symptoms. Nevertheless, we obtained a CT scan, with little expectation of seeing an abnormal finding. To this day, I still remember the peculiar feeling of coldness that washed over me as I scrolled through the scan and found an intracerebral hemorrhage staring at me from the basal ganglia. Take new headaches in elderly patients seriously

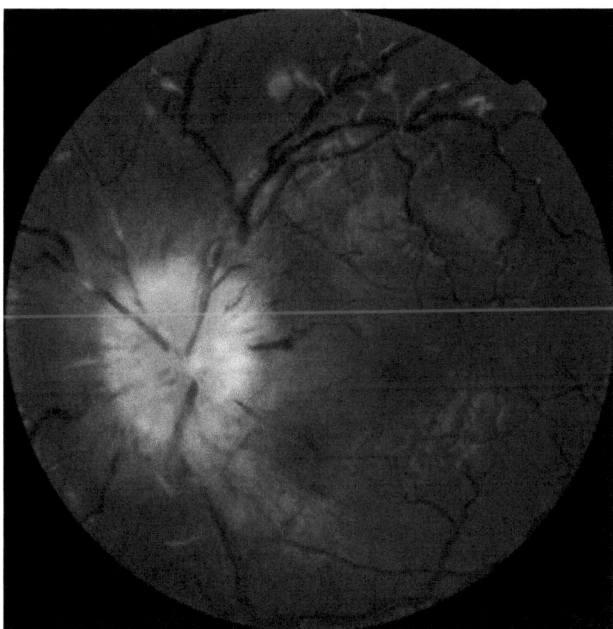

Fig. 9.12 Papilledema

There are a few specific examination maneuvers I want to highlight here:
1. *Do not forget to check for papilledema.* You may not be able to confidently relate what you see through the ophthalmoscope, but attempting this maneuver will improve your skills over time and demonstrates that you are thinking about increased intracranial pressure (■ Fig. 9.12).
2. Pay attention to the vital signs – hypertension can be supportive of a diagnosis of hypertensive emergency or preeclampsia, and fever can be consistent with an infectious cause of headache.
3. Patients are sometimes unsure about whether certain factors – such as positioning or Valsalva - can provoke or palliate their headaches. In these cases, it is acceptable to try to elicit these maneuvers from the patient as part of your examination to see whether the pain changes (while minimizing patient discomfort).
4. Palpate for muscle tenderness in the head, neck, and shoulders. Tenderness in the muscles can be supportive, but not definitive, evidence for a tension headache. In contrast, scalp tenderness may be consistent with giant cell arteritis.

9.4.2.1 Work-Up and Treatment Approach

A key question you will have to address will be whether to obtain brain imaging. In a clinical case that is clearly a tension headache without red flags, imaging is not necessary. Likewise, if the headache is similar in quality to the patient's baseline primary headache, then imaging is not necessary. In contrast, a *new* headache in an older patient is concerning, regardless of the features of the headache. For example, a tumor can cause a new migraine-like headache and would mislead you to diagnose a primary headache.

Protocols for abortive treatment for headache, particularly migraine, vary institutionally. This is particularly the case for acute migraine treatment in the emergency department, which is sometimes referred to as a "migraine cocktail." It can be useful to know what this cocktail is at your institution. Consider the following medication classes for tension and migraine headaches (■ Table 9.8).

■ **Table 9.8** Medications used for migraine and tension type headaches

Headache type	Medication class
Migraine	NSAIDs, acetaminophen, triptans[a], antiemetics, magnesium and IV fluids, steroids[b]
Tension headache[c]	NSAIDs, acetaminophen

[a]The conventional view is that triptans should be avoided in patients with vascular disease, as this medication class may cause vasoconstriction. However, this view is slowly falling out of favor with headache specialists
[b]Typically reserved for more severe cases
[c]Secondary headaches can typically be treated similarly

9.4.3 First Seizure

» I was talking to him in the parking lot when he suddenly stopped responding and collapsed. I think his face may have been twitching, but it was hard to tell in all the chaos.

This excerpt highlights a classic diagnostic challenge in clinical neurology – diagnosis of an unobserved seizure from a history. Taking a detailed history, which means knowing the right questions to ask and report, is essential to distinguishing between a seizure and other causes of transient loss of consciousness. One high-yield tip is to do your best to get *collateral* – that is, an account of what happened from a third-party observer.

There are three key components to the history:
1. Did this patient have a seizure?
2. What could be potential triggers for the seizure?
3. What is the patient's risk for a second seizure?

9.4.3.1 Did This Patient Have a Seizure?

I like to use an evidence-based point system for this clinical scenario. Scoring one or more points on this scale is considered evidence for seizure, and scoring less than one point is more consistent with syncope. The paper [4] that forms the basis for this points system would be a great paper to share with your team and/or present on during your rotation (as are all papers referenced throughout this chapter) (■ Table 9.9).

As you ask these questions, there are additional things to consider. When asking about movements during the episode, make sure your questioning is broader than just asking about generalized tonic-clonic seizures. In particular, it can be helpful to have a "script" asking about the following "automatisms": gesturing, hand rubbing, lip smacking, head turning, and grimacing. On the subject of movements, it is important to note that a few jerks can be seen in a syncopal episode, so it is important to be as detailed a history as possible regarding the pattern and duration of movements.

In your enthusiasm for differentiating seizure vs. syncope, don't forget to consider other potential diagnoses in your differential for a seizure-like episode:
1. In the setting of acute neurological symptoms, you should consider migraine with aura and transient ischemic attacks or stroke in your differential. The former would be more likely in the setting of "positive" symptoms (e.g., tin-

9

🖊 When presenting these patients, try to refer to what happened as an 'episode' or a 'spell.' Without directly observing what happened (especially with an EEG), you should withold a diagnosis of seizure until your clinical assessment.

■ **Table 9.9** Points system for risk stratifying a spell as seizure vs. syncope

Feature	Number of points
Patient woke up with a cut tongue, which is evidence of tongue biting	2
Prodrome of one of the following: Déjà vu - feeling that you have lived through the present situation before Jamais vu - recognizable situation feeling unrecognizable	1
Episode precipitated by emotional stress	1
Head turning to one side during the episode	1
Any of the following: Unresponsiveness Unusual posture Limb movement Amnesia	1
Confusion after the episode	1
Presyncopal symptoms	−2
Sweating before the episode	−2
Episode associated with prolonged sitting or standing	−2

gling, spots in the visual field), whereas the latter would be more likely in the setting of "negative" symptoms (e.g., loss of sensation, visual field deficits).

2. You must also consider whether the patient's episode may be consistent with a psychogenic non-epileptic spell (PNES). Here are some key features that are more consistent with PNES rather than a seizure:
   1. Bilateral movements without loss of consciousness – if the bilateral movements are due to a generalized tonic-clonic seizure, then an impairment in consciousness would be expected. Note that subsequent recall of the events during seizure is further evidence for preservation of consciousness during the event, consistent with PNES.
   2. Asynchronous, variable movements (in contrast to synchronous, consistent movements).
   3. Eyes are closed during the spell (they are generally open in seizures).
   4. PNES typically last longer than epileptic seizures, with some episodes lasting over half an hour.
   5. The manifestation of PNES may not necessary follow a neuroanatomical distribution.

9.4.3.2 Why Did the Patient Have a Seizure?

Once you have worked through the differential diagnosis and have built a case for a seizure, the second step is to determine whether anything precipitated the patient's episode: "why now?" For example, are they an insulin-dependent diabetic patient who is at risk for hypoglycemia? Do they consume illicit substances or are they at risk for withdrawal? Did they have an ischemic stroke which subsequently generated a seizure focus? The following mnemonic (VITAMIN) is helpful in guiding your approach here (▶ Box 9.6).

9

> **Box 9.6   Mnemonic for Causes of Seizure**
> *VITAMIN*
> - *V*ascular: stroke (either ischemic or hemorrhagic), hypertensive emergency
> - *I*nfection: meningitis, encephalitis, abscess, high fever
> - *T*rauma: traumatic brain injury
> - *A*utoimmune: CNS vasculitis, lupus,
> - *M*etabolic: hypoglycemia, hyperglycemia, hyponatremia, hypocalcemia, hypomagnesemia, uremia, hepatic encephalopathy
> - *I*ngestion and iatrogenic: acute intoxication or withdrawal (alcohol)
> - *N*eoplasm: primary or secondary CNS malignancy

9.4.3.3   Is This Patient at Risk for a Second Seizure?

The final step of the history is to determine whether the patient is at high risk for a second seizure. The following are risk factors for having a second seizure that you should ask about in your history (with further details provided in the clinical trials section of this chapter):

1. EEG abnormalities
2. Focal neurological findings on examination
3. Intellectual disability
4. Seizure during sleep
5. Potential remote cause including: history of CNS infection, brain tumor, CNS malformation.

9.4.3.4   Examination

When you examine the patient, be sure to look for evidence of tongue biting and/or trauma consistent with a fall in your general examination. You will then perform a full, careful neurological examination. The goal here is to generate evidence for or against a seizure and to stratify the risk for having a second seizure.

Evidence for Seizure   Admittedly, a postictal examination doesn't generally tell you very much. Alterations in mental status can be evidence for a postictal state but are nonspecific. Indeed, residents and attendings often describe a patient as appearing "postictal"; however as a medical student, I would instead just describe what you see when presenting the examination. Another sign you may see is transient muscle weakness after a seizure, which is also known as Todd's paralysis.

Risk Stratification   A focal neurological deficit is a risk factor for a second seizure, which is helpful evidence for deciding whether or not to initiate an antiepileptic drug.

9.4.3.5   Work-Up

Laboratory studies, including glucose, electrolytes, liver function, and kidney function, help rule in or out metabolic causes of seizure. In some patients, a urine toxicology screen may also be of value to rule out seizure secondary to drug intake.

The key neurological tests to obtain are an EEG and brain imaging – preferably an MRI, as it is the most sensitive imaging modality for determining an etiology. The purpose of an EEG in this setting is not necessarily to capture a seizure, although that is helpful if it happens. Rather, abnormalities on the EEG can provide information to risk stratify future seizures. The MRI provides the same type of information for risk stratification and helps rule out intracranial pathologies potentially triggering seizures (e.g., strokes, tumors, infections).

Table 9.10 Commonly used antiepileptic drugs, comorbidities that favor their use, and important side effects.

AED	Comorbidities that favor use	Side effects
Levetiracetam (Keppra)		Psychiatric disturbances
Phenytoin (Dilantin)[a]		Ataxia, teratogenic
Valproic acid/valproate (Depakote)[a]	Migraine Mood disorders	Teratogenic, liver injury, hyperammonemia, pancreatitis, weight gain, tremor
Lamotrigine (Lamictal)	Mood disorders	Rash, Stevens-Johnson syndrome
Lacosamide (Vimpat)		PR prolongation (obtain EKG)
Topiramate (Topamax)	Migraine	Weight loss, nephrolithiasis
Carbamazepine (Tegretol)[a]		SIADH (hyponatremia)

[a]These medications have prominent drug-drug interactions due to effects on the P450 system

Memorizing these brand names before your rotation can make the transition onto the wards a bit easier.

A key question in management is whether to initiate an antiepileptic drug (AED). Evidence to guide this decision is provided in the clinical trials section of this chapter. There are a few things to consider when picking an AED:
1. Is there an AED that is particularly effective for this type of seizure (e.g., focal vs. generalized seizures)?
2. Are there comorbidities that favor use of a particular AED (Table 9.10)?
3. Are there side effects or medication interactions that are unacceptable?

9.4.4 Bacterial Meningitis

Bacterial meningitis is not a common diagnosis, but it is "bread-and-butter" neurology nonetheless. Indeed, prompt recognition and treatment of bacterial meningitis can save a patient's life.

9.4.4.1 Diagnosis
There are several key symptoms that raise suspicion for meningitis. These include:
1. Fever or hypothermia
2. Altered mental status
3. Nuchal rigidity
4. Severe headache

The majority of patients with bacterial meningitis have at least two of these symptoms. Some of these core symptoms – fever, headache, and altered mental status – can be seen with any infection in an older patient. This emphasizes the importance of maintaining a wide infectious differential and not anchoring early in your approach to meningitis. Focal neurological deficits and seizures can also be seen in bacterial meningitis, therefore warranting a wide neurological review of systems.

9.4.4.2 Examination

There are several important examination maneuvers to elicit from patients with suspected bacterial meningitis. These findings are generally more specific than sensitive, meaning they are better for ruling in the diagnosis. The motivation for the first three maneuvers is to determine whether the patient has meningeal irritation (starred). These examination findings include:

1. Nuchal rigidity. This can be tested by having the patient try to touch their chin to their chest. The relevant parameter here is the range of motion, which is limited in bacterial meningitis.
2. Kernig's sign. The patient must be in the supine position for this maneuver. First, have them flex the knee at 90°. Then, have the patient attempt to fully extend their knees. This sign is positive if the patient is unable to fully extend the knees.
3. Brudzinski's sign. The patient must be in the supine position for this maneuver. The test is positive if the patient spontaneously flexes their hips when you passively flex their neck.
4. Jolt accentuation of headache. Have the patient horizontally rotate their head at a frequency of 2–3 times per second. Worsening headache is considered a positive test.
5. Important non-neurological examination: look for a petechial rash, and assess the vitals for sepsis!
6. Check for papilledema to evaluate for increased intracranial pressure. This should be checked for prior to performing a lumbar puncture.

9.4.4.3 Work-Up and Management

The key elements of the work-up include basic metabolic panels, complete blood counts, blood cultures, and a lumbar puncture. A key question is whether you need to obtain a head CT prior to the lumbar puncture. As a reminder, we are screening for potential causes of increased intracranial pressure that may precipitate a brain herniation in the setting of a lumbar puncture. This should be considered in patients with any of the following:

1. Immunocompromised (e.g., HIV)
2. History of CNS pathology (e.g., stroke, CNS infection, mass lesion)
3. Altered level of consciousness
4. Papilledema
5. Focal neurological deficit
6. New seizure within 1 week of presentation

The *New England Journal of Medicine* has an excellent video tutorial on the procedural steps for a lumbar puncture – watch this at least once prior to starting your rotation. Once the sample is obtained, the following lab studies are typically sent on the CSF.

1. Cell count and differential (expect elevated WBC count with neutrophil predominance)
2. Glucose (low) and protein concentration (high)
3. Gram stain and culture
4. PCR (to rule out specific pathogens, such as HSV)

Make sure you brush up on the changes to CSF expected in different types of meningitis, as this is a commonly asked question on rounds.

Given the potentially devastating consequences of untreated meningitis, one must have a low index of suspicion to treat – antibiotics should not be delayed while awaiting diagnostic results. Broad coverage with vancomycin and ceftriaxone is generally the recommended choice. Addition of ampicillin is recommended for patients who are either immunocompromised or older than

In practice, an extra tube of CSF is oftentimes obtained and saved in case additional studies are later requested.

In practice, an extra tube of CSF is oftentimes obtained and saved in case additional studies are later requested.

50 years old. Dexamethasone is often also administered in pneumococcal meningitis to reduce the risk of hearing loss.

9.5 Evidence-Based Neurology

Justifying your plan with clinical trial data is always looked upon favorably. The following are a few landmark trials that support treatment decisions you will encounter on the wards. Evidence-based medicine is, by nature, constantly evolving. *Thus, while these trials are a good starting point for building your knowledge base, it is important to stay abreast of newer evidence.* Clinical guidelines released by medical specialty groups, such as the American Heart Association, are excellent resources for up-to-date evidence.

9.5.1 *POINT* [5] Trial: Dual Antiplatelet Therapy for Secondary Prevention of Ischemic Stroke

While antiplatelet agents such as aspirin have long been a mainstay of secondary stroke prevention, it has been unclear whether addition of a second antiplatelet agent may confer incremental benefit. This question was most recently addressed by the "Platelet-Oriented Inhibition in New TIA and Minor Ischemic Stroke" (POINT) trial, published in the *New England Journal of Medicine* (NEJM) in 2018. You may have heard of the CHANCE trial, published in 2013, which studied the same question and found evidence of benefit for dual antiplatelet therapy (DAPT) but only recruited patients in China. Given differences in the distribution of stroke risk factors and stroke subtypes in China, as well as potential genetic differences relating to metabolism of clopidogrel, the POINT study sought to replicate these findings with an expanded study population.

The POINT trial enrolled 4881 patients across North America, Europe, Australia, and New Zealand. The key inclusion criteria were onset of a *small* stroke (NIH stroke scale score ≤3) or *high-risk* transient ischemic attack (TIAs; defined as ABCD [2] score ≥4) within 12 hours of randomization. Patients were excluded if they had an indication for oral anticoagulation (e.g., atrial fibrillation). Patients were further excluded if they were candidates for intravenous thrombolysis, endovascular interventions, or carotid endarterectomy. Patients were randomized either to aspirin (50–325 mg) and placebo or to aspirin and clopidogrel (600 mg loading dose followed by 75 mg/d) for 90 days. The primary outcome constituted a composite of ischemic stroke, myocardial infarction, or death from ischemic vascular causes. The primary safety outcome was "risk of major hemorrhage, which was defined as symptomatic intracranial hemorrhage, intraocular bleeding causing vision loss, transfusion of 2 or more units of red cells or an equivalent amount of whole blood, hospitalization or prolongation of an existing hospitalization, or death due to hemorrhage."

DAPT reduced the risk of the primary outcome (HR 0.75), with a number needed to treat of 67. This appeared to be driven by the ischemic stroke contribution to the primary outcome. As expected, DAPT increased the risk of hemorrhagic stroke (HR 2.32), with a number need to harm of 200. Taken together, for every thousand patients treated with this DAPT regimen, 15 ischemic events would be prevented, and 5 major hemorrhages would be caused.

Thus, in carefully selected populations with acute ischemic stroke or TIA that match these criteria, the use of DAPT for the first 90 days after onset appears to reduce risk for a recurrent vascular event, at the cost of elevated bleeding risk.

9

9.5.2 *SPARCL* Trial [6]: Statin Therapy for Secondary Prevention of Ischemic Stroke

You will notice that patients with ischemic strokes are generally started on a daily dose of 80 mg of atorvastatin (sometimes referred to as "Atorva 80"). This treatment approach is justified by results from the "Stroke Prevention by Aggressive Reduction in Cholesterol Levels" (SPARCL) trial, published in the *New England Journal of Medicine* in 2006.

The SPARCL trial enrolled 4731 patients across 205 centers with a TIA or stroke within 1–6 months of study and LDL levels of 100–190 mg/dL (i.e., elevated LDL). Patients were excluded if they had atrial fibrillation or if the stroke was deemed to be cardioembolic. These patients were randomized to either atorvastatin 80 mg or placebo and were followed for a median 4.9 years. The primary outcome was a fatal or nonfatal stroke.

The investigators found a 16% relative reduction in stroke risk, with 45 patients needed to treat (NNT) to prevent one stroke. In secondary analyses stratifying by stroke subtype, a protective effect was observed for ischemic stroke (22% relative reduction in risk), and a potentially harmful effect was observed for hemorrhagic stroke (66% relative increase in risk). Despite this increase in hemorrhagic stroke risk, the net effect when considering both stroke subtypes was consistent with a net benefit from statin use. Unsurprisingly, a protective effect was observed for incident coronary artery disease (42% relative reduction in risk).

9.5.2.1 Takeaway

The bottom line from these data is that treatment with atorvastatin 80 mg/day reduces the risk for a second ischemic stroke. The potential increase in hemorrhagic stroke risk related to statin use is controversial and may be an interesting topic to investigate and present about to your team.

9.5.3 NINDS Trial [7]: Stroke

Patients who present with an ischemic stroke within a particular timeframe are eligible for treatment with tissue plasminogen activator (tPa). As a medical student, you will typically not be involved with the decision to administer tPa. Regardless, once the patient is admitted, there will often be a discussion of the treatment decisions made by the clinicians who made the call to administer tPa. In these discussions, it is essential to know the trial justifying the treatment given to the patient you are caring for.

The National Institute of Neurological Disorders and Stroke rt-PA Stroke Study (NINDS) trial enrolled 624 patients presenting within 3 hours of an acute ischemic stroke (with a hemorrhage ruled out via a non-contrast CT scan). There is a classic list of exclusion criteria designed to minimize risk of intracerebral hemorrhage – including criteria like platelet counts less than 100,000, elevated PT/PTT, and GI bleeding – but memorizing this list is beyond the scope of your rotation (look it up when needed!). Patients were randomized to placebo or tPa and were followed for up to 3 months. The primary outcomes included improvements in functional outcomes, as measured on a variety of scales, at either 24 hours (part 1 of the study) or 3 months (part 2 of the study).

The investigators found no difference in functional outcomes at 24 hours between the tPa and placebo arm. In contrast, there was a consistent benefit in functional outcome at 90 days (70% increased odds for a "favorable outcome" and 30% increased odds for having "minimal or no disability"). This is despite a 5.8% absolute increase in intracranial hemorrhage (ICH) within 36 hours of tPa treatment.

It is worth noting that subsequent studies have investigated extending the 3-hour window and have found a potential benefit up to 4.5 hours. Mechanical thrombectomy – which is sometimes conducted after administration of tPa in certain cases – can sometimes be offered up to 24 hours after the onset of the neurological deficit. A detailed survey of the thrombectomy literature is beyond the scope of this chapter; however I encourage you to read the UpToDate article on the topic once you feel comfortable with management of acute ischemic stroke. This is a rapidly changing field!

9.5.3.1 Takeaway

There are a few key nuances to appreciate from this study. First, the benefit of tPa is primarily an improvement in *long-term* functional outcomes, rather than acute improvements in functional status. Second, despite the increase in hemorrhage risk, there is a net benefit in functional status. Third, the earlier you can treat ischemic stroke, the better the odds of a good outcome for the patient.

> This is where the saying 'time is brain' comes from!

9.5.4 FIRST Trial [8]: Seizures

In patients presenting with an unprovoked first seizure, a key point to address in your plan will be whether to initiate antiepileptic drugs. This question boils down to whether the beneficial effects of preventing a second seizure are outweighed by the side effects of antiepileptic therapy. Luckily, there are several trials that have investigated this question.

The First Seizure Trial Group (FIRST) enrolled 419 patients with a first, witnessed primary or secondarily generalized seizure. The majority of patients were 16–60 years old. Patients were randomized to either immediate prescription of an antiepileptic drug (AED) or were prescribed an AED only after seizure recurrence. Selection of the AED was determined by the treating clinician. The primary outcomes were probabilities of 1 or 2 seizure-free years, as well as long-term seizure remission. Patients were followed up for a minimum of 3 years.

Only 50% of the patients developed a recurrent seizure during the study period. Among the risk factors for a recurrent seizure were abnormal EEG findings and "remote symptomatic causes" (e.g., brain tumor, prior CNS infection, head trauma). The investigators found that treatment with an AED reduced the risk of a second seizure in the next 1–2 years by 50%. However, after 2 years, there was no difference in seizure risk between the two groups. In other words, there was no long-term prognosis benefit conferred by early treatment of a first seizure vs. deferring treatment until the second seizure.

9.5.4.1 Takeaway

The takeaways from this study are threefold. First, patients who are at high risk (i.e., who have any of the above risk factors) for a second seizure should be treated after their first seizure. Second, in patients without these risk factors, it becomes a matter of shared decision-making as to whether to initiate AEDs. The side effect profile should be weighed against potential clinical benefit.

9.5.5 The Optic Neuritis Treatment Trial (ONTT) [9]: Multiple Sclerosis

Optic neuritis is a common initial presentation of multiple sclerosis. The question of whether or not to treat these patients with corticosteroids was addressed by the landmark (ONTT).

The ONTT enrolled 457 patients presenting with a first episode of acute unilateral optic neuritis. Patients were randomized to either (i) intravenous (IV) methylprednisolone (more commonly called "solu-medrol"), (ii) oral prednisone, or (iii) oral placebo. The outcome of interest was the number of patients achieving normal visual acuity at multiple predetermined timepoints, ranging from 4 to 180 days.

The investigators found that, compared to placebo, IV methylprednisolone reduced the time to recovery from the visual symptoms. The difference between treatment arms became smaller with time, but a small benefit persisted at 6 months. In contrast, there was no benefit from oral prednisone. With regard to recurrence of optic neuritis within 2 years, there was a null effect of IV methylprednisolone. However, a worrying signal for increased risk of recurrent optic neuritis within 2 years was observed for oral prednisone compared to placebo.

9.5.5.1 Takeaway

Given the advantages in visual recovery time and risk of recurrence, intravenous methylprednisolone is the preferred treatment option for optic neuritis.

References

1. Inouye SK. Clarifying confusion: the confusion assessment method. Ann Intern Med. 1990;113(12):941. https://doi.org/10.7326/0003-4819-113-12-941.
2. Detsky ME, McDonald DR, Baerlocher MO, Tomlinson GA, McCrory DC, Booth CM. Does this patient with headache have a migraine or need neuroimaging? JAMA. 2006;296(10):1274–83. https://doi.org/10.1001/jama.296.10.1274.
3. Ducros A, Denier C, Joutel A, et al. The clinical spectrum of familial hemiplegic migraine associated with mutations in a neuronal calcium channel. N Engl J Med. 2001;345(1):17–24. https://doi.org/10.1056/NEJM200107053450103.
4. Sheldon R, Rose S, Ritchie D, et al. Historical criteria that distinguish syncope from seizures. J Am Coll Cardiol. 2002;40(1):142–8. https://doi.org/10.1016/S0735-1097(02)01940-X.
5. Johnston SC, Easton JD, Farrant M, et al. Clopidogrel and aspirin in acute ischemic stroke and high-risk TIA. N Engl J Med. 2018;379(3):215–25. https://doi.org/10.1056/NEJMoa1800410.
6. Raymond E, Pisano E, Gatsonis C, et al. High-dose atorvastatin after stroke or transient ischemic attack. N Engl J Med. 2006;355(6):549–59. https://doi.org/10.1056/NEJMoa061894.
7. Chatterjee S. Tissue plasminogen activator for acute ischemic stroke. N Engl J Med. 1995;333(24):1581–8. https://doi.org/10.1056/NEJM199512143332401.
8. Musicco M, Beghi E, Solari A, Viani F. Treatment of first tonic-clonic seizure does not improve the prognosis of epilepsy. Neurology. 1997;49(4):991–8. https://doi.org/10.1212/WNL.49.4.991.
9. Beck RW, Cleary PA, Anderson MM, et al. A randomized, controlled trial of corticosteroids in the treatment of acute optic neuritis. N Engl J Med. 1992;326(9):581–8. https://doi.org/10.1056/NEJM199202273260901.

Pediatrics

Aditya Achanta and Kelly Hallowell

Contents

10.1 Overview

In this chapter, we will be going through an approach for your pediatrics clerkship, a guide to family-centered rounding, a method of evaluation of a child for during a well-child visit, a system to determine if a child is healthy or "sick," and lastly a compilation of some common diseases you will most likely see during your clerkship.

Some key concepts to keep in mind as you read through this chapter:

- Children are not just small adults, and the approach to care needs to be modified based on both their physical age and developmental stage:
  - Children have different and changing physiology, depending on their age.
  - Physical exams should be adapted based on developmental stage.
  - Children are at increased risk for different pathogens and environmental causes for diseases (e.g., foreign body ingestion or aspiration, lead exposure), depending on their age.
  - Medical treatments are often different for children and adults.
  - Children's vital signs need to be assessed based on their age (◘ Fig. 10.1).
- Children are vulnerable but also incredibly resilient.
- Children are a part of a larger web. For instance, they are usually accompanied in medical settings by caretakers, who are often, understandably, concerned; both your patient and their caretakers should understand the medical issues and contribute to medical decision-making.
- History taking is different depending on patient age:
  - Their caretakers contribute to recounting your patient's medical history.
  - Some parts of the history should be taken confidentially with adolescents.

This being said, don't forget your adult medical knowledge! Not everything about children is unique, and a lot of pathophysiology can be applied to pediatrics. If you are unsure what to do, think about how you would start in an adult. If you don't know what is happening, you can say something like, "In adult, I would worry about IBD with her abdominal symptoms and bloody stools, but I don't know how common it is to present in a 15 year old" which shows your medical thinking and can lead to good discussions to fill your gaps in knowledge. Next we will think about some key differences in how to approach kids.

Pediatric Vital Signs

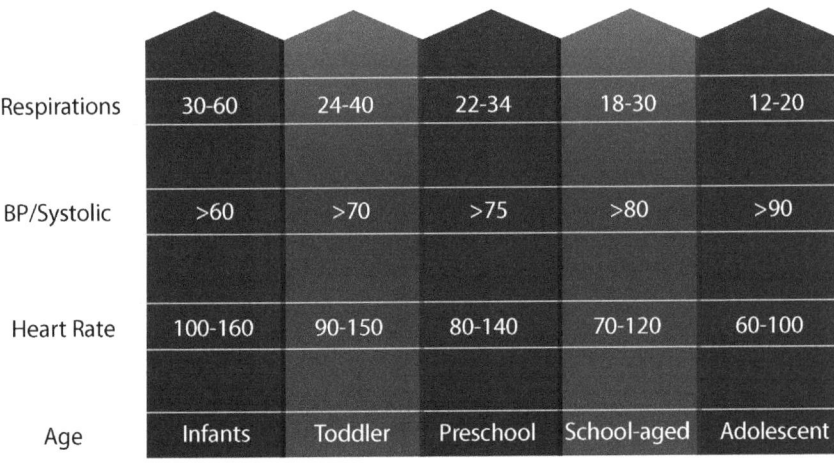

	Infants	Toddler	Preschool	School-aged	Adolescent
Respirations	30-60	24-40	22-34	18-30	12-20
BP/Systolic	>60	>70	>75	>80	>90
Heart Rate	100-160	90-150	80-140	70-120	60-100
Age	Infants	Toddler	Preschool	School-aged	Adolescent

◘ Fig. 10.1 Pediatric vital signs by age

10.1.1 History Taking

Always greet the child first. Ask them to introduce everyone in the room and their relationship to them; it can save you a lot of awkward assumptions. As much as possible, obtain the history from the child if developmentally appropriate. However, if the child is hesitant, it is appropriate to offer their guardian to take over for them. If the child does most of the history, ask the guardian if they have any other concerns the child did not bring up. Try to use their language rather than medical jargon (e.g., period rather than menses).

Adolescence is a transitional stage in medicine. The laws vary state by state, but most states allow treatment of STIs, contraceptive counseling, mental health treatment, and substance abuse treatment without parental consent. In preparation for more sensitive issues and taking care of their own health as adults, parents are asked to step out of the room during visits starting around 11–12 years old. This is done so questions and concerns on topics such as sex and alcohol can be addressed preemptively rather than reactively. When discussing these issues, explain that your conversation is confidential except for concerns of harm to themselves or others. One thing to note is that even though you won't share things without their permission, an insurance bill may list a diagnosis depending on your system.

The HEADSSS exam can be used to obtain a social history in adolescents:
- Home
- Education/eating habits
- Activities
- Drugs (alcohol, marijuana, prescription, recreational)
- Safety (using a seatbelt, riding in a car with a drunk driver, etc.)
- Sex
- Suicidality

This approach starts with easier topics to build rapport before addressing more sensitive topics. One strategy to broach topics is to ask questions first indirectly such as "I know 13 is an age when people start to experiment with alcohol. Do any of your friends drink alcohol?"

10.1.2 Past Medical History

Children typically do not have long past medical histories if at all. However, for young patients, a pregnancy history and birth history can be pertinent. To get a sense of the prenatal course, you can ask how many ultrasounds they had to get a sense if there were any concerns during the pregnancy; generally there are two ultrasounds: one early to confirm the due date and one later for an anatomy scan. Questions such as "was your child able to come home with you right away after they were born?" can give a sense if there were complications after the birth.

10.1.3 Medication Choice

When choosing medications for children, more practical matters might outweigh first-line treatments. A second-line treatment is better than the first-line option the toddler spits out. Certain medications are more palatable than others. Liquids are often available in multiple concentrations; you may have to do some math to find which concentration gives a better result trying to give smaller volume doses or round numbers easier for parents measuring. Giving a bitter medication four times a day is harder than just once. Ask the parent if they think they can handle the frequency of dosing. Medications are given by weight, so make sure you know it. Avoid making math errors by giving recommendations in mg/kg (the latter is often easier).

10.1.4 Medications to Avoid

Many drugs are not as well studied in children as in adults. There is a new list similar to the Beers list for children called the Key Potentially Inappropriate Drugs in Pediatrics (KIDs) list. You will not be expected to know what drugs are preferred but will get a sense of your institution's preferences over your rotation. Here are a few common drugs you may be tempted to use that you should generally avoid in kids that are helpful to know going in:
- Salicylates – risk of Reye's syndrome in children with viral illness
- Tetracyclines – risk of delay of skeletal development and bone growth in neonates, tooth discoloration, and enamel hypoplasia in children without all their adult teeth
- Macrolides – risk of hypertrophic pyloric stenosis
- Benzocaine (in oral pain relief, in the past used in teething products) – methemoglobinemia
- Fluoroquinolones – risk of arthropathy

10.1.5 Labs and Imaging

Children are much less understanding than adults of needles. If you are going to recommend a lab draw – you should have a reason! Pediatricians are much less inclined to draw monitoring labs just to "trend" them. Think ahead so you can draw everything you need at once.

Children have to live with the consequences of radiation for many more years than your elderly patients. Think about the importance of the imaging. Can your question be answered with an X-ray rather than a CT? Is ultrasound a reasonable alternative?

10.1.6 Family-Centered Rounding

Family-centered rounding is a unique form of rounding common in inpatient pediatric settings. The primary goal of this method is to keep families unfailingly up-to-date on their child and allow them to participate more in medical decision, often incorporating their input into the plan. Your responsibility as the medical student in this setting is to ensure that the family – and whenever possible, the patient (child) – understand what is going on and make decisions in line with their values based on this information. Families should and will count on you to follow-up with them, update them, and answer their questions during rounds. As this is a different format for interacting with patients than what you have participated in before, it may be challenging at first. Hence, here is a list of what to do, in suggested order, to best prepare for family-centered rounds:
- Arrive at least 15 minutes earlier than what you anticipate spending on pre-rounding
- Note patient vitals and inputs and outputs (commonly called I/Os and include how much fluid taken by mouth and IV and how much urine, blood, stool, or other fluid is lost over the previous 24 hours).

272 A. Achanta and K. Hallowell

- Check new labs.
- Check if there are any new notes in the electronic medical record.
- Examine the Med Administration Record (MAR) for the past day.
- Attend sign-out (where the night shift tells the day team about overnight events and new admits).
- Touch base with the overnight nurse and/or read the nursing note.
- Think about your assessment and plan: is the patient improving? Worsening?
- Think about how you would explain the patient's condition to family in simple, easy to understand, and age-appropriate terms (if applicable).
- Discuss your plan with your resident before rounds
- If you have time, look online at the clinical management pathway (e.g., at Seattle Children's website and Boston Children's Hospital clinical pathway phone application) for the particular disease for your patient's condition. These clinical pathways can help you suggest an evidenced-based plan.

10.1.7 How to Really Shine

Here are two things that are usually not mandatory but can earn your major bonus points with the patient, family, and team:
- Actually see your patient prior to rounds. For family-centered rounding, it is common for both students and residents to forego this part. If you do this, you will undoubtedly gain better perspective on the child's condition as well as connect to the family and patient on a deeper level:
  - Moreover, eliciting family questions and concerns here gives you time you prepare answers prior to rounding with the team.
  - However, your team may not want you to wake patients. Use other surrogates such as parents or nursing staff to get information about overnight.
- For patients with an out-of-the-ordinary diagnosis, such as Addison's disease, prepare a short "lecture" on one aspect about the disease (e.g., appropriate management) that the team would benefit from. Make sure this presentation is short and sweet. You can also bring along a paper to show the team and allow them to read up more later.

The format of family-centered rounds is institution and team-dependent. Here is one example:

Outside the patient's room:
- Present your one-liner:
  - For new patients, be more detailed about how the team arrived at the differential or diagnosis (e.g., "suspected Crohn's disease due terminal ileitis with phlegmonous changes on CT").
  - For familiar patients, your one-liner should be brief yet updated each day to reflect the most recent developments:
    - On admission: "Mark is a 5-month-old male who presented with 7 days of runny nose and worsening cough, found to have a consolidation on chest X-ray concerning for pneumonia."
    - On day 2: "Mark is a 5-month-old male who presented with 7 days of runny nose and worsening cough, found to have community acquired pneumonia now on day 2 of amoxicillin with minor improvement."
- Present the overnight events.

- Present objective data such as vitals, ins/outs, and labs. Check with the residents prior to your presentation on how much detail to include.

Note that some teams may ask you to do this all inside the room in front of the patient and family.

Inside the patient's room:
- If the patient is new, introduce the idea of family-centered rounding to the family, and introduce everyone on the team and their role:
  - If you are wearing any precautions as you enter the room, briefly explain in a friendly manner.
- Subjective:
  - Ask about how the patient is feeling. A good opening question is "How did Susie do last night?"
    - You want to get a sense of the severity of their illness at that particular moment.
  - Make these questions direct, otherwise families can ramble.
- Objective:
  - Summarize the vitals for the family:
    - Use terms familiar for the family: let them know what the vitals mean (e.g., "A normal heart rate for a baby is much higher than that of adults" or "the heart rate is a bit high likely in response to infection").
  - Perform a focused physical exam, trying to assess if patient is getting better or worse:
    - Let the child and parents know before you conduct each part of the physical exam – "I am going to listen to your child's heart."
  - Explain relevant lab or imaging results if they are pertinent:
    - Give brief explanations of what they mean (e.g., "the white blood count, a measure of her body's response to the infection went, down this morning").
- Assessment/plan:
  - Present your assessment to the family ("[Child's name] was admitted to the hospital for [their diagnosis\], which is [lay person translation])".
  - Discuss if you believe the patient's condition is improving or not.
  - Suggest the plan that you have formulated for their care.
    - Be as specific as you can; families want to know what the plan means for them and their kid that day (e.g., can they not eat because of an upcoming procedure or the vital sign changes are you looking for before discharge)
  - Ask for the rest of the team's, patient's, and family's input.
  - Make sure to ask the family if they have any other questions or concerns.

One of the most difficult parts for many medical students about family-centered rounding is that everyone (the team, the patient, the family) is watching you. One strategy to get over the stage fright is to just focus on the patient. Some specific tips that can help you do this include:
- Sitting down in a chair in the patient's room or kneeling down to get down to your patient's eye level to speak to them
- Avoiding the use of medical jargon that your patient does not understand (afebrile, bowel movement, peritoneal signs, etc.)
  - If you must use medical terminology, always let the patient and family know that you will discuss with your team in medical lingo first and then translate for them.

Pearl: If you have pre-rounded on the patient already, you can reduce the awkwardness of repeating yourself by telling the patient and family that you are getting the team up to speed. Summarize only the key points, and then ask the patient and family to verify if you covered everything.

Pearl: If at all possible, use the child's name and address them directly

Pearl: It can be daunting to propose the plan in front of not only your team but also the family, without necessarily having discussed it with the team (this varies by team). Quickly run your plan by the intern/resident on your team prior to rounds if this is the team's style.

10.1.8 Well-Child Visits

A well visit is a checkup at specific ages for children to make sure that their growth and development is appropriate, prevent problems before they arise, prepare children and caretakers for the child's next stage of development, keep children up to date with vaccinations, and answer a child's or caretaker's questions.

A well-child visit should address the following general components:
- Addressing parents' and patient's concerns about their health and development
- Showing and explaining the growth charts (for height, weight, and when applicable head circumference)
- Evaluating the patient's development and resources that the family has to support their child's development
- Checking for red flags in childcare that deserve further attention
- Counseling for any current issues
- Anticipatory guidance:
  - This helps the family and child start to think about the changes that they will likely experience between this visit and the next. It includes discussing topics such as how to start to feed a 4-month-old baby pureed and solid food, to "baby-proof" a house before a baby starts crawling, or discussing the changes that occur in puberty. The *Bright Futures Guidelines* provides great advice for giving anticipatory guidance to patients.
- Addressing chronic conditions such as asthma or weight management
- Vaccinations
- Labs if necessary
- Referrals if necessary

A great primer on well-child visits in general is the *Bright Futures* guide created by the American Academy of Pediatrics. It has developmental milestones and anticipatory guidance for every well-child visit by age. I recommend keeping a copy at your desk to reference quickly before going in to see a child.

When you do see a child for a well-child visit, you will most likely see note templates in your EMR. Here is an example:

10.2 6-Month-Old Well-Child Visit

10.2.1 Subjective

- Include parental concerns and any relevant interval history (e.g., any injuries, hospitalizations, changes in school performance) since last seen in clinic.
- Diet (what makes up the majority of the patient's diet and what else they are eating):
  - For infants: how many ounces of formula and how many ounces of breast milk?
  - For young children: do they eat their fruits and vegetables? How much milk do they drink?
  - For older children: do they eat a balanced diet? Do they drink sugary beverages or soda?
- Elimination (stool and urine):
  - Especially important for infants, ask how many wet diapers they have each day.
  - Many young children have issues with constipation, so be sure to ask.

— Age-based developmental milestones (social, expressive and receptive language, fine and gross motor).
— Behavioral health assessment (for infants, maternal behavioral health).
— Sleeping (where, how long, with whom):
  – Remember that "co-sleeping" (infants with parents in their bed) is very dangerous and should be discouraged.
— Living situation (Where does the child live and with whom? Is there smoking in the house? Are there guns in the house and if so how are they secured? Who takes care of the child or social needs such as food insecurity?).

10.2.2 Previous Immunizations

— Include dates if possible.

Schedule per the CDC (◘ Fig. 10.2):
— Birth: 1st hepatitis B (HepB)
— 1 month: 2nd HepB
— 2 months: 1st *Rotavirus* (RV); 1st diphtheria, tetanus, and acellular pertussis (DTAP); 1st *Haemophilus influenzae* type B (Hib); 1st pneumococcal conjugate (PCV13); 1st inactivated polio (IPV)
— 4 months: 2nd RV, 2nd DTAP, 2nd Hib, 2nd PCV13, 2nd IPV

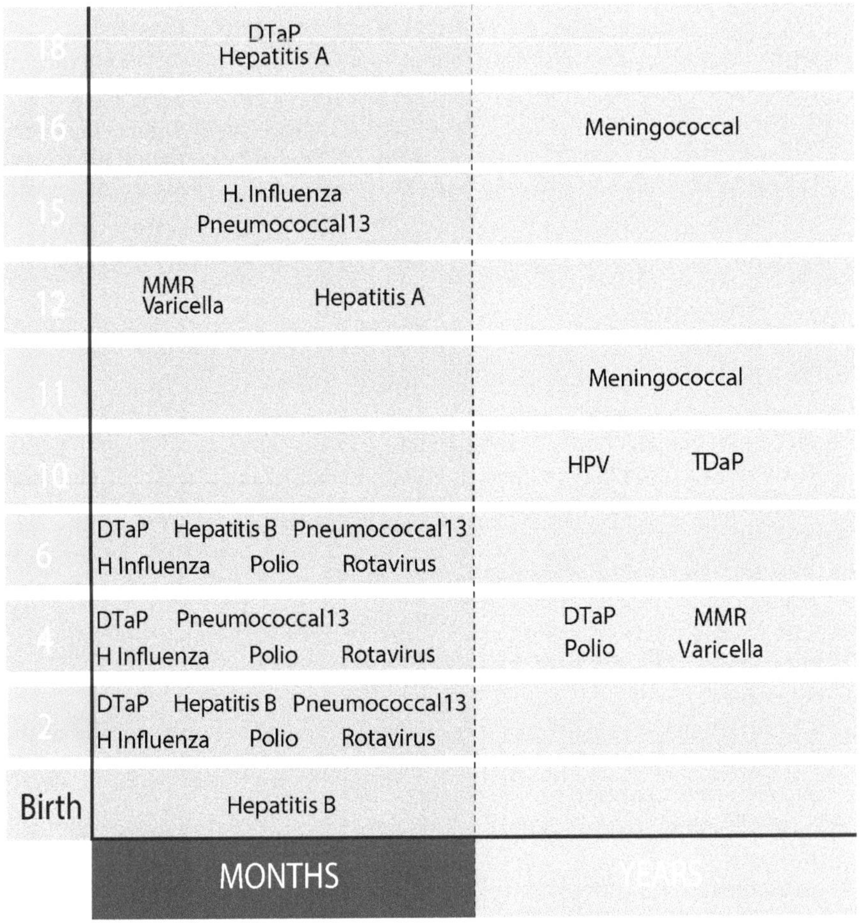

18	DTaP / Hepatitis A	
16		Meningococcal
15	H. Influenza / Pneumococcal13	
12	MMR / Varicella Hepatitis A	
11		Meningococcal
10		HPV TDaP
6	DTaP Hepatitis B Pneumococcal13 / H Influenza Polio Rotavirus	
4	DTaP Pneumococcal13 / H Influenza Polio Rotavirus	DTaP MMR / Polio Varicella
2	DTaP Hepatitis B Pneumococcal13 / H Influenza Polio Rotavirus	
Birth	Hepatitis B	
	MONTHS	YEARS

◘ Fig. 10.2   CDC childhood vaccination schedule

- 6 months: 3rd HepB, 3rd DTAP, 3rd PCV13, 3rd IPV, and possibly RV and Hib depending on the formulation, able to get first influenza vaccine depending on season (need 2 doses 4 weeks apart)
- 1 year: 1st measles, mumps, rubella (MMR); 1st varicella (VAR), 4th PCV13
- 15 months: 4th DTAP, 3rd or 4th HIB (depending on the formulation), hepatitis A (HepA, second dose 6–12 months later)
- 4–6 years old: 5th DTAP, 4th IPV, 2nd MMR, 2nd VAR
- 9 years old: human papillomavirus (HPV, second dose 6–12 months later)
- 11–12 years old: tetanus, diphtheria, and acellular pertussis (TDAP), 1st meningococcal ACWY (MenACWY)
- 16 years old: 2nd MenACWY

Special circumstances:
- Meningococcal B vaccination is recommended for patients who have function or anatomic asplenia and complement component deficiencies and on a case-by-case basis for adolescents at average risk between ages of 16 and 18 (2–3 dose series).
- Pneumococcal polysaccharide (PSV23) vaccination is indicated if patient has chronic heart disease, chronic lung disease, and diabetes mellitus.

General vaccination principles:
- Unconjugated vaccines (such as PPSV23) are less effective for children under 2 years.
- Vaccines are given based on a child's chronologic age; there is no need to delay for premature infants.
- Avoid live vaccines in severely immunocompromised patients.
- Previous severe reaction (e.g., anaphylaxis) to a previous dose or vaccine component is a contraindication to further doses.
- It is okay to vaccine a child with a mild illness (cold, runny nose, cough, otitis media, or mild diarrhea) or fever below 101 F. Children with more severe symptoms should wait until they recover to avoid any diagnostic confusion.

10.2.3 Objective

- Weight, height, and head circumference (if applicable) changes
- Vitals and general appearance
- Head (in infants, check the fontanelles – are they sunken or bulging?)
- Eyes (for young children, have something interesting and see if they can track it)
- Mouth
- Ears (save for last to avoid crying)
- Heart
- Lungs (important to listen to first – maybe even as soon as you walk into the room so you can listen before the baby starts crying)
- Abdomen
- Genitourinary (ask permission from child/parents, and quickly look at the Tanner stage of the child and if testicles are descended; also take a look at the rectum for babies)
- Skin (if a child has a rash, take a look at most of their skin to see where the rash extends)
- Musculoskeletal (opportunity to test a child's motor development – walking and crawling; check Ortolani and Barlow maneuvers for hip dysplasia in infants)

Pearl: The physical exam for a young child is an art. Asking the parents to help position, making games out of exam maneuvers, and having toys in the room can help keep them happy. However, sometimes no matter what, the child will cry and that's not your fault. Know when to come back later in the visit.

Pearl: An ear exam is very important in pediatrics and can be difficult. Positioning is key. One trick to have the parent hug the child chest-to-chest and have them hold the child's head while you look.

Pearl: Important to prioritize what you want to do first for infants and young children who may not like you touching them. Often listening to the lung and heart is a good first step although crying suggests a patent airway!

Pearl: Testicles should be descended by 12 months

- Neurologic (conduct the interview with the child as much as possible, to see how alert and oriented they are)
- Newborn reflexes: Moro reflex (disappears at ~2 months), stepping reflex (disappears at ~2 months), rooting reflex (disappears at ~4 months), suck reflex (disappears at ~4 months), and tonic neck reflex (disappears at ~6 months)

10.2.4 Assessment/Plan

- Overall assessment:
  - Your one-liner will vary from an inpatient encounter – the child may be perfectly healthy!
    - Noah is a 6-month-old healthy male with normal growth and development here for 6-month-old well-child visit.
- Anticipatory guidance
- Counseling
- Problem-based plan
- Vaccines that will be administered today
- Next follow-up

Child development is primarily evaluated using developmental milestones. In clinical practice, it is important to keep in mind that these milestones aren't hard cutoffs but approximations of when most children should develop a certain skill. Children can develop a developmental skill earlier or later than what is endorsed in textbooks and still be within the range of normal. However, if you have any concerns about a child's development, it is important to express these concerns to your attending as the child can be referred to early intervention for further evaluation. Most pediatricians use patient-reported screening tools to assess development:

- Infants and toddlers: ages and stages
- School-aged children: pediatric symptom checklist
- Teenagers or older: PHQ-9 and GAD-7

Early intervention is available for children younger than 3 years old. Early interventions have been shown to improve functional outcomes in children (McManus, Richardson, Schnekman et al. JAMA Network Open 2019). Depending on your setting, keep in mind that there are significant social disparities in the access to early intervention services by race and income.

Here are key developmental milestones before 1 year of age which you should commit to memory:

- Gross motor (■ Fig. 10.3):
  - 2–3 months – holding head up when laying on stomach
  - 6 months – able to sit unassisted
  - 8–9 months – crawling
  - 1 year – walking
- Social:
  - 2 months – social smile
  - 8 months – stranger anxiety
- Fine motor:
  - 6 months – transferring from one hand to another
  - 9 months – pincer grasp
- Language:
  - 2 months – cooing
  - 6 months – babbling
  - 1 year – say a few words such as "dada," "mama," and "uh-oh"

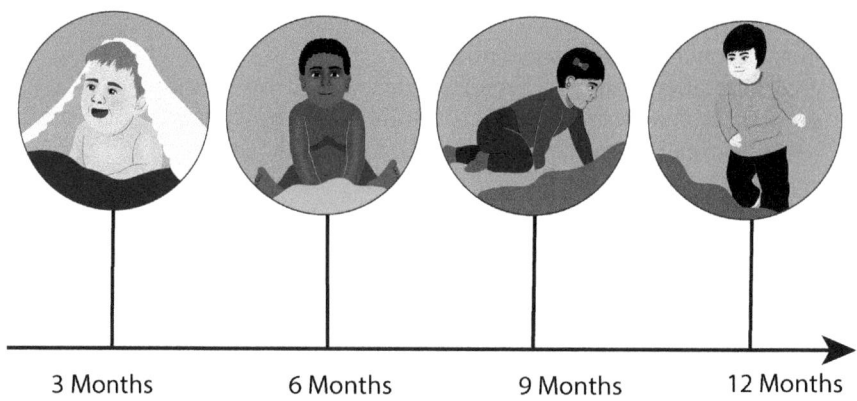

□ **Fig. 10.3**   Gross motor milestones

Here are some red flags that you should think about and rule out if necessary:

General – for all ages:
- Growth changes below two major percentile lines on a growth chart or weight for age falls below the 5th percentile.
- General safety issues:
  - Use seatbelts and age-appropriate car seats.
  - Wear a helmet while riding a bike.
  - Discourage the use of trampolines at home.
  - Discourage storing firearms at home.
- Signs of emotional abuse, which can manifest in developmental delays, changes in behavior, or somatic symptoms although these are not sensitive findings.
- Signs of physical abuse (bruising where there shouldn't be bruising, signs of scalding on the buttocks, signs of shaken baby syndrome).

Infants:
- The position that the baby is sleeping in (children should be sleeping on their back especially before 6 months of age to reduce the risk of sudden infant death syndrome (SIDS))
  - Where baby is sleeping (should be sleeping in their own crib to reduce risk of SIDS)
  - Smoking in the house (secondhand smoke increases the risk of SIDS, acute otitis media)

Toddlers/younger children:
- Signs of sexual abuse (e.g., precocity of sexual knowledge or behavior).
- If the child is obese or you see signs of acanthosis nigricans (this may prompt you to do further testing such as testing for diabetes mellitus with HbA1c, lipid levels, TSH, ALT). Appropriate counseling is to cut down on juices, soda, syrup, and free sugars, and to encourage 30 minutes of exercise per day.
- Signs of autism spectrum disorder such as repetitive, purposeless movements, lack of social reciprocity, inability to relate to others, lack of interest in shared attention, and/or fixation with certain objects:
  - Use the MCHAT screening tool if you have a patient concerning for autism. Most pediatricians use it as an autism screen at 18 and 24 months.

Pearl: Weight categories in children are determined by percentile. Overweight is greater than 85th percentile, obese is greater than 95th percentile.

Pearl: Many parents incorrectly believe that fruit juices are healthy for children. These are extremely high in sugar and should be limited just like sodas and other artificial drinks.

Older children/adolescents:
- Recreational drug use in older children and adolescents – consider screening your patient using the CRAFFT screening interview (Knight et al. *Arch Pediatr Adolesc Med.* 1999;153(6):591–596.):
  - Have you ever been in a **c**ar where the person driving was using drugs?
  - Do you use drugs/alcohol to **r**elax, fit in, or feel better about yourself?
  - Do you ever use drugs or alcohol when **a**lone?
  - Do you **f**orget what you did when using alcohol or drugs?
  - Have your **f**amily or **f**riends encouraged you to stop using or cut down on alcohol or drugs?
  - Have you ever gotten into **t**rouble when using alcohol or drugs?
- Mental health disorders:
  - ADHD – inattention, hyperactivity, and/or impulsiveness in multiple situations.
  - Anxiety – children are more likely to have somatization of anxiety than adults (e.g., stomach aches, headaches, or troubles sleeping).
  - Depression – may have typical adult symptoms but teenagers are more likely to be irritable than have depressed mood.

10.3 Sick vs Not Sick

For a sick visit, it is important to determine when children are very sick and need emergency care or admission and when children are stable enough for you to take further history. One important tool for this determination is the pediatric assessment triangle (◨ Fig. 10.4). The arms of the triangle consist of:
1. Appearance
2. Breathing
3. Circulation

If you are worried about a child's health based on any of the arms of the pediatric assessment triangle, you should call your attending who may send the child to the emergency department or perform life support. Depending on which aspect of the pediatric assessment triangle you are concerned about, you

Pearl: The pediatric assessment triangle is a useful framework to think about the immediate needs of a sick child in a systematic way. There have been multiple studies validating this tool; one well-cited study is "The Pediatric Assessment Triangle: accuracy of its application by nurses in the triage of children" (Horeczko et al. 2013). This is a useful article to reference further on the specifics of the pediatric assessment triangle.

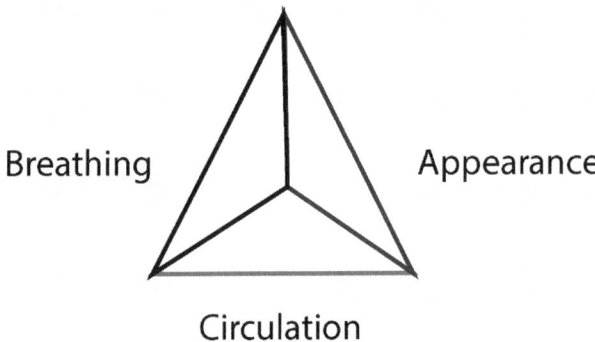

The Pediatric Assessment Triangle

◨ **Fig. 10.4** Pediatric assessment triangle

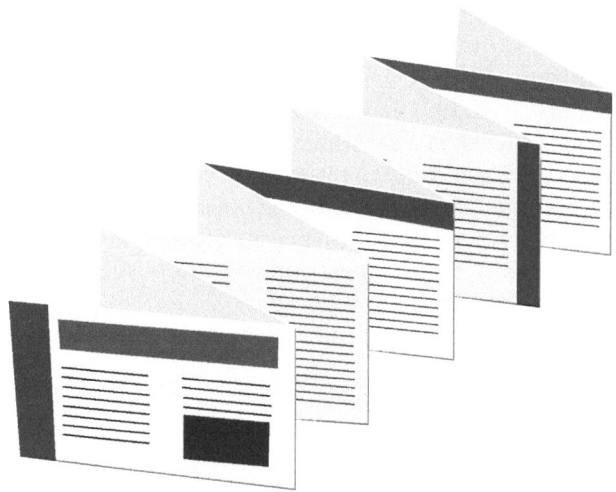

Fig. 10.5 Broselow tape

can narrow your differential. For example, if a child is in shock, you may note marked abnormalities in the appearance and circulation of a child.

Another useful tool in pediatric emergencies is the Broselow tape, which can give you useful information such as medication dosages and level of shock voltage for a defibrillator based on a child's weight and height. It may be helpful to have the Broselow tape on hand if you are expecting to see a very sick child in the near future (■ Fig. 10.5).

10.4 Approach to Acute Fever from Infection

As most children have not yet developed any underlying health conditions, infections are the most common complaints you will see. Most children who are presenting with acute fever (less than 14 days) and are well appearing and stable have a viral illness, but there are serious and important exceptions.

A big exception is for febrile children who are younger than 2–3 months of age. At that age, children may have had their first set of TDAP, Hib, and PCV13 vaccines at their 2-month visit but are not fully immunized as they have not had their second and third set until their 4- and 6-month well-child visit. Their immune systems aren't fully developed, and they are at higher risk of serious bacterial infection. Questions that you would want to ask in your history would be:

- History:
  - Symptoms and duration
  - Pertinent review of symptoms
    - Food and water intake
    - Urination amount and frequency
    - Bowel movements
    - Vomiting
    - Level of alertness and arousability
- Risk factors:
  - Sick contacts
  - Travel
- Past medical history:
  - Prenatal history (e.g., maternal GBS status)
  - Birth history (e.g., prematurity)
  - Other medical history
  - Immunization records

Febrile infants under 60–90 days always need labs:

- All children with unexplained fever under 6 months receive a urine sample and culture:
  - Between 6 months and 2 years: urinalysis and culture should be obtained depending on risk.
  - Females under 2 generally should have urine tested.
  - Uncircumcised males are also at higher risk, as are patients with previous history of UTI or history of vesicoureteral reflux.
- All children under 3 months or younger with a fever receive a CBC with differential and blood cultures x2.
- If a child younger than 1 month has diarrhea or an infant has diarrhea with any concerning features, the child needs a stool culture and WBC count.
- All children younger than 1 month with fever require a lumbar puncture (LP) to test for meningitis and older children if they have symptoms or signs suspicious for meningitis (discussed more later).

There a few different validated clinical tools that are used to evaluate sick children at risk of having a bacterial infection. Common tools include the Rochester criteria (for infants up to 60 days), Boston criteria (for between 28 and 90 days), and the Gomez "Step-by-Step" approach (for under 90 days). These tools are easy to look up on MDCalc. After you take the H&P, take a second to plug the relevant values in the appropriate clinical tool in MDCalc before presenting the patient's case to your attending.

The treatment of bacterial infection generally depends on the etiology and the sensitivities that come back, but there are recommended empiric antibiotic therapies for febrile infants who look "sick" based on suspected etiology. The timing of antibiotics depends on your index of suspicion. It is best to take culture before starting empiric antibiotics if possible, but this is not always done in practice depending on the severity of illness. Some may prefer to wait until culture comes back to direct therapy if they look well and their vital signs besides fever are normal. The decision to admit is based on how sick the child is and whether they would have access to prompt outpatient follow-up.

In older children, some common bacterial infections that you would want to evaluate for include bacterial strep pharyngitis, otitis media, impetigo, and appendicitis. We will delve into some of these diagnoses later.

If you have ruled out bacterial infections in children, the focus is on supportive care and follow-up. It is important to convey to parents that we cannot treat upper respiratory infections (URIs) caused by viruses; URIs most often run their course without harm to the child, and supportive care is the best care. Supportive care includes making sure the child is drinking lots of fluids, able to eat, and not having copious vomiting or diarrhea. As fever is a physiologic response to infection, the use of antipyretics such as acetaminophen or ibuprofen is not necessary for febrile children but can provide comfort if used judiciously.

There are different liquids, suspensions, and tablets for both pediatric acetaminophen and ibuprofen, so double check the dosing for the medication after you have pended it in the EMR with your resident, at least for the first few times (◘ Table 10.1).

Pearl: Aspirin is avoided in children with fever due to concern for Reye's syndrome, which presents with encephalopathy and liver damage.

◘ **Table 10.1** Antipyretic dosing in children

Medication	Acetaminophen	Ibuprofen
Dose and frequency	10–15 mg/kg/dose every 4–6 hours	4–10 mg/kg/dose every 6–8 hours
Maximum daily dose	2600 mg/day	1200 mg/day

10.5 Diseases

We will now go through the most common illnesses you may encounter on your pediatric rotations.

10.6 Infectious Complaints

10.6.1 Meningitis

Bird's Eye View   Meningitis is inflammation of the meninges, or membranes, that cover the brain and spinal cord.

- Presentation
- Infants: Fever, altered mental status, poor feeding (these are nonspecific symptoms; however, make sure you have a high degree of suspicion for meningitis when you see these symptoms)
- Older children: neck pain/stiffness, headache, fever, seizures, photophobia, nausea/vomiting
- Signs: fever, bulging fontanelle, hypotonia, rash, nuchal rigidity, Kernig's sign, Brudzinski's sign, neurologic deficits, Cushing's triad (increased intracranial pressure may lead to bradycardia, hypertension, and irregular breathing), convulsions/seizures (◘ Fig. 10.6)

Differential Diagnosis   Encephalitis, subdural abscess, epidural abscess, brain abscess, CNS leukemia

Pearl: The classic triad for meningitis is headache, nuchal rigidity or tenderness, and fever. However, younger children are less likely to have this triad of signs and symptoms. Even in adults, only around 44% of patients have all three of the classic triad, but 95% have 2/4 symptoms of: headache, nuchal tenderness/rigidity, altered mental status, and fever.

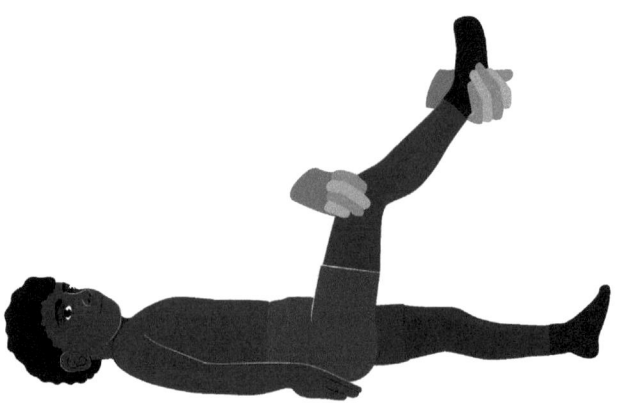

Kernig´s sign

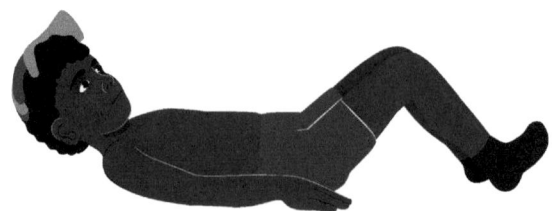

Brudzinski´s sign

◘ Fig. 10.6   Kernig's and Brudzinski's signs

■ Work-Up

When to get a lumbar puncture? All children younger than a month with fever require a lumbar puncture to test for meningitis and older children if they have symptoms or signs suspicious for meningitis.

Lumbar puncture only if there are no signs of increased intracranial pressure, no issues with clotting, and no signs of hemodynamic instability, focal neurologic deficits, or seizures. If any possible contraindications are present, get a CT scan and wait to do a LP 6 hours after if appropriate.

Bacterial meningitis score (Nigrovic et al.) – that helps you decide how likely bacterial meningitis is:

- CSF gram stain
- CSF neutrophils
- CSF protein
- Peripheral blood neutrophils
- Seizures

Other useful labs: CBC, BMP, blood cultures, urinalysis

■ Bugs that Cause Meningitis

Viral: HSV-2 (meningitis), enterovirus (usually summertime and often transmitted fecal-orally), influenza, arboviruses

Bacterial

- Newborns–1 month: group B streptococcus, *E. coli, Listeria*
- 1 month–older children: *H. influenzae* (more common in younger and unvaccinated children), *Neisseria meningitidis* (very common in teenagers), *S. pneumoniae*
- Uncommon causes – Lyme

Pearl: While HSV-1 commonly causes cold sores and can also lead to temporal lobe encephalitis, HSV-2 commonly causes genital sores and cause meningitis.

■ Interpreting the Lumbar Puncture (◘ Table 10.2)

Note that the baseline values for the lumbar puncture may differ by age.

■ Treatment

Always consult with infectious disease for local guidelines.

- Empiric bacterial meningitis:
  - <1 month: ampicillin plus cefotaxime ± acyclovir
  - >1 month old: vancomycin (60 mg/kg IV per day; split up into four doses) plus ceftriaxone (100 mg/kg IV a day; BID)
- Viral meningitis:
  - HSV: acyclovir
  - Otherwise: supportive care (eating as much as possible, drinking lots of fluids or IV fluids, Tylenol, antinausea medications)

◘ **Table 10.2** Meningitis lumbar puncture findings

	White blood cells	Protein	Glucose
Bacterial meningitis	Neutrophil predominance	High	Low (<0.4 CSF:blood)
Viral meningitis	Lymphocyte predominance	Slight increase	Normal
Tuberculosis meningitis	Lymphocyte predominance	Very high	Low (<0.3 CSF:blood)

- Lyme – can give oral or IV treatment:
  - Oral treatment: >8 years old, give doxycycline 4 mg/kg/day BID or amoxicillin 50 mg/kg/day TID
  - IV treatment: ceftriaxone 50–75 mg/kg/day (up to 2 g/dose) once a day

Prophylaxis   Vaccinations; if close contacts with someone with known *Neisseria meningitis*, give rifampicin regardless of vaccination status.

- **Complications**
- Death due to cerebral edema causing herniation
- Hydrocephalus
- Hearing loss (dexamethasone may reduce complication of hearing loss from *H. influenzae* and should be given at the same time as antibiotics)
- Seizures
- Waterhouse-Friderichsen syndrome (adrenal gland failure to due bleeding into the glands, often *N. meningitis*)
- Shock

10.6.2   Urinary Tract Infections

Bird's Eye View   Urinary tract infections are common in young children, especially in females as their urethras are anatomically shorter. The most common causes of UTIs in children are constipation and potty-training issues such as holding in urine.

Presentation   This can manifest with the classic UTI symptoms such as urgency, bedwetting, frequency, dysuria, hematuria, or less obvious symptoms, such as fever, abdominal pain, nausea, and listlessness. If you are worried that your patient between 2 and 23 months has a urinary tract infection yet they don't have the classic symptoms, you can use the UTICalc by the University of Pittsburgh to get a better sense of their pretest probability.

Work-Up   To diagnose a patient, you would get a urinalysis, most likely via transurethral catheterization, and a urine culture. If you have an abnormal urinalysis with at least 50,000 colony-forming units per milliliter, this would be considered a UTI. Furthermore, the current recommendations from the AAFP are that boys, girls under 3 years old, and girls aged between 3 and 7 years old with a temperature of at least 101.3F should have imaging, ultrasound, and voiding cystourethrogram, to evaluate for anatomical abnormalities that may predispose the patient to develop UTIs, such as vesicourethral reflux. Primary vesicourethral reflux is due to an incompetent valve between the urethra and bladder, which normally prevents urine backflow. Urine backflow predisposes to UTI because of upward migration of bacteria and more stagnant urine flow.

- **Management and Treatment**

Admit if child is younger than 2 months, is "sick" (think pediatric assessment triangle), there is no reliable follow-up, or if they have signs of pyelonephritis.

The treatment duration for uncomplicated UTI is controversial. The Cochrane review states that 2–4 days of antibiotics are as effective as 7–14 days of antibiotics in clearing UTI in children. The preferred regimens for uncomplicated UTI are Bactrim dosed at 10 mg/kg/day, split up into two doses q12 hours; amoxicillin-clavulanate can also be trialed; this is dosed at 25–45 mg/kg/day, split up into two doses q12 hours. To prevent future UTIs in young children, it is important to counsel parents to treat their child's constipation with adequate hydration and fiber and to avoid bubble baths.

Complications   If a UTI is not treated, it can progress to pyelonephritis. In addition to UTI symptoms, patients with pyelonephritis may develop fever, chills, costovertebral pain, nausea, or vomiting. If your patient has pyelonephritis, they can be treated with 10–14 days of oral amoxicillin/clavulanate, a third-generation cephalosporin, or IV antibiotics followed by oral therapy.

Discharge if they are tolerating oral fluids, the patient has been afebrile for 24 hours, and the necessary care has been completed or arranged to be completed as an outpatient.

10.6.3 Sepsis

Bird's Eye View   Sepsis is a dysregulated inflammatory response due to bacteremia that may reduce perfusion of vital organs.

Presentation   Symptoms of pediatric sepsis are feeling feverish, cold extremities, reduced activity, and decreased urine output. You should have a high level of suspicion for sepsis when a child meets the systemic inflammatory response syndrome (SIRS) criteria. The pediatric SIRS criteria have been extrapolated from adult literature. The SIRS criteria are as follows:
- Tachycardia or bradycardia (compared to age-based normal)
- Tachypnea (compared to age-based normal)
- Hyperthermia and hypothermia
- Elevated WBC or bandemia (excess of band cells, which are immature white blood cells)

Sepsis defined by the Pediatric Sepsis Consensus Conference is:
- 2+ SIRS criteria (by age category)
- Confirmed invasive bacteremia
- 2+ organ dysfunction

- **Etiology**
- Babies: GBS, RSV, *Listeria, E. coli*
- Older children: infected wounds, UTI, meningitis, pneumonia

- **Differentiating the Differential**
- Anaphylactic shock – acute onset after exposure, hives, GI symptoms, breathing difficulty, rapid improvement with epinephrine
- Cardiogenic shock – in children often occurs in the setting of trauma, arrythmia, or obstructive shock (least common but may occur with trauma, ventilators, or congenital heart disease)
- Hypovolemic shock – in the setting of diarrhea, vomiting, and not being able to take in enough fluids
- Diabetic ketoacidosis – Kussmaul breathing, history of diabetes, high blood sugars, fruity smell to breath, abdominal pain
- Pancreatitis – abdominal pain, high lipases
- Adrenal crisis – presentation with vomiting and shock, if shock is refractory to fluids and pressors but improves with steroid administration
- Hemorrhagic shock

■ Work-Up

Labs and diagnostics:

- Blood cultures x2–3
- CBC
- BMP, LFTs
- UA/UCx
- PT/PTT
- LP if meningitis cannot be ruled out
- Lactate
- CXR if suspicion of pneumonia or respiratory symptoms

■ Treatment

The goals for treatment of septic shock is to maintain perfusion to vital organs, maintain oxygenation and ventilation, and treat the underlying cause. It may be difficult to obtain access and may require IO or central venous access if IV access fails.

The Pediatric Advanced Life Support algorithm for septic shock is helpful to reference for treatment of septic shock in the ICU.

The basics are to give 20 mL/kg NS boluses to raise blood pressure but to stop if the patient develops trouble breathing. If this doesn't work, start an inotrope (to increase myocardial contractility). If inotropes don't work, give hydrocortisone. The last option is extracorporeal membrane oxygenation (ECMO) for maintaining blood pressure. Start empiric antibiotics after drawing blood cultures, and correct electrolyte disturbances.

Empiric antibiotics are based on age-based guidelines:

- Newborns: ampicillin + gentamicin
- Older children: ceftriaxone + vancomycin + clindamycin

10.6.4 Acute Otitis Media

Bird's Eye View   Acute otitis media (ear infections) are one of the most common complaints in young children.

Etiology   Children's eustachian tubes are narrower and straighter than adults resulting in poor drainage that can allow growth of bacteria. The most common causes in children *are Streptococcus pneumoniae, Moraxella catarrhalis*, and non-typeable *Haemophilus influenzae*.

■ Presentation

- Symptoms:
  - Fever
  - Irritability
  - Ear tugging and pulling due to pressure on the tympanic membrane
  - Conductive hearing loss if there is effusion limiting tympanic membrane vibration
- Exam:
  - Erythematous, bulging tympanic membrane
  - Purulent effusion
  - Poor mobility on pneumatic insufflation

■ Differentiating the Differential

- Otitis media with effusion is middle ear fluid accumulation without inflammation. Otoscopic exam will show air-fluid levels behind the tympanic membrane but no bulging or erythema.

- Otitis externa presents with otalgia, pruritis, discharge, and ear canal erythema. The tympanic membrane is normal. It may present with a history of water exposure or trauma.
- Cholesteatoma is due to an accumulation of keratin debris in the middle ear, and the acquired form is common due to multiple episodes of acute otitis media. It would present with hearing loss, painless otorrhea, and a white mass behind the tympanic membrane.

Treatment   Treat all infants under 6 months. Treat children older than 6 months if they have a high fever (>102.2F), severe pain, or bilateral infection. In older children, you can also choose to observe for 48 hours before starting antibiotics.
- First line – oral amoxicillin.
- Second line – oral amoxicillin-clavulanate if symptoms persist after 3 days of treatment or recurrent infection within 30 days of antibiotic therapy.
- If allergic to penicillin, try clindamycin or azithromycin.

- **Complications**
- Tympanic membrane perforation
- Conductive hearing loss
- Mastoiditis
- Meningitis

10.6.5 Conjunctivitis

Bird's Eye View   Conjunctivitis (pink eye) is inflammation of the conjunctiva. There are many causes, but the most common are due to an immune response to allergens, bacteria, or viruses. Red flags such as decreased visual acuity that does not clear with blinking, photophobia, or pain suggest more severe underlying causes and should be referred to an ophthalmologist.

Presentation   Although there are classic descriptions, it is often difficult to determine the etiology. All three forms of conjunctivitis present with red eye, discharge, and the eye feeling "stuck shut."
- Allergic conjunctivitis is bilateral and itchy and may have a dry-eye sensation. Symptoms typically subside within 24 hours. There is often a family or personal history of atopy.
- Bacterial conjunctivitis can be unilateral or bilateral. The discharge is typically purulent and thick.
- Viral conjunctivitis is sometimes preceded by a viral prodrome. There is scant watery and stringy discharge and often a burning or gritty sensation. It can be unilateral or bilateral.

- **Differentiating the Differential**
You are not likely to see other ophthalmologic complaints on your pediatric rotations. Highlighted here are several causes of conjunctivitis due to other diseases that warrant more aggressive management.
- Measles can have a non-purulent conjunctivitis. The prodrome also includes fever, cough, and coryza (runny nose) and presents in unvaccinated children.
- Kawasaki disease classically has bilateral, nonexudative, limbic-sparing (sclera around the iris remains white) conjunctivitis. They will also have a

fever for 5+ days, mucositis, polymorphous rash, extremity changes, and cervical lymphadenopathy.

— Herpes zoster ophthalmicus can cause conjunctivitis with corneal dendritic lesions under fluorescein examination. Consider this diagnosis in a patient with perioral cold sores or vesicular lesions in the trigeminal region. Hutchinson's sign is vesicles at the tip of the nose and strongly predicts eye involvement.

■ **Treatment**

— Allergic conjunctivitis – usually self-limited once removed from environmental allergen. Oral antihistamines can help if taken consistently prior to allergen exposure. Topical agents such as artificial tears can help with persistent symptoms.

— Viral conjunctivitis – self-limited condition.

— Bacterial conjunctivitis – usually self-limited but reasonable to treat to reduce spread and decrease symptoms. No broad spectrum covers all possible causes, but erythromycin or bacitracin-polymyxin B ointment is a good place to start with typical gram-positive causes:
  – Chlamydia – erythromycin drops and oral erythromycin
  – Gonococcus – erythromycin ointment and single-dose ceftriaxone IM

Prophylaxis   All newborns should receive ophthalmic erythromycin to prevent gonococcal conjunctivitis. Note that prophylaxis for chlamydia conjunctivitis is ineffective and not routinely done.

10.6.6 Bronchiolitis

Bird's Eye View   Bronchiolitis, due to RSV, is a very common lower respiratory tract illness in children less than 1 year of age. RSV spreads by direct contact, droplets, or fomites and is especially common in the winter months (November–April). RSV infections typically resolve within 1–3 weeks.

■ **Presentation**
Symptoms (mainly respiratory; worst around days 3–5):
— Wet cough
— Audible wheezing
— Shallow breathing
— Lips, fingers, and/or toes turning blue

Exam (◧ Fig. 10.7):
— Tachypnea
— Crackles
— Wheezing
— Use of accessory muscles

■ **Differentiating the Differential (◧ Fig. 10.8)**
— Bacterial pneumonia will have a more focal, abnormal lung exam and looks "sick." If high suspicion, a CXR may be helpful.
— Asthma is most likely if there is a history or family history of asthma as opposed to the rather acute new onset wheezing in RSV.
— Influenza will present with sudden onset high fevers, chills, myalgias, and fatigue.
— Croup will likely have stridor on exam and be slightly older than your typical RSV patient.

Pearl: Signs of respiratory distress in young children include tachypnea, tracheal tugging, intercostal and subcostal retractions, perioral and extremity cyanosis, grunting, and nasal flaring.

Signs of respiratory distress

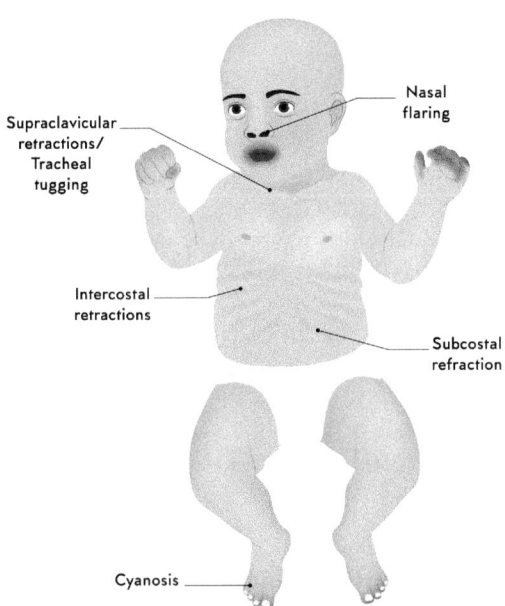

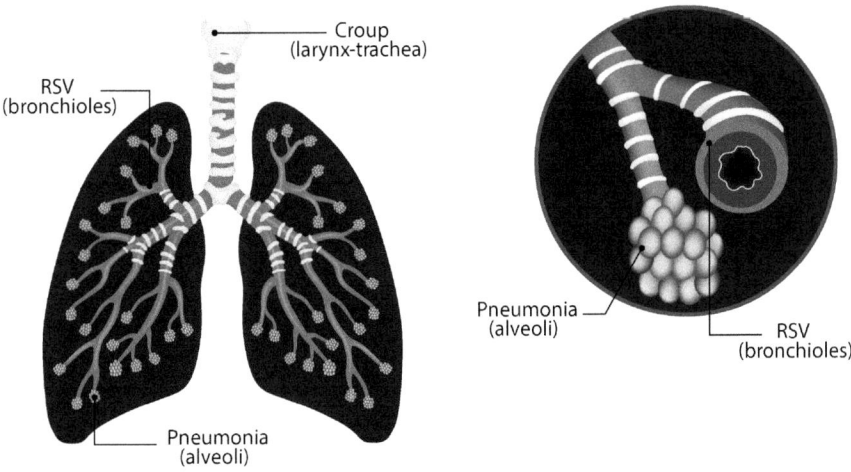

Work-Up   Bronchiolitis is a clinical diagnosis; thus no labs/studies are required, especially if the child does not look "sick." If there is suspicion that something else is going on (e.g., immunocompromise), you may consider a chest X-ray to see if they have RSV pneumonia, a flu swab, and RSV PCR.

Treatment   For the vast majority of cases where patients are stable, the best plan is supportive care at home (e.g., acetaminophen to keep the child comfortable, drinking lots of fluids).

– Admit if the child is unable to feed, looks volume depleted (e.g., capillary refill >2 seconds, dry mucous membranes), is immunocompromised, or if their oxygen saturations drop below 90% on room air.

▬ Treat inpatient by giving supplemental oxygen, IV fluids, and nasal bulb suctioning. For very severe disease (infants who need mechanical ventilation), ribavirin is a nucleoside analog that may decrease mortality and morbidity. Due to concerns regarding safety, it is not routinely used, and the AAP also recommends against routine use of ribavirin.

Prophylaxis   RSV prophylaxis with palivizumab is recommended for premature babies born at younger than 28 weeks gestation or infants younger than 1 year old with chronic lung disease or congenital heart disease.

Complications   Children younger than 6 months of age, premature infants, and immunocompromised children are at especially high risk of co-RSV complications such as apnea or pneumonia.

10.6.7 Croup

Three Ss for your board exams: seal-bark cough, stridor, and steeple sign

Bird's Eye View   Croup, caused most often by parainfluenza, leads to laryngotracheitis (as implied by the name, inflammation of the larynx and trachea).

Presentation   Croup most commonly affects young children between 6 months and 3 years of age. Children's upper airway is narrower than adults, hence predisposing them to develop inspiratory stridor and respiratory distress. Stridor is often worse at night. With severe croup, you may also see signs of respiratory distress such as retractions on physical exam.

The Westley croup score can be used to grade the severity of disease and guide management (however, the criteria are subjective). It includes the following components (definitely look it up on MDCalc):
▬ Chest wall retractions
▬ Stridor
▬ Cyanosis
▬ Level of consciousness
▬ Air entry

Work-Up   For clinical diagnosis, if radiographs are ordered, it is to rule out other conditions (chest X-rays may show a steeple sign or subglottic tracheal narrowing).

■ **Differentiating the Diagnosis**
▬ Bacterial tracheitis may have a viral prodrome and won't improve with croup treatments. A child with bacterial tracheitis looks much more "sick" than a child with croup.
▬ Foreign body aspiration may cause choking and stridor symptoms but will be more sudden onset.
▬ Bronchiolitis (discussed above).
▬ If child has chronic stridor, think laryngomalacia or another anatomic abnormality.

Treatment   Mild: supportive care at home (misting, acetaminophen).
▬ Moderate/severe: nebulized racemic epinephrine (0.05 mL/kg/dose; given over 15 minutes and can be repeated every 20 minutes), dexamethasone (IM), O2 supplementation if satting below 92%, heliox (air with a composition of 21% oxygen and 79% helium), humified air, fluids, acet-

Stridor is a high-pitched sound due to inflammation, narrowing the upper airway. It can be heard during inspiration or expiration depending on the etiology.

10

aminophen, and misting; in very severe cases, intubation may be necessary.
- Children should be admitted from the ED when they are dehydrated, have moderate/severe croup, need supplemental oxygen, or are in respiratory failure.
- Discharge: patients can be discharged when their respiratory symptoms have completely resolved, and they can tolerate food and water.

10.6.8 Influenza

- **Presentation**
- Influenza usually presents with **abrupt** onset of symptoms including fever, URI symptoms, and myalgias.
- In children, the flu may also present as abdominal pain or other atypical symptoms.
- In uncomplicated flu, the disease runs its course over the week.

- **Work-Up**
- May consider Influenza A and B PCR, serology, or rapid antigen testing. The choice of test is likely determined by the options available at your institution:
  - Test if knowing the cause will change your management (e.g., administering treatment, public health monitoring).
- May consider chest X-ray to rule out pneumonia if respiratory symptoms are prominent

- **Treatment**
- The key management for uncomplicated flu is supportive care (making sure the child is drinking lots of water and eating and giving acetaminophen for myalgias and fever).
- Oseltamivir (Tamiflu) can be considered for children 3 months or older who have been symptomatic for less than 48 hours. It is often not considered for mild cases due to its cost and its side effects of nausea and vomiting and minimal benefit (reduces symptoms by 1 day).
- For immunocompromised patients or patients with chronic lung disease, Tamiflu should be strongly considered, even if the patient has been symptomatic for greater than 2 days.

- **Prophylaxis**
- All children 6 months or older should get the flu vaccine annually.
- For high-risk groups, 1 week of a neuraminidase inhibitor in addition to the inactivated flu vaccine for pre-exposure chemoprophylaxis should be considered. However, if a patient gets the live flu vaccine, neuraminidase inhibitors should be avoided for the following 2 weeks.
- Postexposure chemoprophylaxis can also be considered for high-risk groups if the exposure occurred less than 48 hours prior to presentation.

- **Complications**
- Influenza pneumonia
- Post-influenza *Staphylococcus aureus* pneumonia
- Asthma exacerbation
- Otitis media

10.6.9 Pneumonia

Bird's Eye View   An infection of the alveoli of the lungs

Etiology   Pneumonia in children is caused by different pathogens at different ages:
- Neonates: group B strep, *E. coli*, *Listeria*, *Streptococcus pneumoniae*, *Klebsiella*
- Babies to 5 years old: RSV, influenza, other URI viruses
- 5–13 years old: *S. pneumoniae*, *Mycoplasma pneumonia*
- 13–18 years old: *S pneumoniae*, *H. influenzae*, *Mycoplasma pneumonia*, *Legionella*, *Klebsiella*

If children are immunocompromised at baseline, have medical conditions that compromise respiratory epithelium and lining (primary ciliary dyskinesia, cystic fibrosis, etc.), or are exposed to secondhand smoking, they may be at increased risk of pneumonia and atypical bugs.

- **Presentation**
- Symptoms of cough, fever, respiratory distress, abdominal pain, vomiting, and lethargy are typical symptoms of pneumonia.
- Physical exam may show SIRS (see Sepsis section for more info), signs of respiratory distress (such as retractions or tachypnea), abnormal lung exam on auscultation, dullness on percussion of the lungs, or egophony.
- On physical exam, also make sure to look at the upper respiratory system (mouth, pharynx)

- **Work-Up**
- Labs:
  - CBC
  - Blood cultures
  - Sputum cultures (difficult to obtain good-quality sputum and not very sensitive)
  - Lactate (a sign of underperfusion of tissues)
  - Procalcitonin (often shortened to "procal." A high level would suggest this is a bacterial pathogen rather than a viral pathogen – but procalcitonin may not commonly be used at all institutions)
- Imaging: CXR is the most commonly used modality; if there are signs of a complicated pneumonia (with a parapneumonic effusion or an empyema), a CT may be ordered.

- **Treatment and Management**
- Admit if:
  - Hypoxic ($O_2 < 92\%$)
  - Unable to take in fluids
  - In a high-risk group, such as neonates (less than 1 month)
  - Hemodynamically unstable
  - Symptoms or signs of altered mentation
  - Suspicion of sepsis (discussed above)
  - No improvement with outpatient treatment
- Antibiotics:
  - Outpatient treatment (duration of antibiotics, 7–10 days):
  - 60 days to 5 years old: amoxicillin (azithromycin if allergic)
  - 5–16 years old: azithromycin
  - Inpatient treatment (duration of antibiotics, 10–14 days):

- Newborn <6 days old: ampicillin + gentamicin
- Newborn >6 days old: vancomycin (due to increased prevalence of MRSA) and gentamicin
- <5 years old: third-generation cephalosporin (e.g., cefuroxime 150 mg/kg/day q8hrs)
- Consider adding erythromycin 40 mg/kg/day q6hrs if critically ill
- Older children (>5 years): third-generation cephalosporin (e.g., cefuroxime 150 mg/kg/day q6-8hrs) + erythromycin 40 mg/kg/day q6hrs
- Viral/influenza pneumonia: oseltamivir + vancomycin

- Acetaminophen and ibuprofen for comfort.
- O2 if sats are below 95%.
- IV fluids.
- For patients with complicated community acquired pneumonia, follow-up CXR 2 months after is suggested to make sure the pneumonia has resolved.

■ Complications
- Sepsis.
- Parapneumonic effusions – fluid escapes from the lung into the pleural cavity due to pneumonia.
- Empyema – a type of parapneumonic effusion that is characterized by pus in the effusion, respiratory compromise, and lung abscess.

10.7 Atopy

Atopy describes a group of associated diseases with a common allergic component. The most common atopic diseases are allergic rhinitis, eczema, asthma, and food allergies. Children with one atopic disease are prone to develop another due to a shared similarity in the underlying pathophysiology that is characterized by IgE and eosinophils. The commonly referred to "atopic triad" includes asthma, atopic dermatitis, and allergies. While some children affected by diseases achieve remission, many people who have previously had asthma have relapses later in life.

10.7.1 Asthma

■ Bird's Eye View
Pediatric asthma is a common chronic lung disease in children; it affects approximately 8.5% of children in the USA. Risk factors for developing pediatric asthma include other atopic diseases, secondhand smoke, exposure to pollution, and low birth weight.

■ Diagnosis
If a child under 3 has frequent episodes of wheezing and shortness of breath, use the Asthma Predictive Index to evaluate their risk of having asthma. Once you have identified whether a child has asthma or not, you can rate their severity based on their degree of impairment, the frequency at which asthma symptoms disrupt their daily life, and their risk of morbidity and mortality of asthma as measured by number of exacerbations per year.

The degree of impairment and the risk of exacerbation help define the severity grading of asthma per the National Asthma Education and Prevention Program Expert Panel Report 3 (NAEPP EPR3) guidelines. The severity of a child's asthma – intermittent, mild persistent, moderate persistent, or severe persistent – can help guide a stepwise approach to treating and controlling the

Pearl: Check out ▶ asthma.com for easy access to these assessments: ▶ https://www.asthma.com/additional-resources/asthma-control-test.html.

symptoms of a child's asthma without overmedication. For children older than 4 years, asthma control can be assessed using the Asthma Control Test Caregiver Report; for children older than 12, asthma control can be assessed using the Asthma Control Test.

Identifying a trigger for the shortness of breath and spirometry measurements of FEV1 and FVC before and after bronchodilator use may help make the diagnosis for asthma. These measurements can be difficult to obtain in young children. If there is a question about the diagnosis of asthma, signs of chronic hypoxia on physical exam, and unresponsiveness to therapy, a referral to a pulmonologist may be warranted.

- Differentiating the Differential
- Allergic rhinitis occurs more often in the spring to fall and often triggered by environmental allergens such as pollen and dust mites.
- Viral upper respiratory infections occur in the setting of sick contacts and fever and don't have as pronounced respiratory distress as seen with asthma.
- Foreign body aspiration presents acutely with an acute trigger; a chest X-ray can help differentiate if the diagnosis is difficult to make by history alone.
- Chronic diseases such as cystic fibrosis or primary ciliary dyskinesia may also have extrapulmonary symptoms such as pancreatic insufficiency or situs inversus, respectively.
- Reflux may lead to atypical asthma symptoms. Reflux-related atypical asthma symptoms often occur at night rather than during the day and will be associated with GI symptoms such as waking up with a bad taste in the mouth.

- Outpatient Treatment

In a basic framework (Fig. 10.9), you start with a short-acting beta-agonist (SABA, the most commonly used is albuterol) for mild intermittent asthma. For mild persistent asthma, you can start with a SABA and inhaled corticosteroid (ICS, e.g., fluticasone). Then if sufficient control is not achieved, you can add on a long-acting beta-agonist (LABA) to the regiment of ICS and SABA. The doses of ICS can be increased to achieve better control. For aspirin-intolerant asthma, you can consider Montelukast use. The EPR 3 guidelines from NAEPP also give recommendations for controller mediations based on severity.

The keys to asthma management are helping a child and their family understand the asthma triggers and helping the child optimally use their inhalers. Try to clearly identify the triggers driving your patient's asthma if possible and think of strategies with the patient's and their family's input to avoid those triggers as much as possible. A spacer can be used if a child has difficulty coordinating their breath with an inhaler.

If exercise causes asthma symptoms, it is helpful to use a SABA 15–30 minutes before exercise. This can also be done with other known asthma triggers. If you are worried about a patient's compliance with asthma medication, it is also helpful to talk to patients about social situations that may prevent them from using their asthma medications optimally. For example, the child may feel embarrassed using their inhaler at school. Appropriate and supportive counseling can be tremendously helpful in these situations. This information can be put together in an asthma action plan to manage future exacerbations with your patient and family and has been shown to have benefit. An asthma action

Pearl: You should ensure your patient has a strong understanding of how to use an inhaler and can demonstrate proper use to you (form a tight seal around the inhaler, start breathing in, press the button as you breathe in, keep breathing in slowly, hold your breath for 10 seconds, breath out slowly, wait 1 minute between puffs, and rinse your mouth after using the inhaler). Spacers are very helpful in helping children use inhalers well (Fig. 10.10).

Asthma control – step by step increase

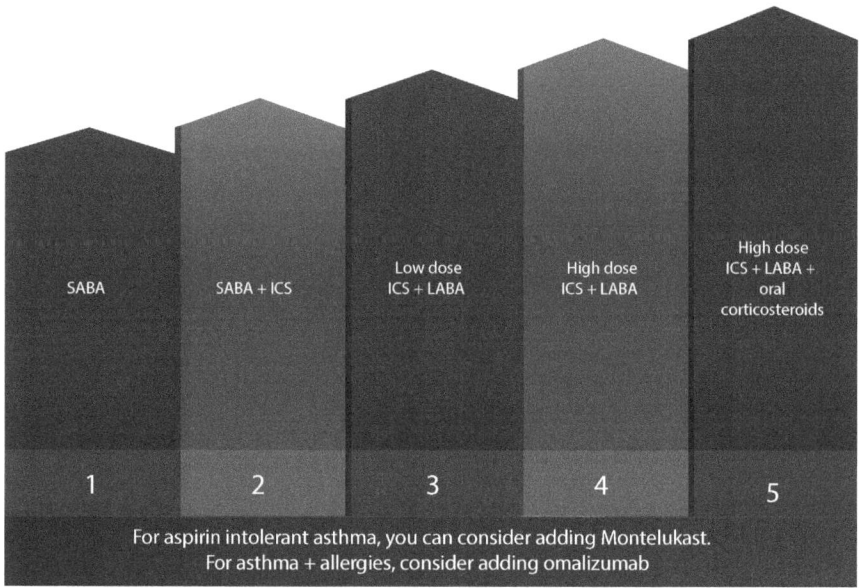

SABA	SABA + ICS	Low dose ICS + LABA	High dose ICS + LABA	High dose ICS + LABA + oral corticosteroids
1	2	3	4	5

For aspirin intolerant asthma, you can consider adding Montelukast.
For asthma + allergies, consider adding omalizumab

Stepwise Approach for Treating
Asthma in Children Older than 6

◘ Fig. 10.9 Asthma controller medications

Asthma Spacer

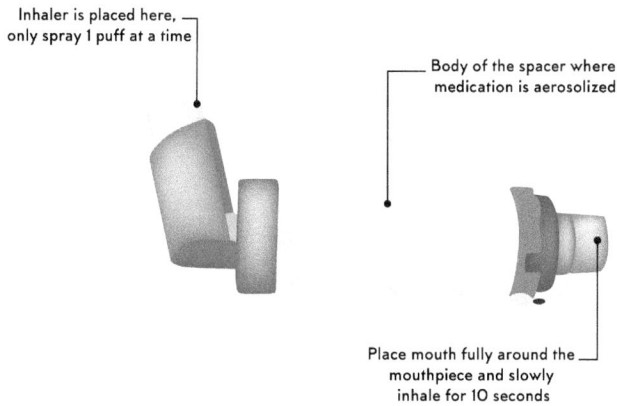

Inhaler is placed here, only spray 1 puff at a time

Body of the spacer where medication is aerosolized

Place mouth fully around the mouthpiece and slowly inhale for 10 seconds

◘ Fig. 10.10 Asthma inhaler and spacer

plan describes what medications patient should take and if they should call the doctor or go to the ER when they have no symptoms, moderate symptoms, or severe symptoms. There are great templates of asthma action plans you can print out and fill out together with patients.

▪ Inpatient Management

Asthma exacerbations can be very dangerous. Many pediatric asthma exacerbations are triggered by viral respiratory illnesses.

■ Diagnosis

Identification of an asthma exacerbation can be done clinically through noting increased work of breathing such as the use of accessory muscles of respiration, retractions, tachypnea, or a low oxygen saturation.

A peak flow meter can be useful if this has previously been recorded; a peak expiratory flow 50% of a patient's personal best is a cause of serious concern.

■ Treatment
– The cornerstone of treatment are "DuoNebs," the combination of albuterol (SABA) and ipratropium (short-acting muscarinic antagonist).
– Systemic steroids – IV or oral dexamethasone if moderate (tachypnea, expiratory wheezing, significant accessory muscle use, oxygen saturations 92–95%) or severe (tachypnea, inspiratory and expiratory wheezing, oxygen saturation <92%) exacerbation.
– If the asthma exacerbation is refractory to DuoNebs and steroids, you can also try:
  – IV magnesium sulfate
  – IV epinephrine
  – Heliox to decrease the work of breathing
  – Intubation is your last resort

10.7.2 Atopic Dermatitis

Bird's Eye View   Atopic dermatitis (eczema) is common (10–20% of children have it). Atopic dermatitis has a complex multifactorial pathophysiology, involving skin barriers, environmental triggers, and IgE.

Presentation   It is characterized by rough, scratchy, inflamed, itchy skin – it is called "the itch that rashes." A common presentation of eczema that you are sure to see is baby eczema. Baby eczema often affects the face, elbows, knees, and other extensor surfaces (in contrast to eczema in every other age group commonly affects the flexor surfaces).

■ Differentiating the Differential
– Seborrheic dermatitis looks like yellow, greasy crusty scales on a baby's scalp ("cradle cap"), near the baby's nose and ears. It is caused by a fungus, most often Malassezia. To treat cradle cap, parents can apply petroleum jelly or mineral oil to the affected areas to soften the areas and then remove the crusty scales using a comb. For refractory cases, antifungal shampoo or topical corticosteroids may be helpful.

Treatment   Eczema is treated by applying moisturizer in the affected areas right after the patient finishes showering to prevent the skin from drying out, every time. For acute exacerbations of eczema, topical steroids are also helpful.

10.8 Food Allergies

Food allergies are a broad group of diseases. Common triggers of food allergies are milk, egg, wheat, peanuts, and fish. Interestingly, even though peanut allergies get a lot of attention in the modern media, milk anaphylaxis is actually more common. Children with eczema should be introduced to peanuts (smear of peanut butter) by age 6 months. If they have severe eczema, they need allergen testing for peanuts first (see below).

Anaphylaxis is the most severe disease in this group.

Diagnosis   Anaphylaxis is diagnosed generally when two out of four or more following systems are involved after exposure to a likely allergen: skin, respiratory system, cardiovascular system (blood pressure), and gastrointestinal system, *or* if a patient presents after exposure to a known allergen and hypotension.

Treatment   If you suspect anaphylaxis, it is a life-threatening emergency – definitely notify your attending as soon as possible. The treatment of anaphylaxis is epinephrine, intubation if necessary, and normal saline boluses as necessary to stabilize blood pressure. Normal saline in children is given in boluses of 20 mL/kg.

10.8.1   Food Protein-Induced Colitis

Bird's Eye View   Food protein-induced colitis is a common food allergy disease that is not IgE mediated; common triggers are cow's milk, egg, and soy.

Presentation   Patients present as healthy infants with bloody stool. It is important to make sure that the patient is not sick – if there is weight loss or a failure to thrive, you should make sure to broaden your differential.

Treatment   The suspected allergens should be removed from the infant's diet or, if the infant is breast feeding, from the mother's diet. Most clinical trials suggest the reintroduction of the allergy-causing food at 1 year of age.

Prevention of Peanut Allergy   For children with atopy, the Guidelines for Prevention of Peanut Allergy recommends early introduction of foods with peanut components, such as peanut butter. With severe atopy, the guidelines recommend 4–6 months having specific IgE and/or skin prick testing and based on those results introducing peanut-containing foods. With moderate atopy, the guidelines recommend starting at 6 months. Children without atopy or any food allergies can introduce peanut-containing foods at age-appropriate times with no need for early intervention. These guidelines are informed by the Learning Early About Peanut allergy (LEAP) trial which showed a reduction in risk of peanut allergy in children exposed early and often to peanut-containing foods.

> Pearl: The LEAP trial (NEJM 2015) is an important trial to read and know – you can counsel the families of your patients with atopy about these new guidelines.

10.9   Strep Throat and Complications

10.9.1   Strep Pharyngitis

Bird's Eye View   Group A strep pharyngitis is an important disease to know because it is very, very common and it is highly tested. You will definitely see it multiple times on your clerkship, especially in outpatient settings. Group A streptococcus, particularly *Streptococcus pyogenes*, is a gram-positive bacterium that commonly causes pharyngitis and impetigo.

■   **Presentation and Diagnosis**

The CENTOR criteria is a clinical tool that is used to assess the probability of a patient having strep throat for adults. There is a modified CENTOR score created by McIsaac that is validated in children. The criteria generally include age, presence of exudate, palpable cervical lymph nodes, fever, and the absence of a cough. The score can help determine your plan: whether further testing by the rapid strep test is necessary, if further testing can be omitted based on pre-test probability, or if empiric antibiotics should be given. Strep throat in children can have a myriad of presentations in addition to a sore or scratchy throat, including abdominal pain and the classic scarlet fever rash which may play a role in your decision. Scarlet fever is often described as a "sandpaper" rash or goose bumps on an erythematous background.

Children under 3 years of age or those with symptoms of viral disease such as coryza, conjunctivitis, cough, and hoarseness should not be tested as it is very unlikely in this age group with signs more consistent with a viral infection.

- ■ Differentiating the Differential
- ─ Viral pharyngitis will present with a viral prodrome (e.g., runny nose, sore throat). The easiest way to differentiate is the rapid strep test.
- ─ Epstein-Barr virus mononucleosis (EBV) has a more insidious time course than the run-of-the-mill viral pharyngitis and may have more prominent pharyngeal exudate and is associated with subacute fatigue; briefly, some common complications of EBV are splenomegaly (patients with EBV should be advised to refrain from sports for at least a month for fear of splenic rupture) and cold agglutinin disease. The diagnosis for EBV is made by testing for antibodies (e.g., anti-VCA antibodies) through the Monospot test.

Treatment   Strep throat can be treated with penicillin V (given orally, 250 mg 2–3 times per day for 10 days) or amoxicillin (50 mg/kg/dose once daily (max 1000 mg/dose) for 10 days).

Complications   Strep throat needs to be treated to prevent rheumatic fever. Another possible sequela is post-strep glomerulonephritis (PSGN), but treating strep pharyngitis with antibiotics has not been shown to prevent PSGN. Each of these is discussed in more detail in the following sections.

10.9.2   Rheumatic Fever

Rheumatic fever is a type 2 hypersensitivity reaction due to molecular mimicry. Your body creates antibodies to defend itself against group A strep bacteria, and the same antibodies also attack your own body tissues.

Diagnosis   Rheumatic fever is diagnosed by the Jones criteria. To diagnose rheumatic fever, you need to have two major criteria or one major criterion in addition to two minor criteria. If a patient is diagnosed with rheumatic fever, the treatment is penicillin.
- ─ Major criteria:
  - – Carditis
  - – Arthritis
  - – Sydenham's chorea – jerky and irregular movements. Patients may have motor weakness. On physical exam, patients may also have "milk maid's grip" – when they are asked to grip a finger firmly, it looks like they are squeezing and relaxing their grip (like someone who is milking a cow)
  - – Erythema marginatum
  - – Subcutaneous nodules

- Minor criteria:
  - Fever
  - Elevated ESR and CRP
  - Prolonged PR interval

Treatment   If your patient has carditis from rheumatic fever, it is important to consider antibiotic prophylaxis to prevent recurrent rheumatic fever carditis. For patients with rheumatic fever with carditis, 10 years of antibiotic prophylaxis is recommended (usually penicillin G every 4 weeks).

10.9.3 Post-Streptococcal/Infectious Glomerulonephritis

Bird's Eye View   Approximately 3 weeks after a streptococcal infection, patients can develop a nephritic syndrome, post-streptococcal glomerulonephritis. It is also called postinfectious glomerulonephritis as it is known now that many other infections besides group A strep can cause it.

Presentation   The symptoms are similar to other nephritic syndromes and include cola-colored urine (hematuria), salt retention and edema, and non-nephrotic range proteinuria.

Treatment   The treatment includes antibiotics and management of volume over-load and blood pressure. If a patient's symptoms are refractory, you are worried, or think it could be something besides PSGN, consider a nephrology referral. Most children recover completely within 6–8 weeks.

10.10 Skin Rashes

We will go briefly over a hodgepodge of common skin diseases that are often seen in pediatrics. A general approach to skin rashes is to think about the terms that you will use to describe the rash to your residents and attending (size, color, raised or flat, etc.). Make sure to take a look at the majority of the patient's skin. When learning about a skin complaint, make sure to search for a picture from a reputable site such as VisualDx or DermNet NZ. Rashes also look quite different on different skin tones, so it would also be useful to google pictures of the same dermatologic complaint on different skin tones (refer to the dermatology section for greater detail).

10.10.1   Tinea Corporis

Etiology   Tinea corporis, or ringworm infection, is a dermatophyte infection caused by fungi such as *Trichophyton rubrum*, *Epidermophyton*, and *Microsporum*. If tinea occurs on the body, it is called tinea corporis; if it is on the feet, tinea pedis or athlete's foot; on the groin, tinea cruris or jock itch; on the scalp, tinea capitis; and on the nails, tinea unguium or onychomycosis – this is much rarer in children than in adults.

Presentation   Tinea looks like an erythematous patch with an elevated, scaly border. It is often pruritic.

Diagnosis   The diagnosis is often made through visual inspection, potassium hydroxide microscopy to visual hyphae, and in certain situations, Wood's lamp examination as only some fungi fluoresce. Tinea is spread by person to person contact, fomites, and contact with animals and pets.

- Treatment
- Tinea corporis is with topical terbinafine, clotrimazole, or butenafine.
- Tinea capitis is usually with terbinafine or griseofulvin; an oral antifungal medication is usually necessary.
- Tinea unguium is difficult as it is often not responsive to medication; it can be treated with oral fluconazole or terbinafine.

10.10.2   Tinea Versicolor

Etiology   Tinea versicolor is another common superficial skin infection caused by the fungus *Malassezia globosa* and *Malassezia furfur*.

Presentation   Tinea versicolor can appear as hypo−/hyperpigmented patches on skin.

Diagnosis   Tinea versicolor is typically a clinical diagnosis. It is often more noticeable in the summertime when your patients are playing outside and the rest of their skin darkens or tans besides those hypopigmented patches. KOH preparation will show a "spaghetti and meatball" pattern due to the presence of curved hyphae and round yeast forms.

Treatment   Topical ketoconazole or selenium sulfide.

10.10.3   Pityriasis Alba

Presentation   Pityriasis alba presents with hypopigmented spots with fine scale but is otherwise asymptomatic.

Diagnosis   Based on clinical appearance, a Wood's lamp shade can also be helpful to help differentiate hypopigmentation (which does not enhance) in pityriasis alba from true depigmentation.

- Differentiating the Differential
- Tinea versicolor would have a positive KOH examination.
- Vitiligo will have more distinct edges and much more depigmented. Often parents will be concerned if pityriasis alba is vitiligo.

Treatment   It is a self-limited condition.

10.10.4   Impetigo

Etiology   Impetigo is a common skin condition that looks like sores that burst and leave "honey-crusted" exudate. It is often caused by *Staphylococcus aureus* or group A strep.

Presentation   Impetigo is a "honey crusted" lesion on an erythematous base (◻ Fig. 10.11).

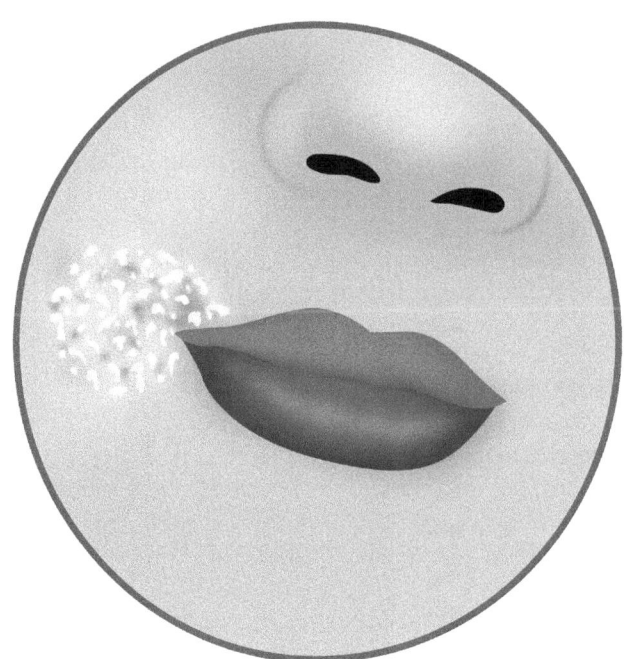

■ **Fig. 10.11** Impetigo

Diagnosis Impetigo is diagnosed clinically, and it may have a bullous appearance or positive gram stain from any exudative discharge. Blood cultures are typically not necessary.

■ **Differentiating the Differential**
▬ Cellulitis is less likely to have crusting/exudate and may be tender and more likely to have systemic symptoms.
▬ Erysipelas will have a well-demarcated, raised border.

Treatment Impetigo can be treated with topical antibiotics such as mupirocin for limited disease or oral antibiotics, such as dicloxacillin, for patients with many lesions or severe disease. Do not lance bullae.

Complications Post-streptococcal glomerulonephritis (see section above)

10.10.5 Erythema Toxicum Neonatorum and Neonatal Cephalic Pustulosis

Both of these are very common and very benign conditions.

10.10.5.1 Erythema Toxicum Neonatorum

Presentation Erythema toxicum neonatorum usually occurs within the first 72 hours of life and is characterized by a maculopapular rash that spares the arms and soles.

Diagnosis This is a clinical diagnosis.

Treatment It is self-limited.

10.10.5.2 Neonatal Cephalic Pustulosis

Presentation   Neonatal cephalic pustulosis, also called "neonatal acne," is characterized by papules and pustules and develops on the face that develops around 2–3 weeks.

Diagnosis   This is a clinical diagnosis.

Treatment   It is a self-limiting condition that is best treated with gentle cleaning of the affected area with soap and water.

10.11 Gastrointestinal Complaints

10.11.1   Physiologic Reflux

Etiology   Reflux occurs because infants have weaker esophageal sphincters that have not fully developed as compared to adults.

Presentation   Physiologic reflux should be suspected in cases when an infant is growing well, gaining weight, and has no other gastrointestinal symptoms. After feedings, infant's "spit up" will resemble what they just ate.

■   Differentiating the Differential

If there are red flags, the child may have gastroesophageal reflux disease or less benign gastrointestinal disease, such as obstruction. Red flags include:
- Weight loss or lack of appropriate weight gain (meaning they fall off their growth curve)
- Ill-appearing child
- Bilious vomiting
- Abdominal pain
- Physiologic reflux lasting longer than 12 months

Pearl: Bilious vomit will appear green or bright yellow due to the presence of bile, and thus the pathology originates below the ampulla of Vater in the duodenum.

Treatment   This is a self-limited condition and generally resolves by 1 year of age. Helpful tips for concerned parents are to keep the infant upright after feeding and thickening the expressed breast milk or the formula with corn starch or rice cereal (the NIH suggests the ratio of 1 tablespoon or rice cereal to 2 ounces of formula).

10.11.2   Pyloric Stenosis

Bird's Eye View   Pyloric stenosis occurs when the pyloric sphincter of the stomach is too tight. It is due to a combination of genetic and environmental factors, but one notable risk factor is macrolide antibiotic administration to young infants.

Presentation   The classic presentation is a 2–6-week-old baby who has non-bilious, projectile vomit after feeds and continues to be very hungry afterward. The symptoms progress as the baby grows unless treated.

Diagnosis   Classically, babies have a palpable olive mass in their abdomen near their liver (right upper quadrant) on physical exam, but it is a finding more reliably observed by ultrasound. Projectile vomiting can be observed after feeding.

Treatment   Manage the baby's metabolic abnormalities from excessive vomiting (a metabolic acidosis) and pyloromyotomy.

10.11.3   Lead Exposure

Etiology   Lead exposure in children is still a fairly common occurrence, as many children may live in older homes (before 1978 when lead-based paint in houses was outlawed) with lead paint. Make sure to ask your patient's parents if there are any places in the house where the paint is chipping off or if they know if their house has lead paint.

Presentation   Lead poisoning symptoms include abdominal pain, delayed growth, and cognitive impairment. Children often present asymptomatically or with subclinical symptoms and signs.

Diagnosis   The screening regulations for lead poisoning are different from state to state. In Massachusetts, children are screened three times at 1 year old, 2 years old, and 3 years old. However, the American Academy of Family Physicians generally recommends against routine screening for children at average risk and instead recommends targeted screening of Medicaid-eligible children and children born outside the USA. Lead is measured through venous blood sampling. If venous blood lead levels are greater than 45 mcg/dL, an abdominal X-ray, UA, and labs should be obtained.

■ Treatment
 － Oral succimer should be initiated, after consultant with a toxicologist, if venous blood levels are greater than 45 mcg/dL (if less than 45 mcg/dL, chelation therapy is not recommended).
 － At all lead levels, educating parents about a child's nutritional needs (calcium intake, vitamin C, and iron) and environmental exposures is recommended.
 － Depending on the level of elevation, further laboratory testing, abdominal X-rays, and an environmental investigation may be indicated.

10.11.4   Foreign Bodies

Bird's Eye View   Foreign body ingestion and aspiration by children is another fairly common occurrence, as children like to put things in their mouths. Anticipatory guidance to avoid choking hazard foods such as whole grapes, seeds, cut hotdogs, and other small foods can help prevent these situations.

10.11.4.1 Foreign Body Ingestion

Presentation   This can present as pain when swallowing, difficulty swallowing, drooling, emesis, and abdominal distention. Most foreign bodies pass without complication. Approximately 10% need to be removed via endoscopy, especially if they are lodged in the esophagus.

Work-Up   Chest and abdominal radiography can be helpful to make the diagnosis, and endoscopy can also be helpful if these tests are inconclusive.

Treatment   Per the recommendations of the North American Society for Pediatric Gastroenterology, Hepatology, and Nutrition (NASPSGHAN – try saying that 10 times fast), the objects that require removal within 2 hours are button batteries regardless of symptoms or symptomatic child who have ingested coins, sharp objects, or any other object causing the child to be unable to manage their secretions. Sharp objects should be removed within 24 hours in asymptomatic children.

10.11.4.2 Foreign Body Aspiration

Presentation This most commonly occurs at 2 years of age. Children have small airways, so even small objects can easily block their proximal airway; children at 2 years of age are also unable to chew optimally which leads to larger chunks of foods blocking their airway. The symptoms would be dyspnea and coughing. The foreign body may lead to atelectasis, pneumothorax, or lung hyperinflation if significant air trapping is present.

Treatment The treatment is rigid bronchoscopy to remove the object.

10.11.5 Viral Gastroenteritis

Etiology Acute viral gastroenteritis is a very common disease often caused by rotavirus (common in fall and winter and occurs in younger toddlers) or norovirus.

Presentation Non-bloody diarrhea, softer stool, or more frequent bowel movements start to occur 1–2 days after inoculation and often resolve within 1–2 weeks. Nausea, vomiting, and fever are also common symptoms.

Work-Up This diagnosis can be made clinically in the absence of red flag symptoms. However, if there are any of the following red flags, children should be evaluated for other causes of their symptoms (such as bacterial causes, parasitic causes, appendicitis, UTI, pneumonia, DKA, strep throat, sepsis, toxic megacolon, first presentation of IBD):
- Fever in babies (younger than 3 months)
- Symptoms lasting longer than 1 week
- Dehydration
- Problems as per the pediatric assessment triangle or children who look "sick"
- Severe abdominal pain
- Acute abdomen
- High fever
- Bloody stool

In the case of red flags, further studies such as CBC, electrolytes, blood glucose, blood cultures, stool leukocytes, stool O&P, stool cultures, and abdominal imaging may be indicated.

Treatment To treat viral gastroenteritis-related hypovolemia, oral rehydration therapy is indicated for most children. If children are too nauseous to drink water, having so much fluid loss that their fluid intake is not able to keep up, or have the red flags listed above, admission for further work-up and IV NS is indicated.

- Complications
- Hypovolemia
- Electrolyte disturbances (hypochloremia, hypokalemia)

10.11.6 Constipation

Etiology In children, constipation most often occurs due to issues with diet or stooling habits.

Diagnosis However, it is important to evaluate for red flags to rule out organic causes. Red flags would include not growing appropriately, not increasing in weight, failing to pass meconium, blood in stool, looking "sick," and severe pain. After a careful history, physical exam (including abdominal and rectal exam), and after ruling out these red flags, you can use the Rome 3 criteria to further evaluate functional constipation.

- Must have two or more of the following:
  - ≤2 defections per week
  - At least 1 episode of fecal incontinence per week
  - History for retentive posturing or excessive volitional stool retention
  - History of painful or hard bowel movements
  - Presence of a large fecal mass in the rectum
  - History of large-diameter stools that may obstruct the toilet

- **Treatment for Functional Constipation**
- If impacted, prescribe medications (polyethylene glycol (MiraLAX), senna, enema) to relieve impaction followed by daily medication regimen with toileting within 30 minutes of meals.
- If not impacted, counsel on dietary changes (lots of fiber, whole grains, legumes, fruits, stay well hydrated, prune juice) and education (healthy toilet training, positive reinforcement for trying).
  - If these changes are ineffective, maintenance medications (polyethylene glycol, sorbitol, senna) may be needed.

- **Complications**
- UTI
- Fecal impaction
- Anal fissures

> Pearl: Meconium is the first bowel movement of an infant and is made of digested intestinal epithelial cells, mucus, amniotic fluid, bile, and water. Unlike later bowel movements, it is sticky like tar, dark green, and almost odorless.

10.12 Acute and Chronic Knee Pain

10.12.1 Acute Knee Pain

Acute knee pain can either result from a fracture, a soft tissue injury, septic arthritis, or an acute flare of a chronic disease like juvenile idiopathic arthritis. When you are initially evaluating a child with acute knee pain, you want to use the pediatric assessment triangle to assess if they need emergency care. Afterward, assess for the following red flags:

- Fever
- Damage to neurovascular structures
- Compartment syndrome – the "6 Ps": pain, poikilothermia (limb is cool to the touch), pallor, paresthesia, pulselessness, and paralysis
- Penetrating injury that extends to the joint
- Gross deformity

If your patient has any of these symptoms or signs, an immediate consult to an orthopedic surgeon is recommended. The general approach to joint pain should be taking a thorough history of the current episode of joint pain and

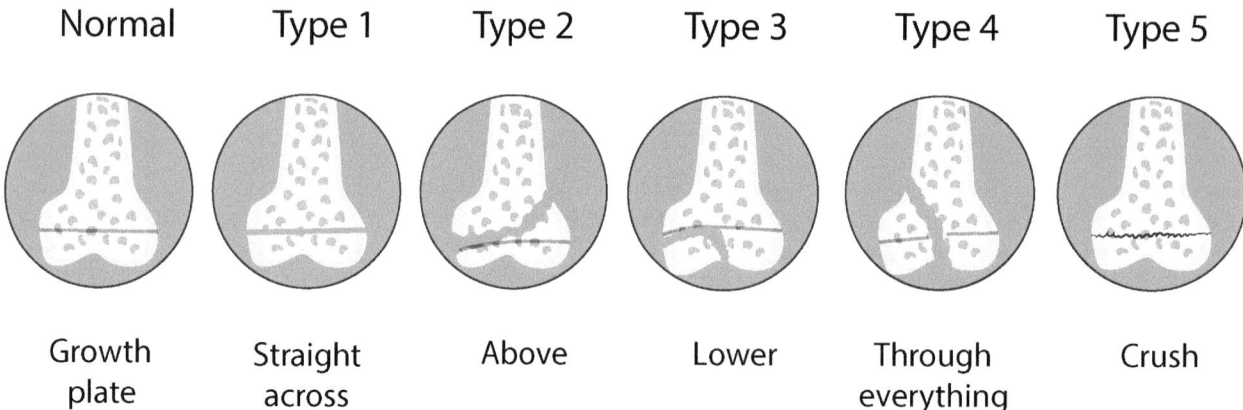

Normal	Type 1	Type 2	Type 3	Type 4	Type 5
Growth plate	Straight across	Above	Lower	Through everything	Crush

Fig. 10.12 Salter-Harris fracture grades

associated symptoms, any past history of joint or bone pain, and a careful physical exam of all joints and bones, carefully looking at the affected joint and bone and the contralateral joint and bone, assessing mobility, and evaluating if this is a problem of the joint or the soft tissues surrounding the joint.

10.12.2 Fractures

Long bones in children that are still growing have a growth plate, which is susceptible to fracture especially during a growth spurt. Knee pain can be caused by a fracture of the physis of the distal femur or proximal tibia. When a fracture involves the growth plate, it can be classified via the Salter-Harris fracture grading system (Fig. 10.12). The greater the Salter-Harris grade, the greater the risk of the fracture affecting the child's growth. Other fractures include fractures of the tibial tubercle or the tibial tubercle apophysis.

10.12.3 Knee Strains and Sprains

A sprain is a tear of or injury to a ligament. A strain is a tear of or injury to a tendon. Common soft tissue injuries that result in acute knee pain are injuries to the acute collateral ligament, medial collateral ligament, lateral collateral ligament, posterior collateral ligament, and menisci. When evaluating a patient for acute knee pain, if possible, make sure to do advanced physical exam maneuvers such as the Lachman test, the anterior and posterior drawer test, and the valgus and varus stress test (refer to the orthopedic chapter).

Less common soft tissue injuries include quadriceps or patellar tendon injuries, which may result in limited knee extension if it is a complete tear. The work-up for soft tissue injuries is MRI or arthroscopy.

10.12.4 Transient Synovitis

Transient synovitis is inflammation of the hip joint that causes pain and a limp. The child is otherwise well or may have a low-grade fever. Ultrasound may show a unilateral or bilateral joint effusion, even if symptoms are limited to one side, while a septic joint will show unilateral effusion. It is a diagnosis of exclusion that must be differentiated from a septic hip.

10.12.5 Septic Arthritis

The most common cause of septic arthritis in children is hematogenous spread of bacteria – most often, *S. aureus*. In adolescents, *N. gonorrhea* is also a common cause of septic arthritis. If the child has sickle cell disease, septic arthritis can be caused by *Salmonella*. The presence of fever is helpful in distinguishing septic arthritis from transient synovitis. Diagnosis is often suggested by ESR and CRP elevation and confirmed by arthrocentesis and culture. The duration of antibiotics is dependent on institutional practice, but generally S. *aureus* septic arthritis is treated initially intravenously and can switch to orals once symptoms are improving and CRP is declining for 2 weeks if uncomplicated or 4 weeks if involving bone or MRSA.

10.12.6 Chronic Knee Pain

Chronic knee pain is defined as knee pain that has been present for longer than **6** weeks. The following common conditions are related to overuse:

- Patellofemoral pain syndrome – not well-defined anterior knee pain that is exacerbated by squatting or rising from a seated position. Management involves a 2-week course of NSAIDS for acute pain and inflammation, avoiding activities that exacerbate pain, and physical therapy.
- Osgood-Schlatter disease – localized anterior knee pain over the tibial tubercle, made worse over time by activity. Preadolescent females are at highest risk. It is a self-limited condition that will resolve spontaneously. Patients are able to continue to play sports and should participate in physical therapy that emphasizes quadriceps exercises. Ice and over-the-counter pain medications should be recommended for pain control.
- Iliotibial band syndrome – gradually worsening lateral knee pain due to overuse, especially with running or cycling. The management generally consists of rest, ice, pain control acutely, and physical therapy to correct muscle strength imbalances.
- Growing pains – characterized by bilateral aching or throbbing that occurs in growing children. Growing pains occur primarily at night and may wake the child up from sleep. Treatment is conservative and supportive through the use of heating pad, elevating the legs, massage, and over-the-counter pain medications.

10.13 Seizures

Bird's Eye View   Seizures are abnormal electrical patterns in the brain that cause temporary dysfunction and can sometimes have long-lasting complications. Epilepsy is a disorder of recurrent seizures. Seizures can present in many ways, and rather than memorizing all the presentations, it is helpful to know the terminology to describe them and basic work-up and management.

- ■ Framework (□ Fig. 10.13)

The first challenge is figuring out if the child is having a seizure or not. Seizures present in a myriad of ways so this can be difficult. Classic symptoms are abnormal body movements (rhythmic muscle contractions), drooling, staring, not breathing for periods of time, tongue biting, and period of confusion following return to consciousness known as a postictal period. If a parent comes in suspecting their child may be acting different in certain situations, doing a lot

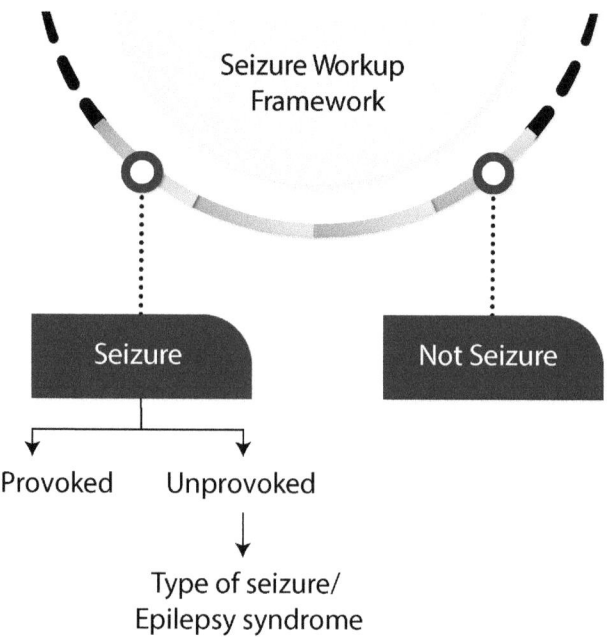

Fig. 10.13 Framework to seizures

of "purposeless movements" or automatisms, losing consciousness, or not paying attention for brief moments of time, they may be having seizures. However, it is often difficult to figure out whether a child is having seizures at home, especially if they are fine in the office or emergency department. Make sure to ask how long this abnormal activity lasted at home, if they have this abnormal activity in the past, and if they have any video recordings of the events.

- **Differentiating the Differential**

The differential for pediatric seizure is vast and includes breath holding spells, meningitis, encephalitis, syncopal episodes, psychogenic seizures, and BRUE (brief, resolved, unexplained events). These conditions can be very difficult to tell apart, but here are some differentiating characteristics that may be helpful:

- Breath holding spells are of two types: cyanotic and pallid. They are usually triggered by stressful events and occur most often when children are 1–2 years old. In both forms, short seizure-like activity may occur after the child passes out.
- Meningitis usually occurs in the setting of fever and nuchal rigidity but may lead to seizures.
- Encephalitis also occurs with fever and focal neurologic deficit.
- Syncope may present similarly to seizure as patients may have convulsions after they pass out.
- Psychogenic seizures have episodes of behavior, movements, or sensation that appear similar to true seizures. They generally lack self-injury and incontinence. They can be diagnosed with video-EEG.
- BRUEs are events that stop within a minute in children less than 1 year old, with one or more of the following symptoms: changes in breathing, changes in oxygenation, altered mental status, and changes in muscle tone. They are a diagnosis of exclusion. If they occur in very low-risk patients, no further work-up is needed, and the infant needs to be reevaluated in 24 hours. In high-risk patients, look for a cause:
  - High risk – age <60 days, gestational age <32 weeks, multiple events, lasted longer than 1 minute, required CPR, or family history of sudden cardiac death

If you have a reasonable suspicion that the child is having a seizure, you should figure out if the seizure is provoked versus unprovoked. The most common cause for provoked seizure for children is febrile seizures.

Febrile seizures or simple febrile seizures last less than 15 minutes, are tonic-clonic, and don't happen more than once in 1 day. They are often triggered by viral illnesses (URI, gastroenteritis, roseola/HSV6). If a child has a simple febrile seizure, neither an EEG nor neuroimaging is necessary for evaluation. Treatment for febrile seizures in the emergency department is with benzodiazepines, acetaminophen, evaluation of the cause of the febrile seizures, and supportive care. Complex febrile seizures – or febrile seizures that last longer than 15 minutes or occur more than once in a day – require further evaluation or prophylactic treatment. While febrile seizures don't mean a child has epilepsy or a seizure disorder, children with febrile seizures have a twice increased risk of developing epilepsy as compared to the general population.

Other causes of provoked seizures are infections such as meningitis and encephalitis, toxins, electrolyte imbalances (including hypoglycemia), tumors, alcohol and benzodiazepine withdrawals, head injury, etc.

Unprovoked seizures, on the other hand, have no identifiable cause and may be due to abnormal neuronal structuring, abnormal signaling, or abnormal electrical activity in the brain. There is a 30–50% chance that someone with an unprovoked seizure will have another within 2 years. EEG and MRI may be warranted for further evaluation of a first-time unprovoked seizure. A first seizure may not be a child's actual first seizure – parents may have missed a previous seizure. The diagnosis of epilepsy or seizure syndrome may or may not be made after a first-time seizure but only after at least two separate seizure instances. The decision to start antiepileptic drugs after a first-time unprovoked seizure is a complicated one weighing risks and benefits, and it is worthwhile and recommended to consult a pediatric neurologist.

Seizure terminology:

- Generalized seizure – begins in both sides of the brain
- Partial/focal seizure – begins in one side of the brain
- Complex seizure – patient loses consciousness
- Simple seizure – patient retains consciousness

In general, this simplifies to simple partial (preserved alertness and awareness), complex partial (preserved alertness, impaired awareness), and generalized seizures (impaired alertness and awareness). Generalized seizures are either primary and lose consciousness from the start or secondarily generalized which start as partial then spreads become general.

Types of seizures:

- Tonic-clonic: generalized complex seizures usually, convulsions, postictal state, incontinence, involuntary scream, tongue biting:
  - Tonic phase: contraction of muscles
  - Clonic phase: convulsions
- Atonic: sudden relaxation of muscle tonicity, no loss of consciousness (patient will suddenly drop to the ground).
- Myoclonic: brief contractions of muscles, no loss of consciousness.
- Absence: generalized seizure that presents as very brief episodes of staring that may occur multiple times with loss of consciousness but no postictal state (may look like a child is distracted at school):
  - Buzzword: 3hz spike and wave complexes on EEG
- Infantile spasms/West syndrome: the spasms may look like a startle (back arches and extremities extend or stiffening of the back or extremities may

occur) and typically start within the first year of life. There may be hypsar-rhythmia on EEG.

Physical exam: for a patient presenting after a seizure, you should do a full physical exam and thorough neurologic and mental status exam. While an EEG is being performed, if absence seizure is suspected, the child may undergo hyperventilation testing to provoke an episode.

■ Work-Up (Evaluate If Your Patient Needs Each Test on a Case-by-Case Basis)
– CBC (to evaluate for infection as a source of provoked seizure).
– Blood cultures.
– Basic metabolic panel (BMP).
– Lumbar puncture (depending on age and clinical suspicion).
– EEG.
– MRI for unprovoked seizure.
– Urinalysis and urine culture, urine tox (depending on age and clinical suspicion).
– Sleep-deprived EEG may be done later.

■ Treatment for Status Epilepticus
Status epilepticus is a medical emergency and potentially lethal complication of seizures. It is defined as a seizure lasting more than 5 minutes or two separate seizures without a return to baseline between the events. This condition can be further divided up into early status epilepticus (5–30 minutes) vs established (greater than 30 minutes) vs refractory (not successfully treated with multiple antiepileptic medications).

Treatment for status epilepticus involves stabilization (think the pediatric assessment triangle), getting labs to be able to fix what may be provoking the seizure (CBC, BMP, glucose, ABG/VBG, blood levels of medications), and establishing IV access. Continuous EEG testing is also helpful to make sure the patient has stopped seizing and not having nonconvulsive seizures (EEG findings of seizure, often with altered mental status, but no obvious motor manifestations of seizure).

Antiepileptic medication should be given along with stabilization, establishing access, and treating any possible underlying causes:
1. Lorazepam (0.1 mg/kg IV, maximum dose of 4 mg) q5–10 minutes as necessary.
2. If that doesn't work, try phenobarbital (15–20 mg/kg IV, maximum dose 1000 mg) or valproic acid (20–40 mg/kg IV, maximum dose 3000 mg).

■ Complications
– Cardiopulmonary complications
– Neurologic sequelae
– Self-inflicted injury

10.13.1 Diabetic Ketoacidosis (DKA)

Bird's Eye View   Diabetic ketoacidosis occurs when the cells of the body don't have access to insulin and thus don't have access to glucose. The body then turns fat into ketones as another energy supply. DKA most often occurs in patients with type 1 diabetes mellitus – where the pancreas does not produce insulin – but may also occur in patients with late-stage (i.e., when the body no longer makes insulin due to organ failure) type 2 diabetes mellitus. DKA is a common way that

patients with undiagnosed type 1 diabetes present to the doctor. In patients with diagnosed type 1 diabetes, common triggers for DKA include:
1. Medication noncompliance, missing doses of insulin, or not administering enough insulin as needed for the child's diet
2. Infections (e.g., gastroenteritis)
3. Pancreatitis

Presentation   Patients commonly present with symptoms of weight loss, polyuria, polydipsia, abdominal pain, nausea, vomiting, change in alertness and consciousness, nocturia, and physical exam findings of Kussmaul respirations (compensatory respiratory alkalosis), dehydration, and tachycardia.

Work-Up   The diagnosis of DKA is confirmed with lab tests: elevated blood glucose above 200, elevated anion gap metabolic acidosis, and ketones in the blood and urine – especially beta-hydroxybutyrate (>3 mmol/L). If a patient has a markedly elevated blood glucose but does not have acidosis or elevated ketones, consider hyperglycemic hyperosmolar state. It is also helpful to get other labs such as CBC, CMP, lipases, lactate, ABG/VBG, and chest X-rays (to rule out a precipitating lung infection).

■ Differentiating the Differential
▬ Asthma – due to respiratory distress and fast respirations; however, wheezing is often heard in asthma, and children with asthma most likely have had previous episodes.
▬ Acute abdomen – can be difficult to differentiate but always keep DKA in mind, and get basic labs and glucose for children presenting with acute abdominal pain.
▬ Hyperglycemic hyperosmolar state – patient will often not have Kussmaul respirations, will not have acidosis or ketonemia, and will often have blood levels well above 200.

■ Treatment
▬ One of the most important components (arguably the most important) of DKA management is fluid management. Initial fluid management should be a 10 mL/kg NS bolus +20 mEq/L K-phos or K-acetate. The patient's total initial fluid resuscitation should not exceed 40 mL/kg.
  – Do not add potassium if patient is frankly hyperkalemic (>5.5 mEq/L).
▬ To calculate how much fluid to give afterward, assume the child's fluid deficit is 5% of their weight. Then calculate how much fluid they need over the next 48 hours by adding their fluid deficit to their maintenance fluids and give them this amount of fluid evenly over the next 48 hours.
  – Use the 4-2-1 rule (◘ Table 10.3) or use the maintenance fluid calculations in MDCalc (Holiday, Segar Pediatrics 1957).

◘ Table 10.3 The 4-2-1 rule for maintenance fluids

Weight	Hourly
<10 kg	4 mL/kg/hr for every kg
10–20 kg	40 mL + 2 mL/kg for every kg over 10 kg
>20 kg	60 mL + 1 mL/kg for every kg over 20 kg

- Potassium should be carefully measured and repleted (initial levels of potassium may be high due to cellular shifts due to lack of insulin and acidosis – insulin usually drives potassium into cells by activating the Na+/K+ pump; without insulin, potassium builds up in the serum, but the total potassium in the body (cellular + serum levels) is low due to diuresis and secondary hyperaldosteronism). As soon as you give insulin, the patient's potassium may tank. Potassium should be >3.3–3.5 mEq/L before you give insulin.
- Insulin should be given carefully as an insulin drip (at the rate of 0.05 units/kg/hour to 0.1 units/kg/hour) to make sure the glucose level does not drop below 5 mmol/L. If the patient's blood glucose is below 250 mg/dl but their anion gap hasn't closed, it may be necessary to give dextrose to keep up the blood glucose. After your patient's anion gap is closed, they should be carefully transitioned to subcutaneous insulin and you should continue to monitor the anion gap to make sure it remains closed.
- Treat precipitating cause.
- Make sure to put the patient on telemetry (due to their shifting electrolyte levels); measure their blood glucose hourly and their electrolytes and VBG at least every 2–4 hours.
- ICU management is required for children with severe acidosis or an altered mental status.

- ■ Complications
- DVT
- Pancreatitis
- Mucormycosis – a rare fungal infection that can present with nasal or sinus congestion and fever and can rapidly progress to necrosis and local spread
- Cerebral edema
- Arrhythmias

10.14 Example Day in Clinic

I arrive at clinic 20 minutes early and let the medical assistant know that I will be working with Dr. X today and later update the medical assistant with the names of the patients I will be seeing. The medical assistant asks patients if they would be willing to be interviewed by a medical student before I walk in the room. I sit at my workstation to go over the schedule for the day and read about the patients for the day in the EMR. In the EMR, the key information to look up is their last well-child visit note, problem list, medications, allergies, birth history, immunization status, growth charts from prior visits, if they are seeing any specialists and why, details of prior hospitalizations if any, relevant labs, as well as the social and family details.

Before clinic starts, I talk with my attending about the appropriate patients for me to see. We identify patients and families of educational value for me and if the family would be willing to and would benefit from being interviewed by a medical student. If the patient I am about to see is one of my preceptor's established patients, I find it valuable to get a sense of who they are from my preceptor. In pediatrics especially, parents can be very anxious about the health of their child. My preceptors have a good idea of where the patient and family are coming from, their concerns, and their expectations for the visit.

While it depends on the attending on your rotation, I usually saw patients first by myself. I think about the age of the patient and decide whether or not to get them a free book or stickers before I walk in the room. In the room, I introduce myself to the child first. I introduce myself to the parents and let them know I am a medical student working with Dr. X and will be taking a history and physical. I make sure to ask for the parents' names as the parents' names are not always in the EMR.

I take the history and with permission and do the physical exam (on average takes 10–15 minutes). For both a well-child visit and for a "sick" visit, it is important to start the history by asking the parents and child what they are most concerned about (sometimes their concerns are completely different from what is listed in the EMR as the purpose of the visit!). For the physical exam, for babies, I make sure to listen to their heart and lungs early before they start crying (in the beginning of the physical exam while they are still on their parent's lap or even before the history). Afterward I find it helpful to think about the physical exam anatomically, head to toe, and then I make sure I didn't miss anything by cross-referencing a pediatric physical exam template on the EMR.

I walk out of the room and then take some time to formulate an assessment and plan. I then present my assessment and plan to my attending. My attending and I walk back into the clinic room where she confirms the key parts of the history and physical and discusses the plan with the patient. If there are orders to place, I pend the orders for the resident to sign. One useful task after the visit that I can do is creating notes for school/work that the patient/family needs, asking the attending to sign these notes, and handing them to the patient. Another useful task is directing the patient to where they need to go next.

When I had downtime between patients, I completed my notes and, with my attending's approval, called patients I have seen in the past few days to communicate laboratory results. After clinic, I check back in with my attending to discuss learning points and feedback.

10.15 Example Day on a General Inpatient Service

I arrive to the resident workroom approximately half an hour before sign-out to review my assigned patients' charts from overnight. Patients would be assigned to me if I had helped admit them or if there was a good learning case that came in overnight. I take notes on any new imaging, testing, lab values (noting trends from previous days), and recommendations from other consultants. I would print lists for the team. During sign-out, I take detailed notes on the patients I was following and more brief notes on the rest of the list. After sign-out we attend morning report, grand rounds, or other educational activities as a team.

Before round, I pre-round on my patients including a focused interval history and relevant physical exam. I always ask if the patient and parents have any questions for the team. If I can't answer them, I let them know I will discuss it with the team and get back to them during rounds.

Before we started rounding, I run my assessment and plan by the resident; it varied if my senior had seen the patient depending on the list. They gave me feedback before I presented to the attending and family. We do family-centered rounds (refer to the Overview section for an example). While seeing patients I was not following, I call the nurse and update the whiteboard in the room with the plan for the day. Between patients as questions came up, the team takes several minutes to discuss teaching points, and the attending sometimes assigns someone to look into topics and present to the team in the afternoon. Rounds take us several hours up until lunch.

In the afternoons, I completed my notes and pend orders. If necessary, I call consults and follow-up on any pending labs. The attending would typically set a time to run the list with the team, and that would be the time to discuss any questions that came up on rounds, or they may do a brief chalk talk. After my work was completed, I would check back in with patients and give any updates. Our team was responsible for any new admissions until the swing shift arrived, and I take their H&Ps. At the end of the day, I would sign-out my patients to the swing shift.

10.16 Review Questions

1. A child who has been playing hooky during gym class is brought in by his mother. His mother states that she notes him wheezing 10 minutes after he starts running outside with his friends and has very recently started wheezing and having shortness of breath even when not exercising. What is your diagnosis for this child? How do you evaluate further and treat this child for his diagnosis?

2. In the EMR, you see that your next patient is 2 years old and coming in for a chief complaint of cough and congestion. You walk into the room and introduce yourself to the child and her parents. The parents say that their child is no longer sick, but she has a white discoloration on her cheek. What questions would you ask? What is your differential diagnosis? How would you counsel this family?

3. A 5-year-old child is in your clinic with vague abdominal pain over the last few days. What do you want to be sure to rule out?

4. A 10-year-old boy presents to your clinic with a history of strep throat 2–3 weeks ago treated with antibiotics and bloody urine and puffy legs. What is the management and treatment?

5. What is a differential diagnosis for the bugs that can cause sore throat?

10.16.1   Answers

1. This child likely has exercise-induced asthma, but make sure you keep a differential diagnosis in mind. Take a thorough history to assess the child's risk of a life-threatening asthma exacerbation and his degree of impairment from asthma. Also make sure to ask about all potential and known triggers, personal history of atopy, family history of atopy/asthma, household or school exposures to pollutants or secondhand smoke, and about bullying at school (which may decrease compliance with prescribed treatment). The most likely general management for this patient would be to prescribe a short-acting beta-agonist (e.g., albuterol) to use 15–30 minutes before exercise. It is important to educate your patient about how to use an inhaler, and make sure your patient is able to teach back to you.

2. This case is based on a clinic visit late in my rotation that was observed by my preceptor. I had no idea what was going on and basically ended up asking the patient's family three times, "Are you sure she doesn't feel sick?" and got thrown way off my game. I hadn't thought about the differential diagnosis for hypopigmented lesions before, so here is a good starting differential: vitiligo, pityriasis alba, tinea versicolor, and post-inflammatory hypopigmentation. There are some zebras you could consider but probably shouldn't in an otherwise healthy child-like ash leaf spots in tuberous sclerosis and sarcoidosis.

3. Depends on other symptoms but generally a good differential to start off with is, in no particular order, intussusception, volvulus, diabetic ketoacidosis, appendicitis, strep throat, testicular or ovarian torsion, hernia, pneumonia, and urinary tract infections.
4. This child most likely has PSGN. You should measure their blood pressure and assess how much edema they have. You can get an ASO titer to confirm their recent history of a strep infection, C3 level, and BUN and creatinine level. You can then give antibiotics, recommend salt and water restriction, and then decide whether or not to give furosemide to reduce the edema and/or antihypertensives.
5. Viral pharyngitis, group A strep, EBV, CMV, HIV.

Radiology

Bliss J. Chang

Contents

© The Author(s), under exclusive license to Springer Nature Switzerland AG 2021
S. H. Lecker, B. J. Chang (eds.), *The Ultimate Medical School Rotation Guide*,
https://doi.org/10.1007/978-3-030-63560-2_11

11

11.1 Overview

The phrase "a picture is worth a thousand words" is quite literally true in radiology, as you will use many words to describe and interpret what you see. As such, the key to excelling in radiology is to be fluent in the language of radiology. Unlike any other radiology resource, in this chapter we will primarily focus on effectively teaching you this language so you can effectively identify and communicate what you see. We will also show you how to correlate what you see with anatomy and physiology rather than simply memorizing clinical correlates. Your ability to clinically correlate radiographic findings will naturally follow with time as you gain more experience in all the fields of medicine.

11.2 Recommended Resources

The best way to learn radiology is to read film after film, using computers that allow for interactive scrolling and other features. Fortunately, there are many good, free, online resources. As such, the goal of this chapter is not to reinvent the wheel but rather provide you with a new perspective of radiology as a new language. After you learn the language basics, we recommend the following three resources:

- *Radiopedia* is an amazing resource that has essentially every image finding you could want. An excellent resource to compare what you're seeing to examples or to read about definitions of special signs (e.g., spine sign) or criteria. The radiology courses on there are also great and broken down into high-yield subjects such as reading neurodegenerative MRIs and even a Pac-Man game that helps with tracking small bowel on CT!
- The *University of Virginia's* Radiology Course (▶ https://www.med-ed. virginia.edu/courses/rad/) is another excellent tool that will walk beginners through the fundamentals of interpreting various imaging studies.
- For ultrasound, *The Pocus Atlas* is by far the best resource for dynamic ultrasound images, just as if you were in a radiology reading room.

Throughout your studies, try to stick with one or two resources, and complete them rather than finding a new resource each day and only completing small portions.

11.3 The Rotation

Unlike all other clinical rotations, the radiology rotation is the most straightforward. Most of your time will be spent with a radiologist in the reading room (it's dark and possibly sleep-provoking, so be sure to bring your coffee!). Your enthusiasm, effort, and ability to effectively communicate what you see in radiologic terms will determine how well you do. Lastly, most radiology clerkships have a case presentation requirement – be sure to ask the radiologists that you work with for feedback and input long before your presentation as they often have very helpful opinions.

11.4 Fundamentals

11.4.1 The Black and White Language

Radiology is a language that centers around interpreting a black to white spectrum of colors (◻ Fig. 11.1). Thus, fluency is predicated on an understanding of what various shades of color on this black-white spectrum represent. This spectrum is practically divided into three portions, black, gray, and white, and each color is described in a unique way among the various imaging modalities.

Let's look at ■ Table 11.1 to better understand what is represented by these colors across the most common imaging modalities. Spend some time comparing and contrasting within this table, as one of the most difficult aspects of starting off in radiology is keeping straight in your mind what the shades of black and white represent.

Notice a few patterns in ■ Table 11.1 to help you when you aren't sure what you're visualizing:

- Gray and gray-white typically represent, among other things, biological tissue regardless of imaging modality.
- Black typically represents air (apart from ultrasound).
- White typically represents the highest density (bone, metal).

Let's practice describing what we see on our four practice images by using this framework. For the sake of practice, we will refrain from describing what the objects are and simply describe what we see.

In ■ Fig. 11.2, we see a large gray-whiteness that is shaped somewhat like a heart in the middle of the x-ray. Since this is an x-ray, we know that this thing must be much denser than air. Surrounding it, we see several gray horizontal projections which are probably something denser than air but less dense the central white matter. Between these gray horizontal projections, we see very faint gray and even light black – this is likely very low density, such as something filled with air. Though we could go on and describe every area on the x-ray, you now have a sense of what real-world correlate you're looking at through these shades of black and white.

The CT scan of the abdomen below can be interpreted similarly. There are four very white linear structures in the lower half of the image. Since these are

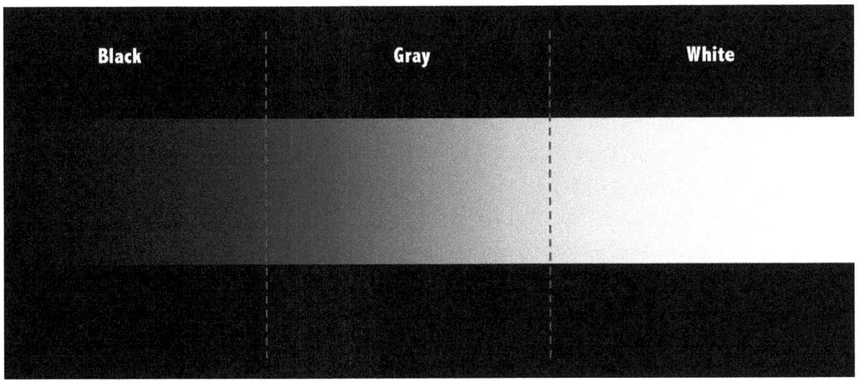

■ **Fig. 11.1** Spectrum of radiographic interpretation

■ **Table 11.1** Black/white correlation for common imaging modalities

Color	X-ray	CT	MRI	Ultrasound
Black	Air	Air	Air, bone	Fluid
Gray	Tissue and fluids	Tissues, fluid, and fat	Tissues	Tissues
White	Bone, metal	Bone	Fat, liquid	Dense tissues, objects (e.g., lines), air

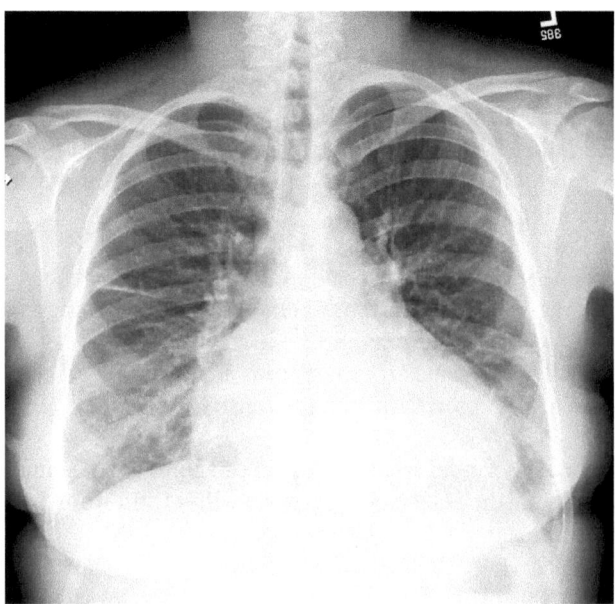

◘ **Fig. 11.2**   Practice CXR #1

◘ **Table 11.2**   Radiographic terms describing black/white shades

Color	X-ray	CT	MRI	Ultrasound
Black	Lucency	Hypodense	Hypointensity	Hypoechoic
Gray	Faint opacity	Dense	Intensity	Echoic
White	Opacity (aka density)	Hyperdense	Hyperintensity	Hyperechoic

When you see an opacity on CXR, you should think of three key causes:
1. Airspace disease
2. Atelectasis
3. Interstitial patterns

On KUB, opacities most commonly represent:
1. Dense fecal matter
2. Foreign bodies

close to true white, they must be very dense. In the upper left, we see a white-gray triangular structure, representing considerable density but less than that of the white linear structures. Interspersed, we can visualize areas of black which represents air (◘ Table 11.2).

Lastly, let's look at ◘ Fig. 11.4. There is a lot of black throughout this ultrasound image, meaning fluid. There is also a prominent white strip in the upper half which likely means either tissue or can be the reflection signifying the interface between air and solid. There are also several areas of gray/white which likely represent structures less dense than fluid.

Now, let's convert these descriptions of black, gray, and white areas of images to more professional terms, which vary by imaging modality (◘ Table 11.2). This is analogous to describing something red as "erythematous." Let's practice with our practice images again (refer to ◘ Figs. 11.2, 11.3, and 11.4), now using more professional descriptors.

◘ Figure 11.2 demonstrates a large opacity in the shape of a water balloon. There are also several fainter linear opacities that line either side of the large opacity. These fainter linear opacities are separated by lucencies that represent a structure likely filled with air.

◘ Figure 11.3 demonstrates linear hyperdensities in the lower half of the image. The upper left corner reveals a dense triangular structure, and we see various scattered hypodensities throughout the image.

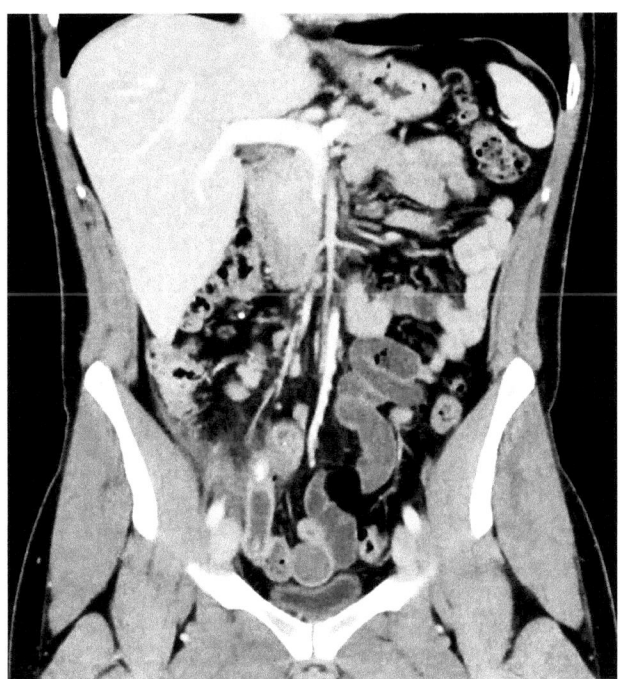

◧ **Fig. 11.3**   Practice CT #1

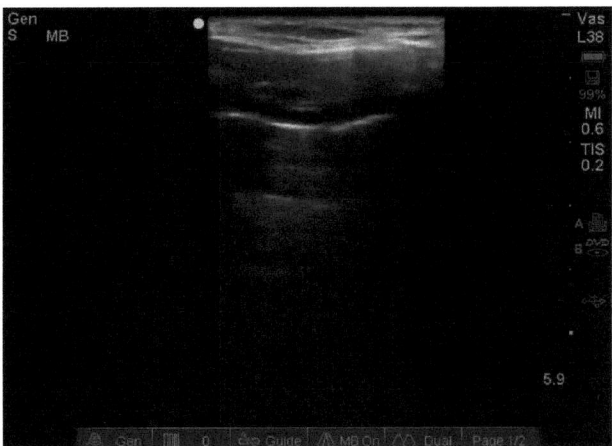

◧ **Fig. 11.4**   Practice Ultrasound #1

◧ Figure 11.4 has many hyperechogenic areas with a prominent hyper-echogenicity strip in the upper half. There are several areas of echogenic material interspersed throughout the image.

Another important aspect of describing the shades of black/white you see is conveying the general appearance (besides color), without naming what exactly it may correlate to clinically. This is similar to presenting the results and saving the discussion (clinical correlation) for later. This allows for a complete and thorough differential diagnosis. ◧ Table 11.3 demonstrates the common appearances on imaging.

□ Table 11.3 Common radiologic descriptors

Descriptor	Common appearances
Shape	Linear, nodular (circular), any geometric shapes (e.g., triangular), reticulonodular (curvilinear on top of circular), ground-glass, dense (solid and continuous without interruption)
Distribution	Unilateral/bilateral, diffuse/hazy, focal

11.4.2 Systematic Reading of CXRs

Though you will see many residents and attendings skip to the "juicy" part of whatever images they're looking at, as a trainee you should always read in a systematic manner. This is particularly true of chest x-rays as they are the most common imaging modality. This will not only help you develop all aspects of your radiology skills consistently but also help you avoid missing key subtle findings. Our suggested method is as follows.

11.4.3 Image Quality (Mainly Applicable to X-rays)

- Exposure: Is the radiograph overexposed (too white) or underexposed (too faint)? Appropriate exposure is critical to ensuring you can see what you need to see on the images. As you view more and more radiographs, you will become naturally good at identifying when there is inappropriate exposure.
- Rotation: Look to see that the clavicles are centered around the vertebral bodies. If there is rotation, it will be indicated by the side with more distance between the clavicle and the vertebral body center. A rotated image can distort the positioning and shape of the heart, making it difficult to properly interpret.

11.4.3.1 Lines/Tubes
Point any lines/tubes on the image. This not only aids in verifying the correct patient but also is useful for confirming appropriate positioning of chest tubes, nasogastric tubes, endotracheal tubes, swan-ganz catheters, and intra-aortic balloon pumps.

11.4.3.2 Bones
Trace the contours of all the bones to ensure that all edges are smooth without interruptions. Small fractures can be picked up by being thorough with this and are always impressive!

Reread the Fundamentals section, and then proceed to our recommended radiology resources to start putting your new language skills to the test!

11.5 Common Images

Though images are best reviewed on a computer with the radiology appropriate software, here are some images of common cases (■ Figs. 11.5, 11.6, 11.7, 11.8, 11.9, 11.10, 11.11, 11.12, 11.13, 11.14, 11.15, 11.16, 11.17, 11.18, 11.19, 11.20, 11.21, 11.22, and 11.23). We recommend using it as a reference throughout your rotation when you have questions on how a clinical case you haven't encountered may present. The ordering is somewhat random so that you may also practice interpreting these images after going through the online resources.

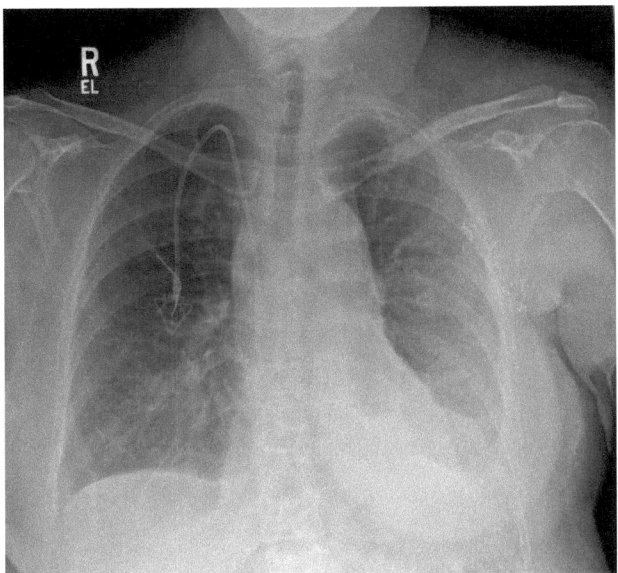

■ **Fig. 11.5** Left-sided pleural effusion. Evidenced by concave opacity blunting the left costo-diaphragmatic recess

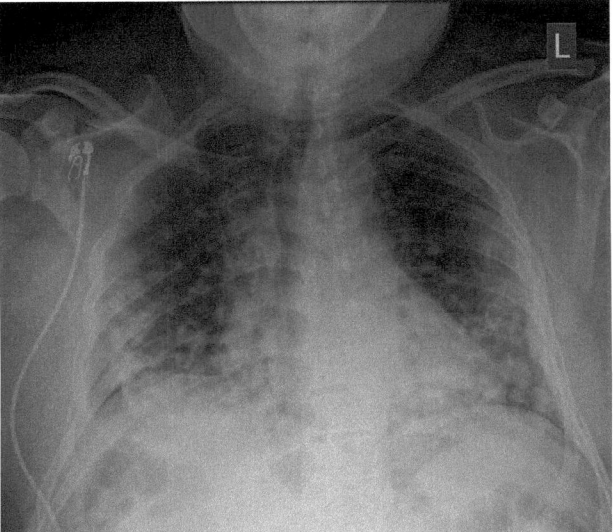

■ **Fig. 11.6** Atypical pneumonia. Bilateral diffuse hazy white opacities

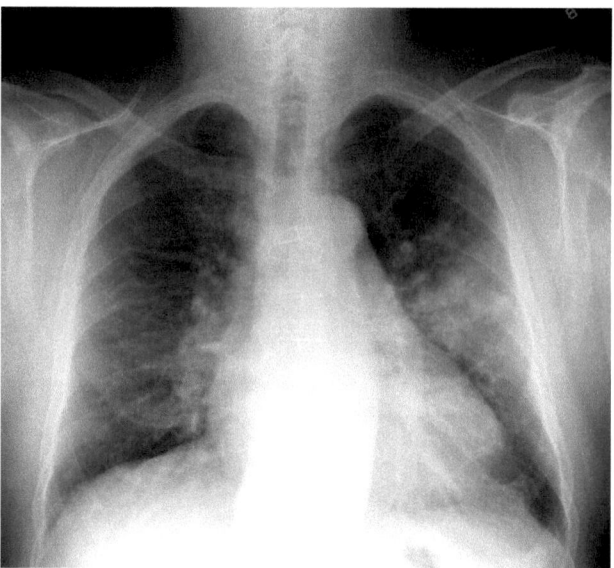

Fig. 11.7 Left upper lobe pneumonia. Large opacity in the left upper lobe area

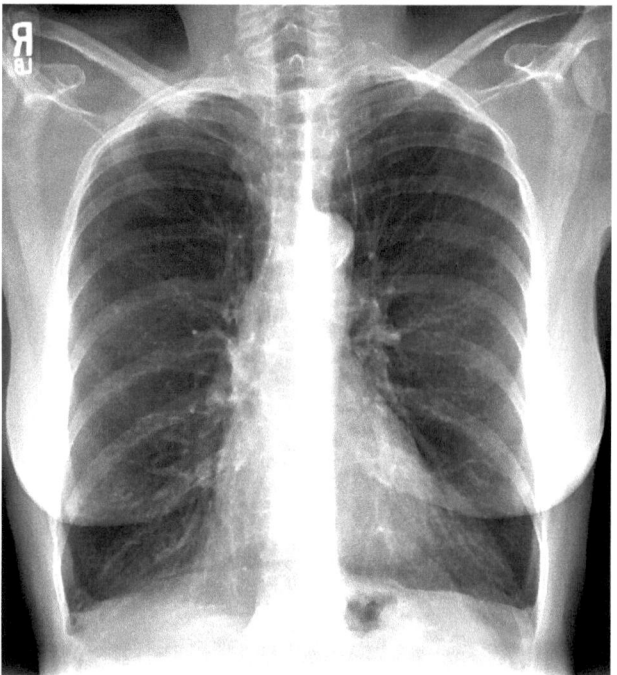

Fig. 11.8 COPD. Increased bilateral lucencies representing increased lung volumes. Cardiac silhouette slimmer than usual. Decreased lung markings

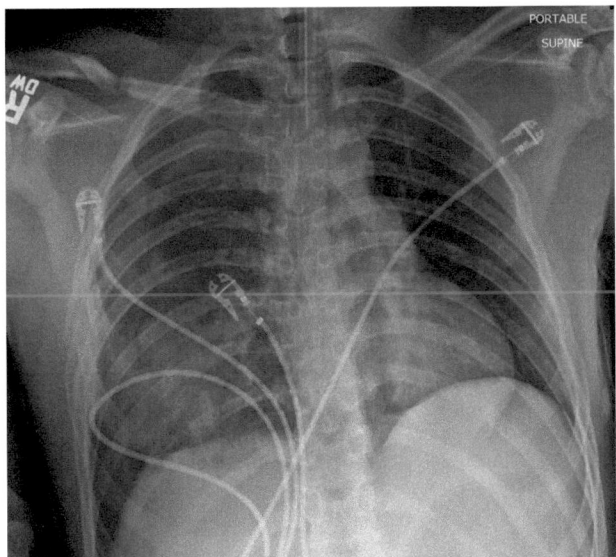

■ **Fig. 11.9** Left pneumothorax. Decreased lung markings and complete lucency of the left lung lobes

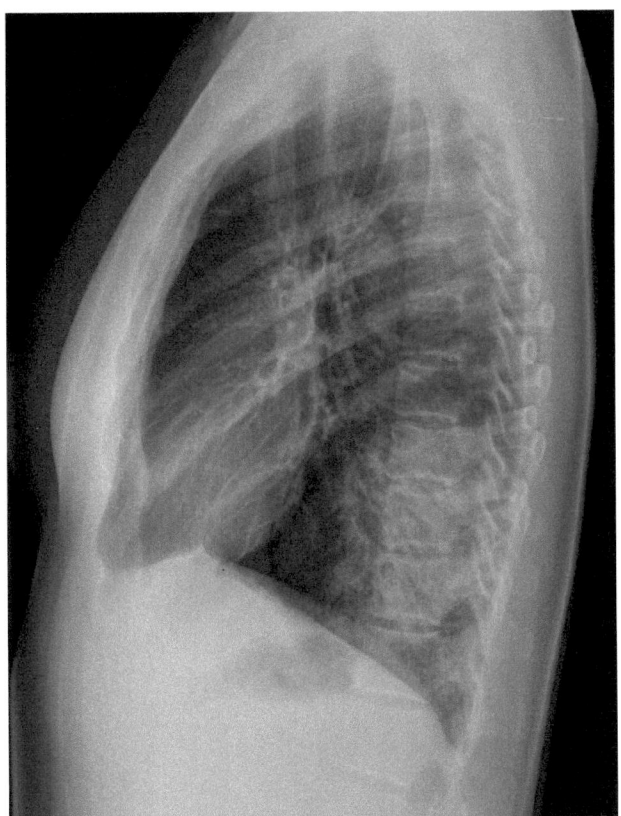

■ **Fig. 11.10** RLL pneumonia with spine sign on lateral CXR

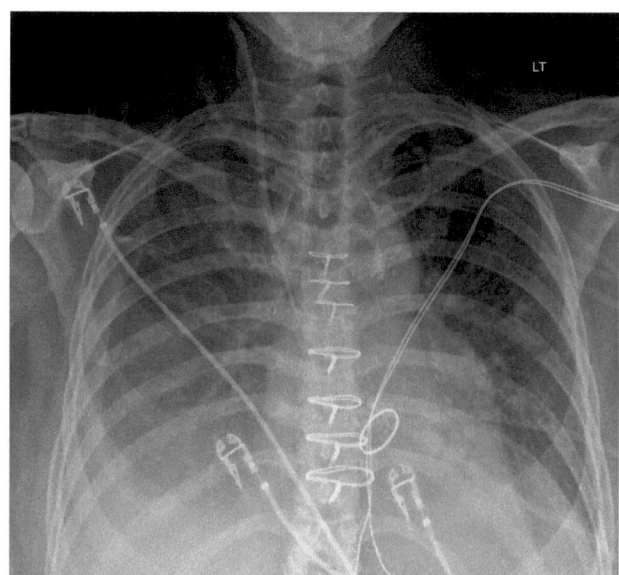

Fig. 11.11   Proper RIJ central line placement. Near the right atrium

11

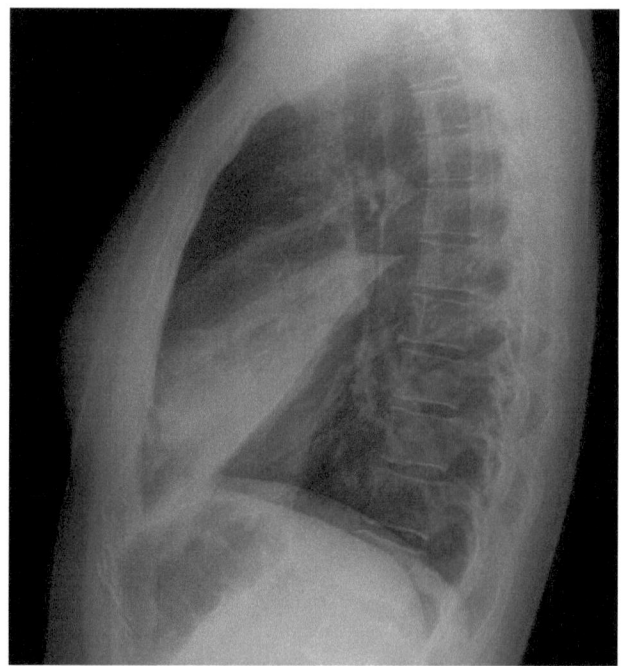

Fig. 11.12   RML pneumonia on lateral CXR

Radiology

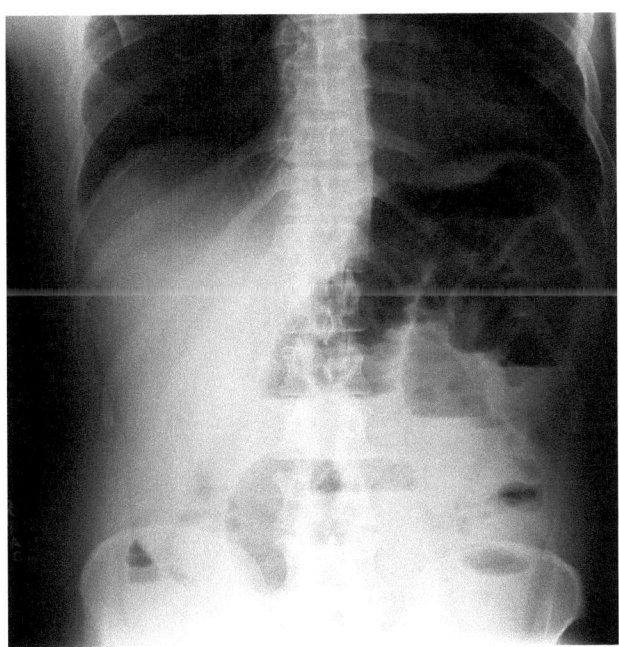

■ **Fig. 11.13** Small bowel obstruction on KUB. Prominent air-fluid levels

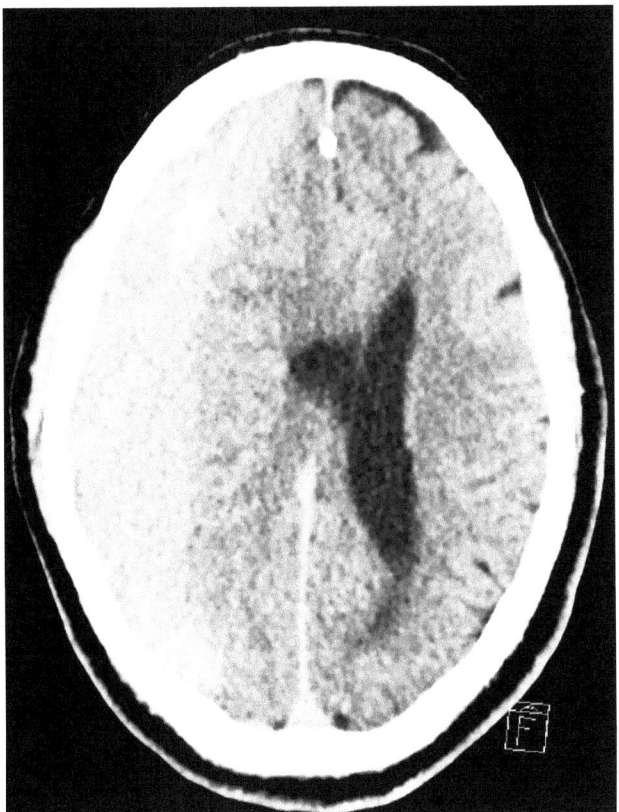

■ **Fig. 11.14** Subdural hematoma axial view on CT. Diffuse crescent-shaped hyperdensity hugging the right cranium

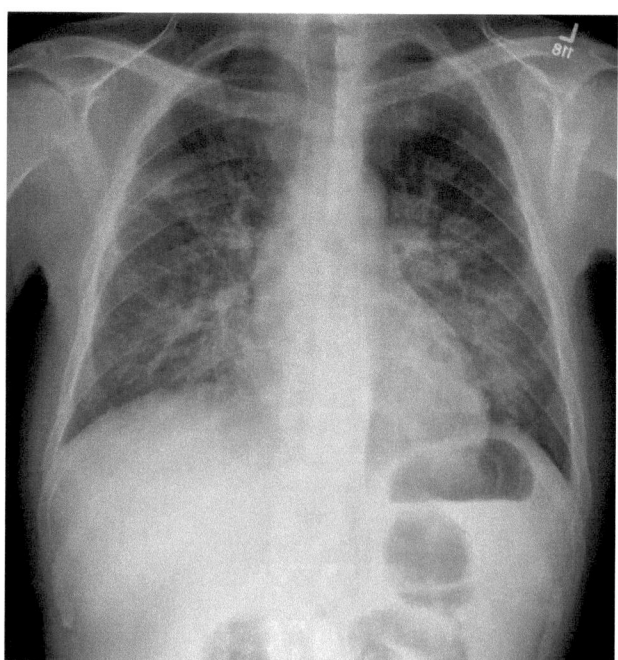

Fig. 11.15 ARDS as evidenced by without pleural effusions diffuse bilateral opacities

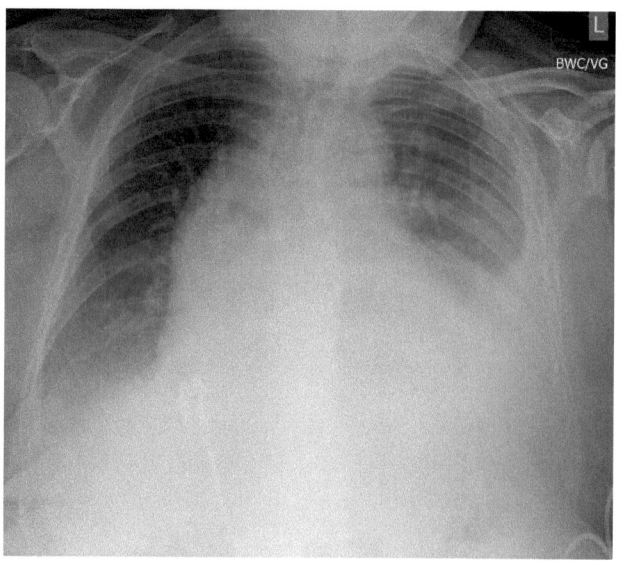

Fig. 11.16 Atelectasis of the LLL with right-sided pleural effusion

Radiology

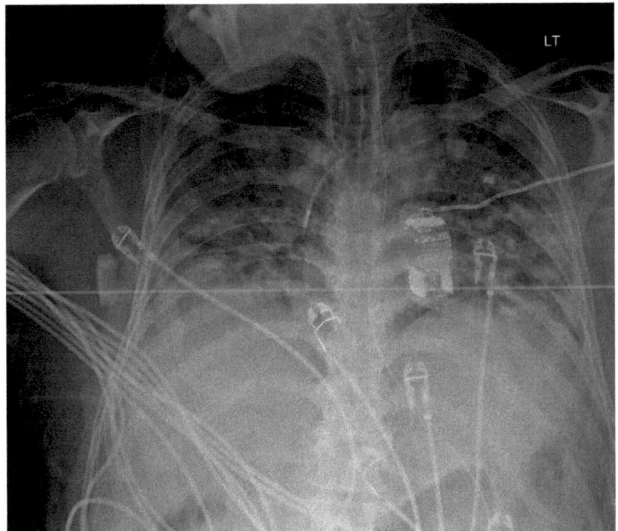

☐ **Fig. 11.17** EKG lines on CXR

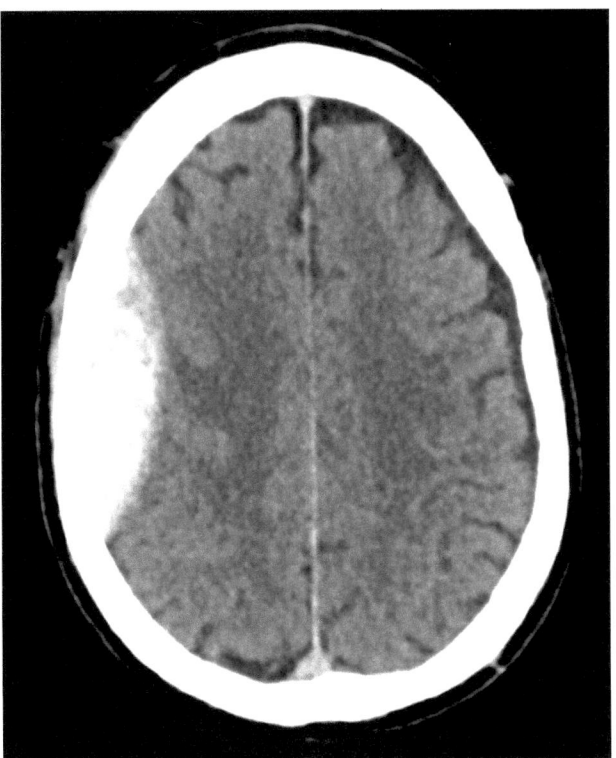

☐ **Fig. 11.18** Epidural hematoma on CXR. R-sided convex-shaped hyperdensity

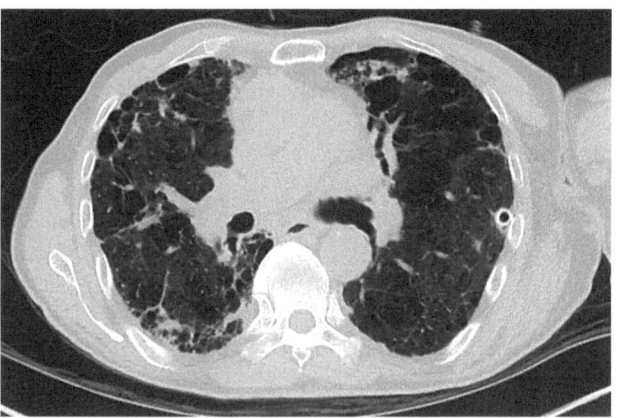

Fig. 11.19   ILD on axial CT. Diffuse honeycombing

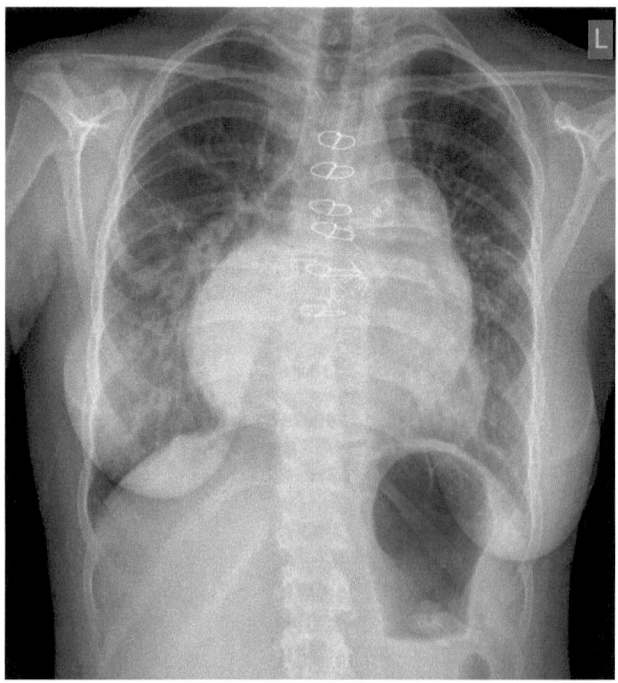

Fig. 11.20   Left atrial enlargement. Carina angle is splayed (>90) with prominent outward curvature of the left atrial heart border

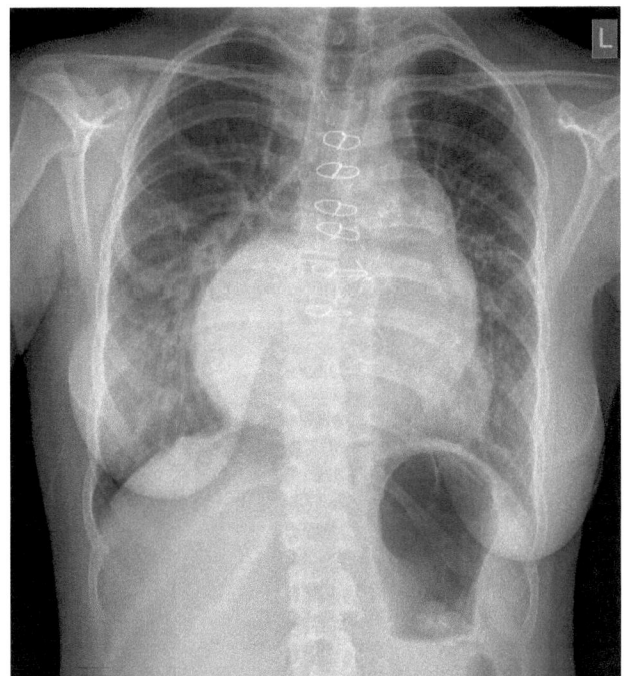

Fig. 11.21   Mitral and aortic valve replacements

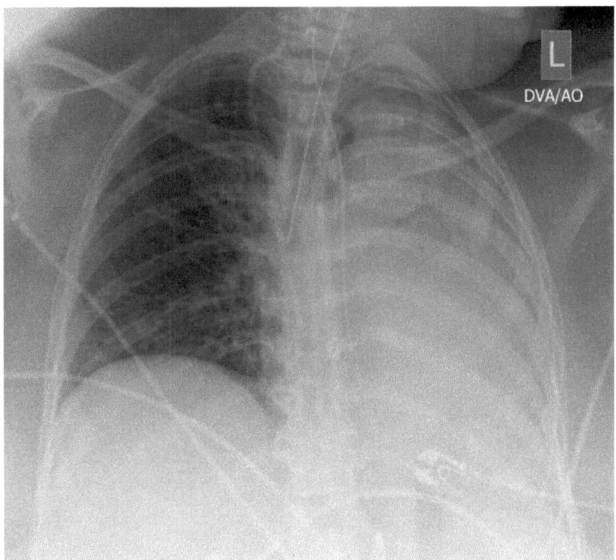

Fig. 11.22   Right mainstem intubation with left lung collapse

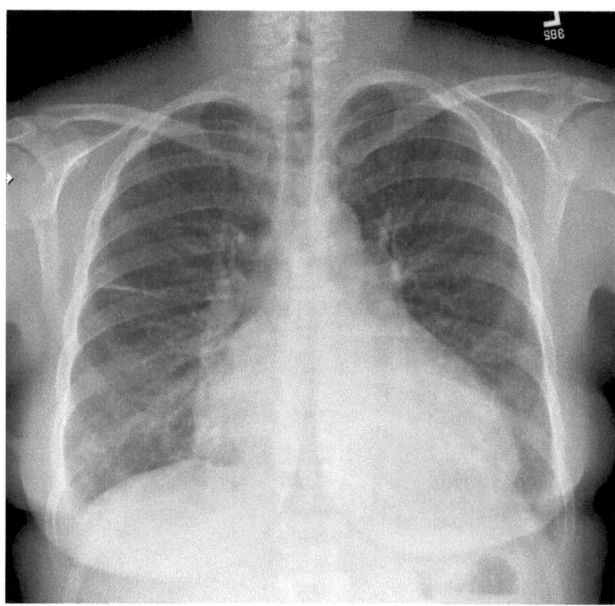

◘ **Fig. 11.23** Moderate pulmonary edema consistent with congestive heart failure. Notice increased bilateral lung markings, increased prominence of pulmonary arteries, and mild blunting of the R costodiaphragmatic recess

11

Psychiatry

Michael Dinh

Contents

© The Author(s), under exclusive license to Springer Nature Switzerland AG 2021
S. H. Lecker, B. J. Chang (eds.), *The Ultimate Medical School Rotation Guide*,
https://doi.org/10.1007/978-3-030-63560-2_12

12.1 Introduction

Psychiatry is a field of medicine in which the therapeutic alliance with patients and an understanding of the biological, psychological, and social underpinnings of their illness are paramount. As such, medical students on psychiatry rotations are judged not only on their clinical competence but also on their *social awareness, psychological mindedness, thoughtfulness, and ability to build rapport*. Furthermore, psychiatry is a highly collaborative setting that involves working with social workers, the legal system, patients' families, and more. In this chapter, we will cover how to think through cases, tips on building a therapeutic alliance with patients, and collaborating effectively with the interdisciplinary team.

12.2 The Interview

Your goal when treating a patient is to answer the following core questions: "What is this patient experiencing now that has brought them here?", "Why now?", and "What can be done to help them?". Ultimately, diagnoses will be assigned as a way to classify the patient's illness and to provide direction for treatment, but it is also important and complementary to have a broader understanding of the patient's experience as a whole person.

12.2.1 The Biopsychosocial Formulation

A common approach to this in psychiatry is the biopsychosocial formulation – it is not a diagnostic approach but rather an *organizational framework for gathering data* and *understanding the factors* influencing the patient's life and course of illness. As you conduct your history and get to know the patient, try to identify biological, psychological, and social factors in the patient's life, and think of ways that you might intervene on these factors to engage them in treatment and to improve their health (◘ Table 12.1).

12.2.2 History

12.2.2.1 History of Present Illness (HPI)

You should begin with a professional introduction and open-ended questions. It is important to maintain a *calm, genuine, and nonjudgmental tone* throughout your interview; the things your patients tell you may be very personal, sensitive, and stigmatized. In fact, there are times when you will be the first person they have ever opened up to. By maintaining respectful curiosity, you will be able to draw out the information you need while building rapport and giving them a positive therapeutic experience.

Phrases to start the open-ended part of the history:
"How have things been for you lately?"
"What's been going on?"
"What brings you here today?"

Informational Cues

There is information you can gather before you even begin talking to the patient, outside of reading the medical record. Speaking with other staff who

◻ Table 12.1 The biopsychosocial formulation

Factors	Biological	Psychological	Social
Predisposing (vulnerabilities that increase the risk for the present problems)	In utero or early childhood Family history Traumatic brain injury Physical and mental illness or disability Exposure to toxins or illness Temperament	Attachment style Emotional (dys)regulation Self-image, self-esteem Family dynamics	Early life trauma, poverty, poor access to health care Education Family structure Work history
Precipitating (acute stressors and life events that led to the current presentation)	Serious illness or injury Drug use	Conflicts in personal identity, relationships, developmental transitions	Interpersonal stress (e.g., loss or separation from loved ones, conflicts) Changes in housing, finances, school, work
Perpetuating (ongoing stressors and conditions that sustain the present problems)	Chronic illness Cognitive deficits	Personality traits Self-destructive coping mechanisms Dynamics (defenses)	Social isolation Chronic family discord Lack of resources (finances, housing, basic needs) Negative work or school situation, stigma, and discrimination Dangerous living conditions
Protective (assets that counteract the present problems)	Intelligence Temperament Good health Response to medications	Health coping mechanisms Positive self-image, self-esteem Good insight Resiliency	Social supports (family, friends) Resources (finances, housing, basic needs) Community cohesiveness Care providers

have already interacted with the patient may give you a sense of how the patient presents. Try to read the affect of the staff: Are they frustrated with the patient, pity them, really like them, or something else?

As you enter the room (and ideally, before the patient notices you), take note of the appearance of the patient and their surroundings. What are they doing, and what are they surrounded by? Books and magazines, flowers and cards, family photos, and other personal belongings may provide information about the patient's hobbies and social support and can serve as starting points for building rapport.

During the interview, the information you gather will come from the words the patient uses (or doesn't use), the way they say those words, and their nonverbal cues. Pay attention to some of the following things (◻ Table 12.2.).

You should refrain from interrupting the patient at the start of the interview. Allow the patient to speak uninterrupted at the beginning of an interview, depending on the amount of time you have with the patient. To gently shape the interview, try using reflective and attentive statements, questions, and gestures to signal to the patient that you are listening and interested and want to hear more.

Phrases/gestures to continue the history:

"Tell me more."

[Nod]

"I see."

[Repeat something that the patient said]

"I can see that this is bothering you a lot."

"What I'm hearing is that…is that right?"

Table 12.2. Informational cues

Language	Speech	Body language and appearance
The words used (and not used)	Tone (emotion, sarcasm, etc.)	Posture
Unusual vocabulary	Volume	Eye contact
Culturally specific vocabulary and slang	Rate	Personal hygiene
	Prosody (expressivity)	Personal belongings (books, family photos, flowers, etc.)
		Dress
		Gestures

Note if the patient is avoiding a topic or evasive towards certain questions. All of this will be captured in the mental status exam later

Phrases to interrupt patients: "I want to hear more about what you're saying, but I also need to hear about a few other things, as well. Can we circle back to this topic later?"

"Excuse me, you mentioned something I want to hear more about. Could you tell me more about…?"

Interrupting Patients

In psychiatry, there will be many times in which you need to interrupt your patients in order to gather information in a timely and organized manner. Examples of this include patients who are tangential and psychotic or have pressured speech. It is important to interrupt in a firm but respectful way that maintains the patient's feeling that you care and are listening.

Do not make assumptions about how a patient feels about a situation For example, a patient may tell you they just lost their job. You could either immediately express your condolences, or you could ask how that went or how they feel about it. Your choice depends on the specific context and tone you receive from the patient. It's possible that the patient is actually elated that they lost their job, and the former response could be received as tone-deaf. In either case, you will gather more information.

Note the connection between what is said and what emotions are expressed. This may be incongruent or congruent. This is important information to be aware of as you get to know the patient and it can point towards important issues with the patient. A common example is when the patient is describing horrible experiences without any expressed emotion.

Remember that while collecting your HPI, you should aim to answer the questions "What is this patient experiencing now that has brought them here?" and "Why now?". It may be helpful to remember or write down some *direct quotes* from the patient to record in the note, especially a chief complaint, report of suicidal ideation or plans, or unusual cognition (paranoid thoughts or report of hallucinations).

Setting Boundaries

The relationship you hold with your patients can be a tricky one. Because psychiatry is a field in which extremely sensitive personal information is shared by the patient to the provider, there exists a clear power dynamic. For this reason, it is inadvisable to have a personal relationship with your patients outside of the clinical setting or to take on people with whom you have a pre-existing personal relationship as a patient. This includes giving them access to your social media or meeting up with them outside the clinical setting.

Good boundaries provide the safe container or "sterile field" for successful psychiatric treatment. Without this, treatment usually derails, and patients do poorly. When a patient attempts to challenge the boundaries of your relationship with them, attempt to understand what this means to the patient, and then help them address the issue in a more appropriate fashion. This happens often, and it may feel uncomfortable. Always discuss boundary challenges with the team and your supervisor.

You may be tempted to reduce the power dynamic in order to build rapport with the patient. This can be good, but remember to strike a balance and also maintain professionality. Here are some factors that can alter the power dynamic and boundaries:

- *Self-disclosure*: Disclosing personal information about yourself to your patient can help build trust with some patients, and harm trust with others. For example, some patients may find hope and solidarity in a provider who has a lived experience similar to their own (e.g., a provider who discloses that they themselves had a substance use disorder), while others may perceive the provider as unqualified/impaired or not interested in listening to the patient.
- *Appearance*: Wearing a white coat may inspire confidence or comfort in some patients' eyes, while in others it may feel cold and unrelatable. The same goes for formal vs. informal clothing, expensive clothing, unconventional dress, tattoos, piercings, gender expression, etc. Feel free to express your own personal identity, but be aware of the way your patients may view this. It's best to appear neutral and professional.
- *Access*: If a patient is asking for your personal phone number or email, ask them why. Sharing this information may create an undue burden on you and create the feeling of a personal relationship to the patient. Instead, give them contact information for the clinic or unit.

If patients ask you a personal question that you are not comfortable answering, ask them why they would like to know, and you could respond with the following: "I don't typically share that personal information about myself with patients. Let's focus on you so that I can learn how I can help."

12.2.3 History Checklist

Be sure to also collect the following information. Some of this will be revealed during the HPI.

Past Psychiatric History
- Hospitalizations: why, when, what happened before, during, and after the hospitalization
- Medication trials and their outcomes
- Treatment providers
- Self-injurious behavior
- Suicidal ideation and attempts
- Homicidal behavior and violence
- Substance use
- Barriers to treatment adherence

Past Medical and Surgical History
- Remember to ask about history of head injuries.

Medications
  Allergies
  Social and Developmental History – this will be much deeper than the social history you have collected in other settings.
- Developmental history
  - Family and home during childhood

- Education
- Trauma history
- Living situation
- Important relationships
- Sexual history/identity
- Work
- Financial situation
- Legal history
- Hobbies and interests

12.2.4 Sensitive Topics

The trauma history, sexual history, substance use, suicidal behavior, and legal history are often very difficult topics for patients to discuss. It is important to remember that patients may feel a wide range of strong emotions surrounding these topics; look out for signs of anger, shame, sadness, regret, resentment, and guilt, to name a few. Also keep in mind that there is a strong *social stigma* surrounding many of these, and that patients may have had negative experiences when trying to share this information in the past.

To approach these topics, decide whether or not you want to *cue* to the patient that difficult questions are about to be asked. Different providers have their own approaches to this. Some use cues to warn the patient that difficult questions are coming and to normalize these questions. Others find that these cues can change the tone of the discussion and perhaps make it uncomfortable and continue into these questions with a continuation of the tone of the rest of the history in order to normalize them. Of course, in either case, if the patient comments on the nature of the questions or asks why you are asking, reassure them that these are normal questions that are asked of all kinds of patients and that they are necessary for developing an appropriate treatment.

Phrases to cue/reassure patients during sensitive topics:

"I have a few questions that I need to ask that may be uncomfortable or difficult. I need to ask to get a better sense of your situation, so that we can figure out how we can improve things from here. Of course, everything you tell me is confidential and will only be used to further your treatment."

"I can see that you find these questions difficult to answer. The reason I'm asking is so that I can understand you better, so that we can develop an appropriate plan for you. I can promise you that I will keep everything you share confidential."

12.2.5 Handling Displays of Emotion

Tears of sadness, angry outbursts, and laughter can be automatic reactions by your patients to the difficult things being discussed. When this happens, the best thing to do is to *validate their feelings* and to *investigate what prompted the emotion*. If the patient is crying, offer them tissues and pause, leaving them room to express their emotion. Then, you can offer words of validation in a gentle tone. Though it may be difficult, take care to regulate your own emotions so that the patient does not have to attend to you during their time to express themselves.

Remember that you don't have to do anything in particular – you don't have to fix the patient or stop the feelings from happening. Just be present, bear witness, and support the patient through them. Feelings are what they are. It's what the patient does with them that will give a clue about how to help.

> You may find that patients are reluctant to share; if it is important that you get a clear answer and understanding of the situation (i.e., current suicidal ideation, plan, and intent) and *probe respectfully and nonjudgmentally but firmly until you get an answer*. It may be that you need to use shorter, more direct questions for this. However, it is also possible to cause harm to patients through an interview. *In particular, bringing up trauma without addressing it or reacting to it in a judgmental or indifferent manner may be re-traumatizing.* If you feel the full, detailed trauma history is not relevant to the current presentation, and the patient is having a hard time discussing their past trauma, it may be better to not probe deeply and readdress the topic at a different time.

12

Phrases to validate emotions:

"I can see this is very hard for you."

"I can't imagine how difficult that [situation] must have been, but I can tell this has affected you a lot."

12.2.6 Safety

Popular media often depicts people living with mental illness as dangerous, which is *highly stigmatizing and inaccurate*. You will find during your rotation that your patients are often quite vulnerable as a result of their mental illness and most are victims, rather than perpetrators, of crime and violence. Nonetheless, it is important that you keep yourself and your patients safe by being aware of potential dangers and knowing what contingencies your hospital has in place.

In most inpatient settings, a patient's belongings, including anything that could potentially be used to harm themselves or others, are stored in a locked closet on admission. If you notice that the patient does have something that could be used to harm, back away and immediately alert the staff.

Positioning is important. During interviews with the patient, especially if you are alone, be aware of the exits to the room. If possible, position yourself so that you are closer to the door than the patient is so that they cannot block your exit. If you are particularly worried, make sure that you are seated/standing far away enough from the patient so that they are a "step and a swing" away from reaching you. The patient may notice that you have taken these measures and be offended by them. Be ready to explain why you are taking these measures, that they are standard and not unique to your patient, and that the safety of both you and your patient is of the highest importance. If you already know the patient and feel safe with them, you can position yourself more freely or strike a balance.

If you are even slightly worried about your safety, do not meet with the patient alone. Discuss this with your team and the patient's nurse. Someone should be available to be with you during the interview. Never meet with a patient alone if you are feeling unsafe with them.

Attire can impact safety. Ties, lanyards, straps, and loose clothing can all be used to grab and hold in a physical altercation. Long loose hair and jewelry can also be easily grabbed by patients. Hospital security officers often wear breakaway ties and badges for this reason. Wear shoes that you can easily run in and that have traction.

12.3 Verbal Aggression

Many psychiatric patients have reduced ability to hold in check their feeling and thoughts. Sometimes they say things that are not part of who they are at baseline. This can include verbal threats, racial slurs, profanity, personal insults, and projections of primitive emotions. First, try not to take it personally. Remember that this is a patient who is suffering from a mental illness. Second, don't retaliate. Remember that you are the professional care provider. Nonetheless, these expressions can be personally very hurtful to everybody present. To address this, you or your team can name the inappropriate nature of the expression and set clear expectations for more appropriate expressions with the patient in the moment. If this is not effective, you can stop the interview immediately and return to the patient later. These are very challenging moments for everybody. Be sure to discuss them afterwards with your team and your supervisors so that you can get the support that you need and so that the team can develop a consistent approach with the patient going forward.

12.3.1 Mental Status Examination (MSE)

During your interview, you will also be gathering information on the patient's *current mental state, which will encompass what the patient says, thinks, and does, and your interpretation of these things.* A thorough mental status examination is a *snapshot* that will allow for other providers listening to your oral presentation or reading your note envision themselves in the room with the patient. It is also helpful to *track mental status over time* to understand disease course and progress in treatment.

The components of the MSE can be remembered using the acronym *ASEPTIC*. Some examples of descriptors accompany each category, but the list is not exhaustive – remember that your goal is to describe the patient vividly and specifically so that others can imagine the patient.

Appearance and Behavior
- Appearance: clothing, gait, posture, level of consciousness (alert, drowsy, fluctuating, etc.), grooming (cleanliness, odor, makeup), personal belongings (especially items that may denote hobbies, family support, or lack thereof)
- Behavior: What the was patient doing before and during the interview, eye contact, gestures, facial expression
  - Note: You will hear the term "psychomotor activity (agitation/retardation)" often. These are changes in level of physical movement, often accompanied by a change in speed of thinking.
  - Psychomotor agitation is an unintentional increase in physical movement, which may manifest as pacing, foot tapping, handwringing, scratching, and more. It may be indicative of anxiety, drug use or withdrawal, manic episodes, and more.
  - Psychomotor retardation is a reduction of physical movement compared to baseline, which may manifest as slow reaction times and abandonment of regular activities including eating and grooming. Everyday tasks that require some physical or mental challenge, such as climbing stairs or planning a shopping list, may be described by the patient as too difficult to tackle. It is often seen in major depressive episodes and as a result of depressant ingestion.
- Attitude: cooperative, guarded, defensive, evasive, apathetic, disingenuous, distracted, sarcastic

Speech
- Rate: fast, slow, normal, pressured (the patient is difficult to interrupt and seems to have some internal pressure to continue speaking rapidly)
- Rhythm: regular, hesitant, slurred, aphasic
- Volume: normal, soft, loud, monotone, mumbled
- Latency (delay) in answering questions

Emotion (Mood and Affect)
- Mood: the patient's stated emotional state. Use the words the patient uses about how they are feeling, i.e., "I've been really down."
- Affect: what you observe about the patient's emotions.
  - Quality: happy, elated, euphoric, sad, despondent, irritable, enraged, anxious, nervous.

- Intensity: blunted (little emotional expression or reactivity), flat (no emotional expression or reactivity, even to normally intense stimuli).
- Range: normal, constricted (stays within a limited range of emotions), labile (rapid shifts between different emotional states).
- If affect matches mood, it is "mood-congruent"; otherwise, it is "mood-incongruent".

Perception (Auditory/Visual Hallucinations)

━ Ask the patient directly, and also observe whether they appear to be responding to internal stimuli (e.g., glancing at points in the room, easily distracted as if they are listening to something else, etc.)

Thought Content and Process

━ Thought process: Are the thoughts expressed logical, coherent, organized, and linear? Or are they slowed, rapid, or incoherent?
  - Key terms:
  - Circumstantial: Thoughts deviate from the original topic but return in a roundabout way.
  - Tangential: Thoughts deviate from one topic to another without ever returning.
  - Loosening of associations: Thoughts move from one idea to another only loosely related idea.
  - Clang associations or "clanging": Thoughts are related by sound, rather than by concept. Speech may be alliterative or rhyming.
━ Thought content.
  - Suicidal and homicidal ideation, plan, and intent.
  - Delusions (false, fixed beliefs).
  - If these thoughts are acceptable to the patient, or compatible with their values, they are described as ego-syntonic. If the patient tis bothered by them, they are ego-dystonic.

Insight and Judgment

━ Insight: describes a patient's understanding of their own illness. Are they aware of whether or not they have a mental illness? Do they recognize their symptoms? Do they seek help appropriately when needed? Do they reject help?
━ Judgment: Have the patient's actions caused harm to themselves or others? Have they been able to care for themselves and adhere to treatment? How do you view their decision-making capability?

Cognition

━ Note the patient's level of education.
━ Includes orientation, attention, concentration, executive functions, memory, language, visuospatial skills, and calculations. Can be assessed at bedside using Montreal cognitive assessment (MoCA) or mini-mental status exam (MMSE).

12.3.2 Other Sources of Information

The nature of mental illness often prohibits patients from providing a detailed, all-encompassing history. *Collecting collateral information from the patient's family, other providers, work, school, or others who see them regularly and reviewing past medical records is one of the most helpful contributions medical students can have.* By doing this you will provide diagnostic clarity and help guide treatment by understanding what has been tried in the past.

12.4 Clinical Vignette and Note Template

Here is an example of an admission note in an inpatient setting. Notes in psychiatry are known for being long and in a narrative style. This allows for the telling of a coherent story that explains the biological, psychological, and social factors surrounding the presentation. You may see more succinct, checklist-style notes from residents and attendings; clarify what is expected of you during the rotation, but generally, medical students have the time to contribute more detailed notes that can be helpful for the rest of the team.

12.5 Inpatient Psychiatry Initial Note

Patient Name: John Doe

Sources of Information: patient, medical record, patient's spouse

Chief Complaint: "I can't take it anymore."

History of Present Illness:

John Doe is a 35-year-old male, living in Boston with his wife, working as a high school teacher, with past medical history of hypertension and ulcerative colitis and past psychiatry history of major depressive disorder, multiple prior hospitalizations, and one prior suicide attempt, who was referred by his outpatient psychiatrist after endorsing suicidal ideation with plan.

Mr. Doe reports that for the past 2 months, he has felt increasingly depressed and lethargic. He notes reduced appetite and endorses 10 pounds of unintentional weight loss in that time. He has been having trouble falling asleep and sleeps 4–5 hours a night. Normal activities which he enjoys, such as hiking and watching football, have not been bringing him joy. Today he felt that he "[couldn't] take it anymore" and had thoughts of hanging himself in his garage. He was distressed by these thoughts and called his outpatient psychiatrist, Dr. Jones, who referred him to our hospital for inpatient admission.

On interview, Mr. Doe reports that "nothing has been going right in [his] life." He notes that his wife has talked of ending their marriage, which came as a surprise to him. "I don't know if I can live without her." They do not have children due to his infertility. Other stressors include social isolation, feeling that he is not progressing in his career as a high school math teacher, and a strained relationship with his mother, from whom he has been estranged for 3 years. He reports that his current symptoms feel similar to previous depressive episodes or perhaps worse.

Several times per day in the past week, he has had thoughts of dying, such as "Maybe the world would be better off if I just disappeared." He has trouble naming things in life that he is looking forward to. Today he reports having repeated thoughts of hanging himself in his garage, saying, "It would be so easy," but denies intent to complete suicide. Patient completed Columbia Suicide Severity Rating Scale (C-SSRS) and is notable for active suicidal ideation with specific plan and intent in the past month, with moderately strong deterrents and controllability.

Mr. Doe has been previously hospitalized for major depressive episodes three times in 2010, 2012, and 2016 at County Hospital. Has one prior suicide attempt by toxic ingestion of acetaminophen in 2012, for which he was treated in the ED without any sequelae. He has been trialed on paroxetine 60 mg (discontinued due to ineffectiveness) and fluoxetine 40 mg (discontinued due to GI side effects) and had been stable on sertraline 200 mg for several years until now.

Clinical Pearl: Include pertinent social and psychiatric history in the one-liner. The mention of his hospitalizations and suicide attempt helps paint a picture of how serious his course of major depressive disorder has been.

Standout Tip: Employ patient quotes in your note.

Clinical Pearl: Remember the biopsychosocial model – include factors from each domain that may be at play in this patient's presentation.

Clinical Pearl: Do not be afraid to ask questions about suicide. It is a common misconception that they make patients more suicidal; on the contrary, asking is critical to patient safety.

Clinical Pearl: Inclusion of a suicide risk assessment tool, such as the Columbia scale, is now required by the Joint Commission on Accreditation of Healthcare Organizations. Become familiar with these scales and their use.

12

On review of symptoms, he denies elevated mood, racing thoughts, increased goal-directed behavior, or other symptoms of mania. He denies anxiety or panic attacks, auditory or visual hallucinations, and thoughts of violence or homicide. He does not have access to firearms in the home.

He endorses drinking 1–2 beers per week and occasionally smoking marijuana and denies other substance use; his frequency of use of either substance has not changed.

Collateral Information

Jane Doe, wife, 111-111-1111, shares during phone call that John has been eating and sleeping poorly and seems distracted and tired all the time and that he is no longer keeping up with his hobbies. She is concerned that his current presentation appears similar to his presentation prior to his previous hospitalizations. She confirms that there are no firearms in the home.

Past Psychiatric History

Diagnoses: major depressive disorder

Past hospitalizations: 2010, 2012, and 2016 at County Hospital for major depressive episodes and once for suicide attempt. Treated and stabilized with medication titration and psychotherapy.

Suicide attempts/self-injury: 2012, by toxic ingestion of acetaminophen. Was treated in the ED followed by inpatient psychiatric admission with no sequelae of ingestion. Denies history of self-injurious behavior.

Violence: denies.

Substance use history: drinks 1–2 beers per week. Denies prior blackouts, withdrawals. Smokes marijuana every few weeks. Denies tobacco use, other illicit drug use.

Family psychiatric history: Maternal uncle died by suicide at age 45.

Psychiatrist: Dr. Jones, since 2008, 222-222-2222

Therapist: none

Additional providers: none

Past Medical History

Hypertension (on amlodipine)

Ulcerative colitis (on mesalamine)

Medications

Amlodipine 10mg daily

Mesalamine 800mg TID

Sertraline 150mg daily

Past medication trials: paroxetine 60mg daily (ineffective), fluoxetine 40mg daily (GI side effects)

Allergies: none.

Social History

The patient was born and raised in Worcester, MA. Raised by a single mother; father left when the patient was an infant and has had no contact with the family. Reportedly normal development, no known history of head injuries, denies history of being abused or trauma. The patient reports being a good student, completed a bachelor's degree, and has been teaching high school math in Boston for 12 years. Lives in an apartment in Boston with his wife of 14 years. Currently about to begin divorce proceedings. Is now estranged from his mother and desires a relationship with her, but he has not reached out. Reports having few friends or close family members. Enjoys hiking and watching football. Denies having access to firearms. No legal history. Financially stable.

Clinical Pearl: Ask about other psychiatric symptoms that will help you distinguish between diagnoses.

{

Standout Tip: It would be very helpful for you as a medical student to call or email Dr. Jones to collect collateral information, update her on her patient's hospital course, and discuss potential medication changes.

Involve the outpatient provider in decisions regarding long-term psychiatric medications whenever possible!

}

Clinical Pearl: A thorough physical exam is warranted in the ED and in the admission. During the admission, regular physical exams are often deferred unless the patient has a physical illness, new physical symptoms, or concern for new physical illness.
Things to look for on physical examination include:
- Signs of organic causes of psychiatric symptoms: head trauma, thyroid, malnutrition, drug use/withdrawal
- Sequelae of mental illness: evidence of self-injury or violence including wounds and scars, evidence of drug use or withdrawal (antecubital fossa for intravenous drug use, nares for cocaine, dilated pupils, etc.)
- Side effects of antipsychotic medications: neuroleptic malignant syndrome, serotonin syndrome, extrapyramidal symptoms

Clinical Pearl: Quotes are great for capturing the patient's mood as accurately as possible. However, it is also important to put down your own interpretation, as sometimes patients won't or can't describe their own mood.

Physical Examination

Vital signs: BP 118/59 | Pulse 78 | Temp 36.4C | Resp 20 | SpO2 100%

General: appears to be in no acute distress

HEENT: normocephalic, PERRL, EOMI, neck supple, non-tender without lymphadenopathy

Cardiac: normal heart sounds, no murmurs, regular rate and rhythm

Lungs: clear to auscultation bilaterally

Abdomen: positive bowel sounds. Soft, nontender, nondistended

Extremities: no edema. No significant deformity

Neurological: CN II-XII intact. Normal gait

Mental Status Examination (Refer to ◘ Fig. 12.1)

Appearance: disheveled, tired-appearing man who appears stated age, lying down in bed staring at ceiling. Appears mildly overweight. Poorly kempt hair and beard. Dark bags under eyes. Wearing hospital garb. On the bedside table, there is a cell phone, biography about a football coach, and get-well-soon card.

Behavior: eye contact kept toward ceiling and limited. Frowning or neutral expression throughout interview, not noted to smile or laugh. Patient cooperative but seems distracted. Psychomotor retardation.

Speech: soft, mumbled speech. Slight latency in response to questions.

Mood: depressed, "I've been really down."

Affect: mood congruent, constricted to despondent and sad, at times tearful.

Thought Process: logical, linear, and goal-directed.

Thought Content: endorses suicidal ideation with plan but no intent. Denies homicidal ideation. No evidence of paranoia or delusions. Denies auditory or visual hallucinations, does not appear to be responding to internal stimuli.

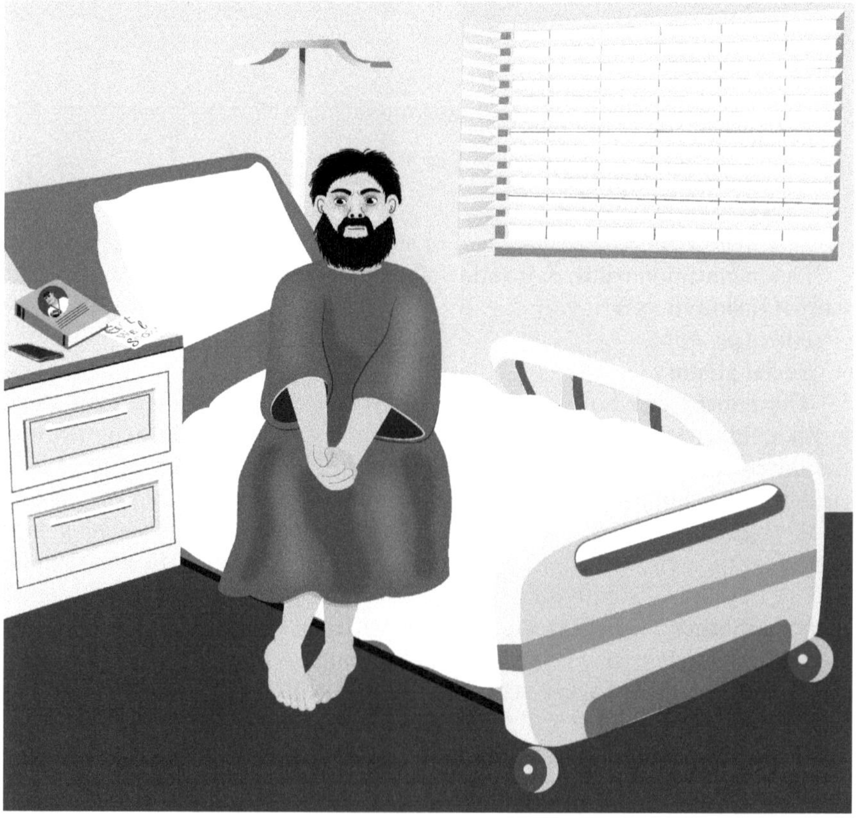

◘ **Fig. 12.1** Example patient

Insight: good. The patient recognized that current symptoms are similar to past major depressive episodes. Able to name social stressors and supports. Accepts help.

Judgment: good. Patient sought help appropriately when he felt he was in danger. Has been adherent to medications. However, patient has not been grooming or eating as he normally would.

Impulse Control: intact on the unit.

Cognitive Exam

Orientation: alert and oriented to person, place, and time

Memory: immediate recall, short-term memory, and long-term memory intact

Attention/Concentration: able to name the days of the week backward

Fund of Knowledge: average, completed college

Language: normal comprehension

Labs/Imaging

Urine toxicology: positive for THC. Per chart review, previous workup showed normal TSH, vitamin B12, CBC, electrolytes. Negative for HIV

Assessment

John Doe is a 35-year-old male with past psychiatric history of major depressive disorder with multiple prior hospitalizations and one prior suicide attempt.

Mr. Doe's presentation is notable for depressed mood and affect; anhedonia; changes in appetite, concentration, and sleep; and suicidal ideation, which are consistent with a major depressive episode in the setting of multiple life stressors, including social isolation and difficulties in his marriage and personal relationships. Given psychomotor retardation and speech latency, there is some concern for catatonia, and this will be evaluated further.

From a safety perspective, the patient is at chronically elevated risk of harm to self-given chronic major depressive disorder, prior suicide attempt, and male sex. The risk is acutely elevated from baseline given current suicidal ideation with plan (without intent), lack of social supports, new interpersonal troubles, feelings of worthlessness, and lack of future orientation. He is protected by his strong relationship with his outpatient psychiatrist, good insight and judgment, medication adherence, and lack of current suicidal intent. He presented voluntarily but would also meet criteria for involuntary hospitalization due to acutely elevated risk of harm to self in the setting of psychiatric illness. He requires inpatient admission for safety, diagnostic clarification, medication adjustment, and coordination of aftercare.

- Axis I: major depressive episode, recurrent major depressive disorder, rule-out catatonia
- Axis II: deferred
- Axis III: ulcerative colitis and hypertension; substance use does not appear to be contributing to current presentation

Standout Tip: Providers often leave the insight and judgment sections vague, writing only "fair," "poor," "good," etc. Your team will appreciate it if you leave a more detailed justification in the note as it will be helpful for tracking symptoms over time and for justifying continued treatment.

Clinical Pearl: This is an extra part of the mental status that may be used on your team. Try to give other providers reading the note a sense of what to expect from the patient, and this is a key element for clinical decisions and treatment planning. Descriptors can include "intact on the unit", "lacking control", "tenuous", etc.

Clinical Pearl: Remember the three questions that we use to approach every patient, and make sure they are answered in the assessment and plan: "What is this patient experiencing now that has brought them here?"

Clinical Pearl: "Why now?"

Clinical Pearl: These laws vary by state – learn your state's law and what criteria must be met for involuntary hospitalization.

Clinical Pearl: "What can be done to help them?". You will also attempt to address the risk factors and leverage the protective factors mentioned above.

This is the DSM multi-axial system that may or may not be used in the notes on your team (it was removed in the DSM-5 but can still be seen at some institutions, and you may see it in old notes). If it is used, here is what to note:

- Axis I: all psychological diagnostic categories except intellectual disability and personality disorder.
- Axis II: personality disorders and intellectual disability.
- Axis III: medical conditions and physical disorders.
- Axis IV: psychosocial and environmental factors contributing to the disorder.
- Axis V: global assessment of functioning – a numeric scale to rate the functioning of an individual. Note that this is subjective and unnuanced and is mostly used for billing and litigation purposes. Generally:
  - 81–100: absent tor minimal symptoms, functioning well.
  - 61–80: mild or transient symptoms with some effect on function.
  - 41–60: moderate to severe symptoms and difficulty with social, occupational, or school functioning.
  - 21–40: problems with reality testing, communication, insight, and judgment that leads to severe impairment in several areas of life.
  - 1–20: Patient is in danger of hurting themselves or others.

If DSM axes are not used, then simply list the problems, including the medical ones.

- Axis IV: lack of friends and social isolation, ongoing divorce from wife, estrangement from mother, sense of worthlessness
- Axis V: 40–50.

Plan:
- Major Depressive Disorder

Diagnostic:
- Urine toxicology positive for THC. Workup from previous hospitalizations notable for normal TSH, vitamin B12, CBC, electrolytes. Negative for HIV.
- Perform bedside Bush-Francis scale to rule out catatonia.
- Continue to track symptoms of depressed mood and affect; anhedonia; changes in appetite, concentration, and sleep; and suicidal ideation.

Treatment:
- Increase sertraline to 200 mg daily.
- Develop a safety plan and recovery plan with the patient.
- Social worker involved; initiate psychosocial interventions.
- Consult psychology for counseling on interpersonal skills and safety planning.
- Encourage participation in groups.

- Ulcerative Colitis and Hypertension
  – Continue home mesalamine and amlodipine.

Legal status: voluntary
  Discharge plan:
- Living situation: lives with wife
- Follow-up: with outpatient psychiatrist
- Anticipated discharge date: TBD

12.6 Differentiating the Differential

Diagnoses within psychiatry are based on the Diagnostic and Statistical Manual of Mental Disorders, Fifth Edition (DSM-5). As a medical student, it is not necessary to purchase or read the DSM (though you may refer to it at times to understand its rationale and layout). Seeing presentations of these disorders during your rotation, as well as currently available test prep and question bank resources, is sufficient for learning about these disorders and doing well on your rotation. Here are some broad buckets of diagnoses to consider and some of the most common ones you will see. Note that this list is not exhaustive and does not include all of the diagnoses that will appear on the NBME shelf exams but rather a sample of what you are most likely to see and should ask about on your rotation as a medical student.
- Affective disorders – major depressive disorder, bipolar disorder
- Anxiety disorders – generalized anxiety disorder, social anxiety disorder, panic disorder, specific phobia
- Trauma-related disorders – posttraumatic stress disorder (PTSD)
- Psychotic disorders – schizophrenia, schizoaffective disorder, delusional disorder, brief psychotic disorder
- Substance use disorders

- Personality disorders – borderline personality disorder, obsessive-compulsive personality disorder, narcissistic personality disorder
- Neurocognitive and neurodevelopmental disorders – autism spectrum disorder, attention-deficit/hyperactivity disorder (ADHD), delirium
- Other things you might see – eating disorders, somatic symptom disorder, conversion disorder, factitious disorder
- With each of these disorders, consider:
  - *What comorbidities exist?* Many of these disorders can coexist. *Even if a patient does not meet diagnostic criteria, they may have traits or characteristics of other disorders that you can inquire about, note in the assessment, and target in the plan.* If something feels "off" or working with the patient feels unusually difficult, explore the possibility of a comorbid diagnosis, especially personality disorders or substance use.
  - Do substances play a role?
    - *Ask about substance use, and if present, does it always precede the depressive/manic/psychotic episode? If it follows the episode, the substance use may be "self-medication" rather than causative.*
    - Withdrawal symptoms may mimic other disorders.
    - Most of your patients should get a urine/blood serum toxicology screen during workup.
  - Do other medical conditions play a role?
    - Discuss with your team the possibility of an organic cause of the presentation. Suspicion should be raised in *unusual presentations*, i.e., new-onset psychosis in an older patient, focal neurologic symptoms, underlying medical illness, history of head trauma, etc.
    - Your investigation may include thyroid function studies, cortisol levels, blood chemistries, complete blood count, STI screening, and pregnancy test. For older patients or those with chronic medical illness, consider folate and vitamin B12.
    - *Head imaging* (CT or MRI brain) for most psychiatric disorders is not common but should be considered in unusual circumstances when there are other symptoms (cognitive impairment, focal neurologic signs) to suggest structural brain disease. One-time head imaging is common for new-onset psychosis.

> Standout Tip: Include the use of a validated screening tool, such as the Hamilton Depression Scale or Beck Depression Inventory. Every patient deserves at least one good tool for quantifying symptoms, and this would be a standout thing for a student to contribute.

> Clinical Pearl: Remember that diagnoses are broad buckets that are often more useful for communication, billing, and research purposes than they are for understanding your patient. If your gut tells you that there is more going on than can be captured in one diagnosis, trust that feeling, and explore the patient's history further. Similarly, even if a history does not perfectly align with a diagnosis, take the parts of the presentation that seem most actionable, and think about how you can treat those symptoms and psychosocial problems. Consider the entire clinical picture before you, as it will be more nuanced than simply a diagnosis.

12.7 A Day in the Life

Here is an example of a typical workday for a medical student on an inpatient psychiatry rotation (◻ Table 12.3). Of course, this will vary by institution and team, so ask your team what is expected of you and how you can best contribute and learn.

12.7.1 Daily Task List

- Before Rounds
  - For each patient, write down significant overnight events, medications and PRNs taken, notable vitals, and lab/imaging findings.
  - For each patient, consider what symptoms to ask about, and have a tentative plan in mind.

◘ **Table 12.3** A day in the life

7:30 AM	Arrive to *pre-round*, which in psychiatry, typically does not involve seeing the patient For each of your patients, check overnight nursing notes (paying attention for changes in symptoms, agitation, trouble sleeping, PRNs given, etc.), labs and vitals if applicable, and medication administration record. Be prepared to briefly discuss this with your team before rounds to "game plan" what will be discussed
8:00 AM	*Round* as a team. Typically done with you, resident, attending, social worker, nurse, and other members of the interprofessional team in a conference room or at bedside. Oftentimes either the resident or attending will conduct the interview while the other writes the note. For the first day or two, observe how the resident or attending leads the interview and then advocate for yourself to lead the interview for your own patients for the rest of the rotation. This is a good chance for you to be observed get feedback on your interview style, so be sure to ask beforehand When rounding, stay open-ended in the beginning. Also be sure to ask about "target symptoms" that you are tracking, such as mood, anxiety, hallucinations, suicidal ideation, etc., that will serve as indicators of clinical progress or decompensation. Once you are done, invite other members of the team and the patient themselves to ask questions, too After all questions have been asked, summarize for the patient what has been discussed and the basic plan for the day, including discharge planning.
12:00 PM	Finish rounding – Yes, rounding on psychiatry can last quite a while! Fortunately, you are usually in a chair. Make sure that you and the team run the list and divvy up all the "to do" items before you break Attend *noon conference*
1:00 PM	*Update notes, assessment, and plans.* Learn from your resident what templates they use and what their style is. Aim to produce notes and plans that are good enough that the resident only needs to skim and sign without major modification *Order labs/imaging and titrate medications as needed* *Call consults and follow up as needed. Call collateral* (outpatient providers, family members), and review past records or outside records for more information. These can be time-consuming but are also some of the most helpful things a medical student can do
3:00 PM	*Spend time with patients.* If further information is needed for diagnostic clarity, try to find a private space on the unit to conduct further interview. If not, just chatting with the patient casually outside of rounds can help build rapport. If you have nothing else to do, just spending time in the unit common space with your patients (chatting, playing board games, drawing, writing, etc.) is both informative and also improves rapport
5:00 PM	*Sign out* to the evening/overnight coverage
Other activities	Didactics Case presentation. Among your patients, keep in mind someone who might be interesting to write up and discuss During your rotation, ask your team if you can join some of the group therapy, skill-building, and activity sessions. It will be helpful for your learning, and if your patient is attending as well, you can gain insight on how they interact with others Ask to observe electroconvulsive therapy (ECT) if your hospital offers it Ask to join a resident doing consult/liaison psychiatry for a morning/afternoon

- During Rounds
  - Take the lead and interview your own patients. Jot down or remember a few quotes for the note later.
  - Note things that are new or surprising to you (about all patients, not just your own) and treatments you would like to learn more about. Look these up and ask your team about them later.
- Afternoon
  - Update the patient note and handoff information.
  - Write discharge summaries for patients who are leaving.
  - Order and follow-up on labs and consults.
  - Call for collateral information.
  - Email/call the outside psychiatrist to discuss the hospital course and plan with them.
  - Spend time with the patient (collect additional history, play games, etc.).
- Outside the Hospital

- Finish up notes left over from the afternoon.
- Study for standardized exams.
- Relax! Psychiatry should be light on prep work.

12.8 The Team

Here are some of the members of the team you will work with as you care for your patients. Push yourself to get to know them and to leverage their expertise, as it will help you stand out as a star medical student.

- The attending: the one in charge. You may see them often, or they may have you report to the resident.
  - Week 1: Watch them interview a patient or defuse a situation (such as agitation) and learn. They are the pros.
  - Rest of rotation: Ask them to observe you interview a patient, and ask for feedback on your interview style.
- The resident: most likely the person you'll report to directly.
  - Week 1: Ask them how they'd like for you to contribute to their workflow, write notes, and volunteer for tasks (calling consults, collecting additional history, checking labs, etc.)
  - Rest of rotation: Ask them for feedback on your notes, interview style, and how you can better contribute to the team and to your patient's care.
- The social worker: a wizard at connecting patients to resources and collecting collateral information.
  - Week 1: Ask them what they know about the patients you're following. They'll likely have been in contact with the patients' families and are working on their disposition (discharge planning). You will stand out if you're able to share with your resident and attending some options for your patients after they leave (outpatient programs, homeless shelters, etc.).
  - You can contribute to the team by reaching out to patients' families for collateral information, but discuss this with the social worker first to make sure you're not repeating work they've already done and to plan your data gathering with the expert.
- The nurse: the person who spends the most time with your patient and sees the most of their behavior.
  - Week 1: Get in a habit of checking in with the nurse every morning or at least once in a while, to hear about how the patient has been doing. They may have a good sense of the patient's sleep, appetite, mood, and behavior.
  - Give them a heads-up about medication changes so that they're not surprised and so that they're ready to help address patients' questions.
- The pharmacist: the expert on all things and drugs.
  - If you have questions about dosing, drug-drug interactions, and the like, ask the pharmacist assigned to your unit.
- Others: You may encounter case managers, occupational therapists, and other members of the interdisciplinary team that can vary by unit and by institution. Learn from your resident and attending how you can work with them constructively.

12.9 Common Errors

- *Not showing an interest in your patients.* Your patients do not necessarily have to like you (and in fact, it is the nature of some disorders that patients may appear combative or apathetic towards you), but *you should demonstrate to the team that you do care about them.* This is reflected in your atti-

Table 12.4 Patient-centered language

Common term	Non-stigmatizing Form
Crazy, lunatic, the mentally ill	Person/people with mental illness
Committed suicide	Died by suicide
Addict, drug abuser, alcoholic	Person with substance (alcohol, opioid, etc.) use disorder, person who injects drugs
Clean	Abstinent, not actively using
Dirty	Actively using
Clean/dirty drug screen	Testing negative/positive for substance use
Mental retardation	Intellectual disability
Schizophrenic	Person with schizophrenia
Manic-depressive	Person with bipolar disorder
Demented	Person with neurocognitive disorder

tude toward the patient (nonjudgmental, concerned), the time you spend caring for them (discussing the case with your team, writing notes, exploring the literature on possible treatment options, collecting collateral information), how you advocate for them, and the way you talk about them (using non-stigmatizing, patient-centered language).

- *Using stigmatizing language.* You will pick this up as you hear it, but in general, remember that patients are people first. Why is this important? Some labels carry a historical connotation that leads to discrimination and shame. This can affect your ability to build good rapport with your patients (Table 12.4).

12.10 How to Stand Out

- *Demonstrate an interest in learning.* Ask questions about patients that you see on rounds even if they aren't the ones you are following. Look up other potential treatment options and discuss them to your team.
- *Spend time with your patients and share what you learn with the team.* Your team will likely appreciate it if, for example, you play chess with your patient in the afternoon and both build rapport and learn some additional things about their social situation.
- *Collect collateral information*, review complicated chart histories, and synthesize this for your team in the note.
- *Collaborate* interprofessionally by discussing the case and receiving input from other members of the team, including nursing, social work, and the patient's outpatient psychiatrist.
- *Be prepared* each morning to report overnight events that may have happened with your patient. If the overnight nurse or provider is still present, discuss with them as well.
- *Be aware* of the subtle differences between medications within the same class. Some examples include:

- Typical/first generation antipsychotics have a greater association with extrapyramidal side effects than do atypical/second generation antipsychotics.
- Among second generation antipsychotics, olanzapine and clozapine carry the highest metabolic risk.
- Clozapine is highly effective but carries a risk of agranulocytosis, so it requires regular blood draws and monitoring.
- Cost is worth considering as patients will not take what is prescribed unless they can afford it. You can compare costs of various medications online.

- Have a basic understanding of the *legal frameworks* that patients pass through in your state. Look up or ask about laws governing involuntary hospitalization and involuntary treatment.
- Develop a basic appreciation for different modalities of *psychotherapy*. As a medical student in the inpatient setting, you will not have the time or supervision to thoroughly develop any skills in psychotherapy, which is often built in the outpatient setting in residents. However, you will likely see elements of psychotherapy being used during the care of your patient. You should ask about basic tenets and about picking up some simple skills.
- Go out of your way to experience other settings of psychiatric care. Ask if you can spend some time observing ECT, and consult psychiatry, outpatient psychiatry, group therapy, and more.
- In psychiatry, you will not be relegated to holding retractors! You will have the opportunity to be the primary clinician for your patients. Own it all and you will stand out wonderfully.

Primary Care

Bliss J. Chang

Contents

© The Author(s), under exclusive license to Springer Nature Switzerland AG 2021
S. H. Lecker, B. J. Chang (eds.), *The Ultimate Medical School Rotation Guide*,
https://doi.org/10.1007/978-3-030-63560-2_13

13.1 Overview

When most people first think about the responsibilities of a doctor, they envision work that is performed by a primary care physician. Primary care is a broad field that is the foundation of modern healthcare. In your primary care rotation, you will have the opportunity to build core competencies that will help you succeed in whatever specialty you ultimately choose.

This chapter begins with various fundamentals from a primary care perspective. We will then delve into the most common cases you will encounter on your primary care rotation. Refer to ▶ Chap. 6 for a great section ▶ Sect. 6.2. Throughout, we emphasize learning how to prepare for primary care visits rather than the exhaustive list of potential cases.

13.2 Fundamentals

In primary care, the ultimate question is "How do we ensure that the patient is healthy physically, mentally, and socially," and its broad nature reflects how primary care covers disease prevention, management of acute conditions, and everything in between. Unlike specialists, who spend most of their time treating already diagnosed conditions, primary care doctors are responsible for primary prevention, that is, preventing a disease from ever developing in the first place.

Please refer to ▶ Sect. 6.3 of ▶ Chap. 6 for complementary reading. Here, we will primarily explore the role of a primary care physician using the key clinic visit types:

- Checkup visits
- Follow-up visits
- New complaint

Importantly, primary care is a rotation that focuses on the complete care of the patient, from when you first meet them to after everything has been taken care of by you and/or other providers. Thus, continuity is key, and caring for your patient sometimes extends beyond clinic hours. Accordingly, for each visit type, we will explore three aspects: before the visit, during the visit, and after the visit.

13.2.1 Checkup Visits

These are the visits that you will think are the most straightforward. However, most patients that are coming in are not healthy 20-year-olds like yourself. They are often older patients with many comorbidities, and it is critical to treat these visits as serious as any other visit – do not let your guard down simply going through a series of motions without critical evaluation. There are a few different categories of checkups: general and disease-specific (e.g., diabetic checkups). We will focus on the general checkup here.

The goal of a checkup visit is to ensure that the patient is in good (baseline) health and to catch anything brewing early (this means reviewing all of the patient's comorbidities). Remember the latter each time you see a patient for a checkup, because that really helps to frame your mind and primes you for the rest of the visit.

13.2.1.1 Before the Visit

Establishing the Baseline

This is generally done the night before your clinic day – this can take time, so you should look up your patients the night before. If you do not have access on your home computer, talk to your preceptors and upperclassmen to figure out how you can gain access – this is a life changer and must do, if allowed at your institution. Start by referring to the prior checkup office note, if it exists. This is a great place to gather the details of what was done previously, whether anything was flagged for follow-up, and the general sense of your patient's health. The following are steps which you should follow to ensure a thorough review of your patient's history prior to showing up to clinic.

Things to Review Since Last Checkup:
- [] Last check-up note
- [] Notes from other providers/hospitalizations since last visit
- [] Current medication list
- [] Procedures since last visit
- [] Labs since last visit, including any pre-visit labs
- [] Social situation (e.g., housing stability, areas for counseling such as smoking cessation)
- [] Patient communications to provider

You do not have to pore over notes from other providers, procedures, and labs in exhaustive detail. This is not a follow-up visit (detailed later), and the purpose of reviewing these is to obtain a sense of how the patient has been faring. One trick is to jot down a quick summary of each thing you review – how does this contribute to the big picture? Specifically, try to (1) obtain a sense of what happened to the patient since the last visit with you, (2) recognize what needs to be done, and (3) identify things that were missed. Always trust but verify – even the best providers miss things here and there in the bustle of their practices, and exceptional care of the patient is a team effort spanning providers and clinic visits.

■ **Example Notes on Patient Chart Review**

Mrs. Johnson, 71F, MRN 123456789

HTN, HLD, T2DM (last A1C 8.9% 01/19/2019, up from 8.1%), HFrEF (last EF 35% on 07/12/2018)

Prior checkup: unclear complaint of fatigue without red flags and obvious diagnosis, opted for watchful waiting, keep malignancy on differential and check weight next visit

Labs: unremarkable last visit and pre-visit

Cardiologist follow-up note 1 month ago: HFrEF stable, adherent to GDMT but occasionally forgoes taking her metoprolol due to subjective notion that it is causing her fatigue; no evidence per our clinic visit

Even if there is a prior note, you should always confirm with your patient if possible the key details you gathered from chart review. If there is no prior note, you will need to do some more extensive chart review, simply because you will need to review (succinctly) all the medical record thus far, not just after the prior checkup. However, sometimes preceptors will want you to see patients without having looked at the chart at all. In these cases, you should be prepared to efficiently review a chart while chatting with the patient (always maintaining a healthy dose of eye contact).

Lastly, if there is no documented electronic medical record for a patient, then you are in luck tonight, but expect to spend more time uncovering the patient's medical history tomorrow.

That's it, you're now ready to see the patient in clinic tomorrow!

13.2.1.2 During the Visit

As a primary care physician, it is arguably even more important to build rapport with your patient than in other specialties because you are the person they are most likely to come to first for their medical problems. Building this relationship is critical to inspire the patient's confidence and trust in you so that they will not hesitate to communicate anything related to their health. Thus, a significant portion of your visit should ideally be unrelated to medicine and simply a conversation with the patient about how they are doing, what's going on that's exciting in their life, and so forth. Keep in mind, however, your time constraints as a clerkship student. Refer to ▶ Chap. 1 for more details. Furthermore, conversation itself is an extremely valuable opportunity for you to make observations that might be relevant to medical care (e.g., cognitive, speech, mood), so you must, on the one hand, engage in great conversation but also be very vigilant for subtle signs requiring further investigation.

Once rapport is built, gradually ease the conversation from general towards their health. Start with open-ended questions, and let the patient drive telling you their story. You should also verify the information that you obtained from the chart review last night. As a student, time is limited (i.e., using it to gather more relevant information or think about your plan versus chatting with patients), but try to incorporate elements of good holistic patient care. Life is not all about evaluations! Common questions for the patient may include:

- How do they feel their health has been since they last saw you?
- Anything specific that they are worried about?
- How have they been doing with their medications? Living circumstances?

For the various visit types, your duties for examining the patient, presenting your patient, and inputting orders remain the same.

13.2.1.3 After the Visit

You should always try to take on the entire role of the PCP. Not all attendings may offer you the opportunity to engage in these post-visit logistics – if they don't, then ask! Managing a patient from start to finish is a great way to be a standout student on the rotation and is very helpful to your team. These after-visit tasks are usually done after clinic when you are out of the hospital, though sometimes these tasks may become apparent prior to leaving the hospital for the day.

Medical information and decisions should be run by your attending, and then your patient should be updated by either phone or message through the EMR.

The following checklist covers common tasks for after the visit:

- [] Follow-up labs and other results.
  - Always INTERPRET the data – suggest to your attending what you think is going on, why, and what you want to do. This can be in the form of a short email to your attending through the EMR (refer to the example below).
- [] If you told the patient you'd get back to them for anything else, now is the time.

- [] Check to make sure all follow-up visits, specialty referrals, etc. are scheduled appropriately.
- [] Complete EMR documentation.

Example Post-Visit Email to Attending:
Subject: Re Patient [Last Name] [MRN]
Hi Dr. Rosa,

It was great working with you in clinic today. I wanted to run Ms. Abigail's lab results by you prior to calling her with updates.

Most of her labs were in the normal range. However, her potassium is slightly elevated at 4.9. Her prior baselines are in the low 4.0 s, and I worry that this is because of her recently initiated Lisinopril 10 mg. We can consider lowering her dose of lisinopril to 5 mg seeing that her blood pressure is under good control. I would also like to advise Ms. Abigail to avoid high dietary potassium intake through over-consumption of potassium rich foods such as bananas.

Looking forward to hearing your thoughts. Thanks so much!

Best,

Bliss

13.2.2 Follow-Up Visits

These are patients who have recently been hospitalized or undergone surgery and were referred to you to ensure that they are recovering well. These are probably the most difficult patients because you will have a wide array of reasons behind their initial hospitalizations, and it is not possible to know everything that a specialist would know regarding that condition. Furthermore, discharge summaries are often poorly written, leaving a lot of work to be done on your end to piece together the story and ensure the patient receives what they need. Thus, we will focus on how you can best prepare for these cases.

13.2.2.1 Before the Visit

This is a focused visit; thus your chart review should be geared towards the specific clinic visit, hospitalization, or surgery the patient recently underwent. Most of the time, the reason is noted in the primary care follow-up referral which you can find in the EMR. It will be rare that the EMR is not already populated with relevant patient information, but if they are, take the initiative, and ask your attending for details before the end of your clinic shift ("I wanted to read up on my patients for tomorrow, but was unable to find any information in the EMR. Would you mind briefly telling me what the patient is coming in for?").

The difficult part of preparing for a follow-up visit, especially as a medical student, is knowing what is important to focus on during the visit. It is hard because you don't know a ton of medicine yet and even basic things may not be obvious to you yet. This means there is a lot of opportunity for thinking critically and learning rather than remembering. Below, we provide you with a framework to help guide you.

- What was the chief complaint (and, if applicable, diagnosis) for the recent visit?
- What was done?
  - The hospital course, clinic visit note, and/or discharge summaries usually have decent summaries of what was done – though as a medical student,

you have the luxury of time and should dig through the primary notes and data to confirm.

— What has yet to be done?

    – What did the provider(s) want checked or done at the follow-up visit?

Here is an example of notes on a follow-up patient to help shed light on what you may wish to consider during your chart review:

Mr. Cole is a 71 M with history of HFrEF, T2DM, and CAD s/p LIMA to LAD CABG in 2018 who was admitted to Cambridge Health Alliance Hospital for a heart failure exacerbation. Under the care of Dr. XXX, he was diuresed down to his dry weight of 71 kg prior to discharge a week ago. During diuresis, Mr. Cole suffered a minor AKI from over-diuresis. He was sent home on Lasix 40 mg PO QD based on his response to diuresis in-hospital.

In the above summary, here is the application of the thought questions and how they can be used to prepare thoroughly even if you had no knowledge of heart failure exacerbation:

— What was the chief complaint (and, if applicable, diagnosis) for the recent visit?

    Heart failure exacerbation. You can now read briefly about this, just to understand the big picture principles (heart is not pumping well, leads to backflow of blood, increase in fluid in lungs and lower extremities; treatment is to remove and keep off the extra volume). This is all you really need to know (!), though knowing more specifics is never a bad idea.

— What was done?

    The patient was diuresed and then discharged on an oral diuretic which may require dose modification.

    – The hospital course and/or discharge summary usually has decent summaries of this – though as a medical student, you have the luxury of time and should dig through the primary notes and data to confirm.

— What has yet to be done?

    I need to recheck the patient's weight and compare it to baseline in order to determine whether the diuretic dose is appropriate. I also need to check basic labs to ensure the patient's kidney function (given AKI and also initiating the PO Lasix) and electrolytes are fine.

    – What did the other provider(s) want checked or done at the follow-up visit?

Congratulations! Now you have a good sense of what the follow-up visit will entail tomorrow.

13.2.2.2 During the Visit

As with any other primary care visit type, you should devote the first few minutes getting to know your patient as a person and building rapport. This is critical especially in follow-up visits where much of the success of a visit hinges on patient compliance. Studies have shown that patients that like you will do what you recommend more often!

Begin to transition towards the medical portion by inquiring how the patient has been since discharge. Briefly recap the highlights of the patient's recent hospitalization or operation to confirm major details. End by summarizing what the recent hospital team wanted out of this follow-up visit. Ask the patient if they have anything that they are worried about, think has been unusual, or have questions about.

Now you are at the point where you can address the major action items for the follow-up visit. This encompasses a variety of possibilities that are too numerous to discuss here, but what is useful to emphasize is the overarching goal you should have during this portion of the visit.

The ultimate question now is "Is the patient doing well after discharge?" and "How do I ensure they keep doing well after today?". Each question that you ask, and each action that you think perform, should be with these questions in mind.

For example, if we had a patient with heart failure exacerbation, even if you didn't know much beyond the basics, you know that the key is to keep the volume off the patient. Thus, you would check for any weight change since discharge and how they've tolerated their diuretic(s), check electrolytes, and discuss risk factors to minimize future exacerbations. These are all things that you can easily think of by thinking about the two questions posed above. Lastly, it's okay to miss something here and there, which you will, and that's how you learn!

If they do not have a specialist and they would benefit from having a specialist who follows them, you should refer them at the end of your visit.

13.2.2.3 After the Visit

There are two main things to do after the visit:
1. Follow-up on any remaining labs/tests.
2. Send a brief update to the provider(s), if not yourself, regarding the follow-up visit. Not only will they appreciate this, but it also helps them to keep track of how their patient is doing.

13.2.3 New Complaint

This is the visit type that you're most likely familiar with from other rotations – a patient presenting with new symptoms for evaluation. These can either be regular scheduled visits or urgent care visits that are typically scheduled no more than a few days out. Refer to the Common Cases section for an overview of the most common topics you'll encounter.

13.2.3.1 Before the Visit

In terms of topics, there are general buckets, but the range of complaints span much wider than in most specialty clinics where most patients come in with a few specific conditions. Thus, it is particularly important to prep in advance for tomorrow's clinic patients. If the patient is coming in for a call the same day, you're unlikely to have had time to prepare. This is tough if your medical knowledge is limited, but you will improve over the course of the rotation as you begin seeing the same cases over and over again.

13.2.3.2 During the Visit

This is similar to clinic visits in other specialties. After pleasantries, you will attempt to characterize what is going on with the patient and what to do about it. If you do not have a systematic approach to these visits, I recommend reading the Deep Diver Approach in the General Skills/Pearls chapter.

Some advices for unfamiliar cases include:

- [] Don't be afraid to take some extra time to read up on the topic after seeing the patient.
- [] You should go back and ask questions or perform exam maneuvers that you forgot.
- [] Let your preceptor know that you want some extra time to collect your thoughts.

13.2.3.3 After the Visit

Ensure that all workup that needs to be completed is either performed or scheduled prior to the patient leaving. Specialist referrals should also be made if applicable. Make a note somewhere to follow up with your patient regarding the status of their chief complaint at the next clinic visit. You may also consider setting a reminder to call and check in with them in a few weeks, prior to their next visit with you.

Note:

Lastly, it is not uncommon for your patients to come to you for truly urgent needs such as chest pain. Because of the relationships they've developed with their PCPs, they come to the office for an urgent care appointment (or sometimes even a regular appointment), rather than to the emergency department. It is critical that you never assume that a patient is coming for a non-acute visit – always take the initiative and rule out the need for urgent interventions. A good proportion of ED visits are of patients sent in by their PCPs.

13.3　Common Cases

13.3.1　Diabetes

The state of having a high blood glucose at an isolated moment in time is not particularly problematic. In fact, this can be a physiologic response at times such as stress and anaerobic exercise. The pathologic effects of diabetes occur specifically during the prolonged, chronic elevation of blood glucose levels known as diabetes. Type 2 (non-insulin dependent) diabetes is one of the most common cases in a primary care clinic. This may present in the form of a new diagnosis or follow-up.

13.3.1.1 New Diagnosis

Goals of Visit

- [] Establish or begin to establish a diagnosis of T2DM.
- [] Assess for complications of DM.
- [] Control the blood glucose.
- [] Establish a longitudinal relationship and engender trust/compliance.
- [] Education about the diagnosis.

Presentation

A diagnosis of diabetes starts with appropriate suspicion based on classic symptoms that speak to the osmotic diuresis effects of high blood glucose. In the USA, it is rare for a new diagnosis patient to present with the long-standing complications of diabetes such as retinopathy, neuropathy, neurogenic bladder, and repeated foot infections.

Key Symptom Checklist

- [] Increased thirst and water intake
- [] Increased urination, including throughout the night
- [] Vision change (blurring)
- [] Nonspecific symptoms: fatigue, hunger, irritability, weight loss

Exam

Early in its course, diabetes does not display many specific physical exam findings. However, there are a number of common complications to screen for both at diagnosis and follow-up visits.

- [] Diabetic retinopathy – funduscopic exam
- [] Peripheral neuropathy (beginning in toes) – monofilament exam, vibration test
- [] Brewing infections (most commonly foot) – examine all aspects of the foot for signs of infection and potential portals of entry (e.g., cuts, scratches)

Labs

An official diagnosis of diabetes can be obtained in two distinct ways, depending on whether the patient presents symptomatically or not. If a patient presents with classic symptoms of osmotic diuresis, all that is needed is a random blood glucose greater than 200 mg/dL. However, if the patient is asymptomatic, the diagnosis may be obtained using one of three specific tests: fasting serum glucose ($\geq$126 mg/dL), hemoglobin A1C ($\geq$6.5%), or an oral glucose tolerance test ($\geq$200 mg/dL 2 hours after a 75 g sugar load). Notably, two positive tests on separate occasions must be made to diagnose asymptomatic diabetes.

Pearl: The HbA1C is the most reliable marker of diabetes as it reflects the average concentration of sugars in the blood over the past 3 months. There are a few factors that may change the A1C level to always consider:

- Underestimation
  - Hemodialysis
  - Shortening of RBC lifespan (e.g., sickle cell)
- Overestimation
  - Anemia
  - Renal failure
  - Recent steroid use

Pearl: The OGTT is rarely used outside of pregnancy due to its inconvenient nature.

Treatment

The management for diabetes can be quite complex, and diabetic specialists exist at many academic centers. However, you should know the basic management carried out in a primary care clinic. We will discuss the (1) treatment goals and (2) treatment options.

Treatment goals are always set with benefit to risk ratios in mind. For diabetic complications, many studies have shown that lowering the A1C leads to significant benefits in clinical outcomes. However, decreasing the A1C below 7% has diminishing clinical returns with increased risk of side effects such as hypoglycemia. Thus, the standard A1C goal for patients is under 7%. However, these goals should always be tailored to the individual patient. For example, elderly patients who are at higher risk of hypoglycemia should receive less aggressive glucose control with a target of 7.5–8.0%. Fasting morning sugar levels should be greater than 75 (lower would suggest risk for hypoglycemia) and ideally under 100. Lastly, diabetes is a progressive disease, and almost all patients' diabetic control will worsen over time, and their goals may need to be adjusted appropriately.

Foremost among treatment options, all patients should begin lifestyle modifications, including diet adjustment and exercise. Diabetic diets focus on minimizing simple carbohydrates and substituting with complex carbs such as whole grains. Patients should be encouraged to carefully track their diet, exercise, and morning fasting blood sugars in a diary. You should review this diary during each follow-up visit to ensure that the patient's blood glucose goals are being met and that they are not becoming hypoglycemic (particularly common in elderly patients).

Pearl: One of the most common side effects of metformin is diarrhea which usually resolves within a few weeks of initiation. Thus, it is worth continuing the metformin and seeing if the diarrhea resolves.

Pearl: SGLT-2 inhibitors have been shown to have a reduction in major cardiovascular events and all-cause mortality, regardless of diabetes status. Refer to the EMPA-REG, DECLARE-TIMI 58, and CANVAS trials for further reading.

Pharmacologic treatment of diabetes can be thought of as either non-insulin or insulin-based management. Type 2 diabetes will always be managed with non-insulin options until the disease progresses to a point where these medications are no longer sufficient. The most common pharmacologic classes are metformin, sulfonylureas, glipizides, and, more recently, SGLT-2 inhibitors. ◘ Figure 13.1 details the most common diabetic pharmacologic agents. Notably, metformin is used either as monotherapy or added to every diabetic regimen unless the patient is unable to tolerate it.

Refer to ◘ Fig. 13.2 for an algorithmic approach to determining glycemic control regimens. In brief, almost all patients receive metformin because of how well tolerated it is and its synergistic mechanism with various other classes. When a patient's A1C is not well-controlled (goal <7%), the next step is to add a second agent from a different class, most commonly a sulfonylurea, glipizide, or more recently SGLT-2 inhibitor. Though there are other classes such as GLP-1 agonists and DPP-4 inhibitors, those are utilized less frequently and more circumstantially. For example, GLP-1 agonists provide the best weight loss among glycemic control agents.

Insulin is reserved for when diabetic management is not effective with other medications. Insulin is typically considered when A1C reaches above 8%, with

Class	Example	Mechanism	Lowers A1C By	Notes
Biguanide	Metformin	Decreases hepatic glucose production and insulin sensitivity	1-1.5	Commonly causes diarrhea which resolves in 1-2 weeks
Sulfonylureas	Glipizide Glyburide Glimepride	Stimulates insulin secretion	1-1.5	Watch out for hypoglycemia!
DPP-4 Inhibitors	Saxagliptin Sitagliptin	Increases incretin (GLP-1, GIP) levels	0.5-1	Best weight loss antidiabetic medication
GLP-1 Agonists	Dulaglutide Liraglutide	Incretins increases insulin secretion	0.5-0.75	Also may promote weight loss
Thiazolidinediones	Pioglitazone	PPAR agonist	0.5-1	Increased risk of heart failure
SGLT-2 Inhibitors	Canagliflozin Dapagliflozin Empagliflozin	Inhibits glucose resorption in kidney	0.8-1.5	Increased UTIs, yeast infections
Insulin	Long-acting Short-acting (basal)	Insulin in its purest form!	2-3	Causes weight gain, usually injectable Highest risk of hypoglycemia

◘ **Fig. 13.1** Common diabetic medications

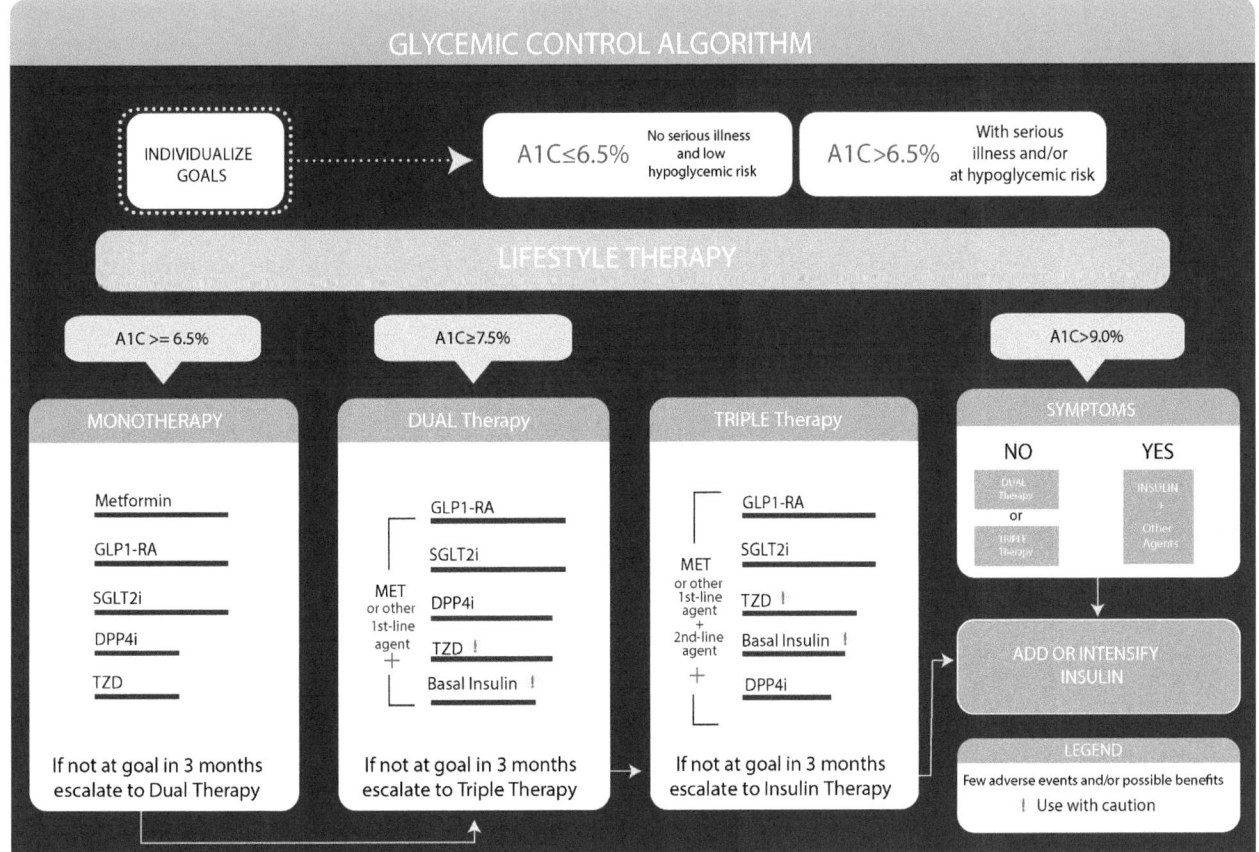

■ Fig. 13.2 Approach to glycemic control

some guidelines suggesting 8.5%. Insulin comes in two forms: basal and meal-time. Basal insulin is the long-lasting insulin used to control levels throughout the whole day, whereas meal-time (postprandial) insulin is to help control the glucose jumps from food intake.

Lastly, diabetes is associated with a strong cardiovascular risk profile secondary to its microvascular effects. Thus, diabetics should be carefully managed with regard to other cardiovascular risk factors such as lipid profiles and blood pressure. In fact, many of these risk factors are treated more aggressively in the presence of diabetes (e.g., when to initiate statin therapy).

Diabetic Treatment Checklist

= [] Lifestyle modifications with daily sugar log
= [] Metformin
= [] Second agent: sulfonylurea, glipizide, or SGLT-2 inhibitor
= [] Consider insulin if A1C >8%

• Fun fact: Insulin is not first-line because it is an invasive medication (injections) and has significant side effects such as weight gain and increased risk of hypoglycemia.

Pearl: Insulin is renally cleared, thus patients with worsening CKD often find that their diabetes naturally improves! You should always consider CKD when dosing insulin.

13.3.1.2 Follow-Up Visits

Goals of Visit
- [] Assess the progress with blood glucose control (lifestyle, medications, compliance).
- [] Assess diabetic complications.
- [] Cardiovascular risk profile management.

The goal for a diabetic follow-up visit is to ensure that the patient's diabetes is being well-managed. Pause here and voice aloud what you think you should do for this visit. It's a great practice on learning how to think based on understanding the overarching premise/goal.

Great! You listed out the following:
- [] Check blood sugar log (for both hypo-/hyperglycemia).
- [] Inquire medication compliance.
- [] Inquire about diet.
- [] Check for diabetic complications on exam.
- [] Diabetic counseling.
- [] Check HbA1C.

If you forgot something above, don't worry; that's expected at this stage. One way to systematically think about the aspects of managing a chronic disease is outlined in the General Pearls/Skills chapter. In our example above, we sort the above into the following buckets:
1. Medications: Check blood sugar Log, and inquire about compliance.
2. Lifestyle: Inquire about diet.
3. Prevention: Check for diabetic complications on exam.
4. Counseling: Continued diabetic counseling.
5. Labs: Check HbA1C.

Checking for Complications of Diabetes

Diabetes is a microvascular (small vessel) disease. This means it also affects the smallest peripheral nerve fibers first which are located at the tips of your extremities, particularly in the toes and feet. This leads to the classic stocking-glove pattern of neuropathy where you progressively lose sensation and/or develop neuropathic pain in an ascending manner starting in the feet and/or fingers. Thus, you want to perform a focused diabetic neurologic exam of the lower extremities (and higher, if advanced diabetes).

The microfilament test is a sensitive test for detecting peripheral neuropathy. Remember from neurology that this same tested tract supplies temperature sensation; thus you don't need to test independently for temperature (which is more subjective anyways). Keep the following in mind as you perform the microfilament test:
- Ask the patient to close their eyes.
- Provide a reference sensation to the patient's fingers.
- The test is validated for use on specific regions of the toes (❏ Fig. 13.3).
- Furthermore, it should always be anticipated that the patient's response is being influenced by visualization of your movements, and so you should pretend to touch areas randomly throughout the test. Alternatively, you can randomly place the monofilament on one of the foot locations, and ask the patient where on the foot you are pressing on.

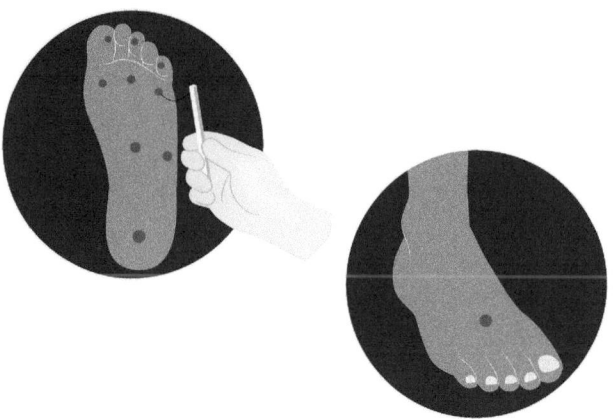

◘ **Fig. 13.3**   Monofilament testing

Diabetic neuropathy also diminishes the sense of proprioception and/or vibration. A tuning fork should be used to check for the patient's sense of vibration, with the result being carefully recorded in the clinic encounter note. The average normal tuning fork test result is at least 10 seconds, but more importantly you should track the changes in vibration sense over time.

13.3.2 Hypertension

Hypertension affects 30% of adults in the USA and is thus no surprise as one of the most common primary care cases. Hypertension is typically managed by PCPs unless severe or refractory, for which patients are referred to hypertension specialists (often nephrologists). As one of the most bread-and-butter topics, you should know this topic inside out.

For the purposes of this book, we will focus only on general hypertension which is defined by the American Heart Association as >130/80 or >150/90 in patients 65 years or older. This discrepancy with age results from the increasing stiffness of the aorta and vasculature over decades which leads to relative hypertension. However, elderly patients often have some degree of autonomic dysfunction and are more prone to hypotensive episodes; thus it was decided that their blood pressure need not be as strictly controlled.

The majority of hypertension results from an entity called primary (essential) hypertension. This means that there is no specific cause that we can find for the hypertension. These patients are usually well-managed with antihypertensive therapy. The remaining cases are termed secondary hypertension, which refers to an underlying cause, such as renal artery stenosis (RAS). These are more likely to be resistant to antihypertensive therapy, and treatment of the underlying cause is essential.

13.3.2.1 Compliance and Why Hypertension Matters

Hypertension is an invisible disease, meaning that patients will not have any symptoms. If they have symptoms due to very high blood pressures, that is known as hypertensive emergency, and they should be directed to the ED immediately. Because chronic hypertension is an invisible disease, some patients may not believe that anything is wrong with them. It is critical to explain to them why we care about hypertension and why they should control their blood pressures. Understanding the why is a huge factor in patient compliance with antihypertensive treatment regimens. Often, I find that patients are able to understand the importance of blood pressure control despite the asymptomatic nature when told about the long-term risks of poorly controlled hypertension such as stroke and MI.

13.3.2.2 New Diagnosis

Goals of Visit
- [] Establish diagnosis of hypertension.
- [] Consider secondary hypertension.
- [] Begin treatment of hypertension, if diagnosed.
- [] Establish therapeutic and longitudinal relationship.

Presentation
You should begin suspecting hypertension if any routine office blood pressures are elevated. This does not mean that the patient has hypertension and simply should pique your attention, particularly the higher the pressures. An official diagnosis of hypertension requires elevated blood pressure readings twice in an ambulatory office setting with readings separated by a minimum of 2 weeks. However, many patients have anxiety that can increase their pressures in a phenomenon known as white coat hypertension. To evaluate patients whom you suspect elevated pressures due to anxiety, we suggest the following steps:
- Remeasure the blood pressure after a while into the office visit after they have had a chance to acclimate to the environment.
- Consider asking the patient to measure their pressures at home.
- Do not trust pressures obtained during an illness, as pain and their acute illness may lead to hypertension.

Once you've confirmed a diagnosis of hypertension, it's worth thinking about whether you suspect primary or secondary hypertension. Generally, patients are assumed to have primary hypertension unless there are clues that suggest otherwise. Clues that make you suspect secondary hypertension include:
- Age <30
- Resistant hypertension (use of three antihypertensives of different classes including a diuretic)
- Electrolyte disorders

Treatment
All patients with hypertension merit lifestyle changes. There have been many studies demonstrating the effectiveness of a variety of lifestyle changes in reducing hypertension, but a few stand out prominently:
- Weight loss: the most effective intervention, with up to a 5–20 mmHg reduction for every 10 kg lost
- DASH Diet: average 8–14 mmHg loss when following a diet rich in fruits, vegetables, and low-fat dairy products
- Exercise: moderately effective at 4–9 mmHg average reduction with regular aerobic exercise

Pharmacologically, here are several antihypertensive therapy classes that may be utilized. Per the latest JNC-8 guidelines, first-line therapy for standard hypertension consists of either an ACE inhibitor, thiazide, or diuretic. This medication is then up-titrated as necessary prior to the addition of a second (or third) antihypertensive, each of which should be in a distinct class. Generally, it is preferred to increase dosages of one class prior to adding a new class. Let's explore the major antihypertensive treatments in ◘ Table 13.1 below.

13.3.2.3 Follow-Up Visits

Goals of Visit
- [] Assess treatment and lifestyle progression.
- [] Tweak treatment regimen as needed.

Although much of the initial management of hypertension can be tried with the antihypertensives in ◘ Table 13.1, there are situational antihypertensives noted in ◘ Table 13.2 that may be considered for patients with comorbidities

◘ **Table 13.1** Key antihypertensive classes

Class	Common examples	Mechanism	Also good for
Ace inhibitors (ACEIs)[a]	Lisinopril	Inhibits conversion of angiotensinogen to angiotensin I	Diabetics, HFrEF
Angiotensin receptor blockers (ARBs)[a]	Losartan	Blocks the binding of angiotensin II to its receptor	Diabetics, HFrEF
Diuretics	Furosemide, Torsemide	Inhibits transporters at different locations in the nephron	Heart failure
Thiazides	Hydrochloro-thiazide	Inhibits the NCC cotransporter in the distal convoluted tubules	Calcium nephrolithiasis

[a]ACEIs and ARBs should NOT be used together due to risk of adverse effects > benefits

◘ **Table 13.2** Alternate antihypertensive classes

Class	Common examples	Mechanism	Also good for
Beta-blockers	Carvedilol, metoprolol, atenolol, propanolol, labetalol	Selective: blocks B1 receptors Nonselective: blocks B1 and B2 +- A1 (carvedilol) receptors	HFrEF, CAD
Calcium channel blockers (CCBs)	Amlodipine	Inhibits L-type calcium channels	Spasms (vasospasm, esophageal spasm)
Smooth muscle vasodilator	Hydralazine	Dilates smooth muscles in arteries/arterioles	Hypertensive emergency, pregnancy
Alpha blockers	Terazosin	Blocks A1 receptors	BPH
Nitric oxide	Imdur	Increases cGMP and leads to both venous and arterial dilation	Angina

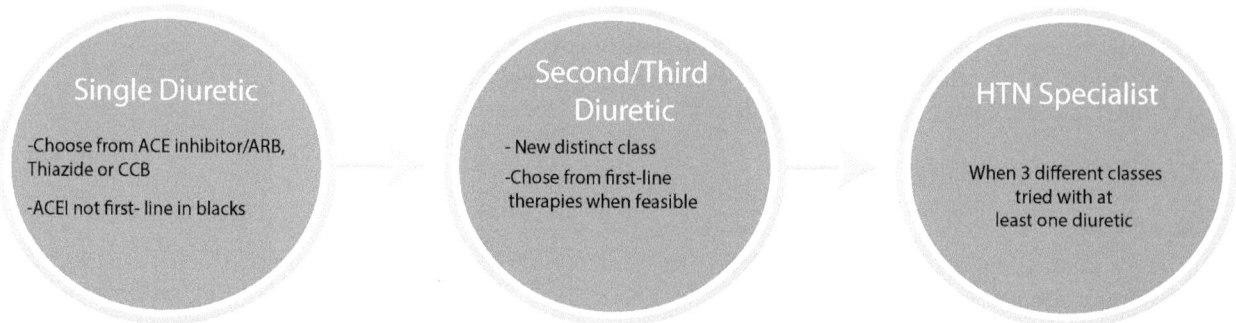

such as CAD. Furthermore, if the patient has been refractory to the typical classes of antihypertensives, it may be worth reassessing and utilizing different classes.

Now that we have an understanding of the antihypertensive toolbox, let's review the antihypertensive escalation ladder (▫ Fig. 13.4) for a better understanding of when and how to escalate therapy.

13.3.3 **Chronic Obstructive Pulmonary Disease (COPD)**

COPD is a very common case that is managed often in the primary care setting. More often than not, you will be managing the chronic symptoms of COPD which has already been diagnosed. Thus we only briefly cover diagnosis, focusing mainly on the chronic treatment.

13.3.3.1 **Diagnosis**

COPD is almost always secondary to a very long (decade+) heavy smoking history. It is a progressive disease, but patients may not notice large differences in their everyday quality of life until the disease is quite progressed. They will present with shortness of breath and classic lung findings such as diminished breath sounds and diffuse crackles. They will be referred to a pulmonologist who confirms the diagnosis with pulmonary function tests demonstrating an obstructive pattern (FEV1/FVC <80%). Another test that support the diagnosis include CXR which demonstrates decreased lung markings, increased lung volumes, and increased AP diameter (barrel chest).

13.3.3.2 **Treatment**

In the primary care setting, your principal role will be to chronically manage COPD treatment regimens based on symptomatic progression of disease. Let's start by looking at how COPD severity is classified according to the GOLD classification system (▫ Fig. 13.5).

The treatment regimen for COPD is based on both symptoms as well as severity classification (which really provides a measure of how likely exacerbations are). The treatment options are best visualized through a stepwise progression as in ▫ Fig. 13.6.

During each follow-up visit, your goal is to characterize their symptoms and adjust their treatment regimen if necessary. Despite the stepwise approach, the easiest way to do this is simply carefully track their baseline. If their baseline is worsening significantly, their treatment regimen likely needs to be escalated (first in dosage amd then adding a medication class).

Classification System

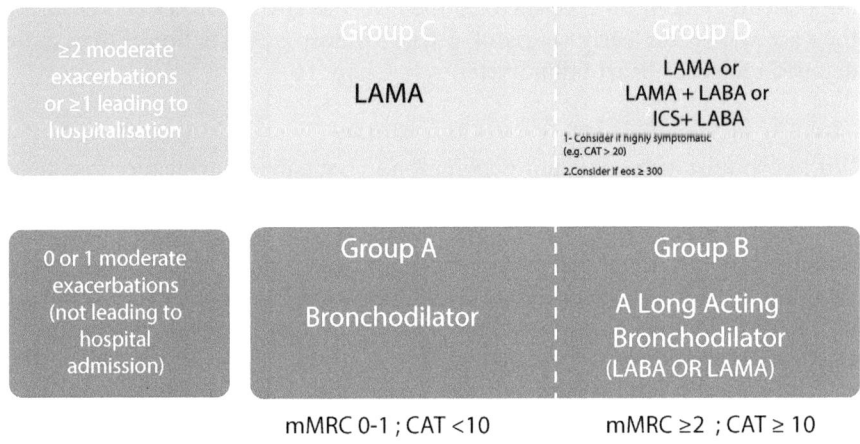

≥2 moderate exacerbations or ≥1 leading to hospitalisation	**Group C** LAMA	**Group D** LAMA or LAMA + LABA or ICS+ LABA 1- Consider if highly symptomatic (e.g. CAT > 20) 2.Consider if eos ≥ 300
0 or 1 moderate exacerbations (not leading to hospital admission)	**Group A** Bronchodilator	**Group B** A Long Acting Bronchodilator (LABA OR LAMA)
	mMRC 0-1 ; CAT <10	mMRC ≥2 ; CAT ≥ 10

■ **Fig. 13.5** GOLD classification system

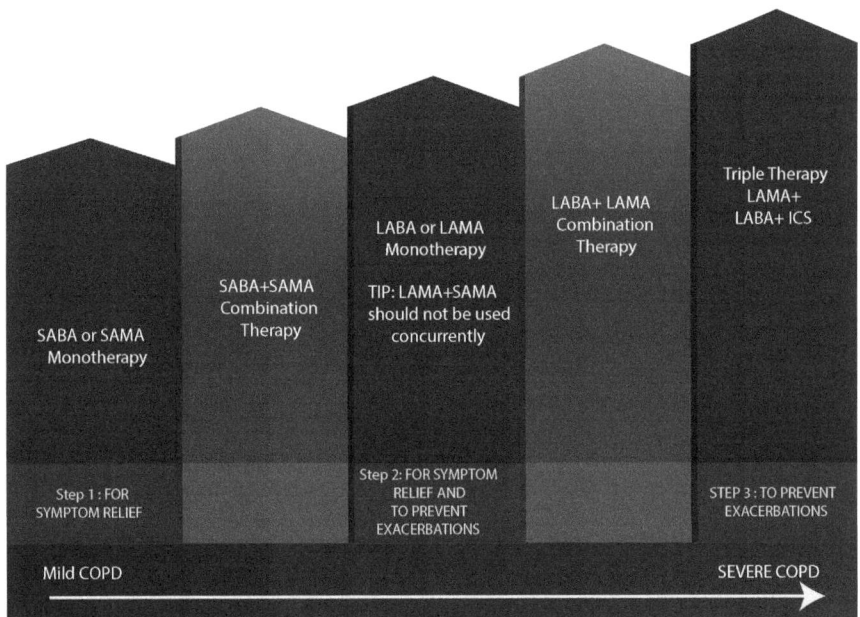

STEPWISE APPROACH:
Use the lowest step that achieves
optimal control based on the severity of COPD

■ **Fig. 13.6** Step-up therapy for chronic COPD

Another common reason for seeing COPD patients is after a recent hospitalization for COPD exacerbation. During these visits, it is critical to try and identify the trigger(s) for their exacerbation. This will help reduce the frequency of future exacerbations. It is also a great opportunity to work further on counseling the patient on lifestyle changes such as smoking cessation.

Pearl: Metoprolol succinate is the form that was shown to have a mortality benefit in HFrEF (MERIT-HF Trial, Lancet 1999). Patients are commonly switched to metoprolol tartrate for fractionation purposes and increased control of dosing while inpatient. Always ensure that the patient is switched back to the long-acting succinate form prior to discharge

Pearl: Carvedilol is favored when the patient also requires blood pressure control. Carvedilol's alpha blocking effects confer greater antihypertensive properties than the other two

Fun fact: Metoprolol is the most common beta-blocker prescribed as GDMT for HFrEF. Though there have not been good head-to-head trials between these three beta-blockers, some people cite the COMET trial comparing metoprolol and carvedilol as evidence of carvedilol's superiority. Unfortunately, this trial was stacked against metoprolol likely with industry motives because (i) metoprolol tartrate was tested and (ii) carvedilol's dose was maximal whereas only half the dose of metoprolol was used

Pearl: Patients on spironolactone may experience breast tenderness and gynecomastia. Eplerenone is an alternative which does not cause those side effects. It is now fairly cheap and much easier to prescribe

Pearl: The original study DAPA-HF only examined HFrEF patients who were type 2 diabetics, but with the DECLARE TIMI 58 study, diabetic status is not required for the mortality benefit.

13.3.4 Congestive Heart Failure (CHF)

This is a common case that is managed together between cardiologists and PCPs. The PCP's primary role in managing CHF (specifically HFrEF) is ensuring patients remain on goal-directed medical therapy (GDMT) and ensuring they are not in the early stages of a heart failure exacerbation. For a more detailed review of heart failure, refer to ▶ Chap. 16.

13.3.4.1 Goal-Directed Medical Therapy

With hospitalizations, it is not uncommon to see patient medication regimens left unchanged prior to discharge. You should always review your patient's medications for heart failure each visit to ensure they are on GDMT which are essentially medications that help slow the progression of disease and have a significant mortality benefit. The exact dosages are less important and usually up to the cardiologist, but your job is to ensure they are taking appropriate classes of medications.

The classes of GDMT for HFrEF are as follows in ◻ Table 13.3. HFpEF does not have data for these same classes though many cardiologists use spironolactone given the limited evidence from a post hoc analysis of the TOPCAT trial and the low cost to potentially significant benefit ratio.

◻ **Table 13.3** GDMT for HFrEF

Class	Examples	Mechanism	Evidence
Beta-blockers	Metoprolol, Bisoprolol, carvedilol	Blocks pathologic heart remodeling	MERIT-HF, CIBIS, COPERNICUS
ACE inhibitors/ angiotensin receptor blockers	Lisinopril, losartan	Blocks pathologic heart remodeling	CONSENSUS, SOLVD, ONTARGET
Mineralocorticoid receptor antagonists	Spironolactone Eplerenone	Blocks mineralocorticoid receptors	RALES, EPHESUS
SGLT2 inhibitors	Dapagliflozin	Inhibits SLGT2 in kidneys	DAPA-HF, DECLARE-TIMI 58
Neprilysin inhibitor – ARB combo	Entresto (Sacubitril-valsartan)	Inhibits the breakdown of BNP	PARADIGM-HF
Nitrates/arterial vasodilator[a]	Isosorbide dinitrate + hydralazine[a]	Arterial and venous dilation	A-HeFT

[a]This combo is specific to African Americans. Current guidelines recommend it for NYHA Class III-IV HFrEF

13.3.5 CAD Primary Prevention

Another common topic is primary CAD prevention. This primarily involves management of a patient's lipid/sugar/blood pressure profiles. Though patients with established CAD will have secondary prevention measures managed by their cardiologists, primary prevention typically falls into the hands of the PCP. Here we will focus on basic lipid management. This is fairly straightforward – you prescribe a moderate to high-intensity statin if the patient is aged 40–75 and their LDL meets the following thresholds:

- Diabetes, regardless of LDL (moderate-intensity) ≥190 (high-intensity)
- LDL 70–189 without diabetes "(moderate-intensity statin with potential for intensification based on risk factors)
- LDL 70–189 with ASCVD ≥7.5% (moderate-intensity with potential intensification for risk factors such as CKD and inflammatory conditions such as HIV)
- All patients with known vascular disease (MI, CVA, PVD) (high-intensity)

In cases where patients are older (age ≥75) or have semi-contraindications such as myalgias, medium-intensity statins may be attempted in lieu of high-intensity regimens. The following two facts are worth remembering for occasional special cases.

- Pravastatin and lovastatin have the lowest risk of myopathy.
- Rosuvastatin and pravastatin have the least CYP3A4 interactions.

> Pearl: African Americans have a higher baseline CK level. Race should be considered carefully in addition to symptoms when deciding to stop/continue therapy.

13.3.6 Musculoskeletal Complaints

MSK issues are a very common source of visits. These issues are most commonly issues with either the lower back, knees, or shoulders/elbows. Here are the most common issues differentiated by their key features (◘ Table 13.4):

> Tinel's sign involves tapping on the carpal Tinel (tunnel).

13.3.6.1 Presentation

The most important elements to elicit in the history for MSK complaints:
- Timing (when did this first occur).
  - True MSK complaints are typically acute onset, with the exception of osteoarthritis.

> Phalen's sign is a maneuver that looks like a Phalen (falling) high five.

◘ **Table 13.4** Common MSK complaints

Pathology	Key differentiating features	Notes
Lower back pain (muscle strain)	Negative straight leg raise (SLR), may have TTP	
Lower back pain (herniated disc)	Positive SLR, may have numbness or shooting pains in distribution of spinal nerve (most commonly L3-S1)	History of heavy lifting activity/exercise with a sudden pain onset
Tennis elbow (lateral epicondylitis)	TTP on lateral epicondyle, Maudsley's test	History of repetitive outward (extensor) motions of forearm
Golfer's elbow (medial epicondylitis)	TTP on medial epicondyle, Golfer's elbow test	History of repetitive flexor motions
Ankle sprain	Swelling, TTP	History of twisting the ankle, misstep
Carpal tunnel syndrome	Positive Phalen & Tinel's signs	History of repetitive wrist motions
Rotator cuff injury	Empty beer can test, drop arm test, liftoff test	History of trauma or unaccustomed/overly strenuous shoulder exercise
Knee pain (osteoarthritis)	Worsens throughout the day	Usually overweight, middle-aged, or elderly

- Context (what were they doing when they first noticed it)?
    - Often involves physical activity (especially unaccustomed strenuous activity) or trauma
- Quality of symptoms (burning, sharp, numb).
    - Numb typically suggests a neurologic cause (though often overlapping with MSK).

The other aspects of OPQRST should also be elicited but are typically not as useful for differentiating your diagnoses.

13.3.6.2 Exam

In addition to a focused neurological exam (◘ Fig. 13.7), these aspects should be investigated closely:
- Inspect and palpate the area for signs of injury and reproducible tenderness
- Active and passive range of motion (if pain exists only during active motion, suspect a muscle problem)
- Strength and neurological testing

Technique	Tests For	
External Rotation Test	Infraspinatus Integrity	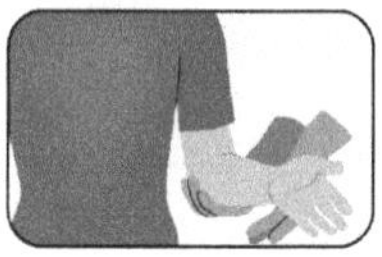
Straight Leg Raise	Lumbar Radiculopathy	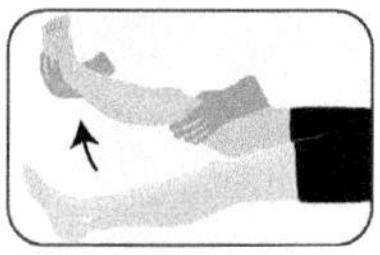
Phalen's Sign	Median Nerve Irritation (Carpal Tunnel)	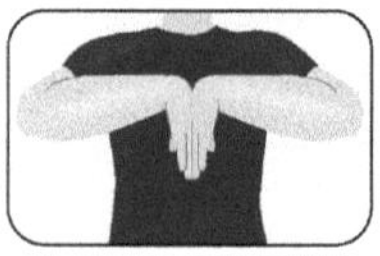
Tinel's Sign	Median Nerve Irritation (Carpal Tunnel)	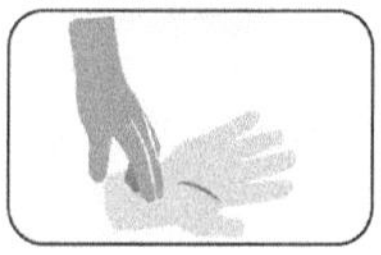
Empty Beer Can Test	Suprasprinatus Integrity	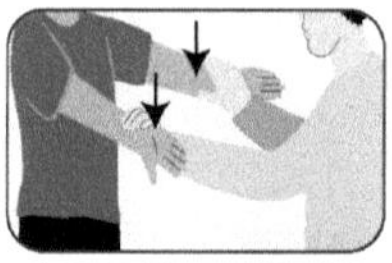
Drop Arm Test	Supraspinatus Integrity	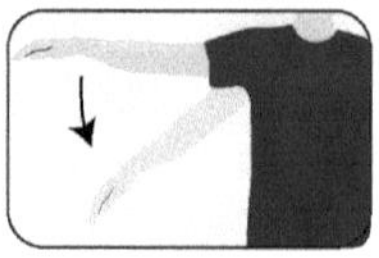
Liftoff Test	Subscapularis Integrity	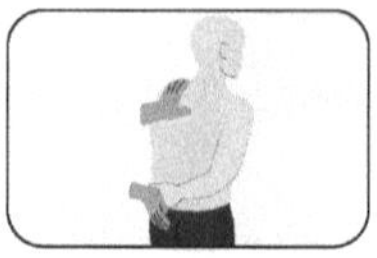
Hornblower's Sign	Teres minor Integrity	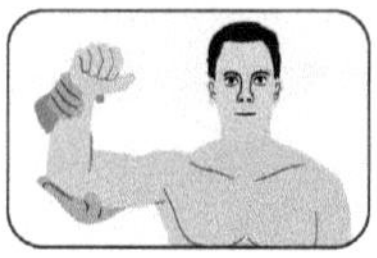

◘ **Fig. 13.7** Common MSK exam techniques

13.3.6.3 Treatment

Most MSK complaints in the primary care setting should first be managed conservatively with rest and NSAIDs. Once these treatments are trialed and found ineffective, the patient may require referral for further workup or treatment. The vast majority of MSK complaints can be treated adequately with conservative management.

13.4 Screening

As a primary care provider, a significant portion of your job is to ensure that all your patients are up-to-date with their required screenings. Many EHR's have systems to help remind you what screenings are due. Some even have alerts that show up when you enter the chart. It is always a good idea to know whether or not your EHR has such a system so that you can efficiently figure out what screening your patient needs for the day. That being said, it is always a good idea to have the more important guidelines memorized and to run through a quick mental checklist before walking into each room.

The main routine screening opportunities to look out for are:

- Malignancy Screening
    - All smokers between ages 55 to 80 who have quit smoking in the past 15 years should receive a one-time CT chest scan.
    - Colorectal cancer screening q5-10y (age 50+).
    - Breast cancer screening q2y (age 50+).
- Aortic aneurysm ultrasound screening once for any patient age 65–75 who has ever been a smoker.
- Lipid screening q5y (age 35+).
- STD screening if appropriate risk factors.
- Depression screening (especially in elderly).

13.5 Vaccinations

In your routine patient population, vaccines will become relevant for the elderly (>60 years old). EMR systems also can help remind you when a patient is due for a vaccine, but you should never rely completely on the information in the EMR. Verbally confirm vaccine history with your patient, and double-check guidelines before going forward with vaccination. Always check for documentation that they have been administered in the EMR, and confirm with the patient.

Emergency Medicine

Alex Bonilla

Contents

© The Author(s), under exclusive license to Springer Nature Switzerland AG 2021
S. H. Lecker, B. J. Chang (eds.), *The Ultimate Medical School Rotation Guide*,
https://doi.org/10.1007/978-3-030-63560-2_14

14.1 Introduction

Emergency medicine (EM) is a multifaceted specialty that provides unscheduled care 24/7; it is often referred to as the "safety net" of the American Health Care System since Federal law (EMTALA) mandates all patients receive an evaluation regardless of ability to pay. The specialty bridges inpatient and outpatient care and has expertise in resource allocation; it focuses on the initial care of the acutely sick patient, who would otherwise experience morbidity or mortality if left untreated. This involves the initial evaluation, treatment, and disposition of any patient presenting to the emergency department (ED). *Medical students often have the misconception that EM focuses on the diagnosis of patients.* While there is an opportunity for diagnosis, the *primary* goals of the emergency physician are to rule out emergent, life- or limb-threatening diagnoses, resuscitate and stabilize patients, and determine disposition.

The practice of EM also involves coordination of care with a diverse team of health care providers encompassing EMS, nurses, physician assistants, physicians, and administrators, as described in ◲ Table 14.1. As such, effective communication, problem-solving, and collaborative and leadership skills are important traits for success in the ED. This skillset places emergency physicians in a unique position to tackle the health care system's most challenging problems with unrivaled leadership and equipoise.

⚠ Warning

Do NOT be rude or condescending to ANY team members (and that goes for anybody in the ED). If you want a positive experience and strong evaluation, you should be polite and professional with ALL team members at ALL times.

◲ **Table 14.1** Role of ED team members (*roles may be site specific*)

Team members	Role
EM Attendings	Board-certified emergency physicians responsible for treating patients, supervising residents, and medical students and midlevel providers managing ED flow and other administrative tasks
Residents (EM, IM, Anesthesia, Ortho)	EM residents are responsible for treating patients, advancing patient care and teaching medical students. Their clinical and administrative responsibilities increase throughout residency. Anesthesia, IM, and Ortho residents may also rotate in the ED to learn about the practice of EM
Physician Assistants (PA)	Responsible for treating patients under supervision of EM attending
Nurses	Advance patient care by triaging, acquiring history, dispensing/administering medications, collecting tests and assisting in procedures. Very involved in patient care and immensely helpful in acquiring patient information
ED Pharmacists	Involved in medication reconciliation, preparing medications, therapeutic monitoring and providing medication information
Registered Respiratory Therapists (RRT)	Assist in management of airways and mechanical ventilation
Social Workers	Perform psychosocial assessment and crisis management. Connect patients with resources to address health care needs
Patient Care Assistants (PCA)/Technicians	Advance patient care by collecting vital signs, assisting in activities of daily living, transporting patients & specimens, serving as chaperones and other tasks
Emergency Medical Services (EMS)	Provide treatment in the out-of-hospital setting and transport patients to the ED. They always give a report on the reason for the 911 call and initial patient assessment

As an EM student and future physician, you will be evaluating patients with undifferentiated complaints from all walks of life, and it will be your job to determine the extent of the immediate diagnostic evaluation and disposition. Ruling out a life- or limb-threatening diagnosis and coordinating next steps are the priority. At times, you will not find a final diagnosis for the patients that you evaluate; this makes following up on your patients a key to building your clinical acumen.

14.1.1 Emergency Medicine Settings

The majority of students will be exposed to EM in the hospital setting; however, EM can also be practiced in other settings, including urgent care, free-standing ED (not physically linked to a hospital), or via telemedicine platforms. Medical students must understand how the setting can impact the clinical practice. Hospital-based EDs are broadly categorized as university, community, and county. They are also categorized depending on the type of care they can provide, such as trauma center, pediatric center, stroke center, geriatric center, etc. A key to successful health center integration is an EMS system that understands the type of care various EDs can deliver, thus ensuring patients are taken to an appropriate ED. Likewise, EDs that lack certain services must be prepared to expediently recognize and transfer patients to hospitals with the services needed.

The *university emergency medicine* setting is typically in an institution with the clinical resources to provide patients with higher subspecialty care. The patients evaluated at university centers are often medically complex (patients with multiple organ transplants, patients on experimental cancer treatments, etc.), well established in the health care system, and may require involvement from several subspecialists. Furthermore, academic centers regularly accept transfer patients from other facilities to provide further interventions, such as complex surgical care, extracorporeal membrane oxygenation (ECMO), etc. Hence, the initial evaluation may be complete in the transfer patient and your primary role may be to coordinate care with other specialists. Consultations, as requested by outside physicians or by institutional policy, are thus a large component of EM practice in these hospital settings. There are generally more ancillary support services available, such as nurses, nursing assistants, patient transporters, pharmacists, respiratory therapists, and 24 h social work. This means that as a student and resident you are less likely to place IVs, draw your own labs, or transport patients to radiology.

County/City emergency medicine most often prides itself in its service to marginalized patients who rely on the safety net of the emergency department. Patients in these settings may face barriers to health care access and, consequently, rely on the ED as their primary source of health care or present with advanced disease processes. Additionally, county settings may be more resource limited and have higher patient volumes. Students and residents may have more autonomy in the initial evaluation of their patients and rely less on consultants given that there may be fewer resources available. In these environments, high patient volumes may strain ancillary resources, so students and residents may regularly start IVs, draw labs, or transport patients to radiology in an effort to advance patient care.

The *community emergency medicine* environment is often somewhere between the university and the county emergency medicine setting. The majority of emergency physicians practice in community settings and most patients are evaluated in community settings. The patients often have reliable access to health care providers and are well known to their providers, so discharging to home with outpatient follow-up may be a more feasible disposition than in other EM settings.

Standout Tip: Introducing yourself and knowing the names of the nurses and support staff can make your life much easier, facilitate efficient patient care, and help facilitate skills practice (start IVs, put on ECG stickers, etc.)!

14

Community emergency physicians have access to some subspecialists, though not always at the level of an academic center. Students and providers will also take responsibility in the initial evaluation of all their patients.

Despite the differences among the broad categories of ED, all three may participate in residency training and academic pursuits. Now that you have a better understanding of EM and the different clinical settings, we can begin with how to maximize your experience – and the patient's experience.

14.1.2 First Day of Your Rotation

The first day of any unfamiliar experience can be challenging. As an EM provider, the last thing you want is unfamiliarity to disrupt the controlled chaos of the ED. As such, it is prudent to show up 30 min early on the first day of your clinical rotation to get a sense of the layout. First, wellness is incredibly important to maintain sustainability in EM, so figure out the location of the restrooms, cafeteria, and water fountains. Next, walk around the ED and locate where the following are stored: ultrasounds (US), interpreter phone or video chat equipment, suture kits, IV starter kits, orthopedic splinting material, and sterile gloves.

Standout Tip: Asking for help from someone who doesn't seem busy can be a good way to introduce yourself and signal your status as an engaged learner – but be ready to be denied if they're working on something else!

14.2 Before the Shift

Investing in the beginning always pays off dividends. To be successful, students should come to every shift prepared with *specific* and *tangible learning goals* to discuss with attendings. Reflect on your past experiences on clinical rotations or shifts and define areas for improvement. For example, this can be your presentation, procedural, or consulting skills. Perhaps you are interested in working on the headache assessment and want to see as many patients with headache as possible during your shift. Another good place to derive goals from is the list of Entrustable Professional Activities (EPAs) that your school uses to assess your clinical competencies. Most of the time, students will be working one-on-one with the attending on shift so identifying these goals demonstrates initiative and allows you to softly guide your attending's evaluation of you.

You should show up 10–15 min before the start of each shift because (1) it is professional and demonstrates interest, but (2) also offers an opportunity to get acquainted to the shift. Each shift is different, so you can get a sense of how busy it is and start to think about patients you are interested in picking up. Always introduce yourself to the attending, residents, physician assistants, nursing and support staff, and other students by your first and last name. Make it clear that you are a sub-intern and, if applicable, that you are applying into EM as this can help you get more involvement in unique learning opportunities. It is also useful to share your learning goals with your residents especially if you are focusing on procedural skills or specific chief complaints. You may not end up getting to see these procedures/complaints during your shift, but having a goal demonstrates engagement and a willingness to learn.

Standout Tip: The ED is a fast-paced dynamic environment that requires flexibility and calmness. Keep an open mind, help out whenever possible, and learn to step aside/call for help.

Additionally, ask your attending about the logistics of picking up patients. Do they want you to pick up patients independently or would they prefer to assign patients to you? This is very attending specific and can depend on patient volume, acuity, and workflow. The last thing you want to do is create more work for your team.

Before shift checklist:
- [] Prepare specific and tangible learning goals
- [] Team introductions
  - If applicable, state you are a sub-intern interested in EM

Clinical Pearl: On the very first day of your rotation, ask your attending and/or residents if you are expected to place IVs or transport your patients. This is more pertinent if you are in a county or high-volume setting.

- [] Discuss learning goals
- [] Clarify logistics with attending
- [] Request specific chief complaints and/or procedures

14.3 During the Shift

14.3.1 Preparing for the Patient Encounter

You should always try to orient yourself to the undifferentiated patient you are about to meet for the first time. Take no more than 5 min to quickly extract relevant information from the patient's electronic medical record (EMR). This will likely be difficult at first, but you will become more efficient with experience. Throughout the process, you should aim for organization and efficiency as you prepare for the patient encounter.

So, what should you do? First, write down the patient's name, age, room number, and chief complaint. Then immediately check the patient's vital signs (VS) to determine urgency. Are they hypotensive, tachycardic, or tachypneic? If so, it's probably a good idea to stop here and go assess the patient in person. You can always come back to the chart after assuring that the patient is stable. Although patients are often triaged by level of acuity, sometimes patients can rapidly deteriorate; so learn to be flexible. After reassuring yourself that you have a few minutes, you can quickly search the EMR for any relevant ED notes or prior hospital discharge relevant to the current chief complaint. The brief hospital course summary in the prior hospital discharge note can offer a wealth of background information to understand the patient's medical history. If your patient is brought in by EMS it would behoove you to be present for the EMS report (you may need to do this first as EMS will be gone shortly after the patient arrives). This is an opportunity to hear EMS talk about the reason for the EMS call and the patient's initial clinical status on EMS arrival. You will quickly learn that the report is especially helpful if the patient is nonverbal, has a history of dementia, or lives in an assisted living facility or nursing home.

Patient preparation checklist:
- [] Patient's name, age, room #
- [] EMS report (if applicable)
- [] Chief complaint
- [] Check VS
- [] Reviewed major comorbidities
- [] Reviewed medications and allergies
- [] Reviewed last ED note or hospital discharge note
- [] Note top must-not miss diagnoses

Clinical Pearl: As you are reading about your patient, start thinking about the top cannot-miss diagnoses pertinent to the chief complaint. At the end of the chapter, we will review the top cannot-miss diagnoses for the most common chief complaints.

Example of Preparation Notes
Room 5

Chief complaint: Shortness of breath (SOB)

Name/age: Ms Z 77F

PMH: COPD (2L home O2), afib (on epixiban), HFrEF on daily Lasix 80 mg, wheelchair bound

Prior relevant admissions: recently admitted 12/29/2019 for CHF exacerbation triggered by influenza

VS:
T – 100.6 F
HR: 105
BP: 105/78 (baseline)
RR: 18
Top differential diagnoses to consider: CHF exacerbation, PNA, PE, ACS

14.3.2 The Patient Encounter

You should limit the patient encounter to less than 10 min. Although it may seem like an impossible task at first, practice and the approaches described in this chapter can improve your efficiency and help to impress your attending(s)/resident(s). Keep your top three to four diagnoses in mind as you progress through the patient interview, as each piece of information will adjust the probabilities of each diagnosis on your differential. Your goals for the patient encounter are to figure out the following:

1. Why the patient came to the ED
2. What life- or limb-threatening illnesses need to be ruled out
3. Where does the patient need to go next (e.g., home vs. admission)

As you progress in your clinical training, you will gain a better sense of differentiating between "sick" versus "not sick" patients. When you walk into the room, keep ◘ Fig. 14.1 in mind as you make a quick visual assessment of the patient, particularly focusing on vital signs, breathing, and mental status. You should be concerned whenever your patient is struggling to breathe or has an increased O_2 requirement, clutching their chest or abdomen, writhing in pain, altered, or the patient looks pale/gray/clammy. If your gut feeling tells you that the patient is very sick and close to passing out or dying, grab your attending or a resident ASAP. No one will ever fault you for being overly cautious.

Clinical Pearl: To maximize building your clinical skills you should see as many patients as possible; if there are no new patients to be seen, ask your attending if you can interview a patient who has already been evaluated and see if you agree with the plan.

Clinical Pearl: Look out for these particular red flags: altered mental status, pale/gray/clammy skin, and acute changes in blood pressure or O_2 saturation, increased oxygen requirement, tripoding, abdominal distension/rigidity, and life-threatening arrhythmias (ventricular fibrillation, ventricular tachycardia, asystole, PEA).

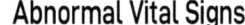

Abnormal Vital Signs

HR > 100 or HR <60
BP > 180/120 or BP <90/60
Temp > 38.3 C or Temp < 35 C
SpO2 < 90%

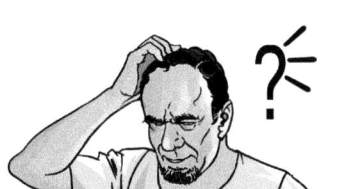

Altered Mental Status

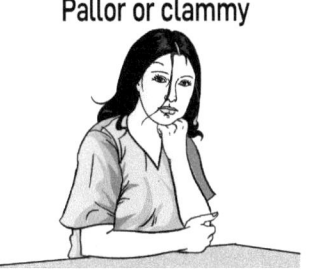

Pallor or clammy

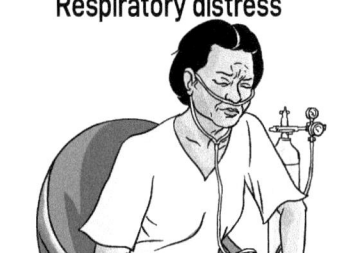

Respiratory distress

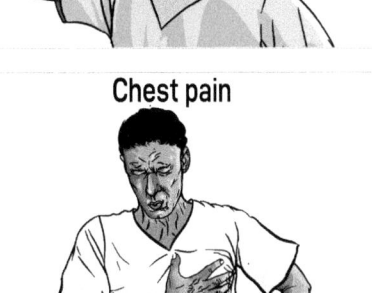

Chest pain

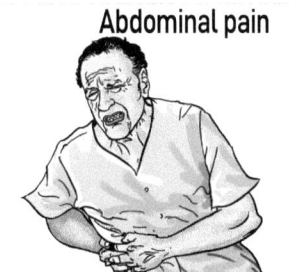

Abdominal pain

◘ **Fig. 14.1** Concerning findings on visual assessment

14.3.3 History of Present Illness

The first step toward accomplishing those goals is to introduce yourself and your role on the team. This goes a long way because although your attending will ultimately make all clinical decisions, your patient needs to think of you as their primary responding clinician. You can say something along the lines of "Hello, my name is Alex Bonilla and I am the medical student on the team of providers taking care of you today." After the pleasantries are out of the way, start the history of present illness and get to the bottom of what is going on: why the patient is in the ED, the patient's concerns, and the questions you need to ask to rule out life-threatening illness. Remember, unlike in other specialties, your primary goal is not to arrive at a specific diagnosis but instead to rule out dangerous conditions and decide on a disposition decision. It is useful to go through the OPQRST (Onset, Provokes/palliates, Quality, Radiates/region, Severity, Time) mnemonic as a starting point, but you should also inquire about risk factors for life-threatening diseases.

Sometimes, your patients will be unable to communicate with you. If you are lucky, they may have a family member or aide at the bedside to help provide information. Otherwise, you will need to rely on the EMR and EMS report to extract relevant past medical history and follow up with their health care proxy (HCP), if the patient has one. The history-taking approach is the same regardless of who provides the history. In these circumstances, it is important that you refer to recent outpatient notes and hospitalization discharge summary to gather the patient's past medical history.

14.3.4 Review of Systems

The review of systems (ROS) is an important toolkit for the EM provider. Here you will ask about symptoms *relevant* to your chief complaint to help you determine the probability of a life-threatening illness. At the beginning of your rotation, it will probably be difficult to determine which systems are relevant to your chief complaint. You should develop an extended ROS covering up to 9 systems that you can use with all patients. As you progress during your rotation, you will start to recognize the ROS questions that are most pertinent to your chief complaint and simplify your ROS. This is called a problem-pertinent ROS. At the end of the chapter, we will review the ROS most pertinent to the most common chief complaints.

Generally speaking, ◘ Fig. 14.2 indicates ROS "positives" to look out for as they may be an indicator of life- or limb-threatening disease.

14.3.5 Past Medical/Surgical History, Family History, Medications, Allergies and Social History

This section is especially relevant for patients without any medical records at your institution or patients who rarely access the health care system. Again, you should acquire and report information that is relevant to your chief complaint and that will help you determine the likelihood of a life- or limb-threatening illness.

Medications can help clue you into a patient's medical conditions, which can be especially helpful for patients who may have low health care literacy. Alternatively, medication adherence/nonadherence can increase your suspicion

Clinical Pearl: The *OPQRST* history can be paired with a *SAMPLE* (Signs/symptoms, Allergies, Medications, Pertinent PMH, Last oral intake/LMP, Events leading to incident/illness) history for a high-yield, well-rounded clinical picture.

Clinical Pearl: If your patient is presenting for a chronic issue, try to understand what has changed to prevent premature closure. Try asking: "what has changed that brought you to the emergency department?" or "how have your symptoms worsened?"

Clinical Pearl: Key to obtaining a good history is gaining the patient's confidence. Your appearance should always be professional: for example, clean pressed well-fitting scrubs, combed hair, etc.; sit down whenever possible, have a warm smile, and look directly in the patient's eyes.

Clinical Pearl: Understanding patients' concern is key to meeting their needs. For example, patients with a headache may be concerned that they have a brain tumor; patients with gastritis may be concerned that they're having a heart attack. Proactively identifying the concern and then making sure the patient understands why you are or are not concerned provides the base for a successful patient encounter.

Common Error: The absence of a history detail or risk factor does not exclude a diagnosis.

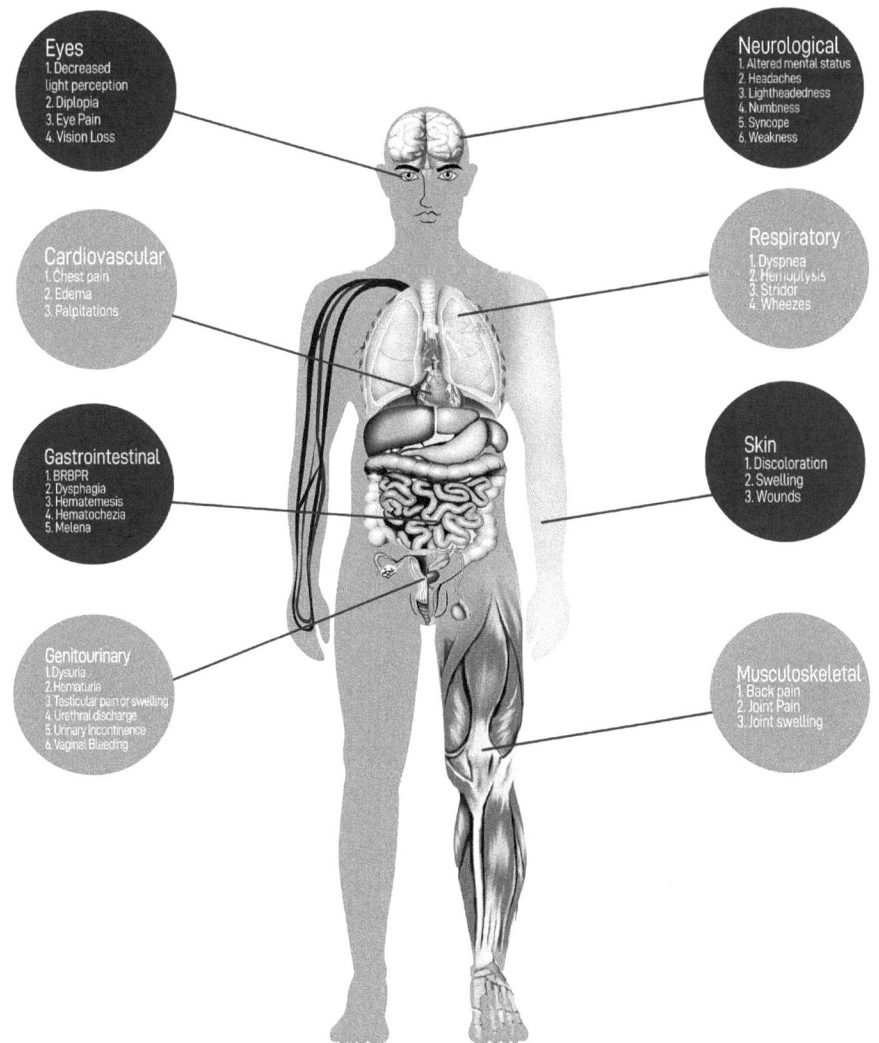

□ **Fig. 14.2** Abnormal ROS "positives" to keep in mind

for an acute illness (e.g., transplant rejection in a patient not taking immuno-suppression or hypertensive urgency in a patient on tacrolimus). Medications can have side effects that may be the cause of your patient's presentation or affect the treatments you can administer. For example, methadone can cause QT prolongation and could explain the patient's new arrhythmia or contraindicate other QT-prolonging agents. Similarly, a history of allergies can help dictate what treatments they can receive.

In the social history, you should ask about the patient's lifestyle choices regarding smoking, alcohol, and substance use. A history of smoking can raise your suspicion for underlying lung disease in a patient presenting with respiratory symptoms. Alcohol use is an important consideration because alcohol withdrawal is a common presentation and cause of altered mental status. Ask the patient whether they consume alcohol and if so, how much and how often. Depending on the route of administration, substance use can place your patient at higher risk of infection (skin, bloodstream, endocarditis, spinal) and other morbidity.

Clinical Pearl: Ask your patient when they had their last alcoholic drink when suspecting alcohol withdrawal

Clinical Pearl: I found it helpful to first ask the patient what they do for work and where they were coming from as this gives more information about the patient's living situation and helps build rapport. Then I would move on to substance use by prefacing my question with "These are questions we ask everyone coming to the ER: Do you drink alcohol? Smoke cigarettes? Use recreational substances?"

Clinical Pearl: Summarize your conversation with the patient to practice your oral presentation and to give the patient an opportunity to add/clarify information.

Try to summarize the conversation (focusing primarily on the HPI and pertinent ROS) with your patient before moving on to the physical exam. This will help confirm the information you have obtained, but also serve as a mock presentation. The information you recall will most likely be the most relevant information.

Background checklist:
- [] PMH
- [] Surgeries (if applicable)
- [] Home medications
- [] Allergies
- [] Social Hx:
  - [] Smoking hx [] EtOH use [] Substance use [] Housing situation [] Social support

14.3.6 Physical Exam

The physical exam is another important tool to help you determine the potential life-threatening illnesses that may be affecting your patient. Your physical exam should be *FOCUSED* and *RELEVANT* to the patient's chief complaint. A useful way to determine what organ systems you need to examine is to ask yourself, *what do I need to examine to assure myself that I am not missing a life- or limb-threatening illness?*

Depending on the chief complaint, you should pay particular attention for the following vital signs physical exam findings given in ◘ Fig. 14.3:
- Vital signs: fevers, hypothermia/hyperthermia, tachycardia/bradycardia, hypertension/hypotension, desaturations, tachypnea/bradypnea

Make sure your patient has a room if you need to perform a breast, genital, or rectal exam or need to undress the patient for a more thorough exam. You can coordinate with the nurse and nurse manager to relocate the patient to a room. Also, let the patient care assistants or nurses know that you will need a chaperone to perform a breast, genital, or rectal exam so they set time for this. These are all small logistical steps that can cause a bottleneck in workflow if you do not anticipate the steps early enough. It is also important to perform these exams under supervision with your attending or residents because they need the exam findings to help guide the evaluation and it also avoids performing the exam twice.

14.3.7 Managing Patient Expectations

Finally, your ability to manage patient expectations will take you far in EM. Realize that the patients coming into the ED are often scared and may be physically, emotionally, and/or mentally overwhelmed. You should respond to your patient's concerns with empathy and aligning statements to gain their trust (highly recommend referring to the Soft Skills chapter). After obtaining your information, ask the patient what questions they have for you. Always try to answer to the best of your ability, but never lie, especially promising a good prognosis without sufficient evidence. It is very reasonable to answer with "I do not know, but I will get back to you about that after we have more lab/imaging results."

Emergency Medicine

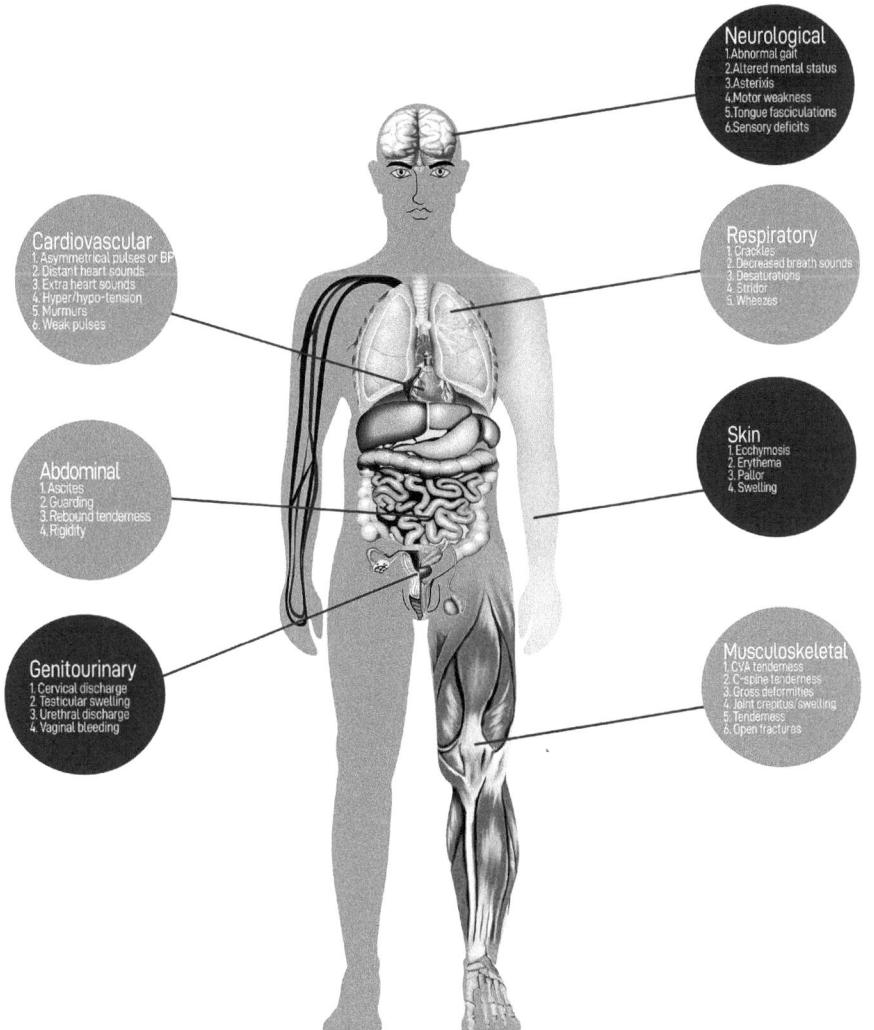

Neurological
1. Abnormal gait
2. Altered mental status
3. Asterixis
4. Motor weakness
5. Tongue fasciculations
6. Sensory deficits

Cardiovascular
1. Asymmetrical pulses or BP
2. Distant heart sounds
3. Extra heart sounds
4. Hyper/hypo-tension
5. Murmurs
6. Weak pulses

Respiratory
1. Crackles
2. Decreased breath sounds
3. Desaturations
4. Stridor
5. Wheezes

Skin
1. Ecchymosis
2. Erythema
3. Pallor
4. Swelling

Abdominal
1. Ascites
2. Guarding
3. Rebound tenderness
4. Rigidity

Genitourinary
1. Cervical discharge
2. Testicular swelling
3. Urethral discharge
4. Vaginal bleeding

Musculoskeletal
1. CVA tenderness
2. C-spine tenderness
3. Gross deformities
4. Joint crepitus/swelling
5. Tenderness
6. Open fractures

◘ **Fig. 14.3**　Abnormal physical exam findings to keep in mind

Once you are done addressing the patient's questions, tell them that you will be touching base with the rest of the team to come up with a plan. Let the patient know that it may take time before test results and more information are available; and then, every hour round on your patient and give them an update.

If your patient is presenting with a chronic condition that has been evaluated by specialists and is otherwise stable with the *same* symptoms, try to preempt them about the possibility of not finding a solution for them today. You can phrase this as "It sounds like this condition has been ongoing and you have seen multiple specialists for this, we will do our due diligence to make sure you are safe and nothing new is brewing, but we may not find a solution today." This by no means a green light to dismiss the patient's chief complaint but rather to manage expectations and prepare the patient for treatment or disposition they may be disappointed with. You still want to take the patient's complaints seriously and rule out severe illnesses that may hide under the guise of a chronic illness.

! Common Error: NEVER make any promises that you cannot keep because this will not bode well for you when the patient is frustrated or angry. This is also unprofessional and unethical.

Clinical Pearl: Avoid discounting a patient's complaint no matter how chronic it is; chronic complaints may acutely decompensate or have been missed/dismissed in prior evaluations.

I once evaluated an elderly patient presenting with chronic dry mouth (xerostomia). He did not have worsening dry mouth or any fevers, pain, difficulty breathing or swallowing symptoms that would suggest an infection or airway obstruction. Likewise, his vital signs were normal, and the physical exam was unremarkable for lymphadenopathy, salivary gland, and tooth tenderness. He had been evaluated by his primary care doctor and multiple specialists in the past with specific treatment recommendations, but unfortunately the patient was frustrated with his poor quality of life due to dry mouth. He was hoping the ED would finally find a treatment for his chronic ailment. My suspicion for sialolithiasis and sialoadenitis was low. Sadly, there was nothing else the ED could do besides advise the patient to follow up with his outpatient medical team and continue the maximum therapy he was already on. ◀

Patient encounter checklist:
- [] Introduction (name and role in team)
- [] HPI
- [] ROS
- [] VS/physical exam
- [] Summarize conversation
- [] Manage expectations

14.3.8   After the Patient Encounter

Now is the time to take a few minutes to gather your thoughts and prepare for your oral presentation. You should already know the history and physical exam so it would be prudent to spend this time on creating an assessment and plan. If applicable, review your patient's ECG and compare it with prior ECGs available in the EMR. Depending on your clinical rotation, you may have EMR privileges to enter and save lab, imaging, and medications orders. These orders can be edited and cosigned by your attending or residents. Entering your orders demonstrates initiative but also helps your attending understand your thought process.

Standout Tip: During my rotations, I noticed that my attendings were more impressed when I presented without notes because it demonstrated that I knew my patient to an exceptional degree. Furthermore, this approach forced me to recall only the PERTINENT details for my patient, yielding a more concise presentation. This will not be easy at first, but your presentation skills will improve significantly the more you practice this approach. As mentioned in the General Pearls/Skills chapter, one way to help yourself present without notes is to practice presenting to the patient by summarizing what you have talked about with them prior to ending the patient encounter.

14

14.3.9   The Oral Presentation

The oral presentation is your opportunity to SHINE! EM physicians value clear and concise presentations. Your ability to provide a succinct presentation will make you a rock star on your rotation. Briefly, the goals of your presentation are to:
1. Convey why your patient is in the ED
2. Concisely deliver your thought process
3. Propose an action plan

Common Error: Oral presentation skills are critical for a STRONG evaluation. Your oral presentation should be as clear and concise as possible – try to keep it under 3 min!

In the HPI, you will provide a one-liner with the patient's PMH and comorbidities relevant to the chief complaint. Quickly go through the OPQRST of the chief complaint and talk about why the patient finally decided to present to the ED. Then mention the pertinent ROS, both positive and negative. This demonstrates to your attending that you are actively thinking about the differential diagnosis without you explicitly mentioning each diagnosis. Your attending will be less impressed if you are reporting negative eye pain for a chief complaint of dyspnea. The EM oral presentation is also unique in that all relevant information, be it past medical history, medications, and social history, is reported in the HPI. This is feasible because only relevant information is mentioned.

Mr. L in room 8 is stable. He is a 40-year-old male smoker with no known PMH presenting with new-onset left-sided chest pain. He first noticed a dull chest pain after a football game, approximately 3 days ago. This morning, the pain changed to a sharp quality with radiation to the back, which is worse with movement. He thinks the pain may be related to collisions during the football game but is now concerned this pain has changed. He has not tried any treatment for the pain. He otherwise denies fevers, cough, hemoptysis, dyspnea, abdominal pain and unilateral lower extremity swelling, discoloration, and pain. Denies prolonged immobilization or long-distance travel. ◀

You do not need to repeat the past medical and surgical history because you have already mentioned the pertinent details in the opening one liner. The complete medication and allergy history does not need to be presented but you should always have that information handy in case your attending asks. This should be followed by the vital signs, pertinent physical exam findings, and any available diagnostic studies.

> Standout Tip: Start your presentation by briefly mentioning the patient's acuity status to help determine the sense of urgency. This can be stable, sick but stable, or unstable. Ideally, you have already told your team about the unstable patient.

▶ Example

Vital signs are notable for a Temp of 99.9, HR of 74, BP of 145/72 in both upper extremities and O$_2$ sat of 99% on RA.

Exam is notable for an individual with obesity resting comfortably. Cardiovascular exam is notable for a normal S1 and S2 without murmurs or extra heart sounds. The lungs are clear to auscultation bilaterally. There is tenderness to palpation along the L sternal border. No evidence of lower extremity DVTs.

His ECG is notable for normal sinus rhythm without ST segment or T wave changes, which is unchanged from a prior ECG in 2015. ◀

14.3.10 Assessment and Plan

Your attendings will likely perk up at the assessment and plan because they want to know what YOU think is going on with the patient. Therefore, you should spend the post patient encounter polishing your assessment and plan. If the first part of your presentation is presented as a well-crafted, convincing story, then they will already have some sense of your clinical intuition. It is up to you to drive the point home and avoid hedging. The assessment can be broken down into a synthesized one liner of the information just discussed and your impression of the patient.

> Standout Tip: Make sure you spend time preparing your assessment and plan before presenting. Feel free to reference medical guides/resources as you prepare.

▶ Example

A 77-year-old female smoker with a history of COPD on 2L of home O$_2$, HFrEF secondary to ischemic cardiomyopathy, CAD, and atrial fibrillation presenting with 1 week of worsening dyspnea, increasing oxygen requirement and weight gain, and new-onset fevers for 1 day can be synthesized as a *"77F with significant lung disease and cardiac comorbidities presenting with subacute dyspnea in the setting of fever, volume overload, and increased O$_2$ demand. I am worried she is very sick and will require close attention."* ◀

In the impression, provide at *least three* differential diagnoses and their supporting evidence, in the following order:

- Most likely diagnosis
- Cannot-miss life- or limb-threatening diagnoses
- Less likely diagnoses to consider

The key here is to provide your differential diagnosis in a coherent and organized manner to demonstrate your thought process. When discussing any diagnosis, be sure to back it up with data based on the history and physical, risk factors, and any available diagnostic results. Be confident and report the diagnosis that you think is most likely because hedging may hurt your oral presentation. Next, discuss the "cannot miss" diagnoses, regardless of whether you truly believe the patient has it or not. The point is to demonstrate that you are actively thinking about dangerous diagnoses. Again, use the available data and risk factors to argue for or against the diagnoses. Integrate clinical risk calculators (e.g., PERC Rule) where possible, as this is another form of evidence and demonstrates your understanding of the literature (more on this later).

▶ Example

In summary, this is a 40-year-old-male with no known PMH presenting with 1 week of worsening reproducible chest pain i/s/o contact sports. His symptoms are *most likely* due to costochondritis given temporal relationship to contact sports and reproducible chest pain on exam. I am *also worried* about an MI given the patient's smoking hx and strong paternal hx of MI, though he is hemodynamically stable, and the current ECG is unchanged from prior ECGs. Aortic dissection is *another important consideration* for sharp chest pain with back pain radiation, especially in the setting of hypertension though the BPs are symmetric in the UEs. I have a *low suspicion* for PE in the absence of dyspnea, hypoxia, and DVT. He is PERC negative so I will defer d-dimer testing for (Pulmonary Embolism (PE). ◀

After discussing your differential diagnosis, move on to the plan, which consists of diagnostic tests, treatments, and presumed disposition. The goal is to discuss what you want to do to rule out certain diagnoses. In your diagnostic plan, list the lab and imaging studies that you plan on ordering. The key here is to justify *WHY* you want to order the studies by tying it back to your differential diagnosis.

▶ Example

I want to order a CBC for an Hgb baseline and evidence of infection, BMP to assess for renal baseline in case the patient needs contrast imaging or further intervention, ECG and q3h troponins to rule out MI, BNP for evidence of heart failure exacerbation and a CXR for evidence of pneumonia, heart failure exacerbation, and dissection. ◀

In your treatment plan, discuss therapeutics you want to administer to the patient, how you will monitor response to therapeutics and what you will do if the patient does not improve. Feel free to refer to landmark EM studies to help support your treatment decision and impress your attendings with your fund of knowledge. Do not worry about knowing this on day 1 as you will find it easier to integrate these studies when you encounter that clinical scenario. Furthermore, this is the time to discuss any consultants you may want to involve in the patient's care. We will review some indications for consulting a subspecialist but note that this will sometimes depend on your attending's preferences and comfort level and institutional policies.

14

Standout Tip: Integrate calculators to determine imaging utilization (NEXUS Criteria, Canadian, Ottawa, etc.), but be cognizant of the inclusion criteria for these calculators.

Table 14.2 Disposition definitions and options (*may be site-specific*)

Disposition option	Definition and who is eligible
Home	Self-explanatory here. Stable patients without a need for further inpatient evaluation or treatment can be discharged home.
Rehabilitation center/Skilled Nursing Facility (SNF)	Institutions that provide physical rehabilitation support and medical and nursing support. Patients who arrived from a rehabilitation center of SNF usually return to the SNF if they are stable.
Observation unit	Unit for patients who are anticipated to need more than 8 h but less than 24 h of care.
General ward	Inpatient unit for stable patients requiring further workup and treatment.
Step down unit (SDU)	Unit for patients requiring an intermediate level of care. This means they are too sick for the general ward, but not sick enough for the ICU. These patients have a higher degree of nursing needs than general ward patients.
Intensive Care Unit (ICU)	Location in the hospital that delivers intensive treatment to high acuity patients. Patients require close monitoring and a higher level of nursing support. If your patient is intubated, needs intensive hemodynamic monitoring, or has drips, then they are likely going to the ICU.

Finally, discuss the patient's disposition plan, which boils down to "*where is the patient going after this evaluation?*" The disposition plan depends on two factors: the patient's social background AND clinical status; the latter being subject to change as you administer treatments and acquire more data. Your disposition options vary depending on your institutional and regional resources, but generally include discharge home, observation, general ward, stepdown unit and ICU, as evident in ◘ Table 14.2.

Patients eligible for a discharge out of the ED are stable and do not require further inpatient evaluation or treatment. Additionally, they may have excellent outpatient follow-up and can see a provider relatively soon. Patients requiring further evaluation and treatment need to be admitted to the hospital. The patient's social background may impact whether the patient needs to be admitted for safety reasons in the home/community or inability to complete treatment in the outpatient setting – these patients may benefit with an admission to an observation unit for coordinated planning with case management and social work. For example, a patient experiencing homelessness may require an admission to complete antibiotic treatment for cellulitis or to obtain a referral to community resources that could assist with outpatient treatment. Refer to ◘ Fig. 14.4 to gain an understanding of a patient's clinical status and disposition options.

Oral Presentation Example

I would like to tell you about Ms. Z in room 5. She is currently stable. This is a wheelchair-bound 77F with h/o COPD (on 2L of home O_2 at baseline), HFrEF 2/2 ischemic cardiomyopathy, afib (on rivaroxaban) presenting with dyspnea. She reports a 1-week history of worsening SOB requiring increased supplemental

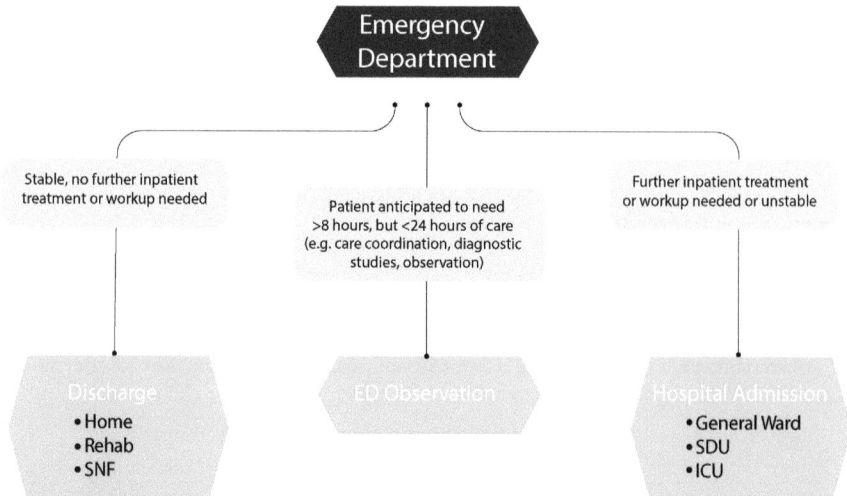

■ **Fig. 14.4**   ED disposition flow based on clinical status

O$_2$ to 4L. Throughout the week, she has also noticed worsening cough with increased sputum, different from her baseline, and fevers. Despite doubling her furosemide dosage to 80 mg PO, she noticed a 10-lb weight gain and peripheral edema. She decided to present today because of a persistent fever to 101.2 F this morning. She otherwise denies syncope, chest pain, palpitations, hemoptysis, abdominal pain, and unilateral extremity swelling or pain.

On exam, she is febrile, tachy to 105 and sating at 92% on 4L O$_2$ on NC. Notably, she is mildly uncomfortable with a JVD to the earlobe, 2+ pitting edema in the bilateral lower extremities, and scattered wheezes and wet crackles at the lung bases.

Her ECG is notable for afib without ST segment changes and unchanged from her previous admission ECG.

In summary, 77F with significant lung disease and cardiac comorbidities presenting with subacute SOB in the setting of fever, volume overload, and increased O$_2$ demand on exam. She is very sick and will require close monitoring.

My top differential diagnosis for the patient's SOB is a CHF exacerbation secondary to underlying PNA given the history of fevers and worsening productive cough along with evidence of volume overload. I would also seriously consider a COPD exacerbation as she reports worsening cough, sputum production, and increased O$_2$ requirement. I have also considered ACS as a cause of HF exacerbation though she does not report chest pain and her EKG is without ST segment changes and unchanged from baseline. PE is an important consideration given the chronic immobilization and tachycardia and hypoxia, although she is currently on anticoagulation treatment and does not have evidence of DVT on exam.

In terms of diagnostics, I would like to order a CBC with differential to assess for evidence of infection, BMP for renal function, BNP for HF exacerbation and a troponin to assess for underlying ischemia. I want to start with a CXR with two views to look for evidence of PNA or volume overload, such as consolidations or effusions.

For treatment, I will titrate her supplemental O$_2$ requirement to a goal SpO$_2$ of 88–92% and provide a single dose of duonebs for potential COPD exacerbation and 40 mg IV Lasix for diuresis. In terms of antibiotics, I would like to start levofloxacin given our high suspicion for PNA. I will defer steroid treatment for now.

I will follow up diagnostics and monitor her O_2 saturation and respiratory and volume status. I suspect she will need an admission to the medicine floor given her clinical status and significant comorbidities.

Post patient encounter preparation checklist:

HPI	VS/physical exam
[ ] One-liner with CC	[ ] VS
[ ] OPQRST	[ ] Pertinent physical Exam
[ ] Risk Factors	
[ ] Pertinent ROS	

Assessment and plan	EMR
[ ] One-liner	[ ] Review ECG
[ ] Top three differential	[ ] Save medication orders
[ ] Diagnostics	[ ] Save imaging orders
[ ] Treatment	
[ ] Disposition	

14.3.11 After the Oral Presentation

Congratulations! You have completed your presentation and can now breathe. Your attending at this point will likely finalize your assessment and plan with you. They may ask clarifying questions if they have not already and may probe your thinking by asking additional questions. Depending on time constraints, this is also an opportunity to ask clarifying questions if your attending has a plan that is different from yours. Do not be afraid to ask your attending for their thought process on the plan because it demonstrates curiosity, but also provides a wealth of information. In fact, it may be advantageous to ask some astute questions if you can!

After you have confirmed the final plan, let the nurse on the team know what to expect. EM is a fast-paced, team sport that requires constant communication among all team members. The nurses will appreciate you updating them on the plan and they, in turn, will be more likely to see you as the responding clinician and trust you with new information as it comes in, which in turn helps you shine. Next, update your patient on what they should expect using simple language. Let them know if they need more lab testing, imaging, or evaluation by another specialist. Your patients will appreciate the updates and attention you give them.

Post oral presentation checklist:
- [] Ask questions
- [] Finalize plan
- [] Update nurse
- [] Update patient

Clinical Pearl: Your attending's plan may not be finalized until they examine the patient. If that is the case, ask them when you can pass along the plan to the patient and the nurse. Corollary: Keep the nurse caring for the patient appraised of plan – this builds teamwork and a partnership in care.

Standout Tips:
- Whenever possible, always try to avoid medical jargon with patients
- Depending on your clinical setting, it may behoove you to place an IV and draw labs or take the patient to imaging
- If you have never placed an IV before, ask nursing staff to help you place one while offering to help them moving forward

14.3.12   The Patient Note

The EM patient note serves as a form of communication with health care providers and a record for reimbursement and medicolegal purposes. The note should be concise and clearly outline what you observed and how you worked up your patient for specific diagnoses. Your patient note should follow the same template as your oral presentation, though with more detail.

Clinical Pearl: Ask your residents or attendings to share a patient note template during your first day of the rotation. Save it and edit it as needed to suit your needs.

⊘ Warning

NEVER record a statement or finding that is not true; never document an action that was not done, e.g., reflexes, rectal exam, fundoscopic exam. This is fraud! Do not enter information that is not directly related to patient care, e.g., frustration with a consultant or process. Never copy someone else's note to auto-populate.

Patient note components:
- Chief complaint
- History of present illness
- ROS
- PMH
- Past surgical history
- Allergies
- Family history
- Social history
- Vital signs
- Physical exam
- Diagnostics (if any are available)
- MDM with assessment and plan
- Disposition

The HPI should contain the OPQRST of the chief complaint and why the patient decided to present to the ED. As previously described, the ROS should be pertinent to the chief complaint and cover both positive and negative findings. It is helpful to create and use an ROS template with all the systems auto-populated, as long as you remember to delete symptoms you did not explicitly ask about. Remember you NEVER want to document something you did not explicitly observe or ask about. Your EMR may auto-populate the patient's past medical and surgical history, family history, and social history, otherwise you should note any pertinent information in these sections.

Document the vital signs and physical exam findings you noted during your evaluation of the patient. You can auto-populate a physical exam template as long as you remove systems and findings you did not examine. In the diagnostics section, add any labs, EKGs, and imaging study results available. Always document whether the EKG has changed from prior EKGs available.

The *Medical Decision Making (MDM)* section contains the patient's diagnosis and clinical reasoning in the form of an assessment and plan. This section follows the same format as your oral presentation so we will not repeat it here. However, you should also include any relevant clinical risk scores (PERC rule, HEART score, NEXUS/Canadian CT Head Rules, etc.) in your assessment as this helps reinforce your decision making. We will briefly discuss the clinical risk scores at the end of the chapter. You do not need to go into the thought process for ordering labs and diagnostic studies as you did in the presentation. Finally, you should document the treatment and follow-up plan and disposition.

Patient Note Example

CC: chest pain

History of Present Illness:

Mr. L is a 40-year-old male with no known PMH presenting with new-onset left-sided chest pain. The patient reports he was in his usual state of health when he noticed onset of dull chest pain after a football game, approximately 3 days ago. However, the pain changed to a sharp quality with radiation to the back this AM. Reports the pain is exacerbated by movement and has not tried any medications. He thinks pain may be related to collisions during the football game but is concerned this pain is now different. He otherwise denies fevers, cough, hemoptysis, dyspnea, abdominal pain, and unilateral lower extremity swelling, discoloration, and pain. He denies prolonged immobilization or long-distance travel. No hormone use or recent surgery.

Review of Systems

Constitutional: Negative for fevers, night sweats, chills

Cardiovascular: Positive for chest pain, Negative for palpitations, peripheral edema

Respiratory: Negative for cough, hemoptysis, dyspnea, wheezes

Gastrointestinal: Negative for abdominal pain

Musculoskeletal: Positive for back pain. Negative for lower extremity pain

Neurologic: Negative for syncope, confusion

Endocrine: Negative for heat or cold intolerance

Skin: Negative for lower extremity skin changes

Past Medical History:

- No known PMH
- Denies prior PE or DVT

Past Surgical History:

- No prior surgeries

Family History:

- Father with h/o MI at age 45, DM, CAD
- Paternal father with multiple MIs
- Mother with h/o PE iso OCP use

Social Hx

Works as a trucker

Smokes 1ppd for last 20 years

Denies EtOH or substance use

Vital Signs:

T- 99.9 F

HR: 74

BP: 145/72 (symmetric in upper extremities)

RR: 12

O2 Sat 99% on RA

Physical Exam:

General: in no apparent distress, obese, comfortably resting on the stretcher

Cardiovascular: normal S1 and S2, no m/r/g, no extra heart sounds, JVP 8cm at 45 degrees, no peripheral edema, +2 radial, DP and PT pulses

Respiratory: clear to auscultation bilaterally, no wheezes, rhonchi or rales

Abdominal: soft, obese, nontender without rebound or guarding

Musculoskeletal: tenderness to palpation along L sternal border and without deformities

Skin: warm without lower extremity skin changes

Neurologic: alert and following commands

Psychiatric: affect appropriate to mood

Diagnostic Studies:

ECG notable for normal sinus rhythm without ST segment or T wave changes. Unchanged compared to ECG dated 4/2015

MDM:

Assessment and Plan

40M w/no known PMH presenting with 1 week of worsening reproducible chest pain i/s/o contact sports. Symptoms are most likely 2/2 costochondritis given temporal relationship to contact sports and reproducible chest pain on exam. Also considering MI given the patient's smoking hx and strong paternal hx of MI, though hemodynamically stable and ECG at triage unchanged from prior ECGs. Aortic dissection is another consideration for sharp chest pain with back pain radiation i/s/o hypertension though BPs are symmetric in the UEs. Low suspicion for PE in the absence of dyspnea, hypoxia, and evidence of DVT. He is PERC negative so will defer d-dimer testing for PE.

Ddx: costochondritis, MI, aortic dissection, PE

Dx:

- CBC, BMP, CXR
- Troponin q3h

Plan:

- F/u diagnostics
- Provide ibuprofen and acetaminophen for pain control; will reassess for pain relief
- If diagnostics are negative then will discharge home

Disposition: likely home pending evaluation

ED Course:

- 1210 Labs drawn
- 1225 CXR without widened mediastinum, normal sized heart, no evidence of infection
- 1245 CBC wnl, w/o leukocytosis
- 1300 BMP within normal limits
- 1300 Troponin <0.4
- 1300 HEART Score 2 point corresponding to 0.9–1.7% risk of major adverse cardiac event
- 1315 Patient reporting improvement in pain s/p acetaminophen
- 1345 Patient stable
- 1450 2nd troponin drawn, awaiting results
- 1500 Troponin <0.4
- 1503 Pain improved will discharge patient given low suspicion for ACS and aortic dissection and HEART score of 2. Will educate patient on return precautions

14.3.13   Follow-Up and Reassessment

Your responsibilities do not end after presenting your patient. The ED is a great place to learn as a medical student because it often grants more autonomy and ownership than most clinical rotations. Make it a goal to demonstrate ownership and interest in the ED, regardless of whether this is a field you are intending to pursue. Always complete the tasks set in your plan, unless your attending says so. The plan your attending helped you put in place is NOT a suggestion and you are expected to put it into action.

Always confirm that labs have been drawn and sent to the lab. You can do this by checking the lab order status in the EMR or asking the nurses. However, give the nurses time (10–15 mins) to complete the lab draws before asking about the labs. You can always draw the labs yourself if there are significant delays.

Additionally, check the EMR for any new test or imaging results and pay attention to any *critical* lab values, such as low blood glucose, elevated troponin, etc. The EMR will often highlight abnormal values that require attention. Your preclinical knowledge base and clinical acumen will help you determine which abnormalities need to be addressed urgently with your attending. For example, blood glucose of 49 requires urgent treatment, whereas a potassium level of 3.6, though abnormal, does not need to be addressed as urgently.

If you ordered imaging for your patient, you can review the imaging yourself to develop your radiology skills. Additionally, you should talk to your local friendly radiologist to ask them specific questions to advance your patient's care and disposition plan. This proactive approach is needed when the radiology report stalls the patient's disposition, such as a patient awaiting a pelvic ultrasound to rule out an ectopic pregnancy or abdominal imaging to rule out complicated diverticulitis/appendicitis, to mention a few examples. If you are unsure about something in the radiology report, you can also ask the radiologist to review specific images to confirm any uncertainty. Surgeons do this all the time when there is a question of free air or perforations on abdominal imaging.

Follow up on any treatments administered to the patient. First, confirm the patient received the treatment and wait for the treatment to take effect (on average ~15–30 mins). Then, ask the patient if their symptoms (pain, wheezing, shortness of breath, etc.) have improved. This can take the form of a simple, "How is your *Insert symptom here* now that you have received the medication?" You should think about repeating or escalating treatment if symptoms do not improve. Think outside the box when the patient's symptoms persist or worsen. Depending on your bandwidth, it can be helpful to reassess your patient every 15–30 min to check in on their symptoms, update them with results, and answer any questions they may have.

Use the combination of your patient reassessments and incoming diagnostic data to update the plan and follow up with your attending. Your attending will often be busy evaluating all the other patients in the ER, so ask to touch base with your attending when they have a few minutes. I usually asked for their time once the first batch of lab results was available, unless something needed to be addressed urgently. This demonstrates that you are considerate of their time constraints but are also taking initiative to follow up on your patient. When you are updating your attending, take the lead on interpreting the data and providing next steps for treatment or workup. These conversations will challenge you to think and open up learning opportunities with your attending. Again, do not forget to update the nurses and patients when there are changes to the plan or you anticipate a disposition.

Lastly, remember that it is your responsibility to advance patient care and discharge your patients to the appropriate setting. Prioritize the disposition before assuming care of more patients (unless told otherwise by your attending).

Common Error: Never worry alone. If you think something needs urgent attention, grab your attending or residents nearby.

Standout Tip: Call radiology for a "wet read" on any imaging holding up a disposition; always collate a wet read report with the final report. Patients must be made aware of any abnormal finding even if not directly related to the presenting complaint.

Standout Tip: Consult the literature relevant to the patient's symptoms and management whenever there is downtime. You can discuss the literature with your attending during follow-ups to guide management and ask clarifying questions.

Standout Tip: As a sub-intern, you are not there to just report and record information, but should be anticipating next steps and preparing treatment plans.

Presenting 10 patients is less impressive if your patients are stalling in the ED without appropriate treatment and your attending/resident(s) need to complete your work.

Follow up checklist:

- [] Follow up labs and imaging results
  - [] Address critical results
- [] Update treatment and disposition
- [] Reassess clinical status
  - [] 15 min [] 30 min [] 45 min [] 60 min
- [] Follow up with attending
  - [] Discuss plans
  - [] Ask questions
- [] Update nurses

14.4 End and Beyond

14.4.1 Calling Consults

Remember, EM physicians are trained to resuscitate and stabilize acutely sick patients. This means that EM physicians are experts at dealing with the most difficult initial critical moments of every specialty, but at times this comes at the cost of not being an expert in the management of some nonacute illnesses. As such, EM allows you to interact with all sorts of specialists in order to advance patient care. This is also a great opportunity to learn from many of your specialty colleagues. Depending on your clinical setting, you may be interacting with very niche subspecialists to make sure your patient is getting the best medical care possible.

Calling a consult is an art in itself. If you are considering ordering a consult, then make sure that you have *actually* evaluated the patient and ordered applicable studies to aid the workup. Consultants hate nothing more than hearing that you have not evaluated the patient or that you have no studies ordered. You should formulate a *specific* question for the consultants with your attending's input. The Clinical Tips and Pearls chapter also contains a general overview of calling consults which can be a nice supplement to this section.

In preparing for the consult, it is very important for you to gather all relevant information, including HPI, physical exam findings, lab and imaging studies, and, most importantly, the specific clinical question related to patient care. Be sure to confirm your clinical question with your attending and ask if the attending would like to supervise the consult call.

General format for the consult:

- Introduce yourself
- Start with the *clinical question or request*
- Patient one-liner with relevant PMH and recent admissions
- Concise HPI
- Vital signs and relevant physical exam
- Relevant lab and imaging findings
- Treatments attempted if any

! Common Error: Never call a consult without examining the patient and at least starting your workup

Never call a consultant without having a focused question you need addressed.

14

Sample Consult

Hello, this is Alex Bonilla the sub-intern in the ED. I'm calling about patient Mr. W in ER bed 5. We would like a surgical evaluation for a small bowel obstruction. He's a 45-year-old male with hx of SBO in 2017 with several days of increased bloating and now presenting with nausea and vomiting. He is currently afebrile and stable with abdominal distension and voluntary guarding. He has a leukocytosis of 16.5 with a lactate of 3.5 and evidence of SBO on CT abdomen/pelvis. We have placed an NGT set to suction with 50 cc of output and are working on pain control with morphine. Do you have any other questions for me?

All consults follow the same general format described above, but the content of your consult will obviously vary with the specialty. ◘ Table 14.3 contains pearls that will guide tailoring your consult to each specialty.

◘ Table 14.3   Guide to consulting subspecialists

Gastroenterology	Common reasons	GIB, SBP, IBD exacerbation, choledocholithiasis, cholangitis
	One liner	Pertinent history of GI disease. If GIB, mention whether the patient is stable or unstable and IV access status
	Physical exam	Abdominal exam looking for tenderness, distension, and fluid wave. Any sequelae of cirrhosis (if relevant)
	Diagnostic studies	Labs – CBC, BMP, AST/ALT, total and direct bilirubin, alkaline phosphate, lipase, lactate Imaging – abdominal ultrasound, CT Abdomen
General Surgery	Common reasons	Appendicitis, acute cholecystitis/cholangitis, esophageal rupture, LBO/SBO, bowel perforation, complicated diverticulitis, and incarcerated hernias
	One liner	Significant comorbidities and abdominal surgical history and anticoagulation status
	Physical exam	hemodynamic stability, abdominal exam looking for tenderness, rigidity, guarding, or signs of peritonitis
	Diagnostics	Labs – CBC, BMP, lactate, type and screen Imaging – Abdominal US or CT abdomen
Neurology	Common reasons	Stroke/TIA, complicated migraines, seizure management, multiple sclerosis flare
	One liner	All relevant neurological history and risk factors for neurological disease
	Physical exam	Complete neurological exam including CN II-XII, motor strength, sensory exam, cerebellar, reflexes. ALWAYS try to walk the patient
	Diagnostics	Imaging – usually noncontrast CT head
Neurosurgery	Common reasons	ICH, SAH, subdural/epidural hematoma, cauda equina syndrome, spinal epidural abscess
	One liner	Mechanism of injury and anticoagulation use
	Physical exam	Focused neuro exam focusing on mental status, CN II-XII and motor/sensory exam, GCS
	Diagnostics	Labs – CBC, BMP, PT-INR, type and screen Imaging – noncontrast CT head
OB-GYN	Common reasons	Vaginal bleeding, preeclampsia/eclampsia, ectopic pregnancy, PID, trauma during pregnancy, ovarian torsion
	One liner	Include gravidity and parity and for pregnant patients, the gestational age and method by which LMP was determined
	Physical exam	Abdominal exam, supervised pelvic exam (look for bleeding, discharge or tissue in the cervical os)
	Diagnostics	Labs – CBC, BMP, AST/ALT, uric acid level and beta-hCG, type and screen Imaging – abdominal ultrasound and transvaginal ultrasound

(continued)

Table 14.3 (continued)

Orthopedic Surgery	Common reasons	Fractures, dislocations, tendon ruptures, hardware infection, joint infection, surgical complications, compartment syndrome
	One liner	Mechanism of injury. For an upper extremity fracture, mention whether the patient is right- or left-hand dominant (RHD or LHD)
	Physical exam	Note gross deformities, open fractures, and neurovascular exam (pulses, sensation, motor strength) For femur fractures, note whether one extremity is shorter than the other
	Diagnostics	Labs – CBC, BMP, PT-INR, type and screen (if anticipating surgery) Imaging – X-rays or CT imaging for relevant extremity
Vascular Surgery	Common reasons	Critical limb ischemia, aortic dissection, abdominal aortic aneurysm, severe DVT, acute mesenteric ischemia, arteriovenous fistula malfunction
	One liner	significant cardiovascular comorbidities, prior vascular surgeries, and current anticoagulation status
	Physical exam	Pulses! Use a doppler for nonpalpable pulses. On abdominal exam look for a pulsatile mass. Perform a neurovascular exam on the affected limb and always assess skin temperature (e.g., cold vs. warm to touch)
	Diagnostics	Labs – CBC, BMP, lactate, type and screen, PT-INR Imaging – CT abdomen (if relevant), US

Standout Tip: If you have the bandwidth, it can be extremely educational to join the consultant during the evaluation to learn important skills, such as physical exam nuances or procedures. Ask your attending and consultant if this is fine with them before disappearing into the room though!

Common Error: Be courteous and professional with the consultants. A positive attitude really goes a long way when working with other providers.

Depending on the institution, consultants may be obligated to respond to all ED consult pages within a predetermined amount of time (institutional dependent). If they don't contact you within that time period, check with the patient and nurse to confirm whether the consultant has evaluated the patient. Sometimes, consultants perform the evaluation before calling back. Let your attending know that you are paging the consultant again. If you still do not have a response after the second page, then you should let your attending know. At this point, your attending may need to reach out directly or escalate to the supervising attending on the consultant team.

Consult checklist:
- [] Order relevant labs and imaging
- [] Review studies
- [] Prepare clinical question
- [] Prepare succinct HPI with relevant VS and physical exam
- [] Page consultant
- [] Page again
- [] Notify attending if consultant doesn't respond to the second page
- [] Follow up recommendations

14.4.2 The Discharge

At this point, you have reviewed all diagnostic results, completed the patient's evaluation for life- or limb-threatening disease and determined (with your attending) that the patient is stable and safe for a discharge home. Now it is time to prepare the discharge paperwork, which serves to educate the patient about their visit, symptoms, and next steps. If you have EMR access, you can

prepare written discharge instructions and attach patient education material to help the patient understand their underlying symptoms and diagnosis. The written discharge summary consists of the following:
1. The patient's reason for the ER visit
2. Diagnostics performed
3. Presumed diagnosis and treatment plan
4. Follow-up instructions
5. Return precautions

The written discharge paperwork should be written using layperson language. Try to avoid medical jargon and abbreviations wherever possible. You do not need to go into intricate details about the diagnostics performed but take a generalized approach. The treatment plan should provide clear instructions on medication doses. In the follow-up instructions, make sure to highlight when to visit a primary care doctor, any specialized outpatient care you have scheduled for them, and any lab/imaging findings that require follow-up. Finally, provide clear instructions on when to return to the emergency department (known as return precautions). Return precautions are the symptoms and scenarios that should prompt the patient to seek emergency care. These symptoms are often suggestive of life- or limb-threatening disease. If you provide the patient with preprinted discharge instructions, make sure you read them to ensure it is appropriate for their presentation.

■ **Discharge Written Example**
1. You presented to the emergency department for chest pain.
2. Your labs and chest imaging did not show evidence of infection, blood clot, or heart attack at this time.
3. Your symptoms are likely due to costochondritis, which is inflammation of the chest joints. Please take Tylenol 325 mg every 4 h and ibuprofen 400 mg every 6 h as needed for your pain.
4. Please follow up with your primary care doctor in 2 weeks if the pain does not resolve.
5. Please return to the emergency department if you experience chest pressure/tightness, sweating, shortness of breath, and weakness.

After writing the discharge summary, you should talk to the patient about the evaluation, results and next steps. Let them know that their testing did not show evidence of life- or limb-threatening disease and the most likely cause of their problem. Again, use simple language to communicate what you did during the visit. If you followed up consistently throughout the visit, then this conversation should not take that long. It is also helpful to make time to answer any questions they may have for you. Once you have clarified, you can proceed to discussing the return precautions. Confirm the patient's preferred pharmacy to submit medication orders.

Clinical Pearl: Ideally, you should update the discharge information throughout the patient's stay. In some EMRs, you may be able to save discharge templates or auto-phrases that can be populated and edited in the discharge tab. Ask your attending or residents about this!

Clinical Pearl: Ask your attending if they want to review your discharge summary before discharging the patient.

Discharge Conversation Example
Hello Mr T, I wanted to circle back with you about your ER visit today. When you presented with your symptoms of chest pain, we were worried about dangerous diagnoses, such as a heart attack or blood clot. Based on your lab work and chest imaging results, there is no evidence of these dangerous diagnoses at this time. All of these symptoms are likely due to something called costochondritis or inflammation of the chest joints. However, if you are not improving

within 72 h, it is very important that you return to us or to your primary medical doctor to be reevaluated. What questions can I answer for you? It is safe for you to go home now. In the meantime, you can take Tylenol and ibuprofen as needed. Please do not hesitate to return to the emergency department if you notice crushing chest pressure, profuse sweating, shortness of breath, and weakness. Everything we have discussed today will be in your discharge paperwork.

Discharge checklist:
- [] Prepare discharge summary
  – [] Presumed diagnosis and plan [] Follow-up instructions [] Return precautions
- [] Discharge summary reviewed by attending
- [] Discuss visit and discharge with patient
- [] Answer patient's questions

Clinical Pearl: The only way to build clinical acumen is to follow up all patients from the simplest to the most complex. It can be humbling (yet instructive!) to find the simple costochondritis was actually a PE or aortic dissection; or the gastroenteritis was appendicitis. Many physicians think they are smarter than they are because they never invested the time to get follow-up.

14.4.3 Signing Out Your Patient to Another Team Member/ Pass-off

You may not complete a patient's workup and disposition before the end of the shift and that is totally fine. Depending on the institution, your team may sign out patients to the incoming team by rounding or through individual sign-outs. Regardless of how it is done, you should prepare to briefly present your patients to another team member. Your sign-out should consist of the following information:
- One-liner detailing PMH and reason for ER presentation
- Pertinent vital signs and physical exam
- Lab and diagnostic findings relevant to chief complaint
- MDM – leading diagnosis, alternate potential diagnoses and what you have done so far
- To do:
  – Follow-up tasks
  – Pending studies to look out for
  – Contingency plans

Common Errors: Do NOT pass on tasks, such as consults, procedures, and pelvic exams, to your incoming colleagues unless instructed by your attending.

Again, EM is a fast-paced team sport and we all have a responsibility to look out for each other. Generally, you should avoid passing on consults, procedures, and pelvic exams as tasks for your incoming colleagues to complete. You know the patient better than your incoming colleagues do, so it makes the most sense for you to complete the consult for the sake of patient care. Similarly, you have developed rapport with your patient, so it is easier for you to complete the pelvic exam. Finally, procedures are time consuming to complete and are actually beneficial for your education. Before leaving, try to introduce your patient to the next responsible provider.

Example Sign-Out
HPI: Mr. W in bed 5 is a 45-year-old male with hx lap chole, umbilical hernia repair, and SBO who presented with several days of increased bloating and constipation and nausea & vomiting today. Found to have SBO on CT imaging.

VS and physical exam: afebrile, HDS, abdominal exam notable for abdominal distension and voluntary guarding, no rebound tenderness or peritonitis.

Labs: leukocytosis to 16K, K+ to 3.2, lactate of 3.5. CT A/P demonstrates partial closed loop SBO at the level of the jejunum.

MDM: He is currently receiving 1L of LR for i/s/o poor PO intake and the lactate of 3.5. Received K+ repletion. We placed an NGT to suction with net 75 cc and working on pain control with morphine. Surgery has been consulted and we are currently awaiting further recommendations regarding medical vs. surgical management. If he becomes hemodynamically unstable, I would reevaluate for bowel perforation and page surgery.

Disposition: likely admission to surgery

To do:
- [] F/u surgery recommendations
- [] Repeat lactate after fluid bolus
- [] Monitor VS and abdominal exam
- [] Monitor pain control

Clinical Pearl: Sign-outs carry the highest medical legal risks because of transferred bias or incomplete transfer of information. At sign-out, you should introduce yourself, so the patient knows your name and briefly evaluate the patient.

14.4.4 Final Tips

We covered a lot of information, but you can refer to ▣ Fig. 14.5 for the main takeaways of the shift workflow. Lastly, you should remember to keep a positive attitude and have fun in the emergency department. Your positive approach will take you far in helping patients feel at ease and also energizing your team members. Remember that the feedback you receive in the emergency department is meant to help you improve your skills and you should make an effort to integrate the feedback in real time. This also demonstrates your flexibility in the ED. Although receiving feedback can be difficult at times, try not to take it personally and assume that the person providing it is coming from a good place. NEVER react in a confrontational manner with colleagues or patients as this is unprofessional and will burn bridges. Finally, try to follow up on interesting patients in the EMR, read about your patients' pathology and learn something new after taking the time to decompress from a shift. This will make the learning more memorable and help you expand your fund of knowledge. Good luck!

Before/Start

- Set tangible goals for shift
- Team introductions
- Discuss learning goals & logistics with attending and team

During

- Prepare for patient encounter (chart review)
- Patient encounter (HPI & Physical Exam)
- Post patient encounter (enter orders, oral presentation, finalize plan)
- Patient follow up (diagnostics, treatment, response, & consults)
- Patient discharge (discharge paperwork and discharge conversation)

End & Beyond

- Complete all consults, procedures & pending discharges
- Sign-out remaining patients
- Debrief (discuss goals and feedback with attending)
- Select a patient to read about at home (e.g. workup, management, evidence behind treatment, etc.)

▣ **Fig. 14.5** Summary of ED shift workflow

14.5 Most Common Emergency Department Chief Complaints

The following section is a very brief overview of the most common chief complaints you are likely to see as a sub-intern. This is by no means comprehensive, but rather meant to cover pertinent clinical (e.g., red flags) and diagnostic findings you should keep in mind and the initial ED management. Feel free to refer to other chapters in the book for more on inpatient management. Other helpful resources include: EM:RAP, EM Clerkship Podcast, 5 Minute Sono, WikEM, Rosen's and Tintinalli's. Note that antibiotic regimens and medication doses may vary by institution, so be sure to follow your institution's guidelines.

14.5.1 Chief Complaint: Chest Pain

- General Considerations
  - Most patients receive an ECG at triage – be sure to review the ECG ASAP or request an ECG if one is not available
  - Always compare the patient's ECG with any previous ECGs available (either from EMS or prior hospitalizations)
  - Concerning ECG signs include *new* Q waves, inverted T waves, ST changes, left bundle branch blocks, AV block or arrhythmias (among other findings)
  - Patients with active chest pain are placed on a cardiac monitor and treated with ASA and NTG. They require at least two troponins and must have repeat ECGs every 30 min until their pain resolves
  - Refer to ◘ Table 14.5 for a summary on life-threatening causes you should consider for chest pain

14.5.1.1 Acute Coronary Syndrome
- Key HPI
  - [] Crushing substernal chest pain or pressure ± radiation to the jaw or arm
  - [] Atypical presentations include abdominal pain and general malaise, especially in elderly, female patients and patients with DM
  - [] Sympathomimetic drug use (e.g., cocaine)

- Key risk factors
  - [] Family h/o cardiac disease [] DM [] HTN [] Hyperlipidemia [] Smoking

- ROS
  - [] Diaphoresis [] Lightheadedness [] Syncope [] Palpitations
  - [] Exertional chest pain [] Dyspnea [] Nausea [] Vomiting

- Physical exam findings
  - VS – tachycardia/bradycardia, hypotension, hypoxia
  - Cardiovascular – extra heart sounds, new murmur, peripheral pulses
  - Respiratory – crackles (if HF present)
  - Abdominal – abdominal tenderness
  - Extremities – peripheral edema (if HF also present), lukewarm/cold extremities (suggests cardiogenic shock)

Diagnostics   CBC, BMP, troponin – may not be elevated initially, BNP (if concerned about HF), ECG- compare to EMS strip or prior ECGs

❗ ● Common Error: Textbooks often describe the classic chest pressure with radiation to the jaw and arms presentation, but certain populations, such as women, the elderly, and patients with DM, may have alternate presentations. I recommend you keep an open mind with these populations and work really hard to convince yourself it is not ACS.

✓ Clinical Pearl: Repeat ECG if history is suspicious despite normal ECG
- CXR – look for widened mediastinum (suggests aortic dissection as cause of ACS)

14

- Management
- IV access, cardiac monitor (look for arrhythmias), supplemental O_2 (if O_2 <94)
- Medications: ASA 162 mg PO (crushed), NTG (avoid if suspecting right-sided STEMI), IV pain control (fentanyl vs. morphine)
- Activate the catherization lab
- Consider the HEART Pathway for stable patients in whom you suspect ACS
    - Use HEART Score to risk-stratify patients and guide management and disposition
    - Not to be used for patients already diagnosed with ACS (e.g., ECG changes, new troponin elevation) or high-risk patients

- Considerations
- Aortic dissection can cause ACS if the dissection extends into the coronary arteries – check a CXR
- Pay attention to new arrhythmias and murmurs as these can be complications of ischemia
- Use HEART Score and HEART pathway to risk-stratify and guide management

14.5.1.2 Aortic Dissection

- Key HPI
- [] Sudden-onset tearing/ripping chest pain radiating to the back
- [] Drug use (methamphetamine)

- Key risk factors
- [] Hypertension [] Connective tissue disorders [] Drug use

- ROS
- [] Syncope [] Lightheadedness [] Chest pain [] Palpitations [] Dyspnea
- [] Abdominal pain [] Numbness [] Weakness [] Hematuria

- Physical Exam findings
- Cardiovascular – new murmur distant heart sounds, JVD, asymmetric pulses, asymmetric blood pressure
- Respiratory – crackles
- Abdominal – abdominal tenderness
- Neurological – syncope, weakness or numbness, or other focal neurological deficits

Diagnostics CBC, BMP – assess for renal injury, PT-INR, troponin – elevated if dissecting into coronary arteries or from demand ischemia, ECG (ischemic changes)
- CXR – look for mediastinal widening
- CT with contrast – confirms diagnosis, classifies dissection, and identifies distal complications (e.g., involvement of distal branches or thromboembolism)

- Management
- IV access, cardiac monitor (look for arrhythmias), supplemental O_2 (if O_2 <94)
- Medications for BP and pain control
    - BP control to reduce shearing forces and prevent dissection from extending

Clinical Pearl: Dissection can cause ischemic changes along the aorta and thus can present with neurological deficits (e.g., weakness or numbness) or gut or renal ischemia.

- Start with IV beta blocker (e.g., esmolol) to prevent reflex tachycardia then IV nitroprusside or nicardipine for afterload reduction
- Measure BP in both upper extremities and use higher BP to guide treatment
  - Pain – IV fentanyl as it blunts catecholamine surge and reduces HR and BP
    - Consider morphine
  - Emergent surgery consult for surgical intervention

- **Considerations**
- Type A dissections may cause ACS if dissection extends into the coronary arteries – always check an ECG
- Can present with neurological deficits – perform a thorough physical exam
- Check BP in both upper extremities – use the higher BP to guide BP control

14.5.1.3   Cardiac Tamponade
- **Key HPI**
- [] Dyspnea [] Fatigue [] Peripheral edema [] Anticoagulation use

- **Key risk factors**
- [] Trauma [] Causes of pericardial inflammation (e.g., HIV, malignancy, SLE, TB, uremia)

- **ROS**
- [] Fatigue [] Cough [] Dyspnea [] Chest pressure
- [] Palpitations [] AMS [] Lightheadedness

- **Physical Exam**
- VS – hypotension, tachycardia
- Cardiovascular – distant heart sounds, JVD, peripheral edema, peripheral pulses

Diagnostics   ECG – electrical alternans, low voltage, bedside US – pericardial effusion, diastolic RV collapse, systolic RA collapse

- **Management**
- IV fluid bolus if patient is hypotensive
- Emergent cardiology or surgical consult for pericardiocentesis vs. surgical drainage

14.5.1.4   Esophageal Rupture
- **Key HPI**
- [] Vomiting/retching [] Heavy alcohol use
- [] Recent thoracic procedures (e.g., endoscopy) [] Thoracic trauma

- **Key risk factors**
- [] Alcohol use disorder [] Recent thoracic procedures

- **ROS**
- [] Cough [] Drooling [] Dysphagia [] Hematemesis [] Chest pain [] Nausea [] Vomiting

- Physical Exam
  - VS – fever, tachycardia
  - Generally – very ill-appearing
  - MSK – cervical/mediastinal subcutaneous emphysema (crepitus)

Diagnostics   CBC, BMP, ECG – to rule out ACS, CXR (pneumomediastinum, left-sided pleural effusion)

- Management
  - Make patient NPO and IV fluids – 1L of NS or LR
  - IV broad spectrum antibiotics for aerobic and anaerobic coverage
    - For example, piperacillin/tazobactam 3.375 g q6h
  - Emergent surgical consult

14.5.1.5   Pulmonary Embolism

Key HPI   [] Pleuritic chest pain worse with inspiration [] Associated back pain [] Unilateral leg swelling and pain (DVT)
  - History of syncope or hemoptysis is very concerning

- Key risk factors
  - [] Prolonged immobilization or hospitalization [] Recent surgery/trauma [] Malignancy
  - [] Estrogen-based OCP use [] Hormone replacement therapy [] Pregnancy
  - [] Stroke with motor deficits (implies immobilization)

- ROS
  - [] Syncope [] Cough [] Hemoptysis [] Chest pain [] Palpitations
  - [] Dyspnea [] Wheezing [] Skin discoloration [] Edema/warmth

- Physical Exam
  - VS – tachycardia, hypoxia, hypotension
  - Respiratory – wheezes, crackles
  - Extremities – unilateral lower extremity pain, edema or warmth
  - Neurological – AMS
  - Skin – unilateral lower extremity swelling or discoloration

Diagnostics   CBC, BMP, cardiac markers (troponin & BNP), ECG (right heart strain, S1Q3T3), bedside US (look for signs of right heart strain)
  - Use Wells' Criteria to determine pretest probability and guide potential diagnostics (e.g., d-dimer, CTPA or V/Q scan). See ◘ Fig. 14.6 below
  - Consider V/Q scan in pregnant patients or patients with contraindication to CTPA

- Management
  - IV access, cardiac monitor, supplemental O_2 if SpO_2 <94%
  - IV fluids – especially if the patient is hypotensive
  - Treatment will depend on the severity of disease as determined by hemodynamic stability and imaging findings and/or cardiac biomarkers (see ◘ Table 14.4)

- Considerations
  - Persistent or isolated tachycardia should raise your suspicion for PE.
  - A negative lower extremity ultrasound for DVT does not exclude PE.

Standout Tip: You can download apps, like MD Calc, to help you use these tools at the bedside – no need to memorize every single criterion!

Clinical Pearl: V/Q scans are typically used in patients with renal insufficiency, chronic PE, or allergy to IV contrast. V/Q scans are not as useful in patients with volume overload.

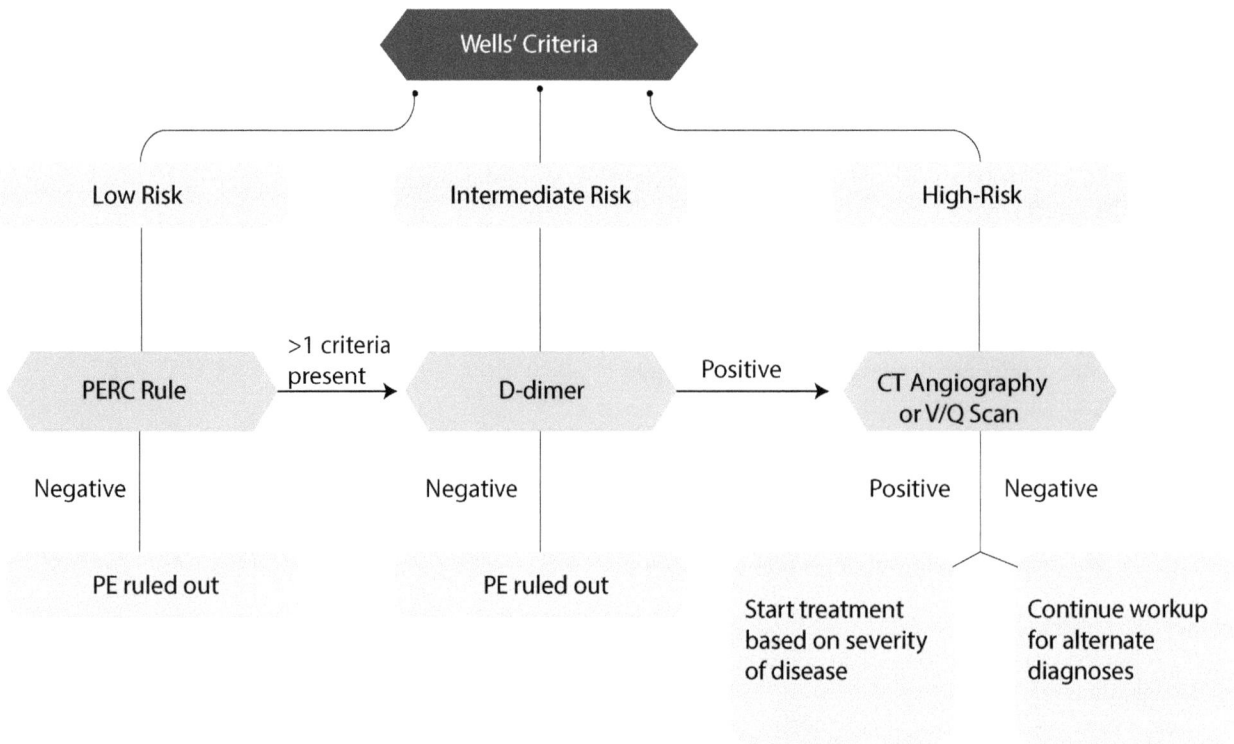

☐ **Fig. 14.6** Risk stratification to determine diagnostic testing

14

☐ **Table 14.4** Treatment of PE based on clinical severity

Severity	Non-massive PE	Sub-massive PE	Massive PE
Clinical Findings	Hemodynamically stable and no evidence of right heart strain	Hemodynamically stable with evidence of right heart strain on echocardiogram or cardiac biomarkers (troponin, BNP)	Systolic BP <90 mmHg
Treatment	Anticoagulation alone	Anticoagulation	Thrombolytics ± anticoagulation or CDT

- Use an age-adjusted d-dimer cutoff for patients over the age of 50 → (age × 10) ug/L.
  - The rationale is that d-dimer increases with age
  - Associated with minimal decline in sensitivity and increases specificity in low-risk patients

14.5.2 Chief Complaint: Dyspnea/Shortness of Breath

- General Considerations
- Before starting the evaluation, observe the patient's work of breathing and O_2 saturation to get a sense of the patient's clinical status
- Always consider cardiac causes of dyspnea
- Monitor hemodynamics, O_2 saturation, and mental status
- Only administer supplemental O_2 if the patient needs it (O_2 sat <94%)
- Refer to ☐ Table 14.6 for a summary on life-threatening causes you should consider for shortness of breath

▢ Table 14.5   Summary of life-threatening and alternate chest pain etiologies

Differential diagnosis	Key history	Key clinical findings	Diagnostic studies	Management
Acute Coronary Syndrome	Classically: diaphoresis, nausea, and radiation to the jaw and upper extremity Watch out for atypical presentations in elderly and female patients (e.g., abdominal pain, malaise, SOB)	New murmur suggests valvular involvement Crackles, JVD & peripheral edema suggests acute heart failure	EKG – compare to priors CBC, BMP, PT/INR & troponin CXR – if concerned STEMI is 2/2 aortic dissection	NTG – relieves anginal pain ASA 162 mg PO (crushed) IV pain medications (fentanyl vs. morphine) Activate the catherization lab
Aortic Dissection	Sudden onset tearing chest pain radiating to the back ± diaphoresis, nausea/vomiting	Check BP in both UEs (use higher BP for management) Pulse deficits, new murmur, JVD Thorough neuro exam	EKG – evidence of ACS CXR – mediastinal widening Bedside US – tamponade CT w/contrast – confirms dx & helps assess for complications	BP control – 1st administer beta-blocker (e.g., esmolol)! 2nd start afterload reducer (e.g., nitroprusside, nicardipine) Pain control – fentanyl vs. morphine Consult vascular surgery for further management
Pulmonary Embolism	Pleuritic chest pain ± SOB, hemoptysis, unilateral leg swelling	Isolated or persistent tachycardia, hypoxia, hypotension DVT	Depends on risk stratification (d-dimer, CTPA vs. V/Q scan) so use Wells' Criteria for guidance V/Q Scan – consider if CTPA is contraindicated or in pregnant patients Bedside echo – look for signs of right heart strain Doppler US – when suspecting DVT EKG – nonspecific findings (sinus tachycardia, right heart strain, S1Q3T3)	Treatment (anticoagulation vs. IV thrombolytics vs. CDT) depends on the severity of disease (massive, sub-massive, and non-massive)
Esophageal Rupture (Boerhaave's syndrome)	h/o retching (e.g., patient's with AUD), recent procedures (e.g., endoscopy) or thoracic trauma	Febrile, Ill-appearing, cervical/mediastinal subcutaneous emphysema (crepitus)	CXR – pleural effusion, pneumomediastinum	NPO, IV broad spectrum antibiotics & IV fluids Emergent surgery consult
Cardiac Tamponade	Acute onset could be 2/2 trauma	Tachycardia, tachypnea, hypotension, JVD, distant heart sounds	Bedside US – shows tamponade	IV fluid bolus Pericardiocentesis vs. surgical drainage

Other diagnoses to consider: costochondritis/MSK, cholecystitis, GERD, herpes zoster, myocarditis, pericarditis or PNA

14.5.2.1 Asthma

- Key HPI
- [] Rescue/maintenance medications use
- [] Number of times the patient has used rescue inhaler since onset of symptoms

Clinical Pearl: A history of volume overload (or weight gain), unilateral leg swelling/pain, or pleuritic chest pain should point you toward an alternate diagnosis such as CHF or PE.

- [] Last hospitalization [] Previous intubation/ICU admission for asthma exacerbation
- [] Potential triggers (allergies, exercise, infection, medication nonadherence, etc.)

- **Risk factors**
- [] Asthma [] Poor living conditions

- **ROS**
- [] Fevers [] Chest pain [] Cough [] Dyspnea [] Sputum [] URI symptoms [] Wheezes [] Myalgias

- **Physical Exam**
- VS – fever, tachycardia, hypotension, decreased O_2 saturation
- Cardiovascular – any evidence of volume overload should point you toward another diagnosis (e.g., CHF)
- Respiratory – difficulty speaking, tripoding, wheezes

Diagnostics   CBC – leukocytosis (i/s/o infection), ECG – if chest pain concerning for ACS
- CXR – usually normal in patients with asthma but could be useful if suspecting underlying infection as trigger or alternate diagnoses

- **Management**
- Bronchodilators – three doses of albuterol (5 mg) + ipratropium (0.5 mg) q20 min
  - This is sometimes referred to as "stacked" nebulizers
- Steroids – prednisone 40–60 mg or methylprednisolone 125 mg IV
  - ED use within the 1st hour is associated with reduced admission rates and relapses
  - Discharge patients with an additional 4 days of prednisone for a total of 5 days of treatment
- For very severe cases consider escalating to magnesium, terbutaline, ketamine, epinephrine, or intubation
  - Considered severe if symptoms are unresponsive to bronchodilators and/or severe respiratory distress
- Disposition –
  - After 1 h, monitor for improvement in chest tightness, dyspnea, and wheezing or PEF
    - Discharge patients with a PEF >80% predicted
    - 60% < PEF <80% requires further monitoring and treatment
    - PEF <40% requires admission
  - FEV1 and PEF are most helpful if you know the patient's baseline and ED has access to PFTs
  - Patients without improvement (declining PEF or PEF <40%) or comorbidities should be admitted

- **Considerations**
- Keep a very watchful eye on patients with previous ICU admission or intubation history
- Asthma exacerbation can be diagnosed clinically, but you should consider further diagnostics if suspecting alternate diagnoses (e.g., ACS, CHF, PE)
- Patient with improvement in symptoms can be discharged home with medications and close PCP follow-up

= Don't forget to address any potential triggers (e.g., influenza)

14.5.2.2 COPD

- **Key HPI**
= [] Worsening dyspnea [] Increased productive cough [] Increased O_2 requirement
= [] Home O_2 requirement and changes in baseline requirements
= [] Medication regimen & adherence [] Triggers (medication nonadherence, infection, etc.)
= [] History of intubation/ICU admission [] Recent hospitalization

- **Risk factors**
= [] Smoking

- **ROS**
= [] Fever [] Chest tightness [] Dyspnea [] Productive cough [] AMS

- **Physical Exam**
= VS – fever, tachycardia, decreased O_2 saturation (likely decreased at baseline, so assess change from baseline)
= Respiratory – difficulty speaking full sentences, pursed lip breathing, tripoding, accessory muscle use, diffuse wheezes
= Neurologic – altered mental status (very concerning finding!)
= Skin – cyanosis

Diagnostics   CBC – leukocytosis, ABG/VBG – monitor pH and CO_2 levels for acidemia and hypercapnia, ECG – may see multifocal atrial tachycardia
= CXR – hyperinflation, flattened diaphragm, may find evidence of pneumonia or pulmonary edema
= CT chest – consider if history and physical is suspicious for PE

- **Management**
= Oxygen – provide oxygen supplementation and titrate to a goal O_2 88–92%
  – Consider NIPPV if concerned for respiratory failure
= Bronchodilators – three doses of albuterol (5 mg) + ipratropium (0.5 mg) q20min
  – AKA "stacked" nebulizers
= Steroids – prednisone 40–60 mg or methylprednisolone 125 mg IV
  – Discharge patients with an additional 4 days of prednisone for a total of 5 days of treatment

- **Considerations**
= Keep a very watchful eye on patients with previous ICU admission or intubation history
= Monitor O_2 saturation – should aim for 88–92%
= Don't forget to address any potential triggers (e.g., influenza)

14.5.2.3 Congestive Heart Failure

- **Key HPI**
= [] Chest pain [] Dyspnea [] PND [] Weight gain (quantify and determine over what period of time)
= [] Swelling [] Exercise intolerance [] Triggers (atrial fibrillation, infection, ischemia, medical nonadherence, etc.) [] Home diuresis regimen

Clinical Pearl: Figure out whether the symptoms are new or chronic. New acute CHF should prompt further workup for potential ACS, myocarditis, valvular disease, or toxicologic causes.

- Weight gain is due to excess volume – ask the patient for baseline weight or check the EMR for the last recorded weight from the last hospital discharge
- Check last available echocardiogram for ejection fraction, valvular disease, or hypokinesis

■ Risk factors
- [] CAD [] DM [] HTN [] Valvular disease

■ ROS
- [] Fevers [] Chills [] URI symptoms [] Cough [] Sputum [] Chest pain
- [] Palpitations [] Dyspnea [] Wheezes [] Edema [] Abdominal pain

■ Physical Exam
- VS – tachycardia, hypotension, tachypnea
- Cardiovascular – S3, elevated JVD, weak pulses, bilateral peripheral edema (usually lower extremities, but may see abdominal, scrotal, or sacral edema)
- Abdominal – RUQ tenderness 2/2 hepatic congestion
- Extremities – lukewarm or cold skin (check inner thighs – above the knees, not the shins or feet)

Diagnostics   BMP – hyponatremia, hypokalemia, and elevated BUN/Cr; BNP – compare to baseline as it may be chronically elevated; troponin – if concerned about ischemia; lactate – for cardiogenic shock; ECG – look for arrhythmias or ischemia
- CXR – if worried about infection, otherwise may see cardiomegaly pleural effusion or pulmonary edema
- Bedside US – quick check for cardiac function

■ Management
- Breathing – start with O_2 supplementation if O_2 saturation <94%
  - Escalate to NIPPV if the patient is in respiratory distress or i/s/o hypercapnia or hypoxia
- Diuresis – administer the patient's daily dose of PO furosemide in IV form as a starting dose
  - Furosemide PO to IV is a 1 to 2 conversion so the patient is actually receiving a higher dose
  - Consider a higher dose if the patient does not respond to the initial dose
  - Monitor oxygen requirement, respiratory status, and UOP for response to treatment – do they feel better?
- NTG IV – indicated for patients with cardiogenic pulmonary edema
  - Doses start at 5 mcg/min and can uptitrate by 5–10 mcg/min (max dose is 200 mcg/min) every 3–5 min based on response
  - Confirm presence of contraindications such as aortic stenosis, RV infarct, recent phosphodiesterase use
- If applicable, address the underlying trigger (atrial fibrillation, influenza, ischemia, pneumonia, etc.)
- More often than not, patients with heart failure exacerbation need to be admitted

14

Clinical Pearl: NIPPV can cause hypotension so be mindful in patients with hypotension or preload dependence (e.g., aortic stenosis).

- Considerations
- Try to identify a trigger for the heart failure exacerbation
- Exercise caution with aggressive diuresis, NIPPV, and nitroglycerin in patients with hypotension or preload dependence
- Avoid beta-blockers during acute heart failure exacerbations

14.5.2.4 Pneumonia

- Key HPI
- [] Dyspnea [] Cough [] Fever [] Sick contacts [] Recent viral illness [] Recent hospitalizations
- [] Immunosuppression status (helps guide disposition and antibiotic treatment)

- Risk factors
- [] Age [] Cardiac/lung disease [] Immunosuppression
- [] Alcohol use disorder [] Smoking

- ROS
- [] Fever [] Fatigue [] Chills [] Hemoptysis [] Pleuritic chest pain [] Dyspnea
- [] Productive cough [] Abdominal pain [] Nausea [] Vomiting [] Myalgias

- Physical Exam
- VS – fever, tachycardia, hypotension, tachypnea, decreased O_2 saturation
- Respiratory – increased WOB, decreased breath sounds, crackles, rhonchi
- Abdominal – abdominal tenderness may be an atypical presentation, particularly in elderly patients

Diagnostics   CBC – leukocytosis, BMP – electrolyte abnormalities, consider lactate, blood gas (ABG or VBG) and blood cultures for very sick patients
- CXR – may see consolidations, infiltrates, pleural effusions, or abscesses
  - Not the most sensitive or specific test
- CT – not a routine test, but consider if you have high suspicion for pneumonia despite normal CXR

Clinical Pearl: Dehydrated, elderly, and immunosuppressed patients may not have any findings – don't rely too heavily on CXR to make the diagnoses and use your clinical judgment.

- Management
- Antibiotic treatment – dependent on disease severity, risk factors, and local resistance patterns
  - CAP
    - Outpatient – azithromycin single dose of 500 mg PO followed by 250 mg PO for 4 days OR doxycycline 100 mg PO q12h for 5–7 days
      - For patients with comorbidities (e.g., DM, heart/lung disease, immunosuppression) add on amoxicillin/clavulanate 2 g PO q12h for 5 days to above regimens OR
      - Consider monotherapy with levofloxacin 750 mg PO q24h for 5 days OR moxifloxacin 400 mg PO q24h for 5 days
    - General inpatient – ceftriaxone 1 g IV q24h AND azithromycin 500 mg PO or IV q24h
      - Add on vancomycin if concerned about MRSA colonization
  - HAP
    - Consider cefepime 2 g IV q8h AND levofloxacin 750 mg IV q24h AND vancomycin
- Disposition –
  - CURB-65 Score to risk-stratify patients with CAP

☐ Table 14.6 Summary of life-threatening and alternate dyspnea etiologies

Differential diagnosis	Key history	Key clinical findings	Diagnostics	Management
Asthma Exacerbation	Chest tightness, dyspnea, medication adherence, triggers, h/o ICU admission or intubation	Tachycardia, decreased O_2 saturation Accessory muscle use, tripoding, wheezes AMS	Clinically diagnosed Consider CBC, BMP, CXR	Supplemental O_2 if O_2 <94% Bronchodilators and steroids Severe exacerbations require escalation of tx
COPD Exacerbation	Increased cough, sputum production, wheezing	Tachycardia, decreased O2 saturation Accessory muscle use, tripoding, wheezes AMS	CXR – flattened diaphragm, hyperinflation, PNA CT – if concerned about alternate diagnosis	Supplemental O_2 with goal O_2 saturation 88–92% NIPPV for respiratory failure Bronchodilators and steroids Monitor AMS and O_2 saturation
Congestive Heart Failure	Chest pain, dyspnea, weight gain, potential triggers, home diuretic regimen	S3 heart sound, elevated JVD, peripheral edema, peripheral pulses	CXR – cardiomegaly, pleural effusion, pulmonary edema	Oxygen supplementation Diuresis – start with total daily dose of furosemide in IV form NTG for cardiogenic pulmonary edema
Pulmonary Embolism	Pleuritic chest pain ± SOB, hemoptysis, unilateral leg swelling	Isolated or persistent tachycardia, hypoxia, hypotension DVT	Depends on risk stratification (d-dimer, CTPA vs. V/Q scan) so use Wells' Criteria for guidance V/Q Scan – consider if CTPA is contraindicated or in pregnant patients Bedside echo – look for signs of right heart strain Doppler US – when suspecting DVT EKG – nonspecific findings (sinus tachycardia, right heart strain, S1Q3T3)	Treatment (anticoagulation vs. IV thrombolytics vs. CDT) depends on the severity of disease (massive, sub-massive, and non-massive)
PNA	Fever, dyspnea, pleuritic chest pain, abdominal pain Comorbidities & risk factors	Fever, tachycardia, decreased O_2 saturation AMS, increased breath sounds ± increased WOB	CBC, BMP, lactate CXR – not the most sensitive/specific CT – if CXR negative + high suspicion for PNA	Supplemental O_2 if O_2 <94% Antibiotic treatment – dependent on health care exposure and severity of disease CURB-65 may guide disposition

Alternate causes of dyspnea to consider: ACS, airway obstruction, anemia, GI bleed, reactive airway disease, myocarditis, pericarditis, pneumothorax, pulmonary embolism, toxicology

    – May not be helpful for patients residing in nursing homes, SNFs or other health care facilities
– Always consider the patient's social situation and risk factors when planning the discharge
    – Specifically, reliable access to antibiotics and outpatient follow-up

■ Considerations
– The patient's risk factors and social situation can guide management and disposition
– Use clinical judgment and available data to make diagnosis – don't anchor heavily on diagnostics
– Consult your hospital antibiogram to determine appropriate antibiotic regimen

14.5.3 CC: Abdominal Pain

■ **General Considerations**

= Break up the abdomen into quadrants and think about the organs and adjacent structures in each quadrant (see ◘ Fig. 14.7)

= Abdominal pain PLUS an additional chief complaint (e.g., lightheadedness, SOB, back pain) should prompt you to cast a wider net of potential diagnoses outside of GI origin

= Assume all female patients of child-bearing age with abdominal pain are pregnant until proven otherwise

= Always keep ectopic pregnancy on your differential for female patients presenting with abdominal pain and/or vaginal bleeding

= All patients with abdominal pain should be instructed to see their PMD or to return to the ED in 24 h if not improved

= Abdominal pain can be a symptom of ACS, PNA, DKA, or renal colic. Do not limit your ROS and physical exam to just the abdomen, especially in elderly patients

= Refer to ◘ Table 14.7 for a summary on life-threatening causes you should consider for abdominal pain

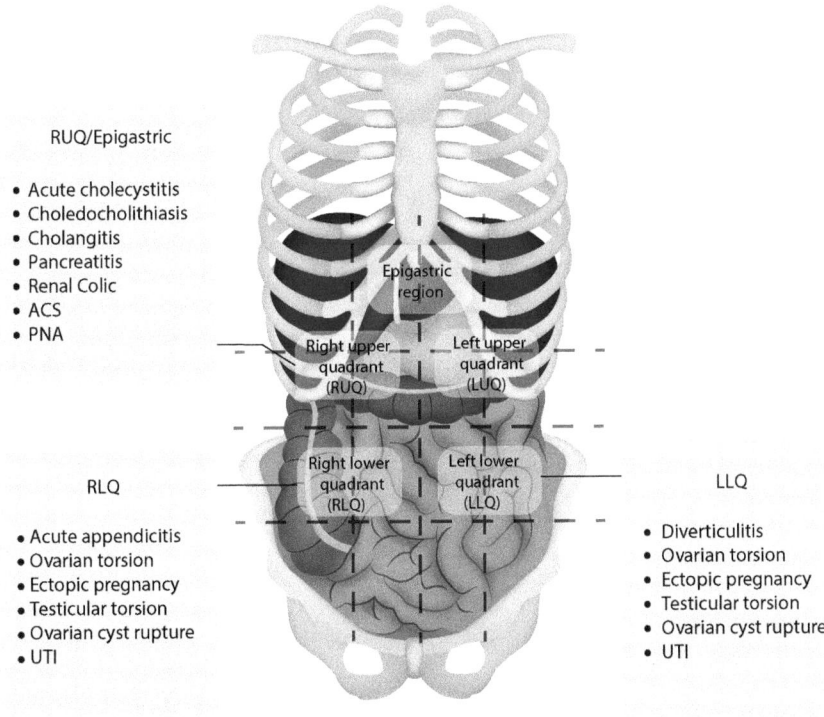

RUQ/Epigastric

- Acute cholecystitis
- Choledocholithiasis
- Cholangitis
- Pancreatitis
- Renal Colic
- ACS
- PNA

RLQ

- Acute appendicitis
- Ovarian torsion
- Ectopic pregnancy
- Testicular torsion
- Ovarian cyst rupture
- UTI

LLQ

- Diverticulitis
- Ovarian torsion
- Ectopic pregnancy
- Testicular torsion
- Ovarian cyst rupture
- UTI

Epigastric region

Right upper quadrant (RUQ)

Left upper quadrant (LUQ)

Right lower quadrant (RLQ)

Left lower quadrant (LLQ)

◘ **Fig. 14.7**　Abdominal quadrant-guided differential diagnoses

Table 14.7 Summary of life-threatening and alternate RUQ/epigastric abdominal pain etiologies

Differential diagnosis	Key history	Key clinical findings	Diagnostics	Management
Acute cholecystitis	RUQ abdominal pain, nausea, vomiting	Fever, Murphy's sign, RUQ abdominal pain referred shoulder pain	LFTs TB/DB – if elevated consider choledocholithiasis RUQ US – sonographic Murphy's sign, pericholecystic fluid, gall bladder wall thickening	IV fluids, pain control, antiemetics IV antibiotics Consult surgery
Cholangitis	RUQ abdominal pain, nausea, vomiting	Fever, hypotension, very sick looking, AMS, RUQ abdominal pain, jaundice	LFTs, TB/DB – elevated ALT/AST, alkaline phosphatase, hyperbilirubinemia RUQ US – intrahepatic ductal dilation, acute cholecystitis CT abdomen – intra/extrahepatic ductal dilation, identifies cause of obstruction	IV fluids, pain control Broad-spectrum antibiotics Emergent GI consult for decompression or surgery consult for cholecystectomy
Pancreatitis	Persistent RUQ/epigastric abdominal pain ± anorexia, back pain, nausea, vomiting	Fever, tachycardia, hypotension Epigastric tenderness, jaundice	Lipase – 3x ULN RUQ US – determine presence of gallstones CT abdomen – if dx uncertain	Antiemetics, IV fluids, pain control Consider antibiotics for underlying infection Monitor for EtOH withdrawal

Alternate causes of RUQ/epigastric abdominal pain to consider: abdominal aortic aneurysm, acute mesenteric ischemia, ACS, aortic dissection, biliary colic, choledocholithiasis, cholangitis, gastritis, obstruction (SBO/LBO), PNA, pyelonephritis, renal colic.

14.5.3.1 Acute Cholecystitis
- **Key HPI**
  - [] RUQ/epigastric abdominal pain [] Scapular pain (referred pain)
  - [] Prior self-resolving episodes [] Post-prandial pain

- **Key risk factors**
  - [] DM [] Gallstones [] Obesity [] OCP use

- **ROS**
  - [] Fevers [] Chest pain [] Nausea [] Vomiting [] Back pain

- **Physical Exam**
  - VS – fever, hypotension
  - Abdominal – RUQ abdominal tenderness, rebound or guarding, Murphy's sign

Diagnostics CBC – leukocytosis, BMP – electrolyte abnormalities, LFTs – elevated ALT/AST (though not always)
  - RUQ US – sonographic Murphy's sign (most sensitive for acute cholecystitis), pericholecystic fluid, gallbladder wall thickening, gallstones (though not always)

- **Management**
  - IV fluids (e.g., LR or NS) + electrolyte repletion
  - Pain control (acetaminophen, ketorolac, morphine, fentanyl) and antiemetics (Zofran, 4 mg IV)

- Antibiotics – regimen will depend on the severity of disease
    - Mild/Moderate – Metronidazole 500 mg IV q8h and ceftriaxone 2g IV once daily
    - Severe – Metronidazole 500 mg IV q8h and cefepime 2g IV q8h ± vancomycin (if suspecting MRSA)
- Consult surgery to determine need for cholecystectomy vs. medical management

- Considerations
- Take extra care with diabetic, elderly, or immunocompromised patients
- Patients with DM are at higher risk of emphysematous cholecystitis
- Elevated total/direct bilirubin should raise your suspicion for choledocholithiasis or cholangitis

14.5.3.2 Cholangitis
- Key HPI
- [] RUQ/epigastric abdominal pain [] Fevers [] Hx post-prandial pain

- Key risk factors
- [] DM [] Gallstones [] ERCP or surgery [] Liver transplant
- **ROS:**
- [] Abdominal pain [] Anorexia [] Nausea [] Vomiting [] AMS

- Physical Exam
- VS – fever, tachycardia, hypotension
- Generally – ill-appearing, altered
- Abdominal – RUQ tenderness, guarding, rigidity
- Skin – jaundice

Diagnostics   CBC – leukocytosis, BMP – electrolyte abnormalities, LFTs – elevated ALT/AST, alkaline phosphatase & GGT, TB/DB – hyperbilirubinemia
- RUQ US – acute cholecystitis (may be concomitant), intrahepatic ductal dilation, gallstones
- CT abdomen – intra/extrahepatic ductal dilation, may identify cause of obstruction and complications (abscess, perforation)

- Management
- IV fluids (e.g., LR or NS) + electrolyte repletion
- Pain control (morphine, fentanyl) and antiemetics (Zofran, 4 mg IV)
- Antibiotics – Metronidazole 500 mg IV q8h and cefepime 2g IV q8h ± vancomycin (if suspecting MRSA)
- Consult GI for gallstone extraction (if applicable) or surgery to determine need for cholecystectomy

- Considerations
- Take extra care with diabetic, elderly, or immunocompromised patients

14.5.3.3 Pancreatitis
- Key HPI
- [] Sudden onset severe abdominal pain [] Radiation to the back [] Persistent pain [] Poor PO intake
    - Assess for alcohol use disorder – # of alcohol drinks/day, time since last drink, h/o withdrawal or seizures

- **Key risk factors**
  - [] Alcohol use disorder [] Recent ERCP [] Gallstones (most common cause)

- **ROS**
  - [] Fever [] Anorexia [] Chest pain [] Dyspnea [] Nausea
  - [] Vomiting [] Diarrhea [] Back pain [] Seizures

- **Physical Exam**
  - VS – fever, tachycardia, hypotension
  - Abdomen – epigastric tenderness, guarding, rigidity
  - Skin – jaundice
  - Neurological – AMS, asterixis, tongue fasciculations, tremors

Diagnostics CBC – leukocytosis, BMP – electrolyte abnormalities, LFTs – elevated ALT/AST, Lipase – 3x the ULN

- CXR – consider CXR if suspecting ARDS
- RUQUS – look for gallstones or biliary disease (e.g., concomitant cholangitis, cholecystitis)
  - Has the potential to change management of pancreatitis if there is evidence of biliary disease (ERCP, cholecystectomy, etc.)
- CT abdomen – indicated if the diagnosis is uncertain or suspecting complications (abscess, hemorrhagic pancreatitis, pseudocyst), worsening clinical status, organ failure, or sepsis

- **Management**
  - IV fluids – up to 2–4L of LR over a period of 24 h
    - Avoid aggressive fluid resuscitation as it increases the risk of complications such as abdominal compartment syndrome, respiratory failure, sepsis, and death
    - Monitor HR, BP, UOP (goal >0.5 cc/kg/h)
    - Fluid resuscitation is dependent on the patient's clinical status (e.g., patients with renal injury or hypotension require more fluids)
  - Supportive care with antiemetics (Zofran, 4 mg IV) and pain control (fentanyl 20–50 mcg, IV or morphine 4 mg IV PRN)
    - Titrate pain control to effect and monitor for respiratory depression and oversedation
  - Antibiotics – typically not indicated unless there is an underlying infection (e.g., cholangitis or sepsis)
  - Consult GI or surgery if there is underlying biliary disease (e.g., cholangitis, choledocholithiasis)
  - If the patient has a h/o alcohol use disorder, then assess, monitor, and treat for alcohol withdrawal
    - Use CIWA scale

- **Considerations**
  - Diagnosis requires the presence of two of the following – acute onset of persistent epigastric pain radiating to the back, elevation in serum lipase 3x the ULN or characteristic findings on imaging
  - Severe pancreatitis may cause ARDS – monitor for hypoxia, tachypnea
  - Assess for biliary disease as a cause of pancreatitis
  - Consider CT abdomen if diagnosis is not clear-cut or if clinical status not improving
  - Monitor for EtOH withdrawal if the patient has a history of alcohol use disorder

You may refer to ◘ Table 14.8 for a summary on life-threatening causes you should consider for RLQ/LLQ abdominal pain.

14.5.3.4 Appendicitis

- Key HPI
- [] Nonspecific periumbilical abdominal pain that localizes to the RLQ within 24–48 h

- ROS
- [] Fever [] Anorexia [] Abdominal pain [] Nausea [] Vomiting
- [] Constipation [] Diarrhea [] Back pain [] Dysuria

- Physical Exam
- VS – fever, tachycardia, hypotension
- Abdominal – McBurney's point tenderness, guarding, rigidity, rebound tenderness
  - Can consider checking Rovsing's sign or psoas sign (suggests retrocecal appendix) – both associated with poor sensitivity
  - May present with LLQ tenderness

Diagnostics   CBC – leukocytosis (WBC can be normal during early disease), BMP – electrolyte abnormalities, CRP – elevated, UA – sterile pyuria
- US – noncompressible dilated appendix (outer diameter >6 mm), target sign on axial view of the appendix, wall thickness >3 mm, periappendiceal fluid
  - First-line imaging modality for pregnant patients or children
  - Need to visualize blind ending to confirm that the appendix has been visualized
  - Ultrasound does not exclude appendicitis
- CT abdomen with IV contrast – appendicolith, appendiceal dilation (outer diameter >6 mm), wall thickening (>3 mm), periappendiceal inflammation (fat stranding, extraluminal fluid), complications (abscess, perforation, phlegmon)
  - Consider noncontrast for patients with renal disease or true IV contrast allergy/contraindication

- Management
- Supportive care with antiemetics (Zofran, 4 mg IV) and pain control (morphine 4 mg IV PRN)
  - Make patient NPO
- IV fluids – particularly if patient has poor PO intake and fluid losses (e.g., vomiting or diarrhea)
- Antibiotics – reserved for complicated appendicitis (e.g., abscess, perforation, or phlegmon)
  - Broad-spectrum antibiotics should cover anaerobic and gram-negative rods
    - Consider metronidazole 500 mg IV q8hs AND cefepime 2 g IV q12h or ciprofloxacin 400 mg IV q12h or levofloxacin 750 mg IV once daily
  - Antibiotics typically not recommended for uncomplicated appendicitis, unless administered for surgical wound infection prophylaxis
- Consult surgery for potential surgical management
  - Coordinate antibiotic prophylaxis for uncomplicated appendicitis

- Considerations
- Commonly presents as RLQ pain, but keep appendicitis on the backburner for LLQ abdominal pain

14.5.3.5 Diverticulitis

- Key HPI
- [] LLQ abdominal pain [] Previous episodes of diverticulitis [] Date of last colonoscopy

- Key risk factors
- [] Diverticulosis [] Obesity [] Smoking

- ROS
- [] Fever [] Abdominal pain [] Anorexia [] Nausea [] Vomiting [] Constipation [] Diarrhea

- Physical Exam
- VS – fever, tachycardia, hypotension
- Abdominal – LLQ tenderness, guarding, rebound tenderness, rigidity

Diagnostics   CBC – leukocytosis, BMP – electrolyte abnormalities, CRP – elevated, UA – sterile pyuria from inflammation, lactate, and blood cultures (if concerned about sepsis)
- CT abdomen with IV contrast – bowel wall thickening, pericolonic fat stranding and diverticula, complications (abscess, colitis, fistula, perforation)

- Management
- Dependent on whether the patient has uncomplicated or complicated diverticulitis
- Uncomplicated diverticulitis can be managed with supportive care (clear liquid diet, bowel rest and pain control) and antibiotics
  - 7–10 days of PO antibiotics – amoxicillin-clavulanate 875 mg PO q12h or Metronidazole 500 mg q8h AND ciprofloxacin 500 mg PO q12h or levofloxacin 750 mg PO
- Complicated diverticulitis
  - Requires admission for management of underlying complication
  - Supportive care – IV fluids (if poor PO intake, dehydrated, or hypotensive), pain control, and bowel rest
    - Keep patients NPO if expecting procedural/surgical intervention
  - IV antibiotics – Metronidazole 500 mg q8h AND ceftriaxone 1 g q24h or levofloxacin 750 mg q24h, piperacillin/tazobactam 4.5 g q8h
    - Consider addition of vancomycin if concerned about MRSA colonization
  - Consult with surgery or interventional radiology for management of complications

- Considerations
- Commonly presents on LLQ abdomen, but you should always consider as a cause of RLQ abdominal pain
- Typically, does not present with rectal bleeding (think diverticulosis instead)
- Complicated diverticulitis usually requires admission
- Admit all elderly, patients with high fevers, immunocompromised status, or inability to tolerate PO intake
- Patients with first episode of acute diverticulitis should undergo colonoscopy to exclude malignancy
  - Performed after resolution of diverticulitis

14.5.3.6 Ectopic Pregnancy
- Key HPI
- [] Abdominal pain [] Vaginal bleeding
- [] # of pads/tampons used (quantify bleeding) [] Missed menstrual period?
- [] Gravidity and Parity (Gs and Ps!) [] Pregnancy status & gestational age [] LMP

- Key risk factors
- [] History of ectopic pregnancy [] Infertility [] IUD use [] PID [] Smoking [] Tubal surgery

- ROS
- [] Fevers [] Lightheadedness [] Syncope [] Nausea [] Vomiting [] Pelvic pain

- Physical Exam
- VS – tachycardia, hypotension, decreased O_2 sat
- Abdominal – abdominal tenderness, guarding, rebound tenderness, rigidity
- Pelvic – inspect the cervical os (is it open or closed?), products of conception, quantify blood volume with large cotton swabs

- Diagnostics
- CBC – Note Hgb/Hct and WBC count
  - Hgb/Hct gives you sense of blood losses and potential need for blood product transfusion
- Hgb/Hct, WBC, LFTs and BUN/Cr help you determine whether the patient is eligible for methotrexate treatment. These are sometimes referred to as "methotrexate labs"
- Quantitative beta-hCG – determines pregnancy status, candidacy for methotrexate treatment and also for trending purposes
- Type & Screen determines Rh status and potential need for RhoGAM
- Abdominal and transvaginal US – both can detect free fluid, IUP, and size & location of an ectopic pregnancy
  - Transvaginal ultrasound is most sensitive for detecting an IUP and identifying an ectopic pregnancy
  - IUP can be detected at a beta-hCG level of about 1500 mIU/mL
  - If the patient is unstable, could perform bedside abdominal ultrasound to look for hemoperitoneum (free fluid in the abdomen)

- Management
- Large bore IV placement, monitor VS, and supplemental O_2 (if needed)
- Supportive care with IV fluids or if indicated, blood product transfusion (e.g., hemorrhage, low Hgb/Hct)
- If the patient is unstable, notify your attending and obtain an emergent OB consult
- Stable patients with confirmed ectopic pregnancy require an OB consult to determine medical or surgical management
- RhoGAM – pregnant patients with Rh-negative status and vaginal bleeding should get treated to prevent isoimmunization
- Stable patients without IUP or ectopic pregnancy – management depends on the beta-hCG level
  - At a beta-hCG level <1500 mIU/mL, suggests early IUP so monitor with a beta-hCG at 48 h and ultrasound
    - Beta-hCG should rise appropriately (double)
  - At a beta-hCG level >1500 mIU/mL, should consult OB-GYN to discuss possibility of ectopic and appropriate management
- Stable patients with an IUP and vaginal bleeding can be treated as a threatened abortion
  - Very low likelihood of an ectopic pregnancy though a heterotopic ectopic is always a possibility
  - Arrange outpatient follow-up with OB-GYN and repeat a beta-hCG in 48 h, provide clear return precautions

- Considerations
- IUP can be detected at a beta-hCG level of about 1500 mIU/mL
- Hemoperitoneum and hemodynamically unstable patients require an emergent obstetrics consult for surgical management
  - Hemoperitoneum suggests a ruptured ectopic pregnancy
- Management and disposition should be determined with OB collaboration

- Always confirm outpatient follow-up plan with the OB team and confirm patient understanding
- All Rh-negative women with vaginal bleeding should receive RhoGAM to prevent isoimmunization

14.5.3.7 Ovarian Torsion

- **Key HPI**
  - [] Constant or intermittent pain – abdominal, back, flank, or pelvic pain
  - [] Pregnancy status and OB-GYN history

- **Key risk factors**
  - [] Adnexal mass >4 cm [] Fertility treatment [] Polycystic ovarian syndrome [] Pregnancy [] Tubal ligation

- **ROS**
  - [] Fever [] Nausea [] Vomiting [] Abdominal pain

- **Physical Exam**
  - VS – tachycardia
  - Abdominal – tenderness may not always be present, palpate for lower quadrant mass
  - Pelvic – may detect adnexal masses or tenderness
    - Exam may not be very helpful to make diagnosis

Diagnostics CBC – Hgb/Hct, leukocytosis, serum or urine beta-hCG – determine pregnancy status
  - Abdominal and pelvic ultrasound – reduced or absent arterial and venous flow on color doppler, enlarged ovary or adnexal mass or midline ovary

- **Management**
  - Provide supportive care with antiemetics and pain control
  - Emergent OB-GYN consultation

- **Considerations**
  - Usually does not present with vaginal bleeding
  - Presence of arterial and venous flow or absence of adnexal mass do NOT exclude ovarian torsion

14.5.3.8 Testicular Torsion

- **Key HPI**
  - [] Acute, unilateral scrotal pain & scrotal swelling
  - [] Pain may be constant or intermittent
  - [] Time since symptom onset

- **Key risk factors**
  - [] Puberty [] Blunt trauma

- **ROS**
  - [] Abdominal pain [] Nausea [] Vomiting [] Flank pain

- **Physical Exam**
  - VS – tachycardia
  - Abdominal – lower quadrant abdominal pain, check for CVA tenderness
    - Do not miss renal colic or GI pathology (appendicitis, diverticulitis, etc.)
  - Genital – absent cremasteric reflex, unilateral scrotal erythema or swelling, unilateral tender or hard testicle or high riding testicle and horizontal lie

- **Diagnostics**
- Can be clinically diagnosed
- Consider scrotal US if diagnosis is uncertain
  - Color doppler – decreased or absent blood flow
  - Affected testicle may be hypoechoic, enlarged testicle
  - Torsion of the testicular appendage can have a similar presentation

- **Management**
- Emergent urology consult for surgical intervention, especially if within 12 h of symptom onset
- Manual detorsion can be considered if urology is not immediately available
- Supportive treatment with antiemetics and pain control
  - Keep patient NPO as patient will need surgery

- **Considerations**
- Do not delay an emergent urology consult for further testing if the diagnosis is obvious!

□ Table 14.8 Summary of life-threatening and alternate RLQ/LLQ abdominal pain etiologies

Differential diagnosis	Key history	Key clinical findings	Diagnostics	Management
Appendicitis	Initially nonspecific (diffuse) then localizes to RLQ ± anorexia, nausea, vomiting	McBurney's point tenderness, abdominal rigidity or guarding	WBC, CRP, UA Abdominal US for pregnant or nonobese patients CT abdomen w/IV contrast	NPO, IV fluids IV pain control Surgery consult
Diverticulitis	LLQ abdominal pain ± fever, anorexia, constipation or diarrhea, h/o diverticulosis	Fever, LLQ abdominal tenderness, guarding or rigidity	CBC, lactate Abdominal CT with IV contrast – bowel wall thickening, abscess, fistula or perforation	Complicated – NPO, IV abx, IV fluids, consult surgery Uncomplicated – Liquid diet, close outpatient follow-up, antibiotics
Ectopic Pregnancy	Abdominal pain, vaginal bleeding, LMP h/o ectopic, infertility, IUD use, PID, tubal surgery	Tachycardia, hypotension Abdominal tenderness, rigidity or guarding On pelvic exam – examine cervical os, locate & quantify bleeding	CBC, Type and Rh, quantitative beta-hCG Abdominal US – free fluid, IUP, ectopic location Pelvic US – most sensitive, IUP, ectopic location	Large bore IVs, fluid resuscitation Methotrexate – if stable, w/o CI, b-hCG <5000 RhoGAM – for Rh- patients exposed to Rh+ fetal blood Emergent Ob-Gyn consult if unstable
Ovarian Torsion	Sudden onset severe abdominal, back, flank, or pelvic pain – may be intermittent ± nausea, vomiting h/o adnexal masses, infertility treatment	Abdominal tenderness	Abdominal + pelvic ultrasound – enlarged ovary, decreased or absent doppler flow	Pain control, antiemetics Emergent Ob-Gyn consult
Testicular Torsion	Acute onset unilateral scrotal pain and swelling ± abdominal or flank pain, nausea, vomiting	Unilateral scrotal erythema or swelling Loss of cremasteric reflex, horizontal testicular lie	Scrotal US –enlarged testicle, increased echogenicity & decreased doppler flow	Pain control, antiemetics Emergent urology consult

Alternate causes of RLQ/LLQ abdominal pain to consider: abdominal aortic aneurysm, acute mesenteric ischemia, diverticulitis, obstruction (SBO/LBO), ovarian cyst rupture, renal colic, uterovesical junction stone, UTI

14.6 Additional Skills/Procedures to Learn About

14.6.1 Trauma/Resuscitation

As a sub-intern, you are less likely to *independently* evaluate trauma patients and patients requiring resuscitation. However, there are definitely ways to help out and maximize your learning in the resuscitation bay. Below are some general considerations.

Although you will not be managing these patients on your own, it is still prudent for you to learn about the resuscitation process. You should familiarize yourself with the trauma/resuscitation bay setup and core team members involved as seen in ◼ Fig. 14.8. Learning these crucial steps will help you follow along while you are observing your seniors lead the resus bay. Familiarize yourself with the following topics:

- Primary survey (e.g., airway, breathing, circulation, disability, exposure)
    - The steps are often orchestrated simultaneously by team members and coordinated by the team leader
- Secondary survey
    - In simple terms, a head to toe assessment looking for foreign objects and signs of trauma in the skin and bones
    - Helps determine need for additional imaging
- FAST exam – familiarize yourself with the views to look for fluid where it should not be:
    - Cardiac: subxiphoid is usually the go-to view
        - Consider parasternal long, parasternal short, apical 4 chamber if time allows
    - RUQ: place the probe posteriorly looking for Morrison's Pouch, use the liver tip as a landmark
    - LUQ: place the probe posteriorly looking for the splenorenal recess, use the spleen tip as a landmark
    - Pelvic: look for fluid in the pouch of Douglas in females and rectovesical pouch in males
- Head CT Rules
    - Both the Canadian and New Orleans rules and their exclusion criteria
        - They do not apply to patients on anticoagulation
    - These rules were developed to minimize indiscriminate CT scanning
- C-spine rules
    - Both the Canadian and NEXUS rules and their exclusion criteria
        - The exclusion criteria help you determine when you are not able to apply the rules
    - Rules are only relevant for blunt neck trauma

- **Other helpful tips**
- Grab supplies for your team – ultrasound machine, IV starter kits, arterial/central line kits, sutures, etc.
- If there is a computer nearby and no one needs it, use it to search the EMR for the patient's medical history and medications
    - Look up existing comorbidities, prior hospitalizations, medications, and anticoagulation status
- Maximize your learning by going through the mental exercise of gathering an H&P and developing a treatment plan
    - Think about the questions you would ask and physical exam you would perform

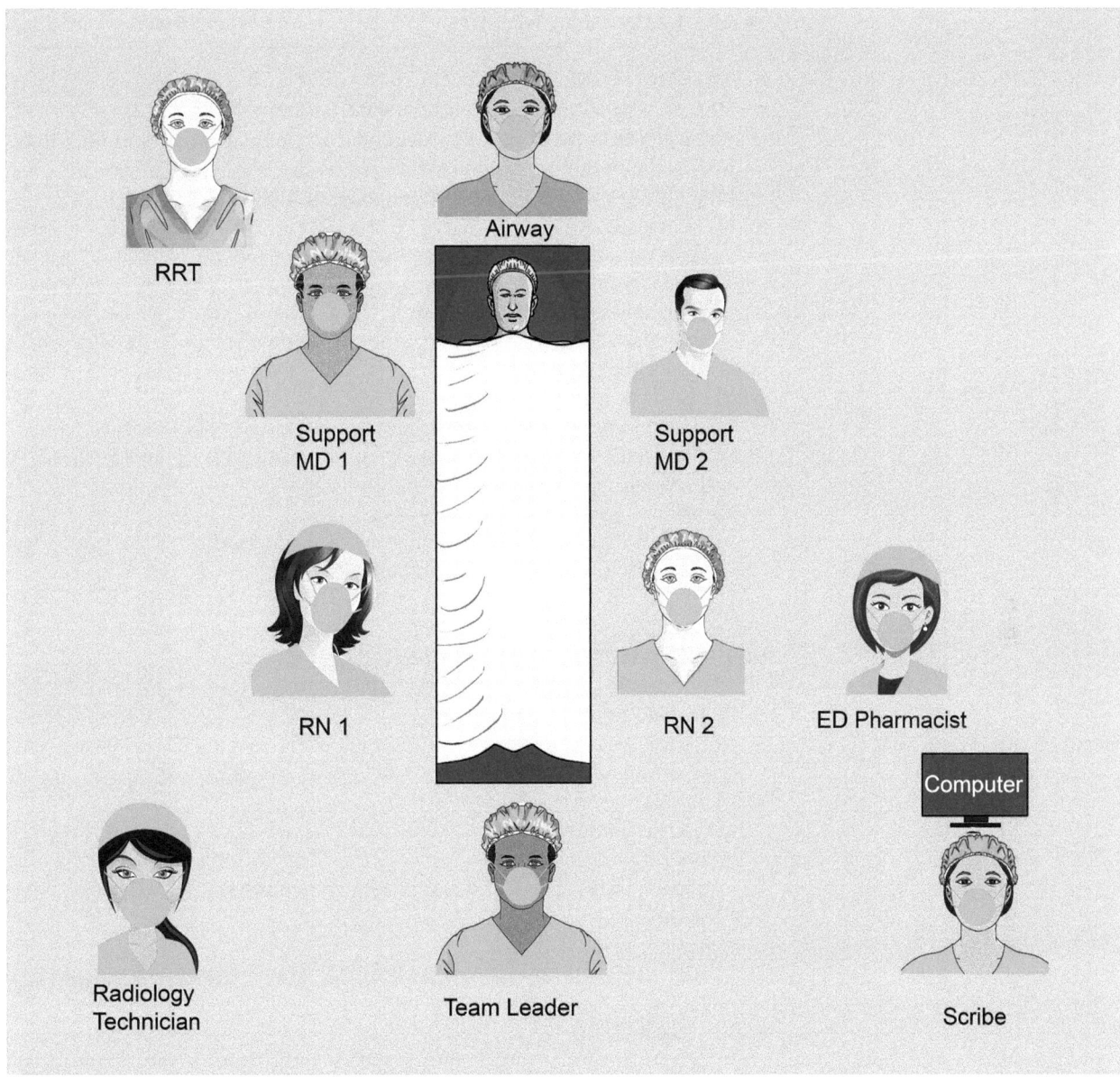

☐ **Fig. 14.8** Trauma/resuscitation room setup and team members (may be site specific)

- Develop an assessment and plan and compare your plan to the team's plan
- Reason through differences and ask questions to show engagement and learn valuable clinical pearls

❗ Common Errors: Ask questions when your supervisors have some bandwidth or there is downtime. Be proactive without being annoying.

14.6.2 Important Procedures

Unfortunately, book explanations will not do procedural skills justice and would actually do you a disservice. Below is a not so extensive list of skills and procedures you should know about. I recommend you watch videos of these procedures at some point before starting your EM rotation. This will help you familiarize yourself with the steps. You can ask your attending/residents to help guide you through the procedures.

14.6.3 Laceration Repairs

- ■ Important considerations
- ▬ HPI: mechanism of injury and patient's tetanus status
- ▬ Physical exam: perform a neurovascular exam, explore wound for foreign bodies, tendon injury, or damage to the bone
- ▬ Imaging: consider XR if suspecting glass or metal in the wound
- ▬ Management:
  - High pressure irrigation (running tap water as effective as sterile water)
  - Consider antibiotic treatment for bite injuries or open fractures/joint
    - No role for topical antibiotics
  - Tetanus vaccine if the patient is not up-to-date
  - Suture the laceration
- ▬ Materials needed:
- ▬ Gloves, do not need to be sterile gloves contrary to popular belief
- ▬ Sterile needle driver, forceps, scissors, lidocaine with epinephrine, towels and syringe
- ▬ Sutures
  - 5-0 or 6-0 for anything involving the face and head
  - 4-0 or 5-0 for anything below the neck

Clinical Pearl: For all lacerations, be sure to ask about mechanism of injury and tetanus status!

14.6.4 Incision and Drainage (I&D)

- ▬ Performed to drain skin abscess
- ▬ I&Ds are a common cause of fluid exposure in the ED so always wear goggles and a face mask.
- ▬ Materials:
  - Goggles and mask
  - Towels
  - Local anesthetic (e.g., lidocaine with epinephrine)
  - Hemostat
  - Scalpel

14.6.5 Splinting

Splinting is used for sprains and closed fractures. You should learn about the most common splint techniques and their indications. Materials:
- ▬ Common splint techniques:
  - Thumb spica splint – 1st metacarpal, thumb, scaphoid, and lunate injuries
  - Radial gutter splint – fractures of the neck, shaft, and base of the 2nd and 3rd metacarpals
  - Ulnar gutter splint – fractures of the neck, shaft, and base of the 4th and 5th metacarpals
  - Volar splint – 2nd –5th metacarpal head fractures
  - Posterior Long arm splint – radial head and neck, humerus, or olecranon fractures
- ▬ Fiberglass and water to activate the fiberglass
  - If your ED uses fiberglass, then you can skip out on the rest of the materials
- ▬ Stocking and undercast padding

- – Both are used to protect the skin from the plaster
- – Use at least three layers of padding
- Plaster
  - – At least 5 layers of plaster
- Elastic bandage (e.g., ACE bandages) to hold the plaster in place
- Scissors
- Warm water in a basin to activate the plaster

14.6.6 Ultrasound-Guided IV Placement

Ultrasounds are commonly used to place IVs in patients with difficult IV access. Use the linear probe to search for veins. Remember, veins are *compressible* on ultrasound!

- ■ Materials
- Ultrasound with linear probe
- Several IVs (in case you miss the first time) and an IV starter kit with gauze
- Ultrasound gel
- Plastic covering for the linear probe (can use transparent film dressings)
- Gloves

Standout Tip: Make sure the padding and cast are not too tight. Always perform a neurovascular exam after the cast has set as casting can result in ischemia, neuropathy, and compartment syndrome.

Common Error: Make sure you completely cover the skin with padding to avoid a thermal injury.

Critical Care

Balakrishnan Pillai

Contents

Ultrasound Images provided by J. Terrill Huggins, MD, Designated Education Officer, Ralph H. Johnson VA Medical Center, Professor of Medicine, Medical University of South Carolina, Division of Pulmonary, Critical Care, Allergy and Sleep Medicine, Charleston*, SC, USA.

© The Author(s), under exclusive license to Springer Nature Switzerland AG 2021
S. H. Lecker, B. J. Chang (eds.), *The Ultimate Medical School Rotation Guide*,
https://doi.org/10.1007/978-3-030-63560-2_15

15.1 Overview

The intensive care unit (ICU) is arguably the site of the highest acuity interventions in modern medicine, contending only with the OR for this title. Since the 1950s, with the commonplace use of positive pressure ventilation, and the growing use of pressors and inotropes, ICUs have grown in their capabilities to provide life-saving care to patients with otherwise fatal disease processes. Needless to say, patients in ICUs are necessarily very ill, harbor a slew of complex medical problems, and require higher-order medical decision making. Consequently, rotations involving critical care medicine are frequently rated as some of the most challenging for medical trainees at all levels, from senior medical students, to residents.

The goal of this chapter is to introduce the reader to the ICU, review common clinical scenarios and procedures encountered in the ICU, and cover the most common topics that confuse medical trainees. This chapter will provide a brief overview of the basic cardiopulmonary pathophysiology involved in the most common ICU admitting diagnoses; however, it is not meant to act as a substitute for primary literature regarding this material, and it is definitely not meant to be an exam-prep chapter. Rather, the fundamental goal of this chapter is to provide the reader with the skills necessary to thrive on critical care rotations – or at least give the reader sea-legs prior to their journey into a critical care rotation.

15.2 ICU Design and Cast of Characters

One of the more confusing and mysterious parts of critical care medicine is the series of acronyms emblazoned above closed doors behind which both medical professionals and patients speak in hushed tones, and the sounds of cardiac monitors and ventilators fill the hallways. The average confused medical student may see acronyms like MICU, NSICU, STICU, CVICU, etc. and simply think "above my paygrade" and move right along. I can assure you that although these names may vary per institution, the organization of ICUs is generally logical and designed such that patients with a diverse array of critical illnesses may be triaged to the appropriate setting specialized to manage their care. In general, the MICU, or medical intensive care unit, manages medical issues that have resulted in an unstable patient such as acute respiratory failure, septic shock, etc. The STICU, or surgical-trauma intensive care unit, on the other hand (in some institutions these may be separate), manages unstable patients postoperatively or following trauma. The CVICU, or cardiovascular intensive care unit (in some institutions CCU or CICU), has patients with acute coronary syndromes, varying degrees of cardiogenic shock, and with advanced mechanical support such as ventricular assist devices or intra-aortic balloon pumps. Finally, the NSICU, or neuroscience intensive care unit, houses patients surrounding neurosurgical procedures with invasive interventions placed for intracranial pressure monitoring or CSF drainage, as well as those with complicated neurologic disease leading to patient instability, such as myasthenic crisis or Guillian–Barre syndrome.

15.2.1 Nursing

ICUs are places of action, where plans are made, and changed, frequently throughout the day. One of the most important parts of ICU level management for dire medical issues is the nursing care and expertise. ICU nurses have extraordinary qualifications to maintain their certification, and they are staffed at a maximum of 1 nurse to 2 patients (compared to general medical-surgical floor nurses who maintain a ratio of 1 nurse to 4 or 6 patients) to allow for optimal attention and frequent reassessment. ICU nurses are not only frequently the eyes and ears of the medical team, but they are also extensively involved in life-saving critical care procedures, titration of pressors, and ensuring the medical plan goes through smoothly.

ICU nurses are also part of many institutions' medical emergency or rapid response teams, and are instrumental in ensuring that unstable patient situations on the floor, or elsewhere, in the hospital are appropriately managed – also to this end, they will be able to tell you the up-to-date events that led to your newest ICU transfer!

> Pearl: One of the most important things to do as a trainee in the ICU setting is to establish and maintain a good rapport with the nursing staff.

15.2.2 Respiratory Therapy

In addition to the unique role of critical care nursing in the ICU, I will mention the vital role of the respiratory therapist in managing critically ill patients. Many medical trainees may have worked with respiratory therapy in passing while taking care of asthmatics, COPD, or bronchiectasis patients. However, in the ICU setting, respiratory therapists manage all positive pressure ventilation devices, ensure airway clearance and patency, obtain STAT arterial blood gases, and conduct spontaneous breathing trials for patients to eventually be extubated. Respiratory therapists frequently stay posted in their ICU, at ratios based on the number of patients requiring mechanical ventilation, with potential to recruit supervisors for help with complex patients.

> Pearl: Similar to ICU nurses, respiratory therapists are critical members of the team. For medical students, they can teach you endlessly about oxygen delivery systems and ventilator mechanics. For interns and residents, they are your primary means of controlling and assessing the patient's respiratory status and are invaluable.

15.2.3 Pharmacy

Many, if not all, ICU medical teams round with a dedicated critical care pharmacist, and potentially a pharmacy resident. These folks are indispensable to the practice of ICU medicine, and are often running the show when it comes to renally or hepatically dosing medications, troubleshooting alternative routes of administration or unconventional treatment methods devised by the team, and being ever vigilant as an expert eye to avoid medication errors.

> Pearl: ICU pharmacists are incredible teachers for medical students to review and add to their pharmacologic knowledge base. They frequently will provide formal, and informal, educational experiences.

15.2.4 Primary Team

Unlike general medicine wards teams in which 2–3 medical students round with 1–2 interns, an upper-level resident, and an attending, in the ICU setting there are generally few medical students, 3 interns, 3 residents, and at least 1 critical care fellow, in addition to the attending physician. The drastically increased team size is largely for the obvious reason that the patients are critically ill and require a higher level of care than can be provided on the floor. In the ICU setting, the intern is largely responsible for being the patient's primary provider and performing all indicated procedures. The resident's role is to ensure that the intern is not overwhelmed, assist with procedures, and to act as safety net for their plans, as well as to carry the medical emergency or rapid response pager (institution dependent). The fellow's role is to act as a sort of in-house attending who oversees the activities of residents and interns, handles all ICU transfers and triages, and leads all emergencies within the unit. The attending largely is there to ensure that no errors are made, assist in complex decision making when appropriate, and to verify that the plan of the day is sound; frequently, ICU attendings conduct both AM and PM rounds. Formal teaching regarding critical care medicine is usually conducted by fellows and attendings, while impromptu teaching is done by all levels of training at any given time.

15.2.5 Medical Students

Last but not least, the role of the medical student cannot be overlooked, even in the ICU. All trainees are learners; however, this word especially marks the role of the medical student in the ICU. Third-year medical students should be focused on gathering the complicated information pertaining to ICU patients, distilling it into a coherent and focused presentation, and orally presenting it to the attending. They should also be reinforcing their knowledge regarding the diagnosis and pathophysiology of their patients, while learning about the preliminary management steps of the most common ICU problems. Fourth-year medical students, building upon the above skills, should be working to increase the number of complex patients they carry, hone their differential diagnoses and plans, and at least first assist – if not attempt – procedures on their patients with supervision.

15.2.6 Schedule

The day-to-day routine of the ICU is that of shift work, typically, in most institutions. For example, the day team of students, residents, and fellows may take on the 6 am to 6 pm shift, while the night team takes the 6 pm to 6 am shift. Ancillary staff typically stagger their shift changes so as to not cause too much turbulence at one point in time on the unit.

15.2.7 Medical Student Routines

From the point of view of the medical student, the day routine is marked by receiving checkout/sign-out by the night team, pre-rounding on your patients, discussing the plan with your residents and fellows, and note writing prior to rounds. Obviously, this is just an ideal routine; it goes without saying that emergencies take immediate precedence and are managed as they arise. There may be an ICU-specific teaching session, led by the fellow or attending, immediately prior to rounds (in lieu of a morning report, since you would be hard-pressed to attend morning report while posted in the ICU). The day then proceeds with rounds, a post-rounds running of the list (discussion and consolidation of plan changes and active management decisions for all patients), and accomplishment of all tasks assigned to your patients (unfinished notes, transfer summaries, consults requests, procedures, etc.). Most attendings frequently round again at the close of the day to see any new admissions and to observe updates on all of the patients as the day has progressed.

The night routine differs significantly from the day routine and depends greatly on the institution that you are training in. There is usually not an in-house attending overnight and there may or may not be an in-house fellow present overnight. Unless there is an in-house attending overnight, the team does not conduct formal rounds, and if questions arise the attending is reached by phone. This difference places a greater amount of autonomy in the hands of the residents, a feature that is passed along to you, as the medical student, as well when it comes time to procedures. ICU night shifts are similar to night float coverage on the general medicine wards, with the exception that the patients are all located geographically and they are critically ill – leading to a low chance for a slow night and odds tending towards frequent emergency patient assessments. The ICU night shift is the time where the intrepid medical student has the highest probability for gaining experience in all aspects of patient care from the workup of a new admission to performing invasive critical care procedures and responding to codes, primarily because most acute indications seem to arise at night, and the team is relatively short-staffed compared to the day team.

So, as you can see, the ICU is a site of a high degree of interprofessional collaboration, as well as a training ground for medical trainees from medical student to fellow. It is a place where rapid actions are undertaken, and the best thing to do is to be in the midst of all of it and always be looking for where to be of help. Please refer to the Soft Skills chapter for further discussion on cultivating these invaluable interprofessional relationships.

> Pearl: One of the best things to do is to station yourself on the unit and NOT in the team room; this allows you to be close to all the action, keep an eye on your patients, and builds camaraderie with nurses and ancillary staff.

15.3 The ICU Patient

As mentioned in the preceding pages, ICU patients are critically ill and have a slew of medical problems that have conspired together to place them in the said ICU. One of the fundamental differences in heuristic – when it comes to thinking about ICU patients versus the floor patient, a consult patient, or an outpatient clinic visit – is that for most critically ill patients you will be using a *systems-based* plan as opposed to a problem-based plan. The benefit of the systems-based plan lies mainly in the fact that it ensures the student will be thorough when thinking through the clinical scenario and minimizes the chance for overlooking problems. The systems-based plan also facilitates communication between the primary team and consultant groups (i.e., nephrology for acute kidney injury (AKI) requiring hemodialysis or continuous renal replacement therapy or cardiology for atrial fibrillation with rapid ventricular response), as it streamlines the charting and increases efficiency of the combined medical effort.

The representative systems of a systems-based plan are as follows:
- Neurologic/sedation/pain
- Cardiovascular
- Pulmonary
- Gastrointestinal
- Renal/genitourinary
- Infectious diseases
- Hematologic
- Endocrine
- Fluids, electrolytes, nutrition, and prophylaxis (FEN/PPx)

While on the topic of plans, I will take a moment for a brief word about oral presentations in the ICU setting. The oral presentation makes up a sizeable chunk of your job, as mentioned previously regarding the roles of third- and fourth-year medical students. It is important, early on, to ask the attending their particular preference regarding oral presentations so that you don't spin your wheels for the duration of your time on service, only to receive a poor evaluation – attendings are always receptive to students who seek this out, if they don't set expectations early themselves. Each attending is different, with some preferring formal presentations on every patient, every day – while others want full formal presentations only for new admissions – it is very important to ask! Once you have organized your plan into systems, most attendings want to see that you are building differential diagnoses for each of the problems that the patient has within each system – this shows that you are reading and putting forth effort to learn, and gives them subjects to educate you on during your rotation. Your plans for each problem within each system should be organized by diagnostic actions to discern which of the differential diagnoses is the leading diagnosis, and therapeutic actions to address the leading diagnosis. Superstar students go ahead and update the patient list in the electronic medical record (EMR) with cross-cover information (contingencies) regarding anticipated changes in the form of conditional "if...then..." statements. Students that really want to impress their attendings frequently do deep dives into the primary literature regarding their patient's problems and share their findings with the team.

15.4 Fundamentals

In this section, I will overview the basic medical knowledge required to succeed in an ICU setting, namely, the patient data available, the ICU assessment of fluid status, oxygen delivery systems and mechanical ventilation, pressors and inotropes, ICU sedation and analgesia, and prophylactic measures deployed in the ICU setting.

15.4.1 A Review of the Data

Another important unique aspect of caring for ICU patients is the amount of relevant data obtained. Here I will overview some figures of merit with their particular relevance to ICU patients (these should be reviewed at least daily, often multiple times per day, and should almost always be reported in an oral presentation on rounds):

- Vital Signs: Important for all patients admitted to the hospital; however, the ICU has a high resolution for *trending* vital signs due to the increased nursing capacity. You can expect to see up to Q1H vitals regularly, and more frequently than in the ICU one can expect vitals to be hourly, versus on the floor where they are usually every 4 hours. Additionally, due to the frequent presence of invasive hemodynamic monitoring, patients are often on continuous heart rate and blood pressure measurement via arterial line placement. When interpreting the blood pressures or mean arterial pressures (MAPs), you must account for the patient's pressor requirement(s) to maintain the measured pressure (often reported in the chart as μg of norepinephrine or units of vasopressin).
- "In's and Out's" (I/Os): Vital to keeping tabs on the patient's overall fluid balance, since the majority of patients are vastly net positive with fluid during their ICU admission in the context of generous fluid boluses – a situation that frequently impedes their respiratory function due to the production of iatrogenic pulmonary edema.
- Ventilator Settings: Namely, tidal volume (V_t), respiratory rate (RR), positive end-expiratory pressure (PEEP), inhaled oxygen tension (F_iO_2), minute ventilation, and ventilator mode. These figures will be discussed in more depth later in the chapter. These settings are frequently altered by respiratory therapists following plan changes by the primary team, or in response to ventilator alarms.

- Basic Labs: ICU patients are subject to a high rate of phlebotomy in efforts to monitor laboratory changes reflective of both disease progression and treatment response. Lab draw frequency varies per situation; however, most ICUs have a maximum frequency of Q4H phlebotomies.
  - Labs of note for ICU patients vary per situation, but in general include the complete blood count (CBC), basic metabolic panel (BMP), liver function tests (LFTs), and coagulation panels (Coags). A brief overview is provided below, highlighting relevance to ICU medicine.
    - Complete Blood Count (CBC):
      - White Blood Cell Count – Relevant to monitor response to antibiotic therapy in the context of infection/septic shock, and to gauge overall degree of inflammation/stress as part of a holistic clinical picture.
      - Hemoglobin/Hematocrit – Relevant to estimate the oxygen carrying capacity of blood and to track its decline in acute blood loss anemia (following volume resuscitation) and hemolysis, as well as to gauge the patient's transfusion response.
      - Platelet Count – Relevant when planning invasive procedures and gauging bleeding risk.
    - Basic Metabolic Panel (BMP):
      - Serum Sodium – Hypernatremia is a core quality measure of an ICU and is avoided by offsetting the free water losses of the critically ill with enteral free water or with parenteral D5W or D5-1/2NS. Hyponatremia is a seizure risk and poses the threat of cerebral edema. See the ▶ Chap. 9 for a more in-depth discussion of water balance. Serum Na is also important in calculating the anion-gap, a heuristic for narrowing the differential diagnosis of metabolic acidosis. And always remember to correct a low serum sodium in the context of hyperglycemia to acknowledge a state of pseudo-hyponatremia $Na_c = Na + (Glucose - 100) * 2.4$.
      - Serum Potassium – Hyperkalemia is very common in ICU patients due to the extremely high prevalence of AKI. Symptomatic (EKG changes) hyperkalemia is an emergency. Hypokalemia is more common overall and frequently occurs in the course of overly aggressive diuresis; however, this is easily corrected with electrolyte repletion to avoid the development of lethal arrhythmias. Hence, hyperkalemia is far more dangerous in the ICU setting.
      - Serum Chloride – Important in calculating the anion-gap as mentioned above.
      - Serum Bicarbonate – A paramount measure of the patient's acid-base status, with deficits implying a metabolic acidosis present, and excesses implying a metabolic alkalosis. This number is also used to calculate the anion gap, and to monitor response to treatment for many ICU admitting conditions (e.g., the anion gap is serially monitored in the management of DKA). Importantly the expected anion gap is largely dependent on the serum albumin, as this is the primary physiologic unmeasured anion and the gap should be corrected if present in hypoalbuminemic individuals.
      - Blood Urea Nitrogen (BUN) and Serum Creatinine (Cr) – Taken together, these components of the BMP can point towards the etiology of AKI (pre-renal associated with BUN/Cr >20, intra-renal associated with BUN/Cr ~10). Note that an elevated BUN/Cr ratio can also be seen in the context of an upper GI bleed (typically a BUN out of proportion to Cr, with ratios >33)). BUN and Cr are used to monitor progression of AKI, and used to gauge need for emergent hemodialysis (symptomatic uremia).

Emergency Measures for Hyperkalemia:

- Calcium Gluconate (IV) for cardiac stabilization
- D50 and Insulin (IV) for intracellular shift
- +/− Albuterol for intracellular shift
- Loop diuretics if renal function is preserved
- Hemodialysis if renal function is compromised

Anion Gap:
Serum Na – (Serum Cl⁻ + Serum HCO₃⁻)

Indications for Acute Hemodialysis:
(*AEIOU*)

- Refractory *A*cidosis
- Refractory *E*lectrolyte Imbalances (hyperkalemia)
- *I*ntoxication with dialyzable substance (Li⁺, Ethylene glycol, methanol)
- Refractory Volume *O*verload
- Symptomatic *U*remia

- Serum Calcium – Hypercalcemia may be seen in the ICU setting in the context of an acute hypercalcemic crisis with severe symptoms (often due to underlying malignancy and PTHrP secretion). Hypocalcemia is less common in the ICU setting unless there is concurrent hypomagnesemia, or overly aggressive diuresis with loop diuretics.
  - Serum Magnesium – Hypomagnesemia is frequently seen in the alcoholic or malnourished individual admitted to the ICU. Always remember that patients with a seemingly refractory hypokalemia or hypocalcemia may require magnesium repletion in order to correct these other electrolyte deficits.
  - Serum Phosphorus – Hypophosphatemia is frequently seen in the refeeding syndrome associated with anorexic or bulimic patients or those with profound malnutrition. In severe cases, hypophosphatemia may result in profound muscle (respiratory) weakness. (i.e., low phosphorus for oxidative phosphorylation and low ATP generation).
- Liver Function Tests (LFTs):
  - Bilirubin – Can be a marker of acute hemolytic processes common in the ICU (drug-induced hemolysis, immune hemolysis, or TTP/HUS/DIC) if you see a rise in the indirect fraction of bilirubin. Can also point towards biliary obstruction as a cause of previously unfocalized infection if you see a rise in direct bilirubin. These are also slower changing markers of hepatocellular damage.

    Corrected Calcium= Serum Calcium +0.8 *(4–Serum Albumin)

  - Serum Aspartate (AST) and Alanine (ALT) Transaminases – Important, and quickly changing, markers of hepatocellular damage, these are followed in all cases of acute hepatitis, drug overdoses (esp. acetaminophen), and any other case of acute liver injury or failure.
  - Serum Alkaline Phosphatase – Relevant to the ICU diagnosis of biliary obstruction, elevations in this parameter in the context of a fever should prompt an abdominal ultrasound in search of extrahepatic biliary dilation with concerns for acute cholangitis (a common ICU condition).
  - Total Protein and Albumin – Due to the long half-life of albumin (21 days) these are not frequently relevant on a day-to-day basis; however, they are important in the context of adjusting serum calcium, and in the estimation of protein gap on admission.
- Coagulation Panel:
  - Activated Partial Thromboplastin Time (aPTT) – Used to titrate the rate of infusion of heparin drips for treatment of thrombotic disease (venous or arterial). The heparin drip is set at a rate to achieve a target aPTT, and due to the erratic pharmacokinetics of this drug, this requires adjustment by nursing in real time. These adjustments are made possible due to unified order sets. Note that the heparin drip is frequently the anticoagulant of choice periprocedurally due to ease of "turning on/off" (half-life of only an hour!) the anticoagulation. Heparin drips are also the anticoagulant of choice in the context of AKI/ESRD.

    DIC:
    If you have a critically ill patient with an elevated aPTT and INR with thrombocytopenia and hypofibrinogenemia, with evidence of fibrinolysis (elevated D-Dimer). Alternatively, one can order a peripheral blood smear (looking for shistocytes); however, this is not necessary in an emergency.

  - International Normalized Ratio (INR) – A normalization of the patient's PT (Prothrombin time) to the laboratory standard, which allows for comparison across labs. Used when titrating a patient's warfarin dosage to get them to a therapeutic level for stroke prophylaxis in atrial fibrillation or for treatment of venous thromboembolic disease in patients with AKI/ESRD, or in the presence of a mechanical heart valve. Relevant when calculating the patient's Model for End-Stage Liver Disease (MELD) score, determining if

    DIC versus Acute Liver Failure Coagulopathy:
    Both will have elevated aPTT and INR with thrombocytopenia to varying extents; however, in acute liver failure factor VIII levels are normal (not a hepatic protein), while in DIC factor VIII levels are decreased.

Pearl: Always question the accuracy of sudden and drastic changes in any piece of laboratory of anthropometric data. The old adage of "trust, but verify" is especially applicable in the ICU.

the patient has acute liver failure, and related to the overall assessment of a cirrhotic patient's Child-Pugh Score.

- Arterial Blood Gases (ABGs): These are labs obtained by either respiratory therapists, residents, or the medical student eager to practice their procedural skills. They list off (in order) the patient's arterial pH, pCO2, pO2, and an inaccurate HCO_3^- at the given F_iO_2 the patient is currently receiving. One should obtain ABGs on patients with acute changes in respiratory status, when an accurate pH is needed for determination of overall acid–base status, and frequently to monitor patients receiving positive pressure ventilation, though this has been replaced largely by end-tidal CO_2 measurements and pulse oximetry.

15.4.2 ICU Assessment of Fluid Status

One of the most important, but challenging, assessments to make on a patient in the ICU is distinguishing between hypovolemia and euvolemia, and volume-responsive states versus volume-unresponsive states. These distinctions are important for a number of reasons. First, they inform you of which patients require fluid resuscitation and which patients do not. Second, they differentiate the patients that are capable of increasing stroke volume concordant with increased intravascular volume, from those that are unable to do so. Third, they prevent the overly liberal administration of fluid in ICU patients, which inevitably makes a comeback as iatrogenic pulmonary edema and frequently leads to increased ventilator dependence, and increased ICU length-of-stay.

Vital signs and their orthostatic changes can point towards hypovolemia, though with low sensitivity and middling specificity. Namely, resting tachycardia and hypotension point toward hypovolemia, obviously after ruling out other common causes of hypotension and tachycardia. A positive test for orthostatic vital signs points toward at least a moderate degree of intravascular volume depletion. To refresh your memory, vital signs are orthostatic if, when moving from supine to standing, heart rate increases by >30 bpm, systolic blood pressure decreases by 20 mmHg, or diastolic blood pressure decreases by 10 mmHg.

With regard to invasive measures of volume status, two points must be made clear. Many studies have shown that measurement of central venous pressures neither correlates with intravascular volume nor changes outcomes – this is why, as alluded to in a previous section, you will not see central lines routinely placed to make decisions about fluid administration. The second point is that arterial blood lactate concentration is an invaluable marker of tissue hypoperfusion in the setting of suspected intravascular volume depletion and hypovolemia and is a useful adjunct in the overall assessment of a patient's fluid status. Arterial lactate is elevated at concentrations of 2 mM and dangerously so at 4 mM concentrations.

Fluid responsiveness is the ability of the body to increase stroke volume, and hence cardiac output and by proxy blood pressure, in response to a fluid bolus. This can be accomplished in one of two common ways. The first method is the passive leg raise, where the patient's legs are quickly raised to 45° by flexing the thigh at the hip. This should have an effect in 30 seconds and is a valuable method of determining fluid responsiveness (sensitivity and specificity >90%). The other method is the administration of a 500-mL bolus of crystalloid over 10 min, which should also see a quick increase in cardiac output and blood pressure if the patient is volume responsive.

A new, popular adjunct to the ICU assessment of fluid status is the ultrasound assessment of the IVC. This method was initially touted as the "silver bullet" to both estimate volume status and fluid responsiveness by measuring the IVC diameter and its change with the respiratory cycle. The thought being that hypovolemic states would have a small diameter IVC, while hypervolemic states would have a plethoric IVC, and that significant collapse of the IVC with inspiration signifies fluid responsiveness. The major benefits of this method lie mainly in its ability to detect the extreme scenarios of hypovolemic and volume responsive (IVC is <1.5 cm and collapses with inspiration), and hypervolemic and volume unresponsive states (IVC is >2.5 cm and no change with inspiration), and the fact that it is a dynamic measure that can be used to assess responses to interventions.

All this to say that there is no one perfect and reproducible method for determining a patient's volume status. The best way to go about things is a comprehensive clinical assessment integrating the history, vital signs, physical exam, as well as objective data such as arterial lactate, response to leg raise and fluids, and IVC imaging.

15.4.3 Oxygen Delivery Systems and Noninvasive Positive Pressure Ventilation

A frequent call for a rapid response or medical emergency team while in the inpatient setting is new-onset hypoxemia. I will discuss the causes of hypoxemia in a later section; however, I will briefly overview the methods of noninvasively correcting hypoxemia as a segue into a discussion of invasive mechanical ventilation.

The simplest of noninvasive oxygen delivery systems is the nasal cannula (◼ Fig. 15.1), which consists of two prongs that fit within the nares of the patient and provide 100% supplemental oxygen flowing at a set rate; however, due to the poor seal or patient mouth breathing, this obviously does not provide 100% F_iO_2. There is a common variant of this that incorporates a reservoir for oxygen (the reservoir cannula) that fits between the two prongs of the nasal cannula and is widely available; however, the same caveats apply. Analogous to the nasal and reservoir cannulas are the facemask and nonrebreather masks (◼ Fig. 15.1). These were initially designed to allow for higher oxygen flow rates and a better seal to prevent air-leaks, and they do indeed provide higher F_iO_2 than their cannula counterparts. Note that the nonrebreather mask requires a minimum of 10 L/min of flow in order to keep the 100-mL reservoir bag filled with supplemental O_2. The importance of this bag, with one-way valve, is that it enables the nonrebreather to cycle out the exhaled CO_2 (versus the simple facemask) thus increasing oxygen delivery. Although these methods have less air-leak than the nasal cannula methods mentioned above, they are still imperfect and thus the F_iO_2 is only approximated. However, an interesting variant of the facemask, known as the Venturi mask (used frequently in pre-hospital settings) (◼ Fig. 15.1), uses the principle of jet mixing to ensure a specific F_iO_2 per the nozzle size placed on the mask.

The newest oxygen delivery system to arise in the past 20 years is the high-flow nasal cannula (HFNC). The HFNC is arguably the most efficacious way to deliver oxygen without invasive mechanical ventilation; it provides humidified oxygen at *extremely* high flow rates (up to 60 L/min) directly into the upper airway that not only provides oxygen, but also washes out dead space, reduces

◻ Fig. 15.1 Noninvasive oxygen delivery methods

airway resistance (and hence work of breathing), and provides some degree of positive airway pressure during expiration that further increases oxygenation and even corrects alveolar hypoventilation in patients with chronic lung disease. Of the oxygen delivery systems, this is the only one noninvasive method that may require ICU admission for initiation of therapy.

The noninvasive positive pressure ventilation (NPPV) systems are those of continuous positive airway pressure (CPAP) and bilevel positive airway pressure (BiPAP). These systems work to correct hypoxemia by providing PEEP, but they additionally decrease dead space ventilation and reduce airway resistance, thus increasing alveolar ventilation at any given work of breathing. Conversely, they can be used to decrease the patient's work of breathing if patients are tiring out. CPAP is simply a machine that provides humidified, oxygenated or atmospheric air at a continuous level of PEEP (typically 5–10 cm H_2O), attached to the patient's face via tightly sealed facemask. BiPAP is a similar machine to CPAP that provides a baseline constant positive airway pressure (approximately 5 cm H_2O, the expiratory pressure) and then a coordinated inspiratory positive airway pressure (approximately 10 cm H_2O). These pressures are all adjustable and are titrated to affect the clinical situation. Importantly, BiPAP machines vary on whether the inspiratory pressure is *in addition to* the baseline pressure or if it is *the total pressure*–always ask the respiratory therapist in charge of the machine if you have any questions. Note that in order to qualify for CPAP or BiPAP, the patient *cannot have altered mentation* and *must be able to protect their airway*. The reason for this is that if the patient were to vomit, the mask would almost ensure aspiration, which would be very, very bad to say the least.

Finally, if these methods of oxygen delivery and NPPV do not seem to be correcting the respiratory failure, the patient should undergo endotracheal intubation and be placed on invasive mechanical ventilation.

Final points about oxygen delivery systems (■ Table 15.1):

- Typically, when managing acute hypoxemia, the first delivery system (and the last when weaning) is the nasal cannula titrated up to 10 L/min.
- If the nasal cannula is failing to correct the hypoxemia, then you go big with the nonrebreather mask to provide the maximum amount of F_iO_2 without intubation or HFNC (which requires respiratory therapy to do an assessment and program the machine, which takes time in an emergency).
- If the nonrebreather mask is failing, or the hypoxemia is only partially responsive, clinical judgment is used to decide between HFNC or intubation and mechanical ventilation.
- BiPAP has been shown to be effective in COPD exacerbations, severe asthma exacerbations, and volume overload states associated with exacerbations of congestive heart failure, specifically to decrease the need for intubation and ventilation in these settings; it is not the first-line therapy for otherwise uncomplicated hypoxemia – and it is not a substitute for intubation if the patient is decompensating.

■ **Table 15.1** Oxygen Delivery Systems

Method	Mechanism	Flow Rate	FiO_2	Location
Nasal Cannula	Nasal prongs delivering supplemental O_2	1–10 L/min	24–40%	Home, EMS, Floor, ICU
Facemask	Facemask delivering supplemental O_2	5–10 L/min	35–60%	EMS, Floor
Venturi Mask	Facemask with nozzles for jet mixing of supplemental O_2 with room air (Venturi effect)	>60 L/min	24–50%	Floor
Nonrebreather Mask	Facemask with ~100 mL reservoir bag and one-way exhalation ports	>10 L/min	60–80%	EMS, Floor
HFNC	Special nasal prongs with warmed and humidified O_2	Up to 40–60 L/min	Up to 100%	Floor or ICU
CPAP	Increases FRC by providing PEEP	5–10 cm H_2O typically of PEEP	Variable	Home, Floor, ICU
BiPAP	Provides pressure support for breaths and PEEP	Inspiratory pressures of ~10 cm H_2O. Expiratory pressures of ~5 cm H_2O	Variable	Home, Floor, ICU

Table Reference: Marino, Paul L. *Marino's the ICU Book*. Fourth edition. Philadelphia: Wolters Kluwer Health/Lippincott Williams & Wilkins, 2014

15.4.4 Basics of Mechanical Ventilation

A full understanding of mechanical ventilation is beyond the scope of this text and, in fact, the scope of a medical student in general – as specific training afforded in anesthesiology residency or critical care fellowships is generally required to attain mastery of this topic. Rather, my goal in this section is to describe the basics of mechanical ventilation, overview common ventilator modes, and review the figures of merit one should be able to interpret on the monitor.

First, a brief word on the patient requiring mechanical ventilation. There are a variety of indications for invasive positive pressure ventilation, such as hypoxemic or hypercapnic respiratory failure, GCS <8, or loss of adequate airway; however, *the most common indication is general clinical gestalt wherein the clinician anticipates that the patient will imminently decompensate from a respiratory standpoint.*

Importantly, this entails that, unlike in the operating room where patients are under general anesthesia and paralyzed with neuromuscular junction blockade, patients are at varying degrees of consciousness and synchrony with the ventilator and continue to ventilate on their own at some respiratory rate and pattern put out by their brainstem. This is a fact that is important when discussing ICU sedation and analgesia (see later on) and the patient ventilator system.

The ventilator–patient circuit is a closed circuit where the airflow at a fixed oxygen tension (FiO_2) is passed from the machine into the patient's airways and alveoli. This passage of air creates a flow in the tubing of the ventilator and the patient's airways and alveoli that is generated by forces produced by the machine and the patient's diaphragm. The logic behind this being that the ventilator offloads the patient's work of breathing to facilitate appropriate gas exchange (correcting hypoventilation and respiratory acidosis) and the ventilator also acts as an oxygen delivery system (correcting any hypoxemia). As the disease process that resulted in mechanical ventilation is reversed, the amount of mechanical support is decreased through adjusting ventilator modes and settings and the amount of diaphragmatic work increases (the patient starts to "work out" their own ventilatory muscles), and eventually the patient receives a spontaneous breathing trial (which they hopefully, eventually pass) and is eventually extubated.

Ventilator modes describe the relationship between breaths in the ventilator–patient circuit. Again, a full discussion is beyond the scope of this text; however, two important modes, assist-control (ACV) and pressure support (PSV) ventilation (◧ Table 15.2) will be described as they are quite common and are the basis of most ICU ventilatory strategies. The first is the AC mode wherein the ventilator both assists the patient's native breaths at the patient's native respiratory rate and pattern but also sets a safety ventilatory rate to control the overall ventilation of the patient, hence "assist-and-control." Note that the overall work of breathing in this mode, and in all modes, is minimized when there is synchrony between the positive pressure administration of the machine and the negative inspiratory portion of the patient's native breath and when the breath is terminated at the onset of the patient's native positive pressure expiration.

The breaths in an AC mode are either pressure controlled (PC) or volume controlled (VC), meaning that the machine is set to deliver a breath at a constant pressure for a predetermined amount of time, or a breath at a constant inspiratory flow to reach a predetermined tidal volume. Note that in a PC breath, the flow and volume of the breath will be variable and dependent on the underlying respiratory physiology and pathology, while in a VC breath, the pressure of the breath will be variable and in general more peaked than in a PC breath leading to increased patient discomfort (◧ Table 15.3).

▣ Table 15.2   Ventilator Modes

Assist-Control Ventilation	Pressure Support Ventilation
Starting ventilator mode	Weaning ventilator mode
Pressure or volume controlled breaths	Constant pressure over PEEP for patient-initiated breaths
Set V_t or pressure, and RR, F_iO_2, PEEP	Set Pressure Support, PEEP, and F_iO_2
Provides baseline ventilation in absence of patient activity	Does not provide baseline ventilation in absence of patient activity

Table Reference: Marino, Paul L. *Marino's the ICU Book*. Fourth edition. Philadelphia: Wolters Kluwer Health/Lippincott Williams & Wilkins, 2014

▣ Table 15.3   Ventilator Breaths in AC Modes

Volume Controlled Breaths	Pressure Controlled Breaths
Triggered by patient negative pressure or time elapsed between breaths	Triggered by patient negative pressure or time elapsed between breaths
Flow in system held constant during inspiration to deliver a preset tidal volume	Flow in system dependent on underlying respiratory physiology and compliance
Pressure in system variable and peaked	Pressure in the system is held constant during inspiration for preset amount of time
Tidal volume is guaranteed and fixed	Tidal volume is variable, determined by pressure and underlying respiratory compliance
Passive expiration	Passive expiration

Table Reference: *Fishman's Pulmonary Diseases and Disorders*, 5th ed. Editor-in-Chief: Michael A. Grippi. Editors: Jack A. Elias, Jay A. Fishman, Robert M. Kotloff, Allan I. Pack, Robert M. Senior. Video Editor: Mark D. Siegel. 278 contributing authors from 12 countries.New York: McGraw-Hill Medical; 2015

The trigger variable in an AC mode is the signal to the ventilator to deliver a positive pressure breath into the system. This variable is either a negative pressure detected in the system (i.e., the patient is initiating a breath through the normal means of negative pressure ventilation), or time between breaths to ensure a preset respiratory rate. The breath is then terminated either after a certain amount of time has passed (PC breaths) or after a certain amount of volume has been delivered (VC breaths).

The second important mode is PSV. This is a very common ventilator weaning mode, as it provides a set amount of positive pressure triggered by the negative pressure in the system marking the onset of the patient's native breath. Hence, it acts as a bit of a boost for the patient's own breaths as they ventilate at the rate and rhythm determined by their brainstem. This mode is not a control mode like ACV, thus not guaranteeing a respiratory rate, and is hence not used unless there has been a reversal of the underlying pathophysiology. This mode is exactly like BiPAP, but via endotracheal tube.

(Currently, there are hybrid modes of ventilation that are becoming more and more common, the most prevalent of which is pressure-restricted volume-controlled ACV (PRVC-ACV). This mode essentially takes the best of both worlds when it comes to VC-ACV and PC-ACV by having computers that are able to optimize both flow and pressure in the system while delivering positive pressure breaths such that a fixed tidal volume breath may be delivered while maintaining airway and alveolar pressures under a threshold that would result in ventilator-induced lung injury. This will likely be the most common mode that you will see in modern ICUs.

There are four important variables that you must be able to interpret and to manipulate on the ventilator machine: V_t, RR, F_iO_2, and PEEP. The first two of these variables affect the alveolar ventilation and hence alter the P_aCO_2 of arterial blood and overall acid–base status.

Alveolar Ventilation = $(V_t - \text{dead space}) \times RR$

With P_aCO_2 being inversely proportional to the alveolar ventilation.

$$P_aCO_2 \propto 1 / \text{Alveolar Ventilation}$$

The third of these variables affect the oxygen delivery of the ventilator as related by the alveolar gas equation:

$$P_AO_2 = FiO_2 \left(P_{atm} - \text{Water Vapor Pressure} \right) - 1.25 \times P_aCO_2$$

(note that P_A stands for alveolar, while P_a stands for arterial; this is an important distinction because in general $P_ACO_2 = P_aCO_2$ due to rapid diffusion and no physiologic shunting, while $P_AO_2 \neq P_aO_2$ due to physiologic shunting, a topic we will revisit during our discussion of hypoxemia).

The fourth of these variables is the PEEP, which refers to the positive pressure in the system held at the end of the expiratory phase of the ventilatory cycle (◘ Table 15.4). This pressure works to splint the small airways and alveoli open and vastly improves oxygenation.

These four variables V_t, RR, FiO_2, and PEEP are the variables that are very frequently adjusted in response to ABGs obtained to monitor the patient's degree of ventilation and oxygenation to ensure appropriate physiologic support while receiving mechanical ventilation.

The main risks of invasive positive pressure ventilation are ventilator-associated pneumonias and ventilator-induced lung injury (VILI). The former is a result of impaired mucociliary clearance, a bypass of intrinsic protective mechanisms, and the addition of a foreign body subject to biofilm formation in a patient that is already critically ill, while the latter is the result of overly aggressive ventilatory strategies. The three main types of VILI are: volutrauma, atelectrauma, and barotrauma. Volutrauma arises from overdistension of alveoli and damage to the alveolar-capillary interface resulting in an inflammatory edema similar to that seen in acute respiratory distress syndrome (ARDS) (see further on). Atelectrauma occurs in the absence of PEEP and is the result of repeated collapse and reinflation of small airways and alveoli. Barotrauma is

◘ **Table 15.4** Altering Arterial Blood Gases Using the Ventilator

P_aCO_2	P_aO_2
Decrease by increasing RR or increasing V_t	Decrease by decreasing FiO_2 or decreasing PEEP
Increase by decreasing RR or decreasing V_t	Increase by increasing FiO_2 or increasing PEEP

Table Reference: Marino, Paul L. *Marino's the ICU Book*. Fourth edition. Philadelphia: Wolters Kluwer Health/Lippincott Williams & Wilkins, 2014

due to the use of excessively high positive pressures during ventilation and manifests as a pneumothorax, pneumomediastinum, or subcutaneous emphysema. All of these risks can be mitigated by use of a lung protective ventilation strategy (▶ Box 15.1) (medical students are always interrogated on this) and liberation from the ventilator as soon as possible.

Ventilators frequently alarm for elevated pressures and the best thing to do when assessing the patient with the pressure alarm ringing is to perform an inspiratory hold procedure on the machine in order to measure the peak pressure and plateau pressure. The peak pressure is the maximum pressure (in cm H_2O) achieved in the circuit, while the plateau pressure is the pressure (in cm H_2O) in the alveoli at the end of inspiration. The relationship between peak pressure and plateau pressure informs you of what the underlying cause of the increased pressure is. If the peak pressure is significantly elevated but the plateau pressure is relatively normal, then there is a problem of airway resistance (mucous plugging, bronchospasm). If the plateau pressure is elevated and almost as high as the peak pressure, then there is a decrease in lung compliance (pulmonary edema, tension pneumothorax, alveolar hemorrhage, etc.).

I will provide one final note, before closing this section, regarding spontaneous breathing trials. These may vary slightly from institution to institution, and are almost uniformly conducted by the respiratory therapist, but just so the reader has some idea what to expect I will provide you with a description of the SBT used in the ARDSnet protocol. This is likely representative of nationwide standard of care.

With the patient receiving $F_iO_2 < 0.5$ and PEEP < 5 cm H_2O, they are placed on a pressure support mode with support of <5 cm H_2O (or on T-piece, tracheostomy collar, or with CPAP <5 cm H_2O). The patient is then assessed for up to 120 min for "tolerance" based on the following variables:

- $P_aO_2 > 60$ mmHg and/or $S_aO_2 > 90\%$
- Spontaneous V_t of >4 mL/kg ideal body weight
- RR < 35 breaths per minute
- pH >7.30
- No distress (defined as >2 of the following)
  - HR $> 120\%$ of baseline
  - Hemodynamically unstable tachycardia or bradycardia
  - Significant hypotension or hypertension
  - Accessory muscle use
  - Paradoxical abdominal motion
  - Diaphoresis
  - Dyspnea

If a patient maintains these variables, on the minimal ventilatory settings outlined above, without respiratory distress *for 30 min or longer* they should be trialed with extubation. If they are unable to maintain these variables, or show respiratory distress, they should be maintained on their prior ventilatory settings.

> **Box 15.1 Lung Protective Ventilation**
>
> V_t of 6–8 mL/kg of ideal body weight with permissive hypercapnia (so long as pH >7.3) to reduce risk of volutrauma, noting that in ARDS patients pH as low as 7.15 is usually well tolerated
>
> Plateau pressure maximum <30 cm H_2O to reduce risk of barotrauma
> Minimum PEEP of 5 cm H_2O to reduce risk of atelectrauma
> Table Reference: Marino, Paul L. *Marino's the ICU Book*. Fourth edition.
> Philadelphia: Wolters Kluwer Health/Lippincott Williams & Wilkins, 2014

15.4.5 Pressors and Inotropes

One of the most daunting features of the ICU setting for medical students, apart from the mechanical ventilation, is the slew of IV drips infusing hemodynamic drugs into the patient. This section is meant to demystify the common pressors and inotropes and help the medical student make sense of all these drips.

Both pressors and inotropes are used to provide pharmacologic support of MAP; recalling that MAP is the product of cardiac output (CO) and total peripheral resistance (TPR), it makes sense that pressors do this by causing peripheral vasoconstriction and increasing TPR, and inotropes do this by increasing cardiac contractility and hence CO.

The pharmacologic support of MAP is *incredibly* commonplace in the ICU setting as one of the reasons for admission to the ICU is hypotension refractory to fluids and other conservative measures. Note that in the MICU setting, it is far more common to use pressors as the etiology of hypotension is usually not a primary cardiac issue; while in the CCU it is more common to use inotropes as the hypotension is due to a primary cardiac pathology.

Note that the goal of using pressors and inotropes is to maintain MAP at a certain level, to maintain tissue perfusion. Needless to say, when patients are requiring these drugs they are in dire straits and their potential life-saving nature outweighs their serious risks. Namely, the risks of most vasoconstrictive pressors are local tissue necrosis from extravasation and organ dysfunction due to peripheral vasoconstriction (lost in favor of perfusing vital organs such as the brain, the heart, and the kidneys). The risks of most positive inotropes are cardiac arrhythmia and myocardial ischemia in those with ischemic heart disease.

- MAP rule of thumb: 65 mmHg to perfuse the kidneys, 55 mmHg to perfuse the brain, and 45 mmHg to perfuse the myocardium.
- Generally speaking, when using pharmacologic support of blood pressure, one orders the specific agent to be used as a drip and informs the nursing staff of a specific MAP goal to reach.
- In order to mitigate the risk of peripheral tissue necrosis and ensure adequate drug delivery, high doses of vasopressors require central venous access for infusion.

Pressors and inotropes fall into two categories, catecholamines and noncatecholamines (vasopressin). Below is a table of the relevant adrenergic receptors, and their hemodynamic effects, targeted by the catecholamines (◘ Table 15.5).

The catecholamines used in hemodynamic support are norepinephrine, epinephrine, dobutamine, dopamine, and phenylephrine. The table below compares their receptor binding and the primary hemodynamic effect of use (◘ Table 15.6).

◘ **Table 15.5** Adrenergic Receptor Types

Alpha1 Receptors	Beta1 Receptors	Beta2 Receptors
Peripheral vasoconstriction	Increased cardiac inotropy, dromotropy, and chronotropy	Vasodilation (skeletal muscle primarily) Bronchodilation

Table Reference: Marino, Paul L. *Marino's the ICU Book*. Fourth edition. Philadelphia: Wolters Kluwer Health/Lippincott Williams & Wilkins, 2014

Table 15.6 Catecholamines Used in Pharmacologic Hemodynamic Support

Catechol-amine	Receptor Binding	Primary Effect	Initial Dosages (Titrate to MAP goal)
Norepineph-rine	Alpha 1 and Beta 1 agonism	Vasoconstriction, mild positive inotropy	8–10 µg/min.
Epinephrine	Alpha1, Beta1, and Beta2 agonism	Vasoconstriction Positive inotropy	0.1–0.5 µg/kg/min
Dobutamine	Beta1 agonism primarily, weak Beta2 agonism	Positive inotropy	3–5 µg/kg/min
Dopamine	Beta1 and B2 agonism primarily, with Alpha1 agonism at high doses	Vasodilation and positive inotropy	3–10 µg/kg/min
Phenylephrine	Only Alpha1 agonism	Vasoconstriction	0.1–0.2 mg/min

Table Reference: Marino, Paul L. *Marino's the ICU Book*. Fourth edition. Philadelphia: Wolters Kluwer Health/Lippincott Williams & Wilkins, 2014

- Norepinephrine is the pressor of choice for use in septic shock primarily due to fewer adverse events when compared to other pressors, and some positive outcome data to support its use.
- Epinephrine is the drug of choice during cardiac arrest, anaphylactic shock, and following VA ECMO or surgery requiring cardiopulmonary bypass (a physiologic state equivalent to cardiac arrest).
- Dobutamine is the inotrope of choice in situations of cardiogenic shock due to an intrinsic cardiac pathology.
- Dopamine is largely not a first-line agent anymore, while phenylephrine is used primarily in patients with spinal cord injury and neurogenic shock.

Vasopressin is the primary noncatecholamine pressor that is used in the ICU setting. Its use is very common and primarily it acts as a norepinephrine sparing drug (to reduce norepinephrine dose and hence side effects) in septic shock. Additionally, vasopressin has been shown, in combination with norepinephrine in patients with septic shock, to improve cardiac output and renal perfusion in the treatment of septic shock. Vasopressin acts as a vasoconstrictor by binding to V_1 receptors on vascular smooth muscle cells (note that this is a nonadrenergic receptor). Vasopressin is given via continuous infusion of 0.01–0.04 units/h and, similar to other pressors, is titrated by nursing to achieve the desired MAP goal.

15.4.6 ICU Sedation and Analgesia

A commonly overlooked aspect of critical care medicine from a medical student's perspective is the fact that patients admitted to the ICU are generally in intense pain and discomfort from a variety of causes including their primary disease process, procedures, inactivity, and mechanical ventilation. ICU patients are not only under intense physiologic stress, but also psychological-cognitive stress that contributes to the common conditions of ICU anxiety, agitation, and delirium.

It is important to diagnose and treat the primary disease process, but it is also your job to minimize the pain and suffering experienced in the course of

□ Table 15.7   Richmond Agitation–Sedation Scale

Description	Score	Terminology
Violent; danger to staff	+4	Combative
Aggressive; pulling out lines	+3	Very agitated
Purposeless movements; desynchronized with ventilator	+2	Agitated
Anxious but not aggressive	+1	Restless
Alert and Calm	0	Alert and calm
Awakens with eye contact, to voice >10s	−1	Drowsy
Awakens with eye contact, to voice <10s	−2	Light sedation
Movement to voice, no eye contact	−3	Moderate sedation
No response to voice, movement to physical stimulation	−4	Deep sedation
No response to voice or physical stimulation	−5	Not arousable

Table Reference: Marino, Paul L. *Marino's the ICU Book*. Fourth edition. Philadelphia: Wolters Kluwer Health/Lippincott Williams & Wilkins, 2014

the critical illness as this leads to shorter lengths of stay, and improved outcomes. You can do this through the judicious use of sedatives (to target stress and anxiety) and analgesics (to target pain).

Mental status in the ICU is quantified by the Richmond Agitation–Sedation Scale (RASS) (□ Table 15.7), giving an objective measure to guide management by sedative drugs. The score is assessed in a standardized way:

- First by observing the patient silently, then addressing the patient by name and asking them to look at you (can repeat one time only).
- Next, by shaking the patient's shoulder, and finally by sternal rub if unresponsive to shoulder shaking.

Ideally, we want all patients at a RASS of 0; however, this is often hard to do and we settle for a score of −1 to −2 which is accomplished through the use of sedative drugs via PRN dosing or infusion. The overall purpose of the use of ICU sedation is to make the experience as comfortable as possible for the patient, and, if mechanically ventilated, to decrease work of breathing by improving synchrony between the patient and the ventilator (□ Table 15.8). You can think of the prescription of ICU sedatives as analogous to the prescription of inotropes wherein the RASS goal of 0 to −1 or − 2 is comparable to the MAP goal of 65 mmHg and is achieved by titrating the sedative infusion in real time.

- First-line agents for ICU sedation are usually Propofol and Dexmedetomidine.
- Benzodiazepines are generally avoided due to prolonged sedation and the promotion of delirium (both leading to worse outcomes), but they are the sedative of choice when treating alcohol and benzodiazepine withdrawal, and sometimes opioid withdrawal.
- Propofol infusion syndrome is characterized by rhabdomyolysis with lactic acidosis, AKI, and bradycardic heart failure. Risk factors are high dose (>5 mg/kg) infusions for prolonged periods, status epilepticus, head trauma or cerebral hemorrhage, pressor use, or steroid use.
- Dexmedetomidine produces a sedated state that theoretically allows for arousal while maintaining deep levels of sedation – what this looks like in

◘ Table 15.8 ICU Sedative Medications

Drug	Mechanism	Advantages	Disadvantages	Infusion
Mid-azolam	$GABA_A$ Agonist	Amnestic and Anticonvulsant	High rates of delirium Prolonged sedation	0.02–0.1 mg/kg/h
Propofol	$GABA_A$ Agonist (?)	Fast onset and offset	Hypotension Respiratory depression Hypertriglyceridemia Propofol infusion syndrome	5–50 μg/kg(ideal)/min
Dexme-detomi-dine	$Alpha_2$ Adrenergic Agonist	Fast onset and offset Cooperative sedation Amnesia Mild analgesia No respiratory depression	Hypotension Bradycardia/Negative Dromotropic Effects	0.2–0.7 μg/kg/h
Haloperi-dol	Dopamine D_2 Antagonist	No hypotension or respiratory depression	QT_c prolongation, Parkinsonism, Dystonia, Akathisia, Neuroleptic Malignant Syndrome	0.5–5 mg q6H

Table Reference: Marino, Paul L. *Marino's the ICU Book*. Fourth edition. Philadelphia: Wolters Kluwer Health/Lippincott Williams & Wilkins, 2014

the ICU is a patient being arousable and following commands without stopping the infusion. It furthermore has some analgesic properties, in addition to its sedative effects.

- Disease of the cardiac conduction system is a contraindication for use of Dexmedetomidine for sedation due to the dose-dependent negative dromo-tropic action of the drug as it acts as a central sympatholytic.
- Haloperidol is not a first-line sedative due to the prominent neuromuscular side effects and the risk for neuroleptic malignant syndrome and polymor-phic ventricular tachycardia. Its main use is as an additional agent for seda-tion in severely agitated patients.

Pain in the ICU is very common and there are a variety of pain rating scales available analogous to the RASS scale to objectively quantify pain; however, the overall clinical impression taking into account patient's facial expression, posturing, ventilator synchrony, and vital signs has proven to be the most widely used and applicable method.

- The most common method of addressing ICU pain is through the opioid pain medications fentanyl and morphine.
- Fentanyl is the favorite due to fast onset and offset, no active metabolites, no renal excretion, and no histamine release (no hypotension). Typical fen-tanyl infusion rates are 0.7–10 μg/kg/h.
- Morphine is contraindicated in renal failure.
- All opioids produce respiratory depression, but unless the patient has underlying hypercapnia (severe COPD), it is uncommon to see clinically relevant hypoxemia at ICU doses of opioids.
- All patients receiving opioids should receive a bowel regimen as well.

Don't forget about pain and agitation in your patients, this is a huge way that you can show empathy toward them and ensure that they have the best outcome possible.

Table 15.9 Prophylactic measures in the ICU

Stress Ulcer	PPI or H₂ Blocker (IV, NG, or PO). This is removed when patient is receiving full feeds due to increased risk of *C. Difficile* infections
Aspiration	Head of bed to 30°, speech/language pathology to follow with diet recommendations
Venous thromboembolism	Low-molecular-weight heparin SQ injections BID or TID or mechanical sequential compression devices depending on patient's bleeding risk
Deconditioning	Early mobilization, physical therapy and occupational therapy to follow. Frequently, a registered dietitian also creates an optimized diet

Table Reference: Marino, Paul L. *Marino's the ICU Book*. Fourth edition. Philadelphia: Wolters Kluwer Health/Lippincott Williams & Wilkins, 2014

15.4.7 ICU Prophylaxis

It is of utmost importance to "dot the i's and cross the t's" when it comes to preventing adverse events in the ICU such as stress ulcers, aspiration, venous thromboembolism, and deconditioning (Table 15.9). Almost all patients in the ICU receive these measures and you should not be surprised when you see them on the medications list in the EMR.

15.5 Common ICU Procedures

As previously alluded to, one of the eminent reasons for a patient to be transferred to the ICU setting is the placement of invasive lines and tubes for both data collection as well as physiologic support. The most common procedures are discussed in the following.

15.5.1 Central Venous Access

This is one of the most important critical care procedures and is referring to accessing the central (i.e., large) veins, namely, the internal jugular veins and the femoral veins. This is done via the Seldinger technique (Fig. 15.2) which involves first accessing the venous site, placing a guidewire and dilating the vein over the guidewire for the eventual insertion of the specific catheter (the central line). A chest X-ray (Fig. 15.3) is then obtained to confirm correct catheter tip placement at the superior end of the superior vena cava. There are many types of central lines varying by brand, number of lumens, how long they can last in the vasculature before they must be removed, etc.; however, I will reserve further discussion about these specifics for other authors.

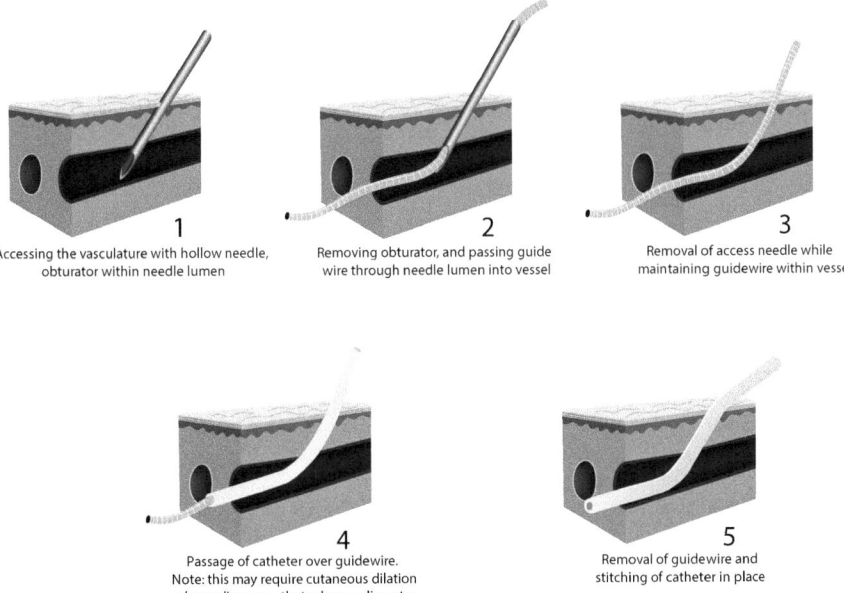

Fig. 15.2 Seldinger technique for central venous access

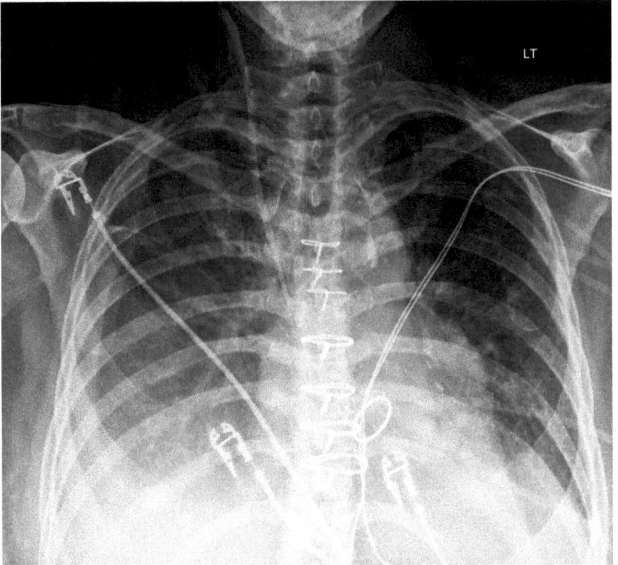

Fig. 15.3 CXR of appropriate right internal jugular vein central venous catheter placement

Central lines are placed for:
- Administration of hypertonic saline, high doses of K^+ replacement, high doses of pressors (norepinephrine, vasopressin) that exceed the peripheral limit
- Administration of fluid resuscitation (not first-line for this indication, as wide bore (<16-gauge) peripheral IVs have been shown to be superior)

- Ascertaining central venous data (venous pressures and oxygen saturations) in specific circumstances
- NOT done to measure central venous pressures for fluid management decisions
- Emergency hemodialysis

Note: *The common adverse events of central line placement are bleeding and pneumothorax, the one that medical students get questioned about is venous air embolism (the reason that central lines are placed in the Trendelenburg position is to reduce the risk of this complication).*

15.5.2 Arterial Access/Invasive Hemodynamics

Obtaining arterial access (placing an A-Line) is another very common critical care procedure. This is performed by either residents, respiratory therapists, or medical students by the same Seldinger technique (◘ Fig. 15.4) as placing a central line; however, the vasculature accessed is typically the radial artery. The arterial line is then connected to a pressurized bag of saline to ensure no hemorrhage, and calibrated to the level of the heart so as to obtain accurate arterial blood pressure waveforms.

Arterial lines are placed for:
- Invasive blood pressure monitoring (shock of any etiology, hypertensive emergency)
- Frequent procurement of ABGs

Note: *The common adverse events of placing an A-line are the same as all arterial access procedures: hemorrhage, hematoma, pseudoaneurysm, aneurysm, and arteriovenous fistula formation. Less commonly occurring is digital ischemia; however, patency of the palmar arterial arch can be tested using the physical exam maneuver of the Allen's Test.*

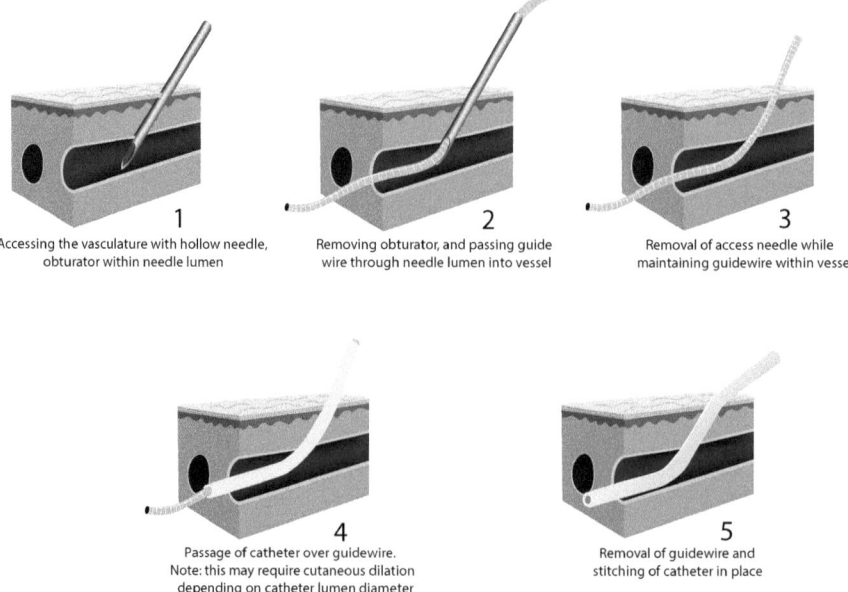

1 Accessing the vasculature with hollow needle, obturator within needle lumen

2 Removing obturator, and passing guide wire through needle lumen into vessel

3 Removal of access needle while maintaining guidewire within vessel

4 Passage of catheter over guidewire. Note: this may require cutaneous dilation depending on catheter lumen diameter

5 Removal of guidewire and stitching of catheter in place

◘ **Fig. 15.4** Seldinger technique for arterial access

15.5.3 Intubation

Endotracheal intubation (■ Fig. 15.5) is common both in the emergency department as well as on the floor in medical emergency/rapid response situations. This is usually done in the emergent setting by an anesthesiologist, emergency medicine physician, or pulmonary/critical care fellow or attending. Endotracheal intubation is the most effective method of securing the patient's airway, which is always the first priority in a medical emergency (remember the ABCs?). A chest X-ray (■ Fig. 15.6) is obtained post-intubation to confirm appropriate placement of the endotracheal tube 3–5 cm above the carina.

The indications for endotracheal intubation are:

- Inability to protect airway due to altered mentation
- Impending airway compromise due to intrinsic or extrinsic pathology
- Acute hypoxemic respiratory failure refractory to other oxygen delivery systems
- Acute hypercapnic respiratory failure

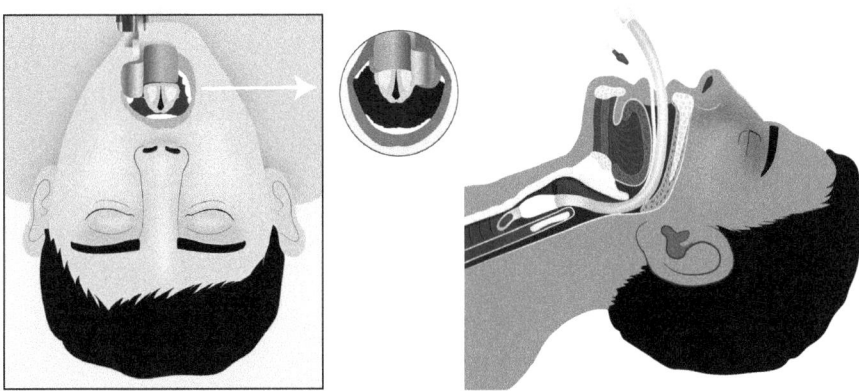

■ **Fig. 15.5** Endotracheal intubation by direct laryngoscopy

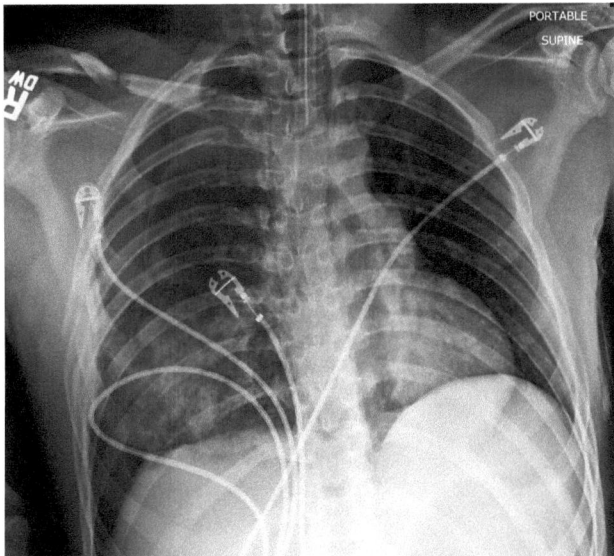

■ **Fig. 15.6** CXR of appropriate endotracheal tube placement

15.5.4 Bronchoscopy with Bronchoalveolar Lavage

This is not an ICU-specific procedure but is commonly done in patients with respiratory failure and concerning findings on chest imaging (e.g., the bilateral pulmonary infiltrates seen on the chest X-ray of a patient with pneumocystis pneumonia) in efforts to diagnose the etiology of the respiratory failure by sampling the alveolar spaces of specific bronchopulmonary segments. This procedure (□ Fig. 15.7) is done under sedation with assistance by a respiratory therapist and nurse; it first involves bronchoscopy with a flexible bronchoscope to inspect the airways leading up to all bronchopulmonary segments for any abnormality. Then a predetermined amount of normal saline is instilled into the region of interest (if a general sampling is required then the right middle lobe is typically used) and aspirated back into a sample collection container using suction. Note that it is normal for there to be residual fluid left in the region that received lavage since aspiration is not 100% effective; this fluid is resorbed into the circulation by the pulmonary lymphatics.

ICU indications (the full list is extensive) for flexible bronchoscopy with bronchoalveolar lavage are:

- Acute hypoxemic respiratory failure with pneumocystis pneumonia
- To determine the infectious pathogen of an otherwise undifferentiated pneumonia
- To define the dominant cell type in an autoimmune process
- To diagnose alveolar hemorrhage or look for source of bleeding
- Uncommonly, to diagnose an eosinophilic pneumonia syndrome, or pulmonary alveolar proteinosis
- Acute hypoxemic respiratory failure of unknown etiology

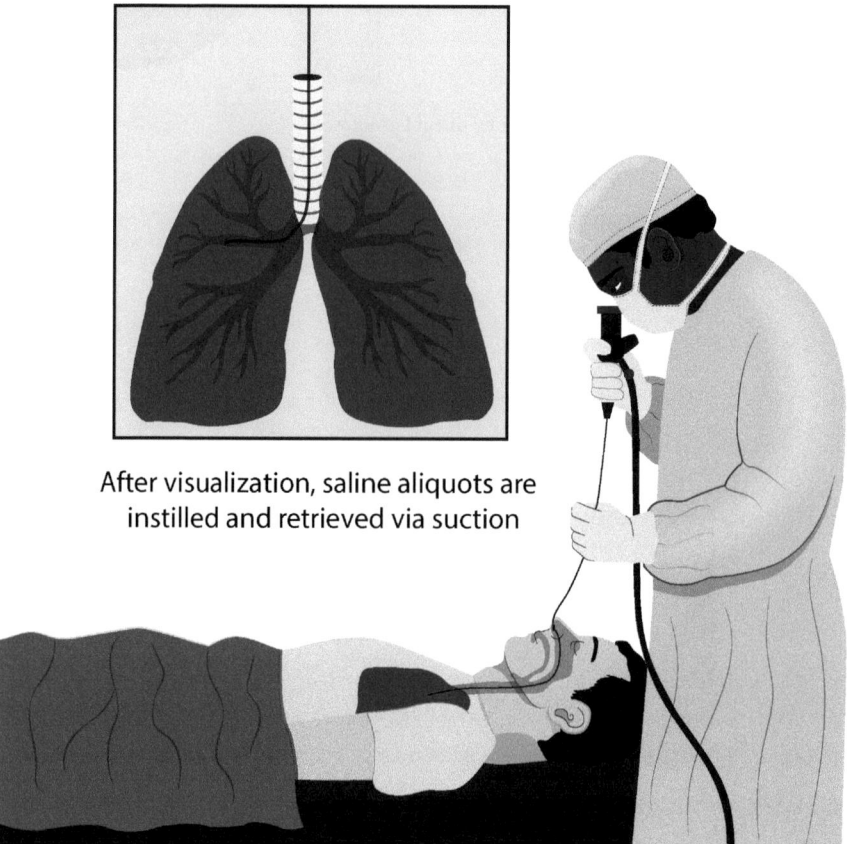

After visualization, saline aliquots are instilled and retrieved via suction

□ **Fig. 15.7** Schematic diagram depicting bronchoscopy

15.5.5 Extracorporeal Membrane Oxygenation (ECMO)

This is one of the most invasive procedures that are performed in the ICU setting. It is equivalent to being on either pulmonary bypass (veno-venous ECMO/VV-ECMO) or cardiopulmonary bypass (veno-arterial ECMO/VA-ECMO) and involves cannulating (via Seldinger technique) central vasculature for infusion of oxygenated blood and drainage of deoxygenated blood (◘ Fig. 15.8). The extracorporeal portion of the circuit allows for oxygenation of the deoxygenated blood. ECMO is the last line, "Hail-Mary," intervention for respiratory or cardiac failure but has been shown to be successful in some disease states. Major complications include hemorrhage (not uncommonly intracerebral hemorrhage) due to the need for continuous anticoagulation, ischemic events, complications associated with vascular access (dissection, pseudoaneurysm, fistulization, hematoma), as well has heparin-induced thrombocytopenia.

- For VV-ECMO, the right femoral vein is cannulated for drainage and the right internal jugular vein (or left femoral vein) is cannulated for infusion, alternatively some institutions use a dual-lumen internal jugular catheter. This procedure is done as the last-line intervention for respiratory failure.

- For VA-ECMO, the right femoral vein is cannulated for drainage, while the right (or left) femoral artery is cannulated for infusion. This procedure is done typically for primary cardiac failure and is analogous to a cardiopulmonary bypass circuit.

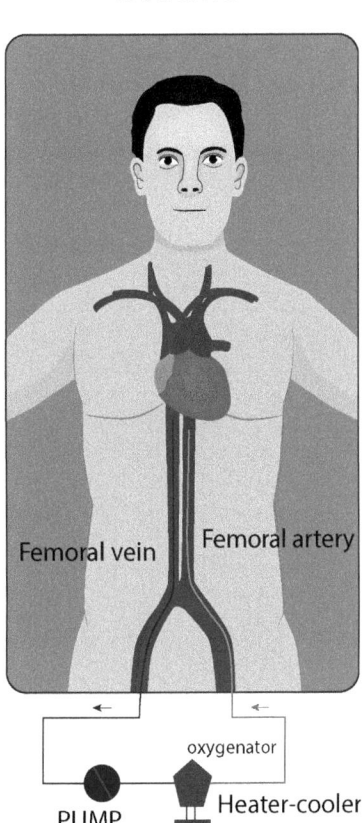

◘ **Fig. 15.8**   Schematic diagram depicting VV and VA ECMO circuits

15.5.6 Lumbar Puncture

Lumbar punctures (aka spinal taps) are fairly common ICU procedures due to the fact that frequently patients with acutely altered mentation are admitted to the ICU for workup and active management. This procedure involves penetrating the dura mater with a spinal needle and entering the subarachnoid space inferior to the termination of the spinal cord. This procedure is indicated most commonly to rule out an intracranial infection and diagnose meningitis (bacterial, viral, fungal, mycobacterial, or spirochetal), but is also used to diagnose a growing list of autoimmune encephalitides by detecting the offending autoantibody (i.e., the now classic anti–NMDA receptor antibody associated with the ovarian teratoma). Please refer to the ▶ Chap. 9 for further discussion.

15.5.7 Thoracentesis

Thoracentesis (aka tapping the pleural space) is common both in the ICU, on the floor, and potentially as an outpatient procedure. The primary indication for thoracentesis is a new or unexplained pleural effusion not in the context of congestive heart failure. This procedure involves identifying the pleural effusion with ultrasound, marking and sterilely preparing the site, and anesthetizing the needle tract with lidocaine. A nick is then made with a small knife that comes with the kit, and a thoracentesis needle is placed into the pleural space and fluid is sampled for analysis, pH, glucose, gram stain and culture, cell count, and cytology usually. Depending on the specific kit, a one-way valve may allow for large volume drainage of pleural fluid into a collection bag by pumping with the syringe. *It is critically important to insert all needles superior to ribs and as lateral as possible (while still accessing the effusion) so as to avoid damaging the intercostal vessels that run inferior to the respective rib and taper as they travel distally from the aorta.*

- Pleural fluid analysis is beyond the scope of this chapter; however, due to the importance (and frequency of medical student interrogation) of differentiating transudative and exudative effusions, the following table is provided (◘ Table 15.10).
- Light's criteria: A pleural fluid is exudative if one or more of the three criteria are met. (sensitivity 97%, specificity 85%)
  - Pleural fluid protein to serum protein ratio >0.5
  - Pleural fluid LDH to serum LDH ratio >0.6
- Pleural fluid LDH >2/3 the upper limit of normal for the serum LDH

◘ **Table 15.10** Characterizing a Pleural Effusion

Transudative	Exudative
Due to imbalance of Starling forces	Due to inflammatory process
All three of Light's criteria negative	At least one of Light's criteria positive
Common etiologies are CHF and Cirrhosis	Common etiologies are malignancy, parapneumonic/empyema spectrum, acute pancreatitis, tuberculosis, and autoimmune diseases

Table Reference: *Fishman's Pulmonary Diseases and Disorders*, 5th ed. Editor-in-Chief: Michael A. Grippi. Editors: Jack A. Elias, Jay A. Fishman, Robert M. Kotloff, Allan I. Pack, Robert M. Senior. Video Editor: Mark D. Siegel. 278 contributing authors from 12 countries. New York: McGraw-Hill Medical; 2015

15.5.8 Paracentesis

Paracentesis (aka tapping the abdomen) is common both on the floor as well as in the ICU. The paracentesis is performed on patients with ascites identified on physical exam and confirmed with abdominal ultrasound. It involves identifying a pocket of ascitic fluid (usually the left lower quadrant), usually under ultrasound guidance, anesthetizing the tract and peritoneum, and inserting a needle for fluid sampling (diagnostic paracentesis) or a catheter for fluid withdrawal (therapeutic paracentesis). Diagnostic paracentesis is significantly more common in the ICU setting due to the fact that when a patient with decompensated cirrhosis and ascites is admitted, spontaneous bacterial peritonitis must be ruled out with ascitic fluid sampling. Further discussion of paracentesis is better served in the ▶ Chap. 17.

15.5.9 Thoracic Ultrasound in the ICU

You would be hard pressed not to notice the ultrasound boom of the last decade, with machines becoming more and more common as a bedside adjunct to the physical exam. With relevance to the ICU, not only are essentially all ICUs equipped with ultrasounds for use in invasive procedures, but they have also become commonplace in diagnosing pleural and pulmonary pathology. I will leave a detailed discussion of ultrasound physics, probe selection, and modalities for other authors, save for one fact: The linear probe provides high resolution and poor penetration, while the phased-array probe provides good penetration and lower resolution, hence most thoracic ultrasound is performed with the phased-array probe (to penetrate deeper into the thoracic cavity). I will briefly discuss the merits of the ultrasound in the ICU, as I can assure you that you will see them there and they will become invaluable tools in your future.

ICU ultrasound makes use of two main imaging modes: B-mode (real-time structures), M-mode (motion), and occasionally color-Doppler mode. It also uses a series of imaging artifacts that arise at the air–tissue, or air–fluid interface, as well as artifacts that arise from the motion of pleural surfaces and chest wall structures, in order to detect, exclude, and diagnose common pathologies (◘ Figs. 15.9, 15.10, 15.11, 15.12, 15.13, and 15.14). Below is a table of artifacts per their ultrasound mode that define a number of common lung-pleural states that are seen in the ICU setting (◘ Table 15.11).

Pearl: A quick word about the terms gauge and French when referring to needles/catheters/sheaths: both refer to the outer diameter of the catheter; however, gauge is inversely proportional to the outer diameter of the catheter and the rate of change per gauge varies per manufacturer, while French is directly proportional to the outer diameter of the catheter and 1 French = 1/3 mm. An example of this terminology is that a 14 gauge is a larger bore than an 18 gauge, while a 10 French is a larger bore than an 8 French.

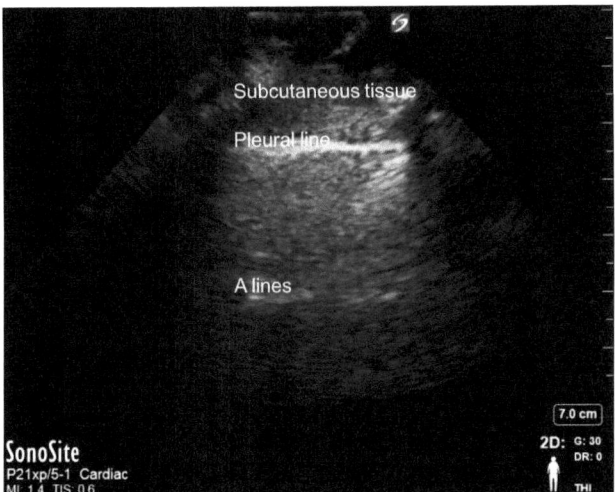

◘ **Fig. 15.9** Thoracic ultrasound image of normal, aerated lung. (Image courtesy of J. Terrill Huggins, MD)

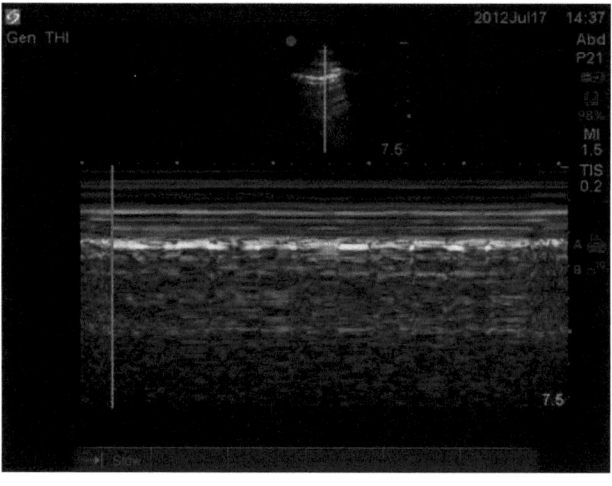

□ **Fig. 15.10** M-Mode ultrasound image showing the seashore sign of normal, aerated lung. I(mage courtesy of J. Terrill Huggins, MD)

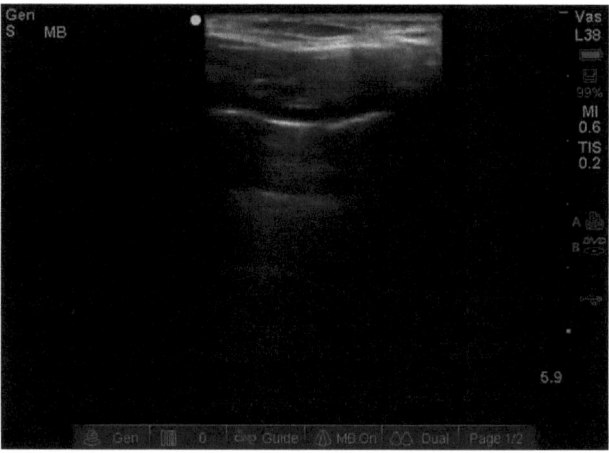

□ **Fig. 15.11** Thoracic ultrasound image depicting Lung Point, a sign of pneumothorax. (Image courtesy of J. Terrill Huggins, MD)

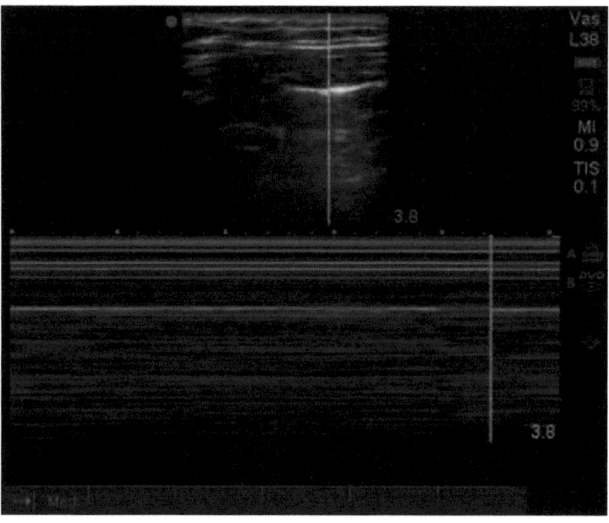

□ **Fig. 15.12** M-Mode ultrasound image showing the barcode sign consistent with pneumothorax. (Image courtesy of J. Terrill Huggins, MD)

15

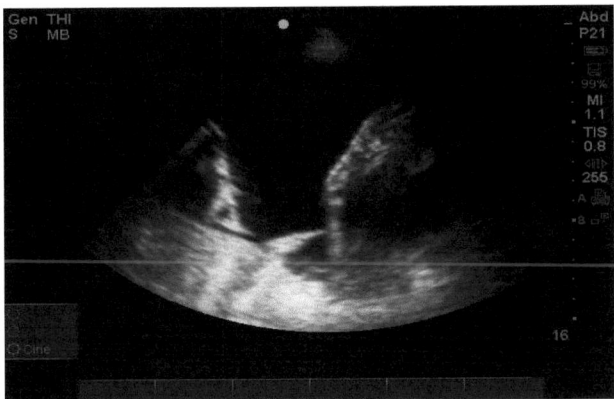

Fig. 15.13 Thoracic ultrasound image depicting Anechoic Region consistent with pleural effusion. (Image courtesy of J. Terrill Huggins, MD)

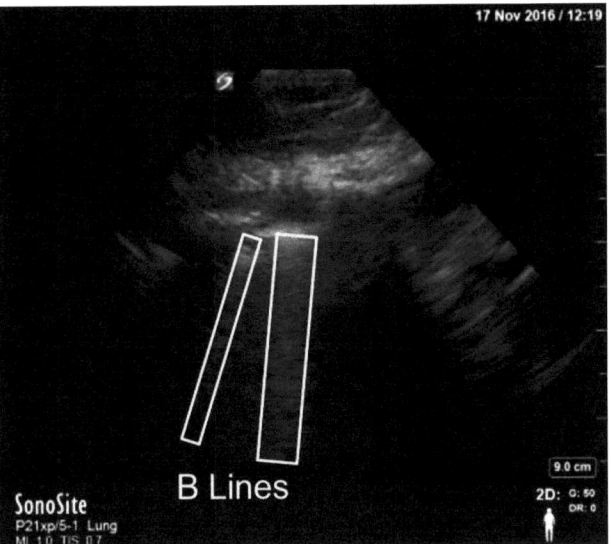

Fig. 15.14 Thoracic ultrasound image depicting B-Lines consistent with an alveolar-interstitial syndrome. (Image courtesy of J. Terrill Huggins, MD)

Table 15.11 Overview of Common Profiles in Thoracic Ultrasound

State of Lung–Pleural System	B-Mode	M-Mode	Note
Normal Lung	Lung sliding (layer of visceral pleura gliding on parietal pleura as two glimmering hyperechoic lines) with A-Lines	Seashore sign	Called A-Profile
Pneumothorax	A-Lines without lung sliding (lung-point being the transition from areas of sliding pleura to pneumothorax)	Barcode sign	Lung sliding excludes this

(continued)

◻ Table 15.11 (continued)

State of Lung–Pleural System	B-Mode	M-Mode	Note
Pleural Effusion	Anechoic areas surrounded by hyperechoic pleura and diaphragm	Sinusoid sign	Can see regions of atelectatic or consolidated lung in the effusion, and posterior acoustic enhancement
Pulmonary Edema (alveolar-interstitial syndrome)	B-Lines/comet tails due to thickened interlobular septae or alveolar edema		The degree of edema is proportional to the number of B-Lines and inversely proportional to the distance between them (i.e., the worse edema would be many B-lines close together)

Table Reference: *Fishman's Pulmonary Diseases and Disorders*, 5th ed. Editor-in-Chief: Michael A. Grippi. Editors: Jack A. Elias, Jay A. Fishman, Robert M. Kotloff, Allan I. Pack, Robert M. Senior. Video Editor: Mark D. Siegel. 278 contributing authors from 12 countries.New York: McGraw-Hill Medical; 2015

15.6 Common Cases

There are a wide variety of specific diagnoses that you can expect to see while rotating through the ICU; I cannot possibly cover each one at length in this chapter – as that would be beyond the scope of this text; however, I encourage you to examine the list below (▶ Box 15.2) prior to the start of your rotation, and read about each of the topics as the rotation progresses. By treating each one of these conditions as a learning objective, you will complete your rotation with a fairly thorough overview of critical care medicine. Nevertheless, due to their ubiquitous nature, and the published data surrounding management, I will discuss the in-depth management of septic shock and acute respiratory failure later in this chapter.

> Pearl: The precise admitting diagnosis for patients in the ICU is part of a vast and varied list; however, the decision to pursue ICU level care is largely one made by clinical gestalt based on increasing nursing demands or requirements for invasive procedures or supportive measures/medications inaccessible on the floor.

Box 15.2   Common ICU Conditions

Acute respiratory failure/ventilator requirement (hypercapnic, hypoxemic respiratory failure, inability to protect airway, neuromuscular weakness, failure to extubate post-op)

  BiPAP requirement

  Pressor or inotropic support requirements

  Shock (septic vs. cardiogenic (intrinsic or extrinsic) vs. neurogenic vs. anaphylactic vs. hemorrhagic/hypovolemic)

  Intoxication or toxic exposure

  Post cardiac arrest

  Acute coronary syndromes

  Acute liver failure

  Acute pancreatitis

  Severe GI bleeds

Quasi stable supraventricular tachycardias requiring IV AV nodal block-
ade (Afib with RVR, A flutter)
Post-op monitoring
DKA/HHS
Thyrotoxicosis or myxedema coma
Adrenal crisis
Acute hemodialysis
Hypertensive emergency
Intracranial hemorrhage
Intracranial infection

15.7 Acute Respiratory Failure

Acute respiratory failure is one of the most common reasons to be admitted to
the ICU; the overall clinical picture of a patient in acute respiratory failure is variable depending on the etiology and ranges from somnolence or altered mentation
to florid respiratory distress with the classical physical exam findings of accessory
muscle use, tripod positioning, and paradoxical abdominal motion. Based on
arterial blood gas findings, respiratory failure can be partitioned into hypoxemic
(generally $P_aO_2 < 60$ mmHg or $S_aO_2 < 90\%$) and hypercapnic ($P_aCO_2 > 46$ mmHg,
without a concomitant primary metabolic alkalosis). Respiratory failure once
carried a high mortality rate; however, with the improved ventilatory support
capabilities of modern ICUs, the prognosis has been drastically improved.

It is important to remember that the decision to pursue endotracheal intubation is not made based solely on numerical data regarding gas exchange and
oxygenation, but is always based in an overall assessment of clinical status as
well as immediate probability for deterioration (i.e., an asthmatic patient tiring
out while in a florid asthma exacerbation).

In all cases, the three goals of managing patients in acute respiratory failure
are:

- Provide supportive ventilation such that hypoxemia and or hypercapnia are
corrected
- Provide disease-modifying therapy, if available, such that the precipitating
insult is reversed as soon as possible
- Provide adequate prophylactic measures for ICU level care, and manage
any complications that arise as a result of the underlying disease process or
as an unforeseen consequence of treatment

For the patient in acute respiratory failure, a full diagnostic workup is performed, guided by the patient's history and physical exam, in order to pin
down the etiology of the hypoxemia and or hypercapnia. This almost always
involves obtaining chest films, EKG's and troponins, arterial blood gases, basic
labs (CBC, BMP, LFTs), and a full infectious workup. It also frequently
involves a contrast-enhanced CT scan of the chest if pulmonary embolism is
on the differential diagnosis.

15.7.1 Hypoxemic Respiratory Failure and Acute Respiratory Distress Syndrome (ARDS)

As mentioned above, the working clinical definition for hypoxemia is
$P_aO_2 < 60$ mmHg or $S_aO_2 < 90\%$. I am using this terminology because it is at
this point that patients of all ages begin to become symptomatic from the low

oxygen tension, but it is relevant to note that the expected P_aO_2 decreases with age due to an ever-increasing A-a gradient, largely as a result of deteriorating efficiency for gaseous diffusion across the alveoli. There are two means by which one can increase the P_aO_2 in a patient: Increase the F_iO_2 or increase the PEEP provided by the ventilatory support device. When providing supportive care, and correcting hypoxemia, one or both of these methods are utilized (see sections regarding ventilator basics and oxygen delivery systems for a discussion of specific modalities).

There are five pathophysiologic processes that lead to hypoxemia:

- Alveolar Hypoventilation
  - As seen in cases of neuromuscular weakness (myasthenic crisis or Guillain-Barre), obesity hypoventilation, opioid intoxication, and part of the pathology of COPD exacerbations.
  - The only most common etiology for hypoxemia that also causes significant hypercapnia.
  - Does not increase A–a gradient.
- V/Q Mismatch
  - As seen in pulmonary pathologies such as pneumonia, pulmonary embolism, cardiogenic pulmonary edema, early ARDS, exacerbations of bronchiectasis, asthma exacerbations, and as part of the pathology of COPD exacerbations.
  - Increases A–a gradient.
- Shunt
  - As seen in, if intrapulmonary, extreme forms of V/Q mismatch wherein large areas of lung are perfused but not ventilated such as in the later stages of severe ARDS or hepatopulmonary syndrome. If intracardiac, this takes the form of any right to left congenital heart defect that had not been corrected, or as a consequence of Eisenmenger's syndrome with an uncorrected left to right shunt.
    - Note that one can discern intrapulmonary versus intracardiac shunting by transthoracic echocardiography with saline bubble study. If it takes >5 heart beats for bubbles to traverse from right heart to left heart, then an intracardiac shunt is excluded.
  - The hypoxemia due to shunts, regardless of etiology, is classically not responsive to increases of F_iO_2 and hence must be treated in unique ways such as liver transplant in hepatopulmonary syndrome, cardiac surgery in intracardiac shunts, and high levels of PEEP with ARDSnet protocol for the management of ARDS (see later).
  - Increases A–a gradient.
- Diffusion Deficit
  - As seen in cases of diffuse parenchymal lung disease such as idiopathic pulmonary fibrosis, scleroderma lung disease, rheumatoid arthritis related lung disease, asbestosis, silicosis, and coal-workers' pneumoconiosis as well as pulmonary fibrosis due to any number of drugs (busulfan, bleomycin, amiodarone, nitrofurantoin) and radiation.
  - Usually not a cause of *acute* hypoxemia, however many of these conditions have exacerbations that may see ICU admission and require supportive care. Unfortunately, these admissions frequently see a deterioration to a new baseline oxygen requirement.
  - Increases A–a gradient
- Decreased inspired F_iO_2
  - As seen typically at high altitudes or in poorly pressurized cabins of aircraft. Not a common cause of ICU admission, but included here for completeness.
  - Does not increase A–a gradient.

After diagnosing a patient with hypoxemic respiratory failure, it is important to next discern the etiology, if not readily apparent from the initial diagnostic workup obtained based on the initial H & P. An elevation in the A–a gradient is useful in this regard, as it points toward V/Q mismatch, shunt, or diffusion deficit as a contributor to the hypoxemia. Note that I say contributor here, as a single patient may have multiple causes of hypoxemia and a mixed picture in aggregate.

Note that the expected A–a gradient increases with F_iO_2. A useful rule of thumb is that for every 10% increase in F_iO_2, the A–a gradient increases by approximately 5 mmHg due to loss of hypoxic vasoconstriction and a relative V/Q mismatching due to a vasodilation of vessels to areas of lung that are relatively poorly ventilated.

Once the specific cause of hypoxemia has been found, the three principles of management (mentioned earlier) for acute respiratory failure are followed until the situation has resolved.

— Note, resolution of respiratory failure may be prolonged and complicated by ventilator dependence/failure to wean in many patients with severe underlying cardiopulmonary disease, and it is important to involve palliative care when appropriate for goals of care discussions.

ARDS is a unique cause of hypoxemic respiratory failure that is extremely common. It is an acute inflammatory response that is widespread across both lungs, and is characterized pathologically by diffuse alveolar damage. The inciting event may be pulmonary (severe pneumonia), or extrapulmonary (sepsis syndromes, aspiration, trauma, pancreatitis, etc.), but the end result is the same – bilateral and multilobar inflammatory injury to the pulmonary parenchyma that results in an exudative, noncardiogenic, pulmonary edema. This manifests clinically as a hypoxemia that acts initially as a V/Q mismatch and is responsive to increased F_iO_2; however, it may progress toward a physiologic intrapulmonary shunt with loss of F_iO_2 responsiveness.

It is important to recognize a patient with ARDS because due to the work of the intrepid researchers of the ARDSnet group, a mortality-reducing strategy for managing the unique hypoxemia of ARDS has been devised: the ARDSnet protocol (◘ Table 15.12). A patient has ARDS by the Berlin Definition if:

— They display bilateral infiltrates on frontal chest X-ray, not fully explained by effusions, nodules, or atelectasis.
— They show a $P_aO_2/F_iO_2 \leq 300$ mmHg while receiving a PEEP of ≥ 5 cm H_2O.

◘ **Table 15.12** ARDSnet Protocol for Mechanical Ventilation (Lung Protective Ventilation)

Goal	Target
Prevent Volutrauma	Low tidal volume ventilation (6–8 mL/kg ideal body weight)
Prevent Barotrauma	Maximum plateau pressure of 30 cm H_2O
Prevent Atelectrauma	Minimum PEEP of 5 cm H_2O

Table Reference: *Fishman's Pulmonary Diseases and Disorders*, 5th ed. Editor-in-Chief: Michael A. Grippi. Editors: Jack A. Elias, Jay A. Fishman, Robert M. Kotloff, Allan I. Pack, Robert M. Senior. Video Editor: Mark D. Siegel. 278 contributing authors from 12 countries. New York: McGraw-Hill Medical; 2015

- They have no evidence of left atrial hypertension (i.e., no fluid overload/left heart failure), or a clinical picture that would not be explained by left atrial hypertension alone. Requires echocardiography or other objective measurement to exclude a cardiac or hydrostatic cause for the edema if no risk factors are present.
- These changes within 1 week of known clinical insult or new/worsening respiratory symptoms.

Note that the P_aO_2/F_iO_2 ratio (pronounced P/F ratio) is a measure of how severely the lungs are shunting, and decreases with increasing severity of shunt – implying worsening hypoxemia in the face of high inspired O_2 tensions.

In addition to the lung protective strategy of ventilation the following goals are targeted in ARDS management (and frequently extrapolated to managing other causes of hypoxemic respiratory failure):
- Arterial pH management
  - Measured on the frequently obtained ABGs in ventilated patients.
  - Goal to keep arterial pH in the range of 7.30–7.45 by adjusting the V_t and the RR. However, patients tolerate a pH of 7.20 down to 7.15 quite well in the context of ARDS.
    - If pH < 7.30, the goal of keeping low tidal volume ventilation trumps respiratory rate and RR is increased preferentially to affect change in pH. V_t is only increased if RR is maximized at 35 breaths per minute.
    - If pH > 7.45, RR is decreased to return the pH to a normal range.
- Oxygenation management
  - Goal P_aO_2 is 55–80 mmHg or SaO_2 of 88–95%.
  - This goal is achieved through incremental increases in F_iO_2 as well as increases in PEEP, with a minimum PEEP of 5 cm H_2O.
- Plateau pressure management
  - Goal of plateau pressures <30 cm H_2O. These are to be checked by inspiratory hold procedures every 4 h and after changes in PEEP or V_t.
  - If plateau pressure > 30 cm H_2O, decrease V_t by 1 mL/kg increments until <30 cm H_2O with a minimum V_t of 4 mL/kg.
- Weaning
  - Approximately daily spontaneous breathing trials when the patient meets the following criteria:
    - F_iO_2 < 0.4 and PEEP ≤8 cm H_2O or F_iO_2 < 0.5 and PEEP ≤5 cm H_2O.
    - F_iO_2 and PEEP requirements less than the prior day.
    - Patient showing effort.
    - Patient has not been given neuromuscular blockade.
    - SBP >90 without high doses of pressors (decreases probability of success).

The lung protective ventilation strategies, as put forth by the ARDSnet group, are some of the most powerful mortality-reducing efforts that we have in treating patients with ARDS resulting in a reduced duration of mechanical ventilation as well as an absolute reduction in mortality of 9% in the original study. In patients with refractory ARDS, the following advanced measures are often attempted:
- *Inhaled* nitric oxide or epoprostenol up to maximum dose of 40 ppm to cause vasodilation directed toward regions of lung that are ventilated in efforts to confront the V/Q mismatch that may be present. This has no proven survival benefit and if there is no benefit at maximum dose this intervention is halted. Note that IV nitric oxide would cause generalized, and not directed, pulmonary vasodilation and would *drastically* worsen V/Q mismatch. Nitric oxide is also an oxidizing agent and may lead to the

development of methemoglobinemia, further reducing oxygen-carrying capacity.
- Prone positioning in order to use gravity's effect to improve V/Q matching, drain dependent portions of the lung, and increase the homogeneity of lung tissue aeration by reducing the pleural pressure gradient from nondependent to dependent regions. This has a survival benefit in patients with a P/F ratio < 100 mmHg.
- VV-ECMO is a last-line therapy for refractory ARDS.

15.7.2 Hypercapnic Respiratory Failure

As mentioned above, hypercapnic respiratory failure is characterized by respiratory failure accompanied by a P_aCO_2 > 46 mmHg without any sort of primary metabolic alkalosis for which a decreased alveolar ventilation would be a compensatory mechanism. There are three pathophysiologic causes of hypercapnia: alveolar hypoventilation (which causes a concomitant hypoxemia and is referenced above), increased production of CO_2 by the body that outpaces ventilatory capacity (overfeeding or hypermetabolic state), and through increased dead space ventilation (e.g., COPD, bronchiectasis).

The unique aspect of supportive ventilation for hypercapnic respiratory failure is that the noninvasive positive pressure ventilatory modes of BiPAP and CPAP are highly efficacious in treating some types of alveolar hypoventilation and increased dead spaced ventilation, and hence these are the supportive ventilatory modes of choice in these patients (unlike hypoxemia which may be treated with sole oxygen delivery systems like nonrebreather mask or HFNC).

Similar to management of hypoxemic respiratory failure, once the specific cause of hypercapnia has been found, the three principles of management for general acute respiratory failure are followed until the situation has resolved.

15.8 Septic Shock

The clinical syndrome of septic shock is one of the most common reasons for ICU admission and still exerts a significant amount of morbidity and mortality. However, due to the successes of modern ICU supportive care and antimicrobial agents, we are able to mitigate more of the morbidly and save more lives from septic shock than ever before. The Surviving Sepsis Campaign has been conducting large-scale analyses regarding the critical care management of septic shock patients and has resulted in a series of practice-defining guidelines that have been adopted worldwide. This section will review the relevant pathophysiology of systemic inflammation and overview the Surviving Sepsis Campaign guidelines regarding the management of septic shock.

Our discussion of the underpinnings of septic shock begins with a more general overview of the body's systemic inflammatory response. When confronted with an acute stressor, the body will respond in a stereotyped fashion with the release of local inflammatory cytokines that stimulate a localized inflammatory reaction and addressing of the initial stimulus. However, the rub is if the acute stressor is sufficiently severe to cause a *global* release of inflammatory cytokines (hepatic acute phase reactants, IL-1, IL-6, TNF-alpha, and others) that cause a *systemic inflammatory response syndrome* (SIRS).

Note that the stressors that can cause a SIRS response are not exclusively infectious in etiology, as acute pancreatitis, burns, major trauma, and other noninfectious causes can also quickly elicit this response. Clinically, the SIRS response affects all organ systems but most significantly it causes a diffuse increase in vascular permeability leading to widespread third-spacing of intra-vascular fluid as well as a massive, global vasodilatory reaction.

These cardiovascular effects of the SIRS response are particularly relevant when turning toward the supportive measures for septic shock that deal with the intravascular depletion/third-spacing by aggressive fluid resuscitation and with the vasodilatation by administering infusions of pressors and potentially steroids (though this remains a controversial topic).

Because questions frequently come up in the ICU, and because it is a good demonstration of the progression of systemic inflammation from vascular permeability to vascular dilatation, I will review the older SIRS classifications. Classically, SIRS is diagnosed based on changes in vital signs and leukocyte count on a CBC, with two of the four above SIRS criteria needing to be present to diagnose a patient with SIRS. Sepsis was once defined by SIRS and the presence of infection (indicating that the systemic inflammation was of an infective etiology and that antimicrobial therapy would be disease modifying). Severe sepsis was sepsis associated with organ dysfunction or hypotension that was responsive to fluids, while septic shock was sepsis with hypotension unresponsive to fluid resuscitation. One will frequently find these terms used in the critical care literature as they are easy to use in order to partition patients in clinical trials. It is useful to keep the SIRS criteria in mind when thinking about patients with systemic inflammation from any cause, and specifically for systemic inflammation due to infection as this is a specific case of a general phenomenon that necessitates specific goal-directed management (□ Table 15.13).

For the reader's reference, though not as clinically useful as the above SIRS criteria definitions, the current definition of sepsis (per the 2016 Surviving Sepsis Campaign) is "life threatening organ dysfunction caused by a dysregulated host response to infection," and the current definition of septic shock is "a subset of sepsis with circulatory and metabolic dysfunction associated with a higher risk of mortality."

It should be noted that the goals for managing septic shock have been loosely adopted and generalized toward managing most systemic inflammatory conditions in the ICU.

In brief, the goals for managing sepsis and septic shock (per the Surviving Sepsis Campaign 2016):

□ **Table 15.13**   Systemic Inflammatory Response (SIRS) Criteria

Heart Rate	>90 Beats per min
Respiratory Rate	>20 Breaths per min or $PCO_2 < 32$ mmHg
Body Temperature	>38 °C or <36 °C
WBC Count	$>12 \times 10^9$/L or $<4 \times 10^9$/L

Two of the above four = SIRS

SIRS + Infective Source = Sepsis

Sepsis + Organ Dysfunction or Hypotension (responsive to fluids) = Severe Sepsis

Sepsis + Hypotension (unresponsive to fluids) = Septic Shock

Table Reference: Marino, Paul L. *Marino's the ICU Book*. Fourth edition. Philadelphia: Wolters Kluwer Health/Lippincott Williams & Wilkins, 2014

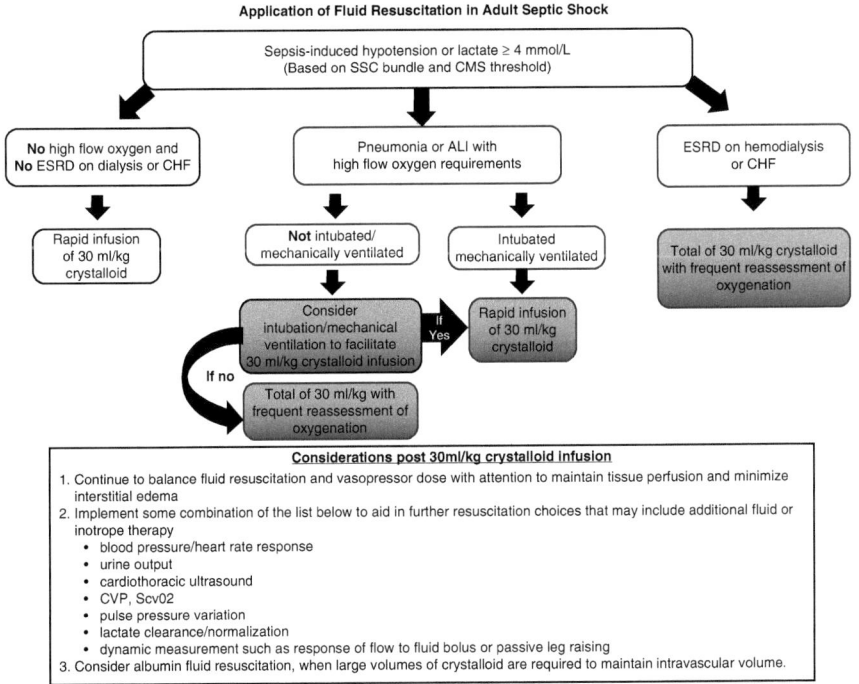

Application of Fluid Resuscitation in Adult Septic Shock

Considerations post 30ml/kg crystalloid infusion
1. Continue to balance fluid resuscitation and vasopressor dose with attention to maintain tissue perfusion and minimize interstitial edema
2. Implement some combination of the list below to aid in further resuscitation choices that may include additional fluid or inotrope therapy
    • blood pressure/heart rate response
    • urine output
    • cardiothoracic ultrasound
    • CVP, Scv02
    • pulse pressure variation
    • lactate clearance/normalization
    • dynamic measurement such as response of flow to fluid bolus or passive leg raising
3. Consider albumin fluid resuscitation, when large volumes of crystalloid are required to maintain intravascular volume.

ALI=acute lung injury; CHF=congestive heart failure; CMS=US Centers for Medicare and Medicaid Services; CVP=central venous pressure; ESRD=end stage renal disease; kg=kilograms; ml=milliliters; oxyhgb=oxyhemoglobin; Scvo2=superior vena cava oxygen saturation

☐ Fig. 15.15 Reproduced with permission from Delling, R Phillip MD, MCCM: Schorr. Christa A. RN, MSN, FCCM; Levy, Mitchell M. MD, MCCM A Users' Guide to the 2016 Surviving Sepsis Guidelines, Critical Care Medicine: March 2017–Volume 45–Issue 3–p 381–385.

- Fluid resuscitation with balanced crystalloids at a dose of 30 mL/kg within the first 3 h, with further resuscitation following volume reassessment (preferably reassessed with dynamic, rather than static variables) (☐ Fig. 15.15).
- Full infectious workup obtained prior to initiation of antimicrobial therapy. Antimicrobial therapy to be administered within 1 h of recognition and deescalation when appropriate.
- Infection source control as soon as logistically possible.
- Initiation of vasopressors to achieve a MAP of >65 mmHg in patients that are no longer fluid responsive, using arterial lactate as a marker of tissue perfusion (☐ Fig. 15.16).
- Norepinephrine is the first-line vasopressor in septic shock, second line is vasopressin as a norepinephrine sparing agent.
- IV hydrocortisone (controversial topic) assessed on a case-by-case basis if and only if patient is refractory to fluid resuscitation and vasopressors.
- Mechanical ventilation in cases of respiratory failure, if sepsis-induced ARDS; the goal is to follow a lung–protective strategy of ventilation (see previous sections regarding specifics for ARDS management).
- Renal replacement therapy in cases of AKI complicated by any of the acute indications for hemodialysis, with continuous renal replacement therapy if hemodynamically unstable.
  A few finer points made clear by the Surviving Sepsis Campaign 2016:
- No evidence supports the use of $NaHCO_3$ in treating academia due to hypoperfusive lactic acidosis.
- Patients should be fed enterally as soon as possible. If there are contraindications to enteral feeds (surgery, etc.), a patient can go up to 7 days without consideration of parenteral feeds.

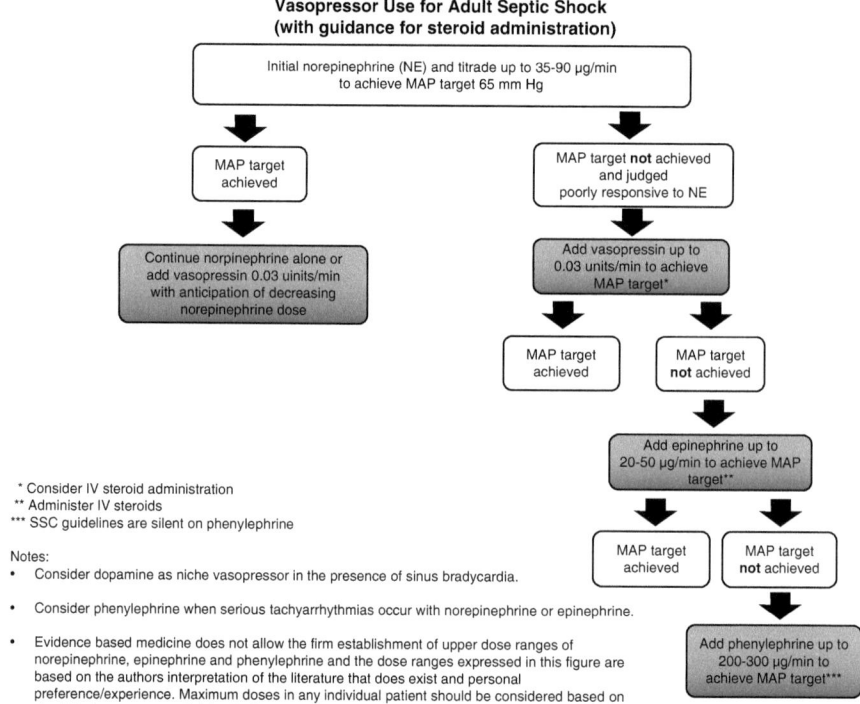

Vasopressor Use for Adult Septic Shock
(with guidance for steroid administration)

Initial norepinephrine (NE) and titrate up to 35-90 µg/min to achieve MAP target 65 mm Hg

MAP target achieved

MAP target **not** achieved and judged poorly responsive to NE

Continue norpinephrine alone or add vasopressin 0.03 uinits/min with anticipation of decreasing norepinephrine dose

Add vasopressin up to 0.03 units/min to achieve MAP target*

MAP target achieved

MAP target **not** achieved

Add epinephrine up to 20-50 µg/min to achieve MAP target**

MAP target achieved

MAP target **not** achieved

Add phenylephrine up to 200-300 µg/min to achieve MAP target***

* Consider IV steroid administration
** Administer IV steroids
*** SSC guidelines are silent on phenylephrine

Notes:
- Consider dopamine as niche vasopressor in the presence of sinus bradycardia.
- Consider phenylephrine when serious tachyarrhythmias occur with norepinephrine or epinephrine.
- Evidence based medicine does not allow the firm establishment of upper dose ranges of norepinephrine, epinephrine and phenylephrine and the dose ranges expressed in this figure are based on the authors interpretation of the literature that does exist and personal preference/experience. Maximum doses in any individual patient should be considered based on physiologic response and side effects.

◘ **Fig. 15.16** Reproduced with permission from Delling, R Phillip MD, MCCM: Schorr. Christa A. RN, MSN, FCCM; Levy, Mitchell M. MD, MCCM A Users' Guide to the 2016 Surviving Sepsis Guidelines, Critical Care Medicine: March 2017–Volume 45–Issue 3–p 381–385.

- There has been no documented mortality difference between patients receiving continuous versus intermittent renal replacement therapy in septic shock related AKI.
- There is no role for the *routine* placement of a pulmonary artery catheter in efforts to monitor hemodynamics during treatment of septic shock.
- In a patient with septic shock induced ARDS, and no more evidence of tissue hypoperfusion (lactate levels have normalized), a *conservative* fluid resuscitation strategy should be used in order to avoid worsening of the noncardiogenic pulmonary edema.
- Transfusion thresholds for packed red blood cells (pRBCs) and platelets are largely unchanged by septic shock. Namely, the transfusion threshold for pRBCs is a hemoglobin of 7, or ~9 if evidence of coronary artery disease/myocardial ischemia or active bleeding, and the transfusion threshold for platelets is 10,000/mL in the absence of bleeding (sometimes 20,000/mL per clinical judgement) and 50,000/mL if actively bleeding or a procedure is planned.

Sepsis syndromes should be treated as medical emergencies with the first goals (after obviously ensuring patent airway and ventilation) to be expedient diagnosis and administration of antibiotics and fluid resuscitation as it has been shown consistently that shorter time between patient contact and antibiotic administration consistently improves mortality, with mortality increasing per hour of antibiotic delay. Additional secondary goals are to be – as listed above – artificial maintenance of MAP >65 mmHg using fluids, vasopressors, and steroids, and management of all other downstream sequelae (ARDS, AKI, myocardial ischemia, atrial fibrillation, acute mesenteric/colonic ischemia, etc.) while maintaining normal ICU supportive measures and prophylaxis. The management of sepsis syndromes is complex and is one of the major accomplishments of the medical ICU; it ties together the supportive care of all organ systems, as well as the specific management of rampant systemic inflammation in the context of an overwhelming infectious process.

15.9 Helpful Tables

A few pearls about hypoxemia that come up in the ICU (■ Table 15.14):

- If a patient is hypoxemic, an ABG should be ordered. Alveolar hypoventilation is the only cause of acute hypoxemia and acute hypercapnia and is best managed with either NPPV (BiPAP) or intubation and mechanical ventilation.
- Shunt is the extreme form of V/Q mismatch where V/Q = 0; it occurs from pathologies on the alveolar side of the alveolar–capillary interface.
- Wasted ventilation/dead space ventilation is the extreme form of V/Q mismatch where V/Q = ∞; it occurs from pathologies on the vascular side of the alveolar–capillary interface.
- V/Q mismatch is a catchall term for everything in between shunt (perfusing nonventilated lung) and dead space ventilation (ventilating nonperfused lung).
- For the hypoxemia associated with a lobar pneumonia, one can decrease the degree of V/Q mismatch (and hence shunting) by placing the patient with the nonaffected lung in the dependent position. Due to gravity, this increases perfusion of good lung, and decreases perfusion of the pus-filled lung. "A patient re-lies on their good lung."
- Hypoxemia refers to low oxygen tension in the blood and low hemoglobin saturation. Hypoxia refers to decreased tissue delivery of oxygen.
- The pulse oximeter is a very useful measure of the oxygen-carrying capacity of the blood and hence will adequately answer the question "is my patient hypoxemic?" provided that the hemoglobin dissociation curve is unaltered. One example to be aware of is carbon monoxide poisoning, which shows a falsely high (100%) hemoglobin saturation, but signs of tissue hypoxia. This is because the carbon monoxide molecule displaces oxygen from the

■ **Table 15.14** Hypoxemia

Causes	A-a Gradient	Corrects with Supplemental O_2?	Examples
Decreased FiO_2	Normal	Yes	High altitude, air travel
Alveolar Hypoventilation	Normal	Yes	COPD exacerbation, opioid overdose, neuromuscular weakness
V/Q Mismatch	Increased	Yes	Pneumonia, PE
Shunt	Increased	No	ARDS
Diffusion Deficit	Increased	Yes	Interstitial lung diseases

Table Reference: *Fishman's Pulmonary Diseases and Disorders*, 5th ed. Editor-in-Chief: Michael A. Grippi. Editors: Jack A. Elias, Jay A. Fishman, Robert M. Kotloff, Allan I. Pack, Robert M. Senior. Video Editor: Mark D. Siegel. 278 contributing authors from 12 countries. New York: McGraw-Hill Medical; 2015

iron moiety of the hemoglobin molecule and concurrently causes a left-shift of the dissociation curve (increased oxygen binding). Taken together, carbon monoxide poisoning causes a drastic reduction in the oxygen-carrying capacity of blood but conventional laser spectrophotometry that is used by pulse oximeters is unable to detect the difference between carboxyhemoglobin and oxyhemoglobin.

A few pearls about anion-gap metabolic acidoses that come up in the ICU (◘ Table 15.15):

- The only ways to generate an anion-gap metabolic acidosis are through consumption of the HCO_3^{2-} buffer in the blood:
  - Increased production of endogenous acids that consume the HCO_3^{2-} buffer in the blood (ketoacidosis or lactic acidosis).
  - Failure to excrete the normal daily metabolic acid load, that then consumes the HCO_3^{2-} buffer in the blood (severe acute kidney injury or end-stage renal disease).
  - Ingestion of toxins that cause production of nonphysiologic acids through the actions of hepatic enzymes (methanol–> formic acid and ethylene glycol–> oxalic acid by the action of hepatic alcohol dehydrogenase). These acids then consume the HCO_3^{2-} buffer in the blood.
- The ketones of all three forms of ketoacidosis come from unopposed glucagon action promoting ketogenesis.
- The lactate in lactic acidosis comes from anaerobic metabolism of cells that are either dying or about to die in the context of local hypoperfusion or systemic hypoperfusion (shock).
- There is a rare form of lactic acidosis (D-lactic acidosis) that manifests in patients with short gut syndrome as an encephalopathy associated with eating carbohydrate rich meals that are fermented in the gut to D-lactic acid, which is absorbed and causes an anion gap but is not measured by arterial lactate measurements. This is usually not relevant in the ICU setting but is mentioned here to point out an interesting phenomenon.
- Classically, ethylene glycol causes oxalate crystals to form in the renal cortices bilaterally while methanol causes bilateral optic neuropathy.

◘ **Table 15.15** Anion-Gap Metabolic Acidoses

Type	Etiology	Diagnosis	Management
Ketoacidosis	Diabetic, Alcoholic, Starvation	Serum beta hydroxybutyrate, urine ketones. Serum glucose	DKA protocol, refeeding. Fluid resuscitation
Lactic Acidosis	Hypoperfusion or mitochondrial/aerobic metabolism toxins	Arterial lactate	Fluid resuscitation, management of underlying etiology (shock, tissue death), toxin removal
Uremic Acidosis	Severe AKI or ESRD	Elevated BUN and Cr	Conservative management or hemodialysis
Acidosis due to Organic Alcohols	Methanol or Ethylene Glycol	Serum levels of methanol and ethylene glycol	Fomepizole or emergent hemodialysis

Table Reference: Marino, Paul L. *Marino's the ICU Book*. Fourth edition. Philadelphia: Wolters Kluwer Health/Lippincott Williams & Wilkins, 2014

A few pearls about shock that come up in the ICU (◘ Table 15.16):
- Patients with both hypovolemic and cardiogenic shock appear pale, cool, diaphoretic, and are likely tachycardic and acutely encephalopathic in the face of their hypotension.
    - JVD is a physical exam measure of CVP and is the best way to distinguish between hypovolemic and cardiogenic shocks by physical exam.
- The three etiologies of a cardiogenic shock picture with elevated CVP, low CO, and elevated SVR, but with *clear lungs* are: acute right ventricular infarction, pericardial tamponade, and massive PE. The common denominator of these three is *right ventricular failure.*
- Patients are under no obligation to fit nicely into one category. In these situations, it is not uncommon to place a pulmonary artery catheter (aka Swan–Ganz catheter) to obtain actual numbers for CVP, CO, and PCWP. Note that this is fundamentally different from obtaining central venous access in efforts to determine CVP alone and make decisions about fluid administration, as a pulmonary artery catheter is able to provide measured CO by thermodilution, calculated CO by the Fick method, and measured PCWP – all of which are used to define shock syndromes and hence guide management.

◘ **Table 15.16**   Classification of Shock Types by Category

Shock– Failing to meet the metabolic needs of the tissues characterized by hypotension and lactic acidosis

Type of Shock	CVP and PCWP	CO	SVR	Examples	Treatment
Hypovolemic	Both decreased	Decreased	Increased	Failure to take PO/profound dehydration. Diarrheal illness.	Volume resuscitation
Hypovolemic–Hemorrhagic	Both decreased	Decreased	Increased	Hemothorax. Hemoperitoneum. Acute severe trauma.	Volume resuscitation then transfusion
Cardiogenic–Intrinsic	Both increased	Decreased	Increased	Acute Coronary Syndromes (ACS). End stage CHF. Viral Myocarditis.	PCI if ACS. Inotropes/ inodilators, diuretics, and mechanical support if non-ACS cardiogenic shock.
Cardiogenic–Extrinsic	CVP increased PCWP normal	Decreased	Increased	Massive PE. Pericardial Tamponade. Tension PTX.	IV tPA for Massive PE. Pericardiocentesis or pericardial window for tamponade. Needle decompression then tube thoracostomy for tension PTX.
Distributive–Septic	Normal to decreased	Increased	Decreased	Any infection eliciting a profound systemic inflammatory response	Source control and antibiotics. Volume resuscitation, then pressors and possibly steroids.
Distributive–Anaphylactic	Normal to decreased	Increased	Decreased	*Hymenoptera* envenomation. Extreme peanut allergy.	Epinepherine (IM), IV Steroids, H_1 and H_2 blockers, volume resuscitation
Distributive–Neurogenic	Normal to decreased	Increased	Decreased	Spinal cord injury	Phenylephrine and management of underlying etiology

Table Reference: Marino, Paul L. *Marino's the ICU Book*. Fourth edition. Philadelphia: Wolters Kluwer Health/Lippincott Williams & Wilkins, 2014

15.10 Common ICU Equations

15.10.1   Alveolar Gas Equation

$$P_A O_2 = F_i O_2 \left(P_{atm} - \text{Water Vapor Pressure}\right) - 1.25 \times P_a CO_2$$

$P_A O_2$ is alveolar oxygen tension

$P_a CO_2$ is arterial PCO_2 measured on ABG

The water vapor pressure is physiologically 47 mmHg

15.10.2   Alveolar–Arterial Gradient

$$A - a = P_A O_2 - P_a O_2$$

$P_A O_2$ is calculated using the alveolar gas equation, while $P_a O_2$ is measured on ABG

15.10.3   Dead Space Ventilation

$$V_D / V_t = \left[P_a CO_2 - P_E CO_2\right] / P_a CO_2$$

V_D is dead space volume

V_t is tidal volume

$P_a CO_2$ is arterial PCO_2 measured on ABG

$P_E CO_2$ is the end – tidal CO_2 measured by capnography

15.10.4   Alveolar Ventilation

$$P_a CO_2 = K \times \left[VCO_2 / V_A\right]$$

$P_a CO_2$ is arterial PCO_2 measured on ABG

K is a proportionality constant

V_A is alveolar ventilation

VCO_2 is the amount of CO_2 produced by metabolism

15.10.5   Ideal Body Weight Equation

$$\text{Ideal Body Weight}_{males} = 50 + 2.3\left(\text{height}\left(\text{in}\right) - 60\right)$$

$$\text{Ideal Body Weight}_{females} = 45.5 + 2.3\left(\text{height}\left(\text{in}\right) - 60\right)$$

15.10.6 Mean Arterial Pressure

$$MAP = (2/3) \times DBP + (1/3) \times SBP = DBP + (1/3) \times \text{Pulse Pressure}$$

15.10.7 Acid/Base Compensations

If the measured value differs from the expected value calculated by these equations, then there is a concomitant acidosis/alkalosis in the direction of that change. The body will never overcompensate. Note that respiratory compensations are fast, while metabolic (renal) compensations take ~48 h to occur and are more efficacious for chronic compensations.

Respiratory compensation for metabolic acidosis (expected P_aCO_2 if metabolic acidosis)

$$(\text{Winter's Formula})\, P_aCO_2 = 1.5 \times \left[HCO_3^{2-}\right] + 8 \pm 2$$

Respiratory compensation for metabolic alkalosis (expected P_aCO_2 if metabolic alkalosis)

P_aCO_2 increases by $0.7\,mmHg$ for every 1.0 increase in $\left[HCO_3^{2-}\right]$

Metabolic compensation for respiratory acidosis (expected $[HCO_3^{2-}]$ if respiratory acidosis)

Acute increase in P_aCO_2:
serum $\left[HCO_3^{2-}\right]$ increases by 1.0 for every $10\,mmHg\, P_aCO_2$

Chronic increase in P_aCO_2:
serum $\left[HCO_3^{2-}\right]$ increases by $3.0 - 3.5$ for every $10\,mmHg\, P_aCO_2$

Metabolic compensation for respiratory alkalosis (expected $[HCO_3^{2-}]$ if respiratory alkalosis)

Acute decrease in P_aCO_2:
serum $\left[HCO_3^{2-}\right]$ decreases by 2.0 for every $10\,mmHg\, P_aCO_2$

Chronic decrease in P_aCO_2:
serum $\left[HCO_3^{2-}\right]$ decreases by $4.0 - 5.0$ for every $10\,mmHg\, P_aCO_2$

Delta Gap Ratio Calculation (to see if there is a concomitant non-gap acidosis or alkalosis present in a patient with an anion gap)

$$(\text{Pt Anion Gap} - 12) \div (24 - \text{Pt HCO}_3^{2-}) = X$$

if $X > 2$ then concomitant metabolic alkalosis

if $X < 1$ then concomitant non $-$ gap metabolic acidosis

if $1 < X < 2$ then pure anion $-$ gap metabolic acidosis

where Pt Anion Gap $= \left[Na - \left(Cl_- + HCO_3^{2-}\right)\right]$

Cardiology

Bliss J. Chang

Contents

© The Author(s), under exclusive license to Springer Nature Switzerland AG 2021
S. H. Lecker, B. J. Chang (eds.), *The Ultimate Medical School Rotation Guide*,
https://doi.org/10.1007/978-3-030-63560-2_16

16.1 Overview

Cardiology is a fast-paced rotation that tests your medical knowledge and critical thinking skills. It is unique in that there is a greater emphasis on understanding physiology and evidence-based medicine than many other specialties. To excel on this rotation, you must have a strong holistic grasp of the basic cardiovascular diseases, including physiology, management, and key evidence for why you're doing what you're doing.

This chapter begins with fundamental concepts from a cardiology perspective. We then delve into practical tips and the most common conditions you will encounter as a medical student on the cardiology rotation (either consult or the general inpatient cardiology service). Notably, you are not expected to know how to manage rare cases such as TB constrictive pericarditis – rather it is the process of reasoning through the physiology in those cases that differentiates the star student. The foundations that you build using this chapter and the rest of the book will sufficiently prepare you to tackle those rarer presentations.

Lastly, I highly recommend reading, if you have not yet already, or refreshing your memory on cardiovascular physiology using *Pathophysiology of Heart Disease* by Dr. Leonard Lilly. It is an amazing and easy-to-use resource, written with the input of medical students. For this chapter, we will assume that you have a basic knowledge of cardiac physiology and will only cover briefly the specific physiology most necessary to excel on your cardiology rotation.

16.2 Fundamentals

Let's start by understanding the vital signs, symptoms, and exam findings from a cardiology perspective. You should not underestimate the importance of actively interpreting these seemingly basic principles for each patient. They are not obtained to be simply jotted down and presented. These basic objective data will guide much of the nuances driving clinical management. Remember, vital signs are vital!

16.2.1 Heart Rate

The heart rate is one of the first pieces of objective data you should check for any patient. It is easy for early trainees to glance at the heart rate and have an oversimplified approach of "tachycardic or not," leading to reassurance if the patient is not tachycardic. This misses a lot of nuances and does not take into account the patient's current state. When available, comparing to a patient's baseline can be very helpful.

Simply put, the conclusion you want to reach when interpreting heart rates is whether it is *physiologic or pathologic* and *appropriate or inappropriate* and whether immediate intervention is required. In addition to stability, consider the following:

- Ask yourself if the heart rate makes sense given the context (states of illness, medications, etc.).
  - For example, a patient may be mildly tachycardic with the flu, but they shouldn't be running in the 160 s.
- The inability of a heart rate to increase as expected under stress (e.g., exercise) may indicate either a medication effect (e.g., AV nodal depressant such as a beta-blocker) or impaired chronotropic reserves (e.g., in heart failure).

Pearl: Sustained tachycardia for a prolonged period of time can cause the heart to become overworked and fail. If a patient has baseline tachycardia, ask them if they know how long this has been going on for.

– Rate of Increase: A heart rate that gradually increases is likely physiologic (e.g., sinus tachycardia), whereas an abrupt jump suggests arrhythmia. The trend, whether physiologic or pathologic, can easily be visualized on telemetry.

16.2.2 Blood Pressure

The most common interpretations of blood pressure are in terms of stability and blood pressure control. Despite this, you should use a systematic approach to interpreting the blood pressure. Each time you read a blood pressure, think about it in four distinct components: systolic pressure (SBP), diastolic pressure (DBP), mean arterial pressure (MAP), and pulse pressure.

16.2.2.1 Systolic Pressure

The SBP is the star of the show. Most of your medical management will be dictated by the systolic blood pressure. Pay particular attention to blood pressure control while caring for your patients – it is often not their primary problem but an important problem to be addressed. Seeing the SBP, you should always think to yourself "Is it too high or low?", and if so, "How would I alter the antihypertensive regimen?". Remember to think about secondary causes of high blood pressure before starting the patient on an antihypertensive medicine. A patient may be hypertensive in the setting of pain or stress, and addressing these symptoms can help lower blood pressure without adding new long-term medications.

16.2.2.2 Diastolic Pressure

You will not often interpret the DBP beyond a superficial check to ensure it is in an appropriate range.

16.2.2.3 Mean Arterial Pressure (MAP)

Defined as

$$MAP = 2/3\,DBP = 1/3\,SBP,$$

it is a marker of organ perfusion. MAP should be kept above 65 at all times. Values below this limit may warrant usage of pressors (refer to the Critical Care chapter).

16.2.2.4 Pulse Pressure

The pulse pressure is defined as

$$Pulse\ Pressure = Systolic\ Blood\ Pressure - Diastolic\ Blood\ Pressure$$

and is a surrogate marker for cardiac output. A normal range is between 40 and 60 mmHg. To a medical student, an elevated pulse pressure should suggest aortic regurgitation or, more commonly, stiffening of the aorta which occurs with aging and atherosclerosis. Other, noncardiac causes of widened pulse pressure include hyperthyroidism and severe iron deficiency anemia. Conversely, a narrow pulse pressure suggests poor cardiac output such as in cardiogenic shock.

16.2.3 Oxygen Saturation

O_2 saturation is distinct from the respiratory rate and patient's reported subjective shortness of breath. It is an objective indicator of how much oxygen is in the arterial blood. In adult cardiology, the O_2 sat is primarily interpreted as an indicator of pulmonary congestion (or lack thereof). When a patient is not volume overloaded, a low O_2 sat strongly points you towards a primary pulmonary issue.

16.2.4 Chest Pain and/or Pressure

Perhaps the hallmark symptom of cardiology, it is critical to understand the ins and outs of chest pain and/or pressure. Note that a significant portion of patients with cardiac disease do not experience true chest pain but rather chest pressure. It is critical to assess using both terms, particularly when they deny chest "pain," as the patient may not admit to one but only the other. Let's look at the different types of chest pain/pressure:

1. *Musculoskeletal:* This type of chest pain is typically focal and varies with physical movement (but typically not with the motion of breathing) and palpation. It is one of the most common causes of chest pain, seen in all age ranges, particularly in the setting of significant/unaccustomed strain on the body such as with exercise or trauma. If the patient admits to chest pressure, this argues against a musculoskeletal cause which is true pain (sharp, dull, sore).
2. *Pleuritic:* Exacerbated by breathing (particularly deep inspiration), this is another common type of focal pain that is usually specific to pericarditis or diseases of the lungs. Pleuritic chest pain may be located slightly away from the chest, such as in the RUQ or LUQ. Ask the patient to take a deep breath, and watch for a grimace that may indicate pleuritic chest pain (always look for objective signs of pain). Chest pressure should not be pleuritic.
3. *Substernal:* The classic chest pain/pressure associated with acute coronary syndrome (ACS), substernal (deep behind the chest) symptoms are often described as an elephant sitting on the chest or as a deep pain. Substernal chest pain is not specific to ACS and can be seen with conditions such as esophageal spasms or gastroesophageal reflux disease (GERD).

Note: The lack of chest pain/pressure does not rule out ACS. This is particularly common in patients known to present atypically (meaning without classic symptoms) with higher frequency, such as women, the elderly, and diabetics. Also, the presence of chest wall tenderness does not exclude more serious etiologies. If you are concerned for ACS (or other serious causes of chest pain, such as pulmonary embolism), do not remove these from your differential diagnosis solely due to the presence of chest wall tenderness.

Let's build on what we just learned. When considering chest pain/pressure, it is important to think about a few different specifics using the *TLDR* mnemonic:

1. *Timing:* How long did the chest pain/pressure last? Has it been intermittent or continuous? Cardiac pain is less likely when symptoms last for a few seconds.
2. *Location:* Is the pain/pressure located in one specific area of the chest or is it generalized? While chest pain obviously raises concern for potential cardiac etiology, pain in the elbow, neck, jaw, and back are also important to elicit as they can be referred cardiac pain (sometimes the only pain the patient experiences). Be sure to inquire how the patient's prior ACS-related pain presented.
3. *Demographics:* This is an important factor for building your pre-test probability of cardiac disease in a patient. Apart from patients with a family history of cardiovascular disease, it is less likely that pain is cardiac in a

Pearl: Although O2 saturation is generally an objective metric, if the obtained reading does not fit with what you would expect for a given clinical picture, ask yourself what could be causing this inconsistency. For example, patient motion and nail polish can be sources of error, while more serious medical problems such as carbon monoxide poisoning can lead to incorrectly normal readings.

healthy young patient with no significant past medical history. Notably, women, elderly, and diabetics are less likely to have classically presenting cardiac disease.

4. *Reproducibility*: Is the pain/pressure reproduced with palpation, breathing, movement, or exercise? Worsening with exercise or stress and improving with rest supports cardiac disease.

16.2.5 Shortness of Breath (SOB)

SOB is ultimately a reflection of inadequate oxygen delivery to tissues. It does not necessarily indicate that there is congestion in the lungs. Poor oxygen delivery to tissues may result from hypoventilation, impaired gas exchange in the alveoli (e.g., due to pulmonary congestion or COPD), a perfusion defect in the blood vessels supplying the alveoli, or poor forward flow of blood (which does not necessarily lead to excess fluid in the lungs). Always interpret SOB jointly with the respiratory rate and oxygen saturation to obtain a fuller insight into the pathophysiology.

Increased shortness of breath is an important symptom to elicit and patients may provide varying answers that mean increased SOB. Be sure to ask in several different ways, particularly if you have a strong prior probability for heart failure:

— How far can you walk without stopping? How many stairs can you walk up without stopping?
— How many pillows do you use when sleeping?
— Do you wake up at night gasping for breath? (Called paroxysmal nocturnal dyspnea).
— Always compare to baseline (e.g., "Is this more (pillows) than usual?").

> Pearl: Be sure to consider musculoskeletal issues that may prevent someone from walking long distances. For example, a patient may say they need to stop once every few blocks because of knee pain.

16.2.6 Volume Status

Jugular venous pressure (JVP) and lower extremity edema are two key tests for volume status. The JVP is a marker of intravascular volume, whereas LE edema represents extravascular volume, though the two are usually correlated.

16.2.6.1 Jugular Venous Pressure

The JVP is a crude indication of the pressure of blood in the right atrium (since there are no valves between the internal jugular vein and right atrium). Thus, when there is increased intravascular volume, or poor forward blood flow through the right side of the heart (e.g., right heart failure), jugular venous distension (JVD) occurs. Remember, a patient can have left-sided heart failure and have a normal JVP if the right side of the heart is not volume-overloaded. Attendings vary stylistically on how they want this reported. Personally, I think the key is to assess whether it is (a) normal or elevated and, if elevated, (b) whether it has changed from the prior measurement. Rough approximations are in ◻ Fig. 16.1. Remember to report the angle at the head of the bed as it significantly effects the perceived JVP (the more upright, the more difficult to see the JVP).

JVP can be confused with the carotid pulse, so make sure to look for an area that pulsates twice in rapid succession. A great way to confirm that you've found the JVP is to augment it using the hepatojugular reflex (HJR) where you apply firm pressure to the right upper quadrant of the stomach for at least 10 seconds. The JVP should elevate in response to the HJR. Normally, the JVP

> Pearl: Conditions such as tricuspid regurgitation may elevate the JVP, providing a falsely elevated sense of volume.

> Pearl: If the JVP is markedly elevated (above level of the mastoid), it can be difficult to see. If you have trouble seeing the JVP, try adjusting the angle of the head of the bed.

> Pearl: When the patient is sitting upright, the distance between the right atrium and clavicle is approximately 12 cm, so if the JVP is visible while the patient is sitting up in bed, you know that JVD is present. This is a good way to assess volume status as soon as you enter the room.

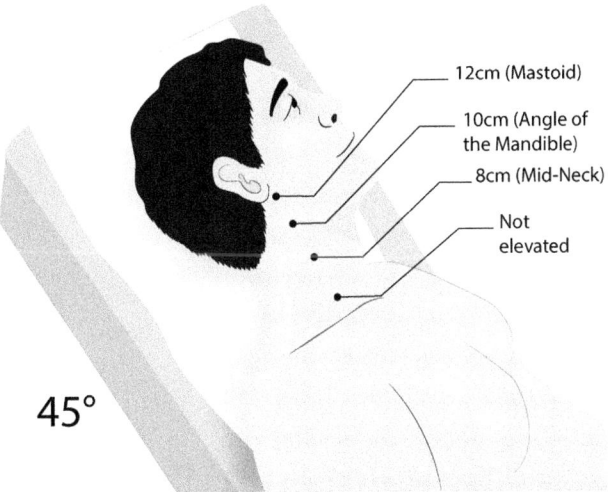

12cm (Mastoid)

10cm (Angle of the Mandible)

8cm (Mid-Neck)

Not elevated

45°

□ Fig. 16.1 JVP approximations by common landmark

should decrease with inspiration due to increased intrathoracic pressure and preload. A paradoxical increase (or absence of decrease) in JVP is called Kussmaul's sign and is indicative of right-sided volume overload.

16.2.6.2 Lower Extremity Edema

Although it is easy to jump straight to the legs, remember to also examine the feet. Be sure to press firmly against a bony surface (typically the shin) for at least 3 seconds. Note how far up the leg the edema is: "marked pitting edema up to the knees." Though the classical teaching is to describe the edema with numbers (e.g., 2+), practically what's important is the dichotomy of "volume up" or "volume down." Remember to ask how long the patient's legs have been swollen for (always compare to prior)!

Pearl: Amlodipine frequently results in LE edema (which can be asymmetric). Check the med list!

16.2.7 Heart Auscultation

At some point, you have undoubtedly been frustrated by the difficulty of putting meaning to heart sounds let alone hearing them at all. On a cardiology rotation, there is no getting by without being able to hear and understand heart sounds. Here, I will attempt to impart what I have discovered through experience to enhance the ability to hear and decipher heart sounds using a traditional stethoscope. Try auscultating without any hypotheses in order to prevent biases. However, as you are learning, it is okay to think about what you might expect.

There are a few important considerations before attempting to auscultate with a stethoscope:
1. Minimize all sources of noise in the room – television, phone, or chatter between your team. Ask your patient to remain silent while you listen.
2. Always listen under any clothing or gowns.
3. Do not create external noise: Stethoscopes are designed to pick up the subtlest of noises. A common source are the fingers touching any part of the stethoscope. It is crucial that you apply a firm but gentle pressure to the area of contact with the stethoscope to prevent sounds from your fingers shifting slightly. An alternative is to allow the stethoscope to rest freely on the patient without touching it (□ Fig. 16.2).

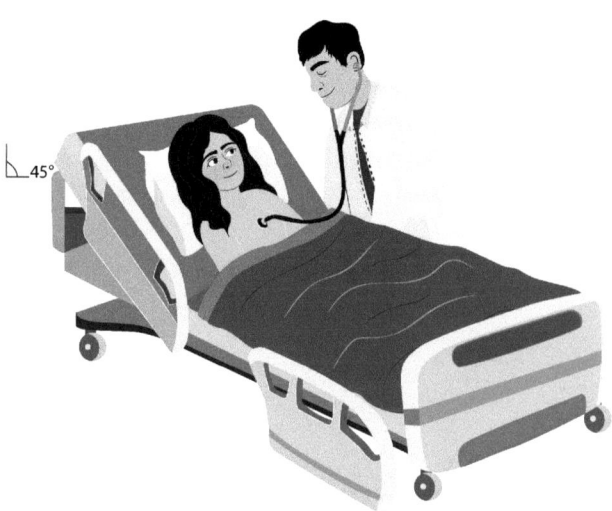

◪ **Fig. 16.2 Using a stethoscope freehand**

4. Ensure proper fit in the ears: First, ensure that the ear pieces are sized appropriately for your ears. Next, when you don a stethoscope, be sure that the ear pieces fit fully and snugly. An ill-fitting ear piece can leak (or let in) a lot of sound!

If you continue to have trouble despite proper stethoscope technique as detailed above, the next step is to adjust your stethoscope position and/or applied pressure.

1. There is abundant space within each classic listening position. Try moving your stethoscope around a bit. Sometimes, a bony prominence or slightly irregular contour of a chest can cause part of the chestpiece to be off the chest, thus disrupting optimal conduction of heart sounds.
2. Attempt a slow escalation of pressure by pressing from almost no pressure to very firm (but not so hard that the patient is in pain!).
3. For patients with a large habitus, pressing firmly often helps.
4. You may ask the patient to exhale and momentarily hold their breath.
5. Lastly, heart sounds can be better heard better if you ask the patient to shift position, as it causes the heart to come closer to your stethoscope:
   (a) For aortic regurgitation, ask the patient to lean forwards.
   (b) For mitral stenosis and S3, ask the patient to roll onto their left side.

> **Memory Aid:** For AR, imagine the aorta leaning forwards and vomiting (regurgitating) blood.

> **Memory Aid:** Remember that rolling into left decubitus is for listening to the heart sounds you'd hear with the bell.

> **Flash Quiz:** What murmur are you checking for using the bell? Answer: mitral stenosis, S3, S4.

If you know what sound(s) you're looking for (or trying to rule out), adjusting the pressure on the chestpiece can help greatly. Heart sounds have varying frequencies, and the pressure that you apply on the chestpiece/diaphragm tunes the pitch that is best heard. Light pressure with the diaphragm favors low-pitch sounds (mitral stenosis, S3, S4), whereas firm pressure *eliminates* low-pitch sounds and enhances high-frequency sounds (most other murmurs). Similarly, placing the bell lightly on the chest enhances low-frequency sounds. In summary, the harder you press, the more you are converting your current auscultation side (diaphragm or bell) to the other.

Lastly, for those like me who are not musically inclined, describing heart sounds can be tough. In fact, reading classic textbook descriptions and even hearing heart sounds a few times online can be difficult to remember or translate into your clinical practice. Thus, I have attempted to communicate in my own words what each major heart murmur sounds like. I hope this is helpful in recognizing and attaching meaning to sounds. If the classic descriptions work for you, feel free to skip this part as it is merely an alternate perspective.

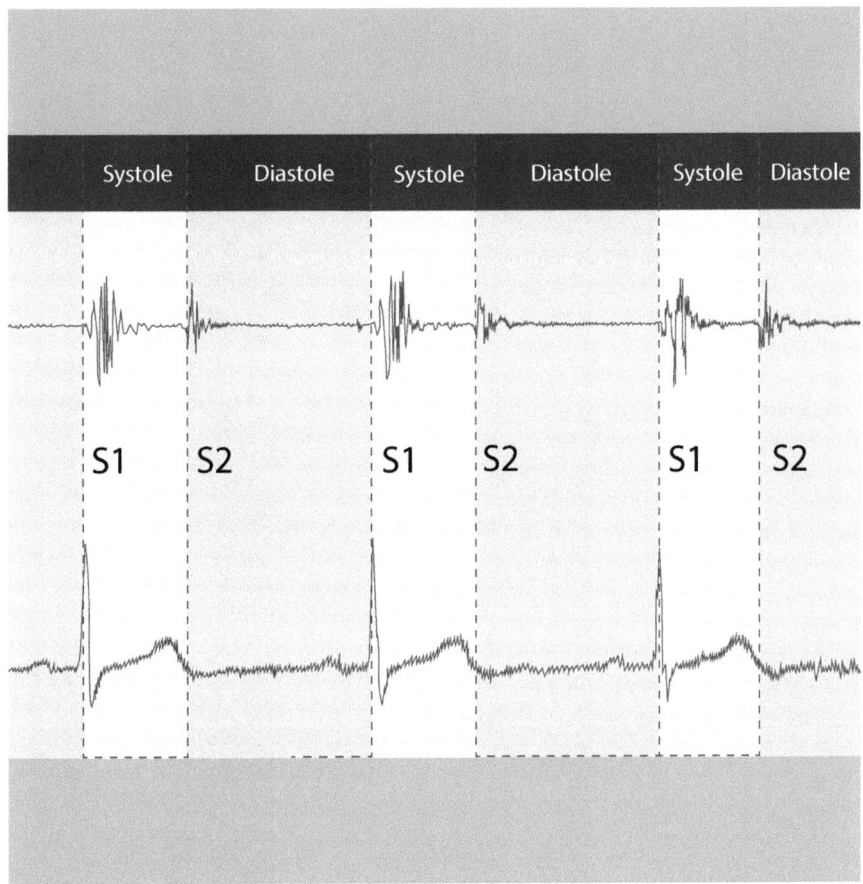

▣ Fig. 16.3 Annotated audiogram of normal heart sounds

16.2.8 Normal Heart Sounds

A structurally normal heart will have an S1 and S2 heard in rapid succession of one another. Systole is between S1 and S2, whereas diastole is between S2 and the next S1 (▣ Fig. 16.3). When you begin listening, start by identifying which sound is S1 and S2 before attempting to identify any extra heart sounds. The easiest way to do this is by finding the pattern of "sound-short silence-sound-long silence." Note that until your ears become accustomed to auscultating, you may find it difficult to identify a clear separation between an early or late murmur and S1 or S2. Your ears will adjust with time and practice, but this should not limit you from deciphering what you hear in a clinically relevant manner.

16.2.9 Extra Heart Sounds

First, identify the sound as either systolic or diastolic. Combined with the auscultation location, this is an easy way to narrow down the possibility of murmurs (▣ Fig. 16.4). For example, a diastolic murmur best heard at the apex is most likely to be mitral stenosis. For your rotation, you will rarely go wrong by identifying it using this method. If you are still unsure, augmentation techniques can be used to aid in identification of the murmur. Although there are maneu-

Pearl: Tachycardia causes the length of systole and diastole to be approximately equal, making it very confusing to identify S1 and S2. Feel the pulse while auscultating – the sound that coincides with the pulse (e.g., radial) is S1.

Pearl: Listen for one thing at a time. Tune out any extra heart sounds, and just listen for the S1 and S2 first instead of trying to listen for everything at once. This really helps your brain and ears pick up one thing. You can then move on to listening for extra heart sounds.

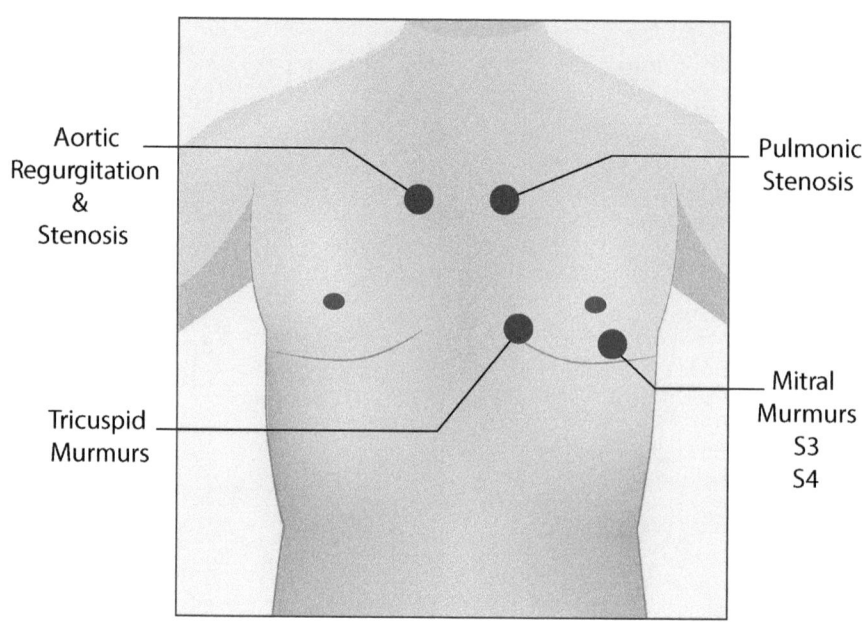

Fig. 16.4 Diagram of common murmurs by location

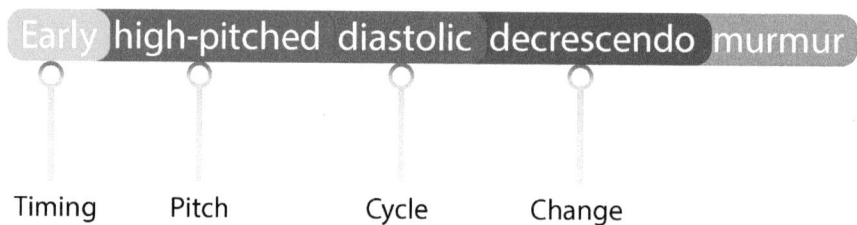

Fig. 16.5 Annotated dissection of extra heart sound description

Pearl: Don't be afraid to listen as long as you need to. The more listening, the better you will become.

vers to decrease the sounds of murmurs, we will focus on the maneuvers that increase the sounds since you may have difficulty hearing the murmurs as is!

16.2.9.1 Concerning Extra Heart Sounds

Not all murmurs are pathologic. Physiologic systolic murmurs are often found in young healthy adults, and states of high output such as pregnancy may produce benign flow murmurs. As a student, you should remember these features which suggest a pathological murmur that requires further workup:
- Diastolic murmurs
- Holosystolic murmurs
- Late systolic murmurs
- Loud murmurs (≥ III/VI)
- New murmurs

16.2.9.2 Describing Extra Heart Sounds

All murmurs can be described by using a series of descriptions as shown in Fig. 16.5.

You should systematically describe all extra heart sounds using the *TPCC* framework below:
- *T*iming: relationship to S1 or S2 (early, late, mid, throughout).
- *P*itch: low, mid, high.
- *C*ycle: systolic or diastolic.
- *C*hange: does the sound become softer or louder or stay the same throughout (crescendo, decrescendo, crescendo-decrescendo)?

Pearl: The pitch reflects the transient gradient between the two chambers surrounding the valves. A high pitch reflects a larger gradient and force.

16.2.9.3 Insufficiency (Regurgitation) Murmurs

Insufficiency murmurs are classically described to medical students as holosystolic "blowing" murmurs. Despite this, be aware that not all "blowing" sounds actually sound alike. Hence, it is preferable to describe the sounds with more specific technical words, since "blowing" is subjective. Lastly, remember that regurgitation murmurs are best differentiated by the location at which the murmur is heard loudest.

- Aortic Regurgitation (Diastolic)
  - Technical Description: early high-pitched diastolic decrescendo murmur
  - Another Description: S1 followed by a blowing sound almost masking the S2
  - Location: left upper sternal border (LUSB)
  - Special Maneuvers: handgrip (increases)
  - Associations: wide pulse pressure with "pulsation" phenomena (fingernail, carotids, uvula, liver/spleen, head bobbing)
- Mitral Regurgitation (Systolic).
  - Technical Description: medium-pitched holosystolic murmur.
  - Another Description: S1 heard almost simultaneously with blowing sound followed by distinct S2.
  - Location: apex.
  - Special Maneuvers: handgrip (increases).
  - Associations: Murmur radiates to the mid axilla (you should always check for this!).
- Tricuspid Regurgitation (Systolic).
  - Technical Description: high-pitched holosystolic murmur
  - Another Description: S1 heard almost simultaneously with blowing sound followed by distinct S2
  - Location: left lower sternal border (LLSB)
  - Special Maneuvers: inspiration (increases)
  - Associations: elevated JVP in the setting of euvolemia if moderate or severe regurgitation

16.2.9.4 Ejection Murmurs

Ejection murmurs are systolic murmurs classically described as harsh or coarse sounds, as you may imagine when fluid is forced through a tight opening. Importantly, the term ejection murmur refers specifically to aortic stenosis and pulmonic stenosis – it is not an alternate term for all stenotic murmurs. Pulmonic stenosis is rare so we will not cover them in this chapter.

- Aortic Stenosis (Systolic)
  - Technical Description: high-pitched diamond-shaped systolic murmur.
  - Another Description: prominent blowing sound almost masking S1 and with a soft S2.
  - Location: right upper sternal border (RUSB).
  - Special Maneuvers: handgrip (decreases).
  - Associations: age, bicuspid aortic valve, SAD (syncope, angina, dyspnea), slow-rising, and weak carotid pulses (pulsus parvus et tardus), radiation of murmur to carotids.
  - Reporting note: If you can, try and determine when in systole the murmur occurs, as more severe disease is associated with a later peaking murmur.

Breaking It Down
Early = starts soon after S2 and thus S2 may be masked as part of the murmur to beginners
High-pitched = prominent, coarse, unpleasant tone.
Diastolic = occurs after S2 and before S1.
Decrescendo = Murmur goes from high to low intensity.

Pearl: When thinking about the effect of maneuvers, think about how the increase or decrease in preload or afterload would affect the gradient across the valve in question.

Pearl: A bounding pulse in the radial arteries is known as a water-hammer or Corrigan's pulse.

Pearl: If mitral valve prolapse is behind the regurgitation, there is often a mid-systolic "click."

Note: Holosystolic murmurs have an even pitch throughout; thus the "change" descriptor is not necessary.

Pearl: Left-sided murmurs should not change notably with inspiration or expiration.

Pearl: The one exception is MR due to posterior leaflet prolapse in which the murmur radiates to the base instead.

Pearl: All right-sided murmurs (except congenital pulmonic stenosis) should increase with inspiration. This is a great way to distinguish between right- and left-sided murmurs.

Pearl: A severe aortic stenosis murmur may be initially perceived as a distinct murmur without clear S1 or S2. Suspect severe AS if you have difficulty hearing both S1 and S2.

Understanding: A soft S2 is due to the stenosis of the valve leading to only partial opening and closing (similar to how shutting a partially closed door makes less noise).

Pearl: It can be confusing trying to remember whether aortic stenosis or regurgitation is best heard on the right or left sides. Keep them straight using the mnemonic SR (senior): "stenosis right."

Recall: Low-pitched sounds are auscultated with the bell or by using very light pressure with the diaphragm.

Pearl: Anticoagulation is required specifically with warfarin for mechanical valves because of lack of current convincing data with DOACs.

Pearl: An S3 is almost always normal in young healthy adults (<age 30).

Pearl: The absence of an S3 cannot be used to rule out volume overload or ventricular dysfunction.

Pearl: In patients under 40 years old, there may be a physiologic gallop that is normal. You should suspect a pathologic S3 when the patient is >40 years old or if they have known ventricular dysfunction.

16.2.9.5 Other Murmurs

– Mitral Stenosis (Diastolic)
  – Technical Description: low-pitched diastolic decrescendo murmur
  – Another Description: quick drum-like sound heart very shortly but distinctly after S2
  – Location: apex
  – Special Maneuvers: patient rolled onto their left side
  – Associations: rheumatic fever (suspect in immigrants), hemoptysis

16.2.9.6 Mechanical Valves

Mechanical valves are composed of a durable material such as metal or carbon which can last several decades. This results in a prominent "click" that can be heard, sometimes even without a stethoscope. Among commonly used valves, several studies have shown that the St. Jude's Medical valve prostheses (refer to ► Sect. 16.8) are among the least audible (great for the patient!).

You should listen to a mechanical valve sound online – it is a very easy sound to recognize and something you should note on exam. For a metallic mitral valve, the click replaces the S1, whereas it replaces the S2 in a metallic aortic valve. This is how you can aid in identifying the click on auscultation, since the click is often quite prominent and may be harder to localize to a specific area.

16.2.9.7 Bioprosthetic Valves

These are valves composed of animal tissue, most commonly from pig (porcine valves). Current bioprostheses have a durability of 10–20 years (>85% durability at 10 years) and do not require anticoagulation as do mechanical valves. These do not have the mechanical click sound of metal valves.

16.2.9.8 Gallops

These are extra heart sounds which come either shortly before S1 (termed S4) or after S2 (termed S3). In fact, "gallop" refers to the sequence of three heart sounds in quick succession. They are named logically in ascending numerical order (◘ Fig. 16.6). Gallops are low-pitched so you should use the bell for auscultating.

An S3, also known as a ventricular gallop, conveys volume overload (from any cause such as heart/renal failure, high-output states). More importantly, the S3 is the *single most sensitive* exam finding for ventricular dysfunction. This sound is created by an increased volume of blood hitting a normally compliant left ventricle. Remember, compliance refers to how well a chamber can accommodate incoming blood. In other words, compliance is the stiffness or rigidity a chamber. Again, S3 is a low-pitched sound in early diastole (so listen for "S1-S2-S3-longest silence-S1-S2-S3-longest silence"). It is best heard (sometimes only heard) using the stethoscope bell at the apex in left lateral decubitus position. People often refer to the cadence of the murmur as "Ken-tuck-y" where the "tuck-y" comes in rapid succession. The best time to practice auscultating for an S3 is when you have a patient with florid heart failure.

On the other hand, an S4, known as an atrial gallop, signals low compliance of the heart (specifically the left ventricle) and is caused by blood hitting the stiff left ventricular wall during atrial contraction. S4 is a low-pitched sound at the end of diastole, right before S1. Similar to S3, S4 is best heard in the lateral decubitus position with light pressure using the bell. To me, this is a bit harder to listen for than an S3, so I find it helpful to first identify S1 and S2. Then I listen for two distinct sounds in the place of S1 – often a very quick succession that is hard to hear particularly due to the low pitch. The sound goes "S4-S1-short silence-S2-long silence." The cadence is similar to "Ten-nes-see", where the "Ten-nes" comes in rapid succession. You should check for these in patients with a significant left ventricular hypertrophy.

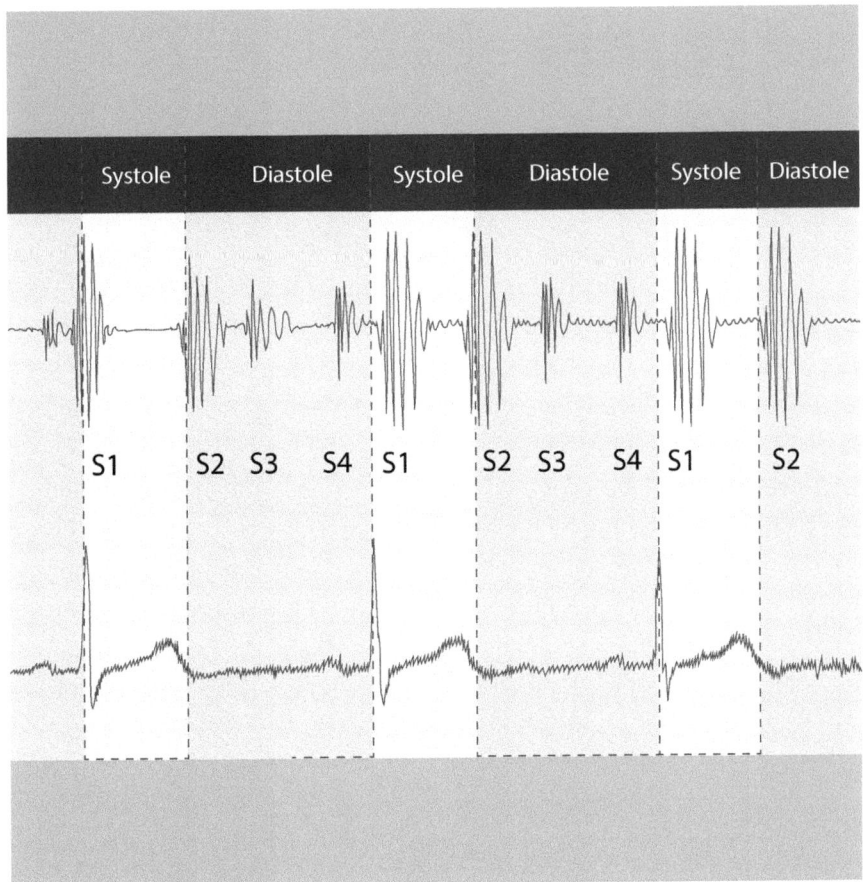

■ Fig. 16.6 S1 through S4 on audiogram

16.2.9.9 Rub

A rub is an extra heart sound synonymous with pericarditis. It is caused by friction between the parietal and visceral layers of the pericardium which typically should be lubricated adequately in the absence of inflammation. Often referred to as a "to and fro" sound, it is a coarse grating sound with up and down intensity. The rub has one systolic and two diastolic components (early and late). Thus, you will appreciate "sound-sound" in quick succession representing the "late diastolic-systolic" sounds with another "sound" afterwards representing the "early diastolic" sound (■ Fig. 16.7). The sound is best appreciated using the diaphragm near the apex. Due to the prominent rub, S1 and S2 may be difficult to appreciate.

16.2.9.10 Grading Murmurs

Lastly, let's look at how to report the intensity of murmurs. Though the official scale is described as I–VI out of VI, practically you will be reporting on a scale of 2 (II) to 4 (IV). Refer to ■ Fig. 16.8.

Now that we've learned about the murmurs you're most likely to encounter, I encourage you to practice with the following:

1. Listen to your heart for a minute each day to begin training your ears to normal heart sounds.
2. Listen to these murmurs using various audios (to account for patient to patient variabilities). I highly recommend EasyAuscultation.com which has a great looping version of extra heart sounds.

Homework Tracker

Tally up each day you practice auscultating here! Hopefully you'll have 30 tallies by the end of your rotation!

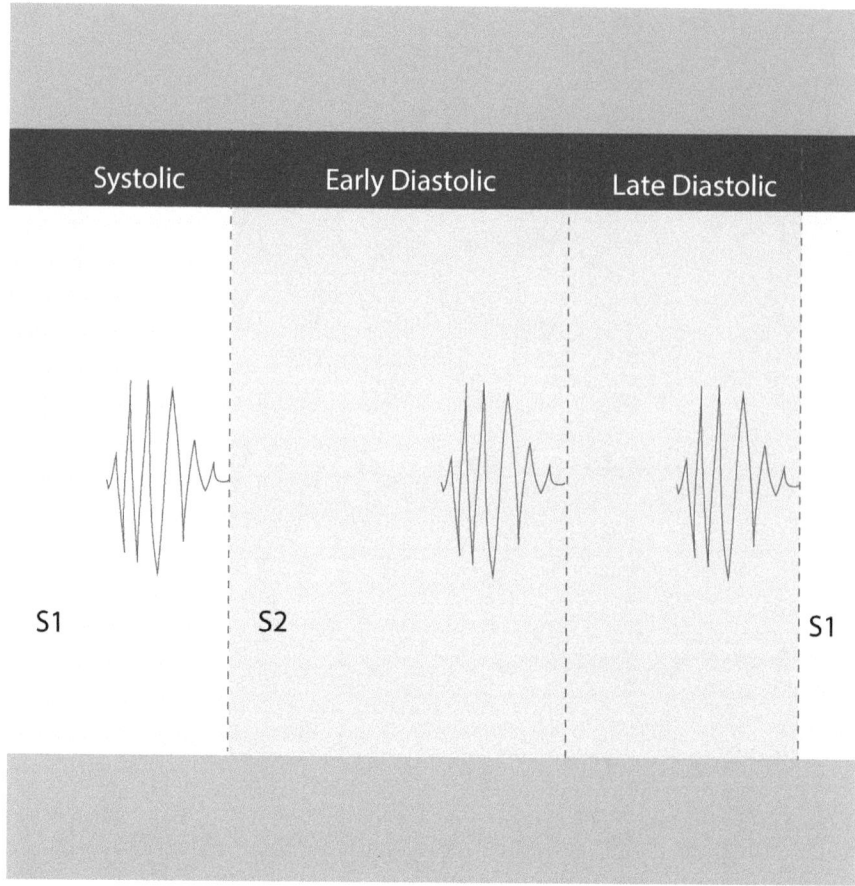

Systolic   Early Diastolic   Late Diastolic

S1   S2   S1

◘ Fig. 16.7 Pericardial rub audiogram

16.2.10 Cardiac Anatomy

There are a few key aspects of cardiac anatomy worth knowing for your rotation. We will start with the coronary vasculature and then go into the structure of the heart itself.

16.2.10.1 Coronary Vasculature

There are two main coronary arteries that immediately arise off the ascending aorta, the right coronary artery (RCA) and left coronary artery (LCA). It is worth learning the following vasculature well as it will come up time and time again (◘ Table 16.1) (◘ Fig. 16.9).

The RCA always gives rise to the right marginal artery (RMA) which supplies the lateral right ventricle. In the majority of patients, the RCA also supplies the sinoatrial node (via the SA nodal artery) and AV node (via the AV nodal artery). Lastly, in most patients, the RCA gives rise to the posterior descending artery (PDA). Note that while the PDA is named "posterior," it really is more inferior.

The LCA gives rise to the left anterior descending artery (LAD) and left circumflex artery (LCx). The LAD supplies the anterior left ventricle and the anterior 2/3 of the interventricular septum. Diagonal branches ("diags") come off the LAD and supply the anterolateral surface. The LCx supplies the left atrium and the posterolateral aspects of the left ventricle. Obtuse marginal branches come off the LCx and supply part of the lateral wall while heading towards the apex. In a minority of patients, the PDA may arise off the LCx.

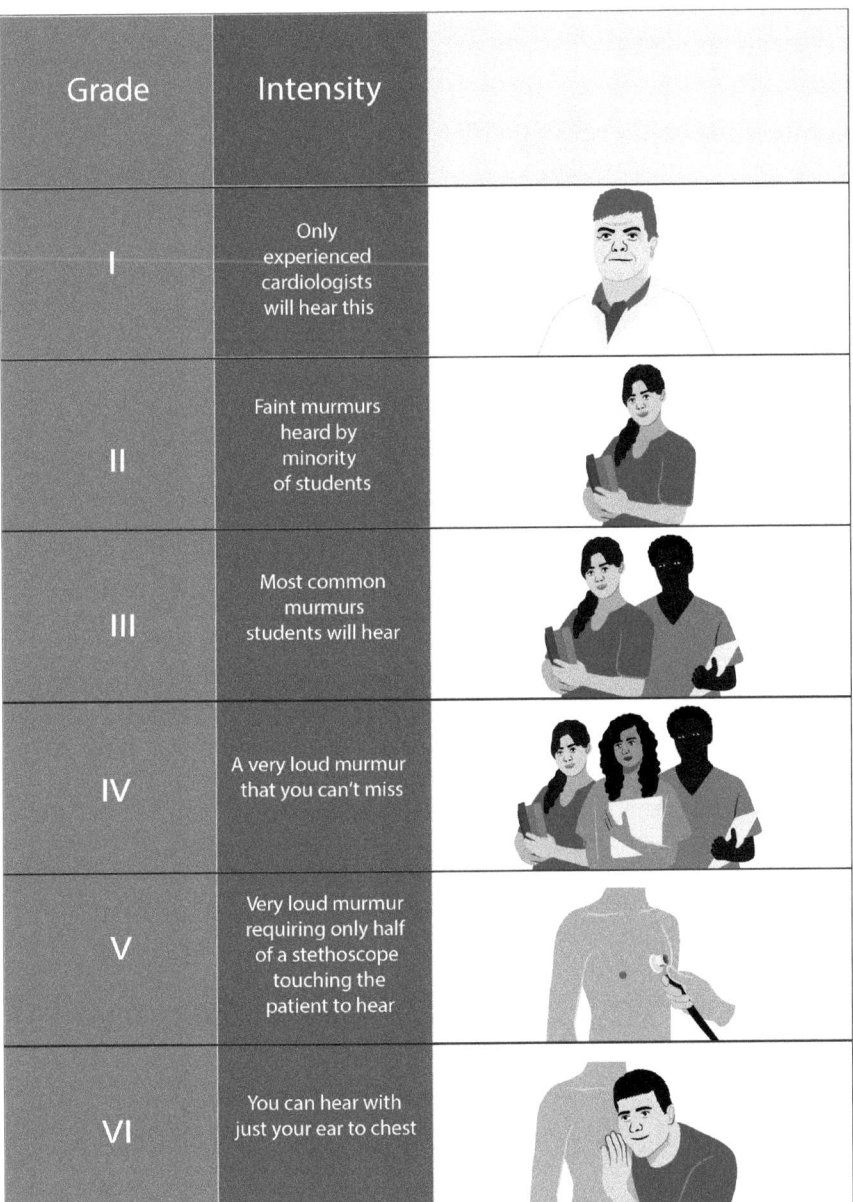

Grade	Intensity	
I	Only experienced cardiologists will hear this	
II	Faint murmurs heard by minority of students	
III	Most common murmurs students will hear	
IV	A very loud murmur that you can't miss	
V	Very loud murmur requiring only half of a stethoscope touching the patient to hear	
VI	You can hear with just your ear to chest	

🔲 Fig. 16.8 Murmur grading

🔲 Table 16.1 Myocardial blood supply

Area	Coronary
Anterior wall	LAD, potential diagonal branch involvement
Lateral (left ventricular) wall	LCx, obtuse marginal branches
Right ventricular wall	RCA, RMA
Inferior wall	PDA
Posterior wall	RCA, LCx
Anterior (2/3) septum	LAD
Posterior (1/3) septum	PDA
Apex	LAD, rarely PDA

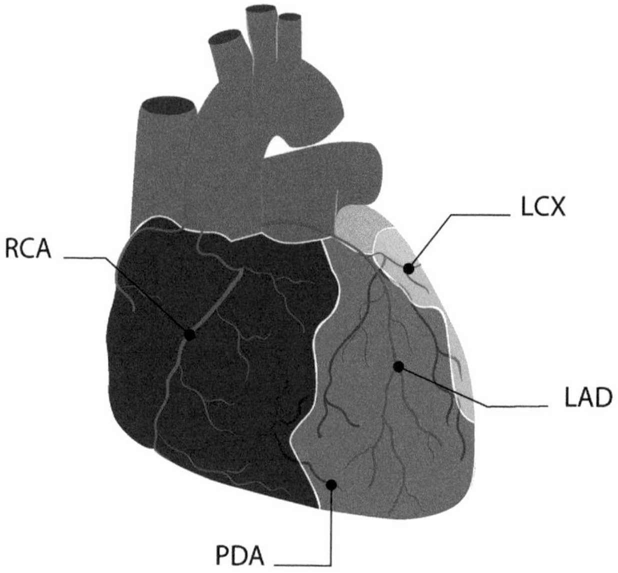

Fig. 16.9 Color-mapped coronary distributions

The PDA is worth knowing for its prominent role in clinical cases. It supplies the inferior wall and posterior 1/3 of the interventricular septum. Moreover, the single branch supplying the posteromedial mitral leaflet originates from the PDA, hence why the mitral valve is prone to papillary muscle rupture in an inferior myocardial infarction (MI).

Each heart has one of three main variants in coronary vasculature, referred to as the *dominance* of the heart. The dominance is determined by the main coronary artery off which the PDA originates. A PDA originating from the RCA is a right-dominant heart, whereas left-dominance is off the LCx, and codominance means off both the RCA and LCx. Most hearts are right-dominant, but you should always check any available cath reports to verify for each patient.

- **Flash Quiz**
1. What coronary artery was most likely occluded if a new ventricular septal defect is found after MI? LAD.
2. Occlusion of which coronary artery is most likely to result in bradycardia? RCA due to its supply to the AV nodal artery.
3. An MI resulting in papillary muscle rupture means which coronary has most likely been occluded? PDA or the parent branch (RCA or LCx).

16.2.10.2 Heart Structure

The *pericardium* is a double-layered sac with fibrous and serous layers. Its function is to lubricate and protect the heart. The serous pericardial layer is further divided into the visceral and parietal layers (■ Fig. 16.10). The potential space in between these two layers of the serous pericardium is known as the pericardial cavity and is where pericardial effusions are located.

The *cavotricuspid isthmus (CTI)* is the most common location for a reentrant circuit causing atrial flutter. The CTI is in the lower right atrium at the junction of the tricuspid valve and inferior vena cava (IVC) (■ Fig. 16.11).

The *tricuspid valve* has three leaflets (hence called tricuspid) (■ Fig. 16.12). Its most common pathology is tricuspid regurgitation (refer to ► Sect. 16.8). Additional details are usually not necessary for this rotation.

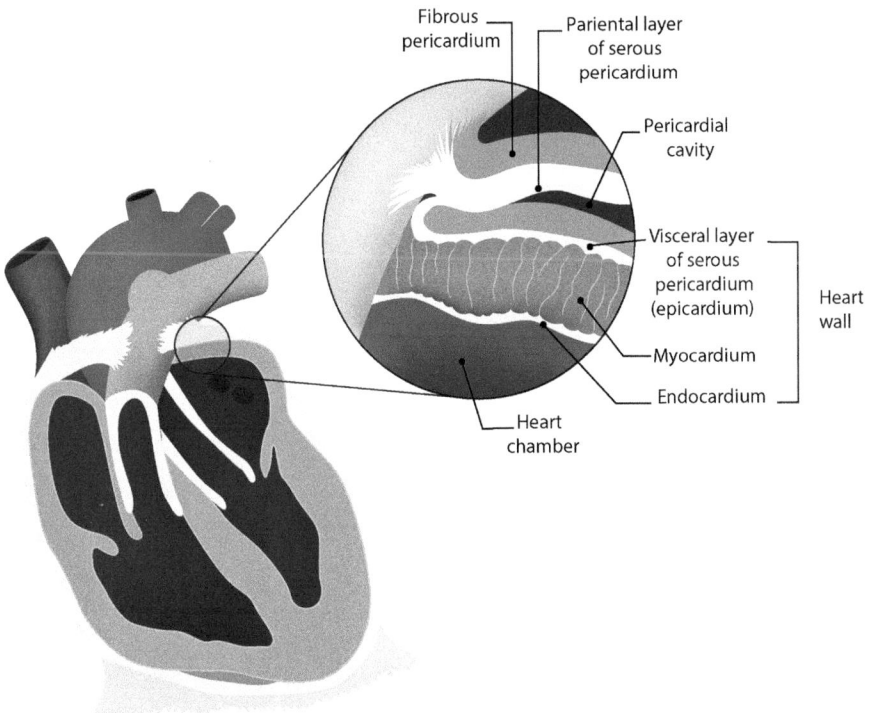

Fig. 16.10 Pericardial structure

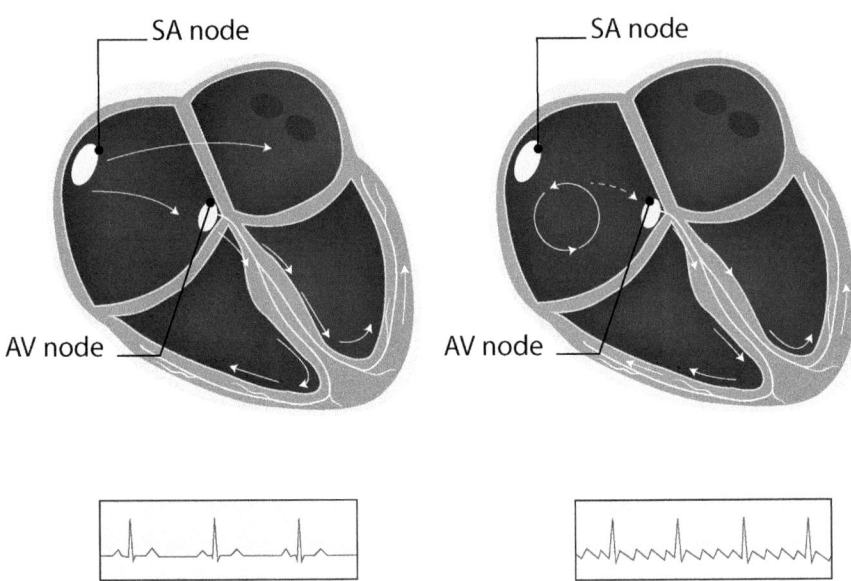

Fig. 16.11 Cavotricuspid isthmus

The *mitral valve* has two leaflets (bicuspid) held by the anterolateral and posteromedial leaflets (Fig. 16.12) and is often described as resembling a fish mouth. Because the posteromedial papillary muscle has a single blood supply from the PDA, it is the most likely to rupture in myocardial infarction. The mitral valve is the most common valve damaged in rheumatic fever, hence the high prevalence of mitral stenosis/regurgitation in patients born abroad.

The *aortic valve* is normally tricuspid (three leaflets) but a common inherited variant is bicuspid aortic valve (Fig. 16.12). A bicuspid aortic valve

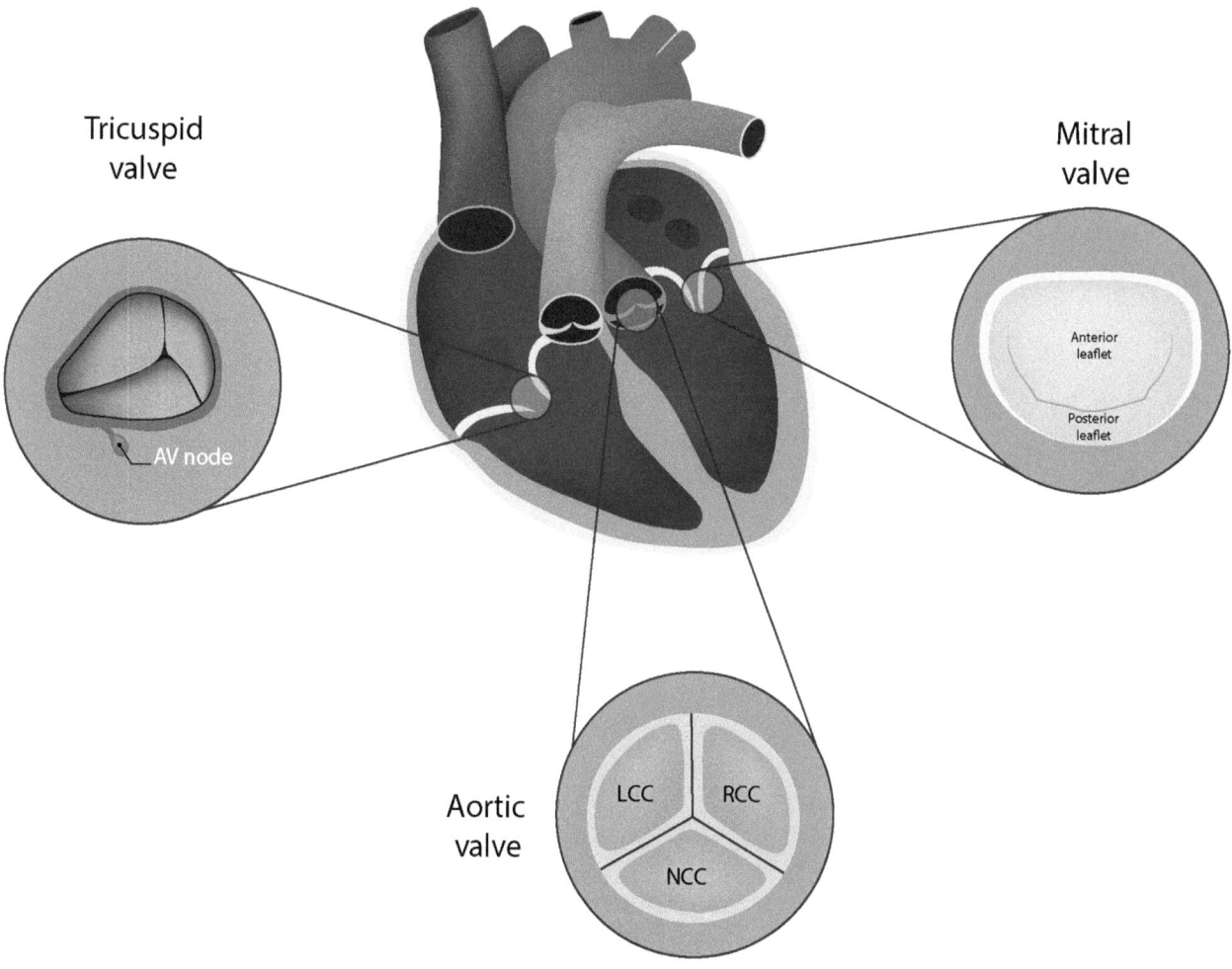

Tricuspid
valve

AV node

Mitral
valve

Anterior
leaflet

Posterior
leaflet

Aortic
valve

LCC   RCC

NCC

◧ Fig. 16.12 Heart valves

predisposes to regurgitation and calcification (leading to stenosis). The aortic valve is anatomically close to the AV node, thus vegetations and/or abscesses in endocarditis that affect the aortic valve may extend into the AV node and cause nodal dysfunction (e.g., AV block).

16.2.11 EKGs

> Remember, one of the most important steps in reading EKGs is by comparing a new EKG to a prior reading: Context is key!

Given that there are several very high-yield EKG books, we will not cover EKGs in detail. Rather, we will highlight some of the most common EKGs you will see. I recommend Dale Dubin's *Rapid Interpretation of EKGs* for a first pass when you have spare time on your rotation for EKG practice.

Let's begin by looking at the relationship of EKG leads to the heart. In ◧ Fig. 16.13, you can visualize which leads best "see" various parts of the heart. For example, the inferior aspect has three leads best covering it (II, III, aVF). Thus, it is no surprise that these leads clue you in to an inferior MI. This way, you won't need to memorize which leads correspond to which portions of the heart!

When interpreting EKGs, it is critical to have a systematic approach. Here we will offer one approach which we call the *PQRSTU* approach. With this method, you will first interpret the rate/rhythm/axis first. The rate and rhythm form the basis for the differential diagnosis for an EKG, and the axis provides

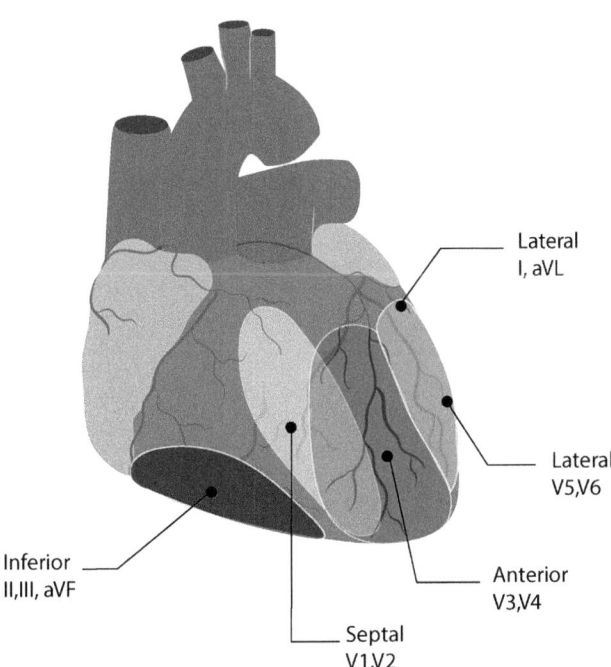

Lateral
I, aVL

Lateral
V5,V6

Anterior
V3,V4

Septal
V1,V2

Inferior
II,III, aVF

□ Fig. 16.13 EKG leads mapped to heart surface

further clues to the diagnosis. Then you will examine the EKG tracing in alphabetical order (e.g., starting with the P wave and then Q, R, and so forth).

16.2.11.1 Rate

There are many methods for determining rate. The easiest is probably counting the number of large boxes in between the R waves and dividing this into 300 (□ Fig. 16.14). For example, four small boxes would correspond to 75 bpm. Similarly, 4.5 small boxes would be around 67 bpm. The goal of these rate calculations is to estimate and quickly tell whether there is profound bradycardia or tachycardia – don't spend forever trying to get the exact number.

However, this only works for regular rhythms. For an irregular rhythm, count the number of R waves on the strip and multiply by 6. For example, 8 R waves corresponds to 48 bpm.

16.2.11.2 Rhythm

The rhythm can be thought of how consistent and appropriate the beating of the heart is, defined in two parts:

$$\text{Pattern} \times \text{Regularity}$$

Regularity refers to whether the atria and ventricles are beating in synchrony. When the atria beat at the same rate as the ventricles, the rhythm is considered regular, and this is reflected in uniform R-R intervals. Conditions such as atrial fibrillation where the atrial rate is differently much greater than the ventricular rate are termed irregular. It follows that the R-R intervals are completely variable.

Pattern refers to the consistency of these intervals. Are the intervals occurring in a uniform manner? For example, in atrial fibrillation, there is no pattern to the QRS complexes and the R-R intervals. This is an irregular pattern. However, in atrial flutter, there is often a fixed pattern and uniform R-R intervals. This is a regular pattern despite abnormal cardiac physiology.

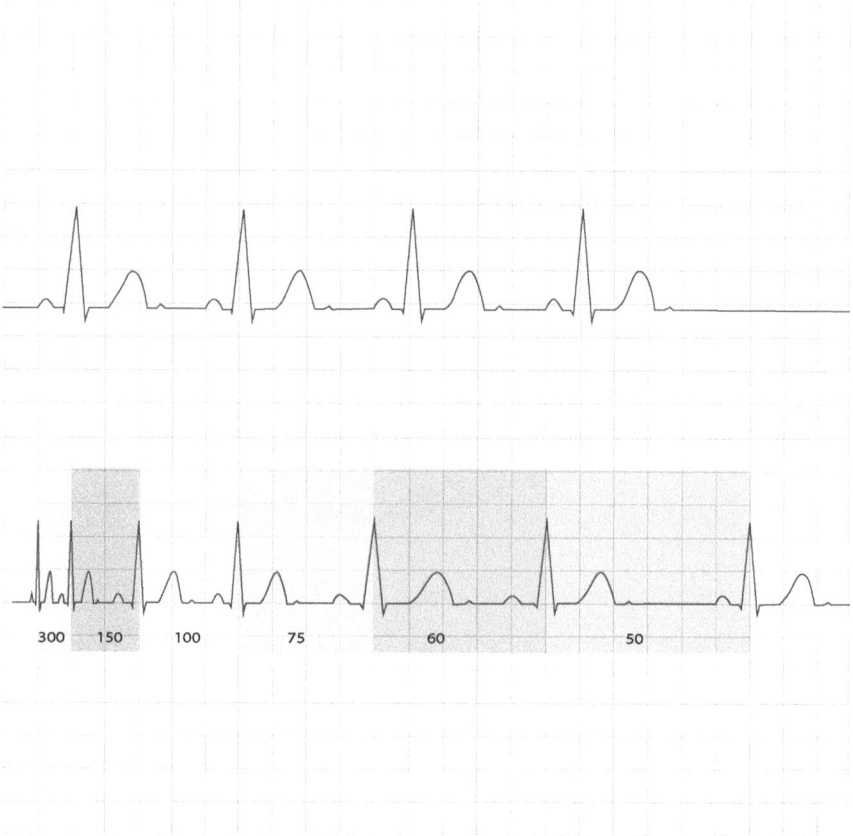

Fig. 16.14 EKG rate calculation methods

Practically speaking, you will likely encounter three variations of rhythm descriptions:
- Regularly regular: sinus rhythm
- Regularly irregular: atrial flutter, sinus arrhythmia
- Irregularly irregular: atrial fibrillation

To determine the rhythm, first look for the presence of P waves. These are best observed in *lead II*. The P wave should *ALWAYS* be positive (upright) in lead I – a negative P wave in lead I should raise concern for mixing of the right and left leads:
- If you find absent P waves in the presence of QRS complexes, you're done – this is usually pathognomonic for atrial fibrillation (look for a narrow QRS) though it may be present in other arrhythmias such as VT (wide QRS) and some junctional tachycardias (retrograde P waves hidden in the QRS complexes).
- If there are P waves, look at the R-R intervals to see if these are equally spaced. Equal spacing means regular intervals and vice versa. Next, check for the presence of a pattern to the R-R interval spacing (regardless of whether it is regularly spaced or not). If there is no variation, this is a regular pattern.
- Just as every P wave should be followed by a QRS complex, every QRS complex should be preceded by a P wave. If either of these conditions are not met, the rhythm cannot be sinus.

16.2.11.3 Axis

Axis is the net direction in which the electrical forces of the heart point. A normal heart's net electrical vector should point somewhere towards −30 and + 90 degrees (◘ Fig. 16.15) because the left ventricle has the most mass (and

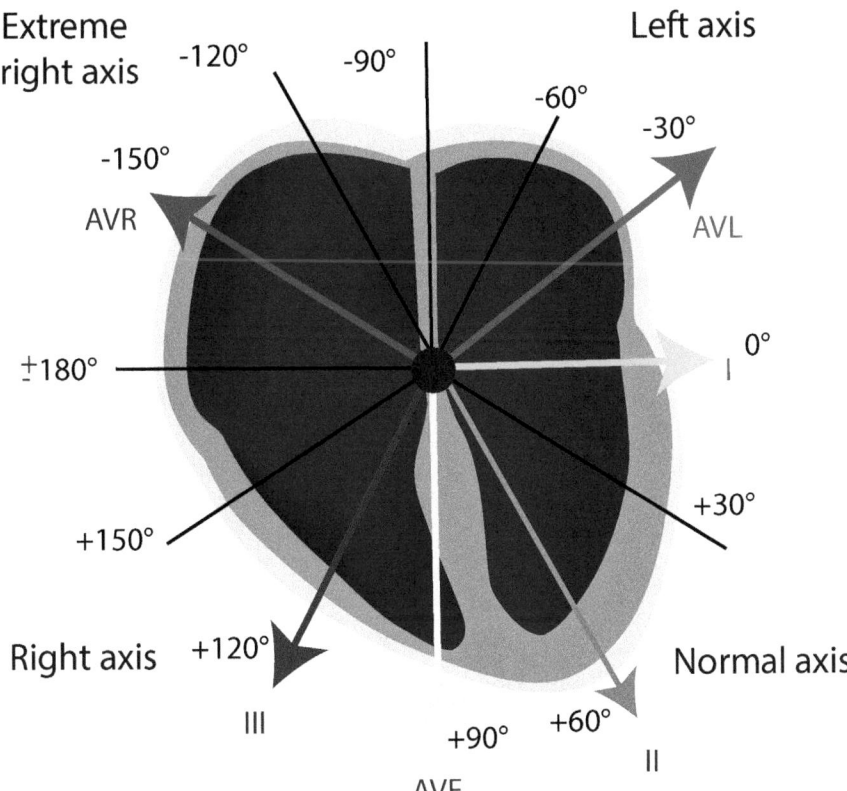

Fig. 16.15 Heart with overlaid EKG axis diagram

thus most electrical activity). If the right ventricle were to become hypertrophied (in the absence of LVH), this would shift the proportion of electrical activity towards the right side of the heart, resulting in right axis deviation. Similarly, LVH may cause a shift towards left axis deviation (many patients with LVH have normal axis). Physiologic hypertrophy (e.g., athletes) can increase LV mass and push the axis closer towards left axis (0 to −30 degrees).

Mass is not the only determinant of the electrical activity's net direction. Anything that causes more electrical activity to go a certain direction can cause axis deviation. For example, if a patient suffered a lateral MI, the dead tissue would contain little to no electrical activity, leading to a greater proportion of the heart's electrical activity based in the right heart (leading to right axis).

When a QRS deflection is positive, the electrical vector travels in the direction of the lead. A negative vector means the opposite direction of the lead. Traditionally, you are taught the quadrant method or three-lead method for determining the axis. However, I like to use a modified quicker version where I simply visualize where the sum of the vectors in leads I and II (and aVF if necessary) would point. Examples are shown in ◘ Fig. 16.16.

Another way to determine the axis is with relation to what defines the normal axis (positive QRS complexes in leads I and aVF). Note: Like many aspects of EKG reading, you will hear different methods depending on who you ask. In this case, it generally depends on what degree you consider to be a positive axis. For example, positive QRS in leads I and II indicate the net axis is between −30 and +90 degrees, while positive QRS in leads I and aVF indicate a net axis between 0 and +90 degrees. According to ◘ Fig. 16.15, if aVF became negative, that would instantly put us into left axis deviation (or rarely extreme right axis deviation). Similarly, if lead I became negative, that would put us into

Shortcut:
Two positives = normal
Two negatives = extreme axis
Negative aVF = LAD
Negative lead I = RAD

LEAD I	LEAD II or aVF	Quadrant	Axis
POSITIVE	POSITIVE (II)		Normal Axis (-30 to +90°)
POSITIVE	NEGATIVE (II)		LAD (-30 to -90°)
NEGATIVE	POSITIVE (aVF)		RAD (+90° to 180°)
NEGATIVE	NEGATIVE (aVF)		Extreme Axis (-90° to 180°)

Fig. 16.16 Example modified axis determination method

right axis deviation. If both leads were negative, we would be in extreme axis deviation. Easy enough to remember, right?

■ Flash Quiz

Identify the rate, rhythm, and axis in the EKGs below. You can check your answers are in the side margin.

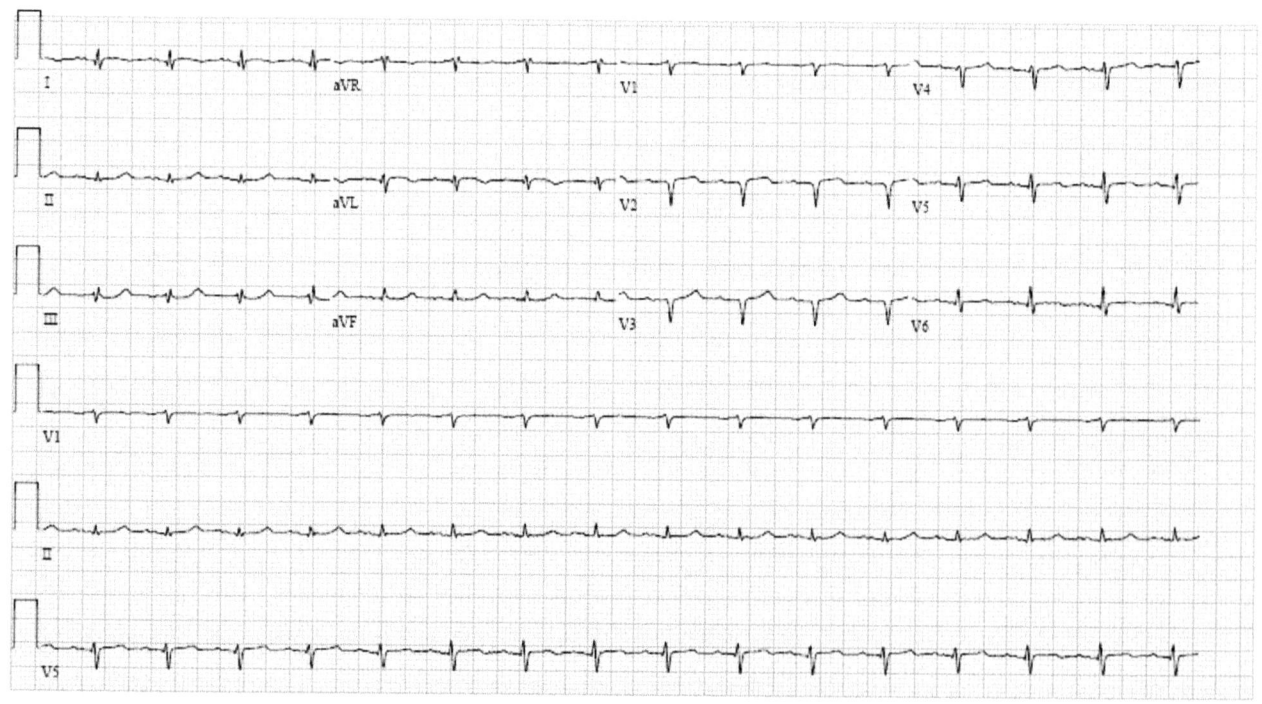

■ Axis Determination Image 1

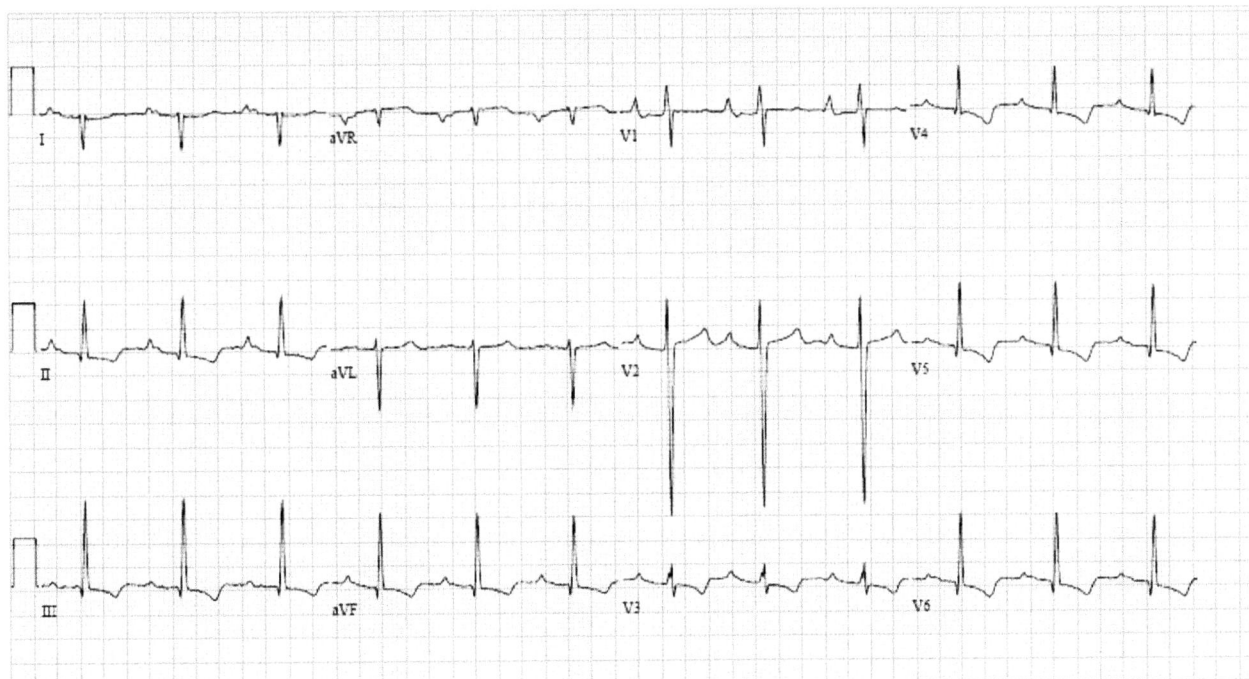

◘ Axis Determination Image 2

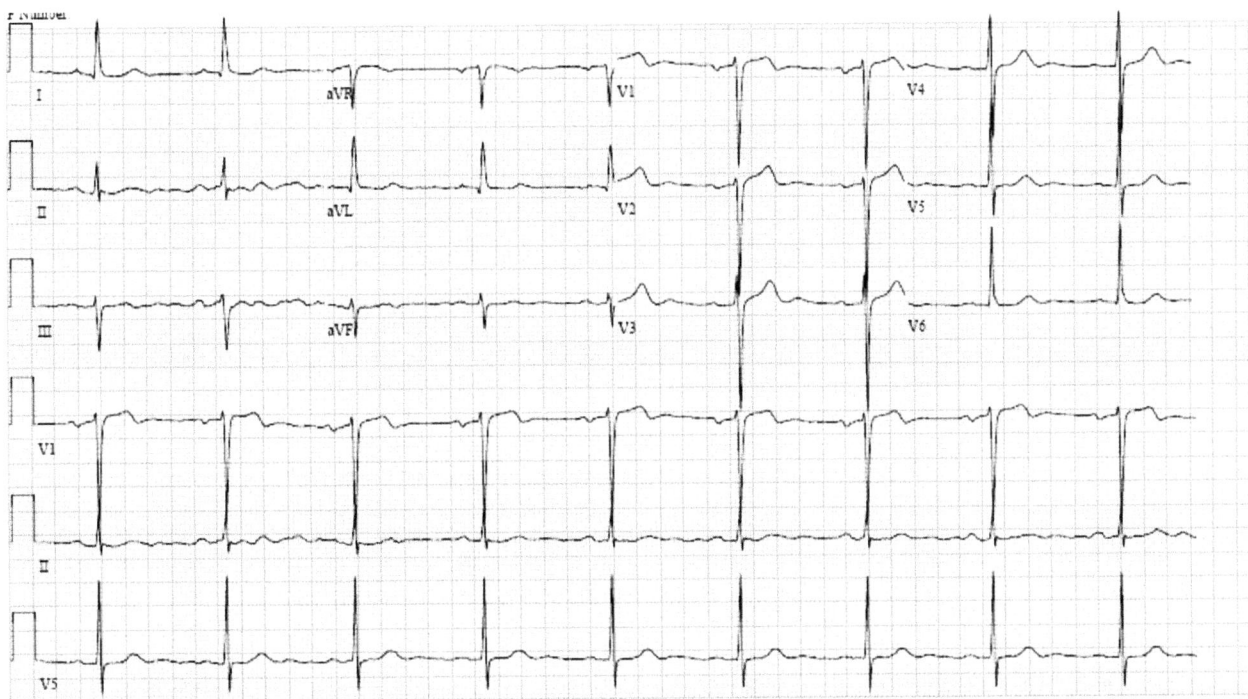

◘ Axis Determination Image 3

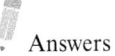
Answers
1. Normal axis
2. RAD
3. LAD

16.2.12 PQRSTU Approach

Let's briefly examine each component of the electrocardiogram tracing (◼ Fig. 16.17):

- P wave: Best visualized in lead II, this represents an atrial impulse causing atrial contraction. Under normal conditions, it is consistently and uniformly generated by the SA node, so the P wave morphology and PR interval remain constant. In pathologies where the integrity of the SA node is not driving the atrial impulses, you may lack a P wave (e.g., atrial fibrillation) or have inconsistent morphologies (e.g., multifocal atrial tachycardia).
- PR Interval: This represents the conduction of electrical impulses through the AV node which acts as a brake and filter. The normal PR interval is <200 msec, and dysfunction such as first-degree AV block will prolong the PR segment.
- QRS Complex: This is a term for the time from the beginning of the Q wave to the end of the S wave, typically less than 100 msec. 100–120 msec is intermediate, and > 120 msec is prolonged. The duration of the QRS complex clues you in on whether a rhythm is atrial (narrow) or ventricular (wide). A narrow complex is the norm; a wide QRS clues you into some form of ventricular dysfunction, either in the conduction system or the presence of a ventricular arrhythmia.
- ST Segment: This is the portion from the *end* of the S wave (QRS) to the *beginning* of the T wave (end to end) representing depolarized ventricles. You will be most interested in the ST segment in cases of suspected myocardial ischemia. ST depression or elevation means that the ST segment is located below or above the J point and TP interval. The ST segment can have one of three shapes:

Pearl: A wide complex tachycardia may represent a supraventricular arrhythmia with aberrancy (refer to ▶ Sect. 16.7).

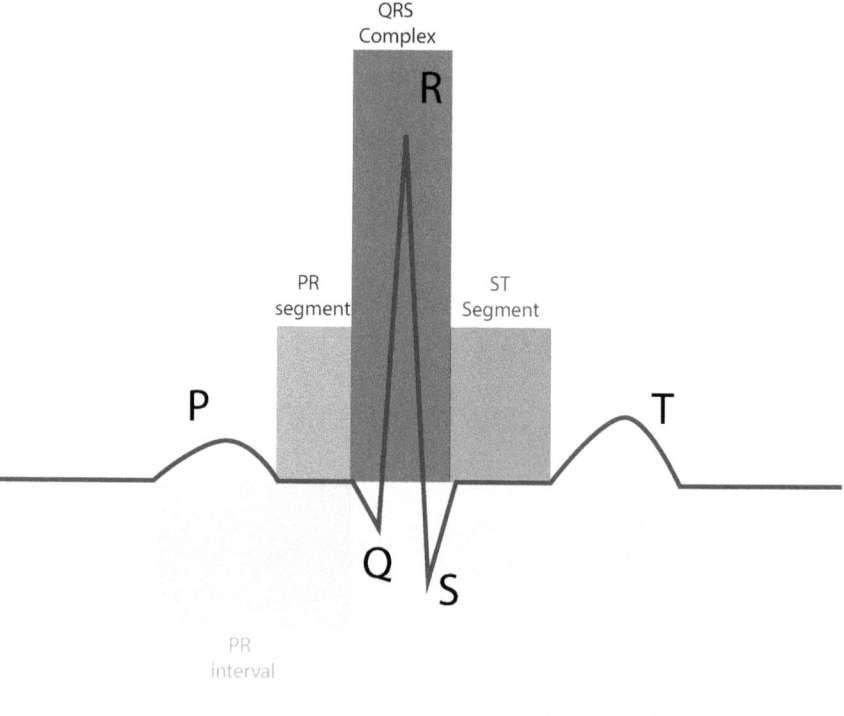

◼ Fig. 16.17 EKG waveform components

- – Up-sloping: Often referred to as a "happy" concavity, this is usually a benign finding such as in benign early repolarization or acute pericarditis.
- – Down-sloping: Sometimes referred to as resembling a "tomb-stone" or "frown," this is concerning for myocardial ischemia.
- – Straight/flat: This is also concerning for myocardial ischemia.
- J point: This is located at the start of the ST segment. It is usually visually distinct from the ST elevation or depression that you will observe; thus, the degree of elevation or depression is measured relative to the J point.
- QT Interval: This represents ventricular contraction and repolarization, typically less than 440 msec (longer in females) but clinically tolerated up to 500 msec. QT interval varies by heart rate (shorter with more rapid rates), so you will often see a QT interval that is corrected for heart rate, or QTc. This is affected by various medications such as antipsychotics, antibiotics, methadone, and even Zofran. When initiating such medications, particularly in patients with cardiac history, always obtain an EKG.
- T wave: This represents ventricular repolarization and is normally asymmetric with the second half demonstrating a steeper downward slope. It may be involved in the early stages of myocardial ischemia. Inverted T waves may be a sign of cardiac ischemia, and peaked T waves may indicate hyperkalemia.
- U wave: This represents late hyperpolarization of the myocardium. It is somewhat useful when present, as it may indicate most commonly hypokalemia.

Pearl: U waves are best visualized in V2–V4.

High-Yield: Draw out the EKG tracing a few times, annotating it with the various components. Think of what each component represents physiologically. This will greatly help develop your familiarity and comfort with reading and interpreting EKGs.

Pearl: Confused trying to remember where these intervals and segments start of end? "Intervals" include waves, whereas "segments" never include waves.

16.2.13 Common EKG Findings

Now we will perform a high-yield review of the most common EKG findings you will encounter.

16.2.13.1 Sinus Arrhythmia

This is an occasional finding that may confuse you if you haven't seen it before. Sinus arrhythmia results from changes in vagal tone that slightly varies the rate, similar to as if you were performing a carotid massage to slow down the heart rate. The R-R interval varies in a regularly irregular pattern consistent with breathing cycles (◼ Fig. 16.18). This is the only regularly irregular pattern you will likely encounter and should be considered pathognomonic for sinus arrhythmia.

16.2.13.2 Non-ST Segment Elevation Myocardial Infarction (N/STEMI)

These are among the most common findings you will encounter. Be sure to use the J point as the reference for determining elevation or depression (◼ Fig. 16.19). Refer to the ACS section for specific NSTEMI/STEMI criteria.

Two common mimics of STEMI that you should always consider are benign early repolarization (BER) and pericarditis. NSTEMI, on the other hand, does not have such convincing mimics:

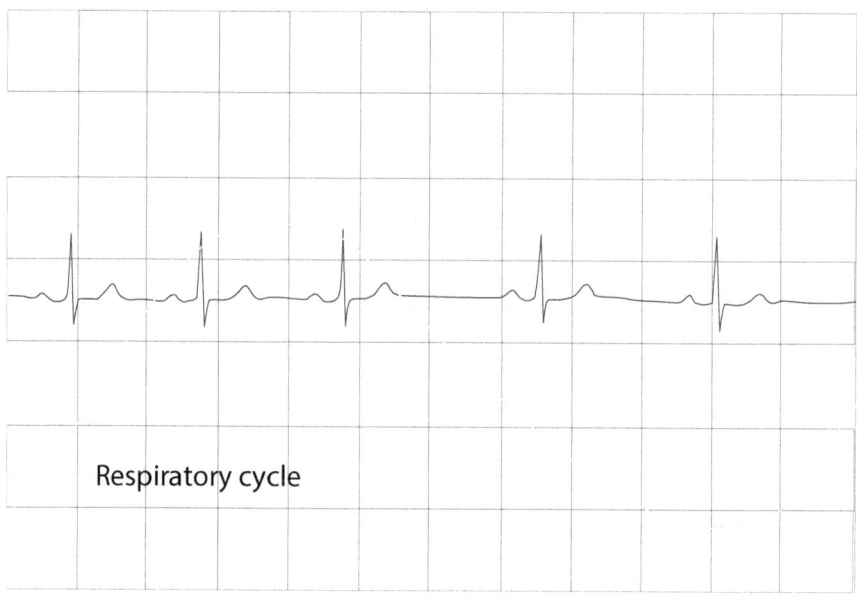

Fig. 16.18 Sinus arrhythmia EKG with overlaid respiratory cycle

- BER: This is a benign variation that occurs mostly in the inferolateral leads in younger men. There are two key differences from STEMI:
  - Lack of reciprocal changes.
  - Concavity is typically up (positive/smile).
- Pericarditis: The ST elevations are diffuse and present in almost every lead except for aVR. If someone had a true MI of this magnitude, they would be dead as that would mean every main coronary is acutely occluded – it is no wonder that this doesn't happen. You can also check for PR segment depressions which are present in pericarditis.

16.2.13.3 T Wave Inversions (TWI)

A negative (downward) T wave is known as a T wave inversion (◻ Fig. 16.20). These can be normal, and the trick is to identify when T wave inversions may suggest pathology, which, for your rotation, will primarily be suggestive of myocardial ischemia, particularly when in the distribution of a coronary territory. Notably, T wave inversions related to ACS are typically symmetric (remember T waves are normally asymmetric, particularly in males, with the latter portion of the wave encompassing a steeper downward slope, ◻ Fig. 16.17). Lastly, deeply inverted T waves are also suggestive of pathology.

Normally, most T waves stand upright (positive). Thus, you should remember which leads contain normal T wave inversions so that you may begin to identify the abnormal presence of TWIs.

Pearl: Wellens syndrome is the finding of large, deeply inverted or biphasic T waves in V2/3 and is very specific for a high-grade proximal LAD stenosis.

Pearl: TWI in lead III, which are normal, is a common consult question.

Normally upright:	Normally inverted:	Variable (nonspecific):
I		
II	aVR	
V3–6	III	aVF
aVL		V1/2

Normal

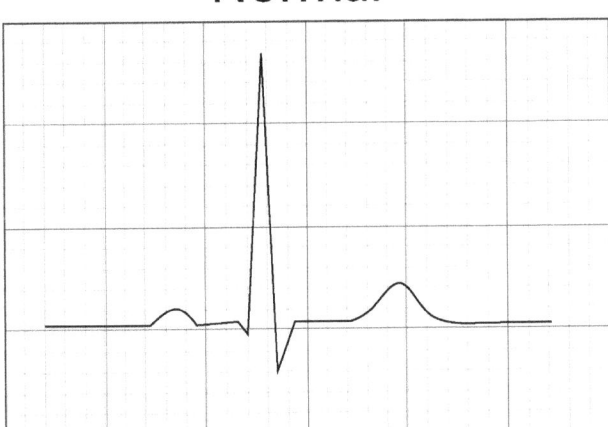

ST Depression

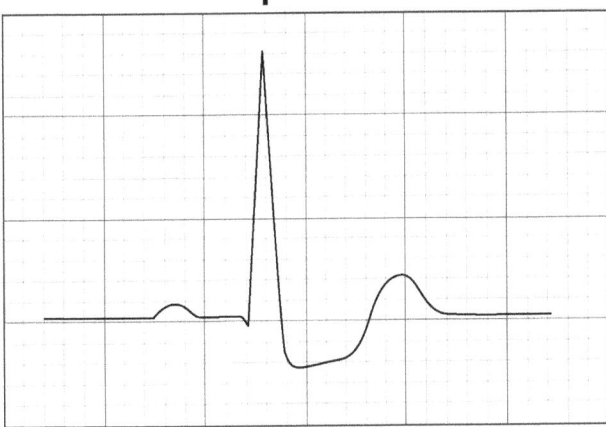

ST Elevation

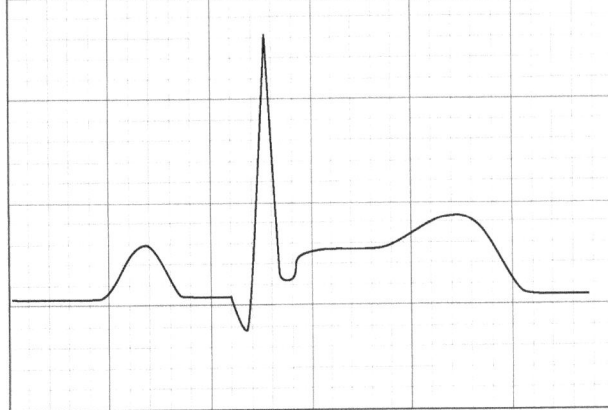

◘ Fig. 16.19 ST depression and elevation

Confusing, right? An easy way to approach TWIs is by thinking of when you should worry that a TWI is pathologic. Simply stated, you should suspect pathology when TWIs are (a) in leads I/II/V3–V6 and (b) in a coronary distribution.

NORMAL

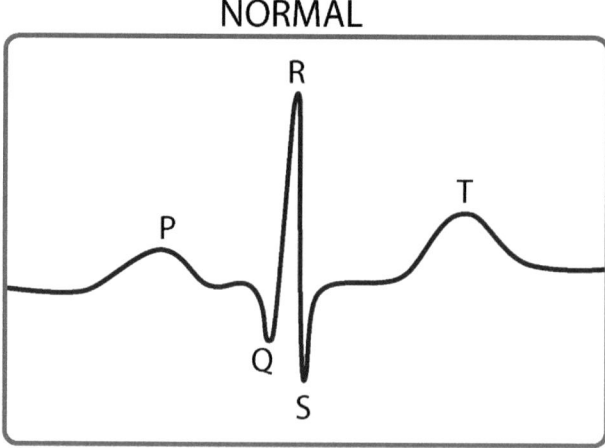

INVERSION

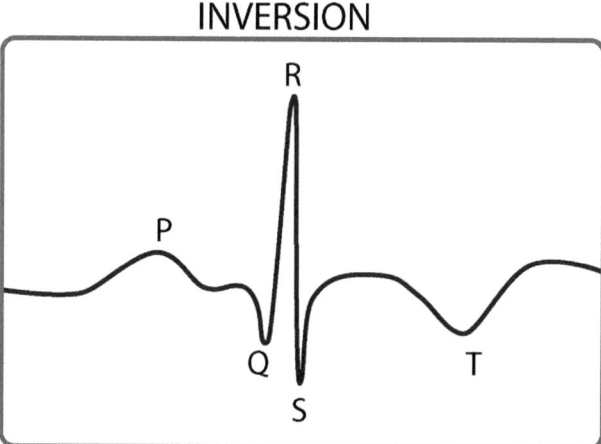

◘ Fig. 16.20 T wave inversion

■ **Flash Quiz**

What is suggested if aVR has an upright T wave? This suggests that the lead placement was mixed up since it should be always inverted.

16.2.13.4 Nonspecific T Wave Changes

This phrase refers to slight alterations in the morphology of a T wave that is not specific for any condition(s). Even drinking a hot or cold beverage can transiently induce these changes. Hence, you should primarily watch for T wave inversions, symmetric T waves, and peaking of T waves (associated with hyperkalemia).

16.2.13.5 Atrioventricular (AV) Blocks

As we learned earlier, the AV node is a rate-dependent brake whose goal is to allow appropriate and well-timed electrical activity to reach the ventricles. Disease of the AV node itself or the His bundle system is known as AV block. There are four distinct types (◘ Fig. 16.21, management is not covered here):

- *First-degree block:* This is a conduction delay (rather than a true block) that results most often from increased vagal tone (e.g. young, athlete, pain) or fibrosis (old). The PR interval is constantly prolonged (>200 msec), but the QRS remains narrow.

First degree heart block

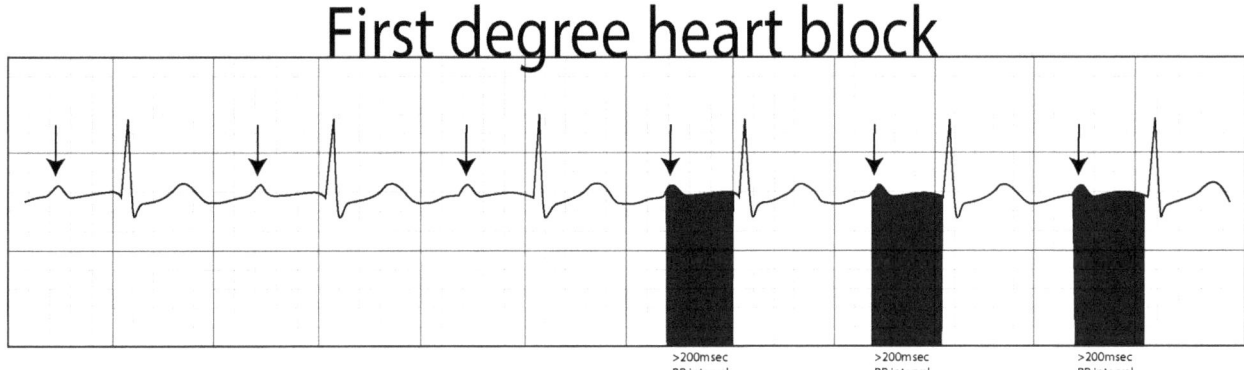

>200msec
PR interval >200msec
PR interval >200msec
PR interval

Second degree heart block, type I

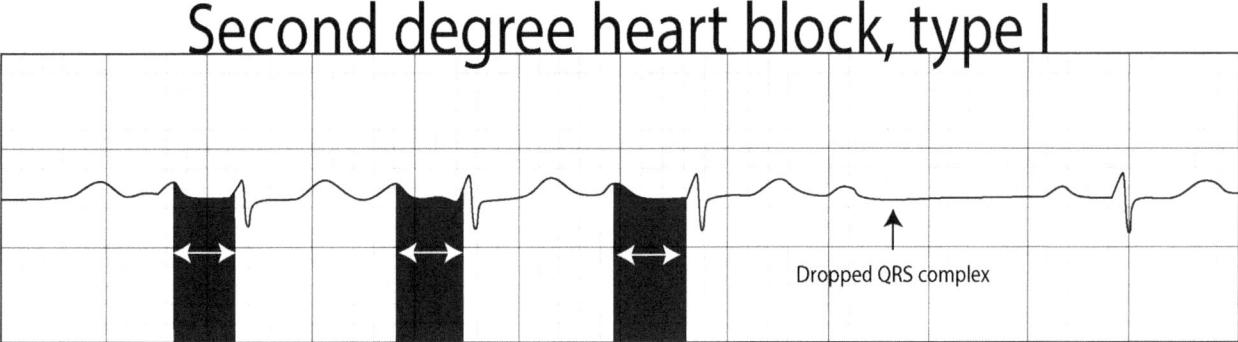

Dropped QRS complex

Progressive prolongantion of PR interval

Second degree heart block, type II

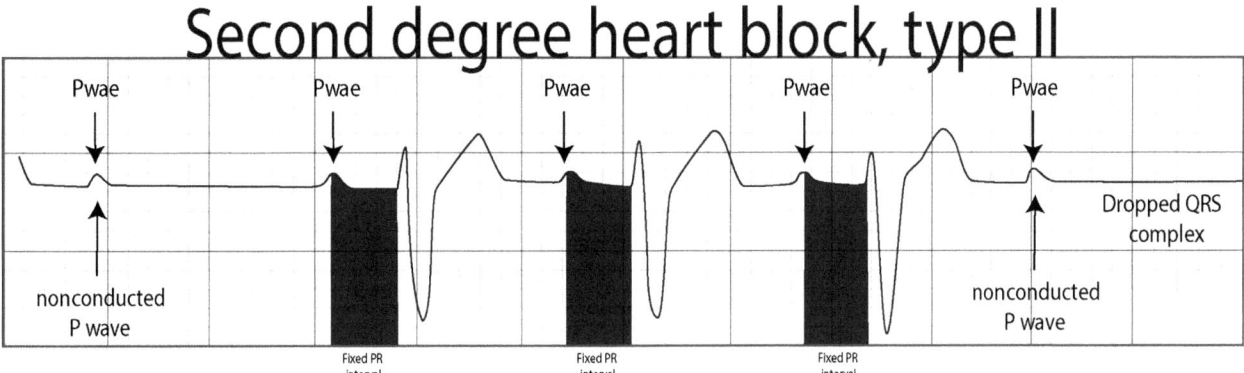

Pwae   Pwae   Pwae   Pwae   Pwae

Dropped QRS complex

nonconducted
P wave

Fixed PR
interval   Fixed PR
interval   Fixed PR
interval

nonconducted
P wave

Third degree heart block

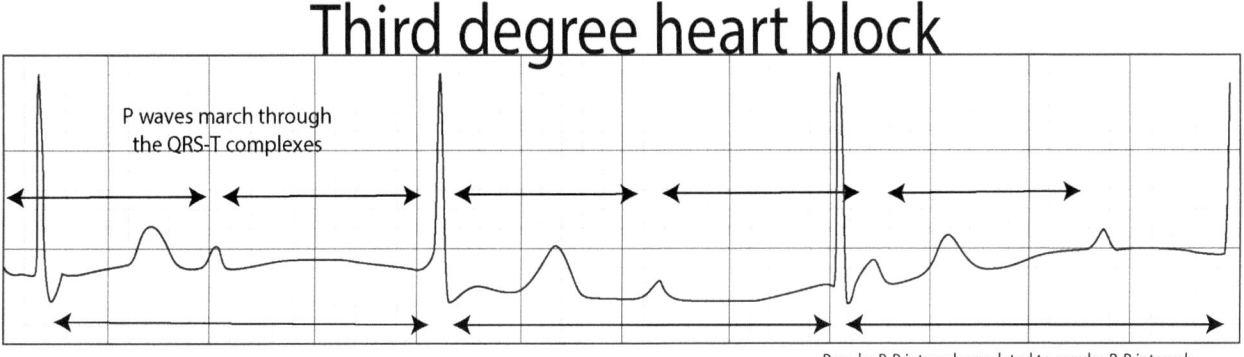

P waves march through
the QRS-T complexes

Regular P-P intervals unrelated to regular R-R intervals

◻ **Fig. 16.21 Atrioventricular blocks EKG**

Pearl: You should note the P to QRS ratios. Higher ratios signify more severe AV block. It is not possible to differentiate Mobitz Type 1 vs Type 2 when in a 2:1 pattern.

- *Second-degree block:*
  - Mobitz Type 1 (Wenckebach): This is the more common and benign type of second-degree block that occurs at the AV node. This presents as a PR interval that progressively lengthens until a QRS complex is dropped. You should also look for constant P-P intervals with shortening RR intervals, a pattern that may result in the appearance of heartbeats in a grouped fashion.
  - Mobitz Type 2 (Hay): This occurs below the AV node in the His bundle and is best remembered as a non-conducted P wave (no following QRS). Think "Hey (Hay)! Where'd the QRS go?!". As such, you should look for constant P-P intervals and constant PR intervals with occasional missing QRS complexes. Type 2 blocks are more likely than Type I to progress to third-degree block and require a pacemaker.
- *Third-degree block (complete heart block):* This is complete dissociation between the atria and ventricles where atrial impulses are not transmitted to the ventricles and the ventricles beat based on their own spontaneous ventricular impulses known as an escape rhythm. The P-P and R-R intervals will remain constant, but there will be no relationship between the P waves and QRS complexes.

16.2.13.6 Bundle Branch Blocks (BBB)

The His bundle divides into a right and left bundle branch, with the left ventricle depolarizing slightly before the right ventricle. With disease, these bundle branches lose their ability to effectively transmit electrical impulses, leading to delays (◨ Fig. 16.22). You should suspect a bundle branch block when:

- Wide QRS complex (>120 msec) (since these are ventricular abnormalities).
- Commonly, increased amplitude of QRS component waves (separated vectors no longer cancel).
- Alterations of QRS most prominently in V1–2 and V5–6 (best views of the right and left heart).
- T Wave Disconcordance: T wave deflected opposite direction to the QRS (specifically in V1 or V6).

Pearl: In the presence of a bundle branch block, you would normally expect T wave disconcordance. T wave concordance in lead V6 may indicate ACS in the setting of LBBB.

It's easy to suspect a bundle branch block but perhaps more difficult for you to identify whether right or left-sided. We'll look at the technical criteria first and then a shortcut which I noticed that seems to work every time (though perhaps technically less valid).

Here are the key additional findings for each:
- Right Bundle Branch Block: "Bunny Ears," "MW"
  - V1–2: RSR' composed of an upward, downward, and then upward deflection
  - V5–6: Widened, slurred S wave
  - T wave disconcordance in V1

Pearl: Though the presence of "bunny ears" is the common medical student teaching, you should look for the criteria below since the bunny ears can occasionally mislead you.

RBBB

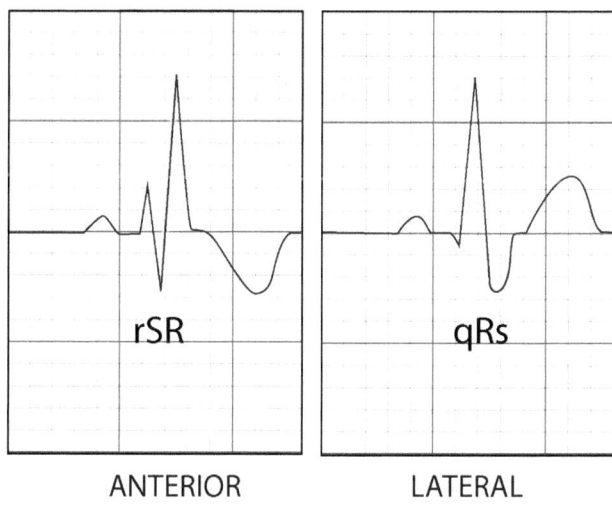

ANTERIOR   LATERAL

LBBB

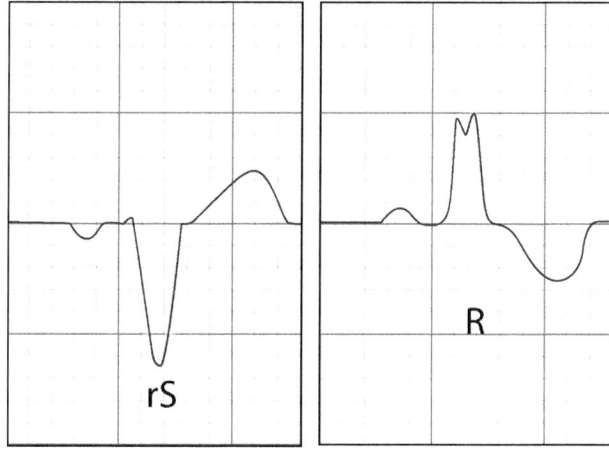

ANTERIOR   LATERAL

◩ Fig. 16.22 Bundle branch blocks EKG

— Left Bundle Branch Block: "[WM]"
  – V1–2: rS Wave – short R followed by side S
  – V5–6: "M"-shaped R wave
  – T wave disconcordance in V6

Shortcut: I term this the rollercoaster method. Simply look at the QRS complexes in V1 and V6 – if you see an M-shape (up-down-up) in V1 and W-shape (down-up-down) in V6, this is a RBBB. The opposite would be true for a LBBB. In order to use this method, pay attention to the occasionally very small subtle initial R waves.

Pearl: Compared to RBBB, the components of the QRS are often less pointy (more rounded).

Pearl: In LBBB morphology, the criteria for detecting STEMIs changes and is known as the Modified Sgarbossa Criteria (you don't have to memorize it and can always look it up, but name-dropping it on rounds will be a very good look).

16.2.13.7 Left Anterior Fascicular Block (LAFB)

The left bundle branch is composed of an anterior and posterior fascicle. Normally, electrical impulses are propagated through both fascicles, but when the anterior fascicle becomes defective (e.g., due to age-related scarring), the impulses travel via the posterior fascicle (■ Fig. 16.23), and depolarization occurs slightly slower, leading to a wider but not necessarily wide QRS. To diagnose a LAFB, you should look for:

- qR complexes: small Q wave with tall R wave in leads I and aVL (lateral leads)
- rS complexes: small R waves with deep S waves in leads II, III, and aVF (inferior leads)

16.2.13.8 Left Atrial Enlargement

The best diagnostic criterion for LA enlargement is a terminal negative P wave in lead V1 that is at least one box wide and one box deep (■ Fig. 16.24). This prominence of the terminal part of the P wave reflects greater LA mass causing the electrical forces to shift posteriorly (remember, LA is the most posterior chamber) and to the left. While board exam resources often emphasize the presence of a "bifid" P wave (P mitrale) in leads II (most prominent) and V1, this is less reliable, and you should always check for the terminal negative P wave in lead V1.

16.2.13.9 Ventricular Hypertrophy

Either ventricle may hypertrophy in response to increased pressures or other rarer physiology such as genetic mutations in sarcomeres. There are many different criteria for hypertrophy, though all have very poor sensitivity. Find one or two that work for you and stick with them. Let's take a look at the most popular:

Pearl: LAFB is one of the few causes of left axis deviation. If you see a left axis deviation, quickly check leads III and aVF. If they have negative QRS complexes, you can quickly diagnose a left anterior fascicular block.

If you're like me, you probably never noticed that there is a small terminal negative portion to the P wave in V1!

LEFT ANTERIOR FASCICULAR BLOCK

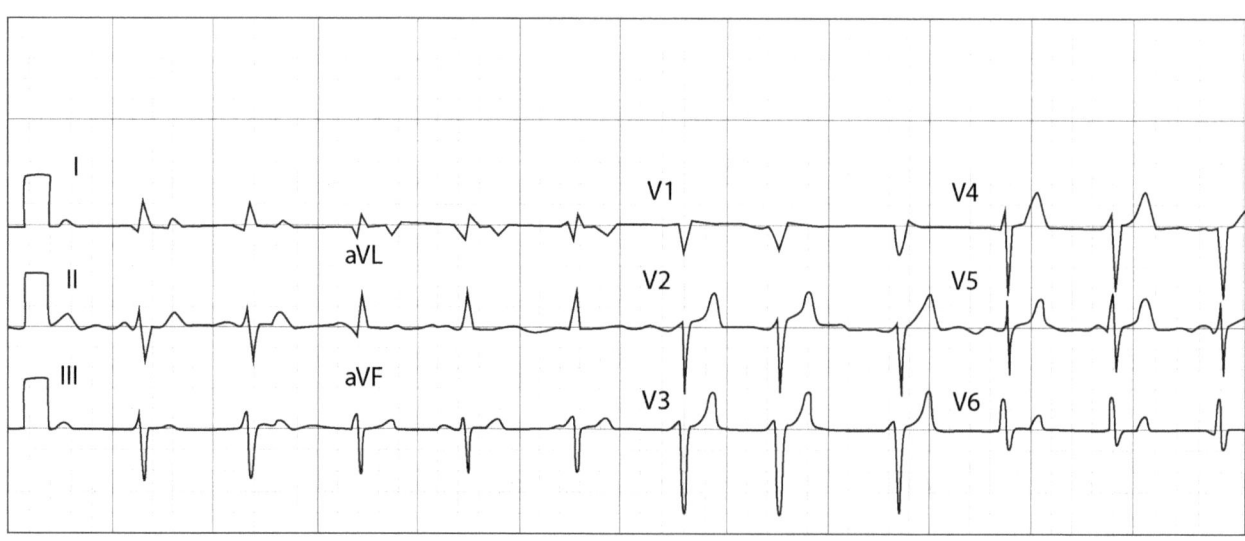

■ Fig. 16.23 Left anterior fascicular block EKG

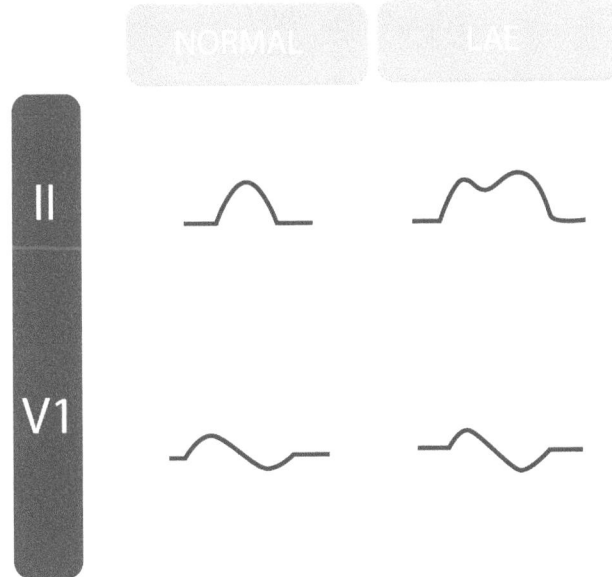

□ Fig. 16.24 Left atrial enlargement EKG

- RVH:
  - [R wave in V1 > 7 mm] OR [R/S Ratio in V1 > 1]
  - With right axis deviation
- LVH:
  - Sokolov-Lyon Criteria:
    - [S wave in V1 + tallest R wave in V5/6] > 35 mm
    - LV strain pattern (ST depression + T wave inversion in lateral leads)
  - Cornell Criteria:
    - [R wave in aVL + S wave in V3] > 28 mm (male) or 20 mm (female)
  - Modified Cornell Criteria:
    - R wave in aVL > 12 mm

16.2.13.10 Atrial and Ventricular Arrhythmias

Here we will focus on keys to identifying these on EKG. These will be described in more detail in the ▶ Sect. 16.7. Atrial rhythms are usually narrow, whereas ventricular rhythms are wide. However, atrial tachycardias may present as a wide complex tachycardia when accompanied by a block (known as aberrancy).

16.2.13.11 Atrial Fibrillation (Afib)

The most common atrial arrhythmia, afib, presents without discernible P waves which indicates that there is no uniform origin of electrical activity coming from the atria. When accompanied by tachycardia, it is known as afib with rapid ventricular rate (RVR). Although the heart is already experiencing poor ventricular filling from incoordination and loss of atrial kick, tachycardia further decreases filling by shortening diastole.

16.2.13.12 Atrial Flutter

Flutter presents in the classic sawtooth pattern (□ Fig. 16.25) due to its reentrant pathophysiology. Typically, flutter will be approximately 150 bpm. The exact block ratio for flutter can be calculated by dividing 300 (the rate at which this rhythm circles around the cavotricuspid isthmus) by the heart rate (e.g., 150 would yield 2:1 flutter).

Atrial Fluter

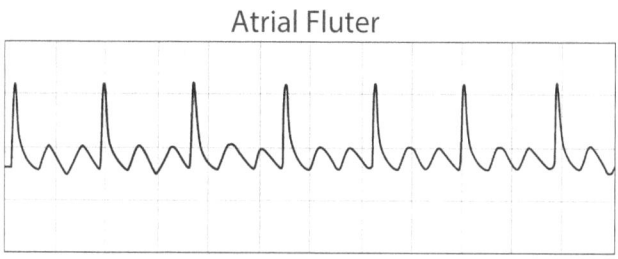

◻ **Fig. 16.25 Atrial flutter EKG**

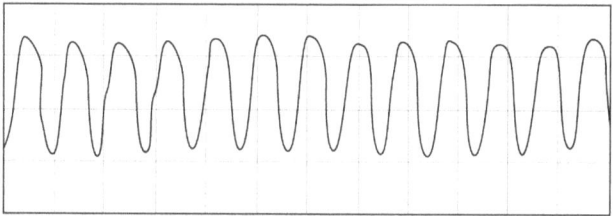

◻ **Fig. 16.26 Monomorphic ventricular tachycardia EKG**

16.2.13.13 Monomorphic Ventricular Tachycardia (Vtach)

To meet the criteria, you will need at least three consecutive wide QRS complexes of the same morphology (◻ Fig. 16.26). When this rhythm persists for greater than 30 seconds, it is referred to as sustained vtach (compared to nonsustained vtach, or NSVT).

16.2.13.14 Premature Atrial/Ventricular Contractions (PAC/PVCs)

As their names suggest, these are extra heart beats that originate from an electrical focus (atrial or ventricular, respectively) other than the sinoatrial node. PVCs are easily recognizable (◻ Fig. 16.27 by their broad QRS of abnormal morphology and premature occurrence.

An occasionally encountered term is *bigeminy*. This simply means that every other heartbeat is a PVC. This can be extended to other patterns such as *trigeminy* for every third beat being a PVC. Lastly a *couplet* simply refers to two back to back PVCs. Using these terms as a medical student can score you some bonus points.

That's a wrap for common EKGs. The key is to see them over and over again, both in isolation and with overlap of various EKG findings. A great resource for EKG practice is Beth Israel Deaconess Hospital's ECG Maven located at ▶ https://ecg.bidmc.harvard.edu/maven/mavenmain.asp.

Pearl: Even though these may seem trivial benign findings, always report exactly what you see on tele!

16.2.14 Telemetry

In the cardiac unit, almost every patient is put on tele. Each morning, you should check the tele strips and print out any notable findings. On the first day of your rotation, you should ask the nurse or intern/resident to show you how to use the tele system. Here's one approach to reviewing the tele:

1. Review the Event Recorder. This is very sensitive and will catch lots of artifact but will likely catch any arrhythmias that the patient experiences.
2. Review the time strip briefly for any abrupt jumps in heart rate that may signal arrhythmia.

Pearl: Motion artifact is very common and presents as a baseline that is shifting up and down.

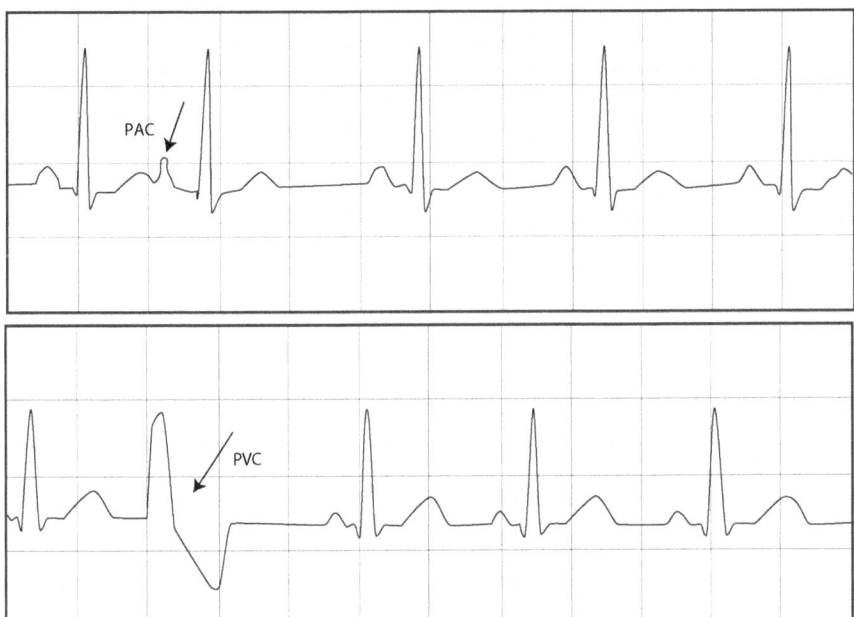

◻ **Fig. 16.27 PAC/PVCs**

Note that telemetry is not sensitive for ST deviations. It is meant for detecting tachy- and bradyarrhythmias. If you suspect ischemia, always obtain a STAT 12-lead EKG.

16.2.15 Pacemakers

This is a topic that often comes up indirectly, and having a basic background can be very helpful. Pacemakers are used to deliver controlled electrical impulses to the heart to restore normal activity and improve heart function. The presence of a pacer will be obvious to you during auscultation as a notable square bump under the skin, most commonly in the left upper corner of the precordium. Each pacer contains a system that will analyze the electrical activity of the heart and only provide electrical impulses during abnormal activity. Pacers contain batteries that typically last 6–7 years but may last as long as 15 years if the pacer isn't used (doesn't fire) much.

The most common pacer indications are as follows:
- Second-degree AV block, type 2
- Complete heart block
- Severe heart failure (EF < 35%)
- Symptomatic bradycardia

You should remember these indications and always be aware of why a patient has a pacer even if they are not coming in for a pacer-related issue, and these indications are also common questions from attendings.

There are several different types of pacemakers (◻ Fig. 16.28):
- Single Chamber: Lead may be placed in either the right atrium (SA node disease) or ventricle (AV node disease).
- Dual Chamber: Leads placed in both the right atrium and ventricle (to synchronize atrial and ventricular activity).

Pearl: Modern pacers are MRI compatible, so always ask your patient as you may be able to obtain MRIs if necessary.

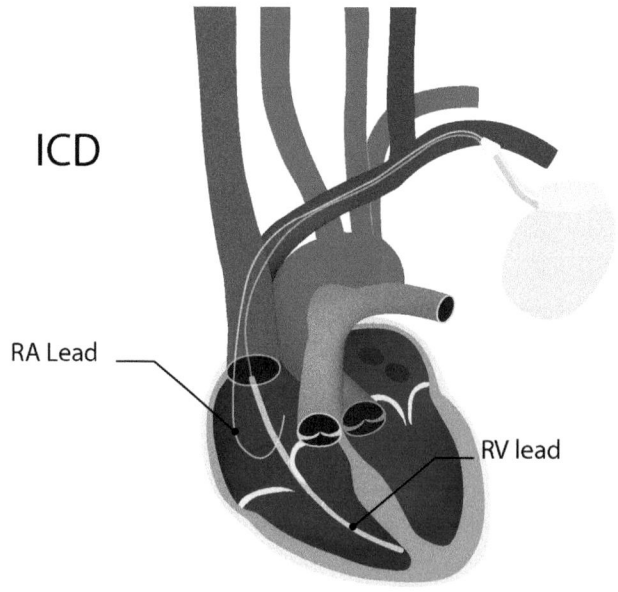

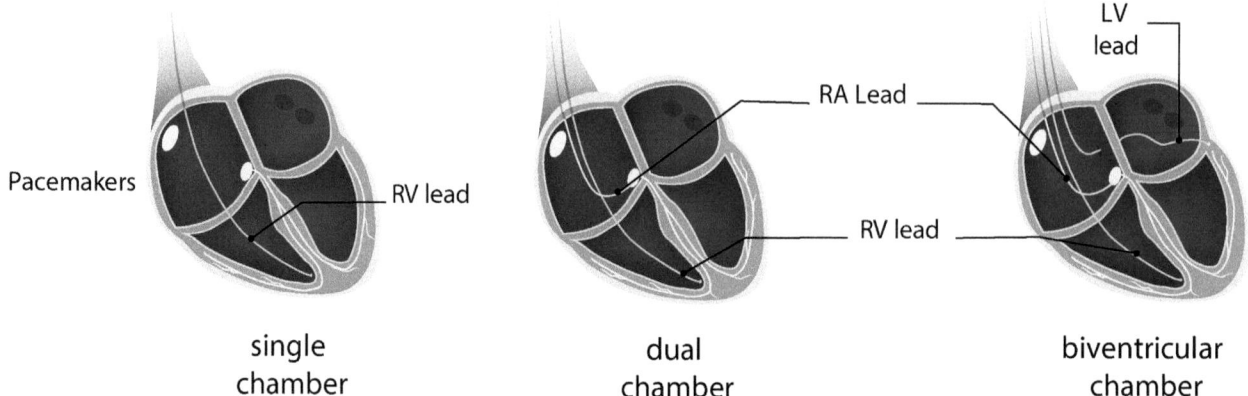

◻ Fig. 16.28 Pacemaker variants

Pearl: ICDs are usually for patients with reduced ejection fractions (<35%) and/or patients at risk for sudden death due to ventricular arrhythmias.

Pearl: Any pacemaker or defibrillator with a lead in the right ventricle can lead to new/worsening tricuspid regurgitation, as the lead needs to traverse the tricuspid valve to enter the ventricle.

– Biventricular: Leads placed in the right atrium as well as both ventricles (severe HFrEF to synchronize all chambers), also known as cardiac resynchronization therapy (CRT).
– Implantable Cardioverter Defibrillator (ICD): Lead placed in the right ventricle (for defibrillation of dangerous rhythms such as ventricular tachycardia/fibrillation).

Take a quick look at these EKGs for a patient with a pacer (◻ Fig. 16.29). Those small vertical "spikes" are a result of the pacer electrical discharges! As you have probably deduced, the location of the vertical spikes clue you in to the type of pacemaker in the patient (◻ Table 16.2).

You may hear the terms "sensed" and "paced" used to describe a patient's EKG. These refer to whether the native heart or the pacemaker is driving the electrical activity of the heart. If there is a pacer spike, it means the heart is "paced," whereas the absence of a pacer spike means the native heart's electrical activity is "sensed" and driving the EKG. For example, the atrial pacer

Atrial Pacer

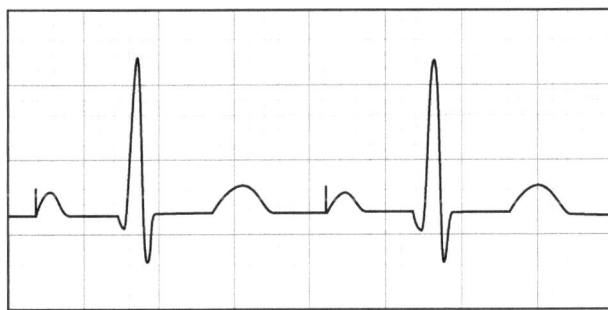

Ventricular Pacer

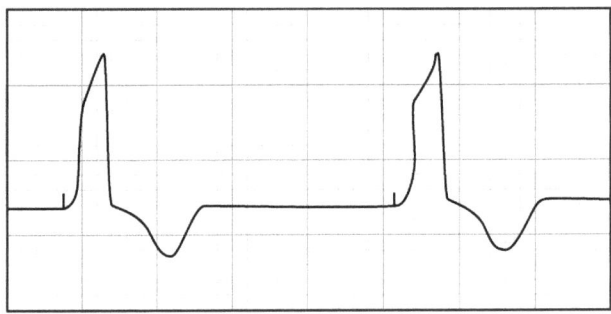

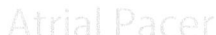 **Fig. 16.29** Pacer spikes on EKG

Table 16.2 EKG clues to pacemaker type

Location	Type
Prior to P wave	Single chamber (Lead in the atrium)
Prior to QRS complex	Single chamber (Lead in the ventricle)
Prior to P and QRS	Dual chamber

EKG in ◻ Fig. 16.29 would be called "A-paced, V-sensed." As you can imagine, there are four possible combinations. Simply put, if you see a pacer spike, the subsequent P wave (representing the atria) and QRS complex (the ventricles) are "paced"; else, they are "sensed".

16.2.16 Echo

Let's briefly compare and contrast the two main types of echocardiography: transthoracic echo (TTE) and transesophageal echo (TEE).

TTE is the easiest to obtain due to its noninvasive nature. Clinically, if a TEE is obtained, a TTE is almost always done first. TTE and TEE should not be thought of as superior or inferior but rather complementary based on the anatomy that each can best visualize (◻ Table 16.3).

Pearl: Remember that the RV is the most anterior chamber, whereas the left atrium is the most posterior.

☐ Table 16.3 TTE versus TEE

TTE	TEE
Better for anterior[a] structures	Better for posterior[b] structures
Low quality if lots of precordial mass (fat, muscle)	Invasive
For native valves	Better for clots, vegetations, and prosthetic valves

[a]Anterior = tricuspid, pulmonic valve, RA, RV
[b]Posterior = mitral valve, aortic valve, left atrial appendage, LA, LV

Lastly, you should be familiar with the main views (☐ Figs. 16.30 and 16.31) on TTE (and less so TEE) so that you can follow along during review of these images. Correlations of some common TTE views with the coronaries are shown in ☐ Fig. 16.32.

16.3 Practical Tips

In this section, we will cover many of the practical and logistical things you will encounter on the rotation. Overall, the cardiology rotation is very similar to the internal medicine clerkship. If you are on the consult cardiology service, your experience will be like being on a consult service for another medical specialty.

16.3.1 Pre-Rounding

This is quite similar to the medicine rotation, so refer to the ▶ Chaps. 6 and 4. This will be the same whether on an inpatient service or consults. For the cardiology rotation, here are a few differences:

- All patients will be on tele. Thus, you should be examining the tele for every patient since after you left the hospital the night before. When examining the tele, print the tele strip(s) of any oddities whether you can identify the abnormality or not. Learn how to identify motion artifact, as you do not need to print these. Check with the patient regarding whether they noticed anything happen around the time of the abnormality. This should all be brought up on rounds.
- As with other rotations, you should be getting overnight events directly from the overnight nurse. The ins/outs are particularly important to obtain accurately in many cardiac patients, and the nurses may not have updated the electronic records.
- Examine any new labs. Perform "electrolyte rounds" where you look specifically at the electrolytes, and identify whether anything needs repletion.

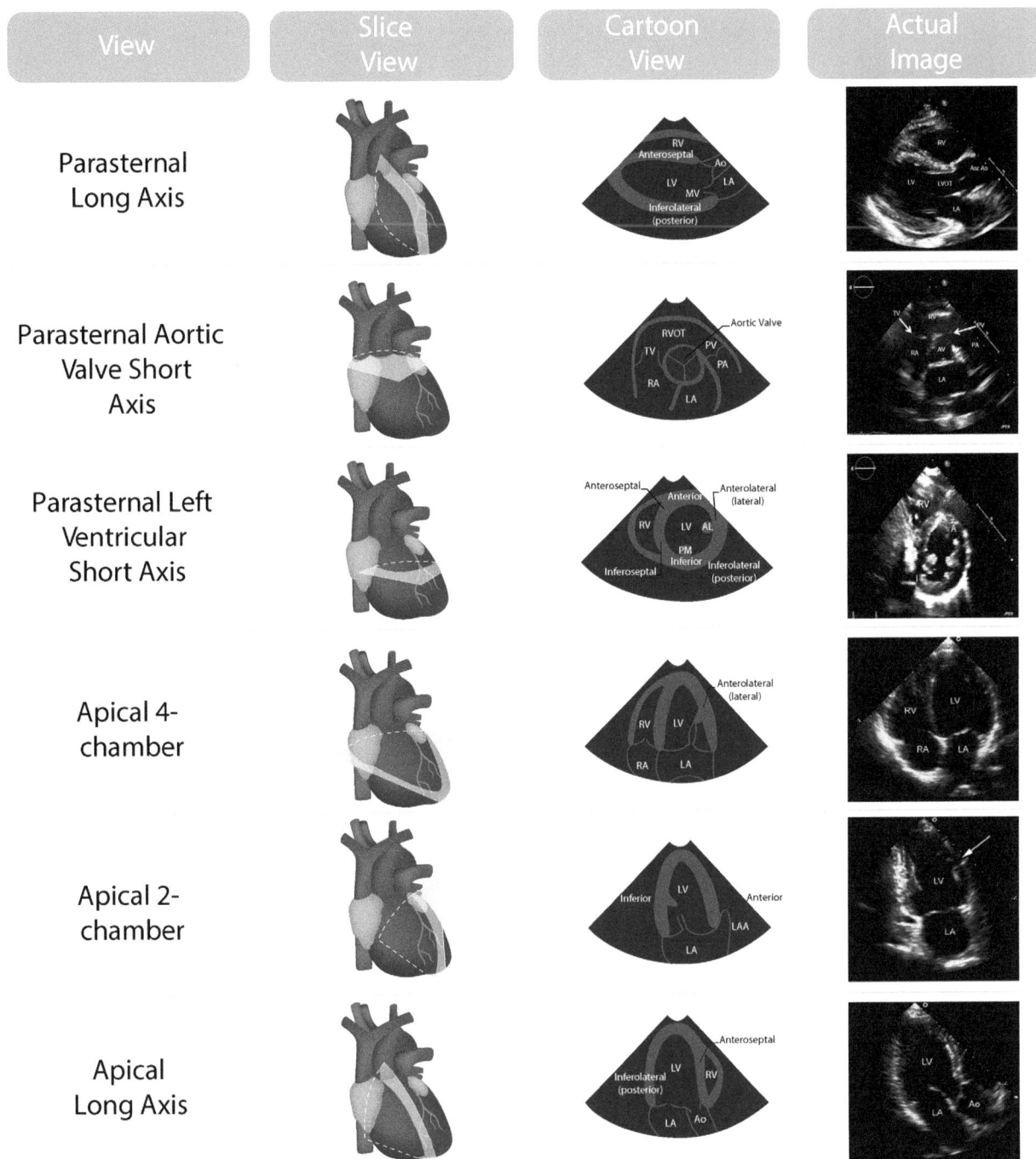

Fig. 16.30 Main TTE views. Echo images (para long, AV short, LV short) courtesy of Maus TM, Nhieu S, Herway ST, editors. *Essential echocardiography*. **Springer Nature. 2016.** ▶ https://doi.org/10.1007/978-3-319-34124-8. Echocardiography in the CCU. Springer Nature ▶ https://doi.org/10.1007/978-3-319-90278-4. Echo images (Apical 4-chamber, Apical 2-Chamber, Apical Long) courtesy of Nihoyannopoulos P, Kisslo J, editors. *Echocardiography*. Springer Nature. 2009. ▶ https://doi.org/10.1007/978-1-84882-293-1

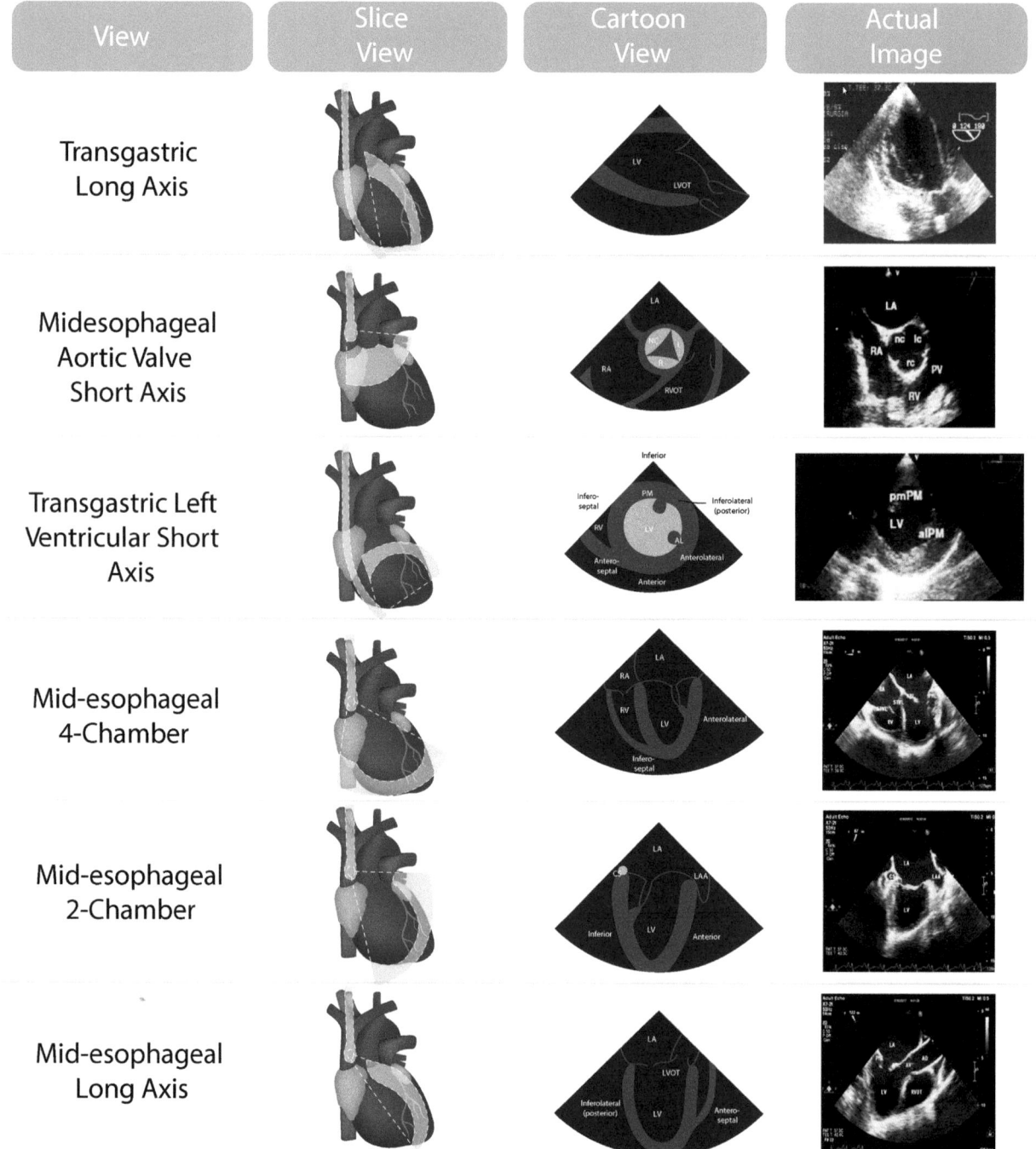

□ **Fig. 16.31 Main TEE views.** Echo images (TG long, ME AV short, TG short) courtesy of Sarti A, Lorini FL, ediotrs. *Textbook of echocardiography for intensivists and emergency physicians.* **Springer Nature. 2019.** ► https://doi.org/10.1007/978-3-319-99891-6. Echo images (ME 4-chamber, ME 2-chamber, ME Long) courtesy of Sadeghpour A, Alizadehasl A, editors. Case-based textbook of echocardiography. Springer Nature. 2018. ► https://doi.org/10.1007/978-3-319-67691-3

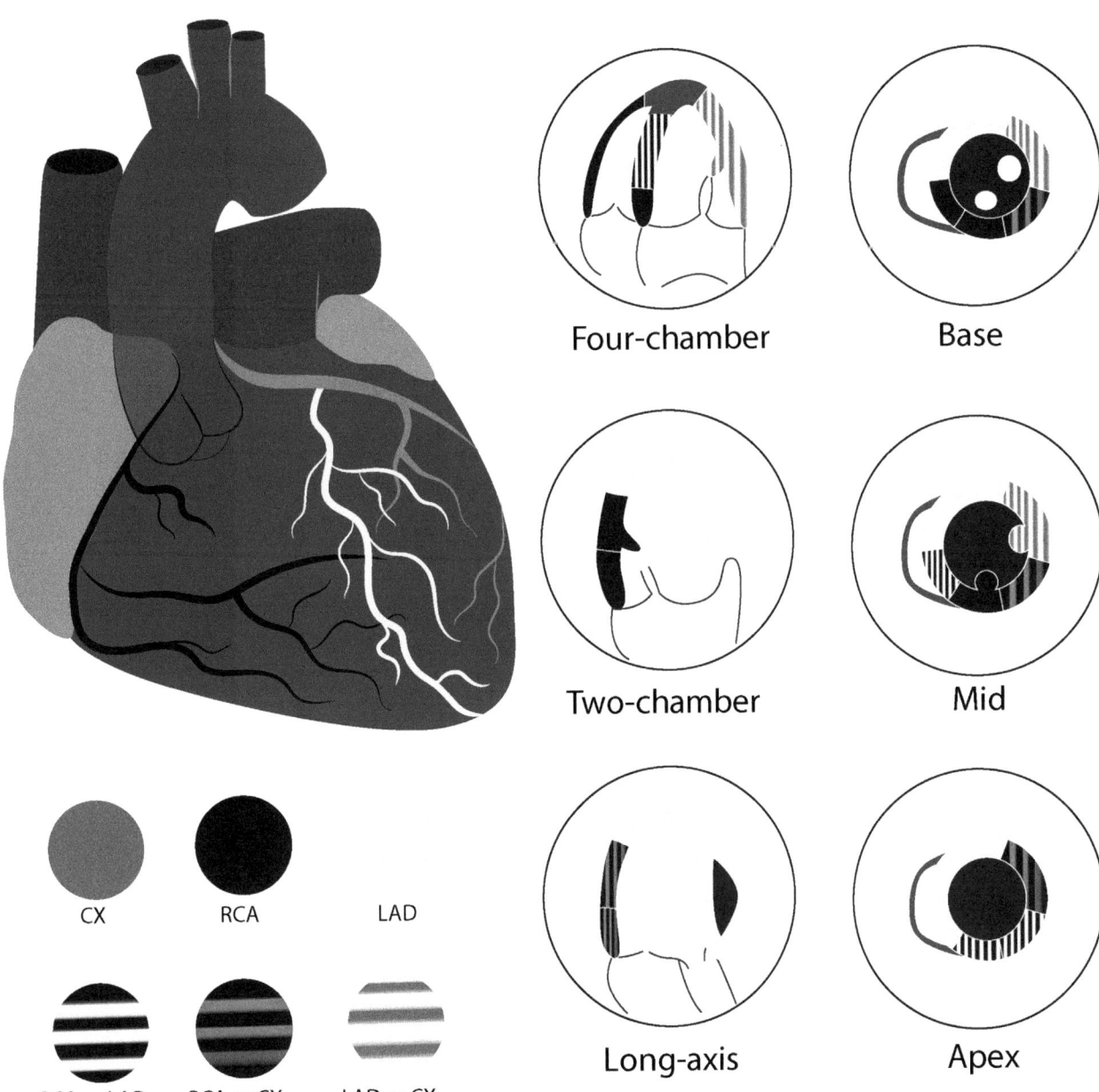

Four-chamber

Base

Two-chamber

Mid

Long-axis

Apex

CX

RCA

LAD

RCA or LAD

RCA or CX

LAD or CX

◻ **Fig. 16.32 Common TTE views correlated with coronaries**

— Read all new notes since you left. Often, consult notes are filed late after you have left the hospital.

— Have a sense for what the patient's day looks like – are they going down for an echo in the morning? Dialysis in the afternoon? These details are very helpful to the team as they will not waste time going to an empty room. As a consultant, it is still important to know the big-picture plan and direction for the patient.

When seeing your patient, your focus should, of course, be on how they are doing in relation to the previous day.

16.3.2 Rounds

The style of rounds will be attending and institution dependent. However, in my experience consult services typically table-round prior to seeing the patients, whereas for inpatient services walk around and discuss patients in the hallway prior to seeing them. Here are some additional pointers:

- Cardiac issues are among the scariest issues for patients. It will be critical to explain everything to them in layman terms.
- Rounds are filled with learning. You learn so much even from patients you are not taking care of. Be inquisitive (ask questions) and jot down all the pearls you learn in a section of your notebook. Asking questions about patients, especially those that are not your responsibility, shows interest and will help you stand out in the eyes of your attendings.
- Find the nurse for each patient so they can join rounds. This is best done as the team is walking towards the next patient's room. It is super helpful to hear directly from them!
- Always update your task list as tasks are delineated to you. You *will* forget something otherwise.

16.3.3 Cardiology-Specific Oral Presentations

Pearl: Always be familiar with the most recent cardiac tests, regardless of whether done inpatient or outpatient, specifically TTE/TEE, stress tests, and LHC.

Much of the oral presentation will be similar to the medicine oral presentation. A sample order for the inpatient service is presented below, with bolding indicating differences from the typical medicine presentation.

New Patients	Follow-Up Patients
HPI	Overnight events
ED course	**Telemetry**
Events since arrival to floor	Subjective
Past history with focus on cardiac	**Active cardiac meds**
All medications.	Vitals/exam (volume status!)
Patient's cardiac anatomy.	Objective data (incl EKG)
Vitals/exam	Plan*
Objective data	Include consultant's thoughts if relevant.
Plan*	

*Cardiology is a very evidence-based field. Try your best to back up your plans with landmark trials. Teams love when you know why you're doing what you're doing!

16.3.4 Tasks

As a consultant, you typically only recommend orders, but this may be institution dependent. On the general inpatient service, a few notable differences are summarized in the task list below (run through it for each patient). Furthermore, if time allows, try to follow your patient to their cardiology-specific interventions (e.g., cath lab, echo, etc.). This will really help paint a better picture of what each subspecialty wants and how to work with them, as well as new learning opportunities.

16.3.4.1 Tasks to Consider

- [ ] Place consults.
- [ ] Review consultant notes.
- [ ] Social work/physical therapy/occupational therapy/nutrition involvement.
- [ ] Email PCP/cardiologist regarding patient's admission.
- [ ] Update healthcare proxy/family.
- [ ] Obtain outside hospital (OSH) records, if applicable.
- [ ] Schedule outpatient follow-up appointments as necessary.
- [ ] If diuresing, check afternoon I/Os with nurse.
- [ ] If diuretic dose changed, consider obtaining afternoon electrolyte check.
- [ ] Late afternoon: Check tele for anything since morning.
- [ ] Later afternoon: Quick check-in with patient and update them with what's going on or planned.
- [ ] Input daily lab orders for tomorrow.
- [ ] Finish notes and sign to resident/attending.
- [ ] Run the list with resident prior to handoff/sign-out.
- [ ] Check with team on any other ways you can help.

16.3.5 Admissions/Consults

For new admissions or consults, use the checklist below to ensure that you don't miss anything when working up a patient. ALWAYS confirm code status.

Prior to Seeing a Patient

Current Admission Data

[ ] Vitals	Prior Admission Data
[ ] EKG	[ ] Old discharge summaries
[ ] Labs +- prior baseline labs	[ ] Old cardiologist notes
[ ] Imaging	[ ] Old PCP notes
[ ] ED notes/handoff	[ ] Prior cardiac tests: TTE, LHC/RHC, stress test
[ ] Create problem list	[ ] Old imaging
[ ] Admit orders, add-on labs	
While Seeing a Patient	*After Seeing a Patient*
[ ] Medications.	[ ] Update ddx.
[ ] Allergies.	[ ] Create plan.
[ ] Code status.	[ ] Run plan by resident.
[ ] Health care proxy.	[ ] Present to attending.
[ ] Summarize history.	[ ] Finish Task List

16.3.6 Sign-Out

The sign-out in Cardiology is very similar to that for General Medicine. Make sure to provide contingencies as things can change especially quick in cardiology!

16.3.7 Discharges

As the patient heals and is getting close to discharge, you should start working on the following:
- [ ] Prep discharge summary.
- [ ] Ensure patient has supply of appropriate medications, including back on home meds.
- [ ] Explain hospital course and future directions to patient in lay person terms.
- [ ] Discharge patient.

Pearl: This is very important! Quite often are patients left on different formulations, such as metoprolol tartrate rather than metoprolol succinate. Check the medications list!

16.4 Approach to Cardiac Disease

Now that we've gathered a solid foundation, let's think about how to think about cardiac disease. Having a framework like this will be particularly useful when you come across pathologies you have not encountered previously.

Whether you're dealing with heart failure, arrhythmias, acute coronary syndrome, or valvular disease, the ultimate question in cardiology becomes "Is the heart pumping blood forwards effectively?" and if not, "How do we help it pump well, now and for the future)?". To answer this question, there are three components which we call the *MEA* system worth thinking about systematically each time you have a cardiac case:
1. *M*echanics
2. *E*lectrical activity
3. *A*daptability (ability to react to stress)

16.4.1 Mechanics

The mechanics of the heart are a well-coordinated act such as ballet dancing – disruption of even the smallest part can have major consequences. Thinking about the key mechanics involved in the forward pumping of blood helps us generate a differential for why the heart may not be pumping effectively. The key mechanics of a heart are as follows:
1. Diastole
2. Systole
3. Valvular function

16.4.1.1 Diastole

Pearl: Rather than memorizing the different etiologies of diastolic impairment, think about how the basic biology (e.g., fibrosis) might lead to increased stiffness.

During diastole, the heart relaxes to accommodate the incoming blood (preload) as does a water balloon. Much like a stiff water balloon, failure of the heart to relax means that there is little blood in the chambers to be pumped forwards, regardless of how good the pumping function. Common conditions that can lead to impaired diastole include heart failure with preserved ejection fraction (HFpEF; you may also see HFpEF referred to as diastolic dysfunction, an older term that is gradually been replaced with HFpEF.), tamponade, and constrictive pericarditis. What these conditions all have in common is something (e.g., hypertrophy, fibrosis, calcification, fluid in the pericardial sac) that you can easily imagine would prevent the LV from filling completely.

Preload dependence refers to a state where the heart's ability to pump enough blood forwards depends on the presence of a threshold volume of blood in the ventricle (the preload). HFpEF as well as other constrictive and obstructive physiologies can all lead to preload dependence. It is critical to factor this into your everyday management, such as when diuresing (attempt a gentler regimen).

16.4.1.2 Systole

All heart chambers must squeeze blood forwards to make way for new venous return. Think about the contraction of a heart as the squeezing of your fist. Impaired contractility is, in the simplest sense, due to impairment in the ability of sarcomeres to contract (i.e., the curling of our fingers to make a fist). When you see a cardiac pathology, always ask yourself whether the pathophysiology leads to an impairment in sarcomere function and therefore in contractility. For example, ischemia to a region of the heart can lead to impairment, as would cardiac remodeling leading to impaired contractility via addition of sarcomeres in series (heart failure with reduced ejection fraction).

For our purposes, there are two primary mechanisms underlying a contraction problem: dilation or scarring (fibrosis after death) of the myocardium. As you might imagine in a rubber band that has been stretched too much, a dilated chamber is unable to pump (contract) effectively. With scarring, there will be reduced or absent movement of portions of a chamber wall, referred to as a wall motion abnormality (WMA). You should consider systolic dysfunction with history or suspicion for an ischemic event (e.g., MI) or a significantly dilated chamber.

16.4.1.3 Valvular Function

Valves are the doors between the different rooms of the heart. Pathology of the valves will typically involve either dysfunctional opening (stenosis) or closing (regurgitation/prolapse). Stenosis of a valve typically occurs due to calcification or fibrosis (imagine a door with glue dumped over the hinges) (◘ Fig. 16.33), though rarer etiologies such as a cardiac tumor can obstruct the outflow

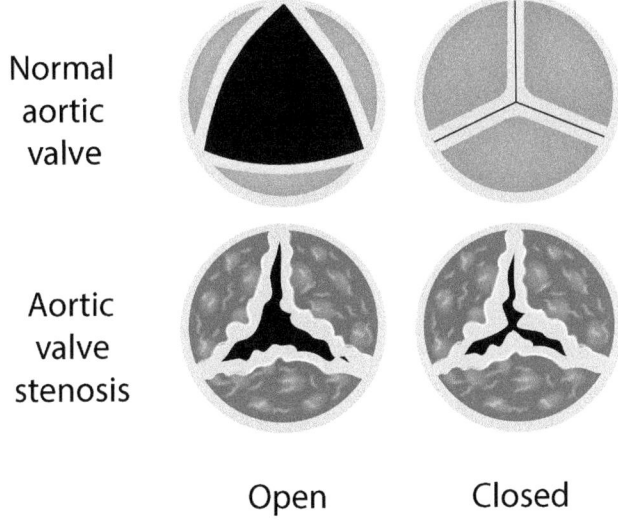

Normal aortic valve

Aortic valve stenosis

Open   Closed

◘ **Fig. 16.33 Valvular stenosis**

of blood. With stenosis, the heart must pump harder to push blood forwards through the stiff doors and can result in several effects including remodeling (e.g., dilated atria and/or ventricles) that participate in a vicious cycle of depressing pump failure.

Regurgitation usually occurs due to improper alignment of the valve leaflets like misaligned doors in a doorframe. Misalignment can result from dilation of where the leaflets are attached called the annulus (using a doorframe too large for the doors), myxomatous degeneration (a misleading term which refers to thickening or elongation of part of the leaflet/door), or from alteration in the positioning of the leaflets (malpositioned hinges). Perforation of a valve, though rare to see as a medical student, can obviously result in regurgitation. Regurgitation decreases forward blood flow by allowing for a backward leak of blood and can also lead to chamber dilation due to higher filling volumes which contributes to pump failure.

16.4.2 Electrical Activity

The electrical activity of a heart is the essence of life. Its fidelity is directly related to the pumping function of the heart. For each case that you encounter, consider (1) the birth of appropriate electrical signals and (2) faithful conduction of those signals through the heart.

16.4.2.1 Electrical Signal Origin

Under normal physiology, electrical signals are born in the SA node. Common alternate sources (known as ectopic foci) include the pulmonary veins and random foci in the atria, AV node, and ventricles. You can determine the rough location of origination by examining the width of the QRS complex – narrow for anywhere above the AV node and wide for below the AV node. You may also check for the presence of a P wave which indicates that the electrical source is in the atria and the morphology of the P waves for consistency (multiple morphologies suggest several foci).

16.4.2.2 Transmission Integrity

Electrical impulses undergo a checkpoint at the atrioventricular (AV) node. This is a way for the heart to protect its star players, the ventricles. Remember that the heart fills with blood during diastole and that the faster a heart beats, the less time there is for blood to fill the heart chambers. Thus, the AV node has a cyclical refractory period to prevent the ventricles from beating too fast. This is very important in conditions such as atrial fibrillation where your atria may be beating at extremely high rates (e.g., 300 bpm) – you would be dead if all those signals made it to the ventricle. Occasionally, accessory pathways exist for the signals to reach the ventricles while bypassing the AV node – this results in the famous Wolf-Parkinson-White syndrome. On the other hand, if the AV node becomes diseased (e.g., fibrotic), it may not transmit signals well to the ventricles – this results in AV blocks.

Pacemaker cells are found throughout the conduction system; in fact there are pacemaker cells in the AV node, which spontaneously depolarize at a rate of 40–60 beats per minute. In healthy individuals, these signals are suppressed by the more rapid impulses arising from the atria. However, if no (or minimal) signals reach the AV node, it can start to fire on its own, leading to what is called a junctional escape rhythm. These rhythms can be appreciated on EKG tracings and are characterized by a rate of 40–60 bpm, narrow QRS complexes, and absence of P waves or any other atrial activity.

16.4.3 Reacting to Stress

The heart has can be thought of as being in binary states: rest or stress. While at rest, the demands of the heart are at their lowest, and many patients (even those with quite sick hearts) may appear asymptomatic despite a significant fraction of heart's maximal potential being tapped. Under conditions of stress (e.g., exercise, infection, pregnancy), the body requires increased oxygen (which is directly linked to energy output). The amount of oxygen delivery can be increased by increasing the cardiac output, defined as

$$CO = \text{stroke volume} \times \text{heart rate}$$

The two variables refer simply to how strong or fast the heart can contract, respectively. In cardiology, the extent to which these factors can be increased is referred to as contractile and chronotropic reserves.

Many patients may not have outright impairment in electrical activity or mechanical function but have subclinical impairment that is only brought out by stress. There are a variety of causes for impaired cardiac reserves, including heart failure and medications such as beta-blockers. If the patient's symptoms worsen with increased stress/demand (e.g., exercise), consider examining their cardiac reserves and any modifiable factors (e.g., beta-blocker dose).

Now let's put this framework into action for a rare case you may see. Imagine you have a 65-year-old female with no significant past medical history who comes in with florid heart failure symptoms. You are unable to figure out exactly what caused the heart failure, but on imaging there is diffuse fibrosis of her pericardium. Using our MEA system, we should think the following, even if we have no idea of the diagnosis:

- Mechanics: Seeing pericardial fibrosis, think of constrictive physiology that may be impairing the patient's diastolic function. This makes sense as to why she is in heart failure – the blood has difficulty entering the ventricles despite its good pumping function. To check out the diastolic, systolic, and valvular function further, obtain a TTE. There are no obvious abnormalities with systolic or valvular function but clear evidence of constrictive physiology. In regard to management, despite the lack of a final diagnosis, utilize this information by diuresing more gently given her preload dependence.
- Electrics: The patient's EKG appears normal without evidence of sinoatrial or AV nodal disease.
- Adaptability: The patient's heart rate is tachycardic to the low 100 s, indicating that the chronotropic reserve isn't severely impaired. This may be compensatory tachycardia for the constrictive physiology. The stroke volume is difficult to interpret given the physiology at play.

If you're wondering, this is a typical presentation of TB constrictive pericarditis. Even if you had no idea to suspect this, using the MEA system, we have much of the information to initially manage the patient while we build a differential.

To recap, always quickly run through the three major components (mechanics, electrical activity, ability to react to stress) of heart function for each patient (there can be more than one involved!). This not only provides you with great practice for understanding the heart but also helps prevent missing key aspects of patient care.

16.5 Acute Coronary Syndrome

Let's begin by breaking down the term acute coronary syndrome. We can see that the term refers to a *sudden* alteration in the ability of the *coronary* vessels to deliver blood effectively to the heart. Each time you are confronted with a potential case of ACS; it is worth considering the underlying mechanism. There are several key mechanisms that can lead to this sudden decrease in blood flow:

1. Plaque rupture: Atherosclerotic plaques rupture and can either transiently or permanently obstruct blood flow.
2. Embolism: A blood clot from elsewhere in the body travels and lodges in a coronary vessel.
3. Vasospasm: The smooth muscles lining the coronary arteries can contract abnormally, leading to diminished blood flow.

We define ACS along a spectrum that mirrors the natural course of atherosclerotic plaques (☐ Fig. 16.34). As you can see below, ACS is an evolution beginning with stable angina and evolving towards STEMI.

Stable angina reflects a fixed stenosis of the coronary that leads to decreased blood flow that becomes clinically significant (appearance of symptoms) when a supply-demand mismatch occurs (i.e., exercise increasing oxygen/blood demand but flow being limited by the atherosclerotic lesion). Traditionally, 70% is used to estimate the degree of stenosis at which angina begins presenting. *Unstable angina* is similar but results from an unfixed (disrupted) plaque that can vary the degree of obstruction; consequently, symptoms may appear at rest when there is no obvious reason for a supply-demand mismatch. *Non-ST-elevation myocardial infarction (NSTEMI)* is further on the spectrum of unstable angina and is distinguished from unstable angina by subendocardial (partial thickness) myocardial damage resulting in troponin leak. *ST-elevation myocardial infarction (STEMI)* is the furthest evolution of ACS and represents complete blockage of blood flow to a region of the heart, leading to transmural (full thickness) damage with elevated troponin and ST elevations.

Pearl: An absent history of CAD and cardiovascular risk factors does not rule out ACS.

Remember: Since the coronary arteries are on the outside of the myocardium, blood supply from the heart goes from the outside to the inside. Therefore, partial thickness ischemia will start at the inner myocardium and work its way outward with subsequent decreases in blood flow.

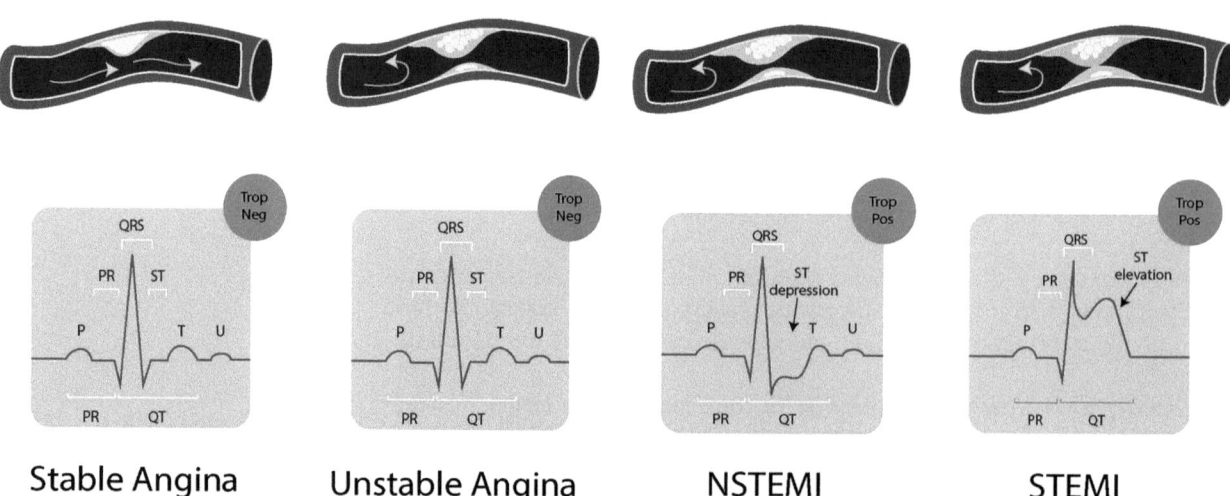

Stable Angina   Unstable Angina   NSTEMI   STEMI

☐ **Fig. 16.34** Natural history of plaques versus spectrum of ACS. ST elevations must be ≥ 1 mm in two contiguous leads (men) and ≥ 1.5 mm (women) for leads V2/V3. ST depressions must be a minimum of 0.5 mm in two contiguous leads. T wave inversions must be greater than 1 mm in two contiguous leads

16.5.1 Differentiating the Differential

These are the primary alternate diagnoses on your differential for ACS when consulted and also for when presenting your patient to your team. Keep in mind the key differentiating factors below during your workup. However, for ACS consult, the ultimate question is really "Is there evidence of ACS?". Alternate diagnoses are typically less urgent and can be dealt with later:

- Musculoskeletal: This pain is usually focal and reproducible with movement or palpation. It differs from ACS pain/pressure in that it changes with position/palpation.
- Aortic Dissection: Most commonly found in elderly smokers (and surprisingly less common in diabetics), blood pressures may be unequal in the upper extremities, and the patient often has significant back pain. CXR demonstrates a widened mediastinum.
- Myocarditis: Nonspecific, but often with heart failure symptoms. Often history of trigger such as recent viral upper respiratory infection.
- Pulmonary Embolism: The patient is tachypnic with shallow breathing. There is also most often no trop leak or EKG changes though possible in larger PEs.

ACS is the primary concern to rule out in patients who present with chest pain or pressure, but be mindful that not all chest pain/pressure is ACS. Your job is to determine the risk of ACS with a quick but thorough workup. However, even before you begin your workup, your mind should be rapidly assessing the pretest probability for ACS:

16.5.2 Chart Review

If the patient has been in your hospital system before, you should always perform a quick but thorough chart review prior to seeing the patient. This should take no longer than 5 minutes initially, but you should spend more time performing a more thorough review as time allows later. As a medical student, you will not be performing a STEMI consult as the primary provider, so taking the time to do this is fine.

16.5.2.1 Chart Review Checklist
- [ ] Review cardiac history
  - [ ] Most recent cardiologist clinic note
  - [ ] Most recent cardiac admission discharge summary
  - [ ] Cardiovascular risk factors: diabetes, HTN, HLD, smoking, recent cocaine, male, age
  - [ ] Family cardiac history
- [ ] Confirm cardiac anatomy (per cath reports or other notes)
  - [ ] Location and degree of blockages
  - [ ] Past interventions
  - [ ] Most recent ejection fraction (look at last echo)
- [ ] Review baseline EKG

Note: We will not include ddx such as pneumonia as it is less likely that you will be consulted for ACS if this was the cause. Rather, we will include the key ddx that are most frequently presented in a student's oral presentation.

Pearl: Always check the blood pressures in both arms during an ACS consult. Though rare, you will catch these.

Pearl: An ascending aortic dissection may cause ACS if a dissection flap extends proximally enough, occluding most commonly the RCA.

Pearl: Always consider the possibility of an atypical ACS presentation. Three factors are strongly associated with greater atypical presentation:
Female biological sex
Increased age (think >80)
Diabetes

Pearl: There are many errors copied and pasted in the modern electronic record that get perpetuated when a more thorough review is not taken. This is an excellent place for medical students to contribute and shine.

Pearl: Prior ACS predicts a high likelihood of recurrent ACS.

16.5.3 History

You should first characterize symptoms into typical, atypical, or noncardiac chest pain/pressure (◉ Fig. 16.35), as this influences the pretest probability of ACS and governs urgency and next steps. Be sure to elicit the time course, setting in which the symptoms first occurred, and review of systems to rule out common mimics (refer to ▶ Sect. 16.6.3). If the patient has had a prior MI with recent stenting, confirm their medication compliance. Though other symptoms such as shortness of breath, nausea/vomiting, and diaphoresis support ACS, the most important history questions are trying to categorize the patient's angina.

> Pearl: Noncompliance with dual antiplatelet therapy is the most common reason within 12 months for restenosis in recently placed stents.

16.5.4 Examination

Though the exam is not particularly specific for diagnosing ACS itself, it is critical to ruling out alternate etiologies of chest pain. It is also very useful in assessing for complications, such as papillary muscle rupture. Heart sounds and JVD are two particularly key elements.

Vital Signs: You are mainly interested in the heart rate and rhythm. Is the heart rate tachycardic? If so, this is something you can consider controlling with a beta-blocker to reduce the cardiac oxygen demand. Is the rhythm sinus or baseline (if patient has a chronic arrhythmia)? You should also confirm that the blood pressure is stable.

> Pearl: The most common cause of death within 24 hours of MI is ventricular arrhythmias.

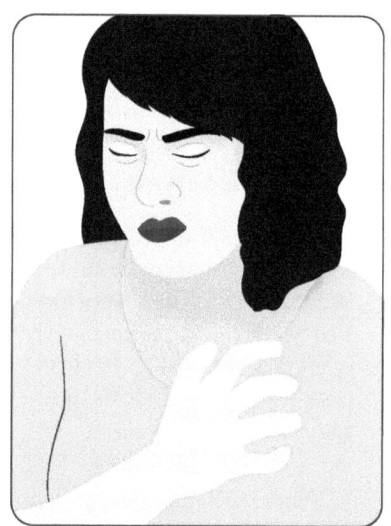

Substernal chest discomfort
with characteristic
quality and duration

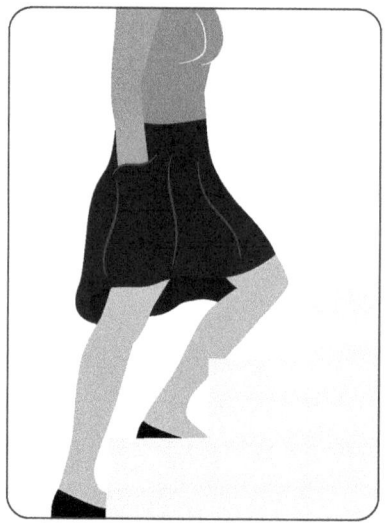

Provoked by exertion
or emotional stress

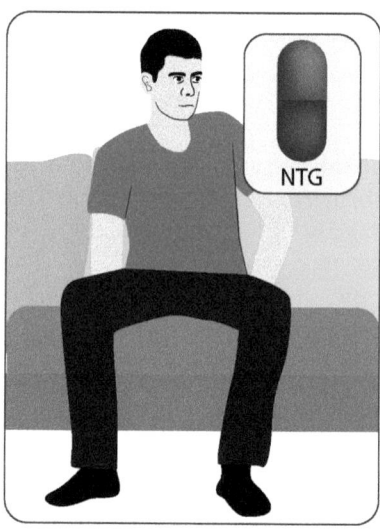

Relieved by rest or NTG

Typical (3/3)
Atypical (2/3)
Noncardiac (1 or none)

◉ Fig. 16.35 Angina classifications

Heart Sounds: Listen carefully for murmurs, particularly new murmurs in the mitral region. The posteromedial papillary muscle supporting the mitral valve is the most common to rupture due to a single blood supply originating off the PDA; thus most often RCA occlusion may lead to rupture although possible with LCx occlusion. Compared to a typical mitral regurgitation murmur (a high-pitched holosystolic murmur), mitral regurgitation due to papillary rupture can be a mid to late systolic murmur. Note, a severe rupture leading to severe acute mitral regurgitation may not produce an audible murmur as there is almost instantaneous equalization of pressure on both sides of the valve throughout the cardiac cycle.

JVP: A newly elevated JVD in the setting of MI signals most commonly heart failure secondary to RV infarction. This is a finding that warrants immediate notification of your team and new echo of the heart.

Precordial Exam: If concern for chest pain of MSK origin, visualize the precordium for signs of trauma. Palpate in the region of pain to assess for reproducible and/or exacerbated chest pain.

16.5.4.1 ACS Physical Exam Checklist

- [ ] Vitals – HR, BP in both arms
- [ ] New heart sounds?
- [ ] JVP
- [ ] Precordial MSK exam, if applicable

16.5.5 Initial Management

We will not delve deeply into the initial management of ACS here as this will be done reflexively by the ED team whenever a patient with chest pain presents, regardless of ACS risk. However, there are a few key points to learn:

- Confirm with the ED team and patient whether they received a full-dose aspirin and/or clopidogrel/ticagrelor.
- Confirm that heparin (unfractionated) was started.
- Troponins begin rising within 4 hours (high-sensitivity troponin T assays rise within 1–3 hours), peak with 12–24 hours, and remain elevated for 7 days.
- Serial EKGs until ACS ruled in or out.

On serial EKGs, one finding you may come across is poor R wave progression. Normally, the R wave height should increase as you go from lead V1 to V6 (◻ Fig. 16.36) – under ischemia, this pattern may be interrupted. Please refer to the ▶ Sect. 16.2.11 in Fundamentals for an overview of EKGs concerning for N/STEMI.

Pearl: All patients with NSTEMI receive DAPT. However, if the patient may receive CABG, clopidogrel should NOT be given as it increases bleeding too much, and cardiothoracic surgery may refuse to take the patient for CABG for several days.

16.5.6 Goals of Admission (Management)

Once you've determined that the patient is likely experiencing ACS, here are the key goals of effective ACS management which should be reflected in your presentation. Keep these in mind at all times:

- [ ] Determine the extent of coronary blockage
- [ ] Revascularize
- [ ] Post-MI heart remodeling prevention
- [ ] Secondary prevention

Pearl: Indications for CABG
- Three-vessel disease (>70% stenosis)
- Severe left main stenosis (>50%)
- In diabetics, two-vessel disease

R-wave Progression

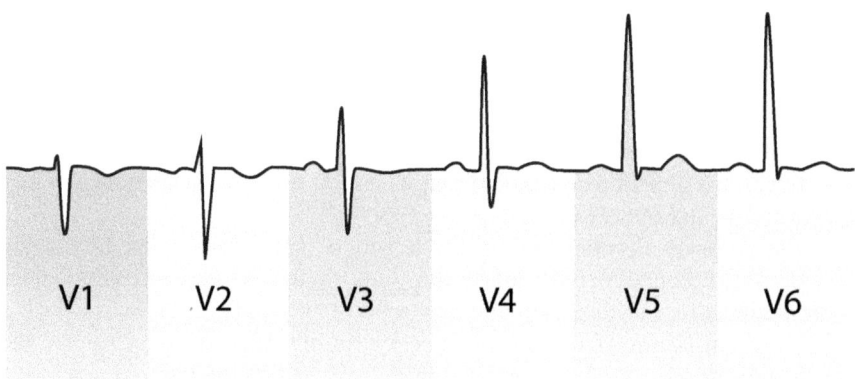

⬛ Fig. 16.36 Normal R wave progression

16.5.6.1 Risk Stratification for Early Invasive Therapy

In STEMI, patients should undergo cardiac catheterization within 90 minutes of arriving at the hospital (door-to-balloon time). However, you may wonder why there is not the same sense of urgency with unstable angina/NSTEMI which may wait up to 48 hours. This is because trials such as TIMACS (NEJM 2009) demonstrated that early invasive therapy (door to cath lab in <24 hours) had no mortality and vascular event benefits if the patient was not high-risk, defined as GRACE score > 140 (TIMI equivalent 5–7). Ask your resident which scoring system is used at your institution, and use MDCalc to quickly calculate it prior to presenting your patient. This score should be included in the assessment and plan.

16.5.6.2 Determination of Coronary Blockage

The primary way to determine the location and degree of coronary blockage is by cardiac catheterization and coronary angiography. Most commonly performed either through the radial or femoral artery, it is a routine and low-risk procedure often pursued diagnostically even when the diagnosis of ACS is less certain. Cath allows for not only determining coronary blockage but also potential simultaneous revascularization.

16.5.6.3 Revascularization

There are a variety of ways to revascularize an obstructed coronary. The most common approach is by using a balloon to open up the lesion and then adding a drug-eluting stent (DES) to keep the artery open. Most stents placed today will be drug-eluting, meaning that a drug such as everolimus or zotarolimus will elute off the drug to reduce rates of restenosis. With DES, patients must be on dual antiplatelet therapy (DAPT; aspirin + clopidogrel) for at least 12 months. Noncompliance with DAPT is the most common cause of stent thrombosis within a year.

Note: Not uncommonly, patients with ACS will have a comorbidity (most commonly afib) that calls for baseline anticoagulation. You will run into the question of whether to continue anticoagulation on top of DAPT (referred to as triple therapy) despite an increased bleeding risk. Many trials have attempted to shed light on this. The WOEST trial (Lancet 2013) demonstrated that anticoagulation plus only clopidogrel resulted in significantly decreased bleeding

> Pearl: Coronary angio will involve the use of contrast dye, so be sure to consider the patient's renal function prior to ordering a cath!

compared to triple therapy, without an increase in thrombosis rates. The ISAR-TRIPLE trial (JACC 2015) saw no benefit in thrombosis rate reduction with 6 months of triple therapy compared to 6 weeks. Given these data, there is provider and institutional variation in how long the average bleeding-risk patient on anticoagulation is on triple therapy. What is important for you is to understand this increased bleeding risk balanced with the risk of stent thrombosis and to bring up this dilemma to your team of how long the patient merits triple therapy. A safe suggestion is for 1 month of initial triple therapy with outpatient follow-up for determination of when to switch to dual therapy (not DAPT) with anticoagulation plus clopidogrel.

16.5.6.4 Post-MI Heart Remodeling Prevention

After an MI, the heart attempts to repair itself and undergoes remodeling driven by pathways such as renin angiotensin aldosterone system (RAAS). Unfortunately, the remodeling is pathologic, and thus preventing this remodeling is of utmost importance. ACE inhibitors (or ARBs if intolerant) and beta-blockers (typically metoprolol) should be started prior to discharge as the number of patients still using the medications after 6 months is significantly higher when initiated while inpatient.

16.5.6.5 Secondary Prevention

Once a patient has demonstrated signs of stable angina, they qualify for intensive secondary prevention measures. This is best learned through ▢ Table 16.4 below. All medications listed have a mortality benefit and decreases cardiovascular events. Insurance is often the barrier to getting patients on some of the newer medications.

16.5.6.6 Other

After an MI, depending on the location and extent, the heart may have significant impairment in function due to hibernating or dead cardiomyocytes. Heart function often recovers over several weeks to months, so it is important to set up outpatient follow-up to reassess the ejection fraction for recovery. There is no urgent need to begin treatment for heart failure based on the acutely depressed EF, particularly without symptoms. There are a variety of acute, subacute, and chronic complications of MI (▢ Fig. 16.37).

▢ Table 16.4 Medications for secondary prevention of major adverse cardiac events (MACE)

Intervention	Dose	Evidence
Aspirin	Baby (81 mg) QD	Various trials, you do not need to know them for the rotation as these are so well established and there is no deliberation
Statin	High-intensity	Various trials, you do not need to know them for the rotation as these are so well established
Ezetimibe (in addition to moderate-intensity statin)	10 mg QD	IMPROVE-IT trial
Vascepa (iscoaspent ethyl)	4 g QD	REDUCE-IT trial; for TCG >150
SGLT2 inhibitor	Variable	2019 Lancet meta-analysis by Marc Sabtatine of EMPA-REG, CANVAS, DECLARE-TIMI 58

Common Post-MI complications

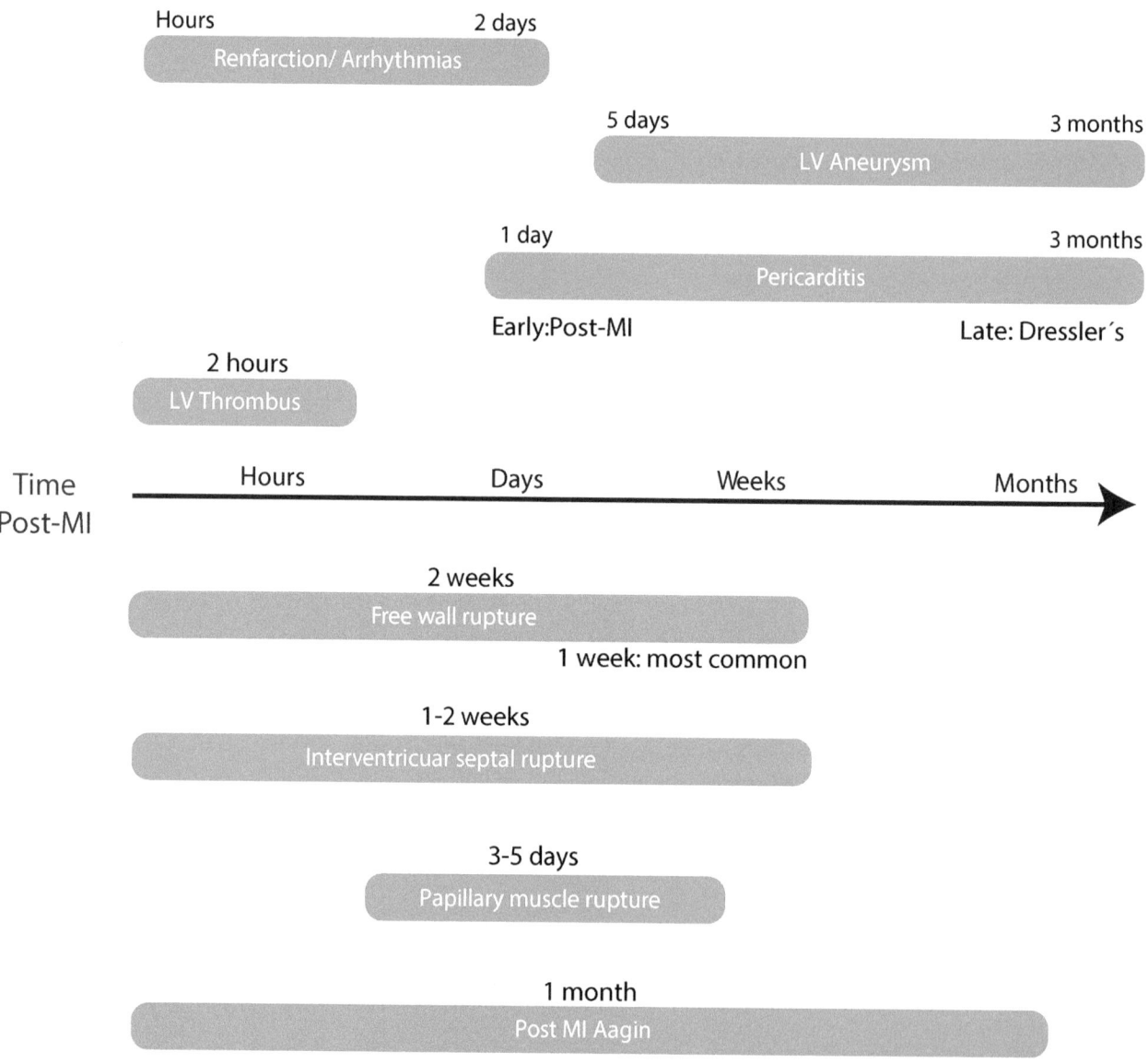

Fig. 16.37 Post-MI complications

16.5.7 **When to Discharge**

The patient can be discharged shortly after revascularization, initiation of the proper medications (anti-remodeling and secondary prevention), and lifestyle counseling. You should actively assess for the suitability to discharge and update your disposition in your presentation.

16.6 **Heart Failure**

You will no doubt see heart failure on your rotation, as it is the most common cause of hospitalizations in patients 65 and older. Heart failure has a terrible prognosis with up to 1/3 of admitted patients being either readmitted or deceased within 90 days of initial discharge.

While there are many ways to classify heart failure, perhaps the most common is based on ejection fraction, a measure of the ventricular pumping function. The two key entities are heart failure with reduced ejection fraction (HFrEF) and heart failure with preserved ejection fraction (HFpEF). For the purposes of this book, we will focus specifically on heart failure referring to left ventricular dysfunction.

HFrEF is the form that you are probably more familiar with from your preclinical studies and results often from an acute insult such as a myocardial infarction leading to weakening, thinning of the heart, and impaired pumping function. Almost all effective pharmacologic therapies for heart failure are specific for HFrEF, specifically targeting two classic neurohormonal pathways: renin-angiotensin-aldosterone (RAAS) and the sympathetic nervous system (SNS).

HFpEF is strongly correlated with age and has become one of the largest unmet needs in cardiovascular and geriatric medicine. As our revascularization techniques improve and as our population ages, HFpEF has steadily replaced HFrEF as the dominant form of heart failure. The biology of HFpEF is not well understood (and increasing evidence suggests HFpEF is quite heterogeneous), but it can be simply thought of as having many properties that is opposite that of HFrEF. Instead of a weak and thin wall, the wall is hypertrophied and thickened leading to impaired relaxation and accommodation of blood entering the ventricles during diastole. Despite a normal ejection fraction, beginning with a small amount of blood results in poor forward blood flow.

The hallmark symptom of heart failure, regardless of classification, is exercise intolerance, a result of poor forward blood flow leading to pulmonary congestion and suboptimal oxygen delivery to tissues. Other symptoms include lower extremity (LE) swelling and cough (◘ Fig. 16.38).

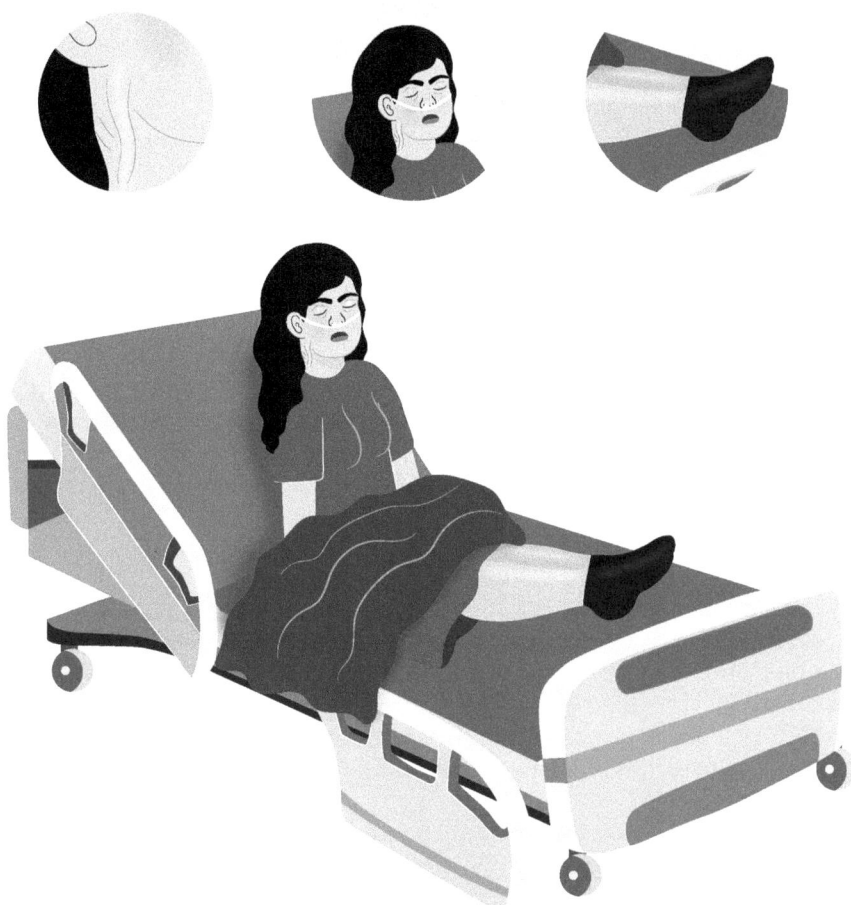

◘ **Fig. 16.38 Heart failure symptoms**

16.6.1 **Heart Failure Exacerbation**

A heart's baseline impaired ability to promote adequate forward flow of blood may be apparent with either stress (e.g., exercise) or at rest, depending on the severity of impairment (refer to NYHA Heart Failure Classification). Patients are generally treated with medications (and sometimes devices) to maintain their baseline heart function and slow the rate of decline. A heart failure *exacerbation* is simply when the patient decompensates from this baseline due to a stressor (refer to the FAILURE mnemonic below) to which the heart cannot compensate due to its impairments. Two fancy terms that refer to this decreased ability to react to stress are chronotropic and contractile reserve. For instance, during exercise, a healthy heart should increase its heart rate and strength of contraction. Similarly, with a reasonable increase in overall volume status, the heart should compensate by adjusting either heart rate or strength of pumping and keeping blood moving forwards, preventing the classic findings of pulmonary congestion, exercise intolerance, and lower extremity edema. With enough volume overload, everyone develops the syndrome of heart failure – it is simply an easier occurrence for patients without the proper pumping and/or relaxation of the ventricle(s).

16.6.2 **Causes of Heart Failure Exacerbation**

A widely used (and good) mnemonic is *FAILURE*. This is worth memorizing now and going through each time you have a heart failure case. By the end of the rotation, you'll know the ins and outs and have learned this by heart rather than memorization.
- *F*orgot meds (most common)
- *A*rrhythmia
- *I*schemia/*I*nfarction/*I*nfection
- *L*ifestyle (diet, exercise)
- *U*pregulation of cardiac output (pregnancy, anemia)
- *R*enal dysfunction
- *E*mbolism

16.6.3 **Differentiating the Differential**

You aren't likely to be consulted for a workup of heart failure exacerbation as that is straightforward. Rather, you are most likely to be consulted for the treatment aspect. If on the general service, you will also be primarily managing the treatment portion. However, it is still worth thinking about the differential:
- COPD Exacerbation: Patient will have a long-standing history of smoking. The best predictor of a COPD exacerbation is prior COPD exacerbation. Though having a classic CXR with COPD findings (increased lung volumes, decreased lung markings, increased AP diameter) nails the diagnosis, often it can be difficult to distinguish if the COPD exacerbation is caused by viral infection (e.g., viral PNA). Many of the same triggers for COPD exacerbation can also lead to heart failure exacerbation, so the best way to distinguish heart failure from COPD is by examining volume status.

- Pneumonia: Will have signs of infection (e.g., fever, cough, pleuritic chest pain). CXR will demonstrate most commonly a lobar opacity as opposed to a generalized process representing pulmonary congestion.
- Pulmonary Embolism: Typically, a sudden development of SOB (as opposed to subacute) with risk factors (immobilization, clotting disorders, procoagulant effect medications).

16.6.4 Chart Review

Prior to seeing the patient, here are the things you should quickly glean from the EMR if possible:
- [ ] Most recent dry weight
- [ ] BNP (baseline and/or prior admission)
- [ ] Home diuretic regimen (confirm with patient)
- [ ] Ejection fraction from most recent echo
- [ ] Baseline heart failure symptoms

> Note: These diagnoses can occasionally overlap, and you should always consider multifactorial etiologies to a patient's presentation. For example, the patient may have right heart failure secondary to COPD (cor pulmonale), a respiratory infection can lead to a heart failure exacerbation, and approximately one out of every four patients requiring hospitalization for a COPD exacerbation may have concomitant pulmonary emboli.

16.6.5 History

Here, your job is first to briefly confirm the history that supports a diagnosis of heart failure exacerbation that has likely already been made. Hallmark features include subacute onset of exercise intolerance, shortness of breath, and increased swelling in the lower extremities. The most specific symptom for heart failure is paroxysmal nocturnal dyspnea (PND; waking up gasping for breath at night), and the most sensitive is dyspnea on exertion. The more interesting aspect for you is to get at the cause of the exacerbation (*FAILURE* mnemonic) so that you can try to help the patient avoid future exacerbations. Furthermore, you should explore for any hints to an exacerbation triggered by new worsening heart failure (e.g., a silent MI).

> Thought Pattern Checklist
> [ ] *New* worsening HF?
> [ ] *HF* symptoms
> [ ] *Exacerbation* etiology
>
> Memory Aid: new HF exacerbation?

16.6.6 Exam

When distinguishing heart failure from other conditions, the two most useful exam findings are jugular venous distension (JVD) and hepatojugular reflux (HJR; a marker of the heart's inability to accommodate increased preload). As a student, this is also a great opportunity to try listening to an S3 (remember, use the bell near the apex). You should of course listen to the lungs and check the lower extremities for pitting edema.

The physical exam is critical for not only the initial diagnosis of heart failure but also each day as you pre-round to guide your treatment. The goal of your pre-rounding exam should be to primarily assess for changes in their volume status using the JVP, lung exam, and lower extremity edema. Of course, you should always be listening to the heart and checking for signs of DVT each day.

> Pearl: Remember to use the hepatojugular reflex to help you verify the JVP. The HRJ is also a great way to distinguish between heart failure and portal venous hypertension.

Pearl: HJR – be sure to hold for at least 10–15 seconds. Textbook answer is 30 seconds. You should not apply unreasonable pressure, but do not be afraid, as many medical students are, to press firmly in the RUQ and hold while assessing for an increase in the JVD. HRJ is particularly useful for differentiating heart failure from portal congestion.

Pearl: NT-proBNP level may be artificially elevated in patients with renal failure. Always compare to baseline and age-adjusted cutoffs.

Why would heart failure be associated with hyponatremia?

Heart failure is a state of low effective circulating volume, leading to RAAS activation and ADH release, both of which exacerbate hyponatremia.

Pearl: Bed weights are usually inaccurate, and daily standing weights can be too, so use your common sense when interpreting these!

- Key Exam Checklist
- [ ] JVP +- HRJ
- [ ] Lung exam
- [ ] Volume exam
- [ ] S3

16.6.7 Objective Data

Though some of the workup may be done prior to you seeing the patient, let's explore them for your knowledge. The N-terminal pro B-type natriuretic peptide (NT-proBNP) is used as a marker to *exclude* heart failure if the value is below an age-adjusted cutoff (■ Fig. 16.39). It is also sometimes checked after treatment as reassurance.

Sodium is a lab value that has significant prognostic value. More severe heart failure exacerbation is associated with more significant hyponatremia, and this has a direct relationship with heart failure mortality.

Creatinine is important to monitor as an increase is a good indicator of when the patient is nearing euvolemia or has been over-diuresed. It can also increase due to cardiorenal syndrome (refer to the ▶ Chap. 18).

Imaging consists of CXR to check for pulmonary congestion and TTE to check ejection fraction if there are no recent echos (some hospitals routinely check a TTE every HF admission). A decrease in ejection fraction may warrant further separate workup (e.g., perhaps there was a silent myocardial infarct leading to a decrease in EF).

For HF cases, you should always pay careful attention to the daily standing weights, the ins/outs, and Cr.

Age	Rule Out NT-proBNP	Rule In NT-proBNP	
<50	300	450	
50-75	300	900	
>=75	300	1800	

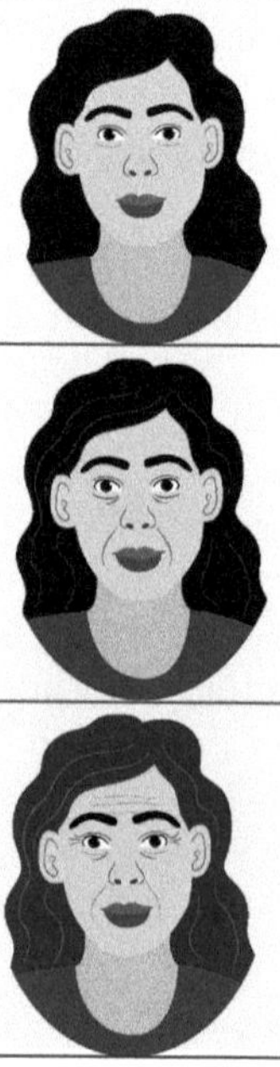

■ Fig. 16.39 BNP levels by age

- Key Objective Data Checklist
- [ ] Daily standing weights
- [ ] I/Os
- [ ] Cr

16.6.8 Goals of Admission

- [ ] Consider the original etiology of heart failure.
- [ ] Determine the cause of current exacerbation.
- [ ] Optimize hemodynamics (treat the exacerbation).
- [ ] Optimize guideline-directed medical therapy (GDMT).

16.6.8.1 Determining the Cause of Current Exacerbation

Prevention refers to our best attempts to keep the patient from developing another exacerbation. This may range from helping the patient adhere to their medications/diet to fixing an underlying arrhythmia. Understanding the most likely etiology of this exacerbation is crucial for this.

Memory Aid: EFGH Approach
Etiology (original)
FAILURE
GDMT
Hemodynamics

16.6.8.2 Optimizing Hemodynamics

Optimization refers to removing the stressful physiology that the heart is dealing with that led to the exacerbation (e.g., removing volume overload) – a common way to phrase this is to say you want to "optimize hemodynamics."

Optimizing hemodynamics begins with diuresis. You will be told over and over that diuresis is stylistic with no right answers. However, that doesn't mean anything flies! You must develop a logical and consistent approach – our approach is detailed and presented in ◘ Fig. 16.40.

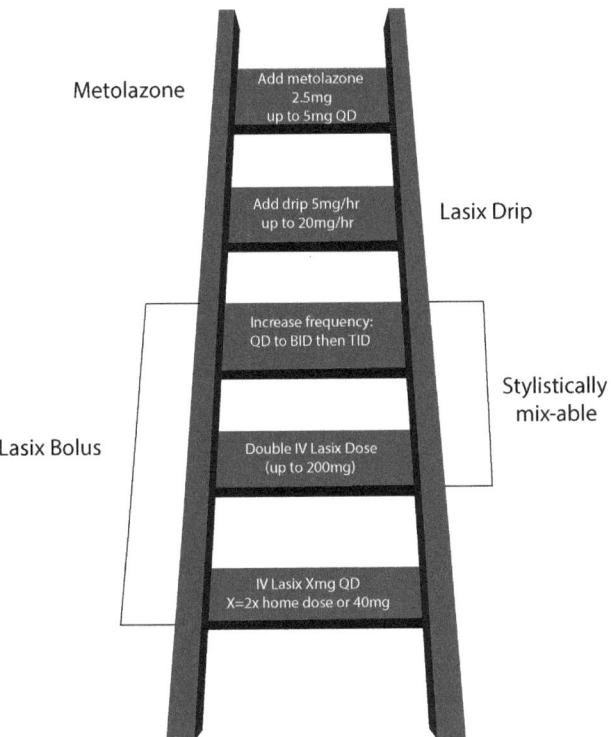

◘ Fig. 16.40 *ADHF* diuresis escalation ladder

Table 16.5 Chart of diuretic conversions

Loop diuret	PO to IV	IV conversion ratios	Duration of effect (h)
Furosemide	1:2	40	6 (Lasix)
Torsemide	1:1	20	~10
Bumetanide	1:1	1	4–6

Pearl: Lasix was named because its duration of effect lasts 6 hours!

Pearl: The IV form is used to increase bioavailability because Lasix absorption is significantly reduced from gut edema during heart failure exacerbation.

Pearl: Some patients will have baseline lower extremity edema: morbidly obese, chronic lymph-edema, post-thrombotic syndrome, etc. It is important to ascertain the baseline swelling – PCP and clinic notes can be very helpful.

Hesitractor: You may see a very slight Cr increase while diuresing. This is very common, and should not cause alarm. A slight bump is acceptable, and you should continue diuresing until the Cr bumps more notably.

Your goal when diuresing in ADHF is to elicit an appropriate decrease in total body fluids, often referred to as the *goal net negative*. In patients without preload-dependent states, the net negative goal is typically 2–3 L/day. In cases such as severe aortic stenosis and constrictive pericarditis, you should diurese gently (goal net negative 500–1000 cc/day). The goal net negative *must be stated every time* you present your patient, whether as a new patient or as follow-up.

Diuresis is often trial and error until you find a dose that meets your daily goal, but beginning with an educated guess is important. If diuretic-naïve (meaning no prior home regimen), Lasix/furosemide 40 mg IV is a good start. Otherwise, double the home PO dose in IV form is used to start. It is thus important to know the basic conversions between PO and IV forms and the main diuretics (Table 16.5). You can convert the Lasix from PO to IV by dividing the dose in half. As an example, if a patient is on Lasix 20 mg QD at home, this is equivalent to 10 mg IV QD, and therefore the admission hospital dose would be double, or 20 mg IV QD.

You should assess the urine output in the morning and in the afternoon. This allows you to adjust the diuresis dose up to twice a day – much more economical time-wise! If you are not meeting your net negative goals, you must escalate your diuresis regimen. There is no one right way to do this, but we suggest our five-step diuresis escalation strategy (Fig. 16.40) each time you do not meet the goal. As you increase your diuretic regimen, pay close attention to the I/Os, Cr, HCO3, and volume exam for signs of either diuresing too quickly or having over-diuresed.

You will typically continue diuresis until a euvolemic exam and/or a noticeable Cr bump, often with an increase in HCO3 due to contraction alkalosis. Although the weight (particularly standing weights) is in theory a good marker of how diuresis is progressing, I've found that it is largely unreliable with significant unexplained variations and would rather rely on other more objective lab data. When the patient's volume status is fixed, always record their "dry weight" for future reference before discharge.

If you've been wondering why we favor diuresing with intermittent boluses as opposed to starting with a continuous drip, consider yourself a very astute student! There is no data so far that demonstrates the superiority of one versus the other. In the DOSE trial (NEJM 2011), no difference was found between the two methods with regard to symptomatic improvement, despite in theory obtaining a more consistent plasma level of diuretic with the drip method. Interestingly, the key finding from the DOSE trial was actually that high-dose diuretics result in faster and greater symptomatic improvement than low-dose regimens. However, this comes at the expense of a mild increase in kidney function impairment. It's important to note that many general medicine floors will not allow for use of Lasix drips, so make sure to check in with your team to see if this will even be an option.

Lastly, a brief note on ultrafiltration. This is rarely used for removing volume, and only done in extreme cases where the patient is completely refractory to medical therapy. This last-approach view is driven by the CARRESS-HF trial

(NEJM 2012) which demonstrated greater renal impairment with ultrafiltration (dialysis), without a significant decrease in weight compared to medical therapy.

16.6.8.3 Clinical Pearls and Exceptions

1. Volume Exam
   (a) Less reliable if baseline LE edema (e.g., varicose veins, prior DVT, amlodipine).
   (b) Moderate-severe tricuspid regurgitation may falsely elevate the JVD.
2. Creatinine
   (a) If the patient has baseline CKD, the absolute Cr change is greater for a proportional change in kidney function. Thus, fluctuations of 0.10 can be quite common and represent normal lab-to-lab variation.
3. Contraction Alkalosis
   (a) A rising HCO3 is another lab finding that can support having diuresed enough.

16.6.8.4 Twice-Daily (Morning, Afternoon) ADHF Diuresis Checklist

- [ ] Check I/Os (and weights, if reliable).
- [ ] Check K, Cr, HCO3, Mg.
- [ ] Volume status exam – JVD, LE edema, lung sounds (crackles or wheezing, i.e., cardiac asthma).
- [ ] Check if diuresis regimen requires escalation.
- [ ] Is it time to stop diuresis? (Cr up? HCO3 up? Euvolemic exam?).

16.6.8.5 Common Knowledge Questions

What role does metolazone play in augmenting diuresis?

With repeated diuresis, the distal convoluted tubules (DCT) becomes hypertrophied to compensate for the salt and water loss. By inhibiting the DCT's newly increased ability to retain water, metolazone augments diuresis. Metolazone should be administered shortly (~30 minutes) *prior* to administration of your main diuretic regimen.

16.6.8.6 Assessment/Plan Examples

Your patient continues to be volume up as reflected by a JVD of 10 cm at 60 degrees, 2 + bilateral pitting edema, and diffuse crackles. The Cr is stable at 0.91 from 0.90, and she was net negative 720 cc yesterday. The following are three variations in how you might approach diuresis:

- Therapeutically, I'd like to escalate her diuresis regimen by doubling the dose of IV Lasix to 80 mg QD for a goal net negative 2 L.
- Given the patient's severe aortic stenosis and resulting preload dependent physiology especially with HFpEF exacerbation, I'd like to diurese gently with Lasix 40 mg QD for a goal net negative 500 to 1000 cc.
- We are already at 200 mg Lasix TID; thus I would like to add a Lasix drip at 5 mg/hr for a goal net negative 2 L. I'll check afternoon labs and urine output, and if she isn't responding, we can consider increasing the drip further to 10 mg/hr.

16.6.9 Optimizing Guideline-Directed Medical Therapy (GDMT)

GDMT refers to medications that have been shown to reduce morbidity and mortality in patients with heart failure. Notably, all current GDMT refer specifically to HFrEF. Each patient you encounter with heart failure should

Fun Fact: The trial was a multinational endeavor, and it was discovered that certain countries were not administering the spironolactone and rather siphoning the research funds.

Pearl: Metoprolol succinate is the form that was shown to have a mortality benefit in HFrEF (MERIT-HF Trial, Lancet 1999). Patients are commonly switched to metoprolol tartrate for fractionation purposes and increased control of dosing while inpatient. Always ensure that the patient is switched back to the long-acting succinate form prior to discharge

Pearl: Carvedilol is favored when the patient also requires blood pressure control. Carvedilol's alpha blocking effects confer greater antihypertensive properties than the other two

Fun Fact: Metoprolol is the most common beta-blocker prescribed as GDMT for HFrEF. Though there have not been good head-to-head trials between these three beta-blockers, some people cite the COMET trial comparing metoprolol and carvedilol as evidence of carvedilol's superiority. Unfortunately, this trial was stacked against metoprolol likely with industry motives because (i) metoprolol tartrate was tested and (ii) carvedilol's dose was maximal, whereas only half the dose of metoprolol was used

Pearl: Patients on spironolactone may experience breast tenderness and gynecomastia. Eplerenone is an alternative which does not cause those side effects. It is now fairly cheap and much easier to prescribe

Pearl: The original study DAPA-HF only examined HFrEF patients who were type 2 diabetics, but with the DECLARE TIMI 58 study, diabetic status is not required for the mortality benefit

Table 16.6 GDMT for HFrEF

Class	Examples	Mechanism	Evidence
Beta-blockers	Metoprolol, bisoprolol, carvedilol	Blocks pathologic heart remodeling	MERIT-HF, CIBIS, COPERNICUS
ACE inhibitors/angiotensin receptor blockers	Lisinopril, losartan	Blocks pathologic heart remodeling	CONSENSUS, SOLVD, ONTARGET
Mineralocorticoid receptor antagonists	Spironolactone, Eplerenone	Blocks mineralo-corticoid receptors	RALES, EPHESUS
SGLT2 inhibitors	Dapagliflozin	Inhibits SGLT2 in kidneys	DAPA-HF, DECLARE-TIMI 58
Neprilysin inhibitor – ARB combo	Entresto (sacubitril-valsartan)	Inhibits the breakdown of BNP	PARADIGM-HF
Nitrates/arterial vasodilator[a]	Isosorbide dinitrate + hydralazine[a]	Arterial and venous dilation	A-HeFT

[a]This combo is specific to African Americans. Current guidelines recommend it for NYHA Classes III–IV HFrEF

be checked for optimization of these medications. For HFpEF, there is some evidence from a post hoc analysis of the TOPCAT trial by Marc Pfeffer that spironolactone may confer some benefits. Therefore, without a contraindication such as hyperkalemia, spironolactone may be considered in HFpEF patients.

Table 16.6 lists the different classes of medications, their mechanisms, and the evidence for use in HFrEF.

When treating patients with heart failure, it is important to be cognizant of the fact that not all heart failure patients have been treated equally. Per the American College of Cardiology, African Americans are 2–3 times more likely to die from cardiovascular disease compared to white patients, African Americans are 33% more likely to die of cardiovascular disease in hospital settings compared to their white counterparts, and a study in Medicare patients found that African Americans were 42% less likely to receive ICDs after MIs than similar white patients. As the next generation of physicians, it is crucial that we explore our biases and attempt to give exemplary treatment to all our patients, regardless of their race, ethnicity, or socioeconomic background.

16.7 Arrhythmias

Before diving into the individual arrhythmias, we should understand why abnormal rhythms are dangerous. Ultimately, abnormal rhythms lead to improper filling of one or more heart chambers (e.g., atrial fibrillation results in loss of atrial kick and thus decreased preload; ventricular tachycardia shortens the length of diastole thus impairing preload while also causing dysfunctional dyssynchronous ventricular contractions). Atrial rhythms are typically less dangerous because the AV node acts as a filter to prevent the ventricles from seeing all the atrial impulses, but occasionally the AV node can be bypassed by accessory tracts such as in Wolf-Parkinson-White (WPW) syndrome via the tract known as the bundle of Kent.

Arrhythmias can be classified based on location: supraventricular (atrial) versus ventricular. Atrial rhythms are narrow (unless coexisting with a bundle branch block) and are generally much faster than the wide complex ventricular arrhythmias. Ventricular rhythms are typically more dangerous and require immediate attention. We will focus on the most common pathologic arrhythmias you will encounter either on the general inpatient or consult service. Of note, we will not delve into a differential diagnosis for these arrhythmias since it is not clinically relevant – the problem will be clear upon checking the EKG.

1. Supraventricular
   (a) Atrial fibrillation
   (b) Atrial flutter
2. Ventricular
   (a) Monomorphic ventricular tachycardia
   (b) Ventricular fibrillation
3. Other
   (a) Atrioventricular (AV) block

For any arrhythmia, you should always categorize as stable or not based on their blood pressure, heart rate, and overall appearance. If unstable, you should immediately notify your team, and the patient will require immediate attention and likely electrical cardioversion/defibrillation. Once stable you may apply the information specific to each arrhythmia in the following sections.

Lastly, arrhythmias apart from afib is often managed in conjunction with the electrophysiology (EP) team. Thus, excelling on these patient cases is slightly different. You will need to defer much of the management to EP but also provide reasonable plans as if you were EP.

Pearl: Use this technique when stating your assessment, and plan regardless of the service. Attendings want to hear what you think optimal management is regardless of the complexity of the problem and the need for specialty consults (it doesn't matter if you are right or wrong, just try!).

16.7.1 Atrial Fibrillation

This is the most common type of arrhythmia you will encounter. You will see more patients with afib as a secondary problem than the principal reason for admission.

To understand the clinical relevance of atrial fibrillation, you should consider the following aspects:
1. Onset: acute (within 48 hours) or chronic (>48 hours)
2. Anticoagulation
3. Ability to conduct to the ventricles

The principal concern of atrial fibrillation is its risk in atrial clot formation which may embolize. You should always calculate the CHA_2DS_2VASc and HAS-BLED scores for patients with atrial fibrillation, regardless of whether it is the primary problem. This will help inform anticoagulation management and is a very common question teams will ask you. While you can use the search feature in the upper right corner of epic to find a previously calculated score, I recommend that you calculate it fresh for each patient – it is not only good practice but more reliable.

Recently, there is a stronger preference to push for anticoagulation in men with CHADSVASC scores ≥1 and in women ≥ 2, de-emphasizing the importance of biological sex. A score of 1 may also be considered for antiplatelet therapy with aspirin.

CHA2DS2VASc Criteria:
*C*HF
*H*TN
*A*ge (1 point ≥ 65; 2 points ≥75)
*D*iabetes
*S*troke/TIA (+2)
*V*ascular disease (MI, PAD)
*S*ex

16.7.2 Chart Review Checklist

- [ ] Home antiarrhythmic regimen (confirm adherence)
- [ ] Any prior notes regarding difficulty controlling the afib

16.7.3 History

Many patients are asymptomatic when it comes to afib, though some people may feel their irregular pulse or occasional palpitations. Your primary objective here is to characterize the effect of afib on their daily life. Do they exhibit symptoms of heart failure?

Fun Fact: The apple watch acts as a one-lead EKG and can detect an irregular pulse. Some patients will present because the apple watch told them they're in afib! You should skim the Apple Heart Study (NEJM 2019) as it is a fun topic to bring up on rounds.

16.7.4 Exam

Your goal here is to verify that the patient has an irregularly irregular pulse, either by feeling the pulse or through auscultation. Note that if the patient has paroxysmal afib, you may not observe an irregular pulse and that the patient may be in afib when you examine the patient again later with the team. Don't freak out – this is the nature of paroxysmal afib! You should also examine for heart failure signs from chronic tachycardia (if afib with RVR).

16.7.5 Goals of Admission

- [ ] Determine the etiology of Afib
- [ ] Control the Afib
- [ ] Anticoagulation

16.7.6 Determining the Afib Etiology

We won't delve into great detail here but simply mention that most afib is primary meaning that for whatever reason, there are some ectopic foci generating electrical activity in the heart. This most commonly occurs in the pulmonary veins for which ablation may be considered. However, sometimes the afib may be secondary to other disease states such as hyperthyroidism, excessive alcohol, or left atrial dilation secondary to mitral valve dysfunction or other causes of chronic left-sided volume overload. As an inpatient team, you will primarily manage chronic afib rather than working up the etiology. Work up.

16.7.7 Controlling the Afib

The primary means of managing atrial fibrillation pharmacologically is either with rate or rhythm control. You should know that the AFFIRM trial (NEJM 2002) demonstrated no difference in mortality between rate and rhythm control for atrial fibrillation, although there was a nonsignificant trend towards decreased mortality with rate control. Given that rhythm control medications may harbor more side effects, rate control is typically attempted first by most clinicians.

Rate control is a method by which the sequelae of atrial fibrillation such as impaired atrial kick are decreased by granting the heart more time in diastole (remember, diastole decreases with increasing heart rate). The two most common agents used are metoprolol and diltiazem. In patients with afib with rapid ventricular rate, the RACE-II trial (NEJM 2010) investigated lenient (<110 bpm) versus strict (<80 bpm) rate control and found no difference in cardiovascular mortality and hospitalizations for heart failure, stroke, systemic embolism, or life-threatening arrhythmic events. In light of increased side effects and more stringent outpatient follow-up, unless the patient is symptomatic, the rate control agent need not be up-titrated if this HR goal is met. Notably, rate control agents are most effective when initiated within a week of afib onset.

Rhythm control aims at converting the atrial fibrillation into sinus rhythm, which would obviously restore the deficits (primarily the loss of atrial kick and thus hemodynamic compromise) caused by atrial fibrillation. The most common drugs include amiodarone, flecainide, dofetilide, and propafenone. Antiarrhythmics are typically laden with more side effects compared to the rate control agents. The other option is to electrically cardiovert the patient. This may be a patient's preferred method if they do not want to take antiarrhythmics. Prior to electrical cardioversion, you must ensure that the onset of afib was acute (<48 hours). If not, there is a risk of clot formation within the left atrium that may dislodge when flipped back into sinus rhythm; thus the patient is anticoagulated for at 3 weeks prior to coming in for an elective cardioversion. If more urgent, DC cardioversion can be performed after TEE or cardiac CT to confirm absence of atrial appendage thrombus.

Lastly, if the afib is originating from a particular region such as the pulmonary veins, that area may be ablated (e.g., pulmonary vein isolation). This has been shown in the SARA (Eur Heart J 2014) and MANTRA-PAF (paroxysmal afib; NEJM 2012) trials to be superior (permanent afib) or equivalent (paroxysmal) to pharmacologic control.

Pearl: For rate control, beta-blockers are likely more effective than calcium channel blockers (see study in Circulation 2015 by Chao TF et al.), also a potential mortality benefit.

16.7.8 Anticoagulation

Due to the risk of stroke and systemic embolism, patients with CHA_2DS_2VASc scores of 1 or greater often require intervention. Notably, the decision to anticoagulate is always dependent on the CHADSVASC and independent of whether the patient is in sinus rhythm or not. Note that there has been a push towards reducing the role of female sex in obtaining this score as it appears to play less prominent of a role than some of the other risk factors. Patients with a CHA_2DS_2VASc of 1 are considered for either antiplatelet therapy with aspirin or anticoagulation based on clinical judgment. A score of 2 or greater indicates anticoagulation.

For anticoagulation, direct oral anticoagulants (DOACs) are preferred due to ease of use (no frequent outpatient INR checks like warfarin). The two key DOACs are rivaroxaban and apixaban, with the ultimate decision on which to use coming down to which the patient's insurance covers. However, apixaban is generally favored as there is moderate evidence that it is superior to warfarin rather than noninferior (as is rivaroxaban). Notably, apixaban is the only DOAC with a lower risk of GI bleeding than warfarin. All DOACs boast a significantly lower risk (~50%) of intracranial hemorrhage compared to warfarin. DOACs should not be used if the patient has mechanical valves. Let's compare these two DOACs and warfarin.

Pearl: Dosing considerations for DOACs are mainly limited to renal function and may be less effective when the BMI is on either extreme.

- Apixaban
  - 5 mg BID dosing
  - Less renal clearance = > favored in setting of renal dysfunction
  - ARISTOTLE trial: seminal trial that demonstrated superiority of apixaban to warfarin in reducing rates of systemic embolism and stroke in nonvalvular afib
- Rivaroxaban
  - 20 mg QD dosing (more convenient for patient, may increase compliance)
- ROCKET-AF trial: seminal trial demonstrating rivaroxaban was non-inferior to warfarin in reducing rates of stroke in nonvalvular afib
- Warfarin
  - Typically started at 5 mg QD with a target INR of 2.0–3.0 (2.5–3.5 for mechanical valves)
  - Requires heparin bridging
  - Requires frequent INR checks
  - Easier reversal
  - Must be used for mechanical valves

Pearl: Rivaroxaban for 30 <= GFR <= 50 merits a reduced dosage of 15 mg QD.

Pearl: Apixaban dosing should be reduced to 2.5 mg BID when any two of the following criteria are met:
- Creatinine >1.5
- Age ≥80
- Body weight < 60 kg

16.7.9 Atrial Flutter

Atrial flutter is a reentrant arrhythmia that results from a continuous circuit of electrical activity. Given this, it is prone to occurrence around areas of scarring, such as that affected by cardiac surgery.

Flutter should be suspected in the presence of a regularly irregular rhythm, particularly around 150 bpm. Unlike afib, flutter is quite hard to control with medications. The gold standard treatment is ablation, depending on where the flutter is located anatomically. Typical (Type I) flutter is located around the cavotricuspid isthmus, while atypical (Type II) flutter is located often in the left atrium. Notably, flutter can have a variable block (e.g. 2:1 followed by 3:1 then 4:1) that causes an irregularly irregular rhythm.

For your purposes, the workup and management for flutter are nearly identical to that in the ▶ Sect. 16.2.13.11 above. However, there are a few notable differences:
- For typical flutter, ablation of the CTI is highly effective.
- Flutter is much more difficult to rate control.
- You should always be seeking the input of the EP (electrophysiology team) for inpatient flutter management.

16.7.10 Monomorphic Ventricular Tachycardia

As the name suggests, monomorphic VT refers to the presence of a wide complex (>120 ms; ventricular) tachycardia (defined as >100 bpm) of the same morphology for at least three consecutive beats. Sustained VT leads to poor LV function and symptoms such as syncope.

The primary differential for vtach is identifying whether the wide QRS complex is a result of true vtach or a supraventricular tachycardia with a bundle branch block, also known as SVT with aberrancy (meaning abnormal conduction). This is best accomplished via the Brugada algorithm (▪ Fig. 16.41). This distinction is critical as the management is very different between the two.

While the Brugada algorithm is useful, there are some general features that alter the likelihood of each that can be used as a quick and dirty shortcut (▪ Fig. 16.42). VT is favored if the patient has a history if ischemic or structural disease, heart failure, or a history of sudden death. SVT with aberrancy is more like if prior EKGs demonstrate a BBB or WPW or if the patient has a history of SVTs without aberrancy.

Pearl: When in doubt, the patient should be treated as if they have VT as it is the more dangerous rhythm.

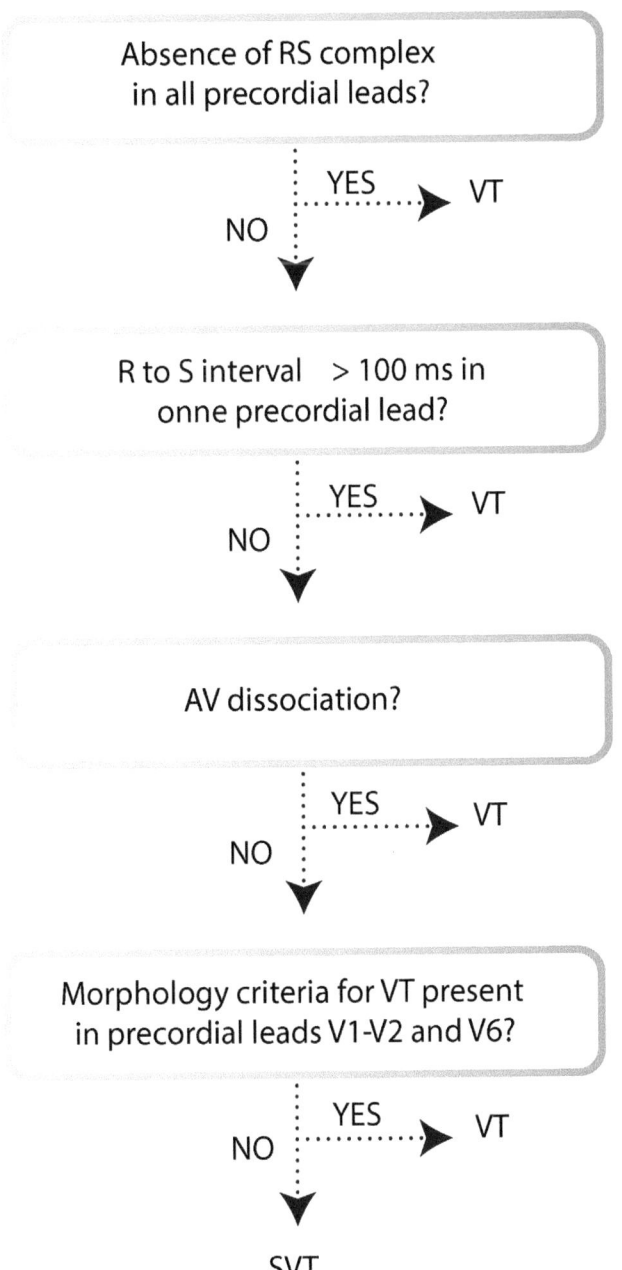

Fig. 16.41 Brugada algorithm for differentiating VT versus SVT with aberrancy

16.7.11 Goals of Admission

The EP team will guide much of the management for cases of VT. As the general inpatient service, you will take care of the patient as the primary team, speculating about what EP wants to do but deferring to them:

▬ [ ] Ensure stability.
▬ [ ] Monitor for VT while hospitalized.
▬ [ ] Appreciate and implement EP recs.

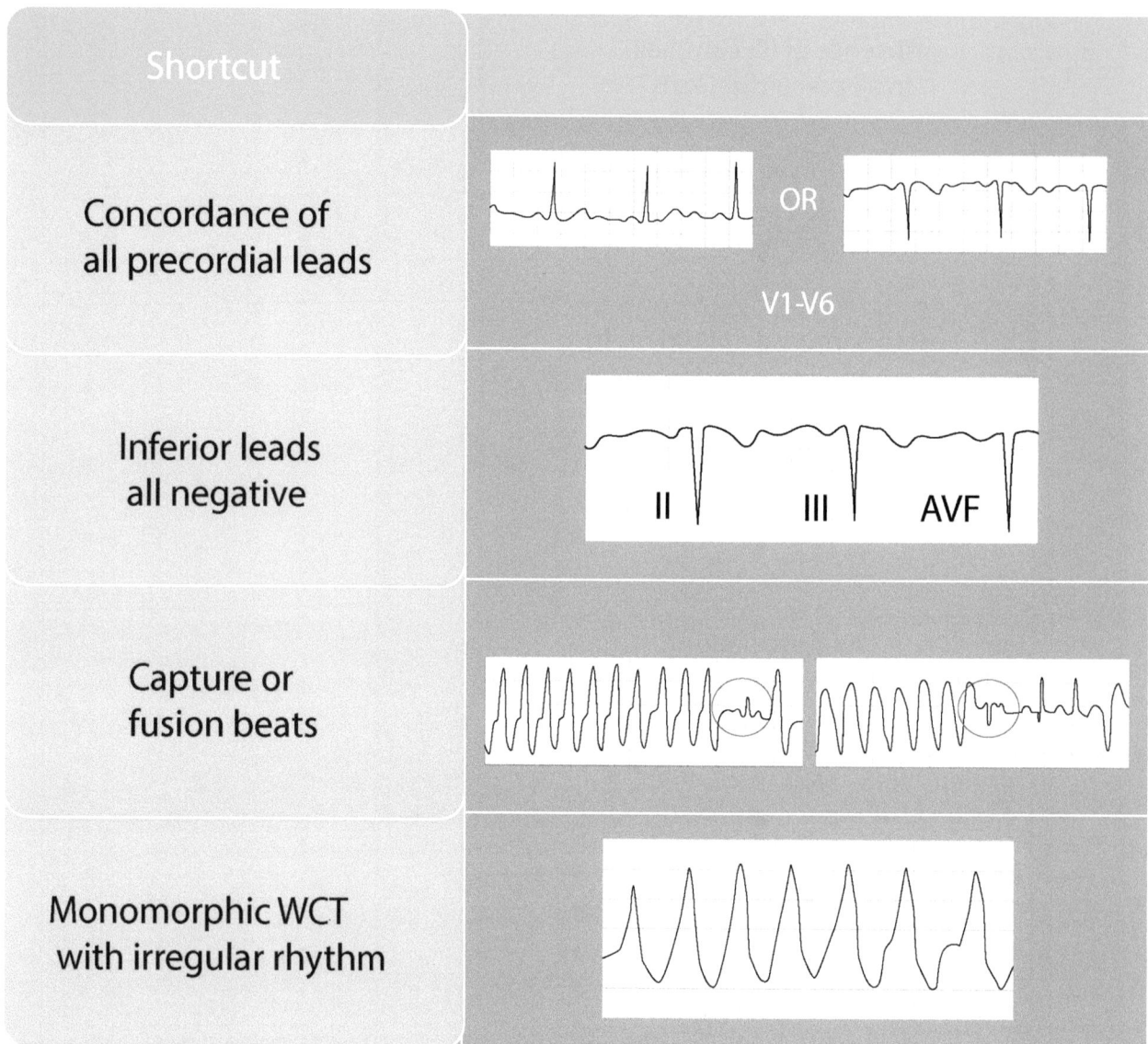

Fig. 16.42 Brugada algorithm shortcut

16.7.12 EP Recs

The treatment of VT is based on the nature of VT. Sustained VT >30 sec first merits an antiarrhythmic agent, usually amiodarone, followed by ablation therapy if necessary non-sustained VT that is more than a few beats may be managed with a nodal agent such as metoprolol.

Notably, the amiodarone must be "loaded" initially with high doses so that it is in the system. During loading, the patient remains inpatient until they have received 10 g. Afterwards, they begin their home dose which is typically between 200 and 400 mg QD.

16.7.13 Ventricular Fibrillation (VFib)

Ventricular fibrillation is one of the most feared arrhythmias and can result in sudden death. Any time vfib is seen on the EKG, the patient should be defibrillated (because there is no clear shockable QRS) immediately. Triggers for vfib are not always clear, though a recent MI is one of the leading causes of vfib.

16.7.14 Atrioventricular (AV) Blocks

AV block refers to a decrease in the transmission of electrical signals from the atria to the ventricles, either at the AV node itself or in the proximal portion of the His bundle system. As such, first-degree AV block is actually a misnomer as it is simply a conduction delay as opposed to a decrease in transmission of signal. Inpatient management of AV blocks will primarily focus on either Mobitz Type 2 or complete degree heart block. First-degree AV block and Mobitz 1 may be secondary findings but rarely, if ever, the principal reason for hospitalization.

Mobitz Type II is an unstable rhythm and can evolve into complete heart block. As such, patients should be kept under close monitoring while hospitalized. As long as the patient is stable, there is no necessity for pacing or immediate pharmacologic intervention. Mobitz II may be caused by a number of reversible etiologies such as ischemia, hyperkalemia, severe hypothyroidism, and AV nodal blocking agents. These should always be investigated prior to the placement of a permanent pacemaker. The preferred type of pacemaker is dual-chamber.

Third-degree AV block, also known as complete heart block (CHB), means that the atria are completely unable to communicate with the ventricles. This results in an independent beating of the atria from the ventricular beating, known as atrioventricular (AV) dissociation. That is, the ventricles are beating due to a ventricular escape rhythm; thus the bradycardia is around 40 bpm. As you can imagine, the coordination of atrial and ventricular contractions is essential to proper forward pumping of blood. As such, complete heart block is typically quite symptomatic. Most patients with third-degree block warrant a temporary pacemaker, with indications for a permanent pacer when the CHB is not reversible (same causes as for Mobitz Type II).

16.8 Valvular Disease

This is a frequent topic that you will encounter on the rotation, yet much of the management is by the interventional cardiology team. Hence, you will not need to know the detailed management of each case but rather a broad overview and some commonly tested facts. In your assessment and plan, you will generally suggest in broad strokes what you think should be done (e.g., TAVR) but include deferral to interventional cardiology on their recommendations. The most common valvular disease you will see while inpatient is aortic stenosis, followed by mitral regurgitation.

16.8.1 Replacement Valve Types

Let's learn briefly about replacement valves. As we briefly mentioned earlier, there are two distinct types.

16.8.1.1 Mechanical Valves

Mechanical valves were the first type of prosthetic valves used. Though sturdy with an average lifespan of 20 years (often the remaining lifespan of the patient), they carry a significant thrombosis risk, and patients must be anticoagulated in warfarin for life. At this point, there is no good evidence for the role of DOACs in mechanical valve anticoagulation.

Pearl: Mechanical valves can shear red blood cells as they pass by the valve, leading to an intravascular hemolytic anemia.

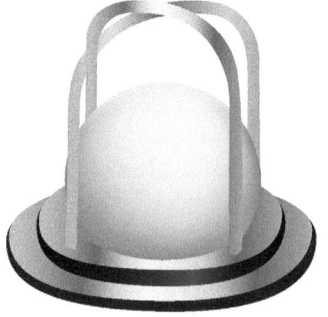

Ball and cage

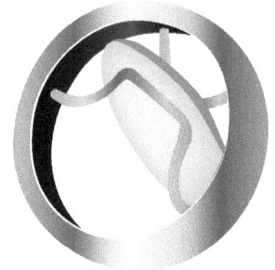

Tilting disc

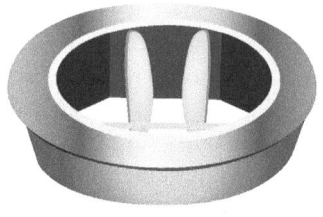

Bileaflet

☐ **Fig. 16.43 Mechanical valve types**

There are three primary types of mechanical valves. These are best learned in ☐ Fig. 16.43. Briefly, the most common type of valve used today is known as the St. Jude's valve, which is composed entirely of a special type of carbon which reduces its predisposition for forming clots and generating immune responses. It has two disks which act as leaflets.

16.8.1.2 Bioprosthetic Valves

These are from animal tissue, usually from pigs (porcine). Modern bioprostheses have lifespans of 10–20 years, and patients need not be anticoagulated routinely for bioprosthetic valves.

Replacement of valves, whether mechanical or bioprosthetic, comes with a small but appreciable risk of infective endocarditis, ranging from 1 to 3%. Since TAVR is minimally invasive, the risk is on the lower end of this range, but the mortality is quite high if the valve does become infected. Infected valves may require replacement (more commonly for mechanical valves; endocarditis with less invasive organisms on bioprosthetic valves may respond to antibiotic therapy alone).

Note: Patients with a prosthetic valve should receive antibiotic prophylaxis prior to invasive dental work.

16.8.1.3 Surgical Versus Minimally Invasive Methods

Valvular disease is treated either with open surgery or minimally invasive approaches. While the exact determination of which method is based on a large number of factors, here is an easy abbreviated way to think about the most common determinants of when to pursue each approach:

- Surgical
  - Other indication for open surgery (e.g., CABG)
- Minimally Invasive
  - Advanced age (think >75)
  - Advanced liver disease
  - Sicker patients

16.8.1.4 Aortic Stenosis

Aortic stenosis is most commonly secondary to either a bicuspid aortic valve (<65 years) or age-related calcification (>65 years old). The classic mnemonic *SAD* for syncope, angina, and dyspnea, particularly with exertion, is great for identifying patients at risk for severe aortic stenosis and in need of replacement.

Clinically, as part of a general cardiology team, you will primarily need to characterize the history, symptoms, and severity of the aortic stenosis. The patient's presentation will likely be syncope, but they may also be admitted for surgical correction or for evaluation and management of diagnoses secondary to chronic stenosis, such as heart failure or afib. Severity is defined as mild, moderate, or severe by echo. A commonly asked question with clinical practicality that is worth remembering are the three criteria for severe aortic stenosis:

- Transaortic pressure gradient >40 mm Hg
- Peak aortic jet velocity of >4 m/s
- Aortic valve area < 1 cm^2

Interventional cardiology is involved when the aortic stenosis is severe and symptomatic, requiring a valve replacement. The most common procedure is a transcatheter aortic valve replacement (TAVR), which involves replacement of the valve through a minimally invasive catheter-based approach through the femoral artery. Due to the minimally invasive approach, these procedures can be performed in older, sicker patients, which happen to be the population most at risk for severe aortic stenosis. Notably, the replacement valve for a TAVR is always bioprosthetic.

16.9 Note Examples

- Cardiology Admission Note

Patient:
Date of admission:
Cardiologist:
PCP:

- Admission Task Checklist
- [ ] ED data
- [ ] EKG
- [ ] Labs
- [ ] Pass-off

- [ ] Pre-admit orders
- [ ] Orders to remember: DVT ppx, lytes repletion, diet, home meds
- [ ] Past DC summary/past notes

- [ ] Note home meds held

■ **When Seeing Patient**
- [ ] Home meds
- [ ] Allergies
- [ ] Code status

■ **History of Present Illness**
- [ ] One-liner (focus on cardiac diagnoses, include most recent ejection fraction if available)
- [ ] Patient's story
- [ ] History from EMR
- [ ] ED course
- [ ] Since arrival to floor
- [ ] Previous cardiac history: EKG, TTE/TEE (EF, valves), ischemia eval (LHC, stress), home cardiac meds

■ **Review of Systems**
PMHx: include HTN, HLD
   PSHx
   Social history
   Family cardiac history
   Physical exam (head to toe, particular emphasis on cardiac)
   Objective data

■ **Assessment and Plan**
Updated one-liner
   Problems ordered by priority

Pearl: Trust but verify. Always confirm and take your own history from the patient. There are too many errors perpetuated in the current era when people rely on the EMR or information gathered by other team members.

Gastroenterology

Emily Gutowski

Contents

© The Author(s), under exclusive license to Springer Nature Switzerland AG 2021
S. H. Lecker, B. J. Chang (eds.), *The Ultimate Medical School Rotation Guide*,
https://doi.org/10.1007/978-3-030-63560-2_17

17.1 Overview

Gastroenterology is a fun and challenging rotation that will demonstrate the importance of a holistic patient evaluation. With so many organs falling within the purview of gastroenterology, you will learn an enormous amount about managing a range of conditions. GI is unique in its breadth: its issues range in severity and acuity, from acute to chronic; patients range from the very young to very old; and inpatient problems differ vastly from outpatient problems. During this rotation, you'll see life-threatening problems requiring urgent management as well as sequelae of chronic disease. You will also start to feel comfortable talking about some of the more "gross" functions of the human body—you may be deep in a discussion about a patient's diarrhea before you've even eaten breakfast, but soon this will start to feel routine! Many of these subjects can be uncomfortable or embarrassing for patients to talk about. That's part of what makes this field special: by providing comfort to patients who feel vulnerable or anxious, you can form a uniquely strong bond.

The GI service will differ significantly by hospital, depending on whether your hospital has a liver/hepatology service, the number and range of procedures you will see (e.g., colonoscopies, endoscopies, variceal banding, EUS, ERCP), and the variation in your patients' problem acuity. This chapter is designed to help you succeed on your GI rotation, no matter where on the spectrum it falls. It will take you through some of the fundamentals of gastroenterology, including how to conduct a GI-focused history and physical, vocabulary unique to GI, as well as diagnostic testing that you may see ordered. We will work through general approaches for common complaints that can prompt a gastroenterology consultation and then introduce several high-yield diagnoses with which you should be familiar when starting your rotation. While we won't be able to cover every problem, this chapter will give you the foundation you need to perform well on your rotation.

17.2 Gastroenterology-Focused History

As in all areas of internal medicine, the history is extremely important in gastroenterology. You may have heard that gastroenterologists are quick to scope patients to figure out what is going on, but this is not necessarily true, as you will soon see on your rotation! As the medical student, you have a bit more time to sit with the patient and ask the right questions. This may eliminate the need for a scope or make your team consider scoping the patient when they otherwise would not have done so.

Later in this chapter, specific, symptom-based history questions will be listed within the relevant chief complaint or suspected diagnosis. However, the following questions may be added for *any* GI consult:

- *GI-focused family history:*
    - Ask whether the patient has a family history of liver disease, peptic ulcer disease, *H. pylori* infection, pancreatitis, GI malignancy (if yes, obtain type, age of diagnosis, and relationship to patient), or inflammatory bowel disease (Crohn's disease or ulcerative colitis).
- *GI-focused social history:*
    - Alcohol use: Obtain a complete history of the patient's history of alcohol use. If they say they don't use alcohol, ask if they ever did in the past. How many drinks a day? What kind of alcohol? At what age did they start? When did they quit? Why did they quit? If they are currently drinking, have they ever tried to quit? Have they joined a support group? Have

they ever felt or been told that they have a problem with alcohol? Alcohol history is extremely important in patients with liver disease—an inaccurate history can lead you down a long road of unnecessary testing if in fact alcohol is the underlying etiology of the patient's disease. So, even if it is uncomfortable, try your best to get answers to these questions.
  - Needle use: Ask about illicit drug use, specifically intravenous drug use. Again, if they deny current use, inquire about previous use and follow the same line of questioning as above, always being gentle and respectful. Ask whether the patient has any tattoos and when they were obtained.
  - Tobacco use: Ask about and quantify the patient's tobacco use. Smoking is a risk factor for many malignancies.
  - Supplement use: Ask whether the patient has been using performance-enhancing supplements or herbal medications. Many of these can be hepatotoxic and patients may forget or intentionally omit these when listing medications.
  - Sexual history: Using sensitive questions, ask whether the patient is currently sexually active, with men, women, or both; whether they use protection; and how many partners they have had in the past year. High-risk sexual activities (in addition to needle exposure, as above) can put patients at risk of infections that can affect the liver, such as hepatitis B and C.
  - Occupational history: Ask about the patient's occupation. Several occupational exposures (e.g., vinyl chloride, used to produce PVC) can put patients at risk for liver pathology.
  - Ask about recent travel and sick contacts, which may be relevant in the case of infectious symptoms.
- *GI-focused review of systems and other questions:*
  - Bowel-related: Change in bowel movement frequency or character, diarrhea (specific diarrhea-focused questions appear later in this chapter), constipation, straining, black/tarry stool, bright red blood in stool, incontinence?
  - Headache, dizziness, difficulty swallowing, shortness of breath, chest pain, heartburn, abdominal pain, nausea/vomiting, urinary frequency, weight loss (intentional or unintentional, how much, over what period of time)?
  - Most recent colonoscopy?
  - Recent medication use including antibiotics, NSAIDs, herbal supplements, or performance-enhancing supplements?
  - Ask about menstrual history in women

17.3 Gastroenterology-Focused Abdominal Exam

Although gastroenterologists have advanced tools for imaging and scoping, your physical exam can provide a great deal of useful information to determine next steps. Perform your physical exam with an emphasis on the following:

17.3.1 Appearance

- *General appearance:*
    Just walking into the room and looking at the patient can tell you a lot. You can get a sense of whether they look uncomfortable, are in pain, or can

distract themselves: Are they reading? Talking to visitors? What is their body habitus? If their symptoms are chronic, they may have signs of malnutrition, such as temporal wasting.

— *Assess the volume status:*

Do they appear dehydrated (dry mucous membranes, concentrated urine in the Foley bag)? Take note of the vital signs on the bedside monitor: Do they suggest dehydration (tachycardia, hypotension)?

Ask the patient to lift up their gown so you can look at their abdomen. If possible, you should expose their chest as well. Take note of the following:

— *Patient's positioning:*

Is the patient uncomfortable lying flat? Does moving into position cause pain? These may be signs of peritonitis, as patients often prefer to lay perfectly still with their knees bent.

— *Distension:*

A distended abdomen is usually the result of accumulated gas or fluid. It is important to differentiate between distention and obesity, however. Ask the patient whether their abdomen looks different from their baseline. If the patient has known ascites, they may always have some degree of distension, but it should not be tense (we will get to this later in the exam).

— *Scaphoid abdomen:*

An abdomen that caves inward can be an indication of long-standing malnutrition. In a patient being evaluated for a gastrointestinal malignancy or chronic mesenteric ischemia, this may support your suspicion.

— *Scars:*

Is there evidence of prior surgery? Ask the patient about their surgical history and look for scars. These may be small if the patient has had laparoscopic surgery.

— *Stigmata of chronic liver disease:*

- Signs of hyperestrogenism and decreased circulating testosterone levels:
  - *Spider angiomata*: Flat, vascular lesions with thin projections branching outward, which blanch (turn skin-colored) when you press on them. These are often found on the upper chest and sometimes on the cheeks and abdomen.
  - *Palmar erythema*: The patient's palms may have a reddish appearance.
  - *Gynecomastia*: Males with chronic liver disease may have enlarged breasts.
- *Jaundice*: A yellowish tint to the skin caused by excess bilirubin in the blood. A general rule of thumb is that jaundice starts in the head and face region and moves downward with rising bilirubin levels. One of the first places jaundice can be seen is underneath the tongue. It can also be seen in the sclera of the eyes (termed "scleral icterus"). If the patient has darker skin, it may be hard to appreciate jaundice in the skin, so make sure you check in these areas.
- *Caput medusae*: Literally, "head of Medusa" in Latin, this is a physical exam sign describing the appearance of engorged epigastric veins surrounding the umbilicus. This is a sign of portal hypertension, a consequence of chronic liver disease.

17.3.2 Auscultation

The utility of auscultation during an abdominal exam goes beyond bowel sounds alone. It can also be helpful to observe the patient's response to pressure placed on the abdomen by the stethoscope. Even this degree of pressure may be painful, which is helpful to know for the rest of your exam. Warm your stethoscope for a few seconds beforehand by rubbing it on your shirt, and place your stethoscope in a few locations around the abdomen—you do not need to follow the four quadrants in this case, as sound travels throughout the abdomen. You can place the diaphragm of the stethoscope on the abdomen and leave it there, without holding it down. This way, there will be no sound interference from your hand.

You should be listening for the presence of bowel sounds, which can be gurgling, bubbling, popping, or squelching. Normally, these occur frequently (every few seconds). Infrequent bowel sounds are called "hypoactive," and more frequent bowel sounds are called "hyperactive." There is no definitive rule for these terms. Once you listen to a few normal abdomens in patients without GI complaints, you'll get a sense of what a hypoactive or hyperactive abdomen sounds like. If you don't hear anything at all, listen for at least 30 more seconds. Absent bowel sounds may indicate a paralytic ileus, or sometimes just constipation. Note any abnormal findings, such as high-pitched bowel sounds, which can indicate an intestinal obstruction, or a splashing or sloshing sound in the left upper quadrant, which can indicate delayed gastric emptying or a gastric outlet obstruction (depending on the timing of the last meal). None of these findings on their own will clinch the diagnosis, but they can be used to support your suspicion.

17.3.3 Percussion

After warming your hands and warning the patient that you'll be tapping on their belly, percuss in several locations around the abdomen. A gas-filled abdomen sounds tympanitic, while a stool-filled abdomen or one filled with fluid will be dull. Expect to hear tympany over the stomach; the rest will be variable. Take note of whether percussion causes the patient pain, which can indicate peritonitis (although you would expect them to have expressed this during auscultation already). Peritonitis is a physical exam sign that indicates inflammation of the peritoneum, usually caused by an infection such as acute pancreatitis, pyelonephritis, appendicitis, or diverticulitis. It may be accompanied by organ rupture.

You can use percussion to estimate the size of the liver or spleen: Starting far away from each of these organs (for the liver, inferior; for the spleen, in the right lower quadrant), percuss and expect to hear resonance or tympany. Gradually percuss your way towards the organ of interest, stopping every centimeter or so. There will be a transition to dullness once you are over the liver or spleen. Take note of whether this occurs below the costal margin—this can occasionally be normal for the liver but is abnormal for the spleen. Organomegaly is a very important finding in the physical exam. The *scratch test* can be used as a helpful correlate to percussion. This is performed by placing the stethoscope over the liver and lightly scratching the skin below the liver with your fingernail, gradually moving upward until you hear a dramatic increase in the volume of the scratching sound. This indicates that you have reached the liver edge. This process can be repeated by lightly scratching the skin just above the stethoscope until the scratching sound suddenly diminishes—this approximates the superior border of the liver. Make sure to move in the midclavicular line whenever assessing a patient's liver span.

You can also use percussion to determine the presence of ascites, using the *shifting dullness technique*, which takes advantage of the fact that the ascitic fluid settles to the most dependent area of the abdomen, while gas-filled intestines are at the surface: Percuss at the umbilicus and continue downward laterally. There should be tympany at first, but when you reach the ascites, the sound should become dull. Mark this transition point (ask the patient if you can draw a line on their belly with a pen or whether you can press your fingernail into their skin). Then, ask the patient to roll onto their side, and begin percussing again, this time starting at the side of their abdomen and continuing towards the umbilicus. The shift from tympany to dullness should change, as the ascites will have moved to a different area, following gravity.

17.3.4 Palpation

You will be palpating in all quadrants plus the epigastric region and umbilicus, with two different levels of pressure. Many clinicians like to place one hand over the other while pressing in each location. Ask the patient where their pain is, if present. Start as far away as possible from this location. Gently palpate by pressing the pads of your fingers into the abdomen. Follow the same technique in all regions. After your gentle palpation, repeat the process, but press down more firmly in each area. This will allow you to feel the deeper organs.

Watch the patient's face (i.e., don't just look at the abdomen) to see if they grimace or express pain when you palpate. Look for signs of peritonitis. These include rebound tenderness or pain upon removal of your hands from palpation as opposed to placement, and guarding, a tensing of the abdominal muscles which can occur voluntarily due to pain, or involuntarily. Involuntary guarding is synonymous with rigidity, which occurs in the setting of peritoneal inflammation. Another way to evaluate for peritonitis is to nudge the bed slightly and see whether this causes pain. In severe inflammation, even this degree of movement will be painful.

If there is only tenderness to deep but not light palpation, note this. Note the quadrant(s) where the pain occurs, as this can tell you which organ(s) may be at play. Keep in mind, however, that there can be referred pain (see ◘ Fig. 17.1), so the source may not be obvious. Feel for any masses or organomegaly, and check whether you can feel the abdominal aorta, which will be pulsating. You should also be getting a sense of whether the patient's abdomen feels distended. If the patient has ascites, determine whether the abdomen is tense: if so, they may need a therapeutic paracentesis to relieve some of the pressure caused by built-up fluid.

If you want to feel the liver edge (e.g., to evaluate for organomegaly or attempt to feel nodularity in a patient with cirrhosis), place your hand under the right costal margin, with your pointer alongside the bottom rib. Ask the patient to take a deep breath in, and as they do so, press your hand into the abdomen. The liver should move downward with inhalation, allowing for easier palpation. This is quite a difficult maneuver, especially if the patient's liver size is normal or fibrotic (often smaller), so don't worry if you are not successful.

If the patient suddenly stops inhaling due to pain with palpation, this is known as a positive *Murphy's sign* and is associated with cholecystitis. The sonographic Murphy's sign is the equivalent response when an ultrasound probe is placed in the same location.

To distinguish abdominal wall pain from pain originating from the abdominal cavity, you can ask the patient to tense the abdominal muscles by performing an abdominal crunch. If the pain remains the same or worsens on palpation, this is known as a positive *Carnett's sign* and points towards an abdominal wall

Note: If you feel a hard mass in the left lower quadrant, this may be stool!

17

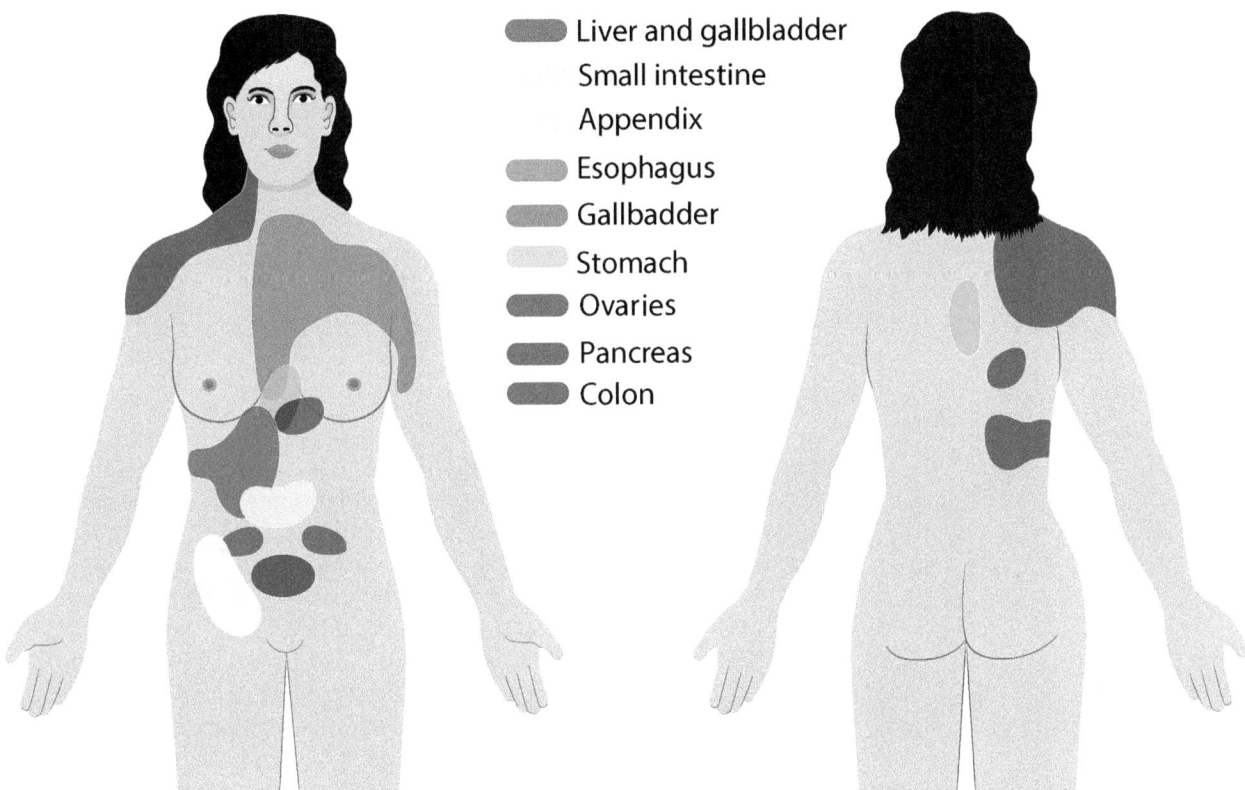

Legend:
- Liver and gallbladder
- Small intestine
- Appendix
- Esophagus
- Gallbadder
- Stomach
- Ovaries
- Pancreas
- Colon

Fig. 17.1 Distribution of referred pain from intra- and extra-abdominal organs

etiology, whereas a negative result (pain with palpation decreasing with abdominal tensing) makes an intra-abdominal cause more likely.

The spleen is not typically palpable in healthy adults. However, if you suspect splenomegaly based on the patient's medical history or your percussion exam, you may be able to palpate it. Start at the right lower quadrant and gently (using superficial and not deep palpation) move towards the left upper quadrant. After you reposition your hand each time, ask the patient to take a deep breath and wait for the spleen tip to touch your fingers. There are several variations to this technique that you may be shown, but it's best to wait for guidance on these as repeated rough examinations can cause trauma to the spleen.

17.3.5 Additions for Liver Disease

For a patient with suspected or confirmed liver disease, there are a few additional components to the physical exam that it is important to include. We already went through the stigmata of chronic liver disease you can see while evaluating the patient's appearance.

■ ■ Hepatic Encephalopathy

Evaluate for *hepatic encephalopathy (HE)*, neurologic dysfunction that occurs with severe liver disease. HE is graded in severity from 0 to 4, and the first sign can be inattention or an altered sleep pattern. It can progress to lethargy and to coma (■ Table 17.1).

- Start with a mental status exam. Ask the patient to tell you their name, the date, and their location. Test attention by asking them to repeat three words back to you immediately. Tell them you'll be asking them to perform a series of mental exercises that might sound silly. Ask them to spell a word

Table 17.1 Grading system for hepatic encephalopathy

Grade 0	No changes in behavior
Grade 1	Mild confusion, disordered sleep, slurred speech, altered behavior
Grade 2	Moderate confusion, lethargy, inappropriate behavior, subtle changes in personality
Grade 3	Confusion, stupor, disorientation, incoherent speech, but responsive to stimuli
Grade 4	Coma, unresponsive to verbal and noxious stimuli

backwards ("WORLD" is commonly used). Ask the patient to tell you the days of the week backwards. If they can do this, progress to the months of the year backwards and then counting backwards from 100 by 7. These tasks test attention and are progressively harder for patients with HE. Inattention is a cognitive component of HE, in contrast to physical components such as asterixis.

- Check for *asterixis*, another manifestation of HE, which is characterized by an inability to maintain tone. Ask the patient to hold up their hands like they're stopping traffic. Their hands should be extended as far back as possible. If you see involuntary quick movements of the hand downward, this is asterixis. Make sure to distinguish this from a tremor. If you are not sure, you can also ask the patient to grasp two of your fingers (pointer and middle finger) on each hand. Tell them to squeeze hard and pull your hands lightly upwards. If asterixis is present, there will be intermittent involuntary release and your fingers will start to come out of the patient's grip.

■■ Check for Edema

Ascites in the abdomen is not the only place where excess fluid builds up in liver disease; the patient may be third-spacing elsewhere. Edema tends to build up in dependent areas. These can include the lower extremities, the back (termed "sacral edema" and especially likely if the patient has been in bed for several days), and the scrotum (termed "scrotal edema"). Take note of how far up the edema goes—you may not be used to this degree of edema. Start at the foot, and press down on a bony area for several seconds. See if your finger leaves an indentation when you release it. If so, it is termed "pitting edema." Not all edema is pitting, but you are more likely to see pitting edema in patients with liver disease as it is caused by fluid retention. In pitting edema, a grading system from 1+ to 4+ is used, for example "3+ pitting edema to the mid-shin." Though each grade does not have an official definition, many clinicians use 1+ to mean a 2 mm depression, 2+ to mean a 4 mm depression, and so on. Take note of the approximate depth of indentation and follow the same process every few inches moving upward along the tibia. The edema may appear to end at the knee, but make sure to check behind the thighs, as well as the lower back, where a lot of fluid may be hiding.

■■ Digital Rectal Exam

See ▶ Sect. 17.8 for indications and steps for the digital rectal exam.

17.4 Unique Vocabulary

As is the case with most subspecialties, gastroenterology has its own unique set of vocabulary. On day 1, when you hear about patients on the GI service, many of these terms will likely be used, and it can feel overwhelming and confusing. For that reason, it can be very helpful to review some of this terminology beforehand. By no means do you need to remember the details of each scoring system or equation, but you should have a general idea of when they are used and what they mean. You can always look up the specifics online if you are calculating a patient's score.

17.4.1 Scoring Systems and Calculations

- *AIMS65 score:* A scoring system to determine the risk of mortality from upper gastrointestinal bleeding. This score takes into account (and gets its name from) the patient's *a*lbumin, *I*NR, *m*ental status, *s*ystolic blood pressure, and whether they are over age *65*.
- *BISAP score*: A scoring system to predict mortality risk in acute pancreatitis, which takes into account the patient's *B*UN, *i*mpairment of mental status, *S*IRS criteria, *a*ge, and presence of *p*leural effusion.
- *Child-Pugh score*, often referred to as "Child Class": A scoring system for prognosis of patients with cirrhosis, which assigns patients a class from A to C with associated life expectancy. This score takes into account the patient's bilirubin, albumin, prothrombin time or INR, presence of ascites, and the presence or absence of hepatic encephalopathy. A helpful memory aid is *ABCDE*, where A is albumin, B is bilirubin, C is clotting (prothrombin time or INR), D is distention (ascites), and E is encephalopathy.
- *Lille score/Lille Model:* A scoring system to predict mortality in patients with alcoholic hepatitis who have been receiving steroid therapy for 7 days and are not improving. This score predicts mortality rates within 6 months, as well as the utility in continuing steroid administration beyond 7 days. It takes into account the patient's age, albumin, bilirubin on days 1 and 7, creatinine, and PT.
- *Maddrey's Discriminant Function*, often referred to as "DF": A number used to evaluate the severity and prognosis in alcoholic hepatitis and to determine whether the patient may benefit from steroid administration. This number takes into account the patient's prothrombin time (PT) and total bilirubin. Scores over 32 suggest a poor prognosis and a potential benefit of steroids.
- *MELD (Model for End-Stage Liver Disease) Score*: A scoring system to stratify the severity of liver disease, typically used for transplant planning purposes. Estimates 3-month mortality. Ranges from ≤9 (1.9% mortality) to 40 (71.3% mortality). This score takes into account the patient's creatinine, bilirubin, INR, sodium, and dialysis status.
- *Milan criteria:* A scoring system that assesses the candidacy of patients with hepatocellular cancer and cirrhosis for liver transplantation. Takes into account the tumor number and diameter, as well as the presence of extrahepatic and vascular involvement.
- *Rome IV criteria:* A scoring system to diagnose irritable bowel syndrome (IBS). To have a positive result, patients must have recurrent abdominal pain 1+ day per week in the last 3 months, associated with 2 of the following: relation to defecation, change in stool frequency, or change in stool

form. Additionally, there should be no warning signs (e.g., unintentional weight loss, iron deficiency anemia) present.

- *SAAG (serum ascites albumin gradient):* A calculation to determine whether or not the likely cause of a patient's ascites is portal hypertension. This number takes into account the concentration of albumin in the patient's serum and ascitic fluid. The equation is as follows:

SAAG = (serum albumin concentration) – (ascites albumin concentration)

If the result is greater than or equal to 1.1 g/dL, it is likely that portal hypertension is the cause of the ascites. Non-portal hypertension-related etiologies of ascites include peritoneal carcinomatosis, hypoalbuminemia, and tuberculous peritonitis, among others (for a more comprehensive list, see ◘ Table 17.8). Within each category, you can further narrow your differential based on the total protein content in the ascitic fluid.

17.4.2 Endoscopy Terminology

Although you will not be directly involved in scoping, it's helpful to know what to look out for when you shadow in the endoscopy suite and to be familiar with the terminology when presenting patients.

- *High-risk stigmata of bleeding from esophageal varices:* Signs on upper endoscopy of either recent bleeding or tendency to bleed. These include:
  - Cherry red spot: circular red marking
  - Red wale sign: red streak overlying a varix
  - White nipple sign: a platelet fibrin clot at the site of a recent variceal hemorrhage
- *Forrest classification for bleeding peptic ulcers:* A scoring system ranging from Forrest 1A (most severe—spurting arterial bleed) to Forrest 3 (least severe—clean ulcer with no evidence of recent bleeding). Used to stratify the severity of upper GI bleeding due to peptic ulcers based on characteristics such as the appearance of the ulcer and the presence of active bleeding. Provides information on the risk of rebleeding and death and can be used to make management decisions.
- *Portal hypertensive gastropathy (PHG):* A condition causing a "snakeskin" appearance of the gastric mucosa, resulting from portal hypertension. This can result in chronic or, less commonly, acute bleeding. Treatment is focused on the underlying portal hypertension. Can be mistaken for GAVE.
- *GAVE (gastric antral vascular ectasia)* or "watermelon stomach": A condition in which the stomach lining develops friable erythematous linear markings, similar in appearance to a watermelon rind. Uncommon cause of UGIB. Associated with cirrhosis and treated with thermoablation. Can be mistaken for PHG.
- *Polyp terminology:* Colorectal polyps can be classified based on histologic features, gross appearance, and malignant potential. Non-neoplastic polyps, which possess no malignant potential, include hyperplastic polyps, hamartomas, lymphoid aggregates, and inflammatory polyps. Contrastingly, adenomas (neoplastic polyps) have a range of malignant potential. They can be classified histologically based on factors such as the amount of villous tissue present: Tubular adenomas have the least amount of villous tissue, followed by tubulovillous adenomas and lastly villous adenomas. Advanced adenomas possess greater degrees of dysplasia, villous components, and a larger size. Adenomas can further be classified based on their gross architecture. Pedunculated polyps possess a narrow stalk connecting the polyp to the colonic wall. Sessile polyps lack this stalk and are flat in appearance on endoscopy.

17

17.5 Lab Interpretation

17.5.1 Liver Function Test (LFT) Abnormalities

In gastroenterology, certain telltale patterns in lab values are very important to recognize. Sometimes, an abnormal liver function test result is the sole reason for a GI consultation. This is a place where you can really shine as a med student. Whereas the other members of the care team may not have as much time to analyze the labs closely each morning, you can take a few extra minutes and notice a certain trend in the numbers, thereby shortening the time to diagnosis and appropriate management for your patient.

One equation that is helpful to calculate is the *R ratio* or *R factor*:

$$R\,ratio = \left(\frac{ALT}{ULN}\right) / \left(\frac{AP}{ULN}\right)$$

where ULN is the upper limit of normal for each respective value and AP is the alkaline phosphatase. The table below outlines some of the patterns you may see, and the *R ratio* can be used to help distinguish between them (◻ Table 17.2).

17.5.2 Viral Hepatitis Antibody Interpretation

Looking at viral hepatitis studies can feel like you are swimming in alphabet soup. The tables and graph below can serve as a helpful guide to interpreting your patients' antibody studies. More background information on viral hepatitis is provided later in this chapter, under "Viral Hepatitis."

◻ **Table 17.2** Patterns of liver function test abnormalities

Type	Labs	Causes	Other considerations
Hepatocellular injury	AST and ALT elevation more pronounced than bilirubin and alkaline phosphatase (AP) elevation *R ratio* > 5	◻ Medications, including acetaminophen, anti-epileptics, statins, antibiotics, illicit drugs, and many others ◻ Alcohol typically causes a modest rise in AST and ALT, usually in a > 2:1 AST/ALT ratio ◻ Other causes include non-alcoholic steatohepatitis (NASH), viral hepatitis (which may also have elevated bilirubin), hemochromatosis, right-sided heart failure causing hepatic congestion, and other less common causes	Consider the degree of AST/ALT elevation ◻ *Mild elevations* (low hundreds) suggest chronic viral hepatitis or acute alcohol related hepatitis ◻ *Moderate elevations* (high hundreds) suggest acute viral hepatitis ◻ *Extreme elevations* (>1000): Importantly, only a few processes can cause extreme rises. These most commonly include ischemic hepatitis (shock liver), acute viral hepatitis, autoimmune hepatitis, drug or toxin induced liver injury, and sometimes biliary obstruction or other rare conditions *Clinical pearls:* ◻ Ischemic hepatitis has a characteristic rise in AST and ALT first, *followed by* a rise in bilirubin about a week later. Look out for this pattern! ◻ Ischemic hepatitis and acetaminophen toxicity often have an ALT:LDH ratio of <1.5
Cholestatic injury	AP elevation more pronounced than AST and ALT *R ratio* < 2	◻ Bile duct obstruction (see ▶ Sect. 17.7.2) ◻ Many of the causes of hepatocellular injury, such as hepatitis, cirrhosis, and medications or toxins	

(continued)

Table 17.2 (continued)

Type	Labs	Causes	Other considerations
Infiltrative process	Isolated AP elevation	☐ Sarcoidosis, amyloidosis, tuberculosis, or malignancy, among others	When an infiltrative pattern is seen, check the GGT to confirm that the source is hepatobiliary. AP elevation can be caused by organs other than the hepatobiliary system, including bone, intestine, and placenta, so make sure to rule out these as causes if the GGT is not elevated. (Similarly, AST is made not only in the liver but also in muscle, kidney, brain, and red blood cells, so an isolated AST elevation may not be hepatic in origin.)
Indirect hyperbilirubine-mia	Elevated indirect>direct bilirubin	☐ Hemolysis, Gilbert's syndrome, resorption of blood after trauma	

Table 17.3 Interpretation of hepatitis A testing

Anti-HAV IgM	Anti-HAV IgG	Possible interpretation
−	−	No current or previous HAV infection, although possibly in incubation period. No immunity
−	+	No active HAV infection. Immunity is present due to either prior infection or vaccination
Not performed	+	Exposure to HAV via either infection or vaccination. Acute infection cannot be ruled out (need negative Anti HAV IgM)
+	±	Acute or recent HAV infection

17.5.2.1 Hepatitis A

Anti-HAV IgM can be detected 2 weeks after exposure and goes away weeks to months after infection (Table 17.3). Anti-HAV IgG appears later, at around 8–12 weeks after infection, and typically remains positive.

17.5.2.2 Hepatitis B

In general, initial tests for HBV antibodies consist of HBsAg, anti-HBs, and anti-HBc (Fig. 17.2). Depending on the results of these tests, you may want to order specific follow-up testing (shaded gray in the table (Table 17.4).)

HBsAg is the hepatitis B surface antigen, which can be detected during acute or chronic infection, and indicates that a patient is infectious. *Anti-HBs* is the hepatitis B surface antibody, produced in response to the presence of HBsAg. It indicates immunity from HBV, either through recovery from a prior infection or successful vaccination.

Anti-HBc is the total hepatitis B core antibody, a nonspecific marker which appears early in HBV infection and persists for life. Its presence indicates prior or current infection but does not establish a time frame. Anti-HBc is absent in patients who are immune from vaccination alone. *Anti-HBc IgM*, in contrast, does provide hints about timing, indicating a recent infection in the past 6 months and acute infection.

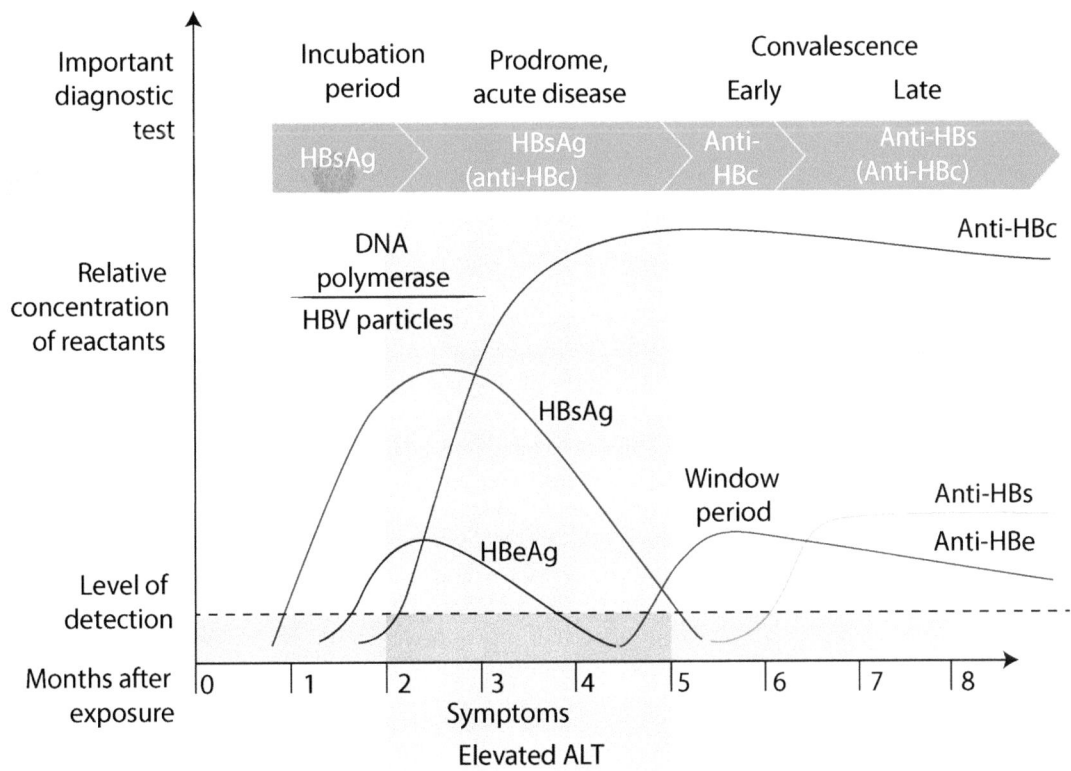

◻ Fig. 17.2 Timeline of hepatitis B testing

◻ Table 17.4 Interpretation of hepatitis B testing

HBsAg	Anti-HBs	Anti-HBc	Anti-HBc IgM	HBeAg	Anti-HBe	HBV DNA	Possible interpretation
–	–	–					No current or prior HBV infection, although may be in incubation period. No immunity
–	+	–					Immunity from successful vaccination
–	+	+					Immunity from prior HBV infection
–	–	+					Four possibilities: resolved infection; false-positive anti-HBc; low level chronic infection; resolving acute infection
+	–	±	+	+	–	±	Acute HBV infection. If no HBV DNA, likely within first month
–	–	+	+	–	+	–	Resolving acute HBV infection
+	–	+	–	+	–	+	Active chronic infection. Likely with liver damage
+	–	+	–	–	+	– or low level	Low level chronic infection. Low risk of liver damage

Table 17.5 Interpretation of hepatitis C testing

Anti-HCV	HCV RNA	Possible interpretation
−	Not performed	Either no HCV infection or too early to detect antibodies. If exposure is suspected, check HCV RNA or retest at a later time
+	−	No current HCV infection (either prior infection or false positive)
+	+	Current HCV infection

HBeAg, or hepatitis B envelope antigen, becomes detectable early in HBV infection and correlates with infectivity. During recovery, levels decrease as *anti-HBe*, the antibody made in response, becomes detectable. In chronic HBV infection, HBeAg can remain positive, indicating viral replication.

HBV DNA is a measure of viral load and reflects HBV virus replication. Levels can be detected by 1 month following infection, peak during acute infection, and disappear in cases that spontaneously resolve. In chronic HBV infection, however, HBV DNA levels may remain high (in chronic active infection) or stay low (in chronic inactive infection). Antiviral treatment decisions are often made with the HBV DNA level in mind.

Keep in mind that there are exceptions to these rules (e.g., HBeAg-negative chronic hepatitis B), but this information should give you the tools you need to start engaging with your team about viral hepatitis lab interpretation.

17.5.2.3 Hepatitis C

HCV RNA can be detected as soon as 2–3 weeks after infection, while HCV antibodies take 4–12 weeks to appear (◘ Table 17.5). There is currently no vaccine for hepatitis C.

17.6 GI-Specific Diagnostic Testing

The range of diagnostic testing in gastroenterology can be particularly overwhelming. There are subtle differences between different types of scopes and confusing combinations of letters that sound similar. Below are some of the tests you may see ordered on your patients.

- *Upper GI series* or *barium swallow*: A series of x-rays using fluoroscopy. Images the esophagus, stomach, and duodenum. The patient swallows contrast (usually barium) and x-ray images are taken during the swallow (◘ Fig. 17.3). This is used to evaluate for structural and functional abnormalities, e.g., dysphagia.
- *MRCP (magnetic resonance cholangiopancreatography):* A noninvasive imaging technique that uses MRI to view the biliary and pancreatic ducts (◘ Fig. 17.4). Used to investigate causes of biliary obstruction and identify structural abnormalities. May include IV contrast.
- *ERCP (endoscopic retrograde cholangiopancreatography):* A diagnostic and therapeutic endoscopic procedure in which the scope is positioned in the duodenum, and contrast and fluoroscopy are used to image structures such as the bile ducts and pancreatic ducts. Indications include diagnosis of ampullary cancer, stone removal, sphincterotomy, relief of biliary obstruction, stent

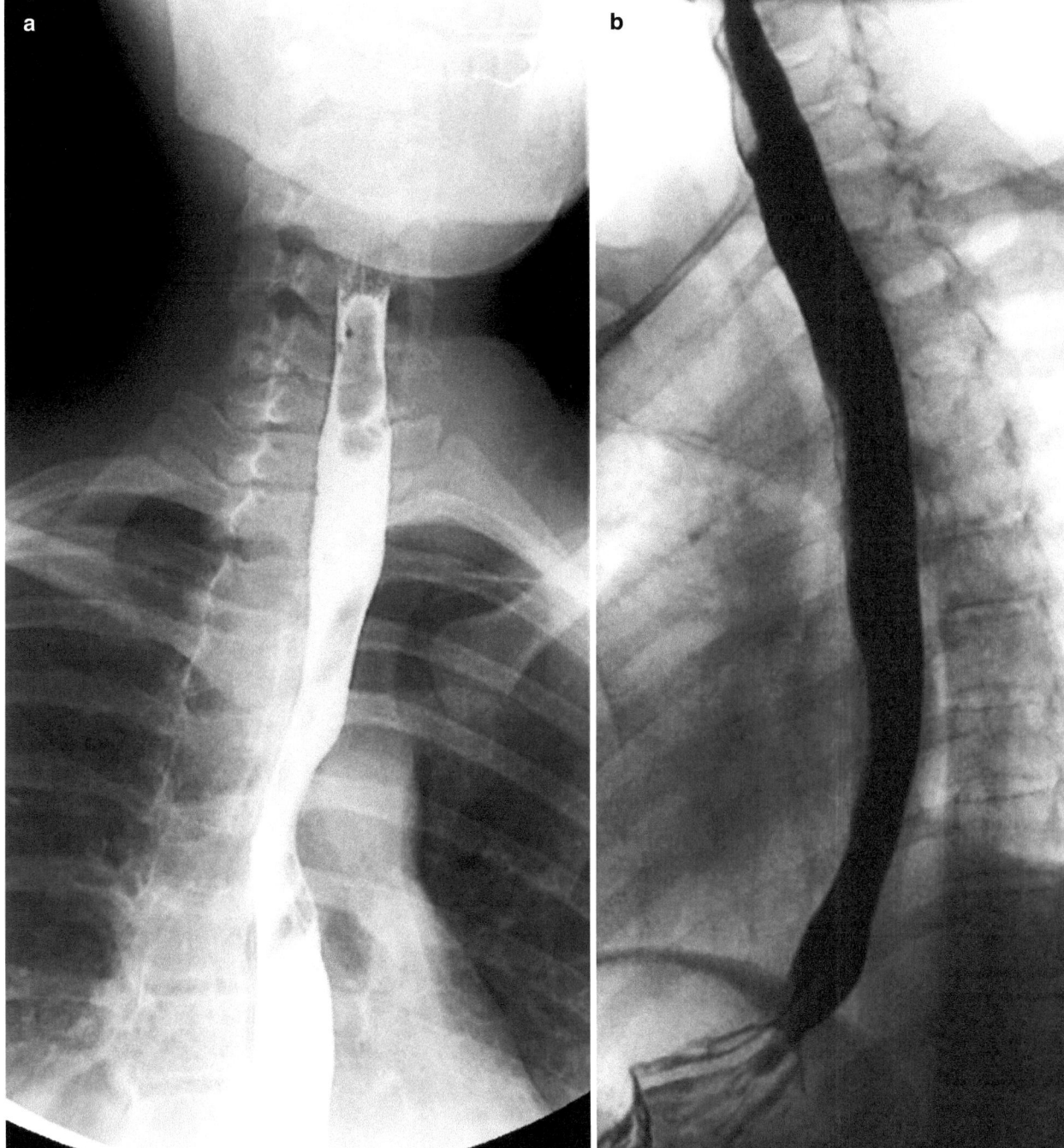

🔲 **Fig. 17.3   a, b** Sample images from a normal barium swallow

placement, and many more. Important complications include post-ERCP pancreatitis and intestinal perforation.

- *CT colonography (CTC,* also known as virtual colonoscopy): A radiologic exam performed for screening every 5 years, in which thin-slice CT is used to construct a 3D image of the bowel (🔲 Fig. 17.5). This test requires the same bowel preparation as a colonoscopy (but is not performed under sedation), and residual stool can appear the same as a mass, requiring further endoscopic follow-up. If a mass or polyp is found on CTC, the patient will require a colonoscopy.

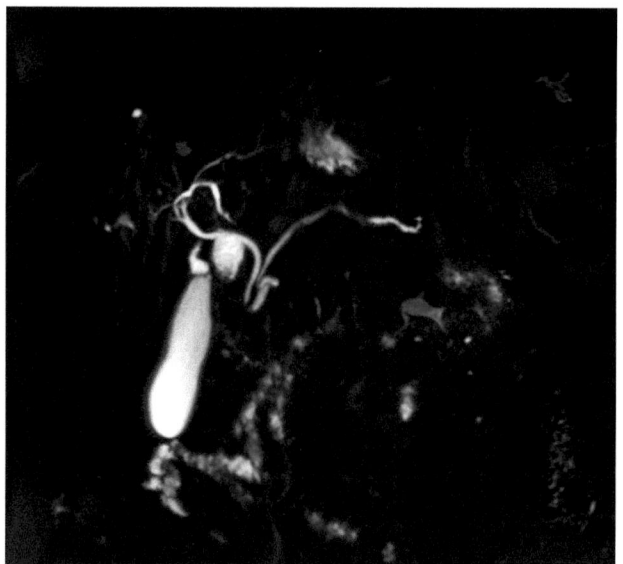

Fig. 17.4 Sample image from MRCP showing gallbladder and biliary tree

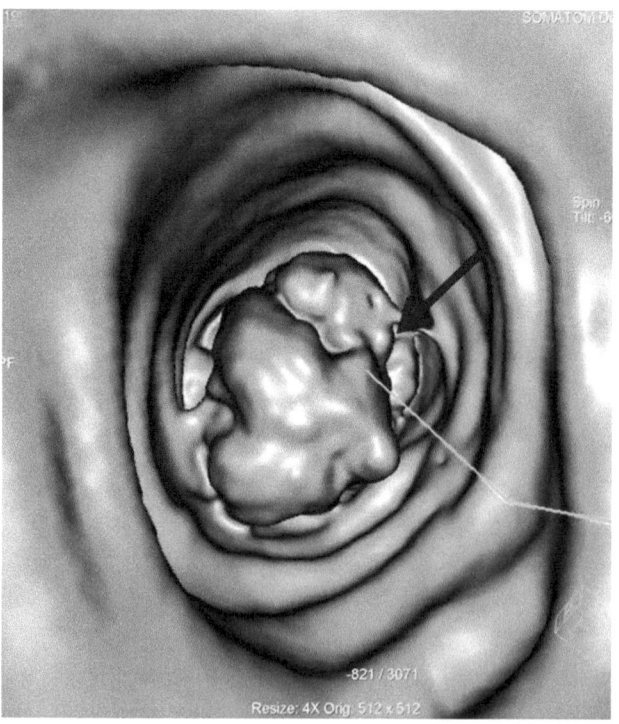

Fig. 17.5 CT colonography image showing adenocarcinoma. (From Sun K, et al. Accuracy of combined computed tomography colonography and dual energy iodine map imaging for detecting colorectal masses using high-pitch dual-source CT. *Sci Rep.* 2018;3790)

- *EGD (esophagogastroduodenoscopy) (upper endoscopy):* A procedure, typically performed under sedation, in which a camera attached to a flexible tube is advanced from the mouth through the esophagus and stomach to the duodenum. The performing physician can perform concurrent procedures including biopsy, resection, variceal banding, electrocautery, or dilation of a stricture. EGD is used for a variety of indications, including unexplained anemia or dysphagia, diagnosis of peptic ulcer disease,

Barrett's esophagus, celiac disease, and malignancy. It can also be used for foreign body removal.

- *Push enteroscopy:* This procedure is similar to an EGD but the scope is longer and thus allows visibility further into the small intestine.
- *EUS (endoscopic ultrasound)*: A minimally invasive imaging procedure whereby an endoscope with attached ultrasound probe is positioned in the duodenum and an ultrasound image is obtained. This is used for imaging the pancreaticobiliary tree and often performed alongside fine-needle aspiration (FNA) or biopsy. EUS can also be used to investigate submucosal masses in the esophagus or stomach and to stage esophageal, gastric, or rectal cancers.
- *Colonoscopy:* A procedure, typically performed under sedation, in which a camera attached to a flexible tube is advanced from the rectum as far as the terminal ileum. Imaged regions include the rectum, sigmoid colon, descending colon, transverse colon, ascending colon, and cecum. The performing physician can perform concurrent procedures including biopsy, resection, or electrocautery. Colonoscopy is used for a variety of indications, including unexplained anemia, diagnosis of inflammatory bowel disease, diverticulosis, and colorectal cancer screening. This test requires the patient to undergo preparation with laxatives to ensure the colon is free of fecal matter.
- *Sigmoidoscopy* (also known as flexible sigmoidoscopy): A procedure in which a camera attached to a flexible tube is advanced from the rectum as far as the sigmoid colon. It is similar to colonoscopy but can be performed without sedation and with a reduced bowel preparation (typically an enema prior to the procedure). Often, it is followed by colonoscopy if there are abnormal findings.
- *Anoscopy:* A procedure in which a rigid tube with a camera attached is inserted several inches into the anus. Indications include rectal bleeding, anorectal mass, and incontinence. No sedation or preparation is required for this procedure.
- *Balloon-assisted/"deep" enteroscopy* (includes double- and single-balloon enteroscopy): Similar to push enteroscopy, but uses balloon inflation/deflation to advance the endoscope far into the GI tract. This procedure generally permits visualization of the entire small intestine and can also be used from below, starting in the lower GI tract, to access the distal small bowel in a retrograde approach.
- *Pill/capsule endoscopy:* A diagnostic procedure in which the patient swallows a camera encased in a pill-shaped capsule. The camera takes images as it is passed through the digestive system. A common indication is suspected small intestinal bleeding if the team has been unable to visualize a source through traditional scoping methods (i.e., EGD and colonoscopy).
- *HIDA scan* (hepatobiliary iminodiacetic acid scan, also known as cholescintigraphy): An imaging procedure in which a radioactive tracer is injected intravenously and travels to the gallbladder. Images are sequentially captured over 2 hours. If there is no obstruction, the gallbladder fills with tracer. This is typically used to diagnose an obstruction in the gallbladder (often used specifically for acute cholecystitis) if ultrasound findings are equivocal.
- *Stool-based CRC screening tests* can be done in the patient's home and do not require bowel preparation. The *fecal immunochemical test (FIT)* is performed annually and detects hemoglobin in the blood. Patients provide one stool sample for this test. The *guaiac-based fecal occult blood test (gFOBT)*, also performed annually, requires patients to apply stool samples to guaiac

cards from three consecutive bowel movements. Lastly, *multitarget stool DNA test with FIT (FIT-DNA)* is a molecular assay to test for DNA mutations associated with colorectal cancer combined with a FIT assay that detects hemoglobin. This test is usually performed every 3 years and the patient provides one stool sample.

17.7 Chief Complaints and Diagnoses: Approach To ...

Now that we've gone through some of the fundamentals, let's move on to chief complaints and diagnoses. We will cover some of the most common reasons you will be consulted and focus on how to approach each category. You will learn an approach to the evaluation of: *abdominal pain, diarrhea, dysphagia, GI bleeding, and liver pathology.* Each of these sections will have subsections covering the presentation, diagnosis, and management of some of the most common associated diagnoses. We won't be able to cover everything you'll see on this rotation, but rather will emphasize the most high-yield information.

17.7.1 Abdominal Pain

Evaluating a patient's abdominal pain is one of the core skills you will learn on this rotation. The character, location, radiation, timing, and severity of the pain can tell you a lot about what is going on. There are three types of pain you should think about when seeing your patient: *visceral, somatic/parietal, and referred pain.* The differences have to do with the type of nerve transmission causing each type of pain, with unmyelinated C fibers causing visceral pain and myelinated A-delta fibers causing parietal pain. Referred pain is caused by an interplay between the two.

Visceral pain occurs when there is activation of the pain receptors on the organs themselves and is diffuse and hard to localize. In contrast, *parietal pain* is due to irritation of the parietal peritoneal wall. This is much easier to localize and generally occurs later in a disease course. An example of the progression from visceral to parietal pain is appendicitis: You may have learned that early in its course, patients may describe a pain around the umbilicus. Later, if things progress without management, they will start to feel pain in the right lower quadrant. The same area is being affected the whole time, but only when the appendix gets inflamed enough to touch the parietal peritoneum do patients begin to feel pain in a localizable place.

Referred pain is another important aspect of abdominal pain. This is a type of pain that is present in one area of the body but actually originating in an entirely different area. This occurs when the organ of interest is innervated by a nerve from the same dermatome as the referred pain. An example is gallbladder pain referring to the right shoulder. There are well-known referred pain locations, which you can see in ◘ Fig. 17.1. Keep this in mind when asking about the patient's pain.

Clinical pearl: Always consider gynecologic causes of pain in women. Ask about the patient's sexual and menstrual history, possibility of pregnancy, and use of contraception.

■ History-Taking for Abdominal Pain

OPQRST mnemonic:
- *Onset*—When did this start? What were you doing at the time of onset?
    - This can give you clues as to the etiology of the pain. For example, epigastric pain while eating can suggest a peptic ulcer, whereas epigastric pain that improves with food is more consistent with a duodenal ulcer (due to release of pancreatic bicarbonate secretions into the duodenum).

- *Provocation/previous episodes*—Does anything make it better or worse (certain type of food or positioning)? Has this ever happened before?
  - For example, fatty foods tend to exacerbate the pain from cholelithiasis, as the gallbladder contracts against an obstruction to release bile in order to help digest the fat. In acute pancreatitis, patients sometimes say that leaning forward helps to relieve the pain.
  - Asking about a previous episode can tell you a lot about the prior workup, if any, as well as therapies that have helped in the past.
- *Quality*—What does it feel like? Is it sharp, dull, burning, shooting, cramping, etc.?
  - A cramping pain suggests that the aggravating factor is intermittent, for example arising from peristaltic waves.
- *Radiation*—Where does the pain start, and does it travel anywhere?
  - For example, epigastric pain radiating to the back can be a sign of acute pancreatitis. This can also be a time when referred pain comes into the picture. Patients may complain of pain in their shoulder when the origin is in the gallbladder. Or, they may say the pain starts in the right upper quadrant area and radiates to the shoulder.
- *Severity*—How would you grade the pain from 1 to 10, 10 being the worst pain of your life?
- *Timing*—Is this happening all the time or intermittently? Is it worse at a certain time of day?
  - If a patient states that the pain is worst at night, this could mean that it is after eating a large dinner, or after laying down horizontally. Try to parse apart these details.
- *Associated symptoms/ROS*—See (▶ Sect. 17.2) for a full list.

See ▶ Sect. 17.3 for guidance on a comprehensive abdominal examination.

- ■ High-Yield Diagnoses for Abdominal Pain

Acute Pancreatitis

Acute pancreatitis ranges widely in severity, from mild edematous to severe necrotizing cases. The mnemonic *I GET SMASHED* can be used to remember some of the causes of acute pancreatitis (*i*diopathic, *g*allstones, *e*thanol, *t*rauma, *s*moking, *m*umps, *a*utoimmune, *s*corpion poison, *h*ypercalcemia/hypertriglyceridemia, *E*RCP, *d*rugs), but the most common etiologies are gallstones (or sludge), alcohol, and hypertriglyceridemia (typically with values over 1000 mg/dL). Patients often present with abdominal pain as their main symptom, typically in the epigastric region and radiating to the back. They may also have nausea and vomiting. Most cases are mild and resolve with supportive care, but 20% of patients have more severe cases and experience complications like those listed below. Many patients develop systemic inflammatory response syndrome (SIRS), the criteria of which include vital sign and laboratory abnormalities. The *BISAP score* (see ▶ Sect. 17.4) can be used to predict mortality in patients with acute pancreatitis.

The most common etiologies of acute pancreatitis are gallstones/sludge, alcohol, and hypertriglyceridemia.

Diagnosis: To diagnose acute pancreatitis, a patient must have *2 of the following 3 criteria*:
1. Consistent clinical picture (acute, severe epigastric pain radiating to the back; nausea and vomiting)
2. Serum lipase (or amylase) > 3x the upper limit of normal
3. Imaging findings consistent with acute pancreatitis

If the first 2 of these criteria is normal, there is no need to obtain imaging to diagnose acute pancreatitis. However, if imaging is required, the first choice should be an abdominal CT with IV contrast. Other labs and diagnostic studies can help determine the cause of pancreatitis. These can include CBC, BMP, LFTs, fasting triglycerides, and right upper quadrant ultrasound (RUQUS).

■■ Treatment

For initial management, remember three things: *fluids, pain control, and NPO.* Patients with acute pancreatitis lose a lot of *fluids* through third spacing and can get hypovolemic quickly. For those with severe volume depletion, guidelines suggest starting with an IV fluid bolus (20 cc/kg) over 30 minutes followed by maintenance rates of 3 cc/kg/hr for the first 12 hours. To ensure you are resuscitating adequately, target a goal heart rate of <120 bpm, MAP 65–85, urine output over 1 cc/kg/hr, and a reduction in hematocrit and BUN. For the patient's *pain*, opioids such as fentanyl are effective, sometimes administered via a patient-controlled anesthesia pump (PCA). Avoid morphine as it can cause increased pressure in the sphincter of Oddi. It is also extremely important to address the underlying etiology and reverse the culprit. (For example, a patient with gallstone pancreatitis should get a cholecystectomy after recovery.) Patients should be made *NPO* initially but can resume a soft diet within 24 hours if pancreatitis is mild. In severe cases in which patients are unable to tolerate a diet after 72 hours of bowel rest, they may require enteral nutrition via a nasogastric (NG) or nasojejunal (NJ) tube. If the cause of the patient's pancreatitis is biliary obstruction or if cholangitis is present, an ERCP may be indicated.

■■ Complications

If the patient has a severe case of acute pancreatitis or is deteriorating, look for pancreatic necrosis (sterile or infected, the latter of which is a major cause of morbidity and mortality) with a contrast-enhanced abdominal CT. Other complications can be thought about in terms of timing: *peripancreatic fluid collections* occur within the 4 weeks following an episode of pancreatitis, while *pseudocysts*, which are well-defined fluid filled sacs, arise after 4 weeks. Vascular complications can occur acutely, including superior mesenteric, splenic, and portal vein thromboses. Lastly, there is a risk for *acute respiratory distress syndrome (ARDS)*, which should be suspected if the patient develops respiratory distress and hypoxia. Importantly, 10% of acute pancreatitis cases will progress to chronic pancreatitis. Chronic pancreatitis will not be discussed in this chapter as it is not likely to be encountered primarily as an acute inpatient issue.

□ Initial checklist for acute pancreatitis

Dx	Tx (varies based on Dx results)
□ CBC, CMP □ LFTs □ Lipase, amylase □ Lipids (fasting) □ Lactate □ RUQUS to rule out gallstones □ Consider CT w/ contrast, MRCP if concern for retained CBD stone	□ Reverse electrolyte abn and underlying etiology □ IV fluids □ NPO for now □ Pain control (consider PCA) □ If gallstone pancreatitis, consult surgery for?cholecystectomy

17.7.2 Biliary Pathology

This section will cover four causes of biliary pathology: *cholelithiasis, cholecystitis, choledocholithiasis,* and *cholangitis (□ Fig. 17.6).* First, let's go over the relevant anatomy: The gallbladder sits underneath the liver and stores bile. Its

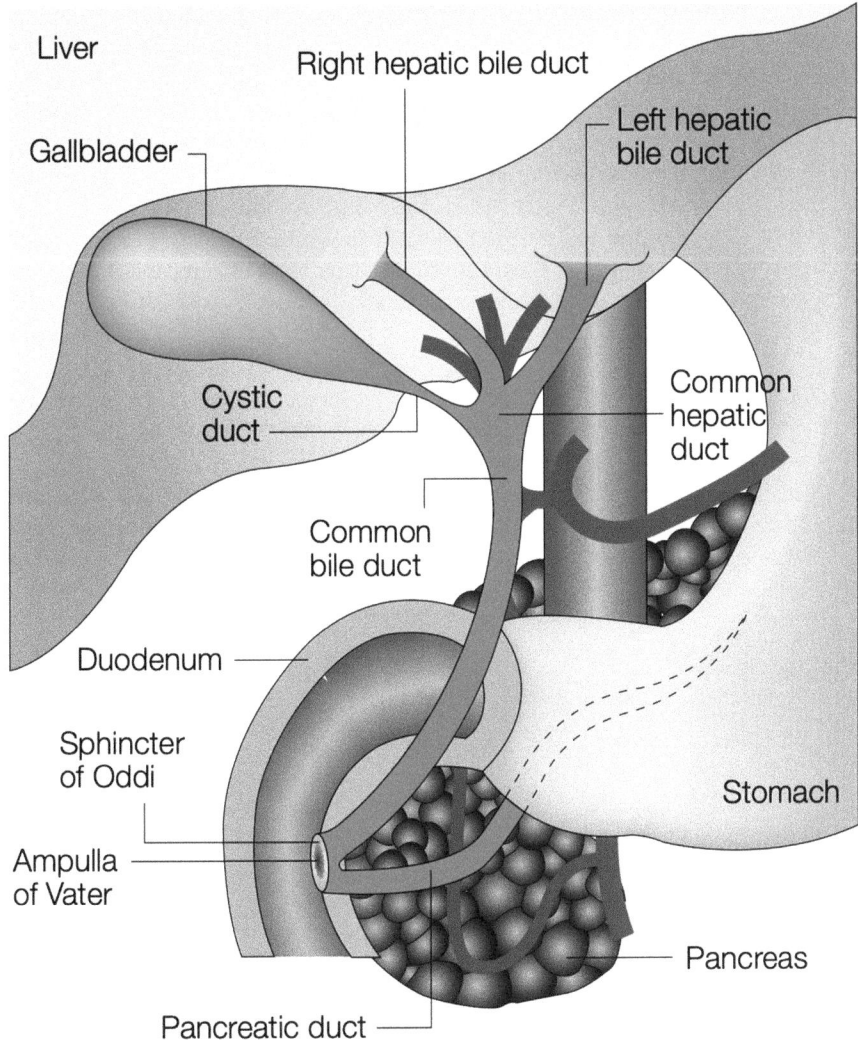

□ **Fig. 17.6** Anatomy of the biliary system. (From Wistuba I, et al: Gallbladder cancer: lessons from a rare tumour. *Nat Rev Cancer*. 2004; 4(9))

contents drain into the cystic duct, which then joins up with the hepatic duct, forming the common bile duct.

Next, let's define these terms: *Cholelithiasis* refers to gallstones, or stones in the gallbladder. These stones can be made from either cholesterol or pigment (or a combination), each of which has a different appearance and associations. Gallstones on their own aren't necessarily problematic—it is only when they cause an obstruction that they become pathologic. When a gallstone obstructs the cystic duct and the gallbladder contracts, patients experience dull abdominal pain (termed biliary colic), usually in the right upper quadrant and lasting up to several hours. Classically, this is felt after eating fatty foods, as the gallbladder contracts against the blocking stone, attempting to release its bile to break down the fatty meal.

Cholecystitis refers to an inflammatory state of the gallbladder wall due to this obstruction (but 10% of cases have no stone, termed acalculous cholecystitis—typically seen in patients who are critically ill in the ICU). Patients present with right upper quadrant pain, fever, and leukocytosis, and may also have nausea and vomiting. On physical exam, they exhibit tenderness in the RUQ and may have *Murphy's sign*, a cessation of inhalation when the examiner deeply palpates the RUQ. Bacterial infection can occur as a secondary process due to obstruction of the cystic duct.

Choledocholithiasis refers to gallstone(s) in the common bile duct, without infection. Aside from abdominal pain, patients may present with jaundice, as a buildup of conjugated bilirubin is absorbed into the blood.

Lastly, *cholangitis* is an infection of the biliary system (i.e., not just the gallbladder), typically due to an obstruction. It presents similarly to cholecystitis with fever and right upper quadrant pain, but patients also have jaundice and may develop mental status changes and shock.

17.7.3 Diagnosis and Treatment

■■ Differentiating the Differential

Cholecystitis and cholangitis can appear similar, with abdominal pain and fever. However, only in cholangitis will the bilirubin and alkaline phosphatase be elevated, except in the rare case of Mirizzi's syndrome, in which a severely distended gallbladder extrinsically compresses the common bile duct (this typically can be distinguished on cross-sectional imaging) (◘ Table 17.6).

◘ Initial checklist for cholecystitis or cholangitis	
Dx	**Tx (varies based on Dx, Dx results)**
☐ CBC, CMP ☐ LFTs ☐ PT, PTT, INR ☐ Blood cultures x2 ☐ RUQUS, cross-sectional imaging if indicated	☐ Antibiotics (GNR, anaerobe coverage) ☐ IV fluids ☐ Pain control ☐ If cholangitis, ERCP ☐ Consult surgery for?cholecystectomy

> Pain during or soon after eating points to an ulcer in the stomach, while pain relieved by eating suggests a duodenal ulcer.

> The most common causes of peptic ulcers are *H. pylori* and NSAIDS.

17.7.3.1 Peptic Ulcer Disease (PUD)

PUD refers to the presence of ulcer(s) in the stomach or duodenum. Although commonly asymptomatic, these ulcers can cause a characteristic abdominal pain which is typically in the epigastric region and described as aching or "gnawing." The timing of the pain can provide clues as to where the ulcer is located. If pain is present during or soon after eating, the ulcer is more likely to be in the stomach, while duodenal ulcers are characterized by alleviation of pain with eating, due to pancreatic secretion of bicarbonate into the duodenum with food. Patients may also experience nausea, vomiting, and early satiety. By far the most common causes of peptic ulcers are *H. pylori* infection and NSAIDs. *H. pylori* causes ulcers by penetrating the stomach's mucus layer and damaging its mucosal lining. The increased acidic output from the stomach can subsequently cause duodenal ulcers as well. NSAIDs (including aspirin) cause ulcers by reducing the production of protective prostaglandins and through local corrosive effects. Be sure to ask the patient about their NSAID use and whether they were raised in a country where *H. pylori* is endemic.

■■ Diagnosis

Visualization via upper endoscopy (EGD) allows for the definitive diagnosis of PUD. Ulcers should be biopsied if there is suspicion for malignancy (malignant ulcers tend to have irregular or thick margins or an associated mass and

17

◻ **Table 17.6** Classification of biliary pathology

Problem	Diagnosis	Treatment
Cholelithiasis	RUQ ultrasound shows stone(s) in the gallbladder	No treatment is necessary if the patient has no symptoms. Elective cholecystectomy is indicated for symptomatic cholelithiasis (biliary colic) to prevent further episodes and/or future complications
Cholecystitis	1. Prolonged biliary pain PLUS [fever, Murphy's sign, and/or leukocytosis] *and* 2. RUQ ultrasound showing gallstones PLUS [gallbladder wall thickening/edema or ultrasonographic Murphy's sign (pain with probe placement over gallbladder)] *Cholescintigraphy (HIDA scan)* can be used if ultrasound findings are equivocal. MRCP is indicated if there is concern for concurrent choledocholithiasis, and CT is indicated in cases with sepsis, peritonitis, bowel obstruction, or abdominal crepitus	Empiric antibiotics (covering gram-negative rods and anaerobes, e.g., ceftriaxone and metronidazole) typically until cholecystectomy; percutaneous cholecystostomy if the patient is not a surgical candidate
Choledocholithiasis	Labs show elevated total and direct bilirubin, alkaline phosphatase. RUQUS does not catch all stones or CBD dilation. If not seen, MRCP or EUS (both diagnostic), or ERCP (diagnostic and therapeutic) is performed	Removal of stone via ERCP (usually with sphincterotomy) followed by cholecystectomy to prevent recurrent episodes
Cholangitis	1. Fever and/or chills OR labs indicating inflammation *plus* 2. Labs indicating cholestasis *and* 3. Imaging showing biliary dilation or underlying obstruction Patients often present with the triad of RUQ pain, jaundice, and fever (*Charcot's triad*). Some may also have altered mental status and shock (*Reynold's pentad*). RUQUS may show biliary dilation and/or the cause of obstruction, but often CT or MRCP is needed to more definitively determine the site of obstruction within the biliary tree	Empiric antibiotics (covering gram-negative rods and anaerobes); biliary drainage usually via ERCP (usually with sphincterotomy) to remove stone and/or place stent; cholecystectomy during hospitalization to prevent repeated episodes

are more common in the stomach than the duodenum). The gastric mucosa should also be biopsied for *H. pylori* testing. In the setting of active GI bleeding from PUD, gastric biopsies are still recommended in most cases, but the yield of histology for identifying *H. pylori* organisms is lower in the setting of bleeding—you may send an *H. pylori* IgG serology as corroborating evidence in these situations. Of note, although the urea breath test and stool antigen test for *H. pylori* are more accurate than serology, these tests are affected by PPI use and thus are typically not options for patients presenting with an upper GI bleed.

■■ Complications
Complications include associated bleeding, gastric outlet obstruction, perforation, penetration into a solid organ, and fistulization.

■■ Treatment
All patients with PUD should be treated with a *proton-pump inhibitor (PPI),* typically for 2–3 months. Addressing the underlying etiology is also para-

mount in treatment and secondary prevention of peptic ulcers. Typically, if the etiology is thought to be NSAID related, patients should discontinue NSAID use. In patients who must continue NSAID use (e.g., for cardiovascular reasons), PPI should be used concurrently. If the patient tests positive for *H. pylori*, a regimen consisting of either three (*triple therapy*) or four (*quadruple therapy*) medications should be initiated. Triple therapy consists of 2 weeks of a PPI (e.g., omeprazole 20 mg BID), amoxicillin, and clarithromycin, while quadruple therapy consists of a PPI, bismuth, metronidazole, and tetracycline. While newer guidelines favor quadruple therapy, this must be balanced with patient compliance, as it can be difficult to take four medications. Follow-up testing for *H. pylori* eradication should be performed with repeat gastric biopsies at the time of the repeat EGD in 2–3 months. In patients who do not require a follow-up EGD, a noninvasive test (urea breath test or stool antigen test) can be performed 4 weeks after completing antibiotics and after 2 weeks of being off PPI. Bleeding ulcers should be treated as a GI bleed (see ▶ Sects. 17.7.7 and 17.7.8). Perforation due to peptic ulcer warrants emergency surgery.

◘ Initial checklist for peptic ulcer disease

Dx	**Tx**
☐ EGD w/ gastric biopsies	☐ NPO for EGD
	☐ PPI BID
	☐ Discontinue NSAIDs
	If +*H. pylori*:
	☐ Triple/quad therapy: PPI + amoxicillin 1 g bid + clarithromycin 500 mg bid *or* PPI + bismuth + metronidazole 500 mg bid + tetracycline 500 mg bid x 2wks
	☐ f/u EGD in 2–3 months (repeat gastric biopsies if initially diagnosed for *H. pylori* to confirm eradication after therapy)

17.7.3.2 Intestinal Ischemia

A very important cause of abdominal pain is intestinal ischemia, which refers to a reduction in blood flow to the intestines. This can occur in the small intestine (termed *mesenteric ischemia*) or large intestine (termed *colonic ischemia* or *ischemic colitis*), with a range of etiologies, including arterial or venous occlusion or vasospasm. Symptoms and sequelae vary largely according to time course.

Acute mesenteric ischemia (which has a mortality rate exceeding 60%) typically presents with abdominal pain "out of proportion to the physical exam." This means that while the patient may be in severe pain, the abdomen is soft, pain does not increase with abdominal palpation, and there are no physical exam signs of peritonitis. It is often caused by an acute embolic event and is typically a surgical emergency. In *acute colonic ischemia* (or ischemic colitis), patients may present with rectal bleeding or bloody diarrhea, and abdominal pain is less pronounced than in acute mesenteric ischemia. Ischemic colitis is usually secondary to a low-flow state at *watershed* areas of the colon (supplied by distal branches of 2 or more arteries, thus making the area particularly vulnerable to ischemia) and is usually managed medically, except in severe cases.

In contrast, *chronic mesenteric ischemia* typically presents with crampy abdominal pain after eating, which resolves after a few hours. These patients often have significant weight loss by the time they are diagnosed and may have developed an aversion to food.

CTA without oral contrast is the initial test of choice in patients with suspected mesenteric ischemia, while colonic ischemia can be diagnosed with colonoscopy or sigmoidoscopy. Definitive treatment depends on the etiology but can consist of pain control, anticoagulation, antibiotics, endovascular revascularization, and/or surgery. We will not go over the full workup and treatment of these conditions here, but it is important to keep these diagnoses in mind as potential causes of abdominal pain.

17.7.4 Diarrhea

Diarrhea is defined as loose stools occurring at least three times a day and is caused by increased water in the stool, typically due to incomplete absorption (osmotic) or increased secretion (secretory) in the intestines. It is typically categorized by its duration: *acute diarrhea* lasts 2 weeks or less, *chronic diarrhea* lasts 1 month or more, and *persistent diarrhea* lasts any duration in between. The most common causes of acute diarrhea are infectious (most cases being viral) and self-limited. Chronic diarrhea is most often caused by irritable bowel syndrome (IBS), inflammatory bowel disease (IBD), malabsorptive syndromes, metabolic causes (e.g., hyperthyroidism), and chronic infections. A discussion of the causes of chronic diarrhea is below. If your patient is hospitalized for diarrhea and GI is being consulted, the case is likely severe and/or persistent or chronic. A detailed history can provide useful clues as to its etiology.

Broadly, chronic diarrhea can be thought about in three categories: *watery, fatty,* and *inflammatory*. Watery diarrhea is caused by secretory or osmotic etiologies, malabsorption causes fatty diarrhea, and inflammatory diarrhea has features of all of the above, typically with blood in addition.

When you present a patient with diarrhea, your team will want you to have asked the questions below to help narrow down the differential.

- ■ History
- ═ How frequent are your bowel movements? How formed are they? What is the consistency?
  - – Considered diarrhea if 3+ watery stools in 1 day.
- ═ How long has this been going on?
  - – See above for timing and associated categories.
- ═ How large are each of the bowel movements? Is there associated abdominal pain, cramping, gas, or bloating?
  - – Large volume, watery stools with cramping and gas are more consistent with a small bowel origin, while small volume, painful bowel movements suggest a colonic origin.
- ═ Is the stool greasy, bulky, and/or difficult to flush?
  - – This suggests fatty stools with malabsorption or maldigestion as the cause, e.g., celiac disease or pancreatic exocrine insufficiency.
- ═ Is there blood in your stool? Quantify amount: streaks, clots, or droplets? Is the blood present in the toilet bowl before wiping or only on the toilet paper after wiping (the latter suggests an anal fissure or hemorrhoid)?
  - – Blood in the stool can be a sign of an invasive infectious cause (e.g., *Salmonella* or *Campylobacter*) or inflammatory bowel disease (Crohn's disease or ulcerative colitis).
- ═ Is there mucus in the stool?
  - – This also suggests an inflammatory source.
- ═ Do certain foods or medications trigger the diarrhea?
  - – Exacerbation with dairy or gluten can suggest intolerance or celiac disease.

- Does it occur more frequently at a certain time of day/night? Does it wake you up from sleep?
  - Nocturnal diarrhea is more characteristic of secretory causes of diarrhea.
- Is there a recurrent sensation of needing to empty your bowels despite just having had a bowel movement (tenesmus)?
  - This is an important symptom of inflammatory bowel disease.
- Any associated weight loss? fever?
  - This can give you an idea of the severity and potential etiology of the diarrhea.
- Have you used antibiotics recently? Any recent medication additions/changes? Any over-the-counter supplements? Recent laxative use?
  - Recent antibiotics brings up the possibility of *C. difficile* as a cause.
  - Many medications can cause diarrhea as a side effect, especially magnesium-containing supplements, antibiotics, and proton-pump inhibitors. Diarrhea and colitis are increasingly commonly recognized adverse effects of checkpoint inhibitors.
- Obtain a full medical and surgical history; obtain a full social history including sexual history, alcohol use, sick contacts, and travel history. Ask about family history of GI problems, including inflammatory bowel disease and celiac disease.
  - Chronic pancreatitis can lead to exocrine pancreatic insufficiency.
  - Dumping syndrome can be a cause of diarrhea after gastric bypass surgery.
  - Certain etiologies of diarrhea (e.g., CMV colitis) are AIDS-defining illnesses.
  - Sick contacts with similar symptoms suggest an infectious etiology.

See ▶ Sect. 17.3 for guidance on a comprehensive abdominal examination.

■ ■ Workup

The workup for each of the following categories differs significantly, and we will use a few examples rather than delving into the details for each diagnosis. Generally, the primary team will likely already have ordered basic labs like a complete blood count, metabolic panel, inflammatory markers, and thyroid function tests. You may wish to order fecal tests such as stool electrolytes and fecal calprotectin. If a chronic infectious cause such as *Giardia* or *C. difficile* is suspected, stool should be sent for microbiologic evaluation.

Also keep in mind that there are two important tools in diagnostic evaluation of diarrhea: endoscopy (including colonoscopy) and imaging. In general, patients require visualization of the GI tract via endoscopy if certain factors are present, including older age, GI bleeding, nocturnal symptoms, worsening abdominal pain, systemic symptoms such as weight loss, family history of inflammatory bowel disease or GI malignancy, worrisome lab abnormalities, or a chronic unexplained history. Abdominal pain along with diarrhea typically warrants imaging.

17.7.4.1 Watery Diarrhea

Secretory diarrhea occurs when electrolytes are secreted into (or not absorbed from) the intestinal lumen, and water follows. Acute secretory diarrhea is most often caused by infections, but chronic causes include endocrine abnormalities such as hyperthyroidism and Addison's disease, amyloidosis, and microscopic colitis. *Osmotic diarrhea* occurs when an exogenous solute (e.g., sugars or ions) is poorly absorbed by the intestine and draws water into the lumen. Common causes include lactose intolerance and osmotic laxative use.

Gastroenterology

Because both secretory and osmotic diarrhea are watery, it can be difficult to distinguish between the two. However, certain components of the patient's history, as well as lab results, can help: Nocturnal symptoms (being woken up at night by the urge to move one's bowels) are present in secretory diarrhea but typically not in osmotic diarrhea. If the patient states that symptoms are brought on by oral intake, this is more consistent with osmotic diarrhea. Lastly, a low *stool osmotic gap* (<50 mOsm/kg) points to a secretory cause while a higher value (>100) suggests an osmotic cause (Table 17.7). A normal gap is between 50 and 100. The osmotic gap can be calculated with the following equation:

$$OsmGap_{Stool} = StoolOsm - 2\left(Na^+_{Stool} + K^+_{Stool}\right)$$

The stool osmolality is assumed to be 290 mmol/L.

Lastly, *functional diarrhea*, of which IBS is a type, also causes watery diarrhea and cannot be explained by an underlying disorder. The Rome IV Criteria are used to diagnose IBS (see ▶ Sect. 17.4).

17.7.4.2 Fatty Diarrhea (Steatorrhea)

Steatorrhea suggests a problem with *absorption* or *digestion*, and is characterized by greasy, foul-smelling, and/or bulky stools that are hard to flush. Symptoms are typically associated with oral intake, and weight loss is common, as nutrients pass through the bowel without being absorbed or digested. The differential diagnosis for steatorrhea differs for malabsorption and maldigestion and includes mucosal diseases such as celiac disease (malabsorption), pancreatic exocrine insufficiency (maldigestion), and others.

If you suspect steatorrhea based on the history, your team may order a *Sudan stain*, which detects excess fecal fat, or *a 24-hour fecal fat test*, which helps to narrow the differential diagnosis based on the weight of excess fat excreted in the stool in 24 hours. Once steatorrhea is confirmed, the underlying etiology should be sought by evaluating the intestines and pancreas.

If the patient endorses symptoms with gluten or has a suggestive family history, you may suspect *celiac disease*. After initial antibody screening (anti-tTG IgA), an endoscopy with biopsy is performed to confirm the diagnosis. If the patient has risk factors for *chronic pancreatitis* (e.g., heavy alcohol use, prior episodes of acute pancreatitis), stool elastase levels may be decreased, and an abdominal CT can demonstrate calcifications and/or atrophy of the pancreas. Therapy depends on the underlying etiology, but for these two examples, celiac disease requires a lifelong gluten-free diet, and exocrine pancreatic insufficiency requires pancreatic enzyme supplementation.

> Secretory causes of diarrhea are suggested by nocturnal symptoms and a low osmotic gap. Osmotic causes of diarrhea are suggested by relationship to oral intake and a high stool osmotic gap.

 Table 17.7 Secretory and osmotic causes of diarrhea

Secretory causes of diarrhea (low stool osmotic gap, <50)	Osmotic causes of diarrhea (high stool osmotic gap, >100)
Bacterial enterotoxins (e.g., cholera) Endocrine abnormalities (e.g., hyperthyroidism, neuroendocrine tumors) Microscopic colitis Bile acid malabsorption Nonosmotic laxatives (e.g., senna, docusate) Others	Carbohydrate malabsorption (e.g., lactose intolerance) Celiac disease Osmotic laxatives (e.g., polyethylene glycol, lactulose) Others

17.7.4.3 Inflammatory Diarrhea

Patients with *inflammatory diarrhea* have frequent episodes of small-volume, bloody diarrhea. They often have accompanying abdominal pain and *tenesmus*, or the sensation of needing to empty one's bowels despite just having had a bowel movement. Symptoms are often present during fasting and at night. Inflammatory diarrhea has a characteristic elevation in fecal calprotectin (a protein found in leukocytes), and patients may have elevated inflammatory markers such as C-reactive protein (CRP). Causes of inflammatory diarrhea include those that alter the mucosa, including IBD and infectious diseases, although the latter more frequently cause acute diarrhea.

Inflammatory bowel disease (IBD) is an umbrella term that includes Crohn's disease (CD) and ulcerative colitis (UC). Both conditions cause abdominal pain and diarrhea, are associated with certain extraintestinal symptoms, and have a genetic predisposition. CD and UC each have unique complications and histologic changes. Distinguishing between the two conditions requires a colonoscopy with biopsy.

Crohn's disease characteristically has *skip lesions* (i.e., the bowel inflammation is not continuous throughout the GI tract) and may involve any part of the GI tract—although most commonly involves the small intestine and/or colon and spares the rectum. Inflammation is present throughout the entire wall of the intestine (*transmural*), histology demonstrates *noncaseating granulomas*, and it is associated with *fistula* formation and *strictures*.

Ulcerative colitis, on the other hand, does cause *continuous inflammation* of the colon, starting from the rectum and moving proximally without involvement of the small intestine. Its inflammation extends to the *mucosa only* and histology demonstrates *crypt abscesses* (in which crypts are filled with polymorphonuclear leukocytes [PMNs]).

Management of IBD is complex and hospitals often have dedicated physicians or multidisciplinary teams for IBD. We will not discuss the pharmacologic management of IBD flares or maintenance here, as this is a more nuanced discussion and options are changing rapidly in recent years. The screening guidelines for colorectal cancer in patients with IBD are discussed below, under "Colorectal Cancer Screening."

As you can see, there is a lot to think about when evaluating a patient with diarrhea. There are overlaps in the categories described above, so take the entire story into account. Treatment largely depends on the underlying etiology and therefore is variable. Beyond determining the cause, it is important to treat the patient's symptoms and any metabolic derangements that have occurred secondary to the diarrhea. Hypokalemia is not uncommon and the patient may be volume depleted, so make sure to replete electrolytes and fluids. Anti-diarrheal agents (e.g., loperamide) should be used with caution, as they can prolong or worsen certain infections, e.g., *C. difficile*.

17.7.5 Dysphagia

Dysphagia is the sensation of having difficulty swallowing. There are multiple ways to classify dysphagia, which can be achieved by taking a detailed history. Here, we will discuss the questions you should ask your patient and how this helps to narrow the diagnosis.

Describe the sensation you are feeling and point to where you feel it most prominently. Do you have any associated choking or coughing? Does it feel like food is getting stuck?

Gastroenterology

Dysphagia can be broken down into *oropharyngeal* and *esophageal* dysphagia. Generally, the former results in difficulty initiating a swallow, which results in choking or coughing. Patients point to their mid-neck region when asked to show where they feel symptoms most prominently. In contrast, esophageal dysphagia causes trouble after initiating a swallow and makes the patient feel as though food is stuck in their chest.

Are you having trouble with solids only or both liquids and solids? Has this changed over time?

Etiologies for both oropharyngeal and esophageal dysphagia can be *neuromuscular* or *structural*. If the patient has always had trouble with both solids and liquids, this points to a neuromuscular cause, whereas trouble with solids only (at least at the start) points to a structural problem. This should make sense intuitively: If there is a mass obstructing the esophagus, liquid should be able to make its way around it, but solids will be obstructed. If both solids and liquids cannot pass from the onset of symptoms, it is more likely a problem with the motility of the esophagus.

Some of the neuromuscular causes of oropharyngeal dysphagia include stroke, ALS, and muscular dystrophy and for esophageal dysphagia include achalasia and scleroderma. Aside from achalasia, it is unlikely that the first and only manifestation of these problems will be dysphagia so we will not discuss these in depth. Some structural causes include masses and strictures. A more detailed discussion follows in the next section.

Is this progressive or intermittent? If progressive, how quickly has it progressed? Has this ever happened before?

Obtain a complete social history including history of alcohol and tobacco use.

Obtain a full medical history including history of GERD, allergies, and radiation exposure.

Have you experienced weight loss? How much, over how long?

When symptoms are progressive and point to a structural problem, causes include esophageal/peptic *strictures/webs* and malignancy, especially if symptoms are progressive. Strictures are more likely in a patient with a history of *gastroesophageal reflux disease (GERD)* or radiation exposure. Esophageal cancer is more likely in a patient with risk factors (tobacco, alcohol for squamous cell, and GERD/Barrett's esophagus for adenocarcinoma) and red flag symptoms such as weight loss. A history of recurrent episodes of food impaction and GERD in patients with preexisting food allergies raises the possibility of *eosinophilic esophagitis*, a chronic condition characterized by an infiltration of eosinophils into the esophageal mucosa. The condition is diagnosed with endoscopic biopsies and can cause strictures and a narrowed esophagus.

Is it painful to swallow?

Obtain a list of current medications.

Odynophagia is pain with swallowing. The presence of odynophagia with dysphagia narrows the differential to infectious and medication-induced causes. Infectious causes should be suspected in immunocompromised patients and include *Candida* (most commonly, though this can also occur in immunocompetent hosts), herpes simplex, and cytomegalovirus (CMV) esophagitis. Each of these has a unique appearance on upper endoscopy. Medication-induced esophagitis should be suspected if the patient is taking a common culprit medication, such as antibiotics (e.g., tetracyclines), bisphosphonates, and NSAIDs.

- **Diagnostic Testing**

The two diagnostic tests likely to provide the most useful information are the *barium swallow* and *upper endoscopy (EGD)* with biopsies. In certain cases

Oropharyngeal dysphagia causes difficulty initiating a swallow. Esophageal dysphagia makes food feel stuck in the chest. Trouble with solids and liquids suggests a neuromuscular cause of dysphagia. Trouble with solids only suggests a structural cause.

The presence of odynophagia narrows the differential of dysphagia to infectious and medication-induced causes.

when there is a significant risk for complex anatomic changes, the barium swallow is performed prior to endoscopy. See 17.6 for more information on the barium swallow and upper endoscopy. If endoscopy is performed first and is normal, a barium swallow can help determine the presence of a mechanical obstruction that was missed on endoscopy, as well as providing a basic description of motility.

If both of these are negative, your patient may require *esophageal manometry*, which measures the strength and coordination of the esophagus and esophageal sphincter. This can help diagnose a motility disorder. Lastly, chest CT can help visualize causes of extrinsic compression that were missed.

■ Treatment

Treatment varies based on the cause of dysphagia. In some cases, empiric treatment can be trialed before pursuing these diagnostic tests. For example, in *Candida* esophagitis, empiric antifungal therapy (e.g., fluconazole) is recommended for immunocompromised patients with dysphagia or odynophagia, particularly if there is evidence of oral thrush; only if symptoms do not improve is an upper endoscopy indicated. HSV esophagitis is treated with acyclovir, with duration dependent on immune status; CMV esophagitis is treated with ganciclovir or valganciclovir. Pill esophagitis is treated with withdrawal of the offending medication.

Esophageal strictures, rings, and webs are treated with *endoscopic dilation* as well as treatment of underlying GERD with PPI (e.g., omeprazole 20 mg bid). Eosinophilic esophagitis is treated with PPI, diet modification, and/or swallowed inhaler steroids—dilation is also indicated in the presence of a stenosis. Esophageal malignancy should prompt a consultation with oncology to determine next steps.

See ▶ *Sect. 17.3 for guidance on a comprehensive abdominal examination. You should also include a HEENT exam, evaluating for lymphadenopathy, which may indicate malignancy or infectious etiologies. Check inside the patient's mouth for clues as well (*e.g., you may be able to see oral thrush, which hints at the possibility of* Candida *esophagitis).*

17.7.6 Gastrointestinal Bleeding

This section will discuss upper and lower gastrointestinal bleeding and some of their most common causes. We will work through how to distinguish the source of bleeding, as well as the workup and management of GI bleeds.

Note: The *fecal occult blood test (FOBT)* should not be used to evaluate the patient for acute GI bleeding. In some cases it is used for colorectal cancer screening, but in the acute setting there are more accurate ways to determine whether the patient has a GI bleed. Additionally, the FOBT can cause false positives due to microtrauma from digital manipulation.

17.7.7 Upper GI Bleeding (UGIB)

Acute upper GI bleeding, occurring anywhere from the esophagus to the ligament of Treitz (at the duodenojejunal flexure), can be alarming and anxiety provoking for providers, so it is important to have a framework when thinking about first steps. About half of cases are caused by ulcers, but several other possibilities exist as well, described below. Depending on the origin, upper GI bleeding can present with hematemesis (with bright red or coffee-ground emesis), hematochezia, and/or vital sign changes like hypotension or orthostasis. *For patients with known varices or portal hypertension, variceal bleeding should be highest on your differential diagnosis. Variceal bleeding carries a mortality risk of 15–20% and requires urgent management. For these patients, unique aspects of care will be in* **bold**.

- **First Steps**

The first thing to think about in a patient with an upper GI bleed is *stability*: is the patient stable or unstable? Take a look at the vital signs, especially blood pressure and heart rate, looking for hypotension and tachycardia. If they are unstable, they should be sent to the ICU for more aggressive care. Assess mental status.

Note: If the patient has *resting tachycardia* (HR >100 bpm), this suggests that they have lost up to 15% of their blood volume. If orthostatic hypotension is present, this suggests that over 15% of blood volume has been lost. If the patient is hypotensive at rest, they have lost >40% of their blood volume.

Next is *resuscitation*. By the time you notice the bleed, the patient has likely already lost a significant amount of volume, so it is important to make sure they have adequate intravenous access. The patient should have *2 large-bore (14–16 gauge) peripheral IVs* (which have better flow than a central line) and receive IV fluids. When you get lab results back, you can then consider *blood transfusion*. For most patients, only transfuse for a hemoglobin of less than 7/dL. The exception to this rule is if the patient is bleeding massively or has had recent cardiovascular or cerebrovascular disease (for whom the Hgb threshold should be more liberal, at 9–10 g/dL).

Consider whether the patient requires *intubation*. The patient should be intubated if they cannot protect their airway, if mental status is altered, or if the bleed is very high volume. **Generally, patients with active variceal upper GI bleeding should be intubated**.

At this point, consider *medication adjustment:* Look at the patient's medication list and make sure you hold any drugs that may exacerbate the risk of bleeding, for example, anticoagulants or antiplatelets. Also consider whether their anticoagulation medications need to be/can be reversed.

For patients with presumed variceal bleeding, your team will be thinking about whether the patient requires *balloon tamponade*. **This is indicated in severe cases (in which endoscopy is not feasible) and involves deploying a balloon into the esophagus and/or stomach and inflating it to stem the bleeding temporarily**.

Clinical pearl: A randomized controlled trial in 2013 found that *less is more*: patients who received blood transfusion for a hemoglobin of less than 7 (termed a "restrictive" transfusion strategy in contrast to a "liberal" strategy) had a mortality benefit compared to patients with a hemoglobin goal of 9. **Importantly, the patients who benefited most from the restrictive transfusion strategy were those with portal hypertension, so this rule applies even more strongly to those with variceal bleeding**. (Villanueva, NEJM 2013)

- **Labs**

Useful labs to send upfront include CBC, CMP, coagulation panel, and type and screen.

- **Etiologies**

When thinking about the source of bleeding, consider the patient's medical history and predisposition to certain causes of GI bleeding. For example, are they on NSAIDs? This may be due to a peptic ulcer. **Do they have known liver disease? This puts them at higher risk for esophageal or gastric varices**.

Now, think anatomically and ask yourself what can bleed in each part of the upper GI tract. Examples include:

- Esophagus—esophagitis, esophageal varices, malignancy
- Gastroesophageal junction, stomach—Mallory-Weiss tear, Boerhaave syndrome, peptic ulcer, gastritis, gastric varices, malignancy

– *Differentiating the differential:* Streaks of blood in the patient's emesis after prolonged vomiting may be from a *Mallory-Weiss tear* or, more rarely, *Boerhaave syndrome*. The former is a superficial tear in the esophageal or gastric mucous membrane. It should be differentiated from Boerhaave syndrome, a spontaneous rupture of the esophagus due to forceful vomiting. In the latter, you may see subcutaneous emphysema (air under the skin) on the physical exam, and pneumomediastinum (air in the mediastinum) on chest x-ray. This should prompt immediate consultation with surgery.

- Small intestine—peptic ulcer, malignancy
- Anywhere—arteriovenous malformation (AVM, angiodysplasia), especially in a patient with aortic stenosis (these comprise *Heyde syndrome*); aortoenteric fistula, especially if the patient has had aortic aneurysm graft repair

> Quick Ddx for Upper GI Bleeding: Esophagitis, varices, malignancy, Mallory-Weiss tear, Boerhaave syndrome, peptic ulcer, gastritis, vascular malformation, fistula

■ ■ Differentiating the Differential

It is important to distinguish upper from lower GI bleeding, as this guides next steps in workup and management (e.g., which type of scope will be used). **For patients with known varices or portal hypertension, assume variceal upper GI bleeding**. For more uncertain cases, the following two rules can be helpful: If the *BUN/Cr ratio is over 30:1*, the likelihood ratio of the bleed arising from an *upper GI source* is about 7. One explanatory theory for this finding is that a high BUN represents the digestion and absorption of blood components from the upper GI tract. The second rule is that if the patient has *blood clots in the stool*, the likelihood ratio of an UGIB is 0.05, highly suggestive that the source is the *lower GI system*.

So, for example, a patient with hematemesis, a Cr of 1.5 and BUN of 65 (BUN/Cr ratio 43.3), and no clots in the stool very likely has an upper GI bleed. Importantly, while nasogastric lavage was used in the past to differentiate between the two types of bleeding (by instilling fluid through an NG tube, washing it out, and looking for blood to confirm an upper GI source), this is no longer recommended due to patient discomfort and more noninvasive means (e.g., BUN/Cr ratio) of localizing the bleed prior to endoscopic evaluation.

■ Risk Stratification

The *AIMS65 scoring system* is used to determine the risk of mortality from upper GI bleeding. See ▶ Sect. 17.4 for more information.

■ Next Steps in Management

Once you've confirmed that this is an upper GI bleed, the next major step in diagnosis and management is an *upper endoscopy*. This procedure is performed both to identify the source of bleeding and treat the lesion. Timing matters here: **if there is concern for a variceal bleed, the endoscopy needs to happen within *12 hours***; otherwise, it can be performed within *24 hours*. Either way, the patient should be adequately resuscitated and hemodynamically stable prior to EGD, as they will be sedated during the procedure, which can induce hypotension.

Note: Performing EGD more urgently has not been shown to be helpful in hemodynamically stable patients.

Prior to EGD, there are a few things to be done to help optimize visualization during endoscopy. First, *administer an IV proton-pump inhibitor* (e.g., pantoprazole 40 mg IV BID) *upfront* to raise the pH in the stomach, so that clots can form over the bleed. Second, consider *administering IV erythromycin*, which has motilin-like properties, 30–90 minutes prior to the EGD. This helps to empty the stomach so that the endoscopist can see the underlying lesion more clearly. **Lastly, if the patient has known cirrhosis, and the GI bleed is assumed to be variceal, administer IV** *octreotide (50 mcg bolus and then a continuous infusion at 50 mcg/hr for 3–5 days after hemostasis is achieved on EGD)* **and IV** *ceftriaxone* **(1 g every day for 5–7d). Octreotide is used to lower portal pressures to help decrease the flow of bleeding and reduce the risk of rebleeding. Ceftriaxone is used as infection prophylaxis (from any infectious complication, not only SBP) and improves mortality in these patients.**

During the procedure, the endoscopist will look for the source of bleeding or **stigmata of recent bleeding (see ▶ Sect. 17.4).** He or she will then treat the bleed accordingly (e.g., **banding if variceal**, clips for ulcers with bleeding vessels, thermal therapy for AVMs, etc.). Afterwards, the patient's medical management will depend on the cause of bleeding. For example, patients with peptic ulcer disease should be kept on intensive proton-pump inhibitor therapy and the underlying cause of PUD should be sought out and treated.

Patients with variceal bleeding should be continued on octreotide for 3–5 days. (Primary prophylaxis for variceal bleeding is discussed in *Liver Pathophysiology***.) Keep a close eye on the patient and watch out for rebleeding, as the risk for this after variceal bleeding is high.**

Note: Expect to see *melena* as the old blood passes through the GI tract; independently, this should not be taken as a sign of rebleeding. Use vital sign and lab abnormalities to support your suspicion if you do think the patient is rebleeding.

Also, take note of the patient's *mental status* after the bleed. Bleeding can cause or exacerbate hepatic encephalopathy, and the patient may need lactulose for a few days during recovery.

Note: Your team may also be considering performing a *transjugular intrahepatic portosystemic shunt (TIPS) procedure* acutely to lower portal pressures and stop the bleeding. See "Screening/Surgery" ▶ Sect. 17.7.9 for more information on TIPS.

If the patient already has known varices, they should already be on primary prophylaxis for variceal bleeding (see *"Bleeding"* ▶ Sect. 17.7.9). However, if this is the patient's first presentation (i.e., they did not have known varices prior to this episode), secondary prophylaxis should be initiated. This consists of both *nonselective beta blockade (e.g., nadolol 40 mg qd)* and *serial endoscopic variceal ligation (banding)*. Serial banding should occur until all varices are obliterated, and the patient should be followed with repeat endoscopies at a regular interval.

◖ **Initial checklist for upper GI bleeding**

Dx	Tx
☐ CBC, CMP, coagulation panel, type and screen	☐ IV fluids
☐ EGD within 12 or 24 hours	☐ Transfuse if Hgb <7–8 (<9–10 in certain cases)
	☐ Pantoprazole 40 mg IV BID
	☐ Erythromycin 250 mg (30 mins before EGD)
	If variceal:
	Octreotide 50 mcg IV × 1 followed by 50 mcg/ hr drip
	Ceftriaxone 1 g IV q24h × 5–7d
	☐ EGD for possible hemostasis

17.7.8   Lower GI Bleeding (LGIB)

Any gastrointestinal bleeding beyond the ligament of Treitz at the duodenum is considered a lower GI bleed. The most common cause of lower GI bleeding is diverticulosis, but as is the case with upper GI bleeding, there are multiple other important etiologies and sources. LGIB can present with *hematochezia* (bright red blood, clots, or maroon colored stool) or *melena*.

Quick Ddx for Lower GI Bleeding: Upper GI bleed, diverticulum, polyp, malignancy, fissures, hemorrhoids, vascular malformation, intestinal ischemia, infection, IBD

■ ■ Differentiating the Differential

The color of the stool can tell you a lot, but should not be relied upon in isolation to determine the source of the bleed. Dark/black stool (*melena*) suggests bleeding in the upper GI system, as the blood becomes darker as hemoglobin becomes oxidized during transit. Fresh red blood (*hematochezia*) in the stool suggests a distal source of bleeding, for example, a diverticulum, polyp, or lower GI malignancy. In cases of very brisk upper GI bleeding, hematochezia may occur. It may also be present with anal fissures or hemorrhoids, so be sure to ask whether the patient notices the blood on the toilet paper after wiping (suggestive of an anal source) or in the toilet bowl beforehand. You can also ask the patient's nurse whether he or she has noted hemorrhoids while helping to clean the patient.

■ First Steps

The first steps in lower GI bleeding are exactly the same as those of upper GI bleeding. See ▸ Sect. 17.7.7 for more specific recommendations on *stability, resuscitation* (with the same transfusion parameters), and *medication adjustment.*

■ Labs

Useful labs to send upfront include *CBC, CMP, coagulation panel,* and *type and screen.*

■ Etiologies

When thinking about the source of bleeding, consider first the rapidity and severity of the bleed. A slow bleed without any lab or vital sign abnormalities is more likely to be caused by a bleeding colonic mass, whereas hematochezia raises diverticular bleeding on the differential.

Also consider the patient's HPI and medical history. Is this an older patient with a history of weight loss? This puts malignancy higher on the list. A younger patient with LGIB and diarrhea may be having a first presentation or flare of IBD. Did the patient recently have surgery or a colonoscopy? This is most likely a complication of the procedure. If the bleeding is painless, suspect diverticular bleeding or, less commonly, an arteriovenous malformation (AVM). If the patient frequently strains with bowel movements or has constipation, hemorrhoids are more likely. Crampy abdominal pain with a history of abdominal radiation raises the possibility of intestinal ischemia causing LGIB. Lastly, if the patient has hematochezia and hemodynamic instability, always consider the possibility of an upper GI source, which is true in about 15% of severe cases. If this is suspected, consider doing an EGD.

■ Next Steps in Management

If you have confirmed that this is a lower GI bleed, the next major step in diagnosis and management is a *colonoscopy*, both to identify the source of bleeding and treat the lesion. This should be done within *24 hours* if possible, and only after the patient is adequately resuscitated and hemodynamically stable. If the patient has hematochezia and hemodynamic instability, administer an IV PPI in case the bleeding is actually originating briskly from an upper GI source.

Prior to the colonoscopy, the patient should complete a bowel preparation in order to clear the colon for proper visualization. The patient needs to be stable in order to tolerate this bowel prep.

During the procedure, the fellow or attending will look for the source of bleeding and treat the bleed accordingly (e.g., clipping for diverticular bleeds, argon plasma coagulation therapy for AVMs). If the source of bleeding is not found on colonoscopy, other diagnostic options include video capsule endoscopy, push enteroscopy, or localizing scans, such as CT angiogram with contrast or nuclear tagged red blood cell scan (see ▶ Sect. 17.6 for more information on these tests). For these scans, the patient must be actively bleeding for any useful information to be gleaned. If either is positive, the next step is typically to go to interventional radiology (IR) for angiography and embolization.

If at any point the patient is unstable, localizing scans are performed first and the patient should go to IR for immediate embolization. Surgery is often consulted for severe lower GI bleeding but typically only operates if the bleeding is not controlled by either GI or IR.

◘ **Initial checklist for lower GI bleeding**

Dx	Tx
☐ CBC, CMP, coagulation panel, type and screen	☐ IV fluids
	☐ Transfuse if Hgb <7–8 (<9–10 in certain cases)
☐ Colonoscopy within 24 hours if stable	☐ Pantoprazole 40 mg IV BID if hematochezia and hemodynamic instability
	☐ Bowel prep for colonoscopy

17.7.8.1 Colorectal Cancer (CRC) Screening

As colorectal cancer can present initially with lower GI bleeding, we will take this opportunity to go over colorectal cancer screening. There are many tools that can be used for CRC screening, which can be divided into *endoscopic visualization, radiologic visualization, and stool-based tests*. We will not go through all of the benefits and limitations of each test here, but it is important to know that *colonoscopy every 10 years is also the most sensitive test for adenomas of all sizes and CRC compared to other testing*. However, it does require going through bowel preparation, which can be uncomfortable (and sometimes unsafe) for some patients. Additionally, any abnormal result from a non-colonoscopy exam requires a follow-up colonoscopy to further investigate the finding.

Endoscopic exams include the colonoscopy, sigmoidoscopy, and capsule endoscopy. CT colonography (CTC) is the only radiologic exam that can be used for CRC screening. Lastly, stool-based exams include the fecal immunochemical test (FIT), the guaiac-based fecal occult blood test (gFOBT), and the multitarget stool DNA test with FIT (FIT-DNA). More information on all of these exams can be found in "*GI-Specific Diagnostic Testing.*"

The frequency of CRC screening depends on the patient's risk factors, medical history, and family history.

- For those at *average risk* (no personal history of CRC, high-risk polyps, IBD, suspected hereditary CRC syndrome, abdominal radiation, or family history of CRC), the United States Preventive Services Task Force (USPSTF) recommends *starting screening at age 50*. If colonoscopy is the chosen method, this should be done *every 10 years through age 75*. From age 76 until 85, the patient should be reevaluated and the decision to screen should take into account life expectancy, personal preference, and medical history. Screening should stop beyond the age of 85.

- For those at *higher risk,* screening begins earlier and should occur more frequently:
  - If a first-degree relative has a history of CRC or advanced adenoma before the age of 60 (or 2 first-degree relatives have this history at any age), screening should begin either *at age 40* or *10 years before the earlier diagnosis,* whichever is earliest. Testing should be repeated *every 5 years.*
  - For patients with *inflammatory bowel disease* (IBD) with colon involvement, colonoscopy should begin *8–10 years after symptom onset* and occur *every 1–3 years.*
  - For those with a personal history of *hereditary CRC syndromes,* recommendations depend on the syndrome but can begin as early as 10 years of age.
- Lastly, patients with a history of abnormal findings on colonoscopy may need their screening schedules adjusted. For example, several tubular adenomas or serrated polyps can decrease the screening interval to every 3 years and even annually in some cases.

You may have heard of *carcinoembryonic antigen (CEA)* as a serum screening test for colorectal cancer. Currently, routine measurement of CEA is not recommended for screening, but can be used in patients who receive colorectal surgery for malignancy to gauge response and guide further management.

17.7.9   Liver Pathophysiology

Hepatology is an enormous and fascinating subject that you will encounter on your GI rotation. Throughout this chapter, we have touched on elements of liver disease in multiple areas, like the physical exam and upper GI bleeding. This section will focus on how to manage a patient with *cirrhosis, acute liver failure,* and *hepatitis.*

17.7.9.1   Cirrhosis

Cirrhosis is a chronic fibrotic state of the liver, which causes *portal hypertension* and problems with normal hepatocellular function. This causes numerous downstream effects that put patients at extremely high risk for complex medical problems. It is definitively diagnosed with a liver biopsy (although this is not always done), which shows characteristic findings such as fibrosis, regenerative nodules, and other architectural changes. *The most common etiologies for cirrhosis are chronic alcohol use, chronic viral hepatitis (HBV and HCV), non-alcoholic fatty liver disease (NAFLD, of which non-alcoholic steatohepatitis [NASH] is a subtype), and hemochromatosis.*

Rarer etiologies include autoimmune conditions like autoimmune hepatitis, primary biliary cirrhosis, and primary sclerosing cholangitis, as well as Wilson's disease and alpha-1 antitrypsin deficiency. Lastly, systemic diseases like congestive heart failure, amyloidosis, and sarcoidosis can cause cirrhosis as well. Whenever a patient with cirrhosis is admitted, make sure to calculate their *MELD score* (see ▶ Sect. 17.4), which gives you a sense of the severity of their disease and urgency for liver transplant evaluation (typically considered when the MELD score is >15). Also keep in mind their *Child-Pugh Score* (see ▶ Sect. 17.4), which estimates mortality.

■   Portal Hypertension and Its Complications

One of the most damaging consequences of cirrhosis is *portal hypertension,* which is abnormally high pressure in the portal venous system. This state leads to high levels of nitric oxide and thus vasodilation of the splanchnic vessels which causes low effective arterial blood volume and causes RAAS to turn on. The increased ADH in this state causes sodium and water retention and leads to edema, ascites, and hyponatremia.

Portal hypertension is the cause of many other sequelae of liver disease such as varices/variceal bleeding, portal hypertensive gastropathy, and hepatic hydrothorax. It is associated with complex pathophysiologic states that are difficult to manage, such as hepatorenal syndrome, hepatopulmonary syndrome, portopulmonary hypertension, and cirrhotic cardiomyopathy (◘ Fig. 17.7). (This interplay of multiple organ systems in cirrhosis physiology is part of what makes hepatology both interesting and difficult!)

You will very likely see *hepatorenal syndrome (HRS)* (or hear it mentioned) while on the liver service during your rotation. This is characterized by acute kidney injury in a patient with liver disease and is caused by renal vasoconstriction due to portal hypertensive physiologic sequelae. This is a diagnosis of

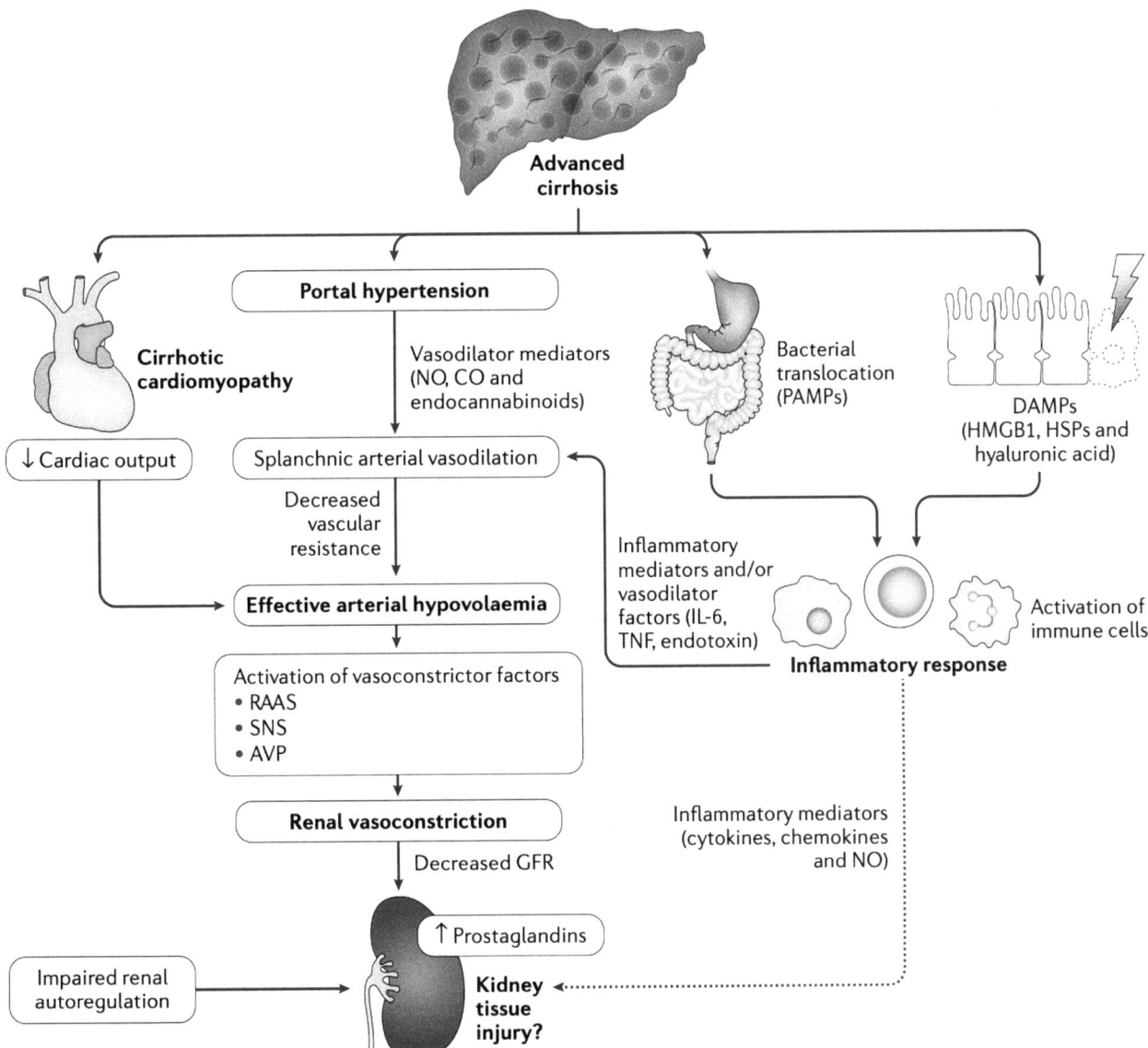

◘ **Fig. 17.7** Factors involved in hepatorenal syndrome (HRS) pathogenesis. (From Ginès et al. Hepatorenal syndrome. *Nat Rev Dis Primers.* 2018;4(1))

exclusion and requires multiple criteria to be met, including a lack of response to 2 days without diuretics, as well as an *albumin challenge*. The albumin challenge (1 g IV per kg of 25% albumin for 2 days with a maximum of 100 g per day) is an attempt to increase oncotic pressure intravascularly.

There are two types of HRS, *Type 1 HRS* involves a twofold increase in creatinine to >2.5 mg/dL in under 2 weeks; there is also usually multiorgan dysfunction. *Type 2 HRS* is less severe and characterized by refractory ascites. *Suspect HRS in a patient with cirrhosis who has had a recent precipitating event (e.g., SBP, GIB) and has a rising creatinine despite stopping diuretics.* Treatment of HRS can be difficult, but the mainstay is a combination of albumin, octreotide (which causes splanchnic vasodilation), and midodrine (which increases mean arterial pressure). If truly refractory, the patient may need renal replacement therapy (RRT). The only definitive treatment is liver transplantation.

■ **History**

Aside from a complete medical, family, and social history, make sure to ask the following questions for patients with known or suspected liver disease:
- Have you been able to take your medications as prescribed (diuretics, rifaximin, lactulose)?
- Do you know your dry weight?
- Have you had any recent changes in your sleeping? (Sleep disturbance is one of the first signs of hepatic encephalopathy.)
- To the patient or someone who lives with them: Have you noticed any inattention or confusion (another sign of HE)?

Decompensated cirrhosis involves the presence of ascites, SBP, jaundice, HE, variceal bleeding, and/or HRS.

■ **Compensated or Decompensated Cirrhosis?**

It is important to determine whether the patient has *decompensated cirrhosis*, as they are at a much higher risk of mortality than those with compensated cirrhosis. Decompensated cirrhosis involves the presence of *ascites, SBP, jaundice, hepatic encephalopathy, variceal bleeding, and/or hepatorenal syndrome*. Decompensated cases should prompt a search for the etiology of decompensation, which can include infection (including SBP), bleeding, alcohol use, malignancy, blood clots, medication changes, and recent surgery. These cases should also be considered for liver transplantation, especially if the MELD score is >15.

In these cases, search for a precipitating cause: infection, bleeding, alcohol use, malignancy, clot, med changes, or surgery.

See ▶ Sect. 17.3 *for specific signs to look for when evaluating a patient with chronic liver disease.*

■ **Labs and Diagnostic Testing**

Initial diagnostic testing (i.e., these do not need to be performed during every hospitalization) to find the cause of cirrhosis includes viral serologies (HBV, HCV), iron studies (transferrin saturation most importantly), antinuclear antibody (ANA), anti-smooth muscle antibody (ASMA) for autoimmune hepatitis, anti-mitochondrial antibody (AMA) for PBC, ceruloplasmin for Wilson's disease, and alpha-1-antitrypsin levels. If all of these are negative and there is no suggestive social history (e.g., heavy alcohol use) that can explain the cause of the patient's cirrhosis, a liver biopsy may be indicated as this can sometimes provide the underlying diagnosis. A noninvasive alternative to the liver biopsy is the FibroScan.

An elevated *INR* indicates that the patient is not producing clotting factors adequately. Importantly, these patients are not only at an increased risk for bleeding but for clotting as well. Low *albumin* also indicates decreased synthetic function as albumin is a protein made by the liver. Less telling labs include AST, ALT, and alkaline phosphatase, and bilirubin, which may be moderately elevated or normal in cirrhosis. *Thrombocytopenia* may occur due to splenic sequestration caused by portal hypertension, as well as decreased hepatic production of thrombopoietin. *Hyponatremia* is common in patients with ascites due to a decreased ability to get rid of free water.

A *diagnostic paracentesis* should be performed for just about every patient with ascites who is admitted to the hospital (see ▶ Sect. 17.8 for guidance on how to perform this). A cell count of *250 polymorphonuclear leukocytes (PMNs) or more is diagnostic of SBP*. To correct for blood in the tap, you can subtract 1 PMN for every 250 red blood cells in the ascitic fluid. The *serum ascites albumin gradient (SAAG)* is calculated by subtracting the ascites albumin concentration from the serum albumin concentration. A value of greater than or equal to 1.1 indicates that portal hypertension is the likely cause of the patient's ascites, whereas a SAAG of less than 1.1 indicates a cause unrelated to portal hypertension. (See ▶ Sect. 17.4 for equation.)

Common causes in both categories are listed below. Within each category, you can further narrow your differential based on the total protein content in the ascitic fluid (◧ Table 17.8).

A *RUQUS* can be used to confirm the presence of ascites and demonstrate a nodular liver contour. The addition of Doppler on RUQUS is helpful in initial presentations of ascites in order to rule out blood clots in the hepatic vein (Budd-Chiari syndrome) or portal vein.

If safe to do so, almost all hospitalized patients with ascites should have a diagnostic paracentesis to rule out SBP.
250+ PMNs diagnoses SBP.
SAAG ≥1.1 suggests portal hypertension as the cause of ascites.

■ Care Plan

Whenever a patient with cirrhosis is admitted to the hospital, whether the reason for admission is GI related or not, GI may be consulted. This is because there will always be a concern that an aspect of their liver disease caused their admission. For example, if the patient is admitted with a hip fracture, was she encephalopathic which caused her to trip? Thus, there are several additional components that need to be on your radar to make sure all aspects of their liver disease are addressed. Use the *"VIBES"* mnemonic in your assessment and plan so that nothing is missed.

■ V: Volume (Ascites, Edema, Diuretics)

Patients with cirrhosis often have low albumin, leading to low osmotic pressure and decreased intravascular volume and water retention through the activation of RAAS. This process causes ascites as well as edema. Ask about the patient's history of *large volume paracenteses* (or thoracenteses for hepatic hydrothorax).

Treatment: Diuretics (administered orally) can help the patient eliminate some of this extra fluid. The magic combination here is *spironolactone and*

◧ **Table 17.8** Causes of ascites based on SAAG value

Portal hypertension-related causes of ascites (SAAG ≥ 1.1)	Other causes of ascites (SAAG < 1.1)
Cirrhosis	Nephrotic syndrome
Cardiac disease (e.g., CHF, constrictive pericarditis)	Peritoneal carcinomatosis
Infiltrative liver disease (e.g., sarcoidosis)	Pancreatic ascites
Hepatic or portal vein thrombosis	Tuberculous peritonitis
Others	Lymphatic obstruction
	Others

furosemide, specifically in the ratio of 5:2. For example, spironolactone 100 mg with furosemide 40 mg works well. Spironolactone is a potassium-sparing diuretic and prevents excess potassium loss from the effect of the loop diuretic, furosemide. These patients should be on a salt-restricted diet (less than 2 g per day). If hyponatremic (Na <125), they should also have a fluid-restricted diet (1.5 L per day limit). Aim for a goal fluid loss of ½ lb per day if the patient does not have lower extremity edema; if edema is present, more weight loss is okay. If the patient continues to have ascites despite diuresis, consider large-volume paracentesis on a regular basis (every 1–2 weeks) with albumin administration following each procedure. See ▶ Sect. 17.8 for more information on performing a therapeutic paracentesis. As a last resort and bridge to more definitive therapy (i.e., transplant), *transjugular intrahepatic portosystemic shunt (TIPS)* can be performed. See *"Screening/Surgery"* for more information on TIPS.

■ **I: Infection (SBP, Hepatitis)**

Spontaneous Bacterial Peritonitis (SBP)

SBP is an infection of ascitic fluid. It is extremely important to think about upfront, as mortality is high and the diagnosis changes the patient's treatment plan and daily medications moving forward. The patient's presentation can range from completely asymptomatic to severe abdominal pain with fever. As discussed above, most patients (as long as they have a large enough pocket of fluid to sample) with cirrhotic ascites admitted to the hospital should undergo a diagnostic paracentesis upfront to check for SBP, and 250 PMNs or greater is diagnostic. The pathogen is usually *E. coli* or *Klebsiella*. If there are more than 50,000 red blood cells/mm^3, this is called "hemorrhagic ascites" and is likely due to trauma of a blood vessel. You can still use the cell count to determine whether the patient has SBP, but must correct the number by subtracting 1 PMN for every 250 RBCs. For example, if there are 60,000 RBCs, you must subtract 240 from the total PMNs that your lab results show.

Treatment: *Stop the patient's nonselective beta blocker*, as it has been shown to increase the risk of hepatorenal syndrome and reduce transplant-free survival (it can be resumed after SBP has been treated in most cases). Treat with *IV ceftriaxone* (2 g daily for 5 days) and *25% albumin* (1.5 g/kg on day 1 and 1 g/kg on day 3, with a maximum of 100 g). If there is no improvement within 48 hours, repeat diagnostic paracentesis to evaluate whether the PMN count is increasing and antibiotics need to be changed.

For anyone who has ever been diagnosed with SBP (or has other specific criteria), secondary prophylaxis must be initiated, which consists of PO ciprofloxacin or sulfamethoxazole/trimethoprim.

■ **B: Bleeding (Coagulopathy, Variceal Bleeding)**

Variceal bleeding is a major risk for these patients. Check to see whether they have ever had an initial endoscopy to evaluate whether varices are present. If the patient does have varices, primary prophylaxis should be initiated. This consists of a *nonselective beta blocker* (e.g., nadolol 40 mg qd, titrate to HR of 50s–60s), which blocks beta-1 heart contractility and beta-2 mesenteric arterial dilation. This results in unopposed alpha vasoconstriction of mesenteric arterioles. There is then a reversal of splanchnic vasodilation, decreased flow into the portal venous system, and overall lowering of portal pressures, thus lessening the risk of variceal bleeding. If the varices are medium or large, the patient may need serial *endoscopic variceal ligation (banding)*. The issue with this is that the underlying portal hypertension is not addressed; rather, the pressure is just transduced elsewhere. Banding requires a follow up endoscopy 3–4 weeks later to make sure these varices have not recurred. Thus, beta-blockade is preferred unless varices are quite large. If there are no varices on endoscopy, the patient does need a repeat endoscopy within 1–3 years depending on the severity of the liver disease and presence of risk factors.

Treatment for variceal bleeding is addressed in "*UGIB.*"

▪ E: Encephalopathy (Rifaximin, Lactulose)

Hepatic encephalopathy (HE) is a condition in which patients have cognitive deficits and impaired neuromuscular function (e.g., asterixis). You can evaluate for the presence of HE on history and physical exam (see ◘ Table 17.1). The onset can be subtle: Sometimes, the only sign of HE is a change in sleeping patterns. HE is graded from I to IV, with the most severe form being coma. Several precipitants can prompt HE, all of which are important to consider throughout the patient's hospitalization. These include infection, bleeding, constipation, hypokalemia, renal failure, and sedative medications. So, if a patient is initially admitted without signs of HE but later develops inattention, you must look for these precipitants and correct the underlying disorder, in addition to treating the HE itself.

Treatment: HE is treated with *lactulose* (30 mL TID) with a goal of 3–4 bowel movements a day. If symptoms persist despite lactulose, *rifaximin* (400 mg TID or 550 mg BID) is typically added. Both of these agents reduce the concentration of ammonia, which is thought to contribute to HE. Lactulose acidifies the colon, donating a proton to ammonia and converting it to ammonium, which is then excreted. Rifaximin is a nonabsorbable antibiotic which clears the colon of ammonia-producing bacteria.

> When a patient is admitted with signs of HE, look for precipitating factors: infection, bleeding, constipation, hypokalemia, renal failure, and sedative medications.

▪ S: Screening/Surgery (Hepatitis, Vaccination, HCC—or—TIPS/Transplant)

Screening: Make sure these patients have received vaccines for hepatitis A and B, the flu vaccine, as well as the pneumococcal polysaccharide vaccine. They should also be offered counseling for alcohol abstention if this is the cause of cirrhosis. Lastly, the risk for *hepatocellular cancer (HCC)* is high in these patients, so they should receive a RUQUS every 6 months to screen for HCC.

Hepatocellular carcinoma (HCC) is the most common primary liver cancer. Screening is indicated in all patients with cirrhosis and certain patients with hepatitis B. Besides RUQUS, some clinicians use serum *alpha-fetoprotein (AFP)* levels as a screening test, though this varies by hospital. Management varies based on staging. Transplant is possible in certain cases, determined by the Milan criteria (see ► Sect. 17.4).

Surgery: This includes *transjugular intrahepatic portosystemic shunt (TIPS)* and *transplantation*. TIPS is a procedure that involves connecting the hepatic vein and portal vein with a stent, allowing blood to bypass the liver. This reduces the high portal pressure and thus largely eliminates many of the complications of portal hypertension, including varices, ascites, and portal gastropathy. The biggest downside of this procedure is that it can worsen hepatic encephalopathy, as the toxins normally causing HE are normally filtered by the liver. TIPS is typically done as a "bridge to transplant" as it does not definitively treat the underlying disorder.

Refer patients for *transplantation* if the MELD score is >15 and there is evidence of decompensation. Other indications include acute liver failure, refractory variceal bleeding, and systemic manifestations of liver-based conditions (e.g., amyloidosis), among others. In most cases, unless there is acute liver failure, the transplant evaluation process is a lengthy one that involves the input of multiple teams such as psychiatry, social work, and transplant surgery. The patient needs to have a social support system in place and cannot have used alcohol or illicit substances for 6 months prior to listing. There is a long list of labs and general health screening exams that need to be performed prior to approving the patient for transplant. It can be helpful to start the process when you are seeing the patient in the inpatient setting if they are potentially eligible for a transplant. In many hospitals, large committees meet on a regular basis to discuss patients' candidacy.

- **Other Things to Keep in Mind**

When caring for a patient with cirrhosis, *avoid NSAIDs, ARBs, and ACE inhibitors* given the risk of precipitating renal injury. Also *avoid narcotics and sedatives*, especially benzodiazepines, as there is a risk of provoking or worsening hepatic encephalopathy (many of these drugs are hepatically cleared). Lastly, it is okay to administer *acetaminophen* for patients with compensated cirrhosis, but limit the dose to 2 g per day. Make sure the patient gets strict daily standing weights and that ins and outs are measured accurately.

- **Presenting a Patient with Cirrhosis**

There are certain components that are important to include when presenting a patient with cirrhosis. These include the patient's Child-Pugh Class, MELD score if relevant (if decompensated and being evaluated for a transplant), whether the cirrhosis is decompensated or not, last endoscopy and findings including the patient's variceal status and whether or not these were banded, history of hepatic encephalopathy, and history of SBP. When presenting a new patient, it may be helpful to frame the one-liner as follows:

» This is Mrs. X, a 52-year-old woman with a history of cirrhosis secondary to Wilson's disease, MELD 29 on presentation, Child Class C, who is admitted with altered mental status. Her liver history is notable for a prior history of SBP for which she is on cipro prophylaxis, as well as hepatic encephalopathy, for which she takes rifaximin and lactulose.

■ **Initial checklist (varies based on the cause of hospitalization)**

Dx	Tx
☐ RUQUS w/ Doppler	☐ Diuretic regimen (e.g., spiro/furosemide 5:2)
☐ Dx para, f/u labs	☐ If HE, lactulose ± rifaximin/titrate to 3–4 BM
	☐ Continue nadolol 40 mg qd
	☐ Goal -1 lb/day
	☐ Strict I/O, daily standing weights
	☐ Avoid NSAIDs, ARBs, ACEi, narcotics, sedatives; 2 g acetaminophen ok

17.7.9.2 Acute Liver Failure (ALF)

Acute liver failure, also called fulminant liver failure, is defined as severe liver injury plus encephalopathy and coagulopathy (INR 1.5 or greater) developing over <26 weeks in a patient who does not have preexisting liver disease/cirrhosis. Acute liver injury, in contrast, involves coagulopathy but not encephalopathy. It can present nonspecifically, for example, with nausea, vomiting, or abdominal pain.

- **Diagnostic Testing**

The following labs should be sent upfront to try and narrow down the causes of the patient's ALF: CBC, CMP, coagulation panel, type and screen, lactate, ammonia, blood glucose, arterial blood gas, HIV, serum toxicology panel, acetaminophen level, viral hepatitis serologies, ceruloplasmin, and autoimmune markers.

Imaging studies should begin with a RUQUS with Doppler to look for Budd-Chiari syndrome (hepatic vein outflow obstruction), malignant invasion, or other reasons for liver failure. Abdominal CT or MRI can also be performed but are limited in utility without intravenous contrast, which is risky in these patients who may also have renal failure.

If a cause is not found after these labs and imaging tests, a liver biopsy may be pursued. Keep in mind that if the patient will have a liver transplantation, there is no need for pre-transplant liver biopsy, as the explanted liver can be analyzed after the surgery.

■ Differential Diagnosis

Etiologies for ALF fall into multiple categories, the most common of which is drug induced (e.g., acetaminophen poisoning). Other potential offenders in this category include herbal supplements, antibiotics, and anticonvulsants. Make sure to get a complete medication history from the patient.

Acetaminophen poisoning is the most common cause of acute liver failure in the United States. *Single doses of 7.5 g are potentially toxic* in adults (for reference, one regular strength tablet of acetaminophen is 325 mg, so 7.5 equates to about 23 pills). Patients are usually asymptomatic during the first 24 hours after ingestion. If patients present within this window, *activated charcoal* administration can help decrease the toxic effect of acetaminophen. Dosing is 1 g per kg, with a maximum dose of 50 g. Use the *Rumack-Matthew nomogram* (available online), which is a diagram that plots the concentration of ingested acetaminophen against time since ingestion. This can help determine the patient's prognosis as well as the utility in using *N-acetylcysteine (NAC)* as treatment. NAC is administered intravenously or orally, with different durations of treatment for each. Make sure that psychiatry has been consulted if this was an intentional overdose as a suicide attempt.

Viral causes of acute liver failure include hepatitis A, B, C, D, and E, as well as herpes simplex virus, Epstein-Barr virus, cytomegalovirus, adenovirus, and varicella zoster virus. *Autoimmune hepatitis* and *Wilson's disease*, as well as *vascular* causes (e.g., Budd-Chiari syndrome/hepatic vein outflow obstruction) or ischemic hepatitis (shock liver) are also potential etiologies. The patient's medical and social history should help point you in the right direction in most cases. For example, was the patient recently transferred to the ICU in septic shock? Ischemic hepatitis/shock liver should be high on your differential. Sometimes, however, you will have to rely on labs alone, or begin management without knowing the underlying cause of the liver failure. These labs can be very telling: For example, only a few processes can elevate the AST and ALT into the 1000s. See ◘ Table 17.2 for more information.

Clinical pearl: If a medication is found to be the cause of the patient's liver failure, make sure to list it in the patient's chart as an allergy—this could save their life and prevent medical errors in the future!

■ Prognosis

One helpful way to think about the causes of ALF is by prognosis: Which etiologies do patients generally recover from and which should prompt a transplant workup? Below is a helpful list:

- *Better prognosis* (transplant-free survival occurs in ~50% of these cases):
  - Acetaminophen poisoning
  - Hepatitis A
  - Shock liver (ischemic hepatitis)
- *Worse prognosis* (transplant-free survival occurs in <25% of these cases):
  - Hepatitis B
  - Other drugs (non-acetaminophen)
  - Wilson's disease
  - Autoimmune hepatitis

■ **Treatment**

Treatment will vary based on the underlying disorder but should also focus on supportive care. Support the patient's hemodynamic status with IV fluids and pressors if needed. Avoid benzodiazepines which can worsen hepatic encephalopathy. If the patient's INR is elevated, administer *IV vitamin K* 10 mg × 3 days. Also initiate GI ulcer prophylaxis.

Watch out for systemic complications from acute liver failure. One of the most worrisome is *cerebral edema or herniation*, a common cause of death in these patients, especially with severe HE. If present, raise the head of the bed to 45 degrees and administer hypertonic saline for a goal sodium of 145–150. Also consider administering IV mannitol. Other systemic complications include renal (e.g., ATN, hepatorenal syndrome), hematologic (severe coagulopathy), infectious, and metabolic (electrolyte derangements) problems. Of course, you will not be making these decisions independently! If a patient is this sick, there will likely be multiple consulting teams involved.

☑ Initial checklist for acute liver failure

Dx	**Tx**
☐ CBC, CMP, coagulation panel, type and screen, FSBG	☐ IVF and pressors if hemodynamically unstable
☐ Acetaminophen level	☐ Consider intubation if severe hepatic encephalopathy
☐ Viral hepatitis serologies (HAV, HBV, HCV, HDV, HEV, HSV 1/2, EBV, CMV, adenovirus, VZV)	☐ Lactulose ± rifaximin if HE
☐ Autoimmune markers: ASMA, ANA, LKM-1 antibody, etc.	☐ Start liver transplant evaluation
☐ Total protein	☐ NAC if acetaminophen poisoning (see nomogram)
☐ SPEP	☐ H2RA for GI ppx
☐ VBG or ABG	
☐ HIV	
☐ Serum tox panel	
☐ Ceruloplasmin, 24-hour urine copper	
☐ RUQUS with Doppler to look for vascular/ischemic causes	

17.7.9.3 Alcohol-Related Hepatitis

Alcohol-related hepatitis is inflammation of the liver associated with heavy alcohol use that occurs over the course of weeks to months. Severe cases carry a very poor prognosis with a 1-month mortality of 25–35%. Patients who develop this condition typically have a history of heavy alcohol use for many years. When taking a history from someone with suspected alcohol related hepatitis, the timing of the patient's last alcohol use can be confusing. They may have stopped drinking several weeks prior, which may make you rule out alcohol as a cause initially. However, it is common for patients to stop drinking precisely because they begin feeling ill from this condition, and they continue to abstain from drinking as the inflammation worsens over time. Therefore, it is important to ask the patient the reason for the recent abstention from alcohol.

■ **Presentation**

Patients with alcohol-related hepatitis may have jaundice, abdominal pain with hepatomegaly, a lack of appetite, and fever. The fever may make you think of an infectious source, but it is relatively common in alcoholic hepatitis. However, you must always rule out SBP and other infectious causes when fever is present. Importantly, patients with this condition may develop all of the sequelae of portal hypertension (e.g., ascites, variceal bleeding) due to acute/subacute liver inflammation, but lack cirrhosis.

■ **Diagnostic Testing**

Liver function tests in alcohol-related hepatitis have a characteristic pattern, which is a moderate elevation in AST and ALT, *usually in a > 2:1 ratio*. They typically do not exceed 500. Alkaline phosphatase and white blood cell count are also elevated in most cases. To rule out other causes of hepatitis/fever, a full infectious workup (including CXR, blood and urine cultures) as well as a diagnostic paracentesis, should be performed. To rule out thrombosis or obstruction as the cause, a RUQUS with Doppler should be performed.

■ **Treatment**

Two unique elements of treatment in alcohol-related hepatitis are *N-acetylcysteine (NAC)* and *glucocorticoids. NAC* is a *possibly* effective treatment that is often used for severe cases and has shown a trend towards increased survival (primarily by reducing the risk of HRS). Hospitals vary in their policies for NAC use. *Glucocorticoids* in the form of prednisolone at 40 mg per day may be indicated in some cases. Calculate the *Maddrey's Discriminant Function (MDF)* to determine whether the patient may benefit from glucocorticoids (see ► Sect. 17.4). If the MDF is 32+, steroids are indicated. If there is a contraindication to steroids, pentoxifylline can be used.

Nutritional status is very important for these patients as they may be chronically undernourished from long-term alcohol use and/or have low albumin due to hepatic dysfunction. Optimize nutrition with a daily multivitamin, as well as thiamine and folate supplementation. Encourage intake of high-protein foods. If the patient is not meeting his or her caloric needs due to anorexia, feeding via an NG tube may be indicated.

After 7 days of steroids, if the patient is not improving, use the *Lille Score* (see ► Sect. 17.4), a system that predicts mortality rates in these patients and utility in continuing steroid treatment. A score of >0.56 indicates a lack of response and an indication to discontinue steroids. If the patient is indeed responding, continue for a full duration of 28 days, followed by a 16-day taper. During this period, the patient is at high risk for infection, GI bleeding, and hyperglycemia.

Abstinence is another extremely important component in treatment and prevention of repeated episodes. Offer the patient abstention counseling as well as medication-assisted therapy. In patients who do not respond to the above therapy, liver transplantation can be considered (in some cases, the 6-month abstinence requirement is waived if certain other factors are present).

🗗 **Initial checklist for alcohol related hepatitis**

Dx	Tx
☐ CBC with MCV, CMP, LFTs	☐ MVI, thiamine, folate, nutrition consult
☐ Iron studies	☐ Consider prednisolone 40 mg qd (if MDF 32+)
☐ Triglycerides	☐ Consider NAC
☐ Blood and urine cultures	☐ Omeprazole 20 mg qd for GI ppx
☐ CXR	
☐ RUQUS w/ Doppler	
☐ Dx para	

17.7.9.4 Viral Hepatitis

Viral hepatitis encompasses any liver inflammation caused by a virus, but this section will only cover hepatitis A, B, C, D, and E. Of these viruses, all can cause acute hepatitis but only hepatitis B and C can cause chronic liver disease. See ▶ Sect. 17.5 for more information on hepatitis antibody interpretation.

Hepatitis A (HAV) is transmitted fecal-orally (person to person or through food or water, often after international travel or eating raw shellfish) and has an incubation period ranging from 2 to 7 weeks. When symptoms arise, they typically start as acute onset nausea, fever, and abdominal pain followed by dark urine and pale stools, and then jaundice. Symptoms can last anywhere from 2 weeks to 2 months. AST and ALT are usually highly elevated first, and bilirubin elevation follows. The diagnosis is confirmed with anti-HAV IgM testing. The illness is most often self-limited and treated with supportive measures but can progress to acute liver failure in a minority of cases, at which point transplantation is indicated. HAV can be prevented with vaccination, which is recommended in certain populations including individuals who use IV drugs, men who have sex with men (MSM), those with chronic liver disease, concurrent HBV or HCV infection, and those with upcoming travel to high-risk areas.

Hepatitis B (HBV) is a double-stranded DNA virus that is transmitted through blood, sexual contact, and vertical transmission. There are an estimated 250 million HBV carriers worldwide and its health effects are profound: HBV is an oncogenic virus and thus can cause HCC even if the patient does not have underlying cirrhosis (whereas most HCC cases arise with underlying cirrhosis). Its incubation period ranges from 1 to 4 months, after which symptoms can include abdominal pain, nausea, jaundice, and malaise. Many patients have mild symptoms in acute infection while about 30% develop more severe cases. In the more severe cases, consider coinfection or superinfection with hepatitis D (HDV). Diagnosis is confirmed with HBsAg and anti-HBc IgM; AST and ALT values rise over 1000. Acute infection does not always need to be treated but if severe (coagulopathy, protracted course), it can be treated with *tenofovir* or *entecavir*. HBV progresses to *chronic infection in < 5% of adult cases* (but much higher for acquisition at younger ages) and is diagnosed when HBsAg is present for longer than 6 months. Treatment of patients with chronic HBV is based on multiple factors including the presence of cirrhosis, the ALT level, and HBV DNA quantification. If treatment is initiated, it usually consists of tenofovir or entecavir. HBV can be prevented with vaccination.

Hepatitis C (HCV) is transmitted primarily through blood, and risk factors include intravenous drug use, blood transfusion prior to 1992, sex with an individual who uses intravenous drugs, and chronic hemodialysis, among others. Acute infection is often asymptomatic but can include symptoms similar to those of HAV and HBV. However, it causes *chronic infection in most (50–85%) cases*, often leading to progressive liver disease over many years. About $\frac{1}{5}$ of patients with chronic HCV progress to cirrhosis. Chronic HCV is the most common cause of chronic liver disease in the United States and can result in many extrahepatic manifestations of disease (e.g., membranous proliferative glomerulonephritis). Treatment of chronic HCV should be initiated in all patients with a detectable HCV viral load. Therapy consists of direct-acting antiviral therapy such as *ledipasvir/sofosbuvir* (brand name Harvoni), with the goal of achieving a sustained virologic response (SVR), considered a cure. The exact choice of therapy regimen depends on the patient's genotype and severity of disease. When you encounter a patient with HCV, it is important to provide counseling on decreasing the risk of transmission. For example, you can guide the patient to avoid sharing grooming equipment and donating blood, consider treatment for substance use disorder, and/or avoid sharing needles.

Hepatitis D (HDV) is endemic in parts of the Mediterranean, Central Africa, South America, and Asia. It requires the presence of HBV to cause infection, so cases represent either coinfection or superinfection with HBV, the latter being more severe.

Hepatitis E (HEV) is transmitted fecal-orally as well as through blood and vertical transmission. Acute infection appears clinically similar to the aforementioned viral hepatitides although tends to be milder. Chronic HEV is rare but can occur in immunocompromised patients. HEV infection during *pregnancy*, especially the third trimester, causes a more severe infection which carries a higher risk of acute liver failure, fetal loss, and mortality. Treatment typically consists of supportive care.

17.8 Procedures

As a medical student on the GI rotation, you may have the opportunity to help with some procedures. These will most likely be the digital rectal exam and the paracentesis (both diagnostic and therapeutic). This section will go over how to perform these procedures. Most other GI procedures, like endoscopies and colonoscopies, will be performed by GI fellows and/or attendings, but you can learn a lot just by observing.

17.8.1 Digital Rectal Exam (DRE)

The DRE is an extremely important part of the physical exam in GI. Often on your rotation, you will be expected to perform a DRE, especially when there is concern for GI bleeding. Although it may be uncomfortable to perform (for both the examiner and examinee), you will be obtaining crucial information that will guide further workup and management.

Indications: Suspected GI bleeding, rule out cauda equina/conus medullaris, fecal incontinence, many others

Contraindications: In general, immunocompromised patients should not have this procedure as there is a risk of bacterial translocation across the bowel wall and resultant life-threatening infection.

Materials: Gloves, lubricant, procedure pad, tissues, +/− guaiac card

Steps:

1. Draw the curtains so that you have privacy. Ask permission from the patient to perform a rectal exam after explaining why it is necessary. Ask if they would like another person from the care team present during the procedure. Tell the patient they will feel a cold finger for a few seconds and that it might feel strange but shouldn't hurt. If the patient is lying in bed, ask them to lay on their side with knees tucked in.
2. Put your gloves on and place the procedure pad under the patient.
3. With one hand, separate the buttocks. Observe the anus for fissures, hemorrhoids, skin tags, bleeding, and any abnormalities.
4. Squeeze about a tablespoon of lubricant onto a gloved finger.
5. With a dry finger, palpate around the anus and ask if the patient can feel this. If not, this may be a sign of spinal cord dysfunction.
6. Gently insert your lubricated finger into the rectum. You can ask the patient to bear down, which should make insertion easier.
7. Next, ask the patient to squeeze, and assess the rectal tone.

8. Rotate your finger clockwise and counterclockwise, palpating the rectal wall and feeling for masses and feces. In males, you should be able to feel the prostate gland anteriorly. If you can, assess its smoothness and size.
9. Remove your finger and examine the glove for feces and/or blood.
10. Clean the patient with tissues (or allow them to clean themselves) and dispose of your gloves.

17.8.2 Diagnostic Paracentesis

In this procedure, you will help accomplish a very important step in the workup and/or management of your patient. You will have guidance from your resident, fellow, and/or attending, so don't worry that you will be completely on your own. The materials and steps for this procedure are similar to those of a therapeutic (large volume) paracentesis. Materials and steps vary by hospital, but the following should give you an idea of what to expect.

Indications: Suspected spontaneous bacterial peritonitis (SBP), new onset ascites (to determine etiology)

Contraindications: Hemodynamic instability, DIC, cutaneous infection or scars overlying intended paracentesis site. Caution in pregnant patients and patients with distended bladders or bowel obstruction. Neither elevated INR nor thrombocytopenia are a contraindication.

Materials: Ultrasound with gel, paracentesis kit (varies by hospital but typically includes iodine/chlorhexidine, sterile gloves and drape, lidocaine, syringes, injection needles, scalpel, alcohol wipes, paracentesis needles), adhesive bandage, appropriate tubes, and culture bottles

Steps:
1. Draw the curtains so that you have privacy. Explain the steps of the procedure and why it is necessary. Obtain consent. Ask if they would like another person from the care team present during the procedure. Have the patient empty their bladder. Ask the patient to lie down flat on the bed with their head resting on the pillow. Prepare all of your materials in advance (e.g., open the specimen tubes and leave the tops on without twisting closed).
2. Use the bedside ultrasound to locate the deepest pocket of fluid (which looks anechoic). The pocket should be at least 3 cm deep and there should be no loops of bowel nearby. The recommended needle insertion sites include slightly under the umbilicus, where there are no blood vessels, or in the RLQ or LLQ, medial and anterior to the ASIS. Care should be taken to avoid the inferior epigastric artery: Use the Doppler mode to find this if using the lateral approach.
3. Mark the intended insertion site and have the patient turn slightly towards the procedure side.
4. Using sterile technique, prep and drape the patient.
5. Make a wheal with lidocaine on the skin over your marking, and, *using a Z-track technique* (described below), continue anesthetizing as you advance the needle to the peritoneum. As you do so, intermittently make sure you are not in a blood vessel by applying slight negative pressure (aspirating) and ensuring that you do not see blood. If this happens, withdraw the needle and change position by 1–2 cm. You will feel a loss of resistance or a "pop" as you enter the peritoneal cavity. Inject an additional 3–5 mL of lidocaine. Remove the needle.

- *The Z-track technique* is a method of minimizing post-paracentesis leakage. Before inserting the needle, pull the skin downward with your nondominant hand. Then, insert the needle while maintaining traction on the skin. Hold the skin in this position until your dominant hand has completed anesthetizing the needle track. Once the needle enters the peritoneum, you can release traction.

6. If using a large-bore needle, use a scalpel to make a small nick at the needle insertion site.

7. Again, using the Z-track technique and intermittent negative pressure, follow the same track you made in Step 5 and insert the paracentesis needle into the peritoneum gradually. Yellowish ascitic fluid should begin to fill the syringe.

8. Fully insert the catheter and remove the syringe with its needle, replacing it with a larger syringe (usually 60 mL) to collect your sample.

   - *Tip*: If you have some advance warning that you will be performing this procedure, it is very helpful to obtain a 60 mL syringe and practice pulling and pushing the plunger with one hand. You may need your other hand to help stabilize the abdomen during the procedure so it is helpful to feel comfortable operating the syringe with one hand only.

9. Remove the catheter and apply gauze to the insertion site with firm pressure. Apply a bandage.

10. Send the fluid for *gram stain, culture, cytology, total protein, albumin, glucose, triglycerides, LDH, and blood cell count with a differential cell count.*

11. Monitor the patient for hemodynamic instability or physical changes, which may signify a complication from the procedure, including bleeding, bowel perforation, arterial aneurysm, or abdominal wall hematoma.

17.8.3 Therapeutic (Large Volume) Paracentesis

Indications: Tense ascites causing respiratory compromise or discomfort, abdominal compartment syndrome, ascites refractory to diuretics.

   Contraindications: Hemodynamic instability, DIC, cutaneous infection or scars overlying intended paracentesis site. Caution in pregnant patients and patients with distended bladders or bowel obstruction. Neither elevated INR nor thrombocytopenia is a contraindication.

   Materials: All of the above plus vacuum bottles (enough to remove 8 L of fluid).

   Steps:

- Steps 1–7 are the same as in the diagnostic paracentesis. You should obtain a diagnostic sample with all of the steps above in addition to the therapeutic paracentesis.

- 8. Fully insert the catheter and remove the syringe with its needle, replacing it with high-pressure connection tubing, which should empty into a collection bottle. Connect the tubing to a new collection bottle when fluid nears the top.

- Steps 9–11 are the same as in the diagnostic paracentesis.

- After a large-volume paracentesis, if over 5 L have been removed, administer 25% albumin at 6–8 g per L removed.

Nephrology

Bliss J. Chang

Contents

© The Author(s), under exclusive license to Springer Nature Switzerland AG 2021
S. H. Lecker, B. J. Chang (eds.), *The Ultimate Medical School Rotation Guide*,
https://doi.org/10.1007/978-3-030-63560-2_18

18.1 Overview

Nephrology is one of the most cerebral rotations, packed with physiology and calculations. Unsurprisingly, nephrologists are on the nerdier side of specialties, and knowing your stuff will really impress them. To excel, you will primarily need a good working knowledge of fundamental concepts and be able to apply physiology to solve cases.

This chapter begins with fundamentals, providing a view into everyday things, like lab values, from a nephrologist's perspective. While these points of discussion may seem routine, you should pay close attention to the nuances that each section discusses.

18.2 Fundamentals

18.2.1 Big Picture

In nephrology, the ultimate question becomes, "Does the patient need dialysis?" And if not, "How do we prevent dialysis?" Given that the function of the kidneys is to filter and prevent accumulation of waste and electrolytes in your body to toxic levels, the last resort is dialysis, an artificial method of filtering the blood, so that one does not suffer from the (often lethal) buildup of toxins. Regardless of what specific disease you're dealing with, always keep this in the back of your mind.

18.2.2 Urine Output (UOP)

You will need to interpret UOP constantly throughout your rotation. A normal UOP is defined as approximately 1.5–2 mL/kg/hr. This translates to approximately 100 mL/hr. or 1–2 L/day for the average patient. You should be familiar with two terms that are frequently used to describe urine output:
- Oliguria/oliguric: <0.5 mL/kg/hr, <500 mL/day
- Anuria/anuric: <100 mL/day

18.2.3 Glomerular Filtration Rate (GFR)

GFR is the primary way by which we define kidney function. Directly proportional to the number of functional nephrons, the GFR, as its name suggests, is a measure of how much blood is filtered through the glomeruli per minute. A normal GFR is usually considered to be >100 mL/min, whereas end-stage kidney disease requiring dialysis is typically less than 10–15 mL/min. Stages of chronic kidney disease (CKD) are classified according to GFR as in ◘ Table 18.1. Whenever you have a patient with known CKD, always use the specific stage descriptor.

GFR calculations differ according to the exact method that you use. The most popular equation for GFR calculation is the CKD-EPI which works well particularly for higher GFRs. This is the equation that most hospitals will use to report GFR in routine labs when applicable. You do not need to know all the various equations and nuances, but you should be aware that certain equations perform better at higher or lower GFRs and that these equations are *estimates*.

18

Table 18.1 CKD stages versus GFR

CKD stage	GFR (mL/min)
I	>90
II	60–89
IIIa	45–59
IIIb	30–44
IV	15–29
V (end stage)	<15

18.2.4 Creatinine (Cr)

This is a very important lab value that is at the center of your nephrology rotation. Let's begin by learning a little about what creatinine is – a metabolite from normal muscle function. As a by-product of muscle function, it is excreted by the kidneys at a constant rate throughout the day. It is used as a marker of kidney function because (1) it is easy to measure in the blood and (2) is approximates GFR well, though not perfectly (overestimates slightly, ~10%).

It is critical to always note a patient's baseline Cr because so many factors can influence it. An easy way to find this is by going through the Lab Flowsheet feature in Epic (or similar process in other EMRs). The normal range of Cr is between 0.6 and 1.2, but clinically the change from baseline is what is most relevant. Though you likely won't need to consciously think about the non-pathologic factors that could elevate or decrease the Cr level each time you see a patient (because again, the change is key), it is a common question from attendings, so it is worth remembering the key modulators:

— Elevate
  - Increased muscle mass (male, bodybuilders, blacks)
  - Medications (cimetidine, trimethoprim, famotidine, cefoxitin)
  - High meat intake, bodybuilding supplements (protein, creatine)
— Decrease
  - Obesity
  - Low muscle mass (elderly, frail, female)
  - Significant liver disease

When interpreting Cr, always keep in mind (1) the magnitude of change from baseline and (2) the rate of change:

— The magnitude of change is not directly proportional to the drop in GFR. Rather, for a doubling in Cr, the GFR drops by 50%, as shown in ▪ Fig. 18.1. Thus, when the Cr is high (e.g., 4.0), a change in the Cr by 0.5 represents only a tiny change in kidney function, potentially even in the range of lab variability. Because of this, you will often see nephrology attendings not concerned about large changes in Cr when in these high territories.

— The rate of change is primarily useful for differentiating between prerenal acute kidney injury (AKI) and acute tubular necrosis (ATN). Prerenal AKI has a gradual climb in Cr, whereas ATN can have much more abrupt changes. We will discuss this later, but it is worth always thinking about as habit.

Pearl: Can mention in your A/P that the GFR doesn't change as much despite this "substantial" change in Cr because of this relationship (mention the graph) – impressive!

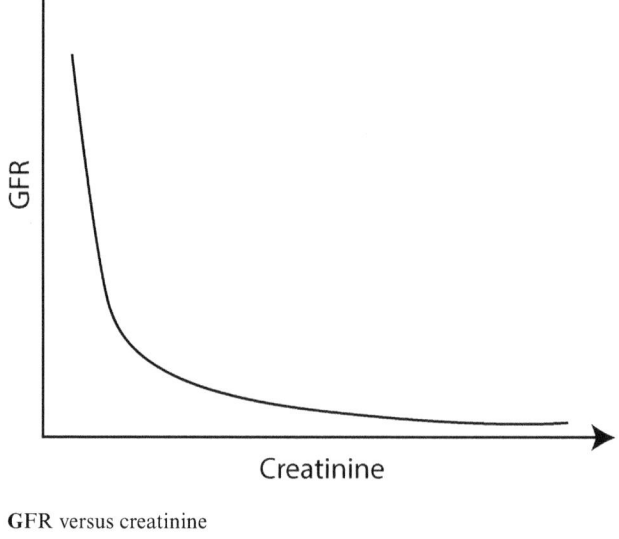

◘ Fig. 18.1 GFR versus creatinine

Lastly, you must know when the Cr is worth using. In other words, what is the purpose of using the Cr value? For instance, in patients on routine hemodialysis (HD), their Cr values will undergo a cyclic pattern of up and down based on their dialysis regimen. As such, it is less important to be focused on the exact value of Cr and keeping it in normal range (which it will never be). Rather, you should simply be reassured when the Cr drops after a dialysis session – evidence that the HD worked.

18.2.5 Blood Urea Nitrogen (BUN)

The BUN is a by-product of protein metabolism. Similar to Cr, it is also renally cleared, meaning that increasing levels will be seen when the kidneys aren't working properly. The BUN is normally under 20. As we will learn later, the BUN/Cr ratio is one tool used for determining the etiology of renal dysfunction. Whenever you interpret the BUN/Cr ratio, you should think about whether the BUN is elevated due to non-renal causes such as a GI bleed or recent steroid use. Conversely, the BUN may be falsely low in cases of malnutrition.

18.2.6 Sodium

 Pearl: Hyponatremia correction for hyperglycemia – use a correction factor of 1.6 per 100 g glucose above 100 g (e.g., a blood glucose of 300 would result in a sodium level of 132 really being 135.2).

Sodium is a routine lab obtained as part of the basic metabolic panel on almost every service. In nephrology, it holds greater meaning. Water always follows sodium; thus, the sodium is a surrogate marker of the intravascular volume. In most cases, the serum sodium level is a better reflection of body water than body sodium. In cases where there is excess body water, sodium levels are low (hyponatremia), and conversely, when there is dehydration, sodium levels rise.

18.2.7 Urine Electrolytes

The electrolytes in our serum are filtered by the kidney into urine. This is a valuable source of diagnostic information. The key urine electrolytes are sodium, chloride, creatinine, and urea:

- Urine sodium (UNa) is an indicator of how much sodium the body is attempting to rid or retain. A low sodium (UNa < 20) indicates that the body wants to hold on to sodium, whereas a high sodium (UNa > 20) indicates a desire to rid sodium. Examples of low UNa conditions include prerenal AKI and hepatorenal syndrome. Examples of conditions that lead to a high UNa most commonly include SIADH (Syndrome of Inappropriate Antidiuretic Hormone) and diuretic usage.
- Urine chloride can be thought of similarly to urine sodium, and also as a surrogate marker for excretion of acid since one Cl- ion is secreted per NH^{4+} secreted into the urine. UCl^- is primarily considered when assessing for metabolic alkalosis (high secretion of acid means the serum pH would increase). Note that urine Cl^- is also increased by diuretic use.
- Urine urea is helpful for a variety of assessments, but we will use it specifically for the FeUrea calculations. Grossly, it can be a marker of your protein intake.

These electrolytes alone provide great information, but their sensitivity and specificity can be increased by using a few formulas that take them into consideration. In particular, you will often use the fractional excretion of sodium (FeNa) and fractional excretion of urea (FeUrea). Both are used to help determine the etiology of AKI as prerenal, intrinsic, or post-obstructive. FeUrea is used when the patient is or has been on diuretics. Since diuretics increase urine sodium even if the kidney should be sodium avid, FeNa is no longer accurate, thus the use of FeUrea. Using the FeUrea appropriately is a great chance to shine!!

You've probably been extremely annoyed at trying to remember the formulas for FeNa and FeUrea. One way to remember is to realize that both the numerator and denominator contain urine and serum values. The trick is to figure out whether the UNa or UUrea belongs in the numerator or denominator. Since we are trying to compute the fraction of excretion of sodium in the urine, it would make sense that the UNa is in the numerator with the serum Na in the denominator. The same rule applies for FeUrea.

$$FeNa = \frac{Urine\,Na \times Serum\,Cr}{Urine\,Cr \times Serum\,Na}$$

$$FeUrea = \frac{Urine\,Urea \times Serum\,Cr}{Urine\,Cr \times Serum\,Urea}$$

Table 18.2 below displays the interpretation associated with these values. The most common use of FeNa or FeUrea is to differentiate between AKI and ATN (acute tubular necrosis). Remember that ATN is an intrinsic process, even though prerenal etiologies often precede ATN.

Table 18.2 Urine electrolytes interpretation

	Prerenal	Intrinsic	Post-obstructive
Urine Na	<20	>40	>40
FeNa	<1%	>1%	>4%
FeUrea	≤35%	>50%	N/A

18.2.8 **Volume Status**

In nephrology, the term "volume" refers specifically to the amount of space occupied by a combination of fluid and dissolved substances such as electrolytes and proteins. Volume is NOT the same as "water" or "fluid." The term "free water" specifically refers to water in isolation, without association with components such as sodium. In other words, volume is made up of free water and everything else dissolved in it.

The volume in our bodies can be thought of as in two primary compartments – intravascular and extravascular. Intravascular volume is that contained inside the blood vessels (vasculature) and is what our organs such as the heart "see." Extravascular volume is that outside the blood vessels and in connective tissues, sometimes referred to as interstitial fluid. Whenever you have a volume problem, consider which compartment is affected.

Fluid shifts between the two compartments in a manner that allows maintenance of equilibrium. If there is too much fluid in the intravascular space, it will shift into the extravascular compartment in a process known as "third-spacing". Conversely, too little intravascular volume and the extravascular fluid will try to shift inward, causing the dry mucous membranes and skin tenting on exam.

When fluid shifts between compartments, the levels of any substance, such as electrolytes and cells, can become concentrated or diluted. For example, when a patient is given copious IV fluid, they will transiently have an increased intravascular volume until the body equilibrates. This means that their blood counts (i.e., RBC, WBC, platelets) may all drop by a notable amount (e.g., Hb drops by 1). This should not prompt concern for an acute GI bleed given that you just administered fluid and there is a congruent decrease across all blood cell types.

Volume status can be approximated by the following exam findings:

- Blood pressure
- Jugular venous distension
- Lower extremity edema
- Mucous membrane moisture

18.2.9 **Fluid Choice**

The administration of IV fluid bypasses the natural mechanisms in place to preserve homeostasis. Thus, careful selection of fluids is critical for preserving the body's equilibrium, particularly with regard to electrolytes. Each time you administer fluid, you should have a clear goal in mind about why you're administering the fluid, and that will inform your choice of fluid. You should NOT be mindlessly administering fluid for patients.

The normal plasma composition is very important to remember for reference during any problem involving fluids and electrolytes (which is all of nephrology). They are as follows:

- Na 135–145
- Cl 100–110
- K 3.5–5.0
- iCa 2.2–2.6
- HCO3 22–26
- Osm 280–295

◪ Table 18.3 IV fluid types

Fluid	Na	Cl	K	HCO₃	Ca	Glucose	Osm	Notes
D5W (dextrose)	–	–	–	–	–	50 g	154	Little remains in the intravascular space
½ (0.45%) NS	77	77	–	–	–	–	154	Some remains in the intravascular space
0.9% NS	154	154	–	–	–	–	308	All remains in the intravascular space
Lactated ringer	130	109	4	–	3	–	273	All remains in the intravascular space
3% (hypertonic) saline	513	513	–	–	–	–	1026	May be used in symptomatic hyponatremia

The most common reason for fluid administration is to replete volume, which typically refers to low intravascular volume (and consequently low extravascular volume). The fluids of choice are either normal 0.9% saline (NS) or lactated ringers (LR). NS is composed of 154 mEq of Na and Cl for a total of 308 Osm. LR is composed of 130 mEq Na, 109 mEq Cl, 4 mEq K, 3 mEq Ca, and 28 mEq lactate for a total of 273 Osm and is thus considered a crystalloid fluid.

Numerous trials have investigated which is the superior fluid choice, and it is worth knowing two key trials. First, the SALT-ED Trial (NEJM 2018) investigated this dilemma in non-critically ill patients in an emergency department setting and found no benefit to either fluid choice. However, the SMART Trial (NEJM 2018) investigated the same dilemma in critically ill ICU patients and found a significantly lower rate of mortality, new renal-replacement therapy, and persistent renal dysfunction with balanced crystalloids (e.g., LR). Long story short, there is not a big difference between which you administer and the choice is often dependent on institution and attending. However, there may be some benefit in careful fluid choice in critically ill patients.

The main fluid options are shown in ◪ Table 18.3.

18.2.10 Renal Replacement Therapy (Dialysis)

Unlike some organs, the kidneys are not essential for survival as long as their function is substituted. Dialysis (also referred to as renal replacement therapy or RRT) has been one of the greatest life-sustaining measures invented, both for acute and chronic kidney dysfunction. It utilizes a semipermeable membrane to filter the blood of toxins and metabolites as would a healthy kidney. Many the patients that you encounter will either require or already be on hemodialysis. Thus, we provide an overview of the different types of dialysis prior to delving into specific diseases.

Chronic dialysis (HD) comes in two major forms: peritoneal and hemodialysis. Hemodialysis is the overwhelmingly more common form that utilizes a dialysis machine with the semipermeable membrane to circulate and filter blood. Access is typically via an AV fistula or graft located on the antecubital fossa, though there are other more temporary options such as a tunneled catheter in the internal jugular vein. HD is performed three times weekly, either on an M/W/F or a T/R/Sa regimen, through 3–4 hour sessions. On the other hand, peritoneal dialysis utilizes the natural peritoneal membrane as a semipermeable filter to perform the same function as a dialyzer.

Dialysis will not filter everything. It would be devastating if things like proteins and red blood cells in your body were dialyzed out! Generally, molecules in size greater than a few hundred Daltons are ineffectively dialyzed.

There are two different dialysate compositions used for CVVH: B32K4 and B22K4. The B refers to the bicarbonate and K, the potassium. The potassium content is the same in both, but the bicarbonate varies so that it can be effective for dialyzing in both acidemic and alkalotic conditions.

Acute dialysis is utilized when the patient has a new condition that leads to imminent danger of complications or death without fixing. Common scenarios include acute intoxications of various chemicals as well as acute renal impairment leading to anuria. Because the patient does not have an established access method for dialysis, a central venous catheter is placed. If hemodynamically stable, such patients can undergo dialysis treatments similar to chronic patients. In the ICU, when many patients are critically ill and hemodynamically unstable, continuous veno-venous hemodialysis (CVVHD) and continuous veno-venous hemodiafiltration (CVVHDF) are more often performed. CVVHD utilizes dialysis using a semipermeable membrane and osmotic gradient, whereas CVVHDF also adds on a convective force (an artificial pulling force) to help take off additional fluid. The convective force is known as ultrafiltration.

18.3 Practical Tips

This section provides a short collection of nephrology-specific practical tips for your nephrology rotation. Please refer to the Practical Tips section of Internal Medicine (▶ Chap. 16) for great tips on general workflow and task management.

18.3.1 Foley Management

As you pre-round in the morning, it is important to always take a look at any Foley bags to check the color and urine output. Do not trust what is recorded in the computer – it is often inaccurate. At the least you should check with the nurse regarding when the bag was last emptied. When you check the bag, hold up the Foley tubing to fully drain the remaining urine in there. This often gives you quite a bit of additional volume that would otherwise be missed.

18.3.2 Urine Sediment

The Foley bag has a knob at the bottom which can be used to drain some urine. Make sure to update the ins/outs recording or notify the nurse.

You should obtain a small amount (~50 cc) of urine and spin for microscopy in just about every patient on the renal consult service. Prior to spinning the urine, use a dipstick to obtain some basic information on the urine, such as pH, presence of blood/glucose/protein, and infection. Next, transfer a pipet-full (~5 cc) of the urine into a clear test tube and spin it for 3–5 minutes at a speed of 1500 rpm. Once the centrifugation is complete, carefully decant off the urine, leaving a small pellet at the bottom along with some urine. Resuspend the pellet in the urine and transfer a drop or two onto a glass plate and add a coverslip to it. Always start with the lowest available power. Common casts are depicted in ◻ Fig. 18.2.

Specific pearls for analyzing the urine sediment:
1. ATN is a low-power diagnosis, meaning that you should be using low-power microscopy to check for the presence of muddy brown casts.
2. Muddy brown casts tend to reside along the edges of the coverslips. Try looking here if there aren't obvious casts everywhere!
3. Always take a picture of what you see on the microscope to show your team. Taking a picture with your smartphone requires obtaining the right angle and stability. This is really trial and error and you'll develop your own system for optimizing the picture quality.

18

Nephrology

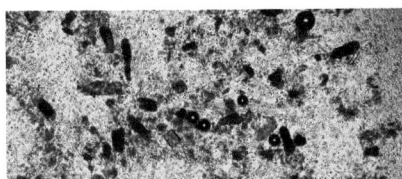

Muddy Brown Casts

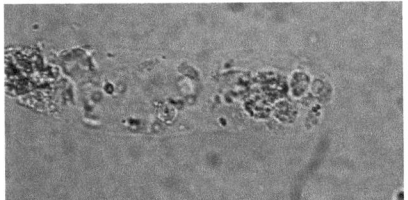

WBC Casts

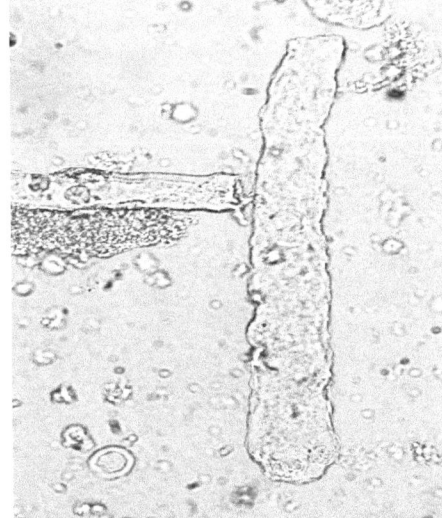

Hyaline Casts

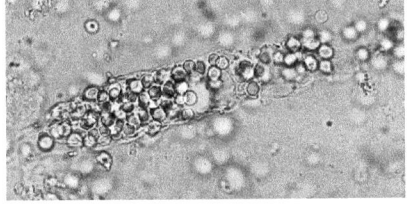

RBC Casts

Fig. 18.2   Common urinary casts

18.4 Common Cases

18.4.1 Acute Kidney Injury

Cr may be elevated for many reasons, but this condition should be treated as an AKI unless proven otherwise. It is critical to thoroughly evaluate all causes of Cr elevation, though the most likely cause is prerenal AKI. Here we provide an approach to evaluating elevated Cr (■ Fig. 18.3).

First, compare the patient's Cr to any baseline values. Certain patients tend to ride on the upper end of normal (high muscle bulk) or live chronically with an elevated Cr (CKD, dialysis patients). Check both the magnitude of the Cr bump and, if applicable, the rate at which the Cr rose. Common medications that artificially elevate the Cr, but do not necessarily decrease the GFR, include IV Bactrim (trimethoprim in particular), famotidine, and cimetidine. These agents block the small amount of tubular secretion of creatinine (~10%) that occurs normally. If one of these medications is taken by the patient, check how long the medication has been taken. If the Cr rise is acute and the medication is chronic, there is likely a different cause.

Once you have established that the Cr is truly elevated from a patient's baseline, our suggested approach is to start checking for acute kidney injury, as that is the most common cause of an elevated Cr. You should systematically think about AKI in three buckets: prerenal, intrinsic, and post-renal. Regardless of the classification, you should always (1) obtain urine lytes (urine Na, urine Cr) and (2) spin the urine sediment for each patient with an elevated Cr.

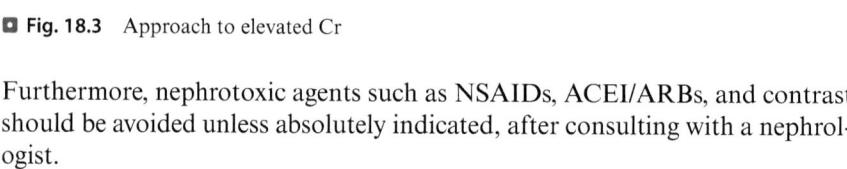

◻ Fig. 18.3   Approach to elevated Cr

Furthermore, nephrotoxic agents such as NSAIDs, ACEI/ARBs, and contrast should be avoided unless absolutely indicated, after consulting with a nephrologist.

- ■ **General AKI Management Checklist**
- ═ [ ] Obtain BMP + urine Lytes
- ═ [ ] Spin urine sediment
- ═ [ ] Avoid nephrotoxins

Prerenal AKI refers to an etiology "before" the kidneys, that is, inadequate blood flow to the kidney. Volume depletion (low intravascular) and poor forward flow (heart failure) are two common conditions that lead to decreased renal perfusion. The patient usually presents with signs of volume loss (dry mucous membranes, flat Jugular Venous Pressure - JVP) and decreased urine output. The BUN/Cr ratio is classically greater than 20 and the FeNa is less than 1%. When the objective data is unclear or borderline, a fluid challenge can be administered to empirically test (and treat) for prerenal AKI. A fluid challenge consists of a 0.5 L–1 L isotonic fluid (NS or LR) bolus to replete the depleted intravascular volume, thereby providing the kidney with newfound adequate perfusion. This should decrease the Cr and improve urine output. The patient should continue to receive adequate hydration to prevent further prerenal AKI.

Nephrology

Intrinsic AKI refers to an elevated Cr secondary to kidney tissue damage. Causes of intrinsic AKI can be divided into three buckets: glomerular, tubulo-interstitial, and vascular.

- Glomerular disease most often refers to glomerulonephritis. Examples include ANCA-positive vasculitis such as granulomatosis with polyangiitis (GPA) and microscopic polyangiitis. Anti-GBM disease is also a common cause in young- to middle-aged adult males.
- Tubulo-interstitial disease refers to dysfunction of the actual tubules in the nephrons, most commonly acute tubular necrosis (ATN) and acute interstitial nephritis (AIN).
- Vascular intrinsic AKI refers to either microvascular or macrovascular dysfunction.
  - Microvascular: the microangiopathic hemolytic anemias (HUS, TTP)
  - Macrovascular: renal artery stenosis

As a medical student, you will not see much glomerular or vascular disease, though possible depending on your institution and particular service. As such, we will not cover those causes in depth here, but if you do encounter those patients, a good resource is *Renal Pathophysiology* by Helmut Rennke and Bradley Denker.

ATN can be thought of as the extreme end of the prerenal AKI spectrum. After prolonged ischemia to the tubules from poor renal perfusion, the tubules die in what is known as acute tubular necrosis. There is no acute recovery possible (though many patients can recover over the course of weeks) for tubules that undergo ATN, so the goal is to identify prerenal AKI as early as possible and prevent the progression. Objective data that support ATN include FeNa >2% and urine osmolality that is close to serum osmolality (without the discerning ability of the tubules, urine is iso-osmolar to plasma). Most helpful, however, is the history (e.g., periods of hypoperfusion) and trajectory of the creatinine rise – ATN often involves significant and abrupt jumps. Classically, muddy brown casts are seen on urine microscopy best at low power.

> Pearl: Check the edges of the coverslip as the muddy brown casts often reside there.

It is not uncommon to have a mixture of prerenal AKI and ATN, with ongoing evolution toward ATN. In these cases, the lab values are in between and microscopy may demonstrate a few muddy brown casts (and more later). This is the critical point in which intervention to improve kidney perfusion can really save a patient's kidney.

> Pearl: The absence of muddy brown casts does not rule out ATN! They are specific but not sensitive.

Acute interstitial nephritis can be due to a variety of causes but most often due to medications. Common medications that can cause AIN are remembered by the mnemonic PND-SR (penicillins, NSAIDs, diuretics, sulfonamide, rifampin). The presence of eosinophilia in the blood is helpful, though its absence does not rule out AIN. The offending agent (typically a newly initiated medication) should be removed immediately.

Post-renal AKI refers to an obstruction distal to the kidney (e.g., in the urethra or ureters) that prevents urine from leaving the urinary system, thus causing a buildup and backup into the kidney. The backup of urine acts as a force against the filtration function of the kidney and thus results in accumulation of wastes such as Cr, BUN as well as electrolyte derangements – the same picture as with any renal dysfunction. Post-renal AKI usually has a BUN/Cr of around 10 and FeNa >2%. Furthermore, using a Foley to cath the patient can be a valuable empiric test for whether there is urine retention/backup and whether an obstruction is the source of AKI.

18.4.1.1 Treatment

Once the type and cause of AKI are determined, the treatment is usually supportive care while addressing the cause of kidney injury. For instance, in prerenal AKI, the solution is IV fluids since volume depletion was the problem. In hepatorenal syndrome, correcting the liver fixes the kidney dysfunction. Removing the obstruction in post-renal AKI does the trick. You get the drift…

18.4.2 Electrolyte Disorders

In this section, we will cover the most common electrolyte disorders and those of sodium, potassium, and calcium.

18.4.3 Sodium Disorders

Remember that in normal physiology, sodium follows water and vice versa. Sodium disorders occur when there is an alteration in the sodium to water ratio. This usually means that the water reabsorption/excretion mechanisms are dysfunctional.

For each sodium disorder, start by establishing the patient's volume status as hypovolemic, euvolemic, or hypervolemic. This greatly aids in narrowing the differential. The best noninvasive markers of volume status are blood pressure, heart rate, JVP, and lower extremity edema.

18.4.3.1 Hyponatremia

Hypovolemic hyponatremia occurs when intravascular volume is reduced triggering antidiuretic hormone (ADH) release and when the patient has fluid intake. Such patients retain this fluid and dilute their body sodium. This is the rarest type of hyponatremia, and you are unlikely to encounter this as a medical student.

In euvolemic hyponatremia, ADH is secreted autonomously, not in response to intravascular volume depletion. The function of ADH is to retain water in the collecting duct via introduction of aquaporin water channels into the tubules. In SIADH, the excess ADH favors a water avid state. In other words, imagine a cup of salt water to which more pure water is added (the effect of excess ADH). Then pour out volume equal to the volume of pure water added (this net excretion of both salt and water is what happens naturally with our kidneys). Since you only took in water but poured out both water and salt, the net effect is euvolemia with hyponatremia.

The diagnosis of SIADH is made based on exam and labs. On exam, the patient appears euvolemic with moist mucous membranes et al. with no signs of volume overload.

■   Workup Checklist for SIADH
–   [ ] Urine sodium (UNa) + urine Osms
–   [ ] Urine output

UNa will be greater than 30–40 and the UOsm will be >100. In severe cases, urine output will be decreased (oliguric), which is another way of saying the urine is very concentrated (lots of ADH around).

The treatment for SIADH centers on (1) treating the underlying cause if known and (2) restricting actions that lead to augmentation of the physiology at work. The vast majority of SIADH cases are of an unclear etiology, but it may warrant consideration of a more worrisome etiology such as small-cell

Pearl for ODS: the studies done examining this risk had no patient experience ODS unless Na change >12 mEq/day.

lung cancer. Given the appropriate demographics (e.g., old male smoker), a case of SIADH should prompt further investigation. Acutely, however, the key is to restrict free water intake because it will worsen the hyponatremia since that fluid cannot be effectively excreted. In acutely symptomatic patients, a 100 cc bolus of hypertonic saline should be administered. If fluids are required, be sure to use normal saline, avoiding any fluids with low osmolality (e.g., D5W, ½ NS). With water restriction, you should perform routine sodium checks (q2h initially to q12h) and closely monitor the urine output, as the transition from oliguria to normal urine output signifies the resolution of SIADH (and may prompt you to stop interventions such as administering hypertonic saline). It is critical not to correct the sodium level too fast (average 6-8 mEq/day) given the risk of osmotic demyelination syndrome (ODS). Adjunctive therapies include providing salt tabs and demeclocycline (rarely used in clinical practice).

Rapid or uncontrolled correction of hyponatremia is a real problem in the management of this condition. An alternate approach to treatment is to use what is known as a DDAVP "clamp." This is a method in which the patient is given synthetic ADH (DDAVP) to fix them iatrogenically in a high SIADH state. Appropriate fluid (usually hypertonic saline) is administered slowly, until sodium levels have normalized. Then the clamp is released. In one of the best studies investigating the clamp, there were no cases of sodium overcorrection utilizing this method. Many institutions have shifted over to this method as it is much less intensive and there have been no downsides shown other than an average of 1-day longer hospitalization.

Hypervolemic hyponatremia is what we classically consider in volume-overload hospital admissions – such as due to heart failure exacerbation and decompensated cirrhosis. In these cases, the hyponatremia is a function of massive volume increase out of proportion to the amount of sodium in our bodies. This water and sodium retention leads to the characteristic lower extremity edema in heart failure patients. The treatment centers on removing the excess water and sodium through diuresis. As the intravascular volume decreases from diuresis, the extravascular fluid will shift into the vasculature, restoring homeostasis. Patients with cirrhosis and heart failure may live with chronic mild hyponatremia. There is no specific need to begin an extensive workup on hyponatremia in these cases when the principal problem (e.g., heart failure) is clear.

18.4.3.2 Hypernatremia

The most common cause of hypernatremia that you will encounter is dehydration. Imagine the nursing home patient with a decreased thirst mechanism and little access to fluid intake. Insensible losses will promote a state in which water is lost in excess of salt. Hypernatremia also results from diabetes insipidus, either central or nephrogenic.

Diabetes insipidus (DI) leads to the inability of the body to retain water, either from a lack of ADH secretion (central) or lack of tubular responsiveness (nephrogenic). Without ADH, the kidney is not able to reabsorb water, leading to free water loss out of proportion to sodium. DI results in hypovolemic hypernatremia. Common causes of DI to ascertain in the history include lithium (nephrogenic) and pituitary adenoma (central).

The management of hypernatremia begins as with all sodium disorders – determination of the volume status. Once you have confirmed that the patient is volume deplete, the treatment is to provide back the missing free water and volume. You read that correctly – both free water and volume. Remember that these are distinct. Volume refers to what specifically the intravascular status is and is a combination of both fluid and osmotic pressure to keep the fluid in the vasculature (without any solutes, water would not stay in the permeable vasculature). Free water is only the water without solutes. Generally, patients with hypernatremia will have lost both free water and volume.

To replete the free water, calculate and administer the free deficit as follows:

$$\text{Free water deficit} = \% \text{ total body water}\left(\text{TBW}\right) \times \text{weight}\left(\text{kg}\right)$$
$$\times\left[\left(\text{current Na / desired Na}\right) - 1\right]$$

where TBW varies slightly with gender (60% male, 50% female). This formula is very logical, and you should be able to reason through this without the use of a calculator (though MDCalc exists). It is a very common thing you will be asked to calculate on the spot, so have the patient's weight handy.

The choice of fluid depends on the extent of hypernatremia. Remember that the osmolality of NS is 154, so it is usually the best choice for correcting significant hypernatremia to avoid extremely quick correction. In very rare situations, you may need to use 1/2NS for a quicker adjustment in very symptomatic patients. The risk of cerebral herniation is not as well known nor evidence-based for lowering the sodium quickly as is osmotic demyelination syndrome for correcting upward. For mild hypernatremia, free water can be provided with PO intake, free water IV flushes (q6h), or small amounts of D5W.

You MUST monitor the sodium level (e.g., q4h checks) while giving back free water. The recommended rate of correction is a maximum of 0.5 mEq/L/h.

Not to be forgotten, the underlying cause of hypernatremia should be addressed. In cases of central DI, the patient will need ADH supplementation. For nephrogenic DI, the patient will typically start with hydrochlorothiazide and/or amiloride.

18.4.4 Potassium Disorders

Potassium resides in both intracellular and extracellular (plasma) compartments, but it prefers to stay inside the cells. Thus, it is no wonder that potassium is the most abundant electrolyte within the cells. The balance of potassium is modulated largely by the sodium-potassium ATPase, which pumps three potassium ions intracellularly for two Na+ ions extracellularly. When looking at a potassium value, always consider the mechanism leading to that value and what, if anything, would happen to this balance of intra- versus extracellular potassium.

Begin by identifying whether the potassium derangement is isolated or in conjunction with other lab abnormalities. The presence of other abnormalities focuses you on a different set of differentials.

18.4.4.1 Hypokalemia

Low potassium levels are most frequently iatrogenic, from causes such as diuresis. They may also result from chronic diarrhea or vomiting. The other causes such as renal tubular acidosis (RTA) are much rarer, and it is unlikely that you will be consulted specifically for a disorder of potassium. Rather it is much more likely to be a secondary problem in patients.

Always check a patient's medication list, specifically looking at recent medication changes. Furthermore, always inquire about patient symptoms of hypokalemia (palpitations, cramping, weakness, constipation). Symptomatic hypokalemia should always prompt urgent intervention, particularly from a cardiac standpoint.

For mild asymptomatic hypokalemia, adjusting medications and/or the underlying cause with observation is the usual management. Potassium supplements are often used for patients who need to be on a potassium-wasting medication but have low potassium. There is no need to pursue an extensive workup in the absence of other indications.

For significant and/or symptomatic hypokalemia, obtain an EKG immediately and look for signs of hypokalemia (flattening of T waves, prolonged QT, ST depressions). If any of these signs are present, the patient should immediately receive IV potassium. Otherwise, oral potassium chloride (KCl) is acceptable as it is absorbed quite quickly without the unpleasant burning sensation through IV. Due to this burning sensation, the maximum rate of IV potassium infusion is 10 mEq/hr. on the floor or 20 mEq/hr. in the ICU.

Lastly, lab potassium levels may be a poor reflection of total body potassium in diabetic ketoacidosis (refer to Critical Care, ▶ Chap. 15). This is because with potassium loss from plasma, the intracellular potassium shifts outward to restore equilibrium. This shift is also caused by low pH and presence of excessive glucose (increases insulin secretion thereby leading to increased cellular uptake of potassium). In these patients, it is important to keep the potassium level in the high range of normal to ensure that there is no acute hypokalemia once the precipitating factors (e.g., pH and glucose) are fixed.

- Hypokalemia Management Checklist
- [ ] Screen for common etiologies
- [ ] Replete (PO > IV)
- [ ] Check Mg and replete if deficient

> Be sure to check magnesium levels and replete if deficient, as low magnesium levels lead to increased excretion of potassium (rendering your potassium repletion efforts ineffective).

> Pearl: Avoid administering solutions containing sugar (e.g., D5W) since this can worsen the hypokalemia via extracellular to intracellular shift.

18.4.4.2 Hyperkalemia

High potassium levels are most commonly caused by renal impairment, ingestions (medications, supplements), and lab artifact (pseudohyperkalemia). Start by ensuring that the potassium value is real, either by rechecking or by ordering a whole blood potassium.

In dialysis patients, potassium levels are chronically high often and thus if the patient is scheduled for dialysis soon, it is reasonable to wait if asymptomatic without EKG findings. I have seen levels as high as the low 6.0's where no acute intervention is taken, though this is stylistic and institution-dependent. Of course, if the patient is symptomatic or the whole blood potassium is sky high (e.g. > 6.5), you should notify your team immediately. Note that potassium may also be elevated in patients with acute renal dysfunction (such as AKI) and varying stages of CKD.

Without kidney disease or pseudohyperkalemia, the principal causes are ingestions and cell lysis. Always check whether it is an isolated hyperkalemia or accompanied by other lab abnormalities. You should also search for common medications that can cause hyperkalemia such as ACEI/ARBs, potassium-sparing diuretics, high-dose Bactrim, succinylcholine, and digoxin.

Management of hyperkalemia is primarily driven by symptoms and EKG changes (peaking of T waves, flattening of P waves, increased PR intervals). When worried about true hyperkalemia, you should always immediately obtain an EKG.

Acutely, the management for hyperkalemia is focused into two parts: stabilization and temporizing measures.

- Stabilization refers to protecting the heart to which hyperkalemia is pro-arrhythmogenic. Administer 1-2 g calcium gluconate every 5 minutes until the potassium is out of the danger zone.
- Temporizing measures are methods of redistributing the potassium between body compartments (i.e., intra/extracellular). There are three common agents used:
  - Insulin (10 U) + D5W (only if blood glucose <250)
  - Bicarbonate (1–2 ampules; only in patients with good renal function)
  - Albuterol (10-20 mg)

Lastly, excess potassium should be eliminated from the body after stabilization and temporizing measures. This is done usually with furosemide, though in certain extreme cases, hemodialysis may be warranted. All the while, treatable underlying causes should be fixed immediately to prevent further worsening or persistence of hyperkalemia.

- **Hyperkalemia Management Checklist**
- [ ] Verify hyperkalemia
- [ ] Stabilize
- [ ] Temporize
- [ ] Check for common etiologies
- [ ] Eliminate

18.4.5 Calcium Disorders

Calcium exists in the body in two forms: ionized and bound. Ionized calcium (iCa^{2+}) is the physiologically active calcium. When you obtain labs on Ca, you are checking the bound form unless you specifically order the iCa^{2+}. The bound calcium is primarily on albumin, and thus can be influenced by albumin levels. When you check reported calcium values, correct for albumin deficiency with the formula below which essentially states that for each 1 g of albumin deficiency, the calcium is underreported by 0.8 mEq.

$$\text{True Calcium} = \text{Measured Calcium} + \left[(4.0 - \text{albumin}) * 0.8\right]$$

18.4.5.1 Hypocalcemia

Common causes of hypocalcemia include parathyroid/thyroid surgery, autoimmune disease, and pancreatitis. Certain medications (cinacalcet, foscarnet, fluoride, EDTA) can be culprits, but they are unusual. Classic signs and symptoms include numbness/tingling around the mouth, cramping of muscles, contraction of facial muscles with tapping over the facial nerve (Chvostek's sign), and curling of the wrist with blood pressure cuff inflation (Trousseau's sign). If consulted for hypocalcemia, your responsibility will primarily be determination of the underlying etiology and treatment.

Your primary workup centers around determining the parathyroid hormone (PTH) state. Causes for low PTH is primarily alterations of the parathyroid (surgery, autoimmune), whereas high PTH hypocalcemia points toward high phosphate states (rhabdo, cell lysis). Always check the levels of PTH, Mg, PO_4, 1,25-$(OH)_2$ Vit D, and 25-(OH) Vit D. The primary team should already have obtained the Ca, iCa, albumin, and Cr levels, but if they have not, you should also obtain these.

Treatment of hypocalcemia is simple: replete the calcium. Repletion is done orally if Ca >7.5 or asymptomatic, whereas IV $CaCl_2$ repletion is reserved for symptomatic hypocalcemia or severely low levels (<7.5). Orally, CaCitrate is better absorbed than $Ca(HCO_3)_2$, particularly for patients on PPIs. However, pay attention to magnesium deficiency as it is the cofactor responsible for PTH secretion (i.e., deficiency causes decreased PTH and thus decreased Ca).

18.4.5.2 Hypercalcemia

The most common cause of hypercalcemia is ingestions, such as calcium supplements, thiazides, vitamin D excess, and TUMs. We will not cover PTH-dependent causes of hypercalcemia as these are in endocrine's territory. If you are consulted for hypercalcemia, your primary role will be to stabilize the patient. The mainstay of therapy is aggressive fluid administration with a high target UOP. Calcitonin may also be given for severe (>14) or symptomatic hypercalcemia. Lastly, bisphosphonates help to chelate the calcium, but they should be avoided for patients with GFR <30.

18.4.6 Diuresis

Though diuresis is usually managed by the primary medical team, there are occasional consults for refractory diuresis. We will delve into the principles of diuresis here as well as into advanced tactics. We will focus on the most common diuretics; thus, we will not cover diuretics affecting the proximal convoluted tubule (PCT).

The nephron is composed of several segments, each with their own set of transporters that tightly regulate the balance of what remains in the plasma and what is excreted. These transporters can be modulated using drugs to take volume off. Importantly, remember that water follows sodium – all diuretic mechanisms ultimately rely on this principle, that is, altering electrolyte handling to induce the outward movement of water. Remember that the amount of sodium in the filtrate (urine) decreases sharply after each segment of the nephron, with as low as 5% of sodium remaining by the time the filtrate reaches the collecting duct. This means that the transporters only have so much sodium to work with to modulate the direction of water, thus diuretics that act later in the nephron are generally less potent.

18.4.6.1 Loop Diuretics

Loop diuretics such as furosemide (Lasix) are named for their action on the loop of Henle. Specifically, they block the sodium-potassium-chloride (Na-K-2Cl) co-transporter. The natural function of the NKCC transporter is to retain sodium, potassium, and chloride. Consequently, this allows the kidneys to hold on to water. Furthermore, the electrochemical gradient from sodium movement that allows for movement of calcium and magnesium is no longer present, and thus calcium and magnesium loss also occurs. You should be comfortable with the conversation ratios for common diuretics (◻ Fig. 18.4).

18.4.6.2 Thiazide Diuretics

Thiazides such as hydrochlorothiazide act in the distal convoluted tubules (DCT) on the sodium-chloride co-transporter (NCC). Like loop diuretics, the reabsorption of sodium into the blood is blocked, leading to water remaining in the filtrate. Despite being a relatively weak diuretic class, they are particularly useful in refractory diuresis. Chronic diuresis can lead to refractoriness via compensatory hypertrophy of the DCT (and its co-transporters) to retain

Loop Diuretic	PO to IV	IV Conversion Ratios	Duration of Effect
Furosemide	1:2	40	6 (La-six)
Torsemide	1:1	20	~10
Bumetanide	1:1	1	4-6

□ **Fig. 18.4**   Loop diuretics

fluid. Blocking the DCT with a thiazide prior to administering another diuretic class such as loop diuretics can augment diuresis by overwhelming the DCT's attempt to retain fluid.

18.4.6.3 Potassium-Sparing Diuretics

K-sparing diuretics are named as such for the unique property of retaining potassium unlike all other diuretic classes. Amiloride and triamterene (which you will rarely see on your rotation if at all) act on the epithelial sodium channel (ENaC) in the collecting tubules. The inward transit of sodium via the ENaC creates the drive for potassium to move out into the urine. Blocking this inward transit leads to diuresis as well as retention of potassium. Spironolactone and Eplerenone are mineralocorticoid receptor antagonists (MRAs) that act in the collecting tubules. Blocking the MRA activity prevents the formation of the luminal potassium channel and the ENaC, leading to the same effect as the ENaC blockers.

Because of their location at the terminal end of the nephron, potassium-sparing diuretics are relatively weak for diuresis purposes, but they provide a very helpful means of balancing potassium in patients who become hypokalemic on the other diuretic classes. Spironolactone is also used in conjunction with Lasix in a 100:40 mg ratio as first-line therapy for controlling ascites.

18.4.6.4 Diuresis Principles

Since standard diuresis is not a reason for consulting renal, we defer discussion on the fundamentals of diuresis to the Cardiology (▶ Chap. 16).

18.4.6.5 Strategies for Diuresis-Refractoriness

If a patient is not urinating adequately to your initial doses of diuretic, first ensure that you are delivering the diuretic intravenously. Certain diuretics such as lasix are significantly less effective in the setting of volume overload due to gut edema and erratic absorption. Next, attempt dose escalation (typically done by doubling the dose, though there is no guideline for this). If pushes of diuretics are ineffective, consider adding a continuous drip on top of the bolus. Remember that a continuous drip alone is no superior to bolusing diuretics as per the DOSE trial (NEJM 2011). Lastly, you may attempt distal convoluted tubule (DCT) blockade with a thiazide diuretic such as chlorothiazide, bumetanide, or hydrochlorothiazide (though this is less common given it is the weakest of the thiazide diuretics). When medical therapy is ineffective for removing volume, dialysis is available as a last resort.

18.4.6.6 Adverse Effects

Pay attention to two specific side effects of diuretics: electrolyte balance and sulfa-allergies.

18.4.6.7 Electrolyte Balance

By modulating the balance of electrolytes, diuresis runs the risk of altering the electrolyte balance beyond what is physiologically tolerated. All patients receiving diuresis should have their basic electrolytes checked, and if started on a new diuretic regimen outpatient, they will need follow-up for a lab check within a week.

Let's start with the non-potassium-sparing diuretics. Overall, think about losing electrolytes. The most common electrolyte abnormality is hypokalemia. Other alterations include hyponatremia, hypomagnesemia, and hypocalcemia (except thiazides which can cause hypercalcemia). Lastly, occasionally in hypercalcemia, lasix is used to help excrete the calcium, taking advantage of its ability to block Ca reabsorption in the loop of Henle.

For potassium-sparing diuretics, you should just remember that sodium and potassium travel in opposite directions in the collecting tubules. Thus, hyperkalemia can be accompanied by hyponatremia. This is the opposite pattern of electrolytes seen in primary hyperaldosteronism (Conn's disease), and that is why mineralocorticoid receptor antagonists are used in the treatment of primary hyperaldosteronism.

If an electrolyte abnormality is found, the decision to continue with a diuretic is dependent on the degree of derangement. A mild abnormality may call for a reduction in dosage or supplementation with potassium tablets, whereas more significant abnormalities indicate that an alternate regimen should be utilized. As a medical student, your role will be to offer your logical opinions on this as there is no right or wrong answer.

18.4.6.8 Sulfa Allergy

Many diuretics contain a sulfonamide moiety which prohibits patients with sulfa allergies from using them, particularly at high doses. To help remember which diuretics contain sulfa, you should consider that all the commonly utilized diuretics except for K-sparing diuretics contain a sulfa group. Patients with a sulfa allergy can use ethacrynic acid (loop diuretic) and potassium-sparing diuretics, though a trial of a sulfa-containing diuretic with the input of allergy is not unreasonable as some patients can tolerate it.

18.4.7 Cardiorenal Syndrome (CRS)

As the name suggests, cardiorenal syndrome involves the heart and kidneys. There are various classifications of CRS, but the two to remember are type 1 (acute heart failure causing renal dysfunction in the form of AKI) and type 3 (AKI leading to heart failure). The end result is a repeated battle between the kidneys and the heart, each trying to compensate and recover at the unintentional expense of the other. Types 1 and 3 become both answers to the age-old "chicken or egg?" question.

You will frequently receive consults asking whether a patient is in cardiorenal syndrome because of an elevated creatinine or diuretic resistance. Most of the time, these consults simply need reassurance that the problem is not CRS but rather over-diuresis leading to AKI and that the kidneys need a diuresis break. The diagnosis of CRS involvement is largely one that is historical in some ways – the Cr should rise prior to the use of diuretics (or if on home diuretics, increasing doses of diuretics) for heart failure treatment.

In type 1 CRS, acute heart failure can lead to AKI in two ways. Most significantly, poor forward blood flow results in backup of fluid from the heart all the way to the afferent arterioles of the kidney. Furthermore, poor forward blood flow leads to lack of adequate perfusion to the kidneys. This lack of perfusion leads to a prerenal AKI. In turn, the prerenal AKI causes activation of the RAAS system which leads to further salt retention, venous congestion, and volume overload.

The treatment of type 1 CRS aims to fix the underlying physiology – renal venous congestion. This is achieved through diuresis, counter-intuitively in light of an increasing Cr, and improving heart function. Most commonly, this involves inotrope-assisted diuresis to help increase cardiac output (thus decreasing venous congestion) while decreasing overall volume. Several trials, of which you do not need to know the names, have come up short studying whether increasing renal blood flow aids in fixing type 1 CRS. Ultrafiltration is also not recommended unless diuretic-refractory.

Type 3 CRS can be thought of as the opposite of type 1 CRS: a kidney problem leading to acute heart failure. A decrease in kidney function leads to decreased urine output and the volume overload leads to heart failure exacerbation. In this case, the treatment is to target fixing the AKI, while managing the symptoms of heart failure as needed.

18.4.8 Hepatorenal Syndrome (HRS)

Unlike CRS, HRS is exclusively the fault of the liver. Poor kidney function does not drive HRS. The pathophysiology involves decompensated liver failure leading to production of vasodilatory substances that cause splanchnic vasodilation which leads to decreased systemic vascular resistance, intense activation of RAAS and renal vasoconstriction, and ultimately poor renal perfusion (◻ Fig. 18.5).

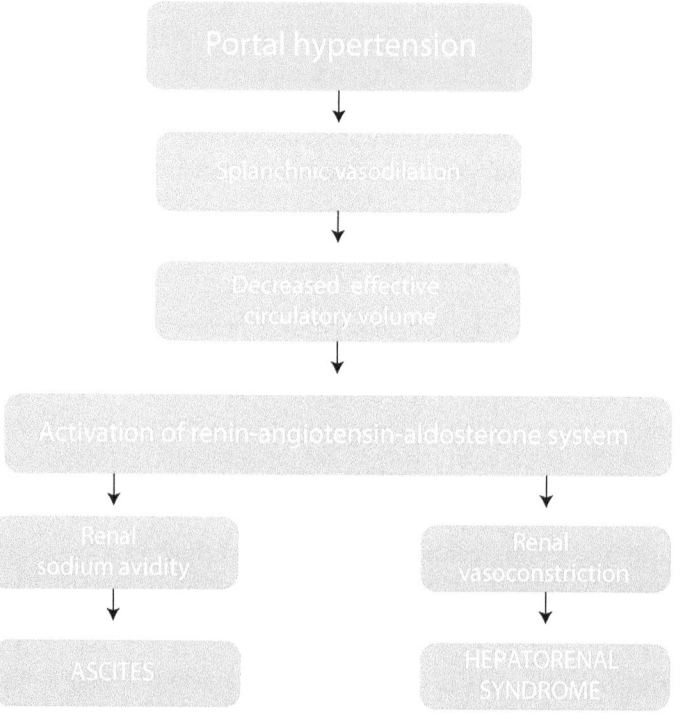

◻ **Fig. 18.5** HRS pathophysiology

The diagnosis of HRS begins with urine lytes. HRS results in a profoundly sodium-avid state, and thus the urine sodium should be <20, often <10.

The treatment of HRS requires a well-functioning liver. This usually means a liver transplant is required, though some causes of liver failure are reversible. However, temporary improvements may be made by addressing the pathophysiology (i.e., splanchnic dilation) with agents such as midodrine, octreotide, and/or albumin.

- Midodrine: 7.5-15 mg q8h PO.
- Octreotide: 50 mcg/hr. IV or SQ.
- Albumin: 1 g/kg/day bolus for 3 days and then 25-50 g/day.

Although stylistic, giving albumin is usually done first prior to considering other interventions.

18.4.9 Acid–Base

This is a topic that will be everywhere on your rotation, and is classically one that students struggle with. Whether it is a primary problem or not, you will be expected to always consider a patient's acid–base status, and free-response-type questions regarding your approach to figuring this out are very common.

Acid–base status simply refers to how the body is dealing with the various components that dictate the patient's pH. The primary components are bicarbonate (HCO_3^-) and carbon dioxide (pCO_2). Both components are part of the buffer equilibrium (remember general chemistry?) as shown below:

$$H_2CO_3 \leftrightarrow H^+ + HCO_3^- \leftrightarrow H_2O + CO_2$$

The bicarbonate acts as a base and the pCO_2 is a surrogate marker of blood acidity. The pH is directly proportional to the amount of protons (H^+) in the blood. As you can see (arrows pointing to CO_2 and HCO_3), increasing CO_2 pushes equilibrum towards acid production and increasing HCO_3 pushes towards more basic conditions via Le Chatelier's principle. This buffer system allows for the body to maintain its tight pH needed for our cellular functions.

Physiologic pH is 7.36–7.44. The usual range for HCO_3 is 22–26 mEq while the pCO_2 is 38–42 mmHg. A high HCO_3 leads to alkalosis, whereas a low HCO_3 (removal of base) leads to acidity. Similarly, an elevated pCO_2 exerts an acidic effect while a low pCO_2 (removal of acid) creates an alkalosis environment.

Your job is to first determine the acid–base status. This status is divided into three parts as in ◻ Fig. 18.6:

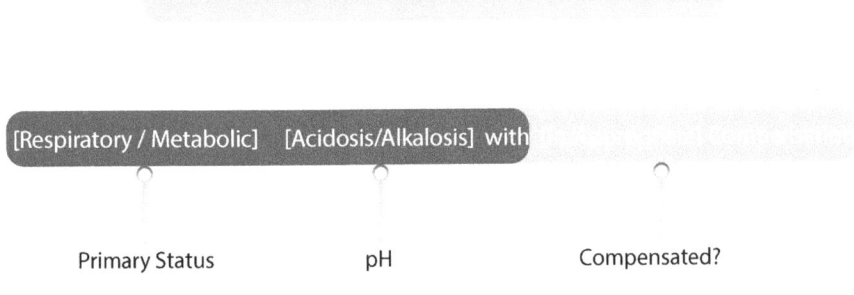

[Respiratory / Metabolic]   [Acidosis/Alkalosis] with

Primary Status   pH   Compensated?

◻ **Fig. 18.6**   Acid–base status dissection

18.4.9.1 Primary Disturbance

The first part refers to whether the acid-base status is primarily driven by changes in respiration (pCO2) or metabolism (HCO_3). All changes in pH are driven by one of these mechanisms. You can determine this by comparing the pH to the bicarbonate and/or pCO_2. Whichever component (HCO_3 or pCO_2) is relatively farthest away from its normal level in a congruent manner as the pH (acidic or basic) will be the primary driver. For example, if the pH is acidic (decreased), check to see if the pCO_2 is elevated. If it is, then we have a primary respiratory acidosis. Otherwise, it would be a metabolic acidosis, confirmed by looking at the HCO_3. This is usually straightforward, though there can be mixed acid–base disorders in which this is more difficult to identify. When a physiologic pH is paired with abnormal HCO_3 and pCO_2 values, this signifies a mixed disorder.

The second part is easy – it simply refers to whether the pH is acidic or alkalic. Now let's practice determining the first two components of an acid–base description with the Flash Quiz below.

■ Flash Quiz
1. pH 7.21; HCO_3 21; pCO_2 89 = > primary acute respiratory acidosis
2. pH 7.55; HCO_3 37; pCO_2 60 => primary metabolic alkalosis

18.4.9.2 Compensation

The third part (◻ Fig. 18.6) refers to whether the body has responded appropriately to the primary disturbance with efforts to adjust the pH in the opposite direction (e.g., increasing base for acidity and vice versa) back toward physiologic range. Notably, respiration can be adjusted much faster than bicarbonate levels, which takes at least a few days for full compensation.

18.4.9.3 Metabolic Acidosis

If you've determined the primary disturbance to be metabolic acidosis, you should check for the presence of an anion gap.

18.4.9.4 Anion Versus Non-anion Gap Metabolic Acidosis

If a patient has a primary metabolic acidosis (a low pH with low bicarbonates), it is important to describe the acidosis as anion versus non-anion gap due to distinct differential and management (which is often treating the underlying cause).

Let's explore the concept of anion gap briefly. Your body must be overall net neutral in charge to avoid various consequences. Thus, it follows that the plasma needs to be near neutral in charge. The number of positive charges (cations) must equal the number of negative charges (anions). The largest sources of positive charges come from electrolytes such as sodium, whereas the most significant sources of negative charges are from electrolytes such as chloride. Thus, the anion gap is the difference between positive and negative electrolytes, specifically the following most abundant electrolytes:

$$\text{Anion Gap} = \left[Na^+ + K^+ \right] - \left[Cl^- + HCO_{3^-} \right].$$

An occasional cause of anion gap metabolic acidosis is oxyproline, the metabolite of tylenol.

A normal anion gap is between 6 and 12. An elevated anion gap suggests that there is an entity in the blood that is unaccounted for. Common causes of anion gap metabolic acidosis can be remembered with the mnemonic MUD-PILES (◻ Fig. 18.7). Causes of non-anion gap metabolic acidosis can be remembered with HARD ASS (◻ Fig. 18.7).

Anion Gap Causes

HARD-ASS

Hyperalimentation
Addison's disease
Renal tubular acidosis
Diarrhea
Acetazolamide
Spironolactone
Saline infusion

MUDPILES

Methanol
Uremia
Diabetic ketoacidosis
Paraldehyde
Iron, isoniazid
Lactic acidosis
Ethylene glycol
Salicylates

Fig. 18.7 Anion gap causes

Distinguishing between the causes of non-anion gap metabolic acidosis in ◘ Fig. 18.7 can be pursued with a urine anion gap (urine AG = urine Na + urine K + urine Cl). A negative UAG represents good urinary NH_4+ excretion which is physiologically appropriate in acidosis. This includes causes such as diarrhea, use of acetazolamide, and excess normal saline. On the other hand, a positive UAG points toward an RTA, hypoaldo state, or early renal failure.

Rarely, metabolic acidosis may be mixed (both anion gap and non-anion gap). To check this, we use a calculation called the "delta-delta." This name is actually quite fitting since we are taking the ratio between two deltas (changes). The two deltas in consideration are (1) difference between the current and a normal anion gap and (2) difference between the current and a normal bicarbonate level:

$$\Delta\Delta = \frac{\Delta \text{Anion Gap}}{\Delta \text{HCO}_3} = \frac{AG - 12}{24 - \text{current HCO}_3}$$

A ratio less much than 1 indicates a concurrent normal AG metabolic acidosis, whereas a ratio much greater than 1 indicates a concomitant AG metabolic acidosis and metabolic alkalosis.

18.4.9.5 Management

The primary treatment for a metabolic acidosis, regardless of cause and gap existence, is to reverse the underlying etiology. However, acute management of severely acidic pH is often attempted. Though there is controversy and attending/institutional preference/guidelines, one potential intervention is administration of bicarbonate at pH < 7.1. For higher pH, bicarb may be considered in the setting of a concurrent AKI due to some data that 28-day mortality and dialysis initiation may be decreased.

18.4.9.6 Metabolic Alkalosis

Common causes of metabolic alkalosis are shown in ◘ Fig. 18.8. Similar to metabolic acidosis, the key is to treat the underlying cause. The primary management otherwise is to provide fluids when appropriate.

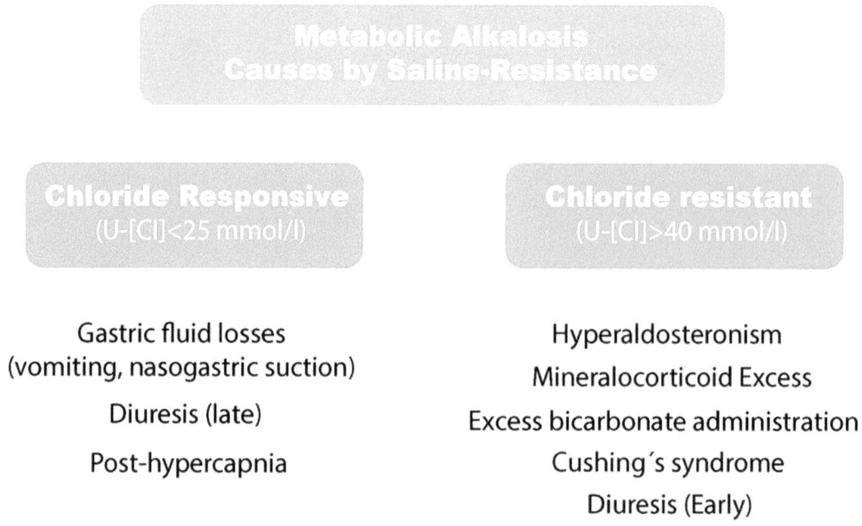

Fig. 18.8 Metabolic alkalosis caused by saline resistance

Similar to differentiating causes of metabolic acidosis, the causes of metabolic alkalosis may be differentiated with a lab value. This is the urine chloride which is an ion that is co-secreted with each molecule of NH_4+ (section of acid leads to blood alkalosis). The urine chloride is thus a surrogate marker for whether there is appropriate or inappropriate secretion of acid into the urine. Note that diuretics will increase urine chloride.

A urine chloride (UCl) of >20 is termed saline resistant whereas UCl <20 is saline responsive. The causes of each are shown in ▪ Fig. 18.8: Saline-responsive causes can be largely thought of as processes that lead to volume loss (remember, this causes contraction alkalosis!). Saline-resistant things are much more heterogeneous but are often inherent defects such as renal tubular acidosis or imbalances in hormones such as hyperaldosteronism.

18.4.10 Glomerular Disease

Though you are unlikely to encounter glomerular diseases as a medical student, it is worth knowing some basics. The overarching theme among all the conditions below is damage to the glomeruli, resulting in renal dysfunction. The mechanisms that lead to glomerular disease are diverse but there is most evidence for autoimmune phenomena. Thus, the mainstay of treatment for all the below involves immunosuppressive therapy, such as with steroids and rituximab.

18.4.10.1 Nephrotic Syndrome

Nephrotic syndrome is a form of nephrotic disease that results from loss of >3.5 g/day of protein in the urine, again without hematuria or hypertension. As a result, patients will have hypoalbuminemia which then leads to decreased intravascular oncotic pressure. This leads to the classic presentation of generalized swelling throughout the body termed anasarca. Unlike other diseases that cause swelling, nephrotic syndrome is unique in that the swelling is not limited to the lower extremities (the face is a very common and noticeable area).

Since the pathophysiology of nephrotic syndrome involves damaged podocytes which normally act as a molecular sieve barrier, molecules smaller than albumin are also lost in large amounts into the urine. Some notable losses include immunoglobulins, lipids, and antithrombin III. These lead to increased infections, responsive hyperlipidemia, and hypercoagulability (leading to increased rates of thromboembolic disease). You should be sure to address these deficiencies in your plan with countermeasures.

18.4.10.2 Nephrotic Diseases

Similar to nephrotic syndrome, nephritic diseases involve losing large amounts of protein. Examples include minimal change disease, focal segmental glomerulonephritis, membranous nephropathy, and diabetic nephropathy. While you are unlikely to manage these cases as a medical student, they may come up in casual conversation or noon conference cases. Thus, it may be helpful to review briefly your step 1 knowledge on these topics.

18.4.10.3 Nephritic Syndrome

Nephritic syndrome is similar to nephrotic syndrome in that there is significant protein loss (however, <3.5 g/day) and is also accompanied by more signs of inflammation and irritation (it is –"itic") such as hematuria and hypertension. Since the magnitude of protein loss is less than nephrotic syndrome, nephritic syndrome does not lead to anasarca.

Infectious Diseases

Bliss J. Chang

Contents

© The Author(s), under exclusive license to Springer Nature Switzerland AG 2021
S. H. Lecker, B. J. Chang (eds.), *The Ultimate Medical School Rotation Guide*,
https://doi.org/10.1007/978-3-030-63560-2_19

19.1   Overview

The Infectious Diseases (ID) rotation is often aptly termed the "chart-review rotation." This stems from each consult requiring an in-depth knowledge of not only current admission data but also prior infectious and medical history. Every little detail plays into the management of ID patients. This is one of my favorite rotations because it teaches you how to be an efficient medical record dissector and pay meticulous attention to details, skills that will be a boon to you regardless of specialty choice. Most of all, this specialty is among the most cerebral where often you must think outside of the routine thought patterns you rely on in many other specialties.

19.2   Fundamentals

The ultimate question in ID ends up being "Is there an infection?" and, if so, "How do we treat it?" If you can answer those two questions well, you'll be the best medical student they've ever seen! Keep these two questions in the back of your mind throughout your consults, and when stuck, ask yourself these questions.

Just because you are consulted on the ID service does not mean that the patient has an infection! In fact, a significant number of cases are noninfectious but still end up with ID consults to *rule out* infection. The following basic principles guide whether one suspects an infection. Do not underestimate how important these basic principles are and how many nuances are associated with a few simple parameters.

Is there an infection? If so, how do we treat it?

19.2.1   Fever

Fever is always induced by something but is not always infectious in nature. The differential should be thought of as infectious vs noninfectious. Common noninfectious causes can be remembered by the mnemonic **DMARD**:

- **D**rug induced
- **M**alignancy
- **A**utoimmune
- **R**heumatologic
- **D**VT/PE

After an extensive workup, a fever of unclear etiology in the developing world is most commonly noninfectious, whereas in low-income countries it is infectious. Notably, patients who are immunocompromised, cirrhotic, or taking antipyretics may have a lower baseline temperature. Thus, always be mindful that a low-grade temp may represent significant fever.

19.2.2   Other Vital Signs

Pearl: Avoid administering beta-blockers or other negative chronotropic agents for sinus tach.

Pay particular attention to the heart rate (HR) and blood pressure (BP) and/or mean arterial pressure (MAP) and oxygen saturation (O2Sat). These can be warning signs before an infection rages its ugly head or evidence for infection in the absence of traditional markers of infection. Sinus tachycardia, for example, is a physiologic response to fever and infection. This is necessary for the body to compensate. The O2Sat may sometimes point you towards a pulmonary infectious source.

19.2.3 White Blood Cell (WBC) Count

The WBC count is a quick and dirty screen for infection. A leukocytosis is technically defined as >10–12 K, depending on your institution. However, an important art to the interpretation of WBCs is to look at levels relative to the patient's baseline, as well as the rate of change. This is particularly useful in immunocompromised patients who have abnormal physiology that may produce inappropriately normal levels. The differential for a massively elevated leukocytosis (think >50 K) is quite unique and you should suspect noninfectious causes. In the USA, severely elevated leukocytosis in adults is most often caused by leukemia (CML, CLL). Strongyloides infections may also cause very high levels.

Pearl: If a patient is immunosuppressed, they are often unable to mount an immune response to infections. Don't be surprised if they do not show prominent leukocytosis!

19.2.4 CBC with Differential

A complete blood count (CBC) with diff (differential) most importantly provides the proportions of your WBC subtypes (e.g., lymphocytes, neutrophils, eosinophils, monocytes). This is often helpful as certain diagnoses are associated with unique patterns.
- A left shift is an increase in the immature neutrophil population that usually occurs due to inflammatory cytokines released during infections. The magnitude of left shift reflects the severity of a bacterial infection.
- Eosinophilia can be seen in drug fevers and parasitic (particularly strongyloides) infections. In the USA, it is very rare to see parasitic infections as an inpatient.
- Atypical lymphocytosis is most often associated with viral infections such as EBV and CMV.

19.2.5 ESR/CRP

The erythrocyte sedimentation rate (ESR) and C-reactive protein (CRP) are two markers of inflammation. It is important to remember that generally ESR is associated with prolonged inflammation (at least several days), whereas CRP represents active inflammation (past 24 hours). This can be quite helpful in establishing the time course of an infectious process. Both may also be used to assess for disease response to treatment.

19.2.6 Antibiotics

Always note the route of administration, dosing, and frequency of antibiotics. Know the start and stop dates of all recent antibiotics! This is hugely important because it provides so much context – perhaps a culture is negative simply due to antibiotics being started prior to drawing the blood! Beware that the fluoroquinolones will require QTc monitoring via EKG (a prolonged QTc increases risk of torsades). Avoid them in people with cardiac issues. Use the checklist below each time you plan to use an antibiotic.

19.2.7 Antibiotics Checklist

- [] Route of administration
- [] Dosing

- [ ] Frequency
- [ ] Start/stop dates
- [ ] Major side effects

19.2.8 Sensitivities (Sensis)

"Sensis" refers to which antibiotics an organism is susceptible. Despite some sensis showing you numerous antibiotics which are effective against an organism, you should still abide by the first-line agents that you learn and are suggested by the IDSA (Infectious Diseases Society of America) as that is what most attendings will follow.

Susceptibility does not mean that all antibiotics are equally efficacious (all the more reason to go with the antibiotics that are recommended as first line and backed by some evidence). A great example is knowing that Nafcillin/oxacillin are superior to vancomycin (despite what the sensis say) for methicillin-susceptible *Staphylococcus aureus* (MSSA) due to their smaller molecular weight that facilitates better cell wall penetration.

One phenomenon to be aware of when reading sensis is the inoculum effect. As a medical student, you should link this particularly to cefazolin in the setting of MSSA. The inoculum effect states that though the bacterium may be susceptible to cefazolin at the low bacterial inoculum in which it is used for testing, at significantly higher concentrations, it may not be susceptible to the antibiotic (cefazolin). This is particularly important when treating infections such as high-grade bacteremia. One clue to high-grade bacteremia is the presence of multiple positive peripheral blood cultures as well as faster positives on blood cultures.

19.2.9 ID-Specific History

Does the patient have a reason to be infected? For nearly every ID consult, you should ask and consider the following:
- Medical history: Recurrent infections? Abnormal anatomy? Conditions that decrease immunocompetence (diabetes, HIV, cirrhosis, autoimmune)?
- Surgical: Any hardware in the body? This includes valves, pacemakers, ventriculoperitoneal (VP) shunts, ostomies, prosthetic joints, plates, screws, Foleys
- Family history: Recurrent infections?
- Medications: Immunosuppressant medications (including steroids)? All antimicrobials should be noted. Also, note any medications that are P450 interactors or QTc prolongers.
- Social: Travels, sick contacts, animals/pets, exposure to water, exposure to wooded areas (depending on your geography), sexual activity, IV drug use, smoking, alcohol, employment exposures, other unusual exposures

The key social exposures listed above for assessing exposure to infectious agents can be remembered with the mnemonic COASTED:
- Contacts (e.g., potentially sick family, friends, coworkers)
- Oral ingestions (e.g., dairy, eating out, seafood) .
- Animal exposure (e.g., pets or animals)
- Sexual history (e.g., recent sexual encounters, sex practices, number of partners, orientation)

19

- **T**ravel history
- **E**mployment exposure (e.g., fumes, pollutants, animals, insects)
- **D**rug history

A good way to learn these is through repeated use. You shouldn't memorize all these but rather understand why each of these raises the likelihood of infection or complicates infections. When I did my ID rotation, I would quickly jot these exposures/risk factors down on paper to ensure I didn't forget. A week in, they come naturally to you, without the effort of sitting down and trying to commit them to memory.

19.2.10   Chart Review

There are many correct ways to review a patient's chart as long as you do so in a logical and efficient manner. However, following a routine for chart reviews can help minimize the risk of missing any pertinent information. Below is one suggestion:
- ☐ Quick screen for potential infection.
- ☐ Review fever curve.
- ☐ Review vital signs.
- ☐ Review WBC trend + − differential.
- ☐ Review microbiology data, if already obtained by primary team.
- ☐ Review antibiotics course (for context to the basic markers of infection).
- ☐ WBC increasing in the setting of antibiotics is worrisome for resistance or lack of coverage.
- ☐ Stable WBC in the setting of antibiotics is concerning for noninfectious cause or resistance (though typically the white count will keep going up).
- ☐ Review other labs.
- ☐ Creatinine (Cr) to check for renal dosing indications.
- ☐ Liver function tests (LFTs) often as a marker of tolerance to common antibiotics.
- ☐ Review imaging with radiology (this gives you a much better sense of infection vs no infection and the differential diagnosis for each lesion on imaging).
- ☐ Review initial presentation.
- ☐ Importantly, do not anchor to the diagnoses suggested by the initial note-writer, no matter how astute a clinician you perceive them!

19.3   Microbes

There are numerous ways to classify bacteria but the most clinically relevant classification is in four major groupings that help to guide antibiotic choice:
- Gram positives
- Gram negatives
- Anaerobes
- Atypicals

Whenever you have a suspected infection, always think about potential sources and into which grouping the bacteria may fall. The other groups of microbes that you will likely encounter include viruses and fungi.

19.3.1 Gram Positives

There are five gram-positive bacteria with which you should be familiar. Gram positives outside of these five are less common cases for a medical student and you can look them up using the Sanford Antimicrobial Guide or UpToDate as needed. These five are *Staphylococcus aureus*, coagulase-negative staphylococci (CoNS), streptococci species, enterococci, and *Clostridium difficile*. The following descriptions of each organism are very clinically focused and do not cover all the extensive details that you learned for Step 1. If you find yourself on a team that pimps you often on those facts, SketchyMicro is your go-to resource.

19.3.1.1 *S. aureus*

This is one of the most common bacteria you will encounter. *S. aureus* are gram-positive cocci in clusters. Remember this characteristic as it is often the first hint on cultures that you may be dealing with *Staphylococcus* species, though this need not be *S. aureus* (could be CoNS described below). In general, *S. aureus* is found on your skin and in your nares. Due to where it inhabits, *S. aureus* is always on the differential whenever the mechanism of infection involves a disturbance in skin integrity (e.g., cuts, joint infections, endocarditis secondary to IV drug use). Note that *S. aureus* is a very "sticky" organism meaning that it produces biofilms which cause difficulty in complete eradication even with potent antibiotics. Thus, antibiotic durations are often longer or involve special ancillary medications to fully rid the *Staphylococcus*. Remember to suggest the addition of rifampin (which helps to penetrate the biofilm) to any infection involving *S. aureus* and prosthetic joints or valves. Since bacteria only require a single mutation to develop resistance to rifampin, it should be added after a week of initial antibiotics.

S. aureus can be either methicillin-resistant (MRSA) or methicillin-sensitive (MSSA). MRSA is resistant to penicillins and is usually covered with vancomycin. Early on without culture data (and even with culture data suggesting gram-positive cocci), you should cover for *S. aureus* empirically. Once culture results come back negative for MRSA, vancomycin may be discontinued and antibiotic therapy tailored.

19.3.1.2 Coagulase-Negative Staph (CoNS)

CoNS include *S. epidermidis* and *S. saprophyticus*. You are more likely to encounter *S. epidermidis*, usually in the setting of bacteremia or endocarditis. CoNS are distinct from *S. aureus* in that they are coagulase negative meaning that they do not produce factors that leads to coagulation of blood products. While *S. epidermidis* colonizes the skin as its name aptly suggests, *S. saprophyticus* is found in the setting of UTIs in young sexually active females. Clinically, you should simply remember that CoNS (though it is not MRSA) is not easily treated with penicillins as is MSSA. Rather, you will typically use vancomycin (which covers all gram positives). Lastly, remember that as *Staphylococcus* species, CoNS are also "sticky" and produce biofilms that are difficult to rid, so remember to use rifampin if there is prosthesis involved.

19.3.1.3 Streptococci

For the ID rotation, strep is most commonly encountered in community-acquired bacteremia or endocarditis cases. We will not discuss their relevance to pneumonia since most strep pneumonia does not lead to ID consults. Strep is a bug that is most reliably covered with a penicillin. You want to pay attention to *S. mutans* of the viridans group as this is a common culprit of bacteremia/endocarditis secondary to poor dentition or after a recent dental procedure. Your first clue to strep infection is gram positive cocci in chains.

19.3.1.4 Enterococci

Simply put, enterococci should be associated with the genitourinary tract and GI tract (particularly the biliary tract). Whenever you are dealing with pathologies in those areas, enterococci is a possibility. Don't forget to screen for a history of recent GU procedures such as cystoscopy. Among the two main types of enterococci, *E. faecium* is the more resistant and deadly type. Ampicillin is the antibiotic of choice though alternatives including vancomycin can be used if susceptible.

19.3.1.5 *Clostridium difficile*

While all clostridium are gram positive, we will focus on *C. diff* as that is the most common *Clostridium* species that you will encounter. You will almost certainly come across *C. diff* in the form of *C. diff* colitis and that is the only infection we will discuss here. A key distinction when dealing with *C. diff* is to determine whether the patient is merely colonized with *C. diff* or whether the *C. diff* is actively producing toxins leading to colitis. This is achieved via the two-tiered testing which tests first for the presence of *C. diff* in stool and then if the results are disconcordant, a reflex PCR occurs for the toxin gene. First-line therapy consists of PO vancomycin.

> Broad-spectrum antibiotics increase the risk of nosocomial infection; thus, a thorough med history is critical!

19.3.2 Gram Negatives

Clinically, gram-negative bacteria are typically found in association with either the GI or GU tracts. We will focus on two rod-shaped gram-negatives that are particularly common and notable.

19.3.2.1 *Pseudomonas (aeruginosa)*

This is one of the most common hospital-associated pathogens that are more difficult to cover with antibiotics, not only due to the limited pseudomonal coverage of many gram-negative antibiotics but also due to high antibiotic resistance particularly to fluoroquinolones. Thus, hospital-associated infections are often covered empirically for *Pseudomonas* with either cefepime or Zosyn (piperacillin-tazobactam). Remember to always keep *Pseudomonas* in your differential when infection is unrelenting in the hospital despite antibiotic therapy. Common associations include uncontrolled diabetes and severe lung diseases (particularly cystic fibrosis). The most common infections caused by *Pseudomonas* are UTI, osteomyelitis, and pneumonia.

19.3.2.2 *E. coli*

This is the most common bacteria in urinary tract infections. Appearing on urinalysis as nitrite and leukocyte esterase positive, *E. coli* can usually be easily treated with a short course of antibiotics. Occasionally, a UTI can evolve into bacteremia (urosepsis). Though rare in the inpatient setting, *E. coli* are also a very common cause of infectious diarrhea.

19.4 Antimicrobials Review

Knowing the most frequently used antimicrobials well is immensely helpful for the ID rotation. If you are limited on time, this is the place to start. Often students approach this topic with a brute-force mentality, but I hope that the way this guide breaks it down will help you understand why each antimicrobial does what it does so that you can take on a more critical problem-solving approach.

19.4.1 Spectrum of Coverage

The most important information for each antibiotic is what organisms it covers, referred to as its spectrum of coverage. In general, there are four major groupings of bacteria that are targeted as we just reviewed and thus we will discuss spectrum of activity by organism type:
- Gram positives
- Gram negatives
- Anaerobes
- Atypicals

Systematically going through each of these four major groupings as you think of the spectrum of coverage for each antibiotic will ensure that you consider all parts of the spectra. Lastly, these spectra focus on what is clinically most relevant. You may assume that if an antimicrobial is said to have activity against a particular organism in this guide, it refers to a clinically relevant level of activity.

19.4.2 Beta-Lactams

The most common class of antibiotics, beta-lactams are so-named due to the presence of a ring-form amide in the chemical formula. This structure is present in penicillins and all penicillin derivatives, including the following common classes: cephalosporins, carbapenems, and monobactams. The integrity of this beta-lactam ring is key to the function of these antibiotics (more on this later). Due to the similar foundational structure around which these classes are built, allergic interactions between beta-lactam classes are increased (e.g., ~15% chance of a penicillin allergy crossover to cephalosporins). However, in general, it is worth obtaining an allergy consult and slowly trialing a dose of a beta-lactam in a different class if it is the first-line antibiotic. Lastly, remember that all beta-lactams share the same core chemical structure. To aid your learning, we cover the beta-lactam classes below in terms of increasing chemical formula complexity, beginning with penicillin which has the maximal gram-positive coverage and adding chemical modifications which increase gram-negative coverage at the cost of gram-positive coverage.

19.4.2.1 Penicillins (The "OG Gram-Positive" Antibiotic)

Penicillins function by binding of its beta-lactam ring to penicillin-binding proteins (PBPs) which are responsible for forming peptidoglycan cross-links in the bacterial wall. As you might imagine, inhibition of peptidoglycan cross-linking is detrimental to the integrity of the bacterial wall. Specifically, the remodeling processes that break down the old bacterial wall continue. Since the wall cannot be remade, leaks begin to occur which eventually leads to bacterial death. Now that you know the mechanism, you know that penicillins are bactericidal. Notably, penicillins are the smallest of the beta-lactams which makes them maximally effective at penetrating bacterial walls. (Remember this for later!)

Gram positives	Strep
Gram negatives	Negligible
Anaerobes[a]	Most oral anaerobes (because oral anaerobes are mostly gram positive)
Atypicals	Spirochetes (for your purposes, *Treponema* and *Leptospira*)
Cidal or static?	Bactericidal (just like all beta-lactams)
Route of administration	IV, IM, PO
Key side effects	Diarrhea (low risk)
First line for	Strep, syphilis, leptospirosis

[a]This is a low-yield fact included for reference sake, but not one that you will utilize clinically

Treatment of syphilis causes release of antigenic debris from the dead spirochetes that may induce a transient inflammatory state with nonspecific symptoms such as new fever, myalgias/arthralgias, and rash. This is known as the Jarisch-Herxheimer reaction and is a common pimp question. Though this is most often associated with syphilis treatment, it can in theory be seen with treatment of any gram-positive bacterium.

- Common Penicillin Types*
  - Penicillin G = IV
  - Penicillin G benzathine = IM
  - Penicillin V potassium = PO

19.4.2.2 Aminopenicillins ("Penicillin 2.0" – More Gram-Positive and Gram-Negative Coverage)

This group is distinguished from penicillins by an extra amino group. This amino group adds some more gram-positive and gram-negative coverage due to better penetration of their outer membranes. Members include ampicillin and amoxicillin. Overall, the gram-positive coverage is the same as that of the penicillins.

Memory pearl: The types of penicillin when put in ABC order as done here goes from most parenteral to least parenteral route of administration

Gram positives	*Strep* (same as penicillins), *Enterococcus*, *Listeria*
Gram negatives[a]	*E. coli* and *H. influenzae*
Anaerobes	Negligible for our purposes
Atypicals	Lyme in pregnancy = amoxicillin
Cidal or static?	Bactericidal (just like all beta-lactams)
Route of administration	Amoxicillin = PO Ampicillin = IV
Key side effects	Diarrhea (low risk)
First-line for	*Enterococcus*, *Listeria*, otitis media (strep, H influenza)

[a]Simplified for practical purposes; overall can be thought of as decent gram-negative coverage including *E. coli, H. influenzae, Klebsiella, Proteus, Salmonella, Shigella*

19.4.2.3   Beta-Lactamase-Inhibitor Combinations ("Penicillin 3.0" – Not Only Do We Get More Gram-Positive and Gram-Negative Coverage, But Most Importantly Anaerobic Coverage!)

As bacteria have been exposed to penicillins for decades, they have realized that the strength in penicillins lies in the beta-lactam ring. As such, some have beta-lactamase enzymes which, as the name suggests, hydrolyzes the beta-lactam, rendering the penicillin useless. Not to be outdone by bacteria, humans have also discovered a way to prevent the activity of these beta-lactamases through inhibitors such as tazobactam, sulbactam, and clavulanate. These inhibitors when combined with piperacillin, ampicillin, or amoxicillin form Zosyn, Unasyn, and Augmentin, respectively. Their routes of administration mimic that of the penicillin. The beta-lactamase inhibitors are often produced by *Staph* and anaerobe species; thus, addition of inhibitors increases activity against them.

Gram positives	MSSA[a], *Strep*
Gram negatives	Broad (covers most) Zosyn covers *Pseudomonas*
Anaerobes	Broad (covers most)
Atypicals	None
Cidal or static?	Bactericidal (just like all beta-lactams)
Route of administration	Zosyn = IV Unasyn = IV Augmentin = PO
Key side effects	Diarrhea (secondary to C diff)
First line for	Fight bites, aspiration + − pneumonia, sinus infections, GI Often one of the best antibiotics for polymicrobial wounds, particularly those which include GN and anaerobic flora! Unasyn/Augmentin[b]

[a]*MSSA* methicillin-sensitive *Staphylococcus aureus*
[b]Unasyn and augmentin are essentially equivalent but in different forms (IV vs PO). Thus, transitioning to a PO antibiotic before discharge is fairly simple!

19.4.2.4   Semisynthetic Penicillins ("The MSSA Drug": Semisynesthetic with Two S's as in MSSA)

These beta-lactams, namely, nafcillin and oxacillin, are so named because of bulky synthetic side chains that are attached to the native penicillin structure. These bulky groups prevent most beta-lactamases from working and thus do not need the aid of a beta-lactamase inhibitor. Despite these bulky groups, semisynthetic penicillins are much smaller than vancomycin which allows for superior penetration into the peptidoglycan cell walls. Thus, nafcillin/oxacillin are the agents of choice for serious MSSA infections.

Gram positives	Just remember MSSA
Gram negatives	Negligible
Anaerobes	Negligible
Atypicals	Negligible
Cidal or static?	Bactericidal (just like all beta-lactams)

Route of administration	IV
Key side effects	Acute interstitial nephritis (nafcillin > oxacillin)
First line for	MSSA (usually for serious MSSA infections such as endocarditis)

19.4.2.5 Cephalosporins

Perhaps the most commonly used class of beta-lactam antibiotics, the cephalosporin family is split into 5 generations. Their spectrum (◻ Fig. 19.1) of activity follows the general trend of good gram-positive coverage with the older generations, moving towards better gram-negative coverage as we get to fourth generation. Fifth-generation cephalosporins are unique and have good broad coverage, including MRSA and excluding *Pseudomonas*. Notably, cephalosporins have ~15% (not too bad!) cross-reactivity to penicillin allergies. Rather than going through the exhaustive list of cephalosporins that you may have seen for your Step 1 exam, we will only focus on the clinically relevant and often-used cephalosporins. Any unique characteristics of each cephalosporin are noted below.

— *1st generation (the gram-positive cephalosporin):* Think common skin flora and surgical prophylaxis. Essentially only covers MSSA and *Strep*. Used mainly for skin and soft tissue infections (SSTIs), but is also sometimes used for MSSA in infections such as endocarditis due to lower risk of nephrotoxicity.
  – Cephalexin (Keflex): PO
  – Cefazolin: IV; nafcillin should typically be used in severe MSSA endocarditis due to risk of inoculum effect
— *2nd generation (the intermediate cephalosporin):* Most frequently clinically used for GI/pelvis infections. As such, they have fairly good gram-negative coverage, covering the typical enteric flora such as *E. coli* and *Klebsiella*
  – Cefotetan: 1 of 2 cephalosporins to have some anaerobic coverage!

Pearl: Cefazolin is particularly prone to what is known as the inoculum effect, where antibiotic sensitivities obtained at normal testing bacterial concentrations are not reflective of sensitivities (measured by minimum inhibitory concentration MIC) at higher inoculum (i.e., bacterial concentrations).

Gram-positive activity

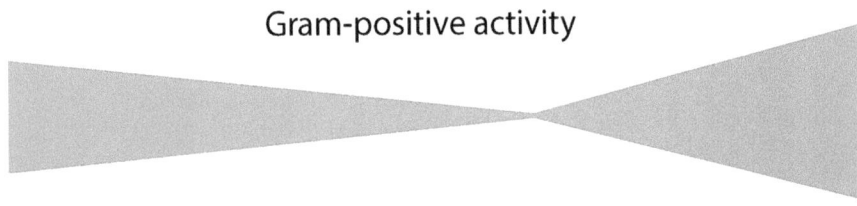

1st Generation   2nd Generation   3rd Generation   4th Generation   5th Generation
(e.g. Cefazolin) (e.g. Cefuroxime) (e.g. Ceftriaxone) (e.g. Cefepime) (e.g. Ceftaroline)

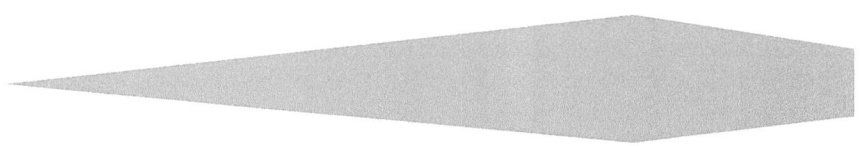

Gram-negative activity

◻ **Fig. 19.1** Cephalosporin spectrum of activity trend

- *3rd generation (the gram-negative cephalosporin):* Overall broad coverage but its gram-positive coverage is not reliable and thus is not usually used to treat gram positives. Notably, third-generation cephalosporins may cause liver function test (LFT) abnormalities due to biliary sludging.
  - Ceftriaxone: Empiric coverage for meningitis; first line for *N. gonorrhoeae*, CNS Lyme, community-acquired pneumonia; convenient once daily dosing
  - Cef**PO**doxime: **PO** but expensive
  - Ceftazidime: Covers *Pseudomonas*
- *4th generation (broad cephalosporins with pseudomonal coverage):* Broad gram negative, *Strep* and MSSA coverage.
  - Cefepime: Covers *Pseudomonas*; also has anaerobic coverage (though not excellent, thus requires Flagyl if suspecting anaerobic infection)
- *5th generation (the MRSA ceftriaxone)*
  - Ceftaroline: Covers MRSA but no *Pseudomonas*; similar gram-negative coverage to ceftriaxone: expensive

To recap the cephalosporins, gram-positive coverage is best with the first-generation cephalosporins and this shifts towards gram-negative coverage for newer generations. Use first-generation cephalosporins such as cefazolin for skin and soft tissue infections (e.g., cellulitis). Cefotetan (second gen) and cefepime (fourth gen) are the only cephalosporins with anaerobic coverage. Broad-spectrum cephalosporins are ceftriaxone, ceftazidime, and cefepime; Ceftazidime or cefepime is the agent of choice when worried about *Pseudomonas*.

Anaerobes	Cefotetan, cefepime
Atypicals	Negligible
Cidal or static?	Bactericidal (just like all beta-lactams)
Route of administration	Cephalexin (first gen) and cefpodoxime (third gen) are the two notable PO cephalosporins; the rest are IV
Key side effects	Later generation cephalosporins have increased risk of *C. diff* Notable unique side effects include 　　Cefotaxime (second gen): 　　Ceftriaxone (third gen): Biliary sludging 　　Cefepime (fourth gen): Inc *C. diff* risk, dec seizure threshold
First line for	First gen = skin and soft tissue infections Third gen = UTIs, meningitis, CNS Lyme, gonorrhea Fourth gen = broad coverage necessitating *Pseudomonal* coverage

19.4.2.6   Carbapenems

Carbapenems are heavy hitters with broad-spectrum activity. They include ertapenem, imipenem, meropenem, and doripenem (not often clinically used). Notably, they all have ESBL coverage and are the agent of choice for those bacteria. Ertapenem does not cover *Pseudomonas* but has a convenient once daily dosing schedule, whereas the other carbapenems have more frequent dosing in exchange for pseudomonal activity. Due to their big-gun nature, carbapenems are reserved until they are really needed; this stewardship is critical in light of increasing resistance rates to carbapenems. Notably, meropenem and imipenem have good CNS penetration.

Gram positives	Broad
Gram negatives	Broad with *Pseudomonas* (except ertapenem) and ESBL coverage
Anaerobes	Broad (would not need Flagyl)
Atypicals	Atypicals with cell walls (due to the beta-lactam mechanism!)
Cidal or static?	Bactericidal (just like all beta-lactams)
Route of administration	IV
Key side effects	Imipenem = dec seizure threshold
First line for	ESBL bacteria Broad coverage when other antibiotics fail or cannot be used

19.4.2.7 Monobactams (The "Second-Line Gram-Negative Beta-Lactam")

As the name implies, a monobactam is a beta-lactam ring that stands alone. An easy way to remember the only monobactam that is clinically relevant is through the "mono" prefix again, as there is only one, Aztreonam. This is a second-line antibiotic reserved for gram-negative bacteria that cannot be treated successfully with other antibiotics or if a patient has a severe allergy to penicillin and related classes. Its spectrum covers almost all gram negatives, excluding atypicals (such as *Legionella*) and anaerobes (such as *Bacteroides* and *Fusobacterium*).

Gram positives	Negligible
Gram negatives	Broad with pseudomonal coverage
Anaerobes	None
Atypicals	Negligible
Cidal or static?	Bactericidal (just like all beta-lactams)
Route of administration	IV
Key side effects	Diarrhea (moderate risk)
First line for	Always second line!

19.4.2.8 Glycopeptides (The "Gram-Positive King")

Vancomycin and dalbavancin are the two glycopeptides to know. These are similar but distinct in their mechanism from beta-lactams. Rather than binding to PBPs, they bind directly to the peptidoglycan via D-alanine-D-alanine moieties, preventing peptidoglycan cross-linking and thus cell death from osmotic imbalance. Notably, vancomycin's bioavailability when taken orally is zero; thus it stays in the GI tract (which is what we want in situations such as *C. diff*!). Dalbavancin is a newer glycopeptides that is similar to vancomycin but is unique in that it may be given in once-weekly infusions. This is great for patients who may fail to follow up or have low compliance rates; however, it is currently very expensive and difficult to obtain insurance approval. Lastly, glycopeptides have large molecular weights, making them inferior to nafcillin/oxacillin in the treatment of MSSA infections.

Gram positives	All (including MRSA), except VRE
Gram negatives	None
Anaerobes	Gram-positive anaerobes only
Atypicals	None
Cidal or static?	Bactericidal (just like all beta-lactams)
Route of administration	IV or PO for vancomycin; PO vancomycin is only used for *C. diff* infection Infusion for dalbavancin
Key side effects	Red-man syndrome (may be circumvented with slow infusion and/or Benadryl pretreatment) High levels cause nephrotoxicity (Acute Tubular Necrosis – ATN)
First line for	Broad gram-positive coverage MRSA

19.4.2.9 Linezolid and Daptomycin (The "Evil Twins of Vancomycin")

These are the evil twins of vancomycin. Almost identical in spectrum of coverage and with more pronounced side effects, these should be used when vancomycin cannot be used or is not effective (e.g., VRE), and only for a limited duration of time (usually no more than 2 weeks).

Linezolid acts by inhibiting the 50S subunit of the bacterial ribosome, inhibiting translation (protein synthesis). You can imagine that the bacterium will not replicate without new protein synthesis but also not succumb until its existing proteins lose their integrity, therefore exhibiting bacteriostatic activity. It's side effect is bone marrow suppression (mainly thrombocytopenia), with the probability increasing directly in proportion to length of use. Weekly CBC monitoring is required. Linezolid also carries a risk of serotonin syndrome if paired with serotonin-reuptake modulators such as SSRIs/SNRIs/MAOIs/TCAs. Always run through the med list to check for interactors before prescribing linezolid, particularly in psychiatric patients!

Daptomycin works by poking holes in the cell membranes of bacteria, leading to disruption of cellular processes and osmotic cell death. Daptomycin leads to myopathies, neuropathy, and pulmonary hemorrhage. Creatine kinase (CK) levels should be monitored twice the week of initiation and once weekly thereafter while on daptomycin. Note: Daptomycin is inactivated by surfactants thus not useful for pulmonary infections.

Gram positives	All (including MRSA and VRE)
Gram negatives	None
Anaerobes	Not used for gram-positive anaerobes, namely, *C. diff*
Atypicals	None
Cidal or static?	Linezolid = mostly bacteriostatic Daptomycin = bactericidal
Route of administration	IV or PO for linezolid IV for daptomycin
Key side effects	Linezolid: Diarrhea, bone marrow toxicity Daptomycin: Alveolar hemorrhage, muscle aches/rhabdomyolysis
First line for	VRE Broad gram-positive coverage when vancomycin cannot be used

19.4.2.10 Clindamycin (The "Gram-Positive and Anaerobe Antibiotic")

Clindamycin is a unique antibiotic with Gram-positive and MRSA coverage as well as broad anaerobic coverage. It acts by inhibiting the 50S (similar to linezolid) bacterial ribosome subunit and inhibiting translation (protein synthesis). It is notably one of the few (and for you, the only) antibiotic that has both gram-positive and anaerobic activity without gram-negative or atypical coverage. Classic medical student teaching goes "Clindamycin for above the diaphragm" and that is true although it is not used very commonly due to its significantly increased risk for *C. diff*. It can be thought of as (1) a convenient drug for outpatient MRSA skin infections and (2) aspiration coverage. It has other niche uses such as for severe babesiosis (seen in the Northeast) and inhibition of toxin production in *S. pyogenes* necrotizing fasciitis.

Gram positives	*Staph* (including MRSA) and *Strep*
Gram negatives	Negligible
Anaerobes	Broad
Atypicals	Severe babesiosis
Cidal or static?	Bactericidal or bacteriostatic based on concentration and organism
Route of administration	IV or PO
Key side effects	Diarrhea (moderate; inc risk of *C. diff*)
Often used for	Outpatient (PO) MRSA SSTIs Aspiration PNA Toxin production neutralization in necrotizing fasciitis (group A *Strep*)

19.4.2.11 Fluoroquinolones

Fluoroquinolones (moxifloxacin, levofloxacin, and ciprofloxacin) are the only antibiotics that inhibit DNA synthesis. They inhibit two key enzymes, DNA topoisomerase II (better known as DNA gyrase) and DNA topoisomerase IV. These enzymes are involved in reducing strain and preventing recombination of strands prior to replication, respectively. As you may imagine, inhibition of these processes disrupts the integrity of cellular DNA, leading to cell death (bactericidal). Spectrum-wise, they vary, with ciprofloxacin being predominantly gram negative while levofloxacin adding more gram-positive coverage. Moxifloxacin has quite a broad spectrum of activity but is expensive and not a preferred agent for most infectious disease physicians.

Ciprofloxacin (the UTI or gram-negative fluoroquinolone) has the narrowest spectra among the three major fluoroquinolones. You can essentially think for practical purposes as just a broad gram-negative antibiotic. Notably, it covers *Pseudomonas* although resistance rates are on the rise and alternate regimens should be explored when possible.

Gram positives	Negligible
Gram negatives	Broad, including *Pseudomonas*
Anaerobes	Negligible
Atypicals	Negligible

Cidal or static?	Bactericidal
Route of administration	IV or PO
Key side effects	QTc prolongation, inc risk for altered mental status/confusion in elderly, tendinopathy (including rupture) in elderly
Often used for	UTIs Intra-abdominal infections

Levofloxacin is famously known as the "respiratory fluoroquinolone" due to its use for various types of pneumonia. It covers the gram negatives as does ciprofloxacin but also adds on better gram-positive and atypical coverage. You can imagine that this atypical coverage is better than nothing to do with the bacterial wall (many atypicals do not have a wall!).

Gram positives	Practically, just remember *Streptococcus pneumoniae*
Gram negatives	Broad, including *Pseudomonas*
Anaerobes	Negligible
Atypicals	Broad (e.g., chlamydia, mycoplasma)
Cidal or static?	Bactericidal
Route of administration	IV or PO
Key side effects	QTc prolongation, inc risk for altered mental status/confusion in elderly, tendinopathy (including rupture) in elderly
Often used for	Pneumonia

Moxifloxacin is the broadest and most expensive of the fluoroquinolones. It builds onto levofloxacin's spectrum of activity (which built upon ciprofloxacin's) to add on better gram-positive and anaerobic coverage. Notably, its coverage of *Pseudomonas* is weaker than cipro and levo and should not be trusted.

Gram positives	*Strep* and *Staph* (though never really used for *Staph*)
Gram negatives	Broad, but NO pseudomonas
Anaerobes	Broad
Atypicals	Broad (e.g., chlamydia, mycoplasma)
Cidal or static?	Bactericidal
Route of administration	IV or PO
Key side effects	QTc prolongation, inc risk for altered mental status/confusion in elderly, tendinopathy (including rupture) in elderly
Often used for	UTIs Intra-abdominal infections

In summary, ciprofloxacin can be thought of as belonging to the genitourinary system, levofloxacin the lungs, and moxifloxacin the whole body. When atypicals are suspected, levofloxacin is the fluoroquinolone of choice. You should be careful when prescribing fluoroquinolones especially to the elderly and patients with high cardiovascular risk profiles. One key advantage of fluoroquinolones is good bioavailability and penetration to everywhere in the body, as well as a PO option. If there is a good alternative, highly consider that!

19.4.2.12 Macrolides

Azithromycin, erythromycin, and clarithromycin are three of the most common macrolides. These drugs inhibit the 50S subunit of bacterial ribosomes, halting protein synthesis and preventing bacterial replication (bacteriostatic). Similar to fluoroquinolones, macrolides prolong the QTc and an EKG should be monitored regularly. Erythromycin is primarily used for either newborn prophylaxis of chlamydia conjunctivitis or increasing GI motility via its motilin-receptor agonist activity. The only thing for you to remember about clarithromycin is that it is part of triple therapy for *H. pylori* treatment.

Pearl: There are several drugs that inhibit the 50S ribosomal subunit. Here's a list to help you keep track:

- Clindamycin
- Linezolid
- Macrolides
- Tetracyclines

The following spectrum of coverage is for azithromycin:

Gram positives	Strep pneumonia
Gram negatives	Respiratory gram negatives – *Moraxella, H. influenzae*
Anaerobes	Negligible
Atypicals	Broad (e.g., chlamydia, mycoplasma, chlamydophila)
Cidal or static?	Bacteriostatic
Route of administration	IV or PO
Key side effects	QTc prolongation, increased cardiac mortality
First line for	Community-acquired pneumonia, atypical coverage (including chlamydia)

19.4.2.13 Tetracyclines (The "King of Atypicals")

These are fraternal twins to macrolides, the key difference being that they inhibit the 30S ribosomal subunit rather than the 50S. Doxycycline is the primary tetracycline that is used on a day-to-day basis. It is an amazing drug for just about any atypical organism and also boasts MRSA activity, all in both IV and PO forms. However, this comes at a cost of increased side effects compared to your typical antibiotic. As a medical student, if you suspect atypical infections, doxycycline is your best friend.

Gram positives	MRSA, *Streptococcus pneumoniae*
Gram negatives	Negligible
Anaerobes	Negligible
Atypicals	Broadest (chlamydia, mycoplasma, Lyme, *Leptospira*, Rocky Mountain spotted fever, certain malaria)

Cidal or static?	Bacteriostatic[a]
Route of administration	IV or PO
Key side effects	Photosensitivity, hepatotoxicity, children <8 years = teeth staining
First line for	MRSA Atypicals

[a]All antibiotics that act on the ribosome (whether 30S or 50S) have bacteriostatic mechanisms!

Tigecycline (the tiger antibiotic – unleash the tiger as a last resort) is another tetracycline antibiotic with an extremely broad spectrum of activity reserved for last-resort use against very multidrug-resistant organisms. This is due to studies that suggest increased mortality relative to other microbials. It is not routinely used for enterococci as might be suggested by the SketchyMicro videos you have watched. Since you will likely never use it as a medical student, we will not discuss it further.

19.4.2.14 Aminoglycosides

Though not a commonly used antibiotic due to its significant nephrotoxic risks, it is occasionally used for difficult-to-treat gram-negative infections and specific indications (such as prosthetic valve endocarditis, tularemia, brucellosis). Aminoglycosides act by inhibiting the 30S ribosome and are usually used in combination with a beta-lactam for synergistic effects. If you do use an aminoglycoside, don't forget to monitor its levels. The peak correlates to its effectiveness and the trough (i.e., the base constant drug level) to its toxicity.

Memory pearl: A-MIN-O
A and O = Aerobes Only
Min = gram-negative

Gram positives	Negligible
Gram negatives	Broad, including *Pseudomonas*
Anaerobes	Negligible
Atypicals	Negligible
Cidal or static?	Bactericidal
Route of administration	IV
Key side effects	Nephrotoxicity Ototoxicity
First-line for	Gentamicin for brucellosis, tularemia, prosthetic valve endocarditis Tobramycin add-on for ventilator-associated pneumonia Amikacin for highly resistant UTIs

19.4.2.15 Bactrim (Trimethoprim-Sulfamethoxazole) (MRSA and PJP Prophylaxis)

Bactrim is a great antibiotic that can be used for a variety of infections though most commonly used for MRSA skin infections, pneumocystis (PJP) prophylaxis, and uncomplicated UTIs. It is composed of two separate antibiotics which act synergistically to produce a bactericidal effect. Trimethoprim inhibits dihydrofolate reductase (DHFR) and thus prevents folic acid production.

19

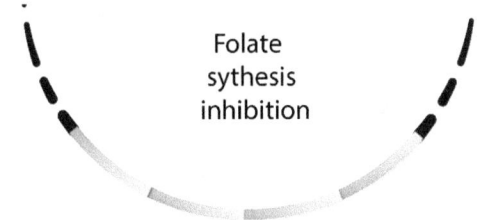

Folate
sythesis
inhibition

Dihydropteroate diphosphate+p-aminobenzoic acid (PABA)

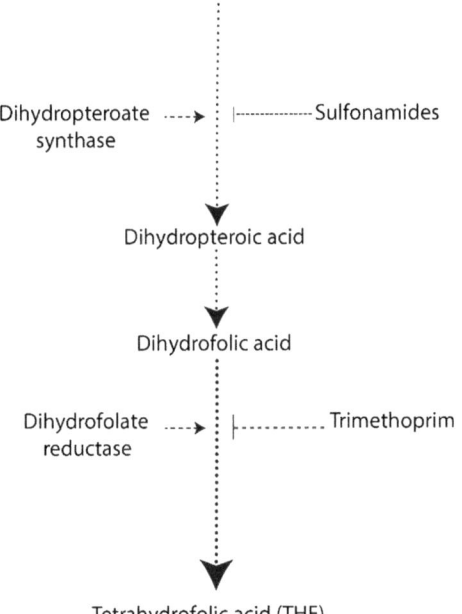

Dihydropteroate ----▶ |------------- Sulfonamides
synthase

Dihydropteroic acid

Dihydrofolic acid

Dihydrofolate ----▶ |----------- Trimethoprim
reductase

Tetrahydrofolic acid (THF)

◨ **Fig. 19.2** Mechanism of Bactrim

One step upstream, sulfamethoxazole inhibits dihydropteroate synthetase
(◨ Fig. 19.2). Avoid this medication in kidney injury since it confounds the Cr
levels and may also prevent your patient from obtaining contrast imaging if his
Cr was borderline high! All in all, it is a great oral option for MRSA coverage.

Gram positives[a]	MRSA/MSSA
Gram negatives	UTI gram negatives
Anaerobes	Negligible
Atypicals	*Pneumocystis jiroveci*, *Nocardia*
Cidal or static?	Bactericidal
Route of administration	IV or PO
Key side effects	Artificial increase in Cr (no effect on GFR) Hyperkalemia (at high doses, esp in HIV patients) Rashes (inc risk compared to other antibiotics)
First line for	MRSA SSTIs Pneumocystis pneumonia or prophylaxis UTIs

[a]Notably poor *Strep* coverage by Bactrim

19.4.2.16 Metronidazole (The "King of Anaerobes")

The king of anaerobic coverage, Flagyl is often added to regimens that have insufficient anaerobic coverage. Common partner antibiotics include cefepime, ciprofloxacin, and ceftriaxone. It functions by creating free radicals that damage bacterial protein and DNA, leading to cell death. Interestingly, it does not impact human cells because it requires reduction for activation, and this occurs primarily in anaerobic cells. Whenever you need significant anaerobic coverage (think intra-abdominal infections, aspiration, gas producing abscesses), add Flagyl!

Gram positives	Negligible (some activity against *C. diff* but not first line)
Gram negatives	Negligible
Anaerobes	Very broad (almost all)
Atypicals	Giardia, *Entamoeba histolytica*
Cidal or static?	Bactericidal
Route of administration	IV or PO
Key side effects	Diarrhea Neurotoxicity Disulfiram-like reaction[a]
First line for	Anaerobic coverage

[a]Disulfiram-like reaction occurs in the presence of alcohol and leads to nausea, vomiting, headache, and flushing similar to hangover symptoms

19.4.2.17 Other Antimicrobials

Briefly, here are some key points regarding a few other antimicrobials you may encounter:
- Nitrofurantoin (PO)
  - This is a great drug for uncomplicated UTIs.
  - It acts by inducing free radicals that damage bacterial DNA.
  - Avoid prescribing to the elderly or for GFR <60.
  - It should NOT be used for pyelonephritis.
- Rifampin (PO)
  - Used for *Staph* infections that involve hardware (prosthetic valve endocarditis, prosthetic joint infections) due to its ability to penetrate biofilms secreted by *Staph*
  - Rifampin has increased vulnerability to resistance due to a single step mutation requirement. Thus, it should always be added after majority of the bacterial load has been dealt with (often added a week after other antibiotics).

19.4.2.18 Antibiotic Interactions Worth Remembering

These are the most common antibiotic interactions worth remembering:
- Vanc/Zosyn: This is a popular combination for broad coverage, including anaerobes and pseudomonas. However, recent data suggest that this combination has a significantly higher risk for nephrotoxicity. Therefore, alternative similar regimens such as Vanc/cefepime/Flagyl are preferred. Note that Vanc/Zosyn may be used in ESRD patients since their kidney function is already at rock bottom.

- P450 interactors:
  - Inducers: Rifampin, though not commonly used aside from tuberculosis treatment, is an important inducer to always keep in mind.
  - Inhibitors: Fluoroquinolones are the most notable P450-inhibiting antibiotic. You should always check the QTc before use and periodically throughout use.

19.4.2.19 Key Antimicrobial Recap

Though the facts below are from above, we will emphasize them again, this time focusing on commonalities to help you remember:

Antimicrobials with significant pseudomonal activity (that you should remember) (◻ Fig. 19.3)
- Ceftazidime
- Cefepime
- Zosyn (piperacillin-tazobactam)
- Fluoroquinolones (PO) excluding moxifloxacin
  - Pearl: The only big PO option with pseudomonal coverage
- Carbapenems (excluding ertapenem)
- Gentamicin
- Aztreonam
  Antimicrobials with significant MRSA activity (that you should remember)
- IV
  - Vancomycin
  - Linezolid
  - Daptomycin
  - Clindamycin
  - Bactrim
  - Doxycycline

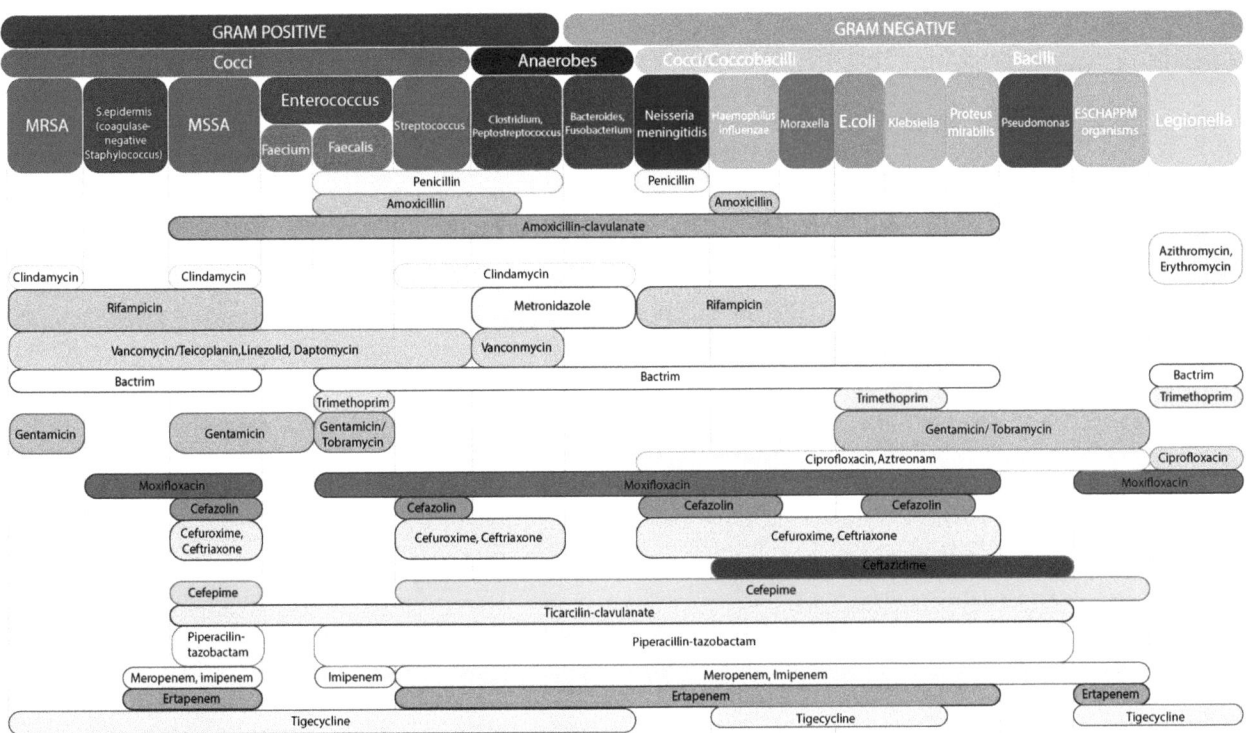

◻ **Fig. 19.3** Antibiotic coverage spectrum

- PO
  - Bactrim
  - Clindamycin
  - Doxycycline
  - Linezolid

19.5 Top Infectious Disease Consults

Your goal should be to become very familiar with the most common consults that will occupy 80% of your rotation. This allows you to do well on most of your consults. For the more esoteric consults, you will have built a strong foundation that will require just a quick skim of those niche topics to do well. Do not spend your time relearning all the Step 1 microbiology or watching all of SketchyMicro. The vast majority of that information will not be used clinically during your ID rotation.

19.5.1 Bacteremia

Bacteremia refers to bacteria in the blood that yields positive blood cultures. This is dangerous not only due to the immediate manifestations such as cytokine and toxin release that can lead to septic shock but also due to downstream complications such as seeding of bacteria leading to abscess formation, endocarditis, septic joints, meningitis, and septic emboli/infarcts. The goals with bacteremia cases are to
1. Identify the organism,
2. Identify the source,
3. Assess for complications.
4. Identify the ideal treatment regimen.

19.5.1.1 Identifying the Organism
Patients are always to be started on antibiotics **AFTER** cultures are obtained, if at all possible. This ensures that you will have data that helps to narrow your empiric antibiotic regimens (don't throw away your answer key!). This is key to reducing rates of resistance, side effects, and cost. At least two blood cultures should be sent from peripheral lines. Any ports that the patient has should also be cultured. Always pay attention to the distribution of positive cultures and where each culture was taken. For example, if the port culture is positive but the peripheral cultures are all negative, it is likely that the port is infected (and may need replacement) with small to no infection of your bloodstream. If multiple peripheral sites return positive, you know that the bacterial burden is quite high.

In addition to blood cultures, you should obtain cultures from wounds or tissues at all potential sources. For example, if a bacteremic patient has a large dorsal burn wound, then that wound should be cultured to see if it reveals the same organism as the peripheral blood cultures. A match would indicate the likely source.

19.5.1.2 Identifying the Source
The location of positive blood cultures can be a good initial hint as to the source. Often, the source is not a visible cut or wound but rather obtained from the history. Common sources include the mouth (ask regarding recent dental work), cuts/wounds/IV drug use sites (thorough skin exam required),

the lungs (check for pneumonia), urinary tract (check for UTI), and lines (assess all line/port sites). High-risk sites should be cultured (e.g., wound culture or respiratory culture) to compare any organism growth with the bacterium in the blood.

Identification of the source itself is not your only task. Other clues to why the patient is bacteremic are important as well. For example, you may want to consider obtaining a full STI workup including testing for HIV (immunocompromise).

19.5.1.3 Assessing for Complications

This is particularly important in the case of sticky bacteria, namely, *Staphylococcus* species. When you have Staph bacteremia, you will always need to assess for signs of endocarditis (see "Endocarditis" section). For most other bacteria (all others that you will need to know as a medical student), you do not automatically pursue an endocarditis workup in the setting of bacteremia. Instead, you wait for suspicion that there is cardiac involvement. Other complications include abscesses that can be located virtually anywhere but more commonly in the psoas, spine, or CNS. Mycotic aneurysm, which simply means an aneurysm due to an infection, is a rare complication with devastating consequences. As a medical student, it is worth bringing up mycotic aneurysm as a potential complication of bacteremia and suggesting head CT if there are signs of CNS involvement. Lastly, septic emboli (collections of bacteria, sometimes from vegetation) can lodge themselves anywhere, from the lungs to the renal arteries, causing infarcts.

Each morning, your job is to carefully interview and examine the patient to assess for signs or symptoms that point to possible complications. This includes assessing for new pains (to be distinguished from chronic pains), new focal neurologic deficits, and changes in baseline basic labs such as creatinine. Interval chest imaging can clue you towards septic pulmonary emboli which are often peripherally distributed.

19.5.1.4 Identifying the Treatment

The ideal treatment is one that covers only all the organisms that need to be covered – no less, no more. Initially, before microbiologic diagnosis, all patients should be put on empiric antibiotics (after drawing cultures!). Empiric regimens are commonly along the lines of vancomycin (to cover MRSA and gram positives) + cefepime (broad gram-negative and pseudomonal coverage) + Flagyl (the best anaerobic coverage) or vancomycin + Zosyn (broad gram-negative, anaerobic, and pseudomonal coverage). Antibiotics can be narrowed as soon as you have some information, such as "Gram-Positive Cocci in Clusters" (signaling a type of *Staph*). However, keep in mind that this is possible since most bacteremia cases are monomicrobial (one organism). It is not possible to narrow as quickly in cases such as open wound infections which may be often polymicrobial since certain bacteria (e.g., anaerobes) grow much slower and may not show up in cultures for a few days.

When choosing an antibiotic, keep in mind the bioavailability of the drugs. Bacteremia is a serious infection and IV administration is required at least initially if not for the whole course of antibiotics. The usual treatment course is 14 days for an uncomplicated bacteremia (some bugs and/or institutions may vary on this; for example, uncomplicated CoNS can often be treated for 7–10 days). Longer treatment is necessary if there are complications such as endocarditis or if the organism is difficult to treat, such as *Staph* species. For *Staph* species, a course of 4–6 weeks is recommended due to its sticky nature and concerns of undiagnosed complications. For prolonged antibiotic courses, once the patient is hemodynamically stable without complications and blood cultures have been negative for >48 hours, they will require a peripherally inserted central catheter (PICC) line for outpatient IV antibiotic administration.

Antibiotic selection is not the only component to treatment. All potential sources of the bacteremia should be dealt with. This means removal of all existing lines (peripheral IV, PICC, hemodialysis lines, etc.) and ports and potentially hardware such as pacemakers.

19.5.2 Endocarditis

Endocarditis, or infection of the inner surface of the heart, is essentially cardiac involvement in the setting of bacteremia. Though there are more esoteric types such as Libman-Sacks and sterile endocarditis; these do not pertain to you as medical students.

■ Workup

The diagnosis of endocarditis is done through the modified Duke Criteria (◘ Fig. 19.4). As a medical student, your job is to perform a thorough physical exam. Many of these signs such as Janeway lesions and splinter hemorrhages are fairly rare given that prolonged bacteremia is required for them to occur. This makes sense given what they are on a molecular level. Janeway lesions are microabsceses filled with neutrophilic infiltration of capillaries, and splinter hemorrhages are embolizations of septic vegetations in distal capillaries.

Almost all patients suspected with endocarditis receive a TTE followed by a TEE. Though some institutions may choose not to follow a TTE with a TEE, clear indications for TEE include organism (*S. aureus*), presence on a prosthetic valve or pacemaker, and presence of persistent bacteremia. The most common valve affected is the mitral valve followed by the aortic valve, both of which are best visualized on TEE, particularly in light of the resolution required to visualize vegetations/abscesses. In IV drug users, the most common affected valve is the tricuspid, and the most common organism is *Staphylococcus aureus*. You should always keep in mind the risk factors for endocarditis (e.g., recent invasive dental procedures, damaged/prosthetic valves, etc.).

■ Treatment

Treatment of endocarditis ultimately comes down to antibiotic choice with or without surgery. Indications for surgery are not worth remembering and can be easily looked up on UpToDate when needed. However, it is worth remembering one: large vegetations (defined as >10 cm for L-sided and > 20 cm for R-sided endocarditis).

Usually requires 2+ positive cultures to ensure that it is not contamination though certain organisms such as *Staph* are considered positive with even 1 positive culture. A "negative" blood culture may be positive for a bacteria or fungus that is not normally known to cause endocarditis.

19.5.3 Meningitis

Meningitis refers to inflammation of the meninges, the thick protective covering around the brain and spinal cord. Many pathologic effects stem from infection of the meninges, most notably swelling induced by the inflammation leading to increased intracranial pressure (ICP) and compression of CNS structures. There may also be other complications such as abscesses.

Major Criteria

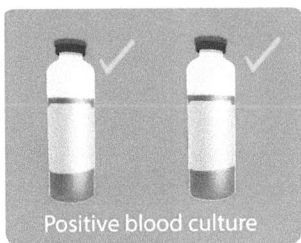

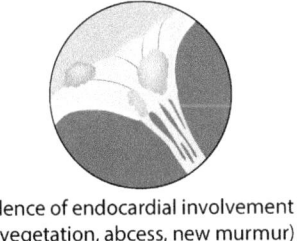

Evidence of endocardial involvement
(eg vegetation, abcess, new murmur)

Minor Criteria

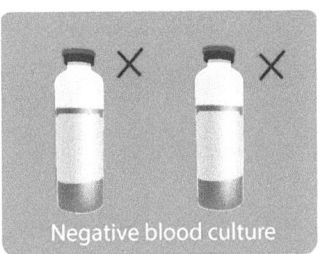

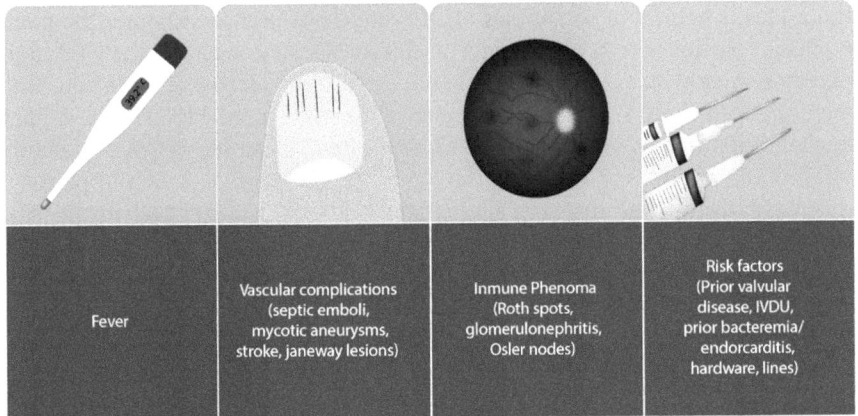

| Fever | Vascular complications (septic emboli, mycotic aneurysms, stroke, janeway lesions) | Inmune Phenoma (Roth spots, glomerulonephritis, Osler nodes) | Risk factors (Prior valvular disease, IVDU, prior bacteremia/ endorcarditis, hardware, lines) |

◧ **Fig. 19.4** Modified Duke Criteria

Please also refer to the meningitis section in the Neurology chapter for complementary information. We will not cover viral, aseptic, or fungal meningitis as those are much rarer than the bacterial meningitis you are likely to encounter.

■ Workup

You probably remember the classic triad for meningitis as fever, AMS, and nuchal rigidity. Clinically, this triad is only present around 40–50% of the time; thus you should never lower your suspicion based on the absence of this triad. On the other hand, greater than 90% of patients will exemplify at least two symptoms from among fever, AMS, nuchal rigidity, and headache.

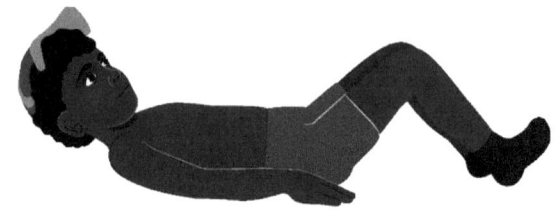

Kernig's sign

Brudzinski's sign

◘ Fig. 19.5 Meningeal signs

When examining the patient, you should perform a head to toe exam each time. This is helpful in sometimes identifying the source, or whether the meningitis is secondary to bacteremia. You should start by assessing the vitals and patient's mental status. The MSE here is really for alertness, attention, and memory; you should not perform the psychiatry-oriented MSE. Shine a light in the patient's eyes and check for photophobia (often it's helpful to simply observe the patient's response to the light being shone). You should perform the classic Kernig and Brudzinksi's maneuvers (◘ Fig. 19.5) which are specific but not sensitive. Listen carefully for the presence of murmurs and examine the skin/nails for changes that may suggest a concurrent endocarditis. A petechial rash may point towards meningococcemia.

If you suspect meningitis based on your exam, obtain blood cultures immediately, prior to administering antibiotics. The primary diagnostic for meningitis will be CSF via lumbar puncture. Obtain a head CT first if you find neurological deficits, evidence of increased intracranial pressure, AMS, immunocompromise, or known CNS disease such as a brain tumor. From the LP, you should obtain the following:

- Opening pressure
- Gram stain
- Culture/PCR (refer to ◘ Table 19.1)
- RBC/WBC/protein

■ Treatment

As soon as blood cultures are drawn, you should initiate empiric antibiotics given the morbidity of meningitis. Empiric regimens are based on risk factors: age, immunocompromise, and potential for involvement of *Staph* or *Pseudomonas* (◘ Table 19.2).

⊡ Table 19.1 Most common bacterial causes of meningitis by age

Adults < 50	Adults ≥ 50
S. pneumoniae	*S. pneumoniae*
N. meningitidis	*Listeria*
H. influenzae	*H. influenzae*

⊡ Table 19.2 Empiric treatment for meningitis

Adults < 50	Adults > 50	Immunocompromised	Nosocomial	B-lactam allergy
Vanc + CTX 2 g q12h	Vanc + CTX 2 g q12h + ampicillin 2 g q4h	Vanc + cefepime 2 g q8h + ampicillin 2 g q4h	Vanc + cefepime or meropenem	Vanc + meropenem 2 g q8h
Streptococcus pneumoniae, N. meningitidis, H. influenzae	*S. pneumoniae Listeria*	*Listeria* GBS	*Pseudomonas* S. aureus CoNS	

Furthermore, steroids (specifically dexamethasone) should be started as soon as meningitis is suspected. While conferring the most benefit in cases of pneumococcal meningitis, it is great for decreasing morbidity due to hearing loss.

19.5.4 Skin and Soft-Tissue Infections (SSTIs)

SSTIs are among the most common consults for your ID rotation. Specifically, you will see cellulitis, diabetic foot infections, and necrotizing fasciitis. Let's take a look at each:

19.5.4.1 Cellulitis

Cellulitis refers to an infection of the dermis (middle skin layer) and the soft deeper tissues. Infection of the middle skin layer is why cellulitis appears as an ill-defined border on examination as opposed to the more superficial infection of erysipelas. When considering cellulitis, you should think about it as either purulent or non-purulent. Purulent is most often due to *Staphylococcus aureus* infection, whereas non-purulent is usually due to *Strep* infection.

- Workup

Cellulitis is a clinical diagnosis meaning that you won't be sending off diagnostics unless there is evidence of systemic toxicity, special exposures, or recurrent infection. Focus on identifying the following features on exam:
- Indistinct border (difficult to draw a margin around the infection)
- Unilateral (bilateral suggests alternate dx such as venous stasis)
- Warm and erythematous with potential drainage

- Treatment

Antibiotic choice depends on whether you find evidence of purulence, which suggests *Staph* involvement. If purulent, you should cover empirically for MRSA with IV vancomycin and then transition to PO with either doxycycline or Bactrim (still covering for MRSA) along with amoxicillin. If a culture was obtained and MRSA is ruled out, you may of course drop the MRSA coverage and opt for dicloxacillin or cephalexin. Pseudomonal coverage should be added if the patient has a hospital-associated infection, has history of prior pseudomonal cellulitis, or has a hematologic malignancy. The overall antibiotic course is typically 5 days though you should begin to see clear improvement within 3 days.

19.5.4.2 Necrotizing Fasciitis

This is a serious and life-threatening infection of the fascia as well as surrounding structures (muscle and skin). It is typically caused by mixed flora (polymicrobial) including many anaerobes but also bacteria that commonly reside on skin such as *Staphylococcus aureus* and *Streptococcus* species.

- **Workup**

Necrotizing fasciitis must be recognized early due to its rapidly progressive nature. Thus, despite many tests that can support this diagnosis, it is practically speaking a clinical diagnosis. The classic presentation is of pain out of proportion to exam meaning that even the slightest touch of the area leads to excruciating pain.

Cellulitis is the most common mimic that may lead to misdiagnosis. Both can present with erythema of indistinct borders associated with mild to moderate (initially, in the case of nec fasc) pain. Clues towards necrotizing fasciitis include evidence of systemic infection (as opposed to cellulitis which is most often localized). This may include fever, elevated lactate, creatinine kinase (from muscle involvement), an elevated WBC, or elevated lactate. On radiographs, gas may be seen in the affected tissues, but this is typically when the infection is caused by anaerobic bacteria and in the later stages of disease.

Since early recognition of necrotizing fasciitis is so important, consideration of risk factors is extremely helpful. These are primarily factors that lead to immunocompromise or reduced vascular perfusion to the area (meaning also a lack of delivery of immune system components to the area). Examples are diabetes (microvascular complications and immunosuppression), HIV/AIDS, and peripheral vascular disease (immunosuppression). Anything that can seed the fascia, such as recent trauma or surgery, also increases risk.

- **Treatment**

This is never a case handled by ID alone! This is a surgical emergency and general surgery should always be involved, as well as vascular surgery in extreme cases. The patient will require debridement of the most severely affected areas and sometimes even amputation.

From an ID perspective, broad-spectrum empiric coverage should be initiated along with clindamycin (or less commonly linezolid) for toxin inhibition (reduces toxin production from *Strep* and *Staph* species via inhibition of translation). An example regimen is vancomycin for MRSA coverage with meropenem and clindamycin.

19.5.4.3 Diabetic Foot Infections (DFI)

While DFIs are a very common outpatient problem, you will see more of the severe DFIs on the inpatient service. Mild DFI is typically managed outpatient.

- **Workup**

DFI is a clinical diagnosis that calls for signs of infection (rubor, dolor, calor, tumor, purulence). While the diagnosis itself is fairly straightforward, a key part of the workup is excluding complications such as osteomyelitis. A radiograph is typically obtained when the infection is at least moderate. Certain features that greatly increase the likelihood of osteomyelitis include a large ulcer (>2 cm^2), subacute or chronic ulcer, and ESR >70. Exposure to bone is, of course, diagnostic of osteomyelitis. With the help of surgery, the patient with moderate or severe DFI also merits evaluation for limb ischemia and/or necrotizing fasciitis.

- **Treatment**

We will focus on the treatment of moderate to severe DFIs here, since mild DFIs need not be hospitalized. Empiric coverage is broad to target the polymicrobial nature of DFIs and usually includes pseudomonal coverage, particularly if involving risk factors such as diabetes and frequent water exposures. Examples of moderate infection regimens include Zosyn, cefepime, and ceftriaxone (no pseudomonal coverage). Severe infections receive anaerobic and MRSA coverage, with examples being vancomycin + meropenem or cefepime/Flagyl.

19.5.5 Osteomyelitis

Osteomyelitis is simply infection of the bone. It can present either acutely with more obvious symptoms or chronically with often less obvious symptoms. The symptoms are fairly nonspecific, such as pain, warmth, erythema, and even systemic signs such as fevers. Furthermore, it is often not possible to clinically diagnose osteomyelitis by a visual inspection because it is the bone is usually not seen. Thus, the diagnosis hinges upon a culture of the causative organism.

- **Workup**

If you're lucky enough to find a draining sinus tract or exposure to bone in diabetics, you have diagnosed osteomyelitis. Otherwise, a step-by-step approach is taken. Plain films are helpful in searching for degenerative changes consistent with osteomyelitis; in particular, lytic lesions appear after approximately 2 weeks and can clue you in on whether this is an acute or chronic osteomyelitis. If plain films are not diagnostic, MRI (preferred) or CT may be used as sensitive but nonspecific diagnostic modalities. The gold standard is to obtain a bone biopsy with culture which is often positive even when the patient has been on antibiotics due to slower and decreased bone penetration.

- **Treatment**

Osteomyelitis is most often chronic and there is no immediate danger to the patient unless they are systemically toxic appearing and unstable. Thus, antibiotics should be delayed until a diagnosis has been made (sometimes until a bone biopsy) if at all possible. As with any infectious disease consult, always obtain blood cultures prior to antibiotics. Due to the need for high bone penetration, IV antibiotics are preferred. Empiric antibiotic regimens include vancomycin + ceftriaxone/cefepime for coverage of gram-positive and gram-negative organisms as well as pseudomonal coverage when risk factors such as water exposure are present. The typical duration of antibiotics is a minimum 6 weeks after any required debridement, though amputation may allow for shorter courses. Lastly, ESR and CRP are commonly checked at the end of the antibiotics course to reassure resolution.

19.5.6 HIV/AIDS

Though you probably won't see someone admitted for complications of HIV, it is a common comorbidity to either see or test for while working up another primary problem. Given the existence of robust antiretrovirals today, the primary concern of HIV is adherence and predisposition for certain infections. Let's explore some of the most relevant inpatient facts for HIV/AIDS.

It's important to understand the distinction between HIV and AIDS. There are three definitions which may classify a patient into AIDS:

- HIV with a CD4 count of less than 200
- HIV with a CD4 count <14% of total lymphocytes
- AIDS defining illness (think of the classic Step 1 bugs such as CMV, PCP, toxoplasmosis, cryptococcus, candidiasis, MAC)

■ Workup

The preferred method of testing is now to use fourth-generation testing which consists of a test against HIV ½ antibody and p24 antigen. This test can detect HIV as early as 10–14 days after infection, much sooner than the prior methods. If the preliminary screen comes back positive, you should always confirm with a HIV RNA PCR viral load, which can detect as early as 17 days after infection. Never tell the patient they have HIV until you confirm with this!

■ Treatment

Once a terminal diagnosis, HIV/AIDs is now a diagnosis that is largely compatible with a normal life, thanks to robust antiretrovirals. If your patient tests positive, antiretrovirals (ARVs) should be initiated early regardless of CD4 count. According to the INSIGHT START trial (NEJM 2015), ARVs initiated early even in asymptomatic patients with CD4 counts >500 led to decreased mortality and complications.

The current treatment regimen consists of 2 nucleotide reverse transcriptase inhibitors (NRTIs) with 1 ARV from a different class, preferably either a protease inhibitor or integrase inhibitor. The first-line regimens are as follows:

- Dolutegravir plus tenofovir (TDF) or tenofovir alafenamide (TAF)/emtricitabine (FTC)
- Elvitegravir/cobicistat/TDF or TAF/FTC
- Ritonavir-boosted darunavir plus TDF or TAF/FTC

As you can see, the 2 NRTIs most commonly used as tenofovir and emtricitabine.

19.5.6.1 Common Knowledge Questions

These are common questions that your team may ask you and suggested responses. Feel free to read up further on these topics!

- What are some common drug interactions with ARVs?
  - The one that comes to mind right away are proton-pump inhibitors and really any medication that is metabolized through the P450 pathway. A good website for checking these interactions is ▶ hiv-druginteractions.org.
- Have you heard of IRIS?
  - This refers to immune reconstitution inflammatory syndrome which is a paradoxical worsening of a patient's symptoms upon initiation of ARVs. However, patients should still be started early on ARVs despite the diagnosis of opportunistic infections.

What are the most common opportunistic infections by CD4 count?

CD4 count	Opportunistic infection
<200	PCP, Candida, Cryptosporidium
<100	Disseminated histoplasmosis, toxoplasmosis, CMV
<50	MAC, Cryptococcus

19.5.7 Recap Questions

- *Compare and contrast the spectrum of cefepime and ceftazidime*
  - Cefepime is a fourth-generation cephalosporin, whereas ceftazidime is third generation. This helps you remember that cefepime has the broader spectrum. Notably, both cover *Pseudomonas*. Ceftazidime is slightly narrower in its gram-negative coverage (particularly for ESCHAPPM* organisms), and it does not have any anaerobic coverage, whereas cefepime has some though it isn't reliable and Flagyl should be added when you are really concerned about anaerobic infections such as in the abdomen.
    *ESCHAPPM = *Enterobacter, Serratia, Citrobacter, H. influenzae, Aeromonas, Providencia, Proteus, Morganella*
- *Compare and contrast the spectrum of ceftriaxone and ceftazidime*
  - Ceftriaxone and ceftazidime are both third-generation cephalosporins. The key difference is that ceftazidime has pseudomonal coverage. Both have excellent gram-negative coverage. Ceftriaxone has better gram-positive coverage for organisms such as *Strep* and MSSA (though not reliable).
- *Compare and contrast the mechanism of action for glycopeptides **vs** penicillins*
  - While both end up leading to osmotic cell death due to losing the integrity of the bacterial cell wall, the specific way they disrupt peptidoglycan cross-linking is different. Glycopeptides such as vancomycin work by binding directly to the peptidoglycan and providing further cross-linking to other peptidoglycan molecules. On the other hand, penicillins inhibit the penicillin-binding proteins (just a fancy name for the enzymes that cross-link peptidoglycan molecules) thus preventing further peptidoglycan cross-linking.
- *Practice determining empiric antibiotic coverage for the following scenarios. Repeat until you can do this rapid fire. (Answers are on the following page.)*
  - Meningitis
  - Sinusitis
  - Pneumonia
    - Aspiration
    - Hospital acquired
    - Ventilator associated
  - Suspected or known intra-abdominal infection (e.g., perforated appendix)
  - Cellulitis/erysipelas
  - Prosthetic joint infections
  - Diabetic foot infection

19.5.8 Answers for Common Empiric Antibiotic Regimens

- Meningitis
  - Vancomycin + ceftriaxone + acyclovir + – ampicillin (if *Listeria* risk)
- Sinusitis
  - Augmentin
- Pneumonia
  - Aspiration
    - Zosyn, augmentin
  - Hospital acquired
    - Vancomycin + cefepime
  - Ventilator associated
    - Add tobramycin to HAP regimen
- Suspected or known intra-abdominal infection (e.g., perforated appendix)
  - Vancomycin + cefepime + Flagyl
  - Vancomycin + ciprofloxacin + Flagyl
- Cellulitis/erysipelas
  - Cefazolin
- Prosthetic joint infections
  - Vancomycin + cefepime + Flagyl.
- Diabetic foot infection
  - Vancomycin + cefepime + Flagyl

We have now covered the most common types of infections you will see on ID consults. When you come across an unfamiliar topic, remember the basic principles that guide infectious diseases. You can always quickly search the diagnostic and treatment modalities, but it is harder to carry out a good consult without the fundamentals.

Anesthesia

Sarah Osmulski

Contents

© The Author(s), under exclusive license to Springer Nature Switzerland AG 2021
S. H. Lecker, B. J. Chang (eds.), *The Ultimate Medical School Rotation Guide*,
https://doi.org/10.1007/978-3-030-63560-2_20

20.1 Introduction

20.1.1 Anesthesiologists' Role

The major role of an anesthesiologist is to provide analgesia and often amnesia during operative procedures, labor and delivery, and areas such as radiology and endoscopy. Anesthesiologists are responsible for the preoperative assessment of the patient, the intraoperative monitoring and control of the patient's cardiovascular, pulmonary, and renal homeostasis, and postoperative care and pain control.

In large hospitals and academic medical centers, departments of anesthesia have sections of acute pain medicine and critical care. Anesthesiologists treat acute postsurgical pain and patients with chronic pain, such as those with malignancies. The field of intensive care medicine was founded by anesthesiologists as an extension of care in the OR. Critical care anesthesiologists staff surgical ICUs and manage patients after extensive surgical procedures often with medically significant comorbidities. Finally, anesthesiologists play an important role on the Labor & Delivery (L&D) floor, partnering with OB/GYN to provide neuraxial and general anesthesia to laboring women.

20.1.2 Anesthesia Training

Anesthesia residency programs come in two varieties: categorical and advanced. The traditional advanced programs offer PGY2–4 training after completion of a PGY1 (or intern year) separately prior to their anesthesia training. PGY1 positions for anesthesia can be fulfilled with a preliminary medicine year, a preliminary surgery year, or a transitional year program. There are increasing numbers of categorical programs that offer integrated PGY1–4 training. Some programs offer only categorical positions, some offer only advanced positions, and many offer both advanced and categorical positions.

After the PGY1 training year, anesthesia-specific training begins and residents are referred to as "Clinical Anesthesia" or CA residents. A CA1 resident is a PGY2; a CA2 resident is a PGY3, and so on.

Anesthesia residency training includes time spent in the operating room, in the ICU, in the Emergency Department, the obstetrics floor, and in chronic pain clinics. Operating room anesthesia is broken down into a few subspecialties: general OR anesthesia, cardiac anesthesia, thoracic anesthesia, neurosurgical OR anesthesia, and pediatric OR anesthesia. Residents generally spend time in Medical Intensive Care Units (MICU) as PGY1s and then transition to rotations in Surgical Intensive Care Units (SICU) in CA years. Residents spend time on the Labor & Delivery floor providing neuraxial and general anesthesia to laboring women. Finally, residents spend time in outpatient chronic pain clinics.

After residency, many want to subspecialize through fellowship training. The ACGME recognizes the following fields for fellowship training: addiction medicine, adult cardiothoracic anesthesia, critical care medicine, clinical informatics, hospice and palliative medicine, pain medicine, pediatric anesthesiology, regional anesthesiology, acute pain medicine, and obstetric anesthesia. Additionally, there are non-ACGME affiliated fellowships offered at some training sites; these include transplant and neurosurgical anesthesia. In general, anesthesiology fellowships are 1 year in length. In academic medicine, many attending physicians frequently have at least one fellowship training. At tertiary and quaternary care centers, it is not uncommon for anesthesiologists to pursue multiple fellowships. For example, a common dual fellowship is adult cardiothoracic anesthesia and critical care medicine. However, fellowship training is not required and upon completion of a 4-year anesthesia residency, you can choose to forgo fellowship training and pursue general anesthesia positions.

As a medical student, fellowship training may feel far off. However, if you have an idea of what you might be interested in, many medical schools offer subspecialty-focused electives within anesthesiology. If you think you might be interested in chronic pain, it might be worth doing a month-long elective in the chronic pain clinic. If you are interested in critical care, an elective in the SICU is strongly recommended. If you're not sure, the general anesthesia elective should provide you with exposure to the different subspecialties throughout your month. If you find you enjoy something, reach out to your clerkship director to attempt to schedule more time in that field.

20.1.3 Exceling on the Anesthesia Rotation

The best thing medical students can do to succeed in an anesthesiology rotation is to have strong situational awareness. Most of the time, anesthesia is relatively relaxed and controlled. However, things can go wrong quickly and it is important as the medical student to be able to recognize when you can step in to help and when it is best to take a step back and get out of the way. This rings true for asking questions as well; anesthesiologists love answering your questions and they will definitely encourage you to ask any and everything you might want to know, but always keep in mind the environment of the room. If you see something that happens during a moment of flurry, bank that question and ask it later when things have settled down.

The goal of this chapter is to introduce you to the basics, but residents and attendings in the field are also happy to teach you the basics in the OR. Feel free to ask any question you might have. Great questions usually focus on why an anesthesiologist is choosing to do one thing over another. For example: why are you choosing to use a Miller blade over the Mac blade for this case? Why did you choose to use etomidate for induction over propofol? These types of questions can be particularly helpful for the learner because they both review the fundamentals (i.e., a Mac vs. a Miller blade) but also help introduce the learner to the niches within the field.

20.2 Fundamentals

The goal of this section is to give you a brief introduction to the different tools anesthesiologists use every day. We've included some tips of how you can shine as a medical student when using these tools.

Everything in this section should be viewed in the context of how we might set up the room for the day, so throughout this section we'll refer back to a useful mnemonic for room setup: MSMAID (◘ Table 20.1).

◘ **Table 20.1**   MSMAID mnemonic

M	Machine
S	Suction
M	Monitors
A	Airway
I	IV Access
D	Drugs

20.2.1 Machine (◻ Table 20.2)

The anesthesia machine is a crucial component of intraoperative anesthesia (◻ Fig. 20.1). The machine supports patient ventilation and provides oxygen and volatile anesthetic agents to the patients via a closed loop system.

The machine needs to be checked every morning to ensure it will function and perform well for the procedures scheduled for the day. Anesthesia residents often get to the OR an hour or two before the first case of the day to set up the room and the machine. Some residents will ask you to come in to help with this portion of the day and some will tell you to arrive after this is complete; be sure to communicate with your resident about expectations for when you should arrive. It can be helpful to ask your resident for their cell phone number (and you should provide yours) so you two can easily communicate throughout the day.

◻ **Table 20.2** MSMAID: M is for Machine

M	*Machine*
	Turn on the machine, computers, and screens
	Run the machine self-test
	Adjust machine parameters for the case and the patient
	Check volatile agent levels
	Check for a bag-valve mask in the room

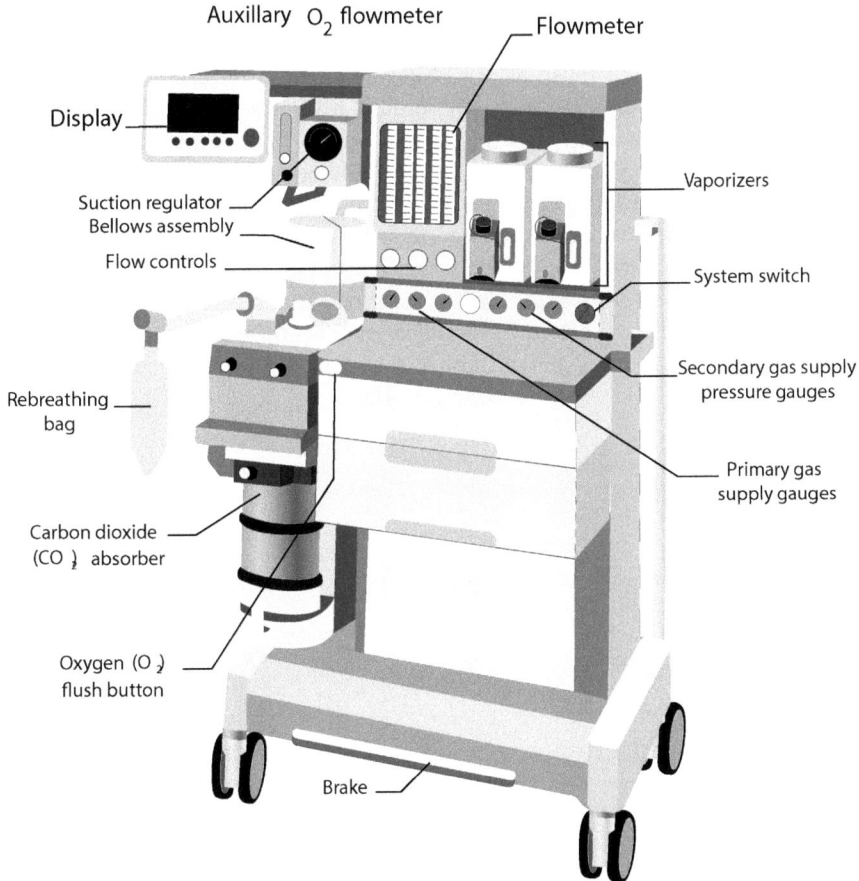

◻ **Fig. 20.1** The Anesthesia Machine

20.2.2 **Suction** (◘ Table 20.3)

Suction is one of the most crucial tools an anesthesiologist has, but it is often undervalued. You should never start a case (or perform an intubation or extubation) unless you are confident you have working suction. Suction is critical for clearing the airway prior to performing an intubation and for suctioning around the cuff of the ET tube prior to extubation to prevent oral secretions from entering the lungs during the extubation.

20.3 **NG and OG Tubes**

Most intra-abdominal surgeries will require the placement of an OG or NG tube. If you aren't sure, it is imperative to ask the surgeon prior to the case starting. In general, the tube should be placed orally after intubation. If the surgeon has requested that the gastric tube stay in the patient postoperatively, it can be placed intranasally.

NG and OG tubes allow us to decompress the stomach, which allows the surgeon to have better visualization of their surgical field. Placement of an OG tube during emergent cases can also be important to decompress the stomach to minimize the risk of aspiration of gastric contents during the procedure.

20.3.1 **Noninvasive and Invasive Monitoring** (◘ Table 20.4)

20.4 **Pulse Oximetry**

The pulse oximetry, or pulse ox, measures hemoglobin saturation using spectrophotometric methods, essentially illuminating the skin and measuring changes in the light absorption of oxyhemoglobin and deoxygenated blood using 660 nm (red) and 940 nm (infrared) wavelengths. The ratio between these two values is then fitted to a curve calibrated against direct measurement of arterial oxygen saturation, producing a measured arterial saturation. The pulse ox also outputs a waveform on the screen, allowing clinicians to better interpret the value and distinguish between noise and true signals (◘ Fig. 20.2).

In the OR, pulse ox is used in similar ways it is utilized on a telemetry unit. The goal is to maintain a patient above a certain threshold, generally greater

◘ **Table 20.3** MSMAID: S is for Suction

M	*Machine*
	Turn on the machine, computers, and screens
	Run the machine self-test
	Adjust machine parameters for the case and the patient
	Check volatile agent levels
	Check for a bag-valve mask in the room
S	*Suction*
	Make sure the suction circuit is connected and a Yankauer suction tip is connected to the end of the tubing
	Prep an OG tube for the case, if necessary (open the packing and lube up the tip)

◘ Table 20.4 MSMAID: M is for Monitors

M *Machine*
Turn on the machine, computers, and screens
Run the machine self-test
Adjust machine parameters for the case and the patient
Check volatile agent levels
Check for a bag-valve mask in the room

S *Suction*
Make sure the suction circuit is connected and a Yankauer suction tip is connected to the end of the tubing
Prep an OG tube for the case, if necessary (open the packing and lube up the tip)

M *Monitors*
Prep EKG pads, temperature probes, O2 sat monitoring, and BP cuff
Gather additional supplies for more advanced monitoring: arterial lines, central lines, BIS monitoring

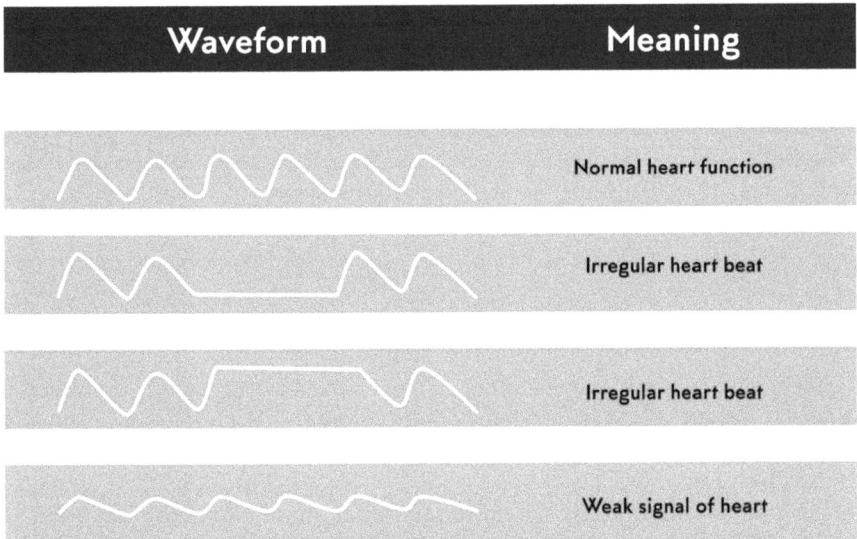

◘ Fig. 20.2 Pulse oximetry waveforms and what they indicate

than 92%. This threshold can be relaxed in patients with severe chronic lung disease, though better oxygenation is a priority intraoperatively. The tone of the beeping that goes with the heart rate corresponds to the oxygen saturation. The higher pitched the tone, the higher the oxygen saturation is. When the oxygen saturation falls in a patient, you will also notice the tone of the beeping fall.

In addition to the percentage and tone, a waveform correlating with the pulse ox will be on the monitor, usually in blue. Different waveforms and what they may represent are shown below:

There is one final high yield bit about pulse ox that may come up during your rotation: If the pulse ox suddenly falls to zero and no waveform is visible, what do you think that represents? While this can represent cardiac arrest, the majority of the time it indicates that the blood pressure cuff and the pulse oximeter are on the same arm and the blood pressure cuff is inflated, preventing an accurate pulse oximetry reading.

20.5 Blood Pressure

Blood pressure is measured throughout the case through either noninvasive or invasive means. In general, most cases will monitor blood pressure through noninvasive means using a blood pressure cuff on one of the arms. This cuff is generally cycled once every 2–5 min depending on the patient and the procedure. For more complex cases, particularly cardiothoracic or neurosurgical cases, patients may have an arterial line placed. This is a flexible catheter placed within an artery that measures blood pressure with every heartbeat.

As a medical student, it is important to watch the blood pressure response to the introduction of certain medications. What medications cause hypotension? What medications cause hypertension? What are the first steps for addressing a hypotensive or hypertensive patient?

20.6 EKG

Continuous telemetry is utilized in every single case. This allows us to observe sudden arrhythmias or ectopy that might occur during the case so that we can respond appropriately.

Medical students can be helpful in the beginning of the case by helping to place EKG pads (◘ Fig. 20.3). A common mnemonic used is "smoke over fire" and "snow over grass," which correspond to the colors of the lead placement. The white lead will be over the green lead (snow over grass) and the black lead will be on top of the brown lead which will be on top of the red lead (smoke over fire) as shown:

20.7 Anesthetic Depth Monitoring

Measuring brain function is important to prevent awareness under anesthesia. Bispectral Index (BIS) and Patient State Index (PSI; Sedline) monitoring are noninvasive means to objectively assess brain function during anesthesia. Specialized electrodes are placed on the forehead and are connected to a processing unit. The BIS uses a proprietary algorithm to calculate a score based on the EEG recording. The score exists on a scale of 0–100, with 0 indicating no EEG activity and 100 indicating wakefulness. Generally, anesthesiologists will aim for a goal BIS score between 20 and 40 during a general anesthetic. With the PSI, four simultaneous channels of frontal EEG waveforms are processed with results demonstrable in spectral waves related to the type of anesthetic and the suppression of cerebral activity. It is important to note that BIS and PSI cannot be used as the only monitor of anesthesia as they are affected by several factors such as the anesthetic drugs used, muscle movement, or artifact from surgical equipment.

20.8 Temperature Monitoring

Temperature is an extremely important vital sign to monitor in the operating room. In the OR, the thermostat is generally set quite low to allow a comfortable environment for surgeons working in heavy gowns under warm lights. Patients can be significantly exposed during cases, leading to loss of body

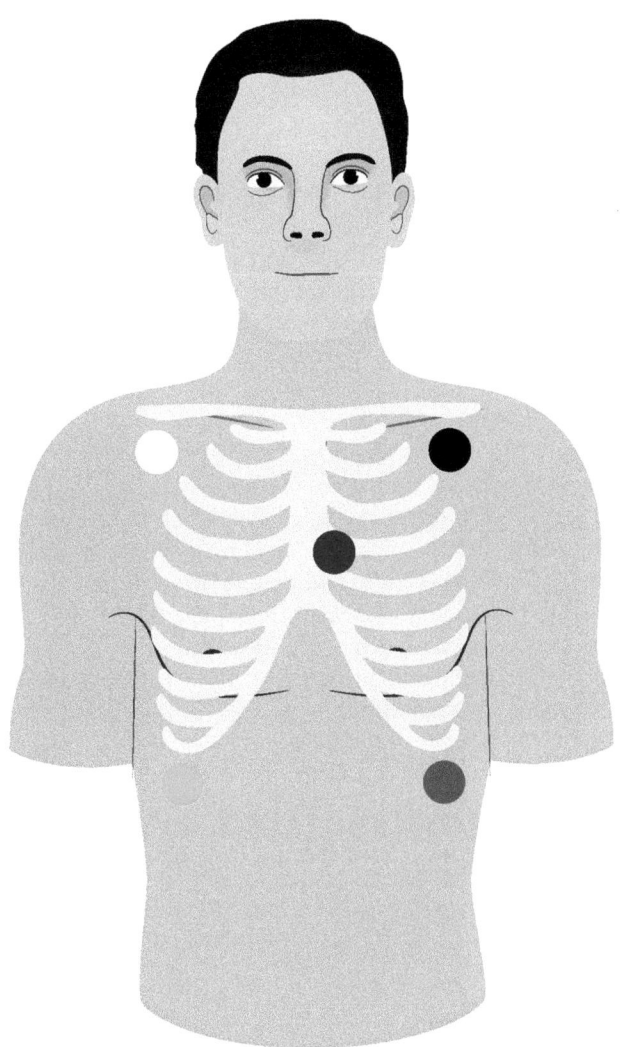

■ **Fig. 20.3** EKG monitoring placement (*snow on grass, smoke over fire*)

heat through insensible losses. Additionally, anesthetics often lead to systemic vasodilation, which can lead to further insensible body heat loss. Maintaining a normal body temperature throughout the case is imperative to maintain patient homeostasis and to provide better hemostasis for your surgical colleagues.

Temperature is often monitored using an intranasal probe, which is placed in the patient after induction and removed from the patient prior to extubation. Anesthesiologists have a few tricks to maintain adequate temperatures in patients. First, placing a Bair Hugger blanket on the patient prior to draping can help keep the patient warm. This unit works by forcing warm air through a blanket attached to the patient's skin, helping to minimize losses through the skin. It is important to place this prior to draping and important to not touch the sterile field when placing these devices. Additionally, anesthesiologists can attempt to modify their anesthetic used to prevent systemic vasodilation. Finally, anesthesiologists can advocate for the thermostat to be set to a higher temperature during the case to keep the patient warmer.

20.9 Train of Four (TOF)

During induction of anesthesia, patients are paralyzed with neuromuscular blockade. It is important to understand how much blockade persists near the end of the case to understand how likely a patient will be able to be appropriately reversed at the end of the case. This is assessed with train of four or TOF (◘ Fig. 20.4). Essentially, two electrodes are placed at the wrist (or another peripheral nerve location such as the face) and an electric current is passed through the electrodes and you measure the twitches. Train of four is discussed in more detail under the "Emergence" section in the drugs category.

20.10 Urinary Catheters

In general, these are placed by the circulating nurse, surgery resident, or surgery medical student. These are placed at the discretion of anesthesia and surgery, and may or may not be placed depending on the surgery type, expected length of the case, and expected blood loss. In general, the more complex the case, the more likely a urinary catheter will be placed.

Once the catheter is placed, urine output monitoring is the responsibility of the anesthesiologist. UOP and urine color are an important way to titrate intraoperative volume resuscitation.

Neuromuscular Blockade

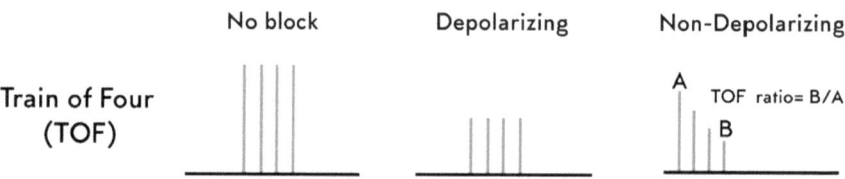

Common Monitoring Sites

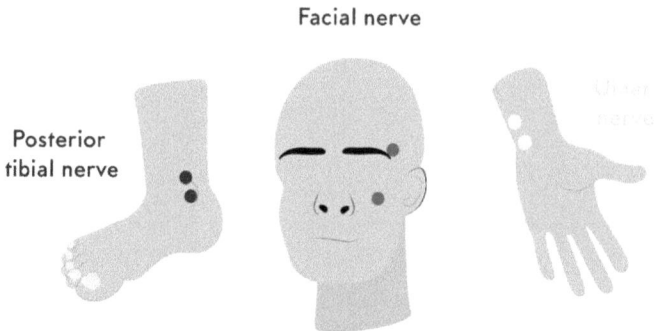

◘ **Fig. 20.4** Train of Four Monitoring

There are many monitors to keep track of during a surgical case. Luckily, many of these monitors are condensed onto one screen that you can quickly reference (◘ Fig. 20.5).

Below is an example of the type of monitoring you might see during a case.

Green represents the telemetry reading and "75" corresponds to the heart rate. The red line is the arterial line waveform with the red number corresponding to the blood pressure; the Mean Arterial Pressure (MAP) is shown beneath the blood pressure in parentheses. The pulse ox waveform is shown in yellow, with the SpO2 value also reported in yellow. End tidal CO2, or the amount of CO2 blown off in each exhalation, is shown in white with the white waveform representing the respiratory flow curve. The temperature is shown in green near the bottom right. In the bottom left, if a cuff was used to measure the blood pressure, this would be displayed here in red where the red dashes are.

20.10.1 Airway Management (◘ Table 20.5)

There are a few ways we maintain patient airways in the operating room when patients are under anesthesia. First, bag-mask ventilation is used to preoxygenate the patient prior to intubation attempts. If the patient is not undergoing full general anesthesia, then an endotracheal tube may not be required, and a laryngeal mask airway (LMA) may be sufficient. In patients undergoing general anesthesia,

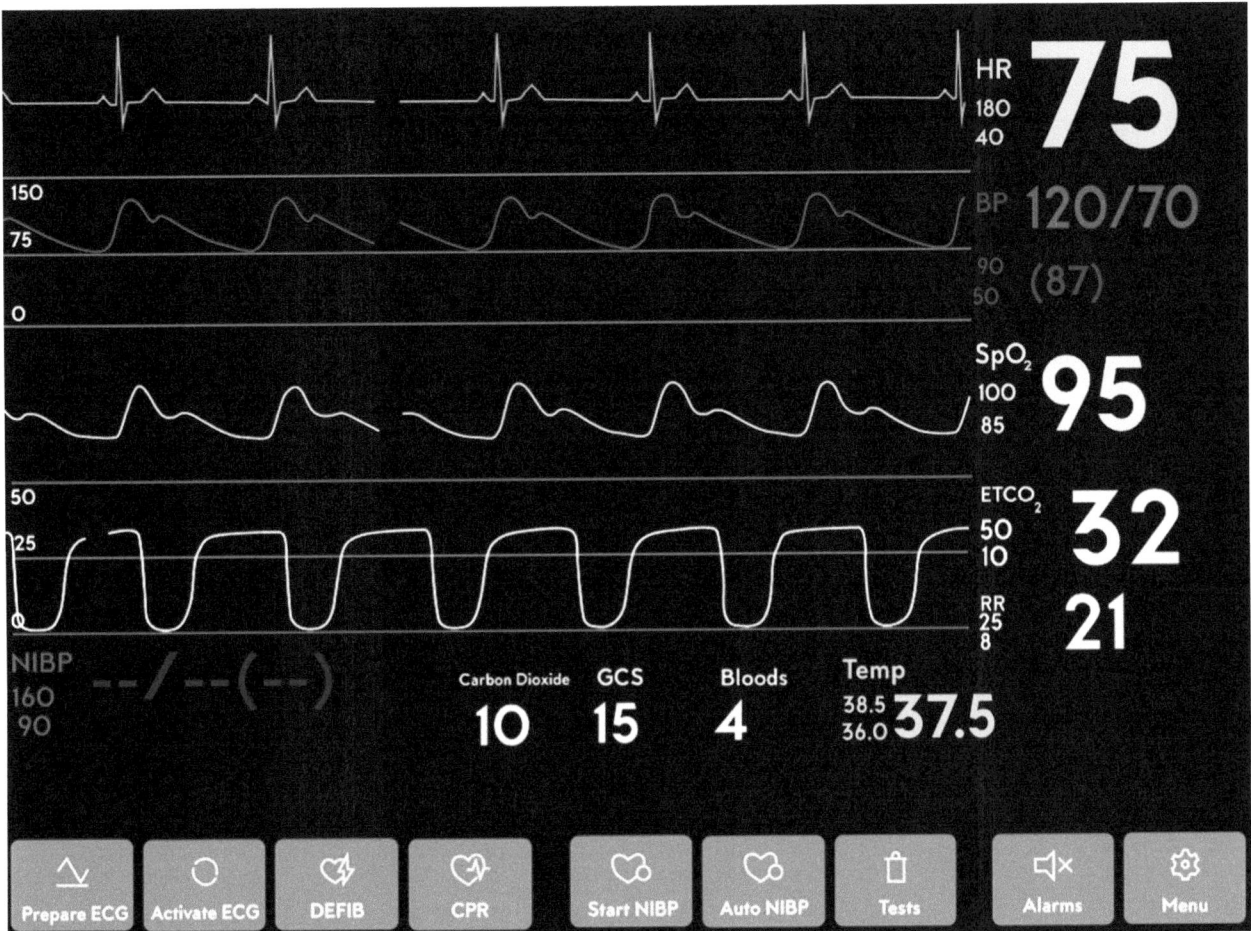

◘ **Fig. 20.5** An intra-op monitor display

◻ **Table 20.5** MSMAID: A is for Airway

M	*Machine*
	Turn on the machine, computers, and screens
	Run the machine self-test
	Adjust machine parameters for the case and the patient
	Check volatile agent levels
	Check for a bag-valve mask in the room
S	*Suction*
	Make sure the suction circuit is connected and a Yankauer suction tip is connected to the end of the tubing
	Prep an OG tube for the case, if necessary (open the packing and lube up the tip)
M	*Monitors*
	Prep EKG pads, temperature probes, O2 sat monitoring, and BP cuff
	Gather additional supplies for more advanced monitoring: arterial lines, central lines, BIS monitoring
A	*Airway*
	Acquire the correct size ETT, check the stylet is in place and check the cuff for leaks
	Prep the laryngoscope, make sure the light is working
	Open an oral airway and place it within reach of where you will be performing intubation
	Make sure a laryngeal mask airway, bougies, or video laryngoscopes are available if you are concerned about a difficult airway

an endotracheal tube is the best means to protect the patient's airway. We'll discuss each of these options and tips for inserting them in the section below.

20.11 Bag-Mask Ventilation

While intubation may be the first thing you think of with airway management, the most important skill to master first is bag-mask ventilation. Bagging is an essential and life-saving skill. Most anesthesiologists will want to confirm you can properly bag-mask before they will allow you to attempt an intubation. Here are some quick tips to help you master the art of bag-mask ventilation:

1. Start with proper positioning of the patient and yourself.
   Your comfort is important during bag-mask ventilation, as you may be expected to hold that position for several minutes. Make sure the height of the bed is at a level that doesn't strain your neck and back. You should be standing at the head of the bed. The patient should be positioned so that their head is near the top of the bed, they should be fully supine, and their neck should be tilted back to open their airway.

2. Make sure all your tools are available and ready to use.
   You're going to need a mask and an Ambu bag or a connection to your anesthesia machine. You should also open and make available an oral airway in case masking is difficult.

3. Place the mask on the patient's face and create a seal with one hand use the C and E technique (◻ Fig. 20.6).
   The anesthesia machine in most ORs will be to the patient's right, therefore, you'll want to make this seal with your left hand so your right hand can be made available to bag. You'll want the C to be composed of your thumb and forefinger with your thumb resting over the nose and your forefinger resting under the bottom lip. Your middle, ring, and pinky fingers will then curl around

Anesthesia

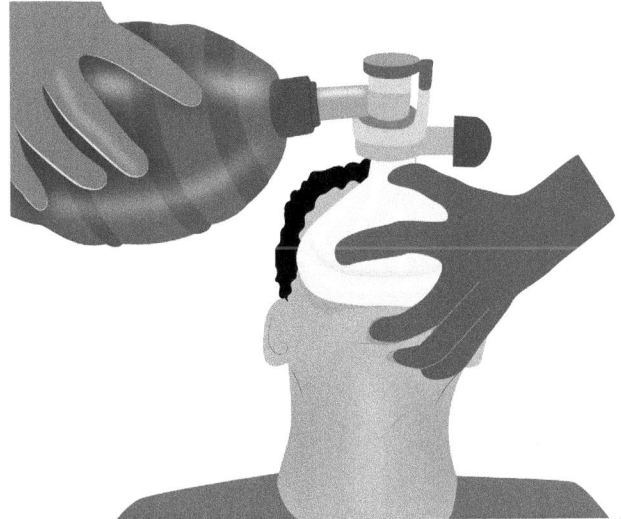

☐ **Fig. 20.6**   The C + E bag-masking technique

the jaw, hooking at the angle of the mandible. These fingers will lift the patient's jaw and face into the mask.

4. Lift the patient's jaw and face into the mask. Do not push the mask down into the patient's face.

   This is crucial. If you apply too much pressure to the patient's face you may cause damage and you may actually make bagging more difficult by collapsing the patient's airway.

5. Deliver a breath. If you feel a leak on exhalation, adjust your hand that is providing the seal.

   With one-handed ventilation you may feel a leak on the opposite side of where your hand is, particularly if you have smaller hands or if the patient is large. One tip to avoid this leak is to gently lean the mask toward that side (i.e., away from your hand). Your left hand will be lifting the patient's face into the mask on that side, so you won't introduce a leak there, but by gently rocking the mask over to the nonsealed (right) side, you will help close that leak.

6. If you are meeting resistance and not able to deliver a breath, you can try inserting an oral airway (☐ Fig. 20.7).

   Oral airways are great adjuncts and can really help with ventilation. These tools help prop the patient's tongue up and out of the way, allowing breaths to reach the lungs. In order to insert the oral airway, have it so the curve points up at you and place in the patient's mouth, then twist the piece 180 degrees so the curve is pointing down and the tongue is swept up and out of the way.

As the medical student, you should ask for the opportunity to pre-ventilate patients who are not undergoing rapid sequence intubation. Ask your resident or attendings to watch your technique and ask for feedback.

20.12 Laryngeal Mask Airways (LMAs)

LMAs are great tools to help protect a patient's airway for short procedures where general anesthesia is not necessary (☐ Fig. 20.8). You will often hear surgeons say they want a procedure done under "MAC," which means Monitored Anesthesia Care. There is no true definition of what MAC means and what it entails, but it is usually meant to refer to lighter sedation, conscious

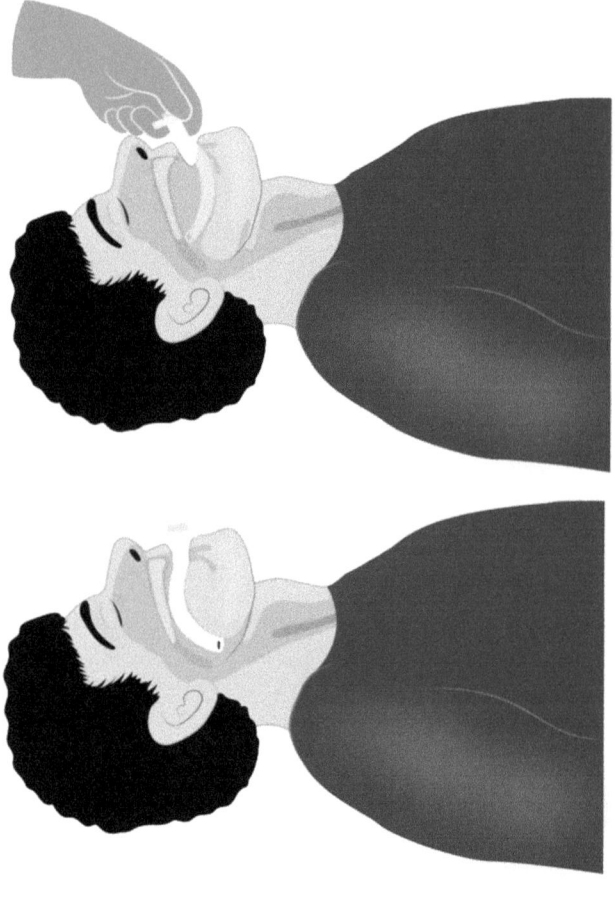

◨ **Fig. 20.7** Oral airway insertion technique

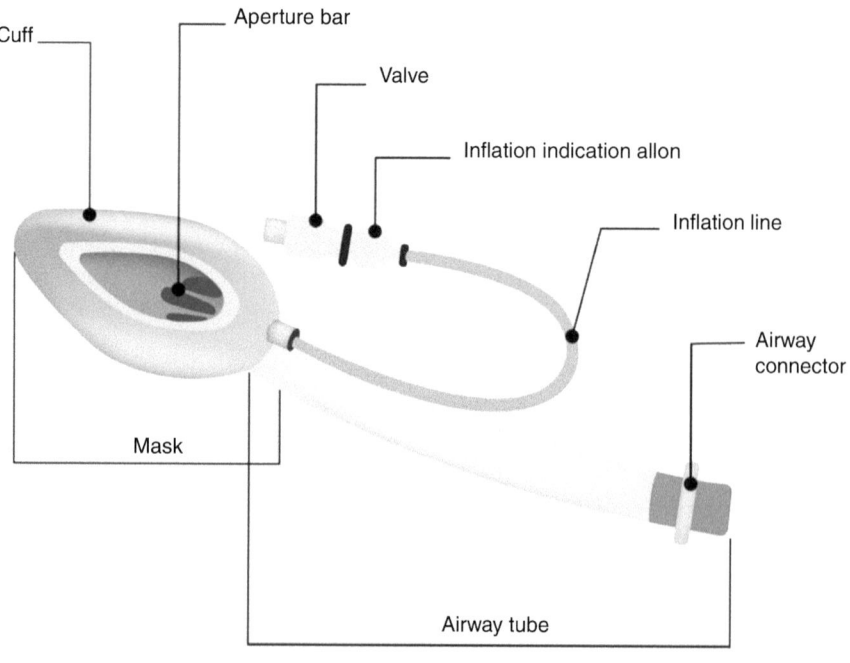

◨ **Fig. 20.8** Parts of a laryngeal mask airway

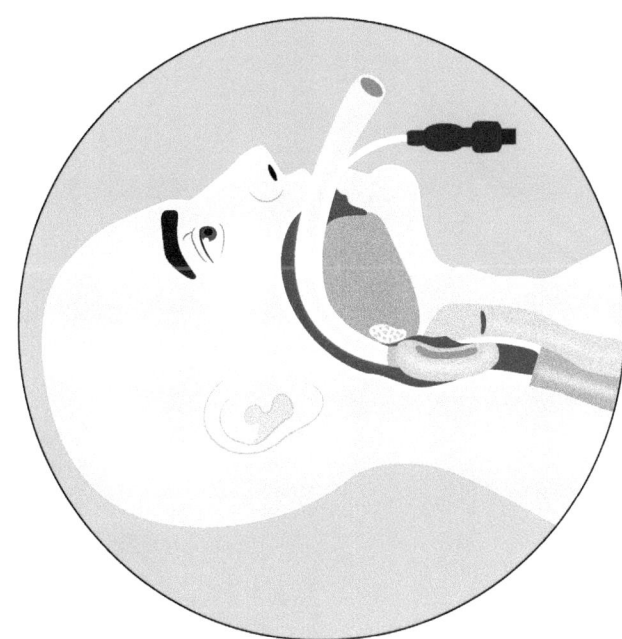

◘ Fig. 20.9 Proper location of an inserted LMA

sedation, or "twilight sleep." During cases where MAC anesthesia is utilized, LMAs are extremely helpful as they protect the patient's airway usually without causing throat soreness after the patient wakes up.

LMAs work by sitting in the patient's pharynx and esophagus and creating a seal over the larynx, so air can go in but oral and gastric secretions cannot (◘ Fig. 20.9). LMAs are reliant on that seal, however, so in patients where a good seal cannot be produced, intubation may be required (along with deeper sedation) in order to adequately protect the patient's airway.

An LMA may be the first thing you are taught to utilize in the OR for more invasive ventilation tools (◘ Fig. 20.10). Here are some tips to keep in mind when trying to insert an LMA:

1. Gather your supplies.

    Pick out the correct sized LMA. Inflate the cuff, make sure there is no leak, and then deflate the cuff. Apply lubricant to the cuff.

2. Positioning is key.

    You should be standing at the head of the bed; make sure the bed is at a height where you do not have to strain yourself. Prop the patient's head up on some blankets and rock their head back, the position is similar to that required for proper bag-mask ventilation.

3. Insert the LMA.

    Open the patient's mouth and slide the LMA in so the top of the mask is facing up toward the patient's palate. Advance the LMA along the palate until approximately 1–2 cm of tube is sticking out of the patient's mouth.

4. Inflate the cuff.

    You must inflate the cuff prior to ventilating the patient otherwise you won't have a proper seal around the airway.

5. Ventilate the patient.

    Check for fog in the tube, end tidal CO2, and bilateral breath sounds in order ensure proper placement. Hint: It is common to be asked how you can verify the tube is in the right spot!

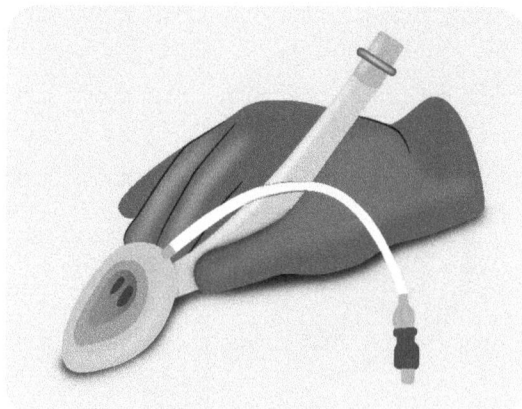

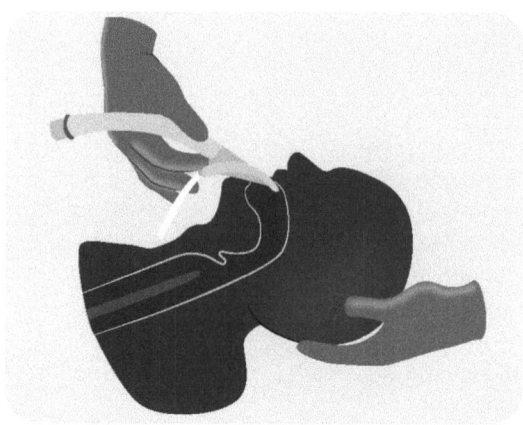

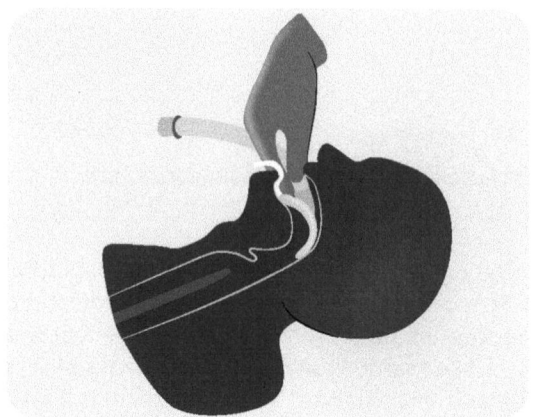

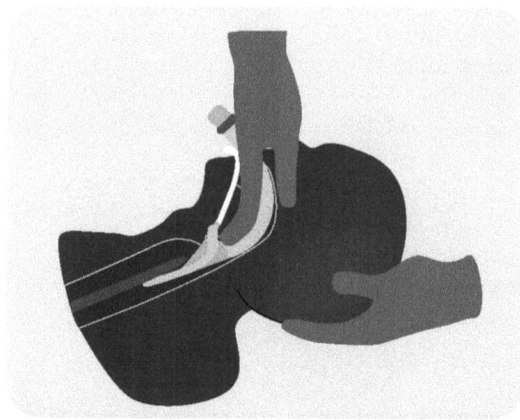

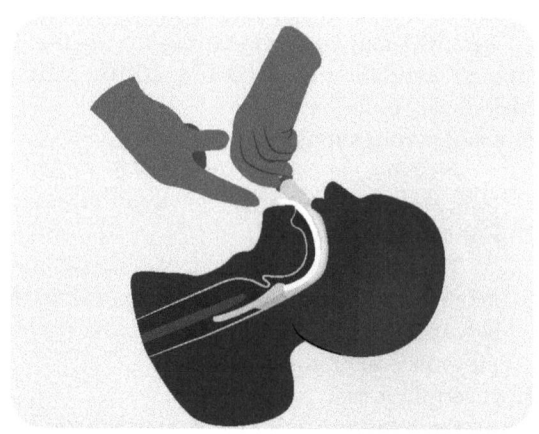

◻ Fig. 20.10   How to insert an LMA

20.13 **Intubation**

Intubation is a critical skill all anesthesiologists must master. There are several different tools we use to lead to a successful intubation, leading to several different branch points in the decision-making process for how to successfully intubate a particular patient. The first branch point is the decision to use direct laryngoscopy (or DL) versus indirect laryngoscopy.

Direct laryngoscopy is the traditional approach and requires the use of a Macintosh (or Mac) or a Miller blade (◻ Fig. 20.12). Choosing between these blades is the second branch point. A Mac blade is curved and the tip is inserted into the vallecula (which is the space between the base of the tongue and the pharyngeal surface of the epiglottis) (■ Figs. 20.11 and 20.12). There are sizes between 1 and 4 for Mac blades, with the majority of adult patients requiring a Mac 3.

The Miller blade is straight and passed beneath the epiglottis such that the epiglottis is lifted to expose the vocal cords (■ Fig. 20.11). The Miller blade provides better visualization than the Mac; however, it decreases the amount of space allowed for passage of the endotracheal tube into the larynx. The size range for Miller blades are from 0 to 4, with most adults requiring a 2 or a 3 sized blade.

Indirect laryngoscopy implies the use of video assistance in order to visualize the vocal cords. Video laryngoscopy has recently advanced significantly and in many teaching hospitals it may be the first way that you intubate a patient. Two commonly used video laryngoscopes are the McGrath and the GlideScope (■ Fig. 20.13). The GlideScope blade is significantly more curved than the McGrath blade. The McGrath curve is comparable to the curve in the Macintosh blade.

In addition, there exists the C-MAC or V-MAC, which both have blades similar to the standard Macintosh blade (■ Fig. 20.14).

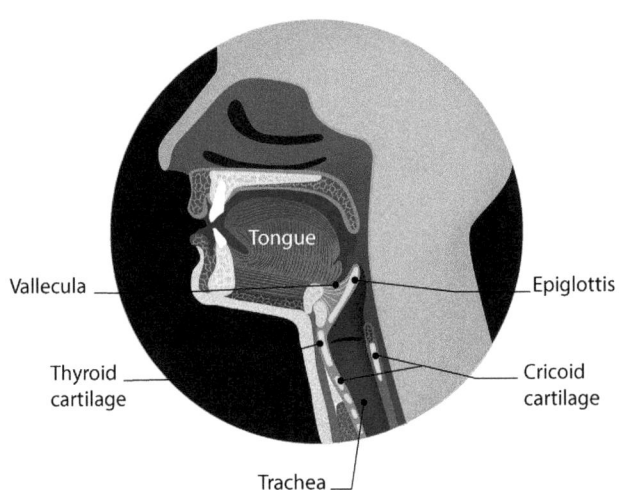

■ **Fig. 20.11** Airway anatomical landmarks (sagittal view)

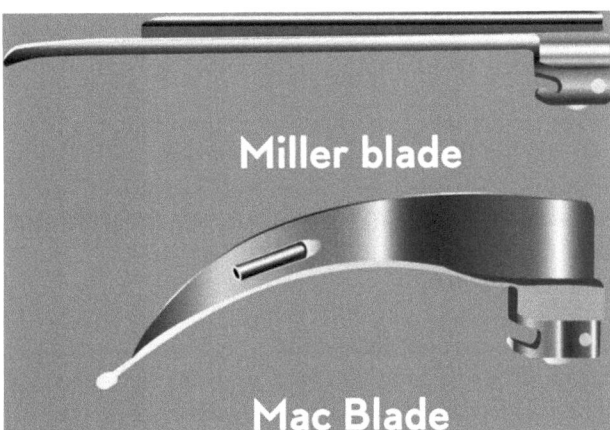

■ **Fig. 20.12** Miller vs. Mac blade shape

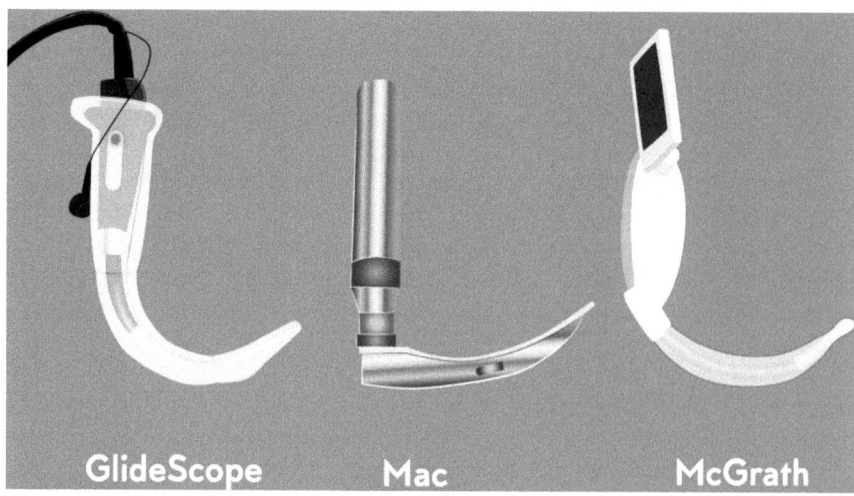

Fig. 20.13 Shape of GlideScope vs. Mac vs. McGrath blades

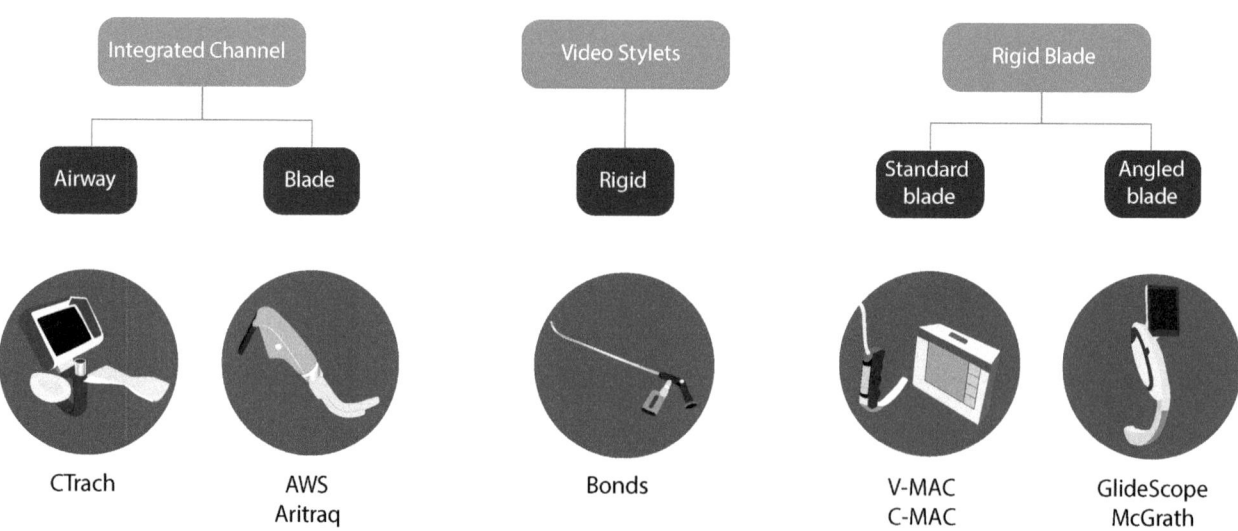

Fig. 20.14 Different types of video laryngoscopes

There are some nuances as to when particular laryngoscopes are better for particular patients, but these nuances are outside the scope of what is expected of a medical student. Your first intubation will likely be with the aid of a video laryngoscope, so the resident can see what you see and assist you throughout the intubation. In general, for elective video laryngoscopy, whatever blade is most readily available at your institution will be used.

Beyond the laryngoscope, the other important piece of equipment for intubation is the tube itself. Endotracheal tubes (ET tubes or ETT) sizes are measured in internal diameter in millimeters and range in size from 2.5 to 10.5 (◘ Table 20.6). The length of the tube also increases with increased diameter. ◘ Table 20.6 provides a quick reference for ET tube sizing for different patient populations.

Table 20.6 ETT sizes by patient type

Infants	2.5–4.0
Young Children	4.0–5.5
Adolescents	5.0–7.0
Adult Females	7.0–8.0
Adult Males	8.0–9.0

Your resident or attending will walk you through the exact steps for intubating your first patient, but the broad steps are as follows:

1. Identify appropriate blade and ET tube size based on patient size.

   Gather your supplies. You will need an ET tube (with stylet), a 10 cc syringe (to inflate the cuff), a laryngoscope and blade. Make sure your laryngoscope and blade are attached correctly and make sure the light on the laryngoscope is working.

2. Positioning is key (◘ Fig. 20.15).

   First, make sure you are comfortable. You should be standing at the head of the bed. Raise or lower the bed so that it is at a height where you will be able to visualize the vocal cords. Next, position the patient. Place the patient in a sniffing position, with their head tilted back. You can use blankets in order to better allow the patient's head to rock back to give you a better position.

3. Hold the laryngoscope in your left hand near the junction between the handle and the blade, with your thumb upright with the handle (◘ Fig. 20.16).

4. Prop the mouth open with a scissoring motion of the right thumb and index finger (◘ Fig. 20.17).

5. Insert the laryngoscope into the right side of the patient's mouth while sweeping the tongue to the left.

6. Move the blade toward the midline and advance until the epiglottis comes into view.

7. *Lift the blade up* (do not rock backwards) to expose the glottic opening. Ideally, you will see a full view of the glottis, arytenoids, and vocal cords (grade I view). You should announce what grade view you visualize to your resident and attending (◘ Fig. 20.18).

   This step requires a bit of finesse. Rocking the blade backward can risk chipping a patient's tooth. To avoid this, keep your wrist rigid and straight as you lift the laryngoscope up.

8. Grab the ET tube with your right hand and advance until the cuff is just beyond the cords. At this time, ask the person assisting you to remove the stylet.

9. Continue advancing the tube until it is in the proper location.

   *For an adult the correct location is ~ 21–23 cm at the teeth (the ET tube has labeled notches on the side). If the ET tube is advanced too far, there is a higher likelihood that it will be pushed past the carina into the **right** mainstem bronchus. This will become clear when you deliver a breath as the airway pressure will be higher than anticipated and you will not hear breath sounds on the left. Hint: This is a frequent pimping question!*

10. Remove the laryngoscope.

    Take care to not damage or chip the teeth when removing the blade.

11. Inflate the cuff.

    Use the 10 cc syringe you grabbed at the beginning to inflate the cuff. Push on the pilot balloon to ensure the cuff is adequately inflated.

**Patient positioning for
optimal intubation**

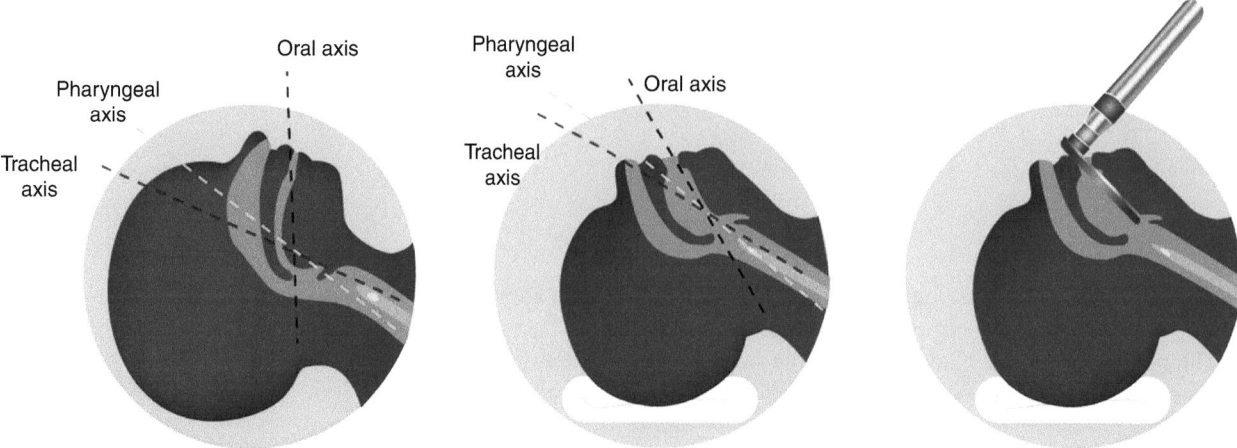

■ **Fig. 20.15**   Optimal patient positioning for intubation

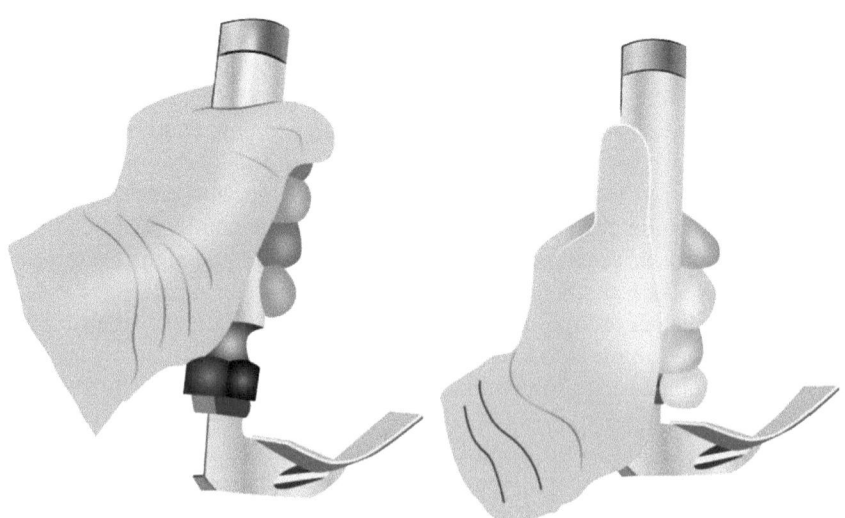

Suboptimal Grip   "Thumb up"-optimal

■ **Fig. 20.16**   How to hold your blade

12. Ensure proper location of tube.
    Give the patient a breath and check for: fogging in the tube, bilateral chest rise, bilateral breath sounds, and end tidal CO2.
13. Secure the tube with tape
    This is crucial. The tube should not move throughout the case, even with changes to patient positioning. Ask your resident or attending to show you how they prefer to tape the tube, as techniques and preferences can vary widely.

Troubleshooting Airway Management

Not every patient will be straightforward to bag-mask ventilate or intubate. Here are a few key features about patients that can make them difficult for bagging or intubation. Keep these in mind when attempting bag-mask ventilation or intubation.

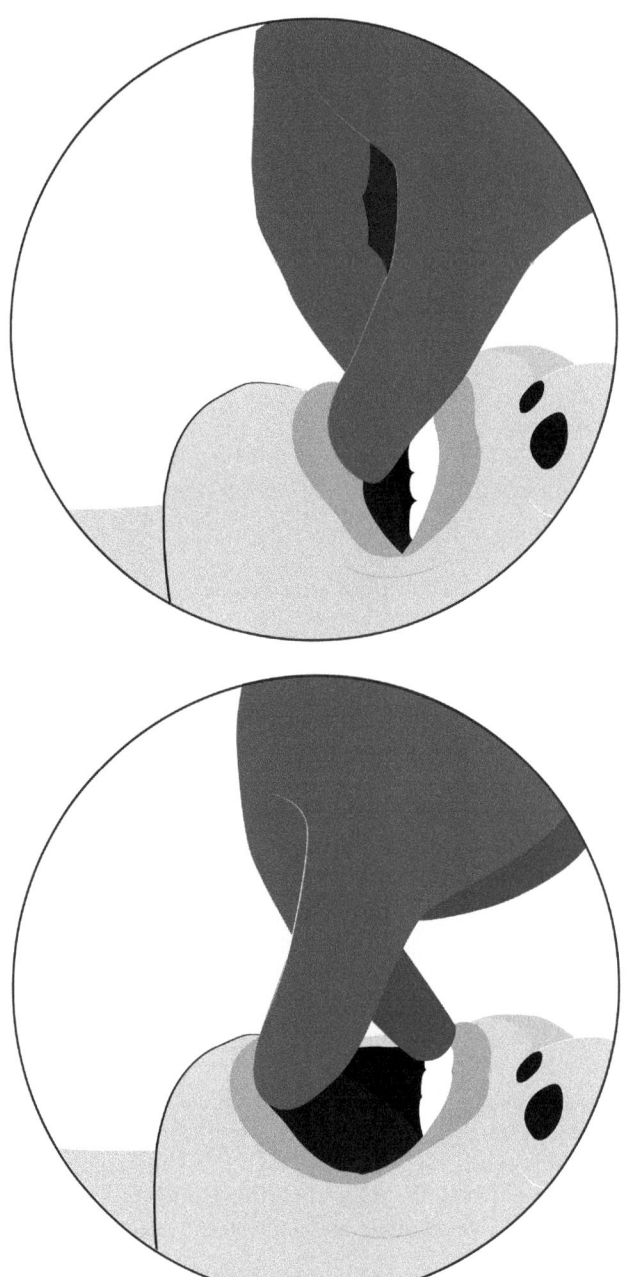

◨ **Fig. 20.17** How to open a patient's mouth using the scissor technique

Patient characteristics that may increase difficulty of bag-mask ventilation:
- Beard and facial hair
- Obesity
- Airway obstruction (i.e., anaphylaxis or angioedema)
- Older age
- Lack of teeth
- History of obstructive sleep apnea
- History of COPD

Troubleshooting tips:
- Reposition yourself
  Make sure you are comfortable and not straining yourself. Ensure your hand is in the proper location on the patient's face and jaw. Make sure you are

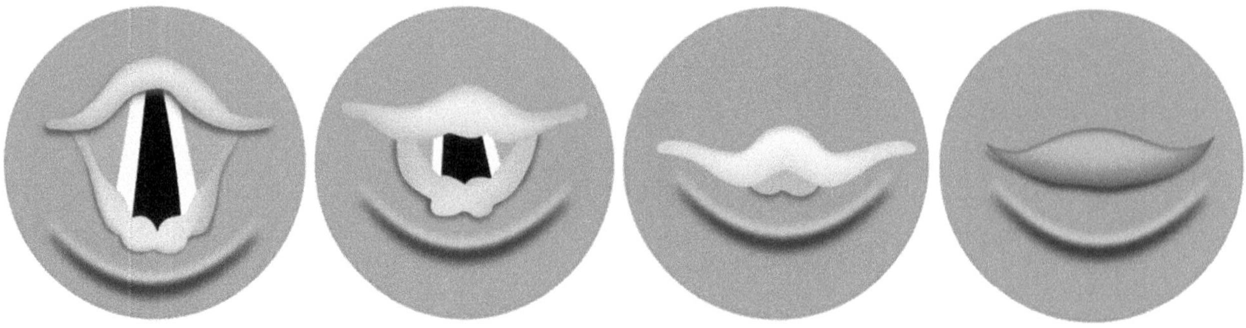

| GRADE I | GRADE II | GRADE III | GRADE IV |

■ **Fig. 20.18**   Cormack–Lehane Classification of Direct Laryngoscopy Views

lifting the patient's face into the mask rather than pushing the mask into the patient's face
- Reposition the patient
    Try tilting their head back further or add pillows under their upper back to help extend the neck.
- Try an oral airway
    If the patient is sedated, they will tolerate an oral airway. Oral airways allow better air exchange by helping to keep the oropharynx open by pushing the tongue and soft tissues out the way
- Ask for help
    If you have multiple hands on deck, ask someone to help bag while you try a two-handed mask technique. This will allow for a better seal and decrease the risk of leaks. If you are still struggling, let your resident or attending know so they can step in to help – remember – patient safety comes first!

Patient characteristics that may increase difficulty of intubation:
- Mallampati score
    – The higher the score the more likely the intubation will be difficult.
- Inter-incisor distance
    – The distance between the incisors when the mouth is fully open. The smaller this distance, the more likely the intubation may be difficult.
- Thyromental distance
    – The distance between the thyroid cartilage and the tip of the chin when fully extended. The shorter this distance, the more likely the intubation may be difficult.
- Degree of head extension
    – The degree to which a patient is able to extend their head. Patients with spinal stenosis, cervical spine arthritis, or spinal fusions may have difficulty extending their neck. Difficulty with neck extension makes the intubation more challenging.
- Prognathism
    – If the patient is unable to advance their mandible past their maxilla, they may be difficult to intubate.
- History of difficult intubation
    – If the patient has a history of a previous difficult intubation, you should always read what strategy worked in prior intubation attempts.

Troubleshooting tips:
- Reposition yourself
  - *Make sure the bed is at a comfortable height and that you are standing behind the patient's head.*
- Reposition the patient
  - *Place blankets under the patient's upper back to help increase neck extension so that you can obtain a better view.*
- Verbally describe what you are seeing
  - *Tell your resident or attending what you are looking at when you are trying to locate the vocal cords. Try to describe what you are seeing in anatomical terms, so your attending and resident can help guide you.*
- Try a different sized blade or ET tube
  - *If the blade is unable to adequately lift the patient's tissues out of the way to allow visualization of the vocal cords, you can try a larger blade. Similarly, if the blade feels cumbersome and like it is taking up too much space in the patient's mouth, try using a smaller blade. If you're having difficulty advancing the ET tube, try again with a smaller tube.*
- Try a different technique
  - *If attempts at direct laryngoscopy fail, you can try video laryngoscopy or bronchoscopy in order to secure the airway*
- Suction the airway
  - *If the patient has a lot of secretions, suctioning the airway can help aid your visualization of the vocal cords*
- Ask for help
  - *When in doubt – ask for help! Remember patient safety always comes first. The first thing someone could do to assist you is to help correct yours or the patient's positioning. Next, they can provide cricoid pressure to help bring the vocal cords into view. Finally, if attempts at intubation are unsuccessful, allow your resident or attending to step in to secure the airway. If your resident or attending steps in to take over, don't be offended! Remember that patient safety is of the utmost importance. Carefully watch what your resident or attending does and ask to debrief with them after the airway is secured to understand what they did differently to secure the airway.*

20.13.1 IV Access (◻ Table 20.7)

Every case you complete will require a peripheral IV (PIV) of some variety. The size of the IV will depend on the case you're completing. Short, ambulatory procedures can likely be completed with just a single 20G PIV. Emergency trauma surgeries, orthopedic procedures, liver procedures, or obstetric procedures may require more peripheral access with larger bore IVs to help with volume resuscitation. For adult patients, at least one peripheral IV should be placed in the preoperative area before the patient is rolled back to the OR. For pediatric patients, the IV is often placed after induction with inhaled anesthetics. Additional IVs can always be placed during the case, but patient positioning and draping can make placement quite difficult.

Peripheral IVs come in a variety of gauges and the higher the number, the smaller is the catheter size (◻ Fig. 20.19). Because flow and velocity through a

◘ **Table 20.7**   MSMAID: I is for IV Access and D is for Drugs

M	*Machine* Turn on the machine, computers, and screens Run the machine self-test Adjust machine parameters for the case and the patient Check volatile agent levels Check for a bag-valve mask in the room
S	*Suction* Make sure the suction circuit is connected and a Yankauer suction tip is connected to the end of the tubing Prep an OG tube for the case, if necessary (open the packing and lube up the tip)
M	*Monitors* Prep EKG pads, temperature probes, O2 sat monitoring, and BP cuff Gather additional supplies for more advanced monitoring: arterial lines, central lines, BIS monitoring
A	*Airway* Acquire the correct size ETT, check whether the stylette is in place and check the cuff for leaks Prep the laryngoscope, make sure the light is working Open a mask to use for bag-mask ventilation Open an oral airway and place it within reach of where you'll be performing intubation Make sure a laryngeal mask airway, bougies, or video laryngoscopes are available if you are concerned about a difficult airway
I	*IV Access* Prep your IV kit (peripheral IV needle, tourniquet, gauze, tegaderm, alcohol swab, IV start tubing, 1–2 cc of lidocaine in a subcutaneous injection needle) Prep your intravenous fluids and lines

D	*Drugs*
	Prep the drugs you will need throughout the case, in general, at a minimum you will want to prep your preinduction and induction drugs:
	  Midazolam
	  Propofol
	  Fentanyl
	  Paralytic (rocuronium or succinylcholine)

tube is reliant on the diameter of that tube squared, increasing the size of the catheter dramatically increases the amount of fluids that can be sent through that catheter in a minute.

$$\text{Pipe Diameter} = \sqrt{\frac{4 \times \text{Flow Rate}}{\pi \times \text{Velocity}}}$$

$$\text{Velocity} = \frac{4 \times \text{Flow Rate}}{\pi \times \left(\text{Pipe Diamter}\right)^2}$$

$$\text{Flow Rate} = \frac{\pi}{4} \times \left(\text{Pipe Diameter}\right)^2 \times \text{Velocity}$$

20.13.1.1 Central Venous Access

Some specialized cases will require the placement of a central venous catheter (or central line). In general, the cases that will require this are open chest cases (particularly open heart surgeries) or cases where a large volume of blood loss is anticipated (such as a liver transplant). The central line is generally placed using sterile

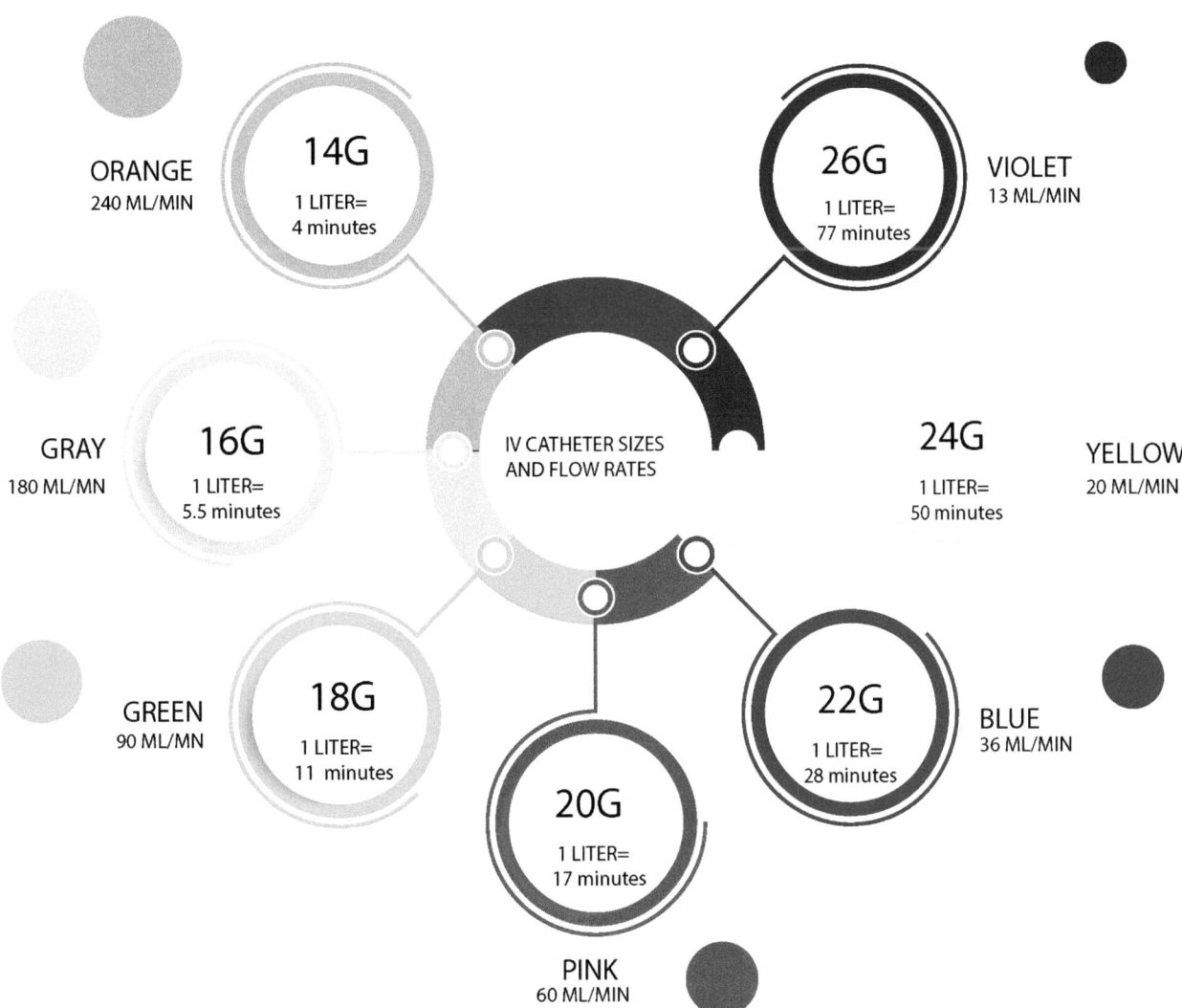

Fig. 20.19 The physics of flow rate and the relationship of needle gauge with max flow

precautions in the OR after the patient has been anesthetized but prior to draping. Most ORs have the capability to place these catheters under ultrasound guidance, which allows for direct visualization of the vessel and the needle. Your resident might ask you how they know the vessel they are looking at is a vein versus an artery. Remember that veins will be compressible and should not be pulsatile. This will help you distinguish the internal jugular vein from the carotid artery.

20.13.1.2 Arterial Lines

Intra-arterial catheters are a critical component of intravascular access for specialized cases. Arterial lines, or A lines, allow for continuous blood pressure monitoring and allow for easy blood gas draws throughout the case. Unless there is a concern about blood pressure monitoring during induction of anesthesia, A lines are generally placed post-induction prior to draping, as A line placement can be quite painful for patients. A lines can be placed with or without ultrasound guidance.

The A line needs to be zeroed at the level of the line; otherwise, blood pressure readings from the line are not accurate. When you see your first intraoperative A line, ask to observe this procedure, as it will be helpful in troubleshooting the line down the road.

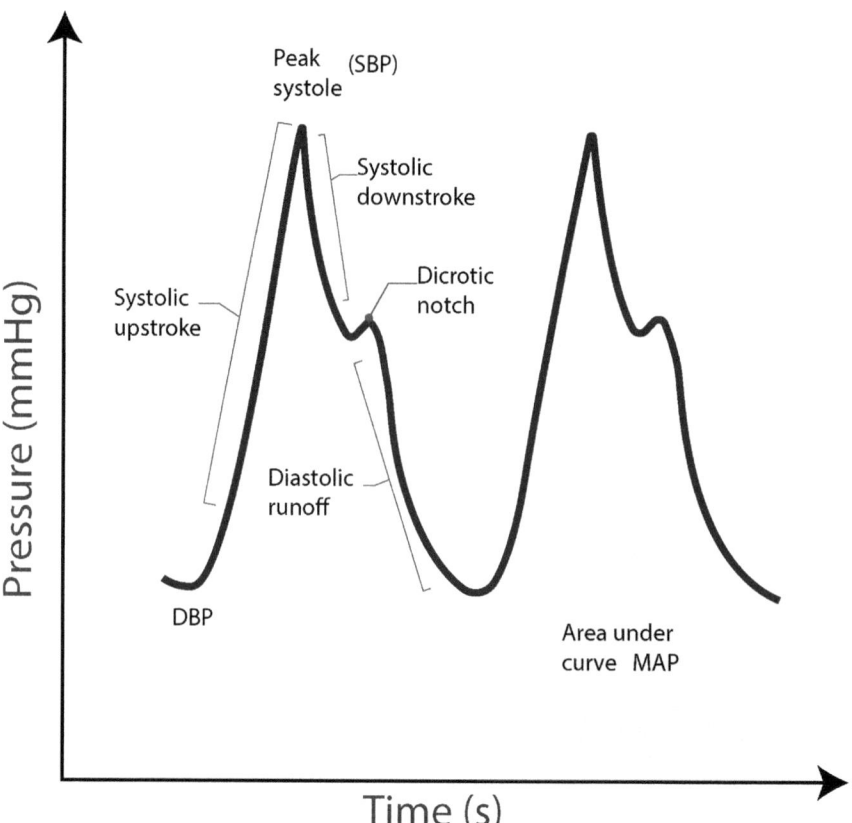

Fig. 20.20 Arterial line waveform

The A line tracing is just as important to look at as the blood pressure number, a good tracing will likely give you an accurate reading but a poor tracing should be viewed with some skepticism (◘ Fig. 20.20). If the tracing of your A line is poor, there are a few ways to troubleshoot it. First, make sure the line is properly zeroed. Next, ensure the line is still in its proper location and that it has not shifted in position. Next, you can try flushing the line to attempt to dislodge any clots that may have formed at the tip of the catheter. In general, these troubleshooting tips will help fix most issues with most A lines, though it is by no means a comprehensive list.

20.13.2 Regional Blockade

Regional nerve blocks and spinal and epidural anesthesia are also important considerations for certain cases. Generally, these forms of anesthesia are administered in the preoperative setting either in the PACU or in the OR. Regional anesthesia allows anesthesiologists to administer less general anesthesia, less narcotic pain medications, and use alternative less invasive airway management.

20.13.2.1 Peripheral Nerve Blocks
Peripheral nerve blocks are extremely common for orthopedic surgery cases. These are usually short acting complete nerve blocks that last for about 4 h (if using bupivacaine) that are placed under ultrasound guidance before the surgery. Beyond bolusing the nerve sheath with local anesthetics, a catheter can also be placed at the site to deliver a continuous infusion of local anesthesia. These catheters can be left in place for several days after the surgery, carrying patients' anesthesia through the most painful postoperative period.

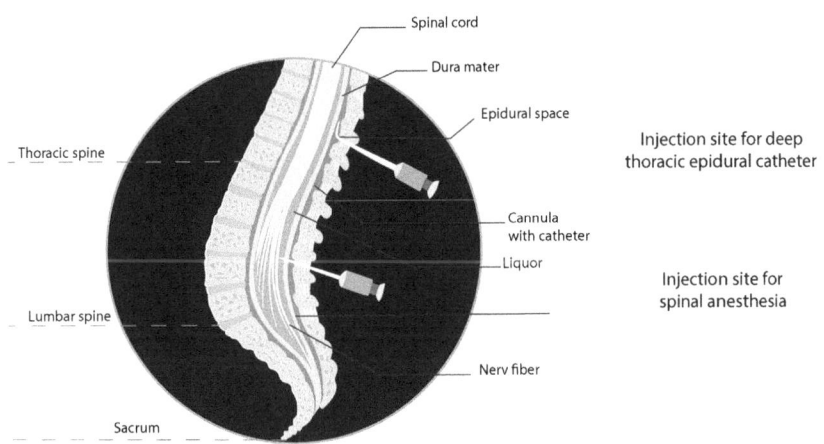

Fig. 20.21 Epidural vs. Spinal Access

20.13.2.2 Spinal Anesthesia

Spinal anesthesia is used less frequently, but is often used in total knee replacement surgeries that are expected to be uncomplicated. Spinal anesthesia provides complete anesthesia and also paralyzes the patient from the level of the blockade down. It generally wears off in ~4 h. Spinal anesthesia allows complex cases like total knee replacements to be performed under twilight sedation, rather than general anesthesia, providing a more comfortable postoperative experience for the patient.

To produce spinal anesthesia, a needle is introduced into the subarachnoid space and a bolus of local anesthetic is introduced, bathing the nerve roots in anesthetic (■ Fig. 20.21). The needle is removed and no catheter is introduced into the space. Compare this to epidural anesthesia, discussed below.

20.13.2.3 Epidural Anesthesia

Epidural anesthesia is usually used for perioperative pain management and is also used for pain management on the L&D floors. Epidurals involve the introduction of a sterile catheter into the epidural space and then anesthetic drugs are infused through the catheter.

Epidurals can be placed at different levels depending on the desired effect. For L&D, they are generally placed around L4 (■ Fig. 20.21). For Cesarean sections, an epidural may be the only form of anesthesia required for the case. For major open abdominal cases, they can be placed in the thoracic spine. Generally, the epidural is placed preoperatively in these patients; they are sedated with general anesthesia for the case, and the epidural is bolused for maximal pain relief prior to emersion and extubation.

Epidurals leave a catheter in the epidural space, so sterile technique is crucial and proper bandaging and care of the catheter tubing is important. Keep in mind that bolusing the epidural can lead to hypotension through blunting of the sympathetic chain and subsequent vasodilation of peripheral vessels.

20.14 Drugs, Drugs, Drugs

The goal of this section is to give you a broad overview of the different pharmacologic agents used in the perioperative setting. It is not designed to be comprehensive. If you have questions, we encourage you to ask your residents or attendings. One great way to learn a lot of pharmacology is to ask the resident you are with to go through their medicine cart throughout the day (or week) that you spend with them.

◻ **Table 20.8** Stages of Anesthetic Depth

Stage I: Analgesia	The patient is conscious and rational, with decreased perception to pain
Stage II: Delirium	Patient is unconscious; reflexes are still intact; irregular breathing pattern with breath holding
Stage III: Surgical Anesthetic	Increased muscle relaxation, patient is unable to protect their own airway
Stage IV: Medullary Depression	Depression of cardiovascular and respiratory centers

Most of the drugs you will see during your anesthesia rotation are used during specific times before, during, or after a case. Here, we will break down for you the different drugs you might expect to see throughout your day.

Before we touch on drugs, it is important to take into consideration the stages of anesthetic depth (◻ Table 20.8). Patients will transition through the stages during induction and emergence and generally the goal is to maintain patients in Stage III. During your rotation, it can be helpful to try and determine what stage a patient is in during the induction and emergence stage. Your attendings and residents can be helpful in assisting you if you have any questions about what stage your patient is in.

20.14.1 Preinduction

Prior to induction of general anesthesia, patients will often receive medications to reduce their anxiety and pain. The most commonly administered medication in this context is midazolam, an anxiolytic and amnestic drug. A dose of 0.5–2 mg is usually administered to the patient before they are transported back to the OR. After patients take midazolam, they remain awake and alert, conversing with providers, but they will not have any recollection of those interactions after emergence from anesthesia.

Prior to induction, the anesthesiologist will talk with the surgeon and discuss dosing a patient with an antibiotic to prevent surgical site infections. Most cases will require a 2 g dosage of cefazolin, but the decision to administer other antibiotics should be a conversation with the entire care team.

20.14.2 Induction

Induction agents are used to put a patient to sleep prior to a procedure. In general, there are three drugs used for induction of anesthesia: a sedative, an analgesic, and a paralytic.

Sedation is the key to anesthesia. There are two main methods that sedation can be delivered: intravenous and inhaled. In general, the initial induction of anesthesia in adults is done with intravenous sedation and maintained with inhaled sedation. In pediatric patients, induction can be done with inhaled sedation, so as to prevent placing an IV in awake pediatric patients.

There are some key exceptions to the above rules. For example, in neurosurgery, the case will often be performed with "total intravenous anesthesia" or TIVA. This is done in order to prevent the increased cerebral vasodilation, resulting in increased cerebral blood flow and increased intracranial pressure (ICP) that is associated with inhaled anesthetics. In patients undergoing craniotomy, increased ICP during surgery from inhaled anesthetics can make surgery more difficult, thereby increasing the risk of ischemic cerebral insults. Using TIVA, thus, has the potential to reduce ICP and improve accessibility of the operative site.

The goal of induction agents is to quickly sedate patients; this is achieved with the use of intravenous anesthetics that have high lipid solubility, hastening penetration into the blood brain barrier and onset of action (◘ Table 20.9). There are three key intravenous induction agents you should be familiar with.

These are the three most commonly used induction agents, with propofol being the most commonly used in the operating room. You may see etomidate used during emergent intubations in unstable patients.

There is one other induction agent you may see during your anesthesia rotation and that is methohexital. Methohexital is a barbiturate that is generally

◘ **Table 20.9** Commonly used induction agents

Drug Name	Useful Information	Advantages	Disadvantages
Propofol	*Induction Dose:* 1–2.5 mg/kg *Half-life:* ~2 min *Duration of action:* 2–8 min	Rapid onset Antiemetic properties Bronchodilatory properties Anticonvulsant properties Suitable for patients with hepatic or renal insufficiency	Dose-dependent hypotension after injection Burning at the injection site Contamination risk given lipid emulsion of drug
Etomidate	*Induction Dose:* 0.15–0.3 mg/kg *Half-life:* 1.6 min *Duration of action:* 3–12 min	Hemodynamic stability (BP and HR remain stable) Rapid onset Anticonvulsant properties	Higher incidence of post-op nausea/vomiting (PONV) vs. propofol Pain at injection site Dose-related involuntary myoclonic movements Absence of any analgesic effect – will not blunt sympathetic response to noxious stimuli (during intubation) that can result in elevated HR and BP Mild increase in airway resistance Transient adrenal insufficiency
Ketamine	*Induction Dose:* 1–2 mg/kg IV; 4–6 mg/kg IM *Half-life:* <1 min *Duration of action:* 9–20 min	Increases sympathetic tone resulting in elevated HR, BP, and CO Bronchodilatory properties Maintains airway reflexes and respiratory drive Rapid onset and recovery Can be administered IM, PO, or PR if necessary	Can lead to cardiac ischemia in patients with underlying cardiovascular disease due to increased sympathetic tone Can worsen right heart strain and pulmonary arterial pressure in patients with PAH Can cause hallucinations, nightmares, and vivid dreams during and shortly after emergence from anesthesia Possibly causes increased cerebral metabolism, though this is debated in the literature Can increase ICP Can confound BIS measurements

used for induction for electroconvulsive therapy (ECT; it works similarly to propofol, however it is the least anticonvulsant of all induction agents and therefore the most ideal to induce a seizure during ECT.

Analgesia for induction is also important, as intubation is a noxious stimulus and can lead to sympathetic activation leading to tachycardia and hypertension. In order to adequately cover a patient's pain during induction, an analgesic agent is commonly administered after the sedative agent. Most analgesia with induction is done with the assistance of an opiate, usually a fast-acting version, like fentanyl. Opiates also help suppress airway reflexes that may result in coughing or bronchospasm during intubation.

The other important component of induction is paralysis. Neuromuscular blocking agents (NMBAs) allow for relaxation of the muscles in the head and neck, allowing ideal visualization of the vocal cords. It is crucial that the patient is fully sedated prior to onset of neuromuscular blockade, as paralysis without sedation can be jarring for patients. There are two classes of NMBAs: depolarizing and nondepolarizing agents.

The only depolarizing agent used in the United States is succinylcholine. Succinylcholine binds directly to nicotinic acetylcholine receptors at the neuromuscular junction and thus produces a prolonged depolarization. Nondepolarizing NMBAs, such as rocuronium or vecuronium, are competitive antagonists, thus they compete with acetylcholine for the binding site on nicotinic acetylcholine receptors thus preventing the initiation of an action potential. This prevents the action potential from spreading, making muscle cells insensitive to motor nerve impulses. Subsequently, muscle paralysis occurs starting with small, fast-twitch muscles in the eyes and larynx and moving to limbs, trunk, airway, intercostal muscles, and diaphragm. Reemergence from neuromuscular blockade occurs in reverse order.

Here are some quick facts about succinylcholine that will be helpful on your rotation:

Succinylcholine
- Dosing: 1–1.5 mg/kg
- Onset of action: 1–2 min
- Duration of action: 7–12 min
- Advantages:
  - Reliable blockade
  - Fastest onset and shortest duration of action
  - Often the go-to for rapid sequence induction and intubation
- Disadvantages:
  - Hyperkalemia
    - This is secondary to muscular depolarization and is exaggerated and can be life-threatening in bed-bound immobile patients who may have upregulation of nicotinic acetylcholine receptors (spinal cord injury patients, burns, prolonged bed rest)
  - Pseudocholinesterase deficiency
    - In patients with the autosomal recessive pseudocholinesterase deficiency, recovery from succinylcholine can be prolonged. Recovery time in heterozygotes can be doubled, whereas homozygous patients can be paralyzed for up to 8 hours after an intubating dose.
  - Trigger for malignant hyperthermia
  - Known to cause myalgias
  - Increased intraocular pressure
  - Cardiac dysrhythmias
  - Allergic reactions

There are numerous nondepolarizing NMBAs available for anesthesiologists to use (● Table 20.10). The most commonly used nondepolarizing NMBAs are vecuronium and rocuronium. Of note, acetylcholine is important in histamine release, muscarinic activation, vagolytic action, and norepinephrine release. Therefore, side effects such as tachycardia, bradycardia, hypertension, bronchodilation, and bronchospasm are seen with their use. Important dosage and onset information is shown in ◘ Table 20.10.

Perhaps the most high-yield information to know is information regarding the use of rocuronium. Rocuronium or "roc" is arguably the most frequently used NBMAs because it can be used as an alternative to succinylcholine for a rapid sequence intubation (RSI). *In patients where succinylcholine is contraindicated, such as someone with a spinal cord injury who may become hyperkalemic with succinylcholine, a dose of 1.2 mg/kg of rocuronium can be used for an RSI.* Additionally, it has a high affinity for the reversal agent sugammadex, which will be discussed in further detail in the emergence section of this chapter.

We have now covered all the key drugs and drug classes you will need to know to understand induction of anesthesia. We will switch gears and now focus on the drugs used to maintain anesthesia throughout the procedure.

20.14.3 Maintenance of Anesthesia

After a patient is intubated and fully sedated, the procedure can begin. Due to the rapid onset and recovery of the pharmacologic agents used for induction, additional medications need to be given to the patient throughout the procedure to keep them properly anesthetized.

The most common means to maintain anesthesia is by using inhaled anesthetic agents delivered by the anesthesia circuit. These drugs are titrated to a goal minimum alveolar concentration, or MAC. *MAC is defined as the minimum alveolar concentration of inhaled anesthetic (at sea level) required to suppress movement to a painful stimulus in 50% of patients. On most anesthesia machines used today, the machine will automatically calculate the MAC and*

◘ **Table 20.10** Commonly used nondepolarizing NMBAs

Drug Name	Classification	Important Information
Vecuronium	Nondepolarizing Intermediate Steroidal	Intubating Dose: 0.10–0.20 mg/kg Onset time: 3–4 min Time to 25% recovery: 20–35 min Elimination: 10–50% renal, 30–50% hepatic
Rocuronium	Nondepolarizing Intermediate Steroidal	r: 0.60–1.00 mg/kg (1.20 mg/kg for RSI) Onset time: 1–2 min Time to 25% recovery: 30–50 min Elimination: Renal 30%, hepatic 70%
Pancuronium	Nondepolarizing Long Steroidal	Intubating Dose: 0.08–0.12 mg/kg Onset time: 2–3 min Time to 25% recovery: 60–120 min Eliimination: Renal 40–70%, hepatic 20%
Mivacurium	Nondepolarizing Short Benzylisoquinolinium	Intubating Dose: 0.20 mg/kg Onset time: 3–4 min Time to 25% recovery: 15–20 min Elimination: Plasma cholinesterase
Cisatracurium	Nondepolarizing Intermediate Benzylisoquinolinium	Intubating dose: 0.15–0.20 mg/kg Onset time: 4–6 min Time to 25% recovery: 30–60 min Elimination: 30% Hoffman elimination, 60% ester hydrolysis

display it based on your input of the patient's age, gender, and body weight. Another value used to titrate volatile agent dosages during a case is the end-tidal anesthetic concentration (ETAC). Typically, an ETAC concentration close to the MAC value is targeted. If you're confused about the MAC during a case, ask your attending or resident why they are titrating to a specific goal MAC.

Volatile anesthetics are ideal for maintenance of anesthesia because they induce a state of hypnosis and sedation required for general anesthesia as well as skeletal and smooth muscle relaxation and bronchodilatory properties (☐ Table 20.11). Disadvantages of volatile agents include dose-dependent decreases in cardiac output and blood pressure, cerebral vasodilation and subsequent increase in ICP (which is contraindicated in some procedures), and the risk of malignant hyperthermia.

☐ Table 20.11 can be helpful for you to distinguish the different inhaled anesthetic agents during your rotation.

☐ **Table 20.11**   Inhaled anesthetic agents

Name	Helpful Information	MAC for response to surgery	Systemic effects	Other effects
Nitrous oxide	Pungency: None Effect on the environment: Least carbon footprint of inhaled options GWP = 289 Cost: <$	105.0%	BP: Negligible Vasculature: Negligible Inotropic: Negligible Chronotropic: Negligible	Nausea and vomiting Very low blood: gas partition coefficient – rapid induction and rapid recovery Very low cost
Isoflurane	Pungency: High Effect on the environment: Medium carbon footprint GWP = 1401 Cost: $	1.2%	BP: Dose-dependent hypotension Vasculature: Vasodilation Inotropic: Slightly negative hronotropic: Tachycardia	Nausea and vomiting Potentially significant tachycardia Lowest cost of the volatile options Moderately high blood: gas partition coefficient – slower uptake and induction and subsequent prolonged emergence High fat solubility – prolonged emergence, particularly in patients with obesity
Sevoflurane	Pungency: Low Effect on the environment: Lower carbon footprint than other volatile agents GWP = 349 Cost: $$	2.0%	BP: Dose-dependent hypotension Vasculature: Vasodilation Inotropic: Slightly negative Chronotropic: Tachycardia at MAC > 1	Nausea and vomiting Most commonly used for inhalation induction Low blood:gas partition coefficient – more rapid uptake and induction as well as rapid clearance and emergence
Desflurane	Pungency: Very high Effect on the environment: Very high carbon footprint GWP = 3714 Cost: $$$	6.0%	BP: Dose-dependent hypotension Vasculature: Initially vasoconstriction, later vasodilation Inotropic: Initially positive, later negative Chronotropic: Tachycardia	Nausea and vomiting Airway irritation Initially a sympathomimetic Very low blood: gas partition coefficient – rapid uptake and induction as well as clearance and emergence Very low oil: gas partition coefficient – minimal uptake in adipose tissue, ideal for use in morbidly obese patients

[a]GWP is the 20-year global warming potential of a gas, scaled based on the impact of carbon dioxide, where the GWP of CO_2 is 1

20

During maintenance of anesthesia, the anesthesiologist is also responsible for monitoring the patient's hemodynamic stability. Surgical manipulation and blood loss can dramatically affect the patient's heart rate, blood pressure, and cardiac output. Luckily, anesthesiologists have a few tools in their toolbox to rapidly address changes to the patient's hemodynamic stability. First, hypotension can be addressed by decreasing hypotensive inducing medications (propofol for example) or through fluid administration. Hypertension can be addressed by increasing the depth of anesthesia. You may see your resident or attending push some medications in order to obtain hemodynamic stability (◘ Tables 20.12 and 20.13). A few of these medications and their key properties are discussed in ◘ Tables 20.12.

◘ **Table 20.12** Pressors used in the OR and in the ICU

Pressor Name	Class	Other Considerations
Epinephrine	Inotrope/chronotrope/vasopressor (alpha 1, beta 1, beta 2 receptor agonist)	First-line treatment for cardiac arrest and anaphylaxis. Low dose – bronchodilatory effects, vasodilation, and decreased BP. Medium dose – increase HR and BP. High dose – vasoconstriction and possible severe hypertension
Phenylephrine	Vasopressor (alpha 1 receptor agonist)	Often the first go-to drug to treat hypertension if HR is normal or elevated
Norepinephrine	Inotrope/vasopressor (alpha 1 and beta 1 receptor agonist)	Often the first-line therapy in noncardiac ORs. Can cause tissue damage if peripheral extravasation occurs
Ephedrine	Inotrope/chronotrope/vasopressor (alpha 1, beta 1 and beta 2 receptor agonist)	Can cause tachyphylaxis with repeated doses. Relies on catecholamine release from adrenals for effect
Vasopressin	Vasopressor (vasopressin 1 and 2 receptor agonist)	Effective for refractory hypotension (nonresponsive to sympathomimetics or catecholamines)
Dopamine	Inotrope/vasopressor/dose-dependent chronotropy (dopaminergic, beta 1, beta 2, and alpha 1 receptor agonist)	Low doses may exacerbate hypotension whereas high doses may cause vasoconstriction, adverse metabolic effects, and arrhythmias
Dobutamine	Inotrope/vasodilator/dose-dependent chronotropy (beta 1 and beta 2 receptor agonist)	Can exacerbate hypotension due to dose-dependent vasodilation secondary to beta 2 stimulation
Milrinone	Inotrope/vasodilator (phosphodiesterase inhibitor)	Can cause exacerbation of hypotension due to vasodilation from phosphodiesterase inhibition
Isoproterenol	Inotrope/chronotrope/vasodilator (beta 1 and beta 2 receptor agonist)	Rarely used in the OR. Can cause exacerbation of hypotension due to beta 2 stimulation and subsequent vasodilation

Table 20.13 Commonly used antihypertensive agents in the OR

Antihypertensive Name	Class	Other Considerations
Beta Blockers – generally avoided in patients with acute decompensated heart failure		
Esmolol	Beta 1 selective receptor blockade	Rapid onset and very short duration of action Clearance is dependent on rapid metabolism my plasma esterases
Metoprolol	Beta 1 selective receptor blockade	Most commonly used if myocardial ischemia is suspected
Labetalol	Postsynaptic blockade of alpha 1 receptors Nonselective blockade of beta 1 and beta 2	First choice for hypertension with tachycardia Avoid in pheochromocytoma surgeries and in patients with severe obstructive or reactive airway disease
Calcium Channel Blockers – used cautiously in patients with increased ICP		
Nicardipine	Selective arteriolar smooth muscle relaxation	Commonly used for neurosurgical patients
Clevidipine	Selective arteriolar smooth muscle relaxation	Rapid onset and duration of action, clearance is reliant on metabolism by plasma esterases
Direct vasodilators – generally avoided in patients with increased ICP		
Hydralazine	Vasodilator of arterial resistance vessels	Minimal effect on venous circulation Relatively slow onset (compared to other options)
Nitroglycerin	Vasodilator reliant on release of NO resulting in smooth muscle relaxation	Ideally only used in patients with A lines or in whom an A line will be placed
Nitroprusside	Vasodilator reliant on release of NO resulting in smooth muscle relaxation	A line monitoring necessary Cyanide accumulation can occur

20.14.4 Emergence

When the case is wrapping up, the anesthesiologist will begin preparing for emergence from general anesthesia. From a pharmacological perspective, there are a few main goals of emergence medications: analgesia, neuromuscular blockade reversal, and postoperative nausea and vomiting (PONV) prevention. In addition to administering medications, the anesthesiologist will decrease and altogether discontinue inhaled and intravenous anesthetic agents.

For analgesia, patients will have received a dose of a short-acting opiate medication during induction and throughout the case they were maintained on a volatile anesthetic agent that had analgesic properties. During emergence, the goal is to provide analgesia for the emergence period as well as in the immediate perioperative period and in the PACU. Thus, longer-acting opiate medications are used prior to emergence, such as morphine or hydromorphone. Depending on the case and surgeon preference, other non-opiate medications, such as ketorolac, may be used. Ketorolac is a nonsteroidal anti-inflammatory drug (NSAID) that is available IV or IM. Because it is an NSAID, there is a theoretical increased risk of bleeding after administration. You may notice on your rotation that some surgeons ask for ketorolac to be administered and some specifically request that the anesthesiologist avoid it. Another pain reliever sometimes used in the postoperative setting is acetaminophen. If acetaminophen is administered, it is usually given IV, which costs significantly more than the PO formulation, so some hospital systems restrict its use.

Antiemetic administration is key to avoiding or minimizing PONV, which can be incredibly uncomfortable for patients. Nearly all patients will receive a combination of medications to prevent PONV from multiple fronts. The most commonly used medications are ondansetron and low doses of dexamethasone and haloperidol.

The final piece of emergence is reversal of the neuromuscular blockade. Full recovery is essential prior to extubation to decrease the risk of weakness of the upper airway muscles and diaphragm. Prior to reversal, one must assess the degree of muscle relaxation using the train-of-four technique (TOF). TOF utilizes electrodes placed on a peripheral nerve and the administration of four successive electrical stimuli given no less than 10 s apart. During nondepolarizing neuromuscular blockade, the response to these stimuli will fade over time. That is, the muscle twitch after the fourth stimulus will be less than the muscle twitch after the third stimulus. With increasing nondepolarizing blockade, the fourth twitch disappears, followed by the third, then the second, and finally the first. For a depolarizing blockade, all four twitches decline in amplitude to a similar extent. If TOF is 0.9 or greater, then the patient has spontaneously recovered and further reversal is not required. However, if TOF is less than 0.9, a reversal agent (or more time) is required prior to an attempt at extubation.

The reversal agent of choice depends on the type of NMBA used. If a depolarizing agent (succinylcholine) was used, an anticholinesterase can be used as a reversal agent. In general, the agent of choice is neostigmine, which is given in conjunction with glycopyrrolate (an antimuscarinic) in order to prevent bradycardia and GI side effects associated with anticholinergic administration. The dosage of neostigmine given to patients depends on the degree of residual blockade. If a patient has four twitches on TOF, then 20–50 mcg/kg can be administered. For fewer twitches, 60–70 mcg/kg can be administered. The combination of edrophonium and atropine can also be used for reversal of depolarizing NMBA, though this is much less commonly used in practice.

For reversal of nondepolarizing NMBAs, a drug called sugammadex is available. Sugammadex is a gamma-cyclodextrin and it essentially works as a sponge: soaking up, encapsulating, and thereby inactivating steroidal NMBAs (like vecuronium, rocuronium, and pancuronium). The affinity of sugammadex is highest for rocuronium, but it will still work for reversal of vecuronium and pancuronium. Sugammadex will not work as a reversal agent for succinylcholine or benzylisoquinolinium NMBAs (cisatracurium). Dosing of sugammadex is dependent on the level of neuromuscular blockade. A deep blockade can be reversed with a 4 mg/kg dosage, whereas a moderate blockage can be reversed with 2 mg/kg.

Sugammadex is a new drug in the anesthesiologist's toolbox and has changed neuromuscular blockade and reversal in the OR. However, it does have some disadvantages. First, it is associated with anaphylaxis in a dose-dependent fashion. Secondly, it can also inactivate hormonal birth control; therefore, patients on hormonal birth control given the drug will need to use alternative methods to prevent pregnancy for their next menstrual cycle. Additionally, given the novelty of the drug, it is quite expensive and not available in every hospital.

20.14.5 Summary (◻ Table 20.14)

There are many medications that anesthesiologists have in their toolbox throughout a procedure, and this list can seem overwhelming at first. One of the best ways to become familiar with these medications is to observe when

◻ **Table 20.14**   OR Pharmaceuticals Quick Reference

Drug class	Commonly Used Drug Name	Dose (adult)
Preinduction		
Anxiolytic	Midazolam	1–2 mg
Antibiotic	Cefazolin	2 mg
Induction		
Sedative Hypnotic	Propofol	1–2.5 mg/kg
	Etomidate	0.15–0.3 mg/kg
	Ketamine	1–2 mg/kg
Analgesia	Fentanyl	100 mcg
Neuromuscular Blockade	Succinylcholine	1–1.5 mg/kg
	Rocuronium	0.6–1.0 mg/kg (1.2 mg/kg for RSI)
	Vecuronium	0.10–0.20 mg/kg
Maintenance		
Inhaled anesthetics		MAC = 1 equivalent
	Nitrous oxide	105
	Isoflurane	1.2
	Sevoflurane	2.0
	Desflurane	6.0
Pressors	Epinephrine	4–10 mcg bolus 1–100 mcg/minute infusion
	Phenylephrine	50–100 mcg bolus 10–100 mcg/minute infusion
	Norepinephrine	4–8 mcg bolus 1–20 mcg/minute infusion
	Ephedrine	5–10 mg bolus Not used for infusions
	Vasopressin	1–4 units bolus 0.01–0.04 units/minute infusion
Antihypertensives	Esmolol	10–50 mg bolus (can be repeated every 5–15 min) 50–300 mcg/kg/min infusion
	Labetalol	5–25 mg bolus (can be repeated every 10 min) 0.5–2 mg/min infusion
	Hydralazine	2.5 mg bolus (can be repeated every 5 min, max 20 mg) Not used for infusions
	Nitroglycerin	10–40 mcg bolus 10–200 mcg/min infusion

■ **Table 20.14** (continued)

Drug class	Commonly Used Drug Name	Dose (adult)
Emergence		
Antiemetics	Ondansetron	4 mg IV
	Dexamethasone	4–8 mg IV
	Haloperidol	1–2 mg IV
Analgesia	Hydromorphone	0.2–0.5 mg IV q5min
	Morphine	1–3 mg IV q5min
NMBA Reversal	Neostigmine + Glycopyrrolate	20–70 mcg/kg 0.2 mg glycopyrrolate for every 1 mg neostigmine
	Sugammadex	2–4 mg/kg

your resident or attending is administering them and to ask questions. One of the most helpful ways a resident can teach you the medications is to go through the medication cart drawer by drawer and discuss the medications in each spot. Once you get a sense of how each medication is used you will be amazed at how quickly you memorize their uses and disadvantages.

The following is a summary chart you can quickly reference while in the OR.

20.15 A Day in the Life

Now that you're familiar with all the tools and medications anesthesiologists use on a daily basis, let us walk through what a day usually entails (with tips where you can be helpful and shine as a medical student on your rotation!).

20.15.1 The Schedule

In general, a normal day for an anesthesiology resident begins between 0600 and 0630 in the OR for setup and the day ends around 1700. For attendings in teaching hospitals, the day can be a bit shorter because they do not have to set up the OR for each case, usually lasting between 0700 and 1600. Depending on the program, residents may be excused from OR duties in order to attend didactics, or didactics may be scheduled before the day begins or at the end of the day. If you're interested in anesthesia, these didactics can be very helpful to add to your knowledge.

As an anesthesiologist, you're responsible for setting up the room between cases and you're required to be in the room during the entire case, which does not leave much time during the day for you to eat or to use the restroom. Because of this, residents will be relieved by their attending, CRNA, or fellow resident for a 15 min break in the morning, a 30 min break for lunch, and a 15 min break in the afternoon. As a medical student, you are usually expected to follow your resident's schedule, though some residents will allow you to go home earlier or take slightly longer breaks than them.

20.15.2 The Night Before

On your anesthesia rotation, your day really begins the night before when you receive your OR schedule for the next day. Anesthesiologists will review the cases on their schedule, look at the patient's chart, and take notes regarding the patient's scheduled procedure, the reason for the procedure, the patient's comorbidities, their daily medications, prior experiences with general anesthesia (if any), and the patient's weight. This information will help the anesthesiologist formulate a plan for the next day in the OR. Residents will discuss this plan with the attending they are partnered with to make sure they are on the same page. Sometimes this is done over the phone the evening before and sometimes this is done the morning before the cases begin for the day. As a medical student, depending on your school curriculum, you may be expected to look up your patients, come up with an anesthetic plan and present your plan to your attending or resident the night before the case.

20.15.3 The Day

An anesthesiologist's day begins well before the first case is scheduled to start. As we mentioned earlier, the day begins by running the MSMAID checklist in the OR and getting everything in the OR ready for the day.

Usually, by the time you have finished setting up the OR your patient has been checked in and can be found in the perioperative area. When you find your patient, introduce yourself and begin to establish rapport. Remember that surgery can be an intimidating experience for anyone, so an anesthesiologist's average day is usually scary and a nerve-wracking day for the patient. Strike up a conversation with your patient and address their questions and concerns. If the patient has not already been consented for anesthesia, obtain their written consent.

You will want to confirm the patient's history you gleaned from their chart. You will also want to ask a few anesthesia-specific history questions:

1. When was the last time you had anything to eat or drink?

   For elective or scheduled procedures, patients are generally informed that they shouldn't have anything to eat or drink after midnight the night before their procedure. This is the most restrictive guideline; however, research indicates it is safe for patients to consume clear liquids up until 2 h prior to their procedure. Patients should refrain from eating food or drinking nonclear liquids for 8 h prior to the procedure.

2. Did you take your medications today?

   It is important to know if a patient has or has not taken their normal daily medications, particularly blood pressure medications. Most medications are safe to continue taking with a sip of water the morning before a surgery.

3. Do you ever get breathless walking up two or more flights of stairs?

   This question is assessing the patient's functional capacity, which helps us understand the patient's risk for major postoperative morbidity or mortality.

4. Have you or anyone in your family ever had issues with anesthesia before?

   This question assesses family history of malignant hyperthermia or pseudocholinesterase deficiency. This question will also give you an idea of the patient's risk for postoperative nausea and vomiting based on their personal history with anesthesia.

5. Do you have any pain, stiffness, or arthritis in your neck or jaw?

   This question is assessing the difficulty level of intubation. If the patient doesn't have adequate range of motion in their jaw or neck, it may be difficult to get an optimal view of the vocal cords for intubation.

6. Do you have asthma or COPD?

   This information is crucial to understand how difficult it may be to ventilate a patient during the procedure and how reactive their airways may be.

7. Do you have any of the following medical conditions: kidney disease, heart disease, liver disease, diabetes, history of stroke, history of epilepsy or seizures?

8. Do you have a history of GERD?

   Severe GERD can be an indicator that this patient may require a rapid sequence induction and intubation to avoid aspiration of gastric contents.

9. Do you have any loose, missing, or removable teeth or dentures?

   Take note of any cracked, chipped, loose or missing teeth. These teeth can be an added challenge during intubation and you'll want to avoid further damaging the patient's teeth. Inform the patient that you will ask them to review any bridges or dentures prior to them being taken to the OR.

In addition to taking a history, you will want to conduct a physical exam of the patient. There are a few anesthesia-specific exam procedures you will want to conduct:

1. Observe the patient.

   Check for characteristics that might make for difficult bagging or difficult intubation.

2. Ask the patient to tilt their head back and touch their chin to their chest.

   This maneuver allows you to understand the patient's neck range of motion, which is important prior to intubation.

3. Ask the patient to open their mouth and stick out their tongue.

   Take note of the patient's Mallampati score (◘ Fig. 20.22), this is one of the indicators of ease of intubation. A Grade 1 view indicates the soft and hard palate, the uvula, and the oropharynx are visible when the patient opens their mouth, this indicates that intubation will likely be easier than someone with a Grade 4 view, since the oral opening is larger and better able to accommodate the blade and ET tube.

4. Listen to the patient's heart and lungs.

   Take note of any irregularities such as an irregular heartbeat, murmurs, or wheezing.

After your exam, ask for the patient's permission to insert an IV.

By now, the attending has likely arrived in the perioperative unit. Catch up with your attending and go through the plan for the day again. Make sure you're in agreement with your anesthetic choices, intubation plan, and pain control plan. If you and your attending agree that your case requires additional lines, such as an A line, epidural, or peripheral nerve block, you should gain informed consent and perform those procedures as well.

While this is happening, it is likely that the surgical team will stop by to check in with the patient. After the surgical team has met with the patient, be sure to introduce yourself to the surgical team. This is also an opportunity to confirm the surgical plan regarding patient positioning, incision location(s), necessary antibiotics, expectation of blood loss, and any other crucial points of information related to the case.

Once the patient has been interviewed, consented, and prepped for the OR, the resident will go check on the status of the OR. If the circulating nurse and scrub nurse, or tech in the room, indicate that they are ready for the patient to be rolled back and the PACU nurse indicates the patient is ready to be rolled back, the resident will go back to the patient and inform them that they are ready to move to the OR. At this point, it is common to give the patient a few moments to say goodbye to their family. If the patient has not already received an anxiolytic like midazolam, then usually the

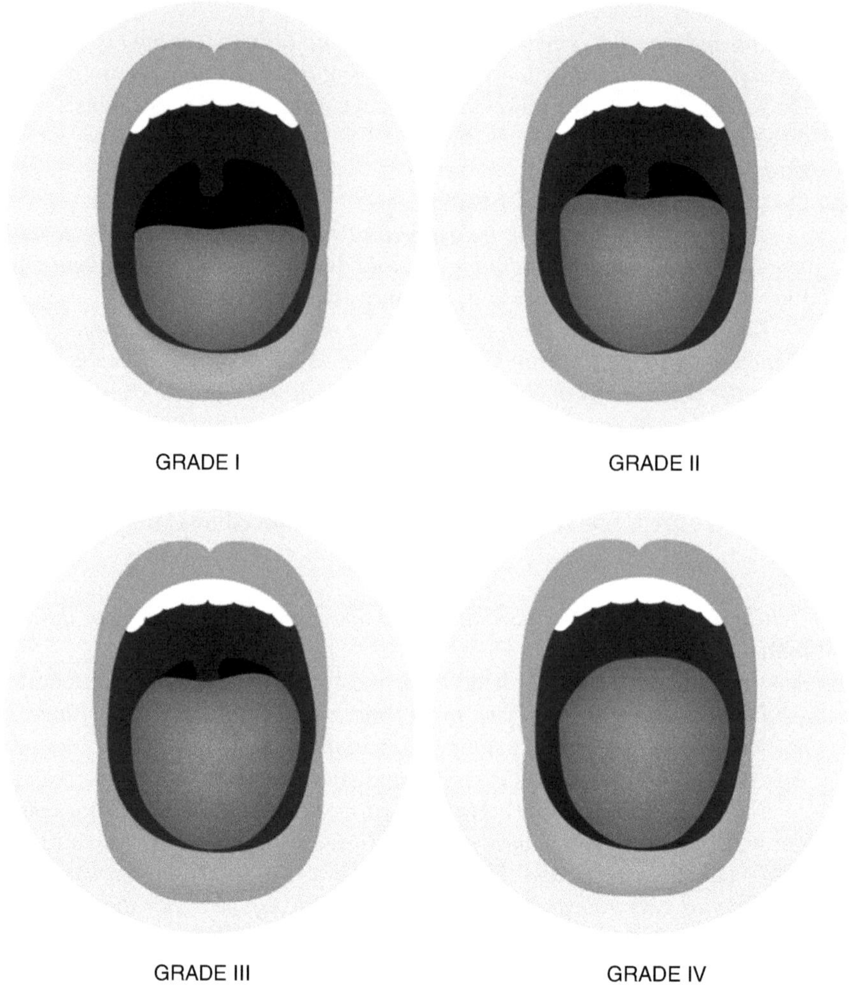

GRADE I   GRADE II

GRADE III   GRADE IV

◘ Fig. 20.22 Mallampati Score Classification

patient will receive this dose. One way to be helpful as the medical student is to double check that the patient's chart and belongings (like eyeglasses and dentures) are traveling with them and double check that the patient has a bouffant to enter the OR space.

Once in the operating room, things can often feel like a flurry, especially for a medical student. There is a lot happening at the beginning of a case, but there are also numerous ways a student can be helpful. When in doubt, take a step back, make sure people are able to move around you and make sure you are not near any blue drapes – the last thing you want to do is contaminate the sterile field! If unsure, ask.

Here are a few ways students can be particularly helpful at the beginning of the case:

- Help the patient shimmy over to the OR table
  - *Hint: make sure the patient's gown is untied in the back so they don't lay on knots for the entire case. Help the patient feel for the sides of the narrow bed and help them get centered.*
- Help place the monitors on the patient
  - *Hint: remember smoke over fire and snow over grass! Help place the sticker for the pulse oximeter and the blood pressure cuff. Keep track of your wires and try to keep everything organized. Always let the patient know what you're doing and warn them about the cold stickers.*

- Double check that all the supplies are ready for induction
  - *Hint: remember to look for: drugs, blade (with functional light), ET tube, oral airway, mask, and suction.*

At this point, a time out will often occur. The surgical time out has been proven to reduce errors in the operating room and it is crucial to ensure that everyone is on the same page.

The timeout checklist will include the following:

1. Room introductions (everyone in the room should announce their name and role)
2. Patient Name and Patient MRN (usually read by the anesthesiologist and checked by the circulating nurse)
3. Procedure confirmation and site confirmation (usually announced by the surgeon and double checked by the circulating nurse)
4. Patient allergies and reactions (usually announced by the anesthesiologist)
5. Consent signature check (usually checked by the circulating nurse)
6. Fire risk (usually announced by the circulating nurse)

Before induction, the patient will be preoxygenated. Ask your resident if you can help with this, it is a great way to increase your skill level and comfort level with bag-mask ventilation. Here are a few tips to help you succeed with this task:

- Keep in mind that the patient is awake! Always ask the patient before you do anything to their body and be aware that a face mask can feel uncomfortable and even claustrophobic to a patient. Gently place the mask down, do not press for a seal. Let the patient become accustomed to the sensation of breathing into a mask, then begin to apply gentle pressure to create a seal. Inform the patient that you are only providing them with oxygen right now. Instruct them to take slow, deep breaths.
- Watch the monitor for the end tidal O2 or etO2 value. You will want to aim for a goal of >80% to confirm that the patient is adequately preoxygenated.

Induction will occur once the resident and attending anesthesiologist are both in the room and feel ready to begin induction. In general, the attending is responsible for pushing the medications and the resident (or medical student!) is responsible for intubation. Once the patient is sedated, remember that they can no longer protect their airway; therefore bag-mask ventilating the patient is crucial. Be sure to apply tape or tegaderm to the patient's eyes to protect them from scratches related to the procedure. Follow the bag masking and intubation tips laid out earlier in this chapter for the best chance at success, and remember to always ask for help if you are struggling!

After induction and intubation, the patient will be positioned, prepped, and draped for their procedure. Volatile anesthetics may be turned on at this time for maintenance of sedation. Medical students can be helpful in a variety of ways during this time:

1. Help place the temperature probe in the nasopharynx and an NG or OG tube if necessary.
2. Help organize lines and tubes so they are up off the floor. One good rule of thumb is to make sure you have easiest access to your ventilator tubing, so all lines should pass under.
3. Help clip the drapes to the IV poles. *Hint: fold over the drape toward you about 3 inches and clip into this fold; this prevents the clip from flying off into the sterile surgical field if it were to come unclipped.*

You will notice that the resident or attending that you're working with will use this time to update their documentation and organize their workstation. When things feel settled out and your resident or attending appears less busy, feel free to ask if now is a good time to ask questions. Throughout the case, ask your resident what they are looking out for and watch to see how they react to changes in the patient's vital signs. Ask questions about things you see that you don't understand.

Throughout the case, the anesthesiologist is continuously monitoring the patient's vitals and monitoring for acute changes. Take notice of what your resident notices and responds to. Feel free to ask questions. You can learn a lot from your resident or attending by asking how they respond to particular things happening to the patient. During the case is your opportunity to learn as much as you can, so take advantage of this time!

As the surgery starts to wrap up, the surgeon will usually let the anesthesiologist and the circulating nurse know that they are close to closing. This helps everyone else in the room get ready for emersion, extubation, and transport to PACU. When the case begins to wind down, you'll notice the anesthesiologist begin to follow the sequence of events laid out in the drugs section of this chapter. They'll begin to wean the patient off the anesthetics and begin providing longer acting pain medications as well as antiemetic drugs. It can be quite difficult to properly time emersion; you want to make sure the patient is still fully sedated through the final skin closure. Listen to your residents and attendings to learn how they approach the timing around emersion.

Just like induction and intubation can feel like a flurry of activity, emersion and extubation will also feel like a lot of action relative to the rest of the case. As the medical student, you should keep your eyes and ears open, look and listen for ways you can help and know when to take a step back and let the resident and attending in your space. Look for opportunities where you can assist and also opportunities where you can observe attendings and residents utilizing different techniques so you can maximize your learning.

The key steps of emergence, as laid out in the drugs section, are reduction of anesthetic agents, addition of analgesic and antiemetic agents, and reversal of neuromuscular blockage. All four of these steps are required prior to beginning to assess for extubation. The patient must be able to follow commands prior to extubation. The ability to follow commands indicates that the patient has intact airway reflexes and will be able to protect their airway. You will notice your resident or attending say the patient's name, tap their shoulder, ask them to open their eyes or squeeze their hand. It can sometimes be jarring to watch this phase of anesthesia. The patient can look quite uncomfortable, sometimes bucking on the tube. It is important to remember that you cannot pull out the tube until the patient is responsive to commands. *Talk to the patient, remind them of where they are, tell them that their surgery is over, and that they are safe.* This can often be one of the easiest ways for you to be helpful as the medical student. Another way to be helpful is to hold the patient's hands. Often patients will try to rub their eyes or pull out their ET tube during emergence, gently hold onto the patient's hand and continue to affirm that they are safe and remind them where they are.

Once the patient is able to respond to commands, you will notice extubation happens quite swiftly. First, the resident or attending will suction deep in the patient's throat, removing all secretions that have built up around the cuff of the ET tube. Next, they will deflate the cuff. In one swift motion, they will gently pull the tube out of the patient's throat. The resident or attending will then quickly apply an oxygen mask to the patient's face. Encourage the patient to take a few deep breaths and ask them not to remove the mask from their face.

Now that the patient is extubated and breathing on their own, the surgical and nursing teams will help roll in the PACU bed to transfer the patient on to.

Moving the patient is a team effort, and you can always lend a hand here as a medical student. Remember that moving the patient is always on the count of the anesthesiologist. Check to make sure no lines, tubes, or monitors will get tangled in the move. Always remember to make sure the bed is in the locked position before moving the patient. These are all small ways you can lend a hand as a medical student.

Once the patient is moved to the PACU bed, be sure to transition the oxygen source from the anesthesia machine to the oxygen tank on the bed. Hook up the plastic tubing and turn the oxygen up to 6 L. Before the patient is transported to the PACU, make sure the patient's chart is with them. Ask the circulating nurse what bay in the PACU the patient is destined for and commit that number to memory. The anesthesiologist will remain at the head of the bed, and you can help pull the bed from the foot. Another way to be helpful is to make sure all the doors are opened for the team as the patient is rolled through the hallways. Be careful not to get your toes run over by the bed!

On arrival to the PACU, you will be met with the patient's new PACU nurse. They (and a colleague if one is available) will begin hooking the patient up to monitors in the room and they will transition the oxygen from the tank to the room supply. Only once the patient is secured in the room will sign out begin, so always offer to lend a hand rather than watching the nurse do all the work!

Sign out is the final crucial piece to the anesthesiologists role with this patient. Both the surgical team and the anesthesia team will need to sign out. The order doesn't particularly matter; it can be a nice gesture to the surgical team to let them go first so they can start what may be their only break for the day.

Here is a checklist of what needs to be covered during sign out:

Patient Name, DOB, MRN

Procedure Performed

Any issues with the case

Paralytics given and reversal provided?

Fluids given:

  Crystalloid total:

  Colloid total:

  Blood product total (with individual product breakdown):

Estimated blood loss

Urine output total

Pain control given:

  Initial fentanyl dose

  Other opiates provided at end of case

  Non-opiate pain meds provided

Antiemetics given

You can definitely ask your resident to help with signing out the case in the PACU. Feel free to make a copy of the above checklist before you start your rotation to have as a quick reference in the event that you are asked to provide sign out.

Next, the resident or attending will go to a nearby computer to finish documenting the case. They will sign orders for the patient in PACU, including pain management and oxygen requirements. If the patient has an epidural, they will also make sure the perioperative pain service is aware of the patient.

Now the case is over! The resident will now go back to the OR to begin setting up for the next case and then see their next patient in the preoperative unit to place an IV and obtain consent. Unlike for the surgical team, there is not as much down time between cases for the anesthesiology team, so they rely on the two 15 min and one half hour break throughout their day to stay hydrated and well fed. If you had any questions about the preceding case, be sure to ask your attending or resident before the next case begins.

20.15.4 Summary

You've just made it through your first case! If it felt like a whirlwind that is okay! You will begin to feel more comfortable with the anesthesiologist role with each new case you see. Always stop, look, and listen for ways you can be helpful and save questions for quieter times in the case.

20.16 Conclusion

This chapter has served as a crash course of the basics of how to succeed during your anesthesiology rotation, but nothing will be more helpful than experiencing it for yourself. If you are at all considering a career in anesthesia, surgery, emergency medicine, or critical care, we highly recommend spending some time with the anesthesia team during your medical school training.

Below is a consolidated list of resources that you can quickly reference while you are on your rotation (◘ Table 20.15). But always remember – it is okay not to know the answers for everything! Ask questions, ask to help, and learn something from each case. Good luck! We hope you find your time with anesthesia as enjoyable as we do!

Machine Check and Room Setup:
Questions in the Pre-Op Setting:

When was the last time you had anything to eat or drink?

Did you take your medications today?

Do you ever get breathless walking up two or more flights of stairs?

Have you or anyone in your family ever had issues with anesthesia before?

Do you have any pain, stiffness, or arthritis in your neck or jaw?

Do you have asthma or COPD?

Do you have any of the following medical conditions: kidney disease, heart disease, liver disease, diabetes, history of stroke, history of epilepsy or seizures?

Do you have a history of GERD?

Do you have any loose, missing, or removable teeth or dentures?

Intra-Op medications (◘ Table 20.16):
PACU sign out

Patient Name, DOB, MRN

Procedure Performed

Any issues with the case

Paralytics given and reversal provided?

Fluids given:

  Crystalloid total:

  Colloid total:

  Blood product total (with individual product breakdown):

Estimated blood loss

Urine output total

Pain control given:

  Initial fentanyl dose

  Other opiates provided at end of case

  Non-opiate pain meds provided

Antiemetics given

◻ Table 20.15 MSMAID mnemonic device

M *Machine*
   Turn on the machine, computers, and screens
   Run the machine self-test
   Adjust machine parameters for the case and the patient
   Check volatile agent levels
   Check for a bag-valve mask in the room

S *Suction*
   Make sure the suction circuit is connected and a Yankauer suction tip is connected
   to the end of the tubing
   Prep an OG tube for the case, if necessary (open the packing and lube up the tip)

M *Monitors*
   Prep EKG pads, temperature probes, O2 sat monitoring, and BP cuff
   Gather additional supplies for more advanced monitoring: arterial lines, central
   lines, BIS monitoring

A *Airway*
   Acquire the correct size ETT, check the stylette is in place and check the cuff for
   leaks
   Prep the laryngoscope, make sure the light is working
   Open a mask to use for bag-mask ventilation
   Open an oral airway and place it within reach of where you will be performing
   intubation
   Make sure a laryngeal mask airway, bougies, or video laryngoscopes are available if
   you are concerned about a difficult airway

I *IV Access*
   Prep your IV kit (peripheral IV needle, tourniquet, gauze, tegaderm, alcohol swab,
   IV start tubing, 1–2 cc of lidocaine in a subcutaneous injection needle)
   Prep your intravenous fluids and lines

D *Drugs*
   Prep the drugs you will need throughout the case; in general, at a minimum you will
   want to prep your preinduction and induction drugs:
     Midazolam
     Propofol
     Fentanyl
     Paralytic (rocuronium or succinylcholine)

■ Table 20.16   OR Pharmaceuticals Quick Reference

Drug class	Commonly Used Drug Name	Dose (adult)
Preinduction		
Anxiolytic	Midazolam	1–2 mg
Antibiotic	Cefazolin	2 mg
Induction		
Sedative Hypnotic	Propofol	1–2.5 mg/kg
	Etomidate	0.15–0.3 mg/kg
	Ketamine	1–2 mg/kg
Analgesia	Fentanyl	100 mcg
Neuromuscular Blockade	Succinylcholine	1–1.5 mg/kg
	Rocuronium	0.6–1.0 mg/kg (1.2 mg/kg for RSI)
	Vecuronium	0.10–0.20 mg/kg
Maintenance		
Inhaled anesthetics		MAC = 1 equivalent
	Nitrous oxide	105
	Isoflurane	1.2
	Sevoflurane	2.0
	Desflurane	6.0
Pressors	Epinephrine	4–10 mcg bolus 1–100 mcg/min infusion
	Phenylephrine	50–100 mcg bolus 10–100 mcg/min infusion
	Norepinephrine	4–8 mcg bolus 1–20 mcg/min infusion
	Ephedrine	5–10 mg bolus Not used for infusions
	Vasopressin	1–4 units bolus 0.01–0.04 units/min infusion
Antihypertensives	Esmolol	10–50 mg bolus (can be repeated every 5–15 min) 50–300 mcg/kg/min infusion
	Labetalol	5–25 mg bolus (can be repeated every 10 min) 0.5–2 mg/min infusion
	Hydralazine	2.5 mg bolus (can be repeated every 5 min, max 20 mg) Not used for infusions
	Nitroglycerin	10–40 mcg bolus 10–200 mcg/min infusion

20

◼ **Table 20.16** (continued)

Drug class	Commonly Used Drug Name	Dose (adult)
Emergence		
Antiemetics	Ondansetron	4 mg IV
	Dexamethasone	4–8 mg IV
	Haloperidol	1–2 mg IV
Analgesia	Hydromorphone	0.2–0.5 mg IV q5min
	Morphine	1–3 mg IV q5min
NMBA Reversal	Neostigmine + Glycopyrrolate	20–70 mcg/kg 0.2 mg glycopyrrolate for every 1 mg neostigmine
	Sugammadex	2–4 mg/kg

Radiation Oncology

Parsa Erfani

Contents

Most medical students step into their radiation oncology rotation with no exposure to the field. This chapter aims to provide a framework for your rotation and is split into three sections:

1. Introduction to Radiation Oncology: reviews basic principles of radiation therapy
2. Steps of Radiation Therapy: outlines the radiation therapy workflow and the ways medical students can engage in the different steps of radiation planning and delivery
3. Disease Site Overview: provides an outline of some of the cancers you may encounter and their primary treatment modality

21.1 Introduction to Radiation Oncology

21.1.1 What Is Radiation Oncology?

Radiation oncology is a branch of medicine devoted to the treatment of malignant and benign disease with ionizing radiation. Radiation oncologists work with a team of nurses, radiation therapists, dosimetrists, and medical physicists who are involved in the evaluation, planning, radiation delivery, and follow-up of cancer patients. They also work within a multidisciplinary team of surgeons, medical oncologists, radiologists, and other specialists to jointly determine the best treatment for each patient.

21.1.2 What Is Radiation Therapy?

Radiation therapy (RT) is a treatment modality that delivers ionizing radiation to treat benign and malignant tumors. RT has been used with surgery and systemic therapies in combined modality approaches for a wide range of malignancies to maximize tumor control and quality of life while minimizing toxicity. Approximately 50% of cancer patients receive RT as a part of their treatment. The goal of RT can be either curative or palliative, if treating metastatic disease that is incurable.

RT may be the sole modality of treatment (definitive), as in some prostate cancers. Alternatively, it may be delivered before surgery (neoadjuvant, e.g., rectal cancers) or after surgery (adjuvant, e.g., breast cancers). It can also be combined with systemic therapies depending on whether combining modalities improves outcomes: systemic therapies can be given prior to radiation (induction), simultaneously with the radiation (concurrent), or after radiation (consolidation). Ablative doses of RT may also be used to treat oligometastatic disease (a state of limited systemic metastatic tumors) for certain cancers types (e.g., non-small cell lung cancer). Finally, RT is also utilized for palliation as it can provide considerable symptomatic relief to patients (e.g., bone metastases, cord compression). The duration of RT can range from a single treatment to multiple weeks of daily RT (called RT fractionation). In each clinical scenario, the technique, dose, expected outcomes, and related toxicities vary depending on the diagnosis and treatment site.

The therapeutic ratio of RT is a balance between the acceptable probability of radiation-induced toxicity and the probability of tumor control. Different types of radiation delivery techniques, RT dose, immobilization, radiosensitizers, and fractionation can help skew the therapeutic ratio in a favorable direction.

21

21.1.3 How Do RT and Fractionation Work?

Fractionation refers to when the total radiation dose is administered over more than one dose (or fraction). Fractionation is thought to cause less damage to the healthy tissue and allow time for tissue to repair between fractions. The most important biological factors influencing the responses of tumors and normal tissues to fractioned RT are often called the "Four Rs" of RT (■ Table 21.1).

Hypofractionation refers to when a specific RT dose is delivered in fewer fractions and larger fraction sizes (often greater than 200 cGy). Hyperfractionation refers to when a specific RT dose is delivered in smaller fraction sizes (usually less than 180 cGy) that are often delivered in two or more fractions per day (generally with a 6 or more hour interval between fractions) [1].

21.1.4 How Is the RT Dose Measured?

RT dose is a measure of the amount of energy from ionizing radiation deposited in a unit mass of a medium. The SI unit used to measure absorbed dose is the gray (Gy).

cGy (centigray) is the modern basic unit of radiotherapy dose.

– 1 Gy = 1 J/kg of absorbed energy
– 1 cGy = 1 rad

There are different types of detectors that can be used to measure radiation, depending on the type and the purpose of the study. For example, ionization chambers detect radiation by measuring the charge that has been liberated when radiation ionizes the gas inside. Solid-state dosimeters are commonly

■ **Table 21.1** The "Four Rs" of RT

"Rs"	Description
Repair (hours)	When radiation enters the patient, ions are produced and cause DNA damage either directly or indirectly through the formation of free radicals and reactive oxygen species. The DNA damage (single- or double-stranded breaks) leads to mitotic cell death. Malignant and normal cells in the treatment field are both affected by RT. However, healthy cells have a distinct advantage because malignant cells often have a deficiency or defect in their DNA repair machinery. Therefore, malignant cells are preferentially damaged by RT
Redistribution (hours)	Cells exhibit differential radiation sensitivity while in different phases of the cell cycle. Cells in mitosis are the most sensitive to DNA damage and cells in late S-phase are most resistant (■ Fig. 21.1). Throughout the different fractions of RT, cells progress through different phases of the cell cycle and become radiosensitive at different times. Therefore, redistribution makes the cell population more sensitive to fractionated treatments as compared to a single radiation dose
Repopulation (weeks)	Repopulation is important in tumors that have stem cells capable of rapid proliferation. As the tumor shrinks from RT, clonogenic cells that survive irradiation can repopulate the tumor and result in decreased local control. Each fraction of RT results in a decrease in the number of surviving clonogenic tumor cells
Reoxygenation (hours to days)	Sensitivity to RT increases with oxygen availability, as more double-stranded breaks occur in cells irradiated in the presence of oxygen than in the absence of oxygen. Tumors <1 mm are fully oxygenated and thus sensitive to RT. However, areas of tumors that are hypoxic are less radiosensitive. Fractionation allows for the hypoxic clonogenic cells to become better oxygenated during the period after irradiation of a tumor and thus more radiosensitive during the next RT fraction (■ Fig. 21.1). In other words, if tumors are irradiated with a large single RT dose, most radiosensitive aerobic cells will be killed, but hypoxic cells will survive. But fractionation allows for reoxygenation of tumor cells, increased radiosensitivity, and a substantial improvement in the therapeutic ratio

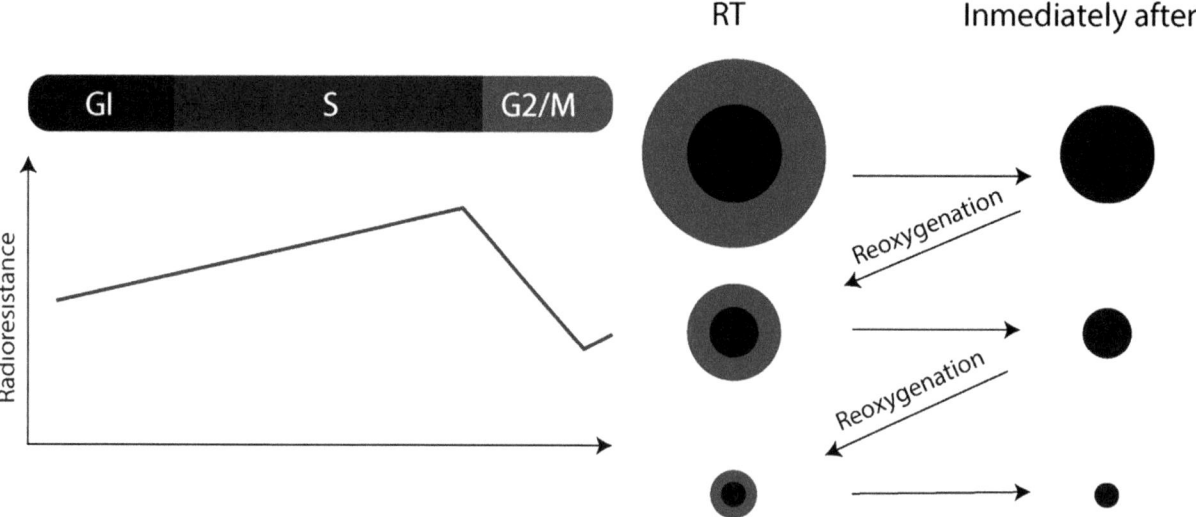

Fig. 21.1 Redistribution and reoxygenation in the "Four Rs" of RT

used in the radiation oncology department, and they measure radiation by storing the energy absorbed during the exposure in "electron traps." Thermoluminescent dosimeters (TLDs) are used to measure patient doses and optically stimulated luminescence dosimeters (OSLDs) are used for personnel dosimetry [1].

21.1.5 What Are the Various Types of Ionizing Radiation?

External Beam Radiation Therapy (EBRT)   The most common form of RT that delivers ionizing radiation from a source outside the body. Forms of ionizing radiation include (□ Fig. 21.2):

- *Photons (X-ray or gamma rays)* – photons are produced electronically by the acceleration of electrons in a linear accelerator (LINAC) or by radioactive decay of a nuclide (e.g., cobalt-60). They are widely used as they can penetrate tissue and reach internal organs more easily than electrons.
- *Electrons* – electrons are also produced by a LINAC and are primarily used for superficial targets (e.g., skin) in order to help minimize radiation to deeper tissues and organs.
- *Protons* – protons penetrate tissue to a variable depth (depending on their energy) and deposit energy in the tissue as a sharp peak, known as a Bragg peak. This rapid dose falloff at a depth allows for decreased radiation to tissue past the Bragg peak and accurate dose delivery to target structures. Presently proton therapy is being investigated for use in pediatric populations and in situations in which normal structures that are in close proximity to the treatment target limit the ability to deliver conventional photon beam therapy (e.g., uveal melanoma, sarcomas of the skull base, and spine). Protons are generated in particle accelerators (cyclotron), which are limited in availability due to cost.
- Neutrons, carbon, etc. are less commonly used.

Radiation Oncology

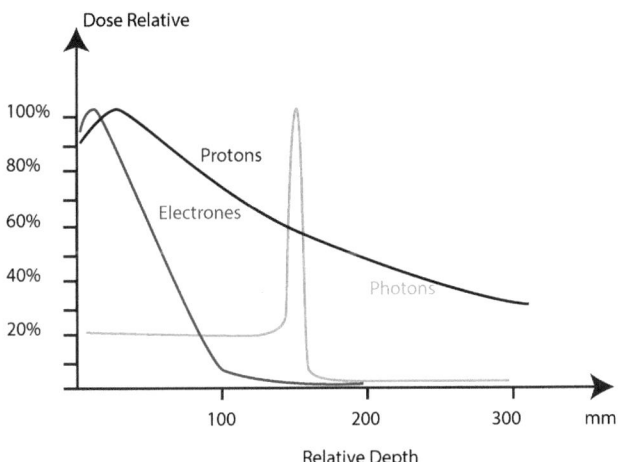

Fig. 21.2 Dose-depth curves of photons, proton, and electrons

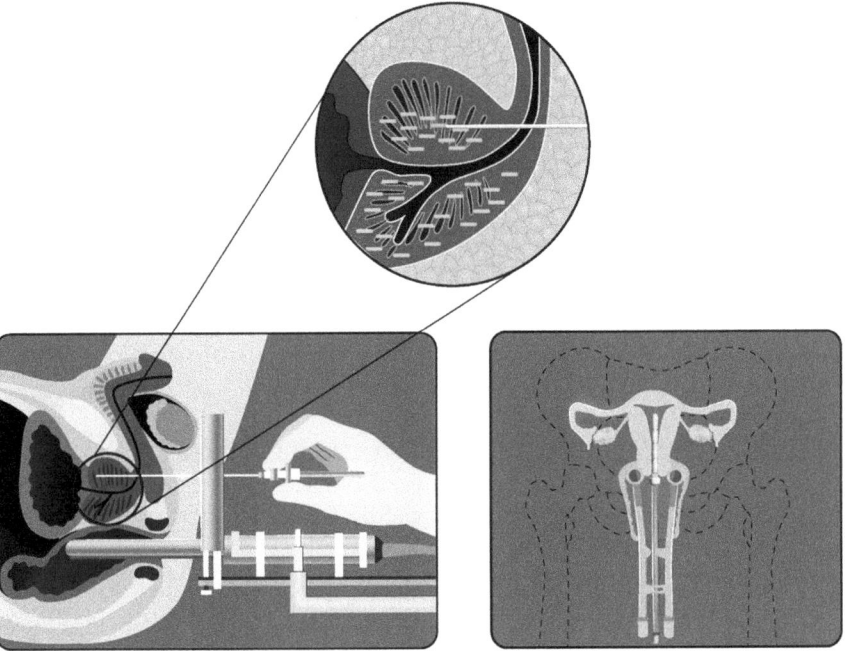

Fig. 21.3 Brachytherapy: Interstitial (prostate seeds) and intracavity (tandem and ovoids for cervical cancer)

Brachytherapy ("Short-Range Therapy") Another form of RT in which the radiation source is placed inside or next to the treatment area and is active over a relatively short distance. The advantage of brachytherapy is that it can deliver high doses of radiation to the tumor while limiting dose to surrounding normal tissues. It can be delivered with either a low-dose rate (LDR: 0.4–2 Gy/hour) or high-dose rate (HDR: >12 Gy per hour) [2]. Brachytherapy (□ Fig. 21.3) may be:

- *Interstitial* – such as prostate seeds
- *Intracavity* – such as tandem and ovoids for cervical cancer
- *Surface* – such as skin brachytherapy

21.1.6 What Are the Various Delivery Techniques for EBRT?

3D Conformal Radiation (3D-CRT) Uses 3D anatomic information to create a dose distribution that matches (or conforms to) the target as closely as possible. The radiation beam exits the EBRT machine at the gantry. Blocks and MLCs (multileaf collimators) are incorporated into the head of the machine to shape the radiation beam. Conformal therapy is used when the target volumes are defined using a high-definition imaging study such as CT, MRI, or PET. 3D-CRT has reduced toxicity compared to 2D-RT and has allowed for dose escalation trials that have allowed for improved long-term tumor control.

Intensity-Modulated Radiation Therapy (IMRT) A high-precision form of RT that improves the ability to conform the treatment volume to irregular tumor shapes. In IMRT, the intensity of photons changes in different parts of a single radiation beam while treatment is delivered. Modern IMRT uses MLCs (multileaf collimators) in the head of the gantry that open or close dynamically to shape the photon beam to the target. This helps maximize the delivery of radiation to the planned treatment volume while minimizing radiation to normal tissue outside the target (especially as compared to older techniques such as 3D-CRT or 2D-RT).

- There are several variations on IMRT including intensity-modulated arc therapy (IMAT) or volumetric-modulated arc therapy (VMAT) in which the MLCs are moving while the gantry rotates as an arc.

Stereotactic Techniques A form of extremely conformal EBRT in which the full radiation dose is given with extreme accuracy and precision in a single or limited number of fractions, often with photons generated by a LINAC or cobalt-60 source. Stereotactic RT includes both stereotactic radiosurgery (SRS) and stereotactic body radiation therapy (SBRT):

- SRS usually refers to a single-fraction treatment of intracranial and spinal targets (e.g., Gamma Knife®).
- SBRT refers to a two- to five-fraction treatment of intracranial, spinal, or extracranial sites, such as the lung, head and neck, liver, pancreas, and prostate, and oligometastatic disease (e.g., SBRT can be curative for Stage I lung cancers).
- Stereotactic techniques are often very well tolerated and have limited side effects because of the extreme accuracy and precision.
- Stereotactic techniques have a steep dose falloff making them incredibly conformal. Therefore, accurate tumor localization (via MRI or CT) and consistent patient immobilization are necessary to optimize the therapeutic ratio.
- Immobilization is critical for high reproducibility: a custom body cast may be used to establish a coordinate system for thoracic, spine, and abdominal tumors. SRS may use rigid headframes.
- Extracranial stereotactic RT such as CyberKnife® can localize and track tumors with implanted fiducial markers during respiratory motion.

- Specialty Techniques
- *Total Body Irradiation (TBI)* – use of conventional photons for preparation of hematopoietic cell transplantation for treatment of leukemias. TBI is used for immunosuppression to allow engraftment of donor stem cells and irradiation of malignant cells. One advantage of TBI over systemic chemotherapy is that it can penetrate sites independent of blood supply.

- *Intraoperative Radiation Therapy (IORT)* – radiation delivery at the time of surgery. In IORT, dose-limiting sensitive structures are often excluded by operative mobilization or direct shielding of these structures. The dose of the IORT is limited by structures that cannot be displaced.
    - IORT can be used when there are areas of high risk for local recurrence noted during surgery (such as positive margins or incompletely resected tumors).
    - A single-fraction treatment of IORT may be insufficient for tumor control and may be followed by post-op EBRT.
    - IORT is most useful for pelvic and abdominal malignancies where normal bowel limits the dose that can be delivered with EBRT.

Many of the aforementioned EBRT techniques (3D-CRT, IMRT, etc.) may be delivered using a technique called image-guided radiation therapy (IGRT). IGRT uses imaging of the target during each treatment, which can allow for reduction in treatment volume and sparing of normal tissue. Normally, clinicians must add margins to target volumes to account for uncertainty around patient positioning (e.g., daily position changes despite immobilization, inherent organ motion secondary to respiration). However, IGRT decreases this positional uncertainty, allowing for smaller margins that reduce the irradiated volumes [2].

21.1.7 What Are the Side Effects of RT?

Side effects of RT vary based on the irradiated area, specifics of the RT (e.g., cumulative dose, dose per fraction, proximity to sensitive tissues), and patient characteristics (e.g., age and genetics).

A common acute side effect of RT is fatigue. Other acute side effects are limited to the area of treatment. For example, upper GI tract RT can cause nausea and vomiting, lower GI tract RT can cause diarrhea, head and neck RT can lead to mouth sores, and thoracic RT can cause esophagitis. These can all lead to dysphagia, poor oral intake, and dehydration. Pelvic RT, on the other hand, can lead to urinary symptoms and bowel changes. With the reduction in tissue swelling and irritation over time, acute side effects largely resolve.

The long-term side effects of RT are often related to irradiated tissue fibrosis. The manifestation of tissue fibrosis depends on the organ involved. For example, infertility can be a sequelae of certain pediatric and young adult cancer patients as ovaries and testicles are very sensitive to RT. Cardiac toxicity (e.g., accelerated atherosclerosis) may also be a late complication of malignancies in which radiation to the heart is inevitable. Finally, and frequently a concern of patients, is the potential of RT to cause secondary cancers in the irradiated field. Although secondary cancers have been associated with prior RT, they are very rare and may take decades to develop. There are multiple models to determine the risk of carcinogenesis, which seem to be a function of dose, sex, age of exposure, and time since exposure. Therefore, secondary cancers are of greater concern for pediatric and younger patients.

The acute side effects and long-term sequelae of RT are always discussed with patients during the consent process. More site-specific sequelae of radiation are included in ▶ Sect. 21.3.

21.2 Steps of Radiation Therapy: Role of Medical Students

21.2.1 What Is the Workflow for Receiving RT?

Overview of steps involved in a patient receiving RT (■ Fig. 21.4):

1. *Consultation* – decision to irradiate based on clinical picture, supporting data, and pre-radiation workup, including staging, dental evaluation (if needed), and nutritional assessment.
2. *Simulation* – custom planning appointment placing patient in reproducible position, with the necessary immobilization.
3. *Contouring* – defining target structures that should be irradiated and normal tissue that should receive the least amount of radiation possible.
4. *Treatment Planning + Quality Assurance* – iterative process in which dosimetrists and physicists create the treatment plan and calculate the radiation dose to the tumor and organs at risk (OARs) while the physician reviews and evaluates the plan. Plan undergoes quality assurance.
5. *Treatment* – RT plan is delivered by the radiation therapists under the guidance of and review of the radiation oncologist. During the course of RT, the patient will meet with physician and staff weekly for an on-treatment visit (OTV).
6. *Follow-Up* – follow-up visits posttreatment with scans.

21.2.1.1 Consultation: How to Prepare

Radiation oncology has both inpatient and outpatient components, although the outpatient component will likely be a large part of your rotation. As a medical student, you will be asked to take on several consultations during a clinical day. The goal of the consultation is to read the patient's chart, perform a full history and physical exam, and present a complete assessment and plan.

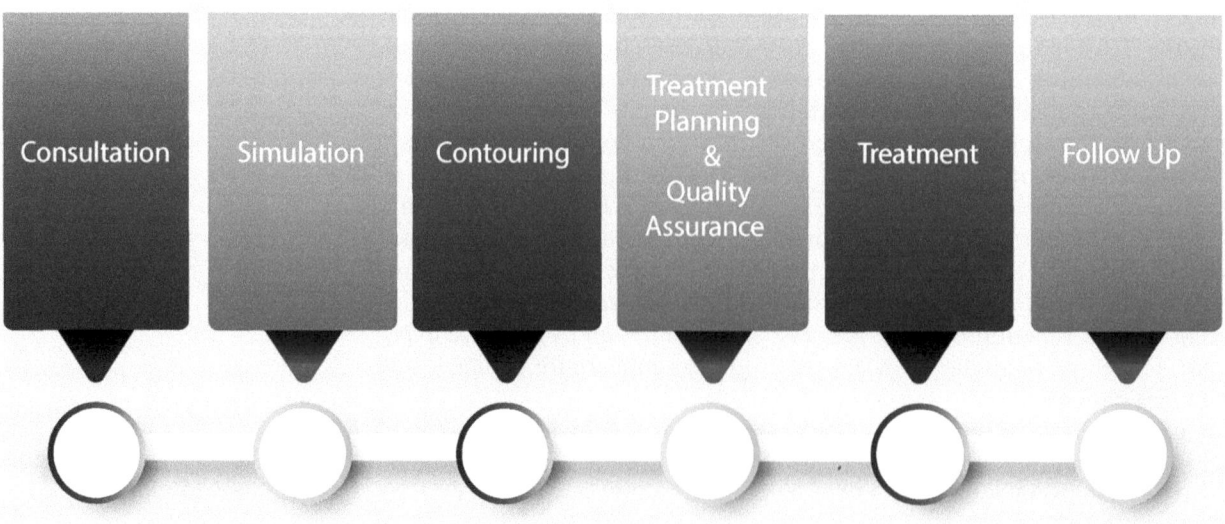

■ **Fig. 21.4** Radiotherapy workflow

21.2.1.2 The Night Before

Given medical student's limited exposure to the field and the mass amount of data and clinical trials that exists for specific disease processes, it is essential to prepare for consultations the day before clinic. Your chart review should include a review of the patient's initial presentation and diagnosis. All laboratory data, pathology, and radiological images should be reviewed (including the primary images). All treatments performed (surgery, chemotherapy, prior radiation) should also be noted. Notes from the referring physician (often medical or surgical oncology) are a good place to begin.

Essential Components of Chart Review

- Laboratory data provides information on the functioning of specific organs that may be affected by the cancer or therapy. Tumor markers can also aid in diagnosis, locating tumor origin, tracking therapeutic response, or determining recurrence.
- Pathology reports are essential to making the diagnosis. One should note how the pathology was obtained, such as via fine needle aspiration, excisional biopsy, or surgical resection. Some key components of a pathology report include size, histology of cancer, grade, margin status (positive, negative, or close), and disease-specific mutations (see ▶ Sect. 21.3).
  - Histology – separated into -sarcoma (derived from connective tissue) or -carcinoma (derived from epithelial tissue). Carcinomas can be further classified as adeno- (glandular epithelial tissue) and squamous- (squamous epithelial tissue), among others. To further describe histologic appearances, terms such as cystic, follicular, papillary, medullary, exophytic, and polypoid are often added. Lymphomas and leukemias are neoplasms derived from hematologic precursor cells.
  - Grade – classification of cell differentiation and mitotic activity. Grading can be expressed using descriptive terms such as well, moderately, or poorly differentiated or using numeric grades. Special grading systems are used for some tumors, such as the Gleason Score for prostate cancer. The pathology report may include immunohistochemistry, flow cytometry, or other more advanced laboratory procedures that may aid in the diagnosis and/or prognosis of a specific tumor (e.g., lymphovascular invasion for gynecological cancers, tumor depth for head and neck cancers).
- Imaging should be reviewed in addition to reading the final report, as there is often an expectation that you can review the primary images with the attending physician. Commonly used radiological imaging for diagnosis, staging, and follow-up includes CT, MRI, ultrasonography, or positron emission tomography (PET/CT).
- Staging of cancer is a systematic method of classifying extent of malignancy. The TNM staging system is used for solid tumors (◘ Table 21.2) [2].

   Several TNM stages may be assigned. The clinical TNM (cTNM) is based on physical exam and imaging, while the pathologic TNM (pTMN) is based on surgical findings. yTNM refers to TNM staging after preoperative therapy (such as neoadjuvant chemotherapy or RT), and rTNM refers to TNM staging at the time of retreatment or recurrence. It is important to designate which TNM stage is being reported.

   Once the TNM numerical values are determined, the patient's disease is classified as either Stage I, II, III, or IV – with increasing stage indicating more advance disease. Staging for certain cancer may include other factors, such as tumor receptor status. The American Joint Committee on Cancer (AJCC) staging system should be referenced, as the assigned TNM and stage differ by each cancer type.

Table 21.2 TNM staging

TNM	Description
T	Represents the extent of the primary tumor and may be measured on depth of invasion, surface spread, or tumor size
N	Represents the presence and extent of lymph node metastases in terms of sizes, numbers, and locations of involved nodes
M	Represents the presence or absence of distant metastases

Preparing the Note

It will also be very helpful if you prepare the notes for assigned consultations the night before clinic. Reviewing prior consultation notes for the specific disease site in your clinic will help guide the structure and level of detail necessary. Similar to an internal medicine note, a radiation oncology note should include history of present illness, past medical/surgical history, family history, social history, physical exam, labs, pathology, and assessment and plan. Notes should also include a section dedicated to "oncological history," which presents a detailed timeline of the patient's initial presentation, final diagnosis (including pertinent imaging and pathology), as well as treatments received and their complications. Most notes also include a "one-liner" that includes TNM staging, details specific to the disease site (e.g., Gleason Score for prostate cancer), and radiation-specific considerations (such as history of prior radiation, connective tissue disease, inflammatory bowel disease, pacemakers or implantable cardioverter-defibrillators [ICD]).

Review of Literature

After preparing the note and understanding the patient's oncological history, much of your time will be spent on learning about the specific cancer and the existing treatments. Scratching the surface of a disease process may be a larger task than expected. A good place to start for a specific disease process is ► Sect. 21.3 of this chapter which will broadly categorize what types of treatment are used (RT, chemotherapy, surgery, or a combination). Next, the UpToDate page and National Comprehensive Cancer Network (NCCN) guidelines should be reviewed as these resources will provide the present standard of care for a specific cancer and will cite the major clinical trials that have established these guidelines (check out the NCCN app!). It is also helpful to review the cited studies in UpToDate to understand their limitations and assess whether the data is relevant for your specific patient. Understanding the trial's various arms, primary outcome, median follow-up, and exclusion/inclusion criteria is integral to assessing whether the data should influence your recommendation. ► Radoncreview.org is another great resource that consolidates material on workup, management, and relevant trials by disease site.

Radiation oncology is a data-driven field, and there is an expectation to apply data to patient care. However, it is important to not get lost in the many studies and technical aspects of radiation as you are preparing your assessment and plan. It will be helpful to use the Other Resources section of this chapter to take a deeper dive into the disease site and better understand and organize the relevant trials. More on preparing our assessment and plan below!

21.2.1.3 Seeing the Patient

An effective evaluation begins with a detailed review of the history and a physical exam. Even though you may have read most of the patient's history before seeing them, it is important to review the complete history as well as labs, imaging, and pathology with the patient. Make sure to confirm history of prior radiation and presence of pacemakers/ICDs. Regardless of whether the patient has a tobacco-related malignancy, smoking history should be reviewed and cessation should be discussed. The social history should also include how far away patients live or work, as RT can require daily treatments for several weeks and may not be feasible in certain circumstances. Finally, future reproductive plans should also be reviewed depending on the patient's age and site of disease.

In the physical exam, it is important to note any weight changes. Functional status must also be assessed, as this has been shown to dictate both treatment decisions and prognosis. The most commonly used scales are the Karnofsky Performance Status (KPS) scale (scores from 0% for deceased to 100% for no complaints) and the Eastern Cooperative Oncology Group (ECOG) scale, which rates from 0 for asymptomatic to 4 if bedridden (and 5 if deceased). A full lymph node exam is also important in most malignancies [2].

21.2.1.4 Assessment and Plan

One of the most challenging parts of a note or presentation in radiation oncology is preparing a comprehensive assessment and plan.

An assessment should start with a comprehensive "one-liner" that includes pertinent medical conditions, the tumor site, histology, and stage, as well as any treatments received thus far. Developing an assessment and plan can be challenging as medical student. Therefore, attending physicians often expect medical students to decide whether this patient would benefit from RT. The assessment should explain whether or not RT is recommended in this patient, based on your search of relevant clinical trials. It is helpful to cite which studies helped you come to the conclusion in order to get feedback on why that trial may or may not apply to this specific patient. Most attending physicians often do not expect medical students to provide a perfect plan for the patient. The most important part of your plan is deciding whether the patient receives RT.

If RT is recommended, the plan should include more specific details on the RT modality, dose, and fractionation. However, attending physicians do not often expect your plan to be entirely accurate – so no need sweat on the specific details! That said, a plan should include whether the radiation used will be external beam or brachytherapy. As explained above, if external beam is used, one must specify whether photons or particles (electron, proton, etc.) will be used. The modality of treatment should also be specified as described above (3D-CRT, IMRT, SBRT, etc.). The total radiation dose planned, number of total fractions, and number of fractions per day should be described.

Furthermore, it is important to note if any further studies need to be performed prior to beginning therapy. For example, some patients require a complete staging workup. Those receiving radiation to the thorax will require pulmonary function tests prior to treatment. In addition, if the patient is receiving chemotherapy or surgery, the timing of chemotherapy or surgery relative to RT should be specified and coordinated with the medical or surgical oncologist. One should also note where the patient is planning to receive RT, as this may not be at the consulted physician's institution. Finally, it is important to note whether consultations are needed prior to RT. For example, referral to a social worker, speech pathologist, dietitian, smoking cessation specialists, or physical therapist may be necessary prior to RT initiation.

21.2.1.5 Simulation

After consultation and mutual decision to start radiation treatment, simulation is the next step in treatment planning. Simulation is a detailed planning session, which "simulates" but does not actually deliver RT. The goal of the simulation is to place patients in an immobilized position on the CT simulator (CT-S) couch that can be reproduced daily during the actual treatment (◘ Fig. 21.5a). The patient's placement on the CT-S is leveled using side room lasers as well as sagittal laser for straightening. Depending on the treatment site and modality, the patient's skin may be marked for isocenter placement. The area to be treated will be localized under fluoroscopy, and images will be taken.

During your rotation, you should ask the physician whether you can join for the simulation of a patient you have seen in clinic. This may not be built into your rotation schedule but will help you gain a more holistic sense of the patient experience and will allow you to learn from radiation oncology nurses, radiation therapists, dosimetrists, and physicists. You can look out for the following factors during the simulation:

Imaging Modality Radiation planning is commonly based on CT, and modalities such as PET and MRI can be used to supplement definition of anatomic and tumor boundaries.

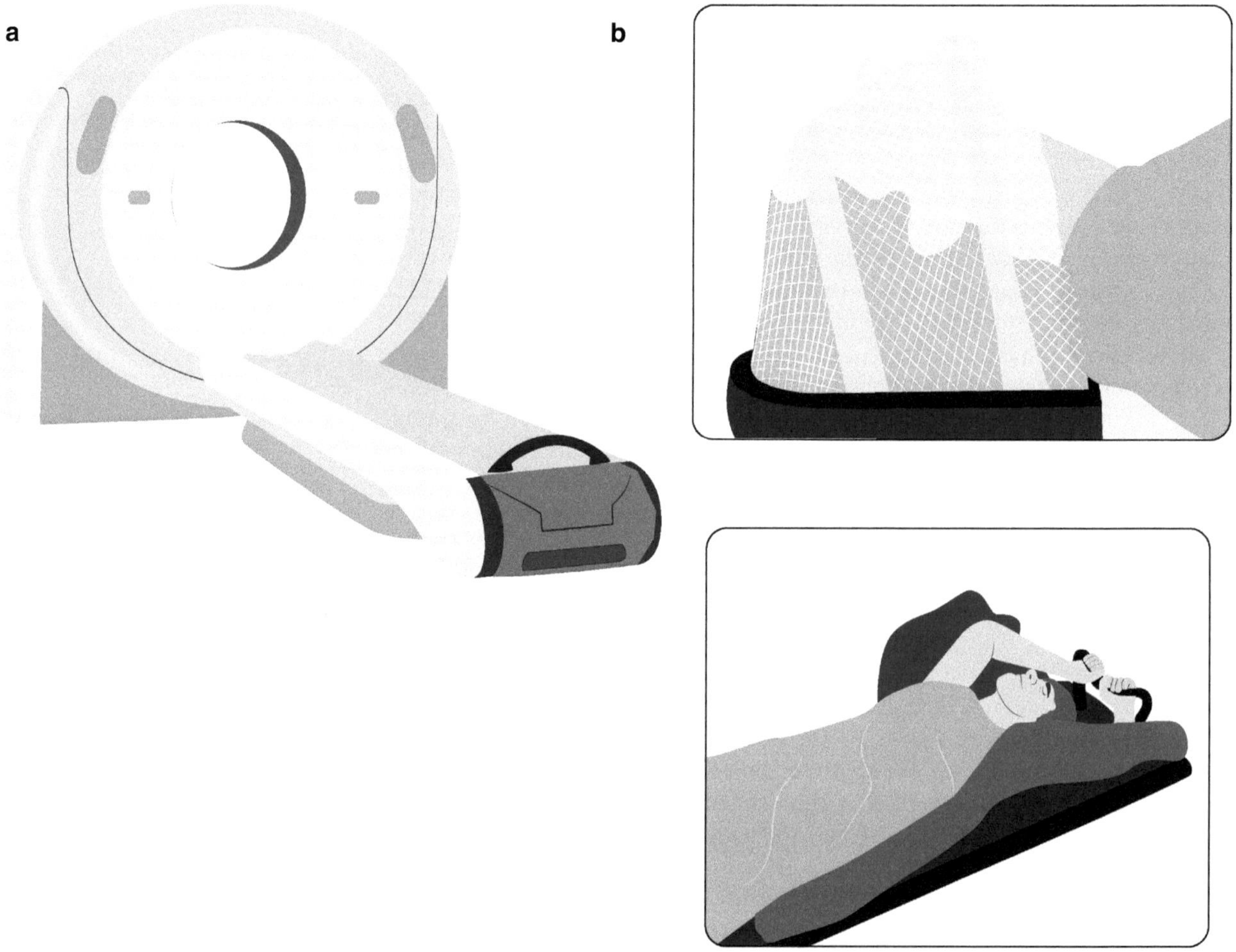

◘ **Fig. 21.5** **a** CT stimulator, **b** immobilization devices (Aquaplast™ face mask and Thorax Vac-Lok™ cushion)

- CT allows for the delineation of target or nearby structures. An algorithm is used to generate Hounsfield units based on the attenuation of structures along the radiation path. The treatment planning software will then measure and correct for the heterogeneity within the radiation beam path and determine how radiation will actually be deposited in the body. During simulation, IV contrast may also be used to aid in target/normal tissue delineation, and oral contrast may be used to determine intraluminal abnormalities (via mouth for upper GI abnormalities or rectum for lower GI abnormalities).
- PET or MRI can be also performed during simulation to improve tumor delineation. PET provides functional imaging of a tumor and reveals the metabolic activity of the tumor. PET/CT fusion approach is often used for head and neck, lung, lymphoma, and GI tumors. MRI can be used to better delineate tumors in the prostate apex or in the brain.

Reproducibility One of the key goals of simulation is to create a setup that is reproducible during and between each treatment fractions. This is accomplished with isocenter placement often using "dot" tattoos or stickers and immobilization devices. Motion during each fraction must also be accounted for.

- *Isocenter placement* – a point in the x, y, and z planes of the body that represents the axis of gantry rotation. It plays an important role when calculating the dose of radiation on a virtual plan. Once the isocenter is determined, the patient may be marked with small tattoos so that the isocenter can be reproduced at the same exact point in space.
- *Immobilization device* (◘ Fig. 21.5b) – a device that is used to minimize *intrafraction* and *interfraction* motion but is comfortable enough for the patient to use for the duration of the treatment (e.g., stereotactic headframes, Aquaplast™ face masks, Vac-Lok™ cushion, BodyFIX®).
- *Accounting for motion* – intrafraction motion may be inevitable due to respiratory motion, as normal cyclical breathing can affect the radiation field in both the thorax and upper abdominal organs (up to 1 cm of change can occur during the respiratory cycle!). Several techniques have been devised to account for respiratory motion (primarily for the treatment of lung cancer):
  - *4D-CT* – a technique used to measure organ motion through 4D cross-sectional imaging obtained during various phases of the respiration cycle. This is used to quantify the range of organ motion. When target volumes are outlined (or contoured), the maximum tumor size is contoured at expiration and inspiration so that the tumor is targeted throughout the respiratory cycle. This inevitably expands the irradiated volume.
  - *Breath hold* – radiation is delivered only during a fixed phase of respiratory cycle when the target volume is in the desired location of the radiation field.
  - *Respiratory-gated treatment* – an external device predicts the location of the tumor based on the respiratory cycle phase, and radiation is delivered only when the target volume is in the desired location of the radiation field.

It is important to note that some patients will undergo other procedures before simulation. For example, some patients may need "spacer" placement for prostate RT (e.g., spacer is injected between prostate and rectum to reduce radiation dose to rectum), ovarian transposition for pelvic RT (surgical maneuver used to protect ovaries from radiation to preserve function), or fiducial marker placement (seeds implanted around soft tissue tumors to act as radiological landmark to increase accuracy and precision of radiation dose).

21.2.1.6 Contouring

After simulation is complete and the CT scan of the patient is obtained, the clinician will outline (or contour) the target volumes (described below) and the organs at risk (OARs) using a specific computer program. During your rotation, you should get your feet wet with contouring as it is part of any radiation oncologist's workflow. You can ask the resident or attending physician whether a case you saw in clinic is simple enough for you to try contouring. It will be helpful to ask a resident physician to show you the basics of how to use the contouring program. The attending physician may use some of your contours but will most likely recontour the case himself/herself in order to optimize patient care.

To begin contouring, it is important to understand the function of different target volumes (🔳 Fig. 21.6) [1].

– *Gross tumor volume (GTV)* – represents the gross tumor volume that contains the visible tumor, either on clinical examination, imaging, endoscopy, laparoscopy, or bronchoscopy. In cases of treating the postoperative bed of a tumor after excision, there is no gross tumor and therefore no GTV.

– *Clinical target volume (CTV)* – represents the additional volumes that might harbor microscopic disease, such as lymph node groups that drain the affected organ. In cases of treating the postoperative bed of tumor after excision, the CTV is an area surrounding the tumor bed possibly containing microscopic disease. CTV – GTV = subclinical malignant disease.

– *Internal target volume (ITV)* – represents the volume that accounts for physiological patient movements that are unable to be accounted for during treatment. This may include movement of the gut, beating of the heart, or respiration. The distance between the CTV and ITV is called the internal margin (IM = movement and variation of CTV). The internal margin may vary in height, breadth, and depth based on the location within the body. The ITV is a newer concept that attempts to divide treatment uncertainties

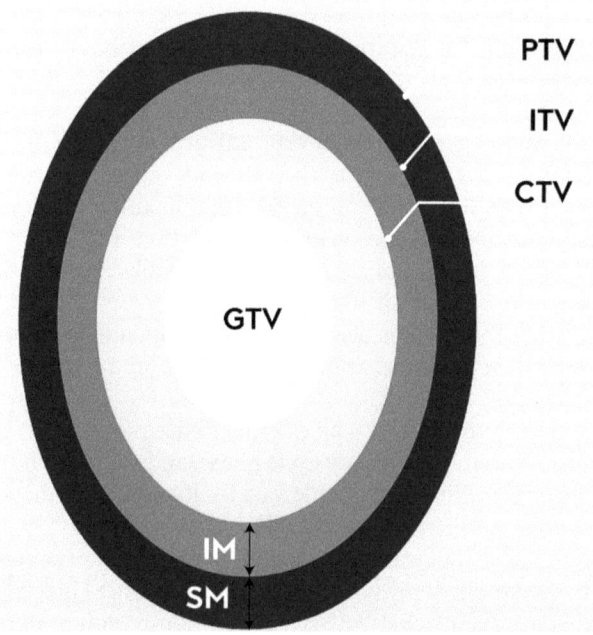

🔳 **Fig. 21.6** Standardized radiation volumes: gross tumor volume (GTV), clinical target volume (CTV), internal target volume (ITV), planning target volume (PTV), internal margin = ITV – CTV (IM, movement and variation of CTV), setup margin = PTV – ITV (SM, uncertainty in positioning and beam alignment)

into internal patient factors and external factors. If a method to reduce the effect of internal movements is used (e.g., respiratory-gated treatment), then the ITV can be substantially reduced.

- *Planning target volume (PTV)* – represents an expansion from the ITV (or CTV if no ITV is necessary) to account for external uncertainties such as patient motion, setup uncertainties, and beam uncertainty. This distance between the ITV and PTV is the setup margin (SM = uncertainty in positioning and beam alignment). Improving the external factors may reduce the external margin and allow for smaller PTV expansions.
- *Organ at risk (OAR)* – the volumes placed on organs which are susceptible to radiation. They place constraints on the beam arrangement and dose that may be delivered. OARs may have different radiation tolerances based on the tissue involved. Examples include the spinal cord, kidneys, and salivary glands.
- ◘ Figure 21.7a shows an example of contours for adjuvant RT of the left breast post-lumpectomy.

It is important to note that not all radiation plans require contouring. For example, in certain palliative cases, the physician draws "blocks" that outline the radiation field. The block takes into account both the setup uncertainty and the region of rapid dose falloff at the block borders (called the penumbra).

21.2.1.7 Treatment Planning and Quality Assurance
Plan Generation

After the target and OAR volumes are complete, dosimetrists, physicists, and physicians work iteratively together to generate a plan based on the volumes, modality of radiation selected, and constraints of the OAR placed by the

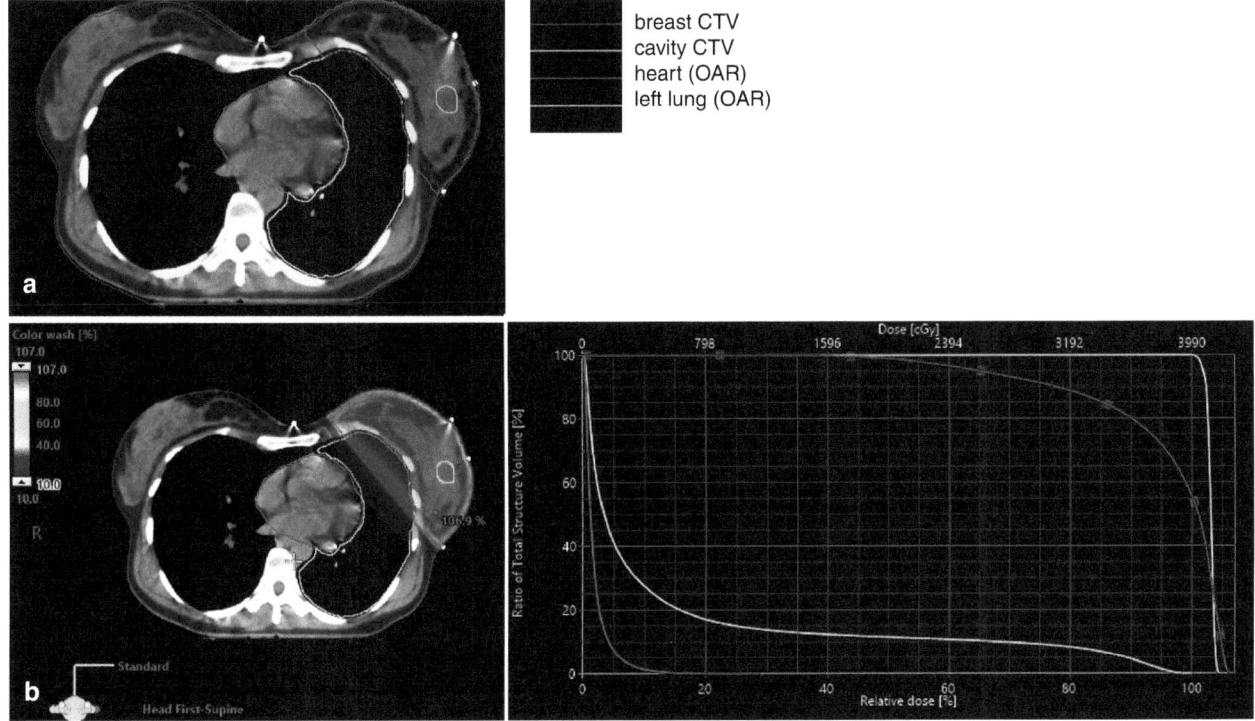

◘ **Fig. 21.7** Adjuvant RT of the left breast post-lumpectomy: **a** Contours: breast CTV (GTV not present as the patient is post-lumpectomy), cavity CTV (lumpectomy cavity receiving boost), heart (OAR), left lung (OAR). **b** Sample plan with isodose distribution on a CT axial slice and dose-volume histogram

physician. In their plan generation, they can account for tissue heterogeneity and other important physical properties. Physician input is integral at this step as clinical knowledge will help guide decisions on what radiation trade-offs are appropriate: achieving full radiation dose to target volume vs. protecting certain structures to meet patient priorities (e.g., fertility preservation). Often, several plans will be generated for evaluation by the physician. It can be helpful to spend some time with physicists and dosimetrists during your rotation to better understand how plans are generated.

Plan Evaluation

After plan generation, physicians evaluate the preliminary plans. Although medical students are often removed from plan evaluation, understanding how plans are evaluated is essential to understanding what a radiation oncologist must think about to make a final decision about the radiation treatment. The physician will evaluate the plan by considering the following [1].

Beam Placement   The arrangement of beams is usually discussed with the planner before planning. When possible, beams are placed in a way to avoid critical structures, and the field placement is confirmed on CT. The CT images with the relevant OARs are viewed as axial, sagittal, or coronal slices as well as in the beam's eye view (BEV) in order to ensure that the relative orientation of the patient and treatment machine is correct. For specific disease sites and radiation modalities, the beam arrangement is well-established (e.g., IMRT for prostate treatment).

Radiation to Target Structures   The dose that various structures will receive can be evaluated through a dose-volume histogram (DVH) or isodose distribution on a CT image (◘ Fig. 21.7b).
- *Dose-volume histogram (DVH)* – a graph of volume vs. radiation dose for each structure (target volume or OAR) in a radiation treatment plan. The DVH is used to evaluate how much dose is given to a certain volume and how much volume is receiving a certain dose. In the histogram, the x-axis is the dose (in cGy or % of prescribed dose) and the y-axis is the volume. The role of the DVH is to visualize the therapeutic ratio in graphical form where the coverage of the target is weighted against risk of toxicity to OARs.
- *Isodose distribution on CT slices* – the isodose distribution should be examined to confirm the dose distribution seen on the DVH. It is used to review coverage of the target volume, sparing of the OAR, as well as the location of hot spots and cold spots throughout the plan.
  - Specific attention should be paid to minimize the dose to OARs in order to reduce acute and chronic side effects of RT. The dose OARs can receive depends on the clinical and anatomic circumstances, and the cost-benefit ratio must be considered. The constraints that are used for OARs have been determined empirically (see QUANTEC: Quantitative Analysis of Normal Tissue Effects in the Clinic), however, they are constantly revised and updated in the disease site-specific literature.

If necessary, the physician will make changes to improve coverage of target volumes and minimize the OAR dose. He or she may do this by changing the weighting of each field, changing the field size (by shielding more of an OAR with an MLC or block), changing the beam arrangement, using a different energy beam, or re-optimizing the plan.

One way to systemically evaluate a plan is to use the acronym *CB-CHOP* (◘ Table 21.3)!

■ **Table 21.3** CB-CHOP acronym

CB-CHOP	Description
Contours	Review target volumes and OARs
Beam arrangement/ fields	Appropriate and reasonable
Coverage	Evaluate on the 3D graphic plan and DVH
Hot spots	Value and location
OAR	Review specific constraints, corresponding isodose lines on plan, and DVH
Prescription	Total dose, dose per fraction, and image guidance

21.2.1.8 Treatment
Radiation Delivery

On the day of radiation delivery, the patient will undergo the same setup as the simulation. The patient will be positioned on the treatment table, which will then be moved to exact position determined at the time of isocenter placement. Before radiation is delivered, it is confirmed that the treatment table and gantry do not collide as it rotates to different positions. The radiation time can range from less than a minute to more than 15 minutes, depending on the treatment plan and modality.

On-Treatment Visits (OTVs)

During their radiation treatment course, the physician will see the patients at least once per week to track side effects. Patients may not have side effects until a few weeks into the treatment, as the effects of radiation are cumulative. When seeing a patient for an OTV, make sure to consider the following.

History

– Management of site-specific side effects.
   – Side effects of RT are reviewed in ▶ Sects. 21.1 and 21.3 of this chapter. Make sure to manage and prophylactically treat side effects with appropriate agents (e.g., antiemetic or anti-diarrheal medication, "magic mouthwash"). Patients receiving concurrent chemotherapy are at increased risk for side effects.
– Track fatigue level weekly.
   – Fatigue is a common cumulative effect of RT irrespective of disease sites. The severity should be tracked, and the patient should be counseled that fatigue can last for weeks to months post-RT.
– Track pain level weekly.
   – Cancer patients often experience pain, either due to their disease or treatment. Their pain should be tracked weekly and appropriately treated (acetaminophen, NSAID, narcotic, gabapentin for neuropathic pain, etc.)

Physical Exam

– Skin Exam
   – Skin reactions to RT range from no skin reaction to erythema to dry or wet desquamation. Skin folds in the axilla or groin regions are especially susceptible when in the radiation field. First-line management includes moisturizers, but desquamation may require medications such as alumi-

num acetate. Rarely, treatment can be stopped for wet desquamation. Pruritus is another side effect that can be treated with corticosteroid creams. The patient should be counseled that hyperpigmentation and fibrosis can be a long-term result of radiation.
- Site-Specific Exam
  - For example, for head and neck cancers, a complete mouth exam is important to check for mucositis.

Laboratory Order

- If the patient is receiving concurrent chemotherapy, complete blood count and comprehensive metabolic panel can be obtained weekly and should be monitored. Radiation may be held for certain blood counts, but this differs based on the disease site and physician recommendation.

21.3 Disease Site Overview

This chapter provides bird's-eye view of the most common disease processes that medical students encounter on their radiation oncology rotation. As discussed above, scratching the surface of a disease site can be overwhelming. This overview is a reasonable starting point that will help clarify what role RT can play in treatment of the cancer. Following this overview, the relevant UpToDate page and National Comprehensive Cancer Network (NCCN) guidelines are a good next step as they provide the present standard of care for a specific cancer and will cite the major studies that have established guidelines. The resources listed in the Other Resources of this chapter delve into more detail about the basic anatomy, pathology, genetics, presentation, workup, treatment, and seminal clinical trials for each cancer [2, 3].

21.3.1 Central Nervous System

21.3.1.1 Glioblastoma

- Disease: Glioblastoma multiforme (GBM) is the most common primary malignant brain tumor in adults and has a poor prognosis (median survival of ~14 months). Genetic factors such as IDH-mutant and MGMT methylation are important prognostic factors.
- Pathology: Glial cells are the cell of origin. GBM falls into the grading category of World Health Organization (WHO) Grade IV (aggressive malignant tumors). WHO defines three distinct GBM subtypes: IDH-wildtype, IDH-mutant, and IDH-not otherwise specified.
- Treatment: Treatment is maximal resection with adjuvant chemoradiation. Adjuvant RT improves overall survival versus observation or chemotherapy alone after surgery and is indicated in all patients who can tolerate treatment.

21.3.1.2 Low-Grade Glioma

- Disease: Low-grade gliomas (LGGs) are a less common and heterogeneous group of primary brain tumors affecting primarily younger adults and at times pediatric patients. Molecular and genomic factors provide some prognostic stratification (IDH1status and 1p/q19 codeletion are important prognostic factors).
- Pathology: LGGs represent a heterogeneous group of WHO Grade I (non-infiltrative) and WHO Grade II (infiltrative/diffuse) glial neoplasms. Generally, oligodendrogliomas have better prognosis than astrocytomas.
- Treatment: Despite new prognostic information, treatment decisions are based on clinical factors and require patient-specific decision-making given the variety of these tumors. After surgical resection, options can include observation, RT, chemotherapy, or combined chemoradiation. High-risk patients should undergo adjuvant chemoradiation (RTOG 9802 defined high-risk patients as those 40 years and older or those below 40 who received a subtotal resection).

21.3.1.3 Meningioma

- Disease: Meningiomas are the most common primary brain tumors in adult populations. Although there is a 2 to 1 female predominance, males are slightly more likely to have atypical or malignant meningiomas. The vast majority of meningiomas are benign, but they may cause morbidity and mortality.
- Pathology: Meningiomas are classified into three WHO grades and the Simpson Grading System depending on the extent of resection (gross total resection, subtotal resection, tumor debulking).
- Treatment: Maximal surgical resection is the standard of care for surgically accessible lesions. Although it often requires a craniotomy, sphenoid wing/skull base lesions can be resected with endoscopic surgery. The tumor's Simpson Grade post-resection correlates with local failure. Based on the extent of resection and grade of the meningioma, postsurgical RT may be indicated. RT dosing depends on WHO grade. Recurrent meningiomas are generally treated with re-resection followed by RT. When meningiomas are unresectable, they are managed with fractionated RT or SRS, depending on size and location. Similar strategies are used for spinal meningiomas. In young patients, the decision to use RT should be based on the likelihood of recurrence and potential long-term sequelae of RT.

21.3.1.4 CNS-Associated Radiation Toxicity

- Acute: Fatigue, headache, exacerbation of presenting neurologic deficits, alopecia, nausea, cerebral edema, side effects related to chemotherapy.
- Late: Cognitive changes, radiation necrosis, hypopituitarism, cataracts, vision loss (rare and location dependent)

21.3.2 Head and Neck

21.3.2.1 Nasopharyngeal Cancer

- Disease: Nasopharyngeal carcinoma is rare in the United States and has higher prevalence in Southern China, Southeast Asia, and North Africa. The majority of cases are related to EBV.

- Pathology: WHO classification divided squamous cell carcinomas into keratinizing, non-keratinizing, or basaloid. Generally, keratinizing pathology has worse prognoses, and EBV-associated pathology has better prognoses.
- Treatment: Stage I disease (T1N0M0) is commonly treated with RT alone. Stage II–IVB disease is treated with concurrent chemoradiation, followed by adjuvant chemotherapy. Surgery is not routine in up-front setting, but rather reserved as salvage option.

21.3.2.2   Oropharyngeal Cancer (OPC)

- Disease: Squamous cell carcinoma (SCC) of the oropharynx is the most common head and neck cancer in the United States. There are two distinct etiologies that are classified as two distinct diseases: cases associated with tobacco and alcohol (often HPV negative) and cases associated with HPV infection.
- Pathology: Approximately 95% of oropharyngeal cancers are SCC. HPV-positive and HPV-negative cancers appear different pathologically. HPV(+) tumors commonly originate from lymphoid tissue of tonsil or the base of the tongue (BOT) and are more likely to be poorly differentiated/nonkeratinizing. HPV(−) tumors do not have a predilection for location and are often keratinizing.
- Treatment: RT is indicated for definitive treatment of OPC or in postoperative setting when surgical resection is preferred. Concurrent chemotherapy is standard for fit patients receiving definitive RT with Stage III–IV disease.

21.3.2.3   Oral Cavity Cancer

- Disease: In contrast to oropharyngeal SCC, HPV infection is not associated with oral cavity squamous cell carcinoma. Alcohol and tobacco (especially chewing tobacco) are primary risk factors for oral cavity squamous cell carcinoma.
- Pathology: SCC make up 95% of oral cavity cancers.
- Treatment: Primary management of oral cavity cancers is surgical resection with selective neck dissection, followed by postoperative RT with or without concurrent chemotherapy. Early-stage lesions can be treated with definitive RT using brachytherapy.

21.3.2.4   Laryngeal and Hypopharyngeal Cancers

- Disease: Laryngeal cancer includes squamous carcinoma originating from the supraglottis, glottis, or subglottis.
- Pathology: Ninety-five percent of tumors are squamous cell carcinoma.
- Treatment: The goal of treatment is to achieve disease control while maintaining a functional voice and intact swallowing. Early-stage glottic cancers can be treated with RT alone or microsurgery. Locoregionally advanced disease (T3–4 or node-positive) often requires either total laryngectomy (with adjuvant RT as indicated) or definitive chemoradiation.

21.3.2.5   Post-op Radiation Therapy for Head and Neck Cancers

- Surgical resection alone is often sufficient treatment for T1-T2N0-1 H&N tumors when resected with negative margins. However, some H&N cancers may require post-op radiation therapy (PORT).
- PORT for mucosal H&N SCCs depends on specific pathologic risk factors including the presence of lymphovascular invasion (LVI), perineural invasion (PNI), positive margins, extracapsular extension (ECE), and size and

number of involved nodes. Concurrent chemotherapy may also be indicated for specific high-risk factors (ECE, positive margins).

21.3.2.6 Head and Neck-Associated Radiation Toxicity

- Acute: Fatigue, dermatitis, mucositis, loss of taste, xerostomia, thrush, dysphagia, odynophagia, weight loss (may require temporary PEG tube placement and/or IV hydration during therapy)
- Late: Xerostomia, dysphagia, neck fibrosis, lifelong need for fluoride prophylaxis, risk for dental caries, osteoradionecrosis, hearing loss, trismus, hypothyroidism, optic neuritis

21.3.3 Thoracic

21.3.3.1 Early-Stage (I–II) Non-small Cell Lung Cancer (NSCLC)

- Disease: Lung cancer is the most common non-cutaneous cancer worldwide and the second most common in the United States.
- Pathology: Adenocarcinoma is the most common histology, and the majority are peripherally located. Squamous cell carcinomas make up ~20% of all lung cancers and are centrally located. Greater than 95% of clinically relevant mutations are found in adenocarcinomas (EGFR, ALK, etc.)
- Treatment:
  - Early Stage (I–II) – Surgical resection when appropriate is the standard of care for operable early-stage NSCLC. Adjuvant RT is not indicated in completely resected Stage I/II patients. For medically inoperable patients, SBRT is a reasonable alternative to surgery. For high-risk operable patients, it is unclear whether surgery or SBRT is superior.
  - Late Stage (III–IV) – The treatment of Stage III NSCLC depends on patient performance, nodal status, and comorbidity and includes a combination of chemotherapy, RT, and/or surgery.
  - Oligometastatic disease – Patients with Stage IV NSCLC with one or a limited number of metastases may have oligometastatic disease that can be treated definitively. Patients with good performance status and one to three metastases usually undergo local therapy (ablative or surgical therapy) with systemic therapy. Local therapy may include RT, including stereotactic techniques such as SBRT.

21.3.3.2 Small Cell Lung Cancer

- Disease: SCLC represents ~15% of all lung cancer diagnoses and occurs almost exclusively in smokers. SCLC is classically described as either limited stage (LS-SCLC – historically defined as fitting within one radiation portal) or extensive stage (ES-SCLC – metastatic). Outcomes are generally poor.
- Pathology: SCLC is of neuroendocrine origin.
- Treatment: Treatment for LS-SCLC includes concurrent chemoradiation followed by adjuvant chemotherapy, with consideration for prophylactic cranial irradiation offered for those who respond to therapy. Treatment for ES-SCLC includes chemotherapy and immunotherapy, with consideration for adjuvant thoracic RT and prophylactic cranial irradiation in partial or complete responders.

21.3.3.3 Thoracic-Associated Radiation Toxicity

- Acute: Fatigue, cough, shortness of breath, pneumonitis, esophagitis
- Late: Pneumonitis, cardiac toxicity, brachial plexopathy, rib fracture

21.3.4 Breast

21.3.4.1 Ductal and Lobular Carcinoma In Situ

- Disease: Ductal carcinoma in situ (DCIS) makes up ~20% of all breast cancers. Up to 30% of DCIS cases can progress to invasive breast cancer over 30 years if treatment is not recieved. Lobular carcinoma in situ (LCIS) is distinct from DCIS.
- Pathology: In DCIS, the basement membrane is preserved despite malignant cells arising from the ductal epithelium. LCIS can be associated with or without atypical ductal hyperplasia or atypical lobular hyperplasia and is not considered a malignancy.
- Treatment: DCIS treatment includes either breast conservation therapy (lumpectomy plus adjuvant RT) or mastectomy. After lumpectomy, adjuvant RT results in risk reduction for local recurrence but no improvement in overall survival. Absolute risk of local recurrence depends on tumor characteristics, such as grade, histologic subtype, size, estrogen receptor status, and margin status. LCIS treatment usually does not require a negative margin excision or adjuvant RT.

21.3.4.2 Early-Stage (I–II) Breast Cancer

- Disease: Breast cancer is the most common cancer and leading cause of cancer death among women. Lifetime risk is one in eight women with a median age of diagnosis at 61. Risk factors include estrogen exposure, family history, or genetics (BRCA1, 60–80% lifetime risk of breast cancer; BRCA2, 50–60% lifetime risk of breast cancer).
- Pathology: Breast carcinomas arise from epithelial elements and consist of a diverse group of tumors. Estrogen receptor (ER) and/or progesterone receptor (PR) is expressed in 70% of tumors. HER2 (a receptor tyrosine kinase) amplification is seen in 25–30% of invasive cancers. Triple negative breast cancer is an aggressive tumor in which tumors do not express ER, PR, or HER2, and accounts for ~15% of cases. BRCA mutation carriers are more likely than non-carriers to have triple negative breast cancer.
- Treatment:
  - Early Stage (I–II): Treatment commonly involves surgical resection followed by adjuvant therapy (CHT, RT, and/or endocrine therapy) depending on pathology. For patients with unifocal cancers who desire organ preservation, breast-conserving surgery + adjuvant RT (whole breast irradiation; WBI) is usually an equivalent alternative to mastectomy. In patients with limited axillary nodal involvement on sentinel lymph node biopsy, a complete axillary lymph node dissection may not be necessary if the patients undergo WBI (although some patients may receive regional node RT). Lower-risk patients (older age, T1N0, ER+, negative margins) may consider partial breast RT, intraoperative RT, or endocrine therapy alone after lumpectomy.
  - Locally Advanced: Locally advanced breast cancer generally includes clinical Stage IIB (T3N0) to Stage III. Treatment includes a combination of chemotherapy (neoadjuvant or adjuvant), surgery, and adjuvant RT. Radiation may include WBI plus regional nodal irradiation.

21

21.3.4.3 Breast-Associated Radiation Toxicity
- Acute: Fatigue, erythema, pruritus, tenderness, desquamation
- Late: Hyper-/hypopigmentation, volume loss, fibrosis, rib fracture, lymphedema, pulmonary fibrosis, and cardiac toxicity

21.3.5 Gastrointestinal

21.3.5.1 Esophageal Cancer
- Disease: Esophageal cancer includes squamous cell carcinomas (SCCs) arising from upper to middle esophagus (often associated with chronic alcohol and tobacco use) or adenocarcinomas arising from the distal esophagus or gastroesophageal junction (often associated with chronic reflux, obesity, and Barrett's esophagus).
- Pathology: SCC accounts for 90% of cases globally, but adenocarcinoma comprises 70% of cases in North America and Western Europe.
- Treatment: External beam RT is utilized in definitive, neoadjuvant, and adjuvant settings. The use and sequencing of modalities in trimodal therapy (surgery, CHT, and RT) remains controversial. Brachytherapy may be beneficial for specific patients (for boost or for palliation).

21.3.5.2 Gastric Cancer
- Disease: Patients with gastric cancer often present with locoregionally advanced or metastatic disease.
- Pathology: Adenocarcinoma is the most common histology (90–95%). MALT lymphoma is the second most common histology.
- Treatment: For cT2-4 or node-positive locoregionally confined disease, the most common treatment is neoadjuvant chemotherapy followed by surgery. Surgery can be either partial or total gastrectomy depending on disease location and burden.

21.3.5.3 Pancreatic Cancer
- Disease: Pancreatic cancer has a poor prognosis. Surgical resection can prove challenging due to nearby anatomy, and tumors are relatively resistant to chemotherapy and RT. Mean survival ranges from 3 to 24 months depending on the stage of disease and the performance status of the patient.
- Pathology: Greater than 80% are ductal adenocarcinoma. Approximately 60% arise from head and 15% in body or tail, and 20% diffusely involve pancreas.
- Treatment: Treatment depends on whether the tumor is resectable, borderline resectable, locally advanced/unrespectable, or metastatic.
  - Resectable: Only about 20% of patients have resectable disease at presentation, and treatment consists of surgery followed by either adjuvant chemotherapy or chemoradiation.
  - Borderline resectable: Treatment often consists of neoadjuvant chemotherapy followed by chemoradiation or SBRT and then reassessment for surgery. Only ~60% of these patients will undergo surgery to a clear margin.
  - Locally advanced/unresectable: Treatment includes a combination of chemotherapy +/− radiation.
  - Metastatic: Treatment includes single or multiagent systemic therapy +/− palliative surgery, biliary stent, or RT.

21.3.5.4 Rectal Cancer

- Disease: Colorectal cancer (CRC) is the third most common cancer in the United States. Patients with familial adenomatous polyposis (FAP) or hereditary nonpolyposis colorectal cancer (HNPCC) have a higher risk of developing CRC at younger age.
- Pathology: Greater than 90% of rectal cancers are adenocarcinomas.
- Treatment: Surgical resection is standard and includes total mesorectal excision (TME). TME is achieved by either low anterior resection (LAR; sphincter sparing) or abdominoperineal resection (APR; not sphincter sparing). Neoadjuvant RT is standard for high-risk patients (either node-positive or cT3-4) and reduces the local recurrence rate.

21.3.5.5 Anal Cancer

- Disease: Anal canal is a relatively rare but highly curable cancer.
- Pathology: 75–80% are squamous cell carcinoma.
- Treatment: In non-metastatic patients, the standard of care is concurrent chemoRT. Select T1N0 patients with well-differentiated anal margin cancers without high-risk features may be treated with wide local excision with 1-cm margins. IMRT has been shown to reduce hematologic, GI, and skin toxicities.

21.3.5.6 Gastrointestinal-Associated Radiation Toxicity

- Acute: Fatigue, dermatitis, gastritis/esophagitis, nausea, vomiting, diarrhea, appetite loss, weight loss, stomach ulcers
- Late: Liver/renal dysfunction, bowel obstruction, stomach/bowel ulcers, strictures, pneumonitis, pericarditis, dry/hyperpigmented skin

21.3.6 Genitourinary

21.3.6.1 Prostate Cancer

- Disease: Prostate cancer is the most common non-cutaneous malignancy in men and second most common cause of cancer death in men. Prostate cancer is stratified into low risk, intermediate risk, and high risk.
- Pathology: Ninety-five percent of prostate cancers are adenocarcinomas. The Gleason Score is a grading system based on the architectural structure of the malignant cells. Two core needle biopsies with the most prevalent and highest grade are summed together for the Gleason Score. The grade for each core needle biopsy ranges from 3 to 5; therefore, the final Gleason Score ranges from 6 to 10.
- Treatment:
  - Low risk: Organ-confined disease typically detected by a screening PSA or on digital rectal exam (T1–T2a), with a PSA <10 ng/mL and Gleason Score (GS) ≤6. Standard treatment options all have prostate cancer-specific survival of >95%. Therefore, treatment selection is guided by side effect profiles and patient preference. Treatment options include:
    - Active Surveillance
    - Prostatectomy

- EBRT or Brachytherapy

Most guidelines recommend treatment only if life expectancy is >10 years.

- Intermediate risk: Intermediate-risk disease includes cT2b-c disease or GS 7 or PSA 10–20 ng/mL. Most patients with intermediate risk are expected to benefit from definitive therapy, compared to active surveillance. Intermediate-risk prostate cancers are further stratified into favorable and unfavorable risk in order to guide treatment (unfavorable risk is defined by 2+ intermediate risk factors or GS 4 + 3, or ≥50% biopsy cores positive). Therapeutic options include:
  - EBRT ± short-term androgen deprivation therapy (ADT; 4–6 months)
  - Brachytherapy alone
  - Radical prostatectomy: consider adjuvant or salvage EBRT for adverse features (+ margins, seminal vesicle invasion, extracapsular extension, detectable postoperative PSA)
- High risk: High-risk disease includes cT3a or GS 8–10 or PSA>20ng/mL. Very-high-risk disease includes T3b-4 or Primary GS 5 or >4 cores with GS 8–10. Nearly all those with high-risk disease are expected to benefit from definitive therapy. Treatment options include:
  - EBRT + long-term ADT (2–3 years).
  - EBRT + brachytherapy boost ± long-term ADT.
  - Radical prostatectomy: consider adjuvant or salvage EBRT for adverse features (+ margins, seminal vesicle invasion, extracapsular extension, detectable postoperative PSA). If lymph node positive, consider ADT and pelvic EBRT.
  - ADT alone in patients who are not candidates for local therapy.

21.3.6.2 Prostate-Associated Radiation Toxicity

- Acute: Fatigue, dysuria, urinary frequency, rectal urgency. Pelvic node treatment may cause diarrhea and cramping.
- Late: Less common but may include radiation cystitis, urethral stricture, radiation proctitis, bowel obstruction, and fistula.

21.3.7 Gynecology

21.3.7.1 Cervical Cancer

- Disease: The disease burden of cervical cancer is much higher in lower-income countries. The incidence of cervical cancers have significantly declined in the United States with use of Pap smears for screening. Vaccines are also available that prevent development of cervical cancer.
- Pathology: Most common types of cervical cancer include squamous cell carcinomas (~70%) and adenocarcinomas (~20%). Adenocarcinomas are more common in younger patients and often present as larger tumors with higher risk of local failure. The majority of cervical cancers are HPV-mediated.
- Treatment: Treatment at early stages often includes surgical excision. Later stages of disease require RT +/− chemotherapy. For definitive treatment, EBRT is followed by an intracavitary brachytherapy boost.

21.3.7.2 Cervix-Associated Radiation Toxicity

- Acute: Fatigue, diarrhea, rectal urgency, bloating or cramping, bladder or urethral irritation, skin erythema, and possible desquamation if inguinal lymph nodes or distal vagina/vulva is irradiated.
- Late: Rectal bleeding, bowel obstruction, hematuria, fistula (GI or urinary), vaginal ulceration/necrosis (generally heals within 6 months with local care), vaginal stenosis (use dilators), infertility, ovarian failure, osteopenia leading to hip and sacral insufficiency fractures.

21.3.8 Palliative

21.3.8.1 Brain Metastases

- Disease: Brain metastases are the most common intracranial tumor.
- Pathology: Most common histologies include lung, breast, and melanoma.
- Treatment: Treatment options include surgery, whole brain radiation therapy (WBRT), or SRS and can be performed in many combinations. Patient selection for varying treatments depends on performance status, number of lesions, size of the lesions, histology, and status of extracranial disease. Surgery is reserved for large or symptomatic lesions.

21.3.8.2 Bone Metastases

- Disease: Approximately 80% of patients with advanced cancer develop bone metastases. Approximately 2/3 of patients experience pain improvement with RT palliation.
- Pathology: Tissue diagnosis may not be needed for patients with metastatic bone disease or pathologic fracture. However, tissue diagnosis may be necessary for patients with solitary bone lesions without a cancer history or as a first metastatic relapse.
- Treatment: The most common RT regimens include 8 Gy in 1 fx, 20 Gy in 5 fx, and 30 Gy in 10 fx. The decided treatment technique depends on the patient's performance status, logistics, tumor size, tumor location, soft tissue component, histology, previous surgery, neurologic deficits, impending fracture, prior RT, and physician preference. For uncomplicated bone metastases, there is no difference in pain control between single and multiple fraction regimens (multi-fraction regimens are used when the patient has a longer prognosis and may benefit from longer-term pain relief). The role for SBRT/SRS is still being determined.

21.3.8.3 Spinal Cord Compression

- Disease: Malignant spinal cord compression is an oncologic emergency and defined as any radiographic compression of the spinal cord or cauda equina secondary to an extradural or intramedullary malignancy. The most common presenting symptom is pain and the severity and reversibility of symptoms vary.
- Pathology: Occurs through two main mechanisms. External compression typically arises from the vertebral body and internal compression through intramedullary metastasis.
- Treatment: Initial treatment usually involves steroids. Surgical evaluation should be obtained, and if surgical intervention is required, postoperative palliative RT should follow. If no surgical intervention is indicated, the patient may recieve RT alone.

21

References

1. Berman AT, Plastaras JP, Vapiwala N. Radiation oncology: a primer for medical students. J Cancer Educ. 2013;28(3):547–53.
2. Hristov B, Lin S, Christodouleas J. Radiation oncology: a question based review. 3rd ed. Philadelphia: Wolters Kluwer; 2019.
3. Ward M, Tendulkar R, Videtic G. Essentials of clinical radiation oncology. New York: demosMedical, Springer Publishing Company; 2018.

Other Resources

Hristov B, Lin S, Christodouleas J. Radiation oncology: a question based review. 3rd ed. Philadelphia: Wolters Kluwer; 2019.
Ward M, Tendulkar R, Videtic G. Essentials of clinical radiation oncology. New York: demosMedical, Springer Publishing Company; 2018.
Radoncreview.org

Dermatology

Connie Zhong

Contents

22.1 Introduction

Congratulations on choosing to do a dermatology elective! Dermatology is a unique field that emphasizes visual inspection, palpation, integration of the patient's medical history, and clinicopathologic correlation. While dermatology is a broad field with many nuances, as a medical student, you should aim to recognize the most common dermatologic diseases and understand their management. This chapter will help you succeed in your dermatology rotation by providing an overview of the structure of the skin and how to approach a History and Physical in dermatology, write a note and present, and distinguish common skin conditions.

22.1.1 Skin Structure

The skin is the largest organ of the body with important functions of maintaining internal homeostasis and providing a barrier to the outside. An understanding of the structure of the skin and the appearance of lesions based on the affected skin level will help you diagnose the condition and determine the type of skin biopsy to perform. Below are descriptions of what skin conditions may look like depending on what level of the skin is affected and an outline of key structures you should know in each layer.

The skin is composed of the epidermis, dermis, and subcutis (Fig. 22.1).

22.1.1.1 Epidermis
Skin conditions that affect the epidermis often look dry and scaly (loose dead skin) or rough (e.g., lichenified). The epidermis is divided into four layers (Mnemonic: "*Come, let's get sunburned!*") (Fig. 22.2).
1. Stratum *corneum*: composed of dead cells (specifically keratinocytes) that act as the major physical barrier.
2. Stratum *lucidum*: thin, clear layer of dead cells, named for its translucent appearance; readily visible under microscopy only in areas of thick skin such as the palms and soles.
3. Stratum *granulosum*: keratinocytes in this layer have distinctive dark granules. *Filaggrin*, a protein that retains water in keratinocytes, is found in this layer. Mutations in filaggrin can cause *atopic dermatitis* (eczema).
4. Stratum *spinosum*: made of keratinocytes, which produce keratin (a fibrous protein). In this layer, there are "spines" (i.e., desmosomes) that hold the

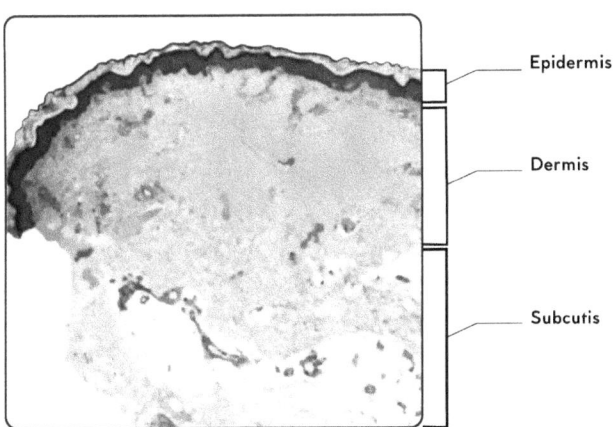

Epidermis

Dermis

Subcutis

 Fig. 22.1   Structure of the skin

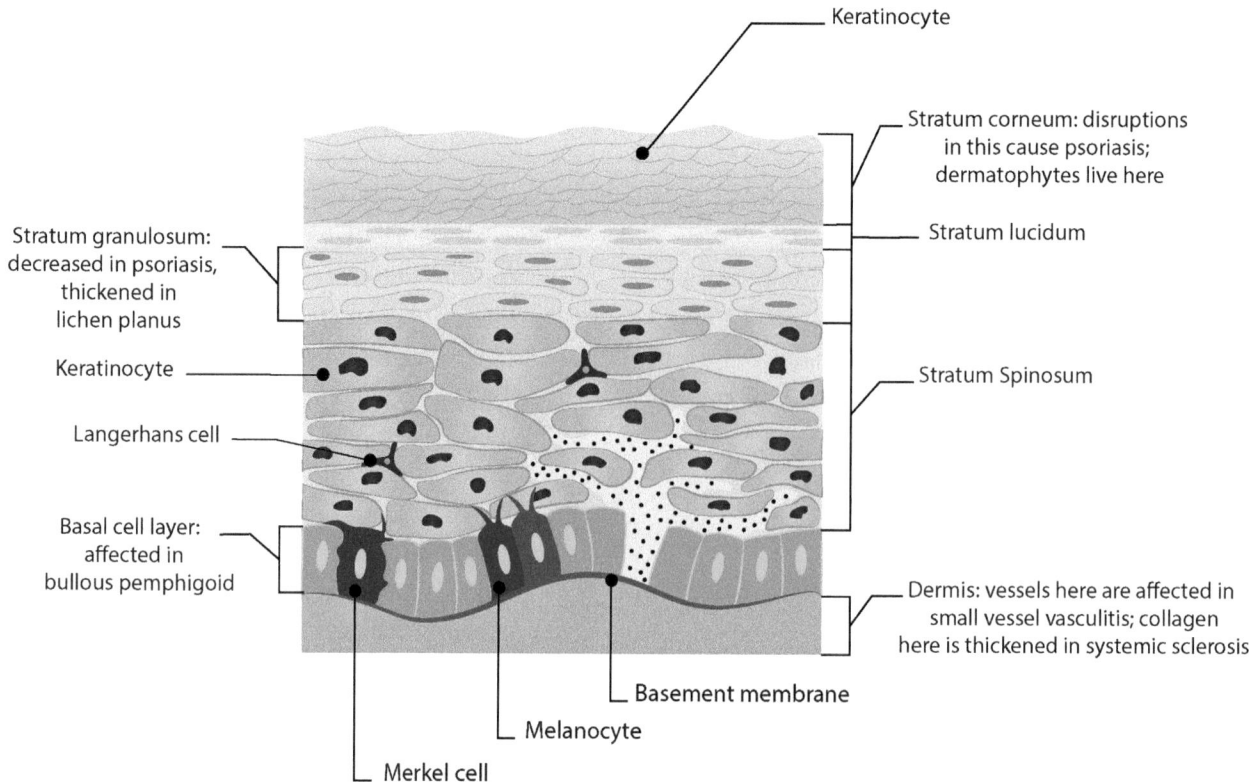

Keratinocyte

Stratum corneum: disruptions in this cause psoriasis; dermatophytes live here

Stratum lucidum

Stratum granulosum: decreased in psoriasis, thickened in lichen planus

Keratinocyte

Langerhans cell

Stratum Spinosum

Basal cell layer: affected in bullous pemphigoid

Dermis: vessels here are affected in small vessel vasculitis; collagen here is thickened in systemic sclerosis

Basement membrane

Melanocyte

Merkel cell

Fig. 22.2 Structure of the epidermis

cells together. *Langerhans cells* are tissue macrophages that live in this layer. These cells are the first line of immunologic defense in the skin.

5. *B*asal cell layer: where skin *stem cells*, *melanocytes*, and *Merkel cells* are located. Melanocytes produce melanin to protect the skin from UV radiation, and Merkel cells act as mechanoreceptors.

22.1.1.2 Dermis

The dermis is situated under the epidermis; the layers are separated by the dermal-epidermal junction, which is a key site of pathology in many diseases that cause blistering of the skin. The dermis is much thicker than the epidermis and provides stability and flexibility for the skin. Skin conditions that affect the dermis can present in a variety of ways, such as cystic, nodular, or blistering, depending on what structure of the dermis is affected.

The dermis is composed of the following components (■ Fig. 22.3). You won't be expected to memorize all of this, but note that the dermis has blood vessels which can be affected in vasculitis, mast cells that can trigger urticaria (hives), and the pilosebaceous unit (see below).

1. Blood vessels
2. Nerves
3. Collagen: provides strength
4. Elastic fibers: provide elasticity

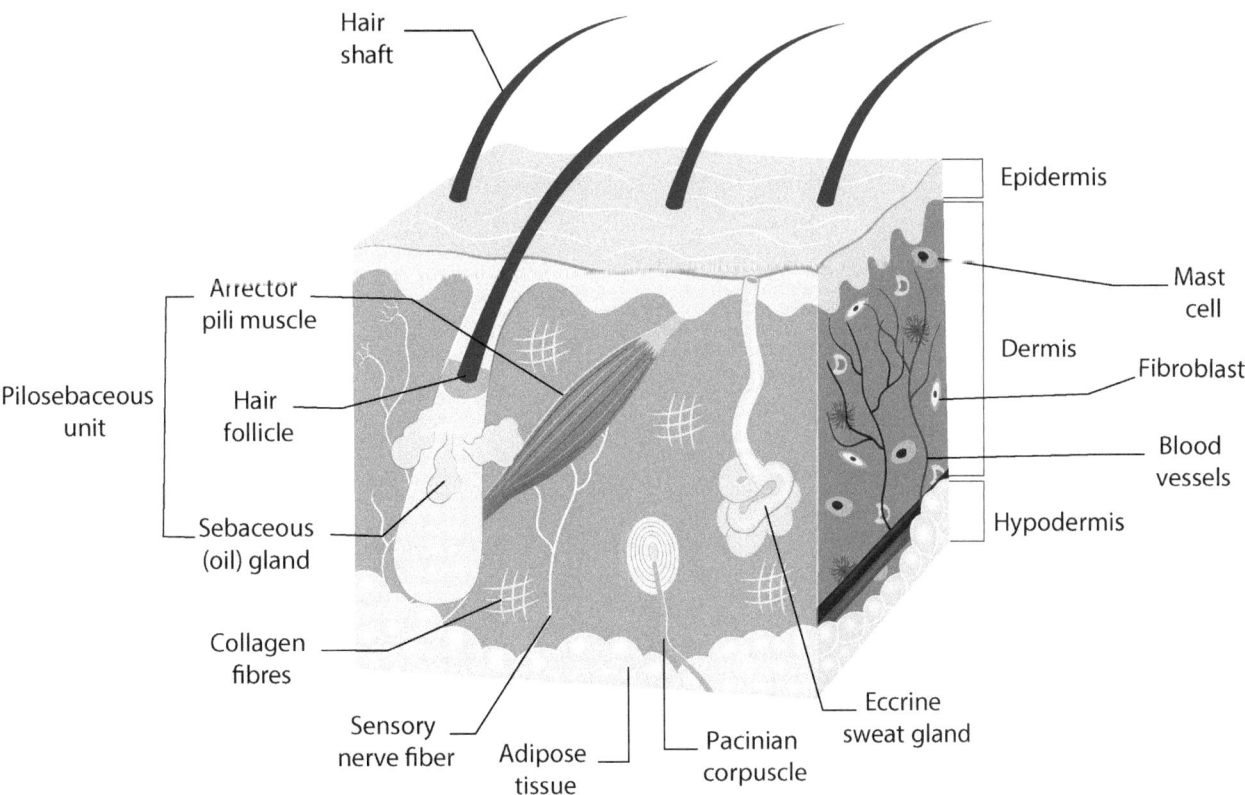

☐ Fig. 22.3 Structure of the dermis

5. Extracellular matrix
6. Mast cells: responsible for immediate-type hypersensitivity reactions; cause urticaria (hives)
7. Fibroblasts: important for wound healing
8. Cutaneous appendages
   1. Eccrine glands: regulate body temperature; under cholinergic innervation.
      1. They are the major sweat glands and are found in all skin, though have the highest density in *palms and soles.*
   2. Apocrine sweat glands: develop in the presence of androgens; bacterial action on apocrine sweat causes body odor.
      1. Found most commonly in the *axilla, nipples, and anogenital region.*
   3. Sebaceous glands.
      1. Located *everywhere except the palms and soles.*
   4. Hair follicles.
   5. *Pilosebaceous units:* composed of the hair follicle, sebaceous gland, and arrector pili muscle (cause hairs to stand on end – goosebumps!).

22.1.1.3 Subcutis

The subcutis is below the dermis and is the "fat layer." It is made of adipocytes and insulates the body. Skin conditions that affect the subcutis are deep-seated and nodular. An example of a disorder of the subcutis is erythema nodosum, a form of panniculitis (inflammation of subcutaneous fat).

Table 22.1 Primary morphology

Characteristic	What the lesion is called if <1 cm in size	What the lesion is called if >1 cm in size
Flat	Macule	Patch
Raised	Papule	Plaque
Serous, fluid-filled	Vesicle	Bullae
Deep-seated and raised	--	Nodule
Filled with white blood cells and bacterial debris	Pustule	Furuncle (if around hair follicle) or abscess (> several centimeters)

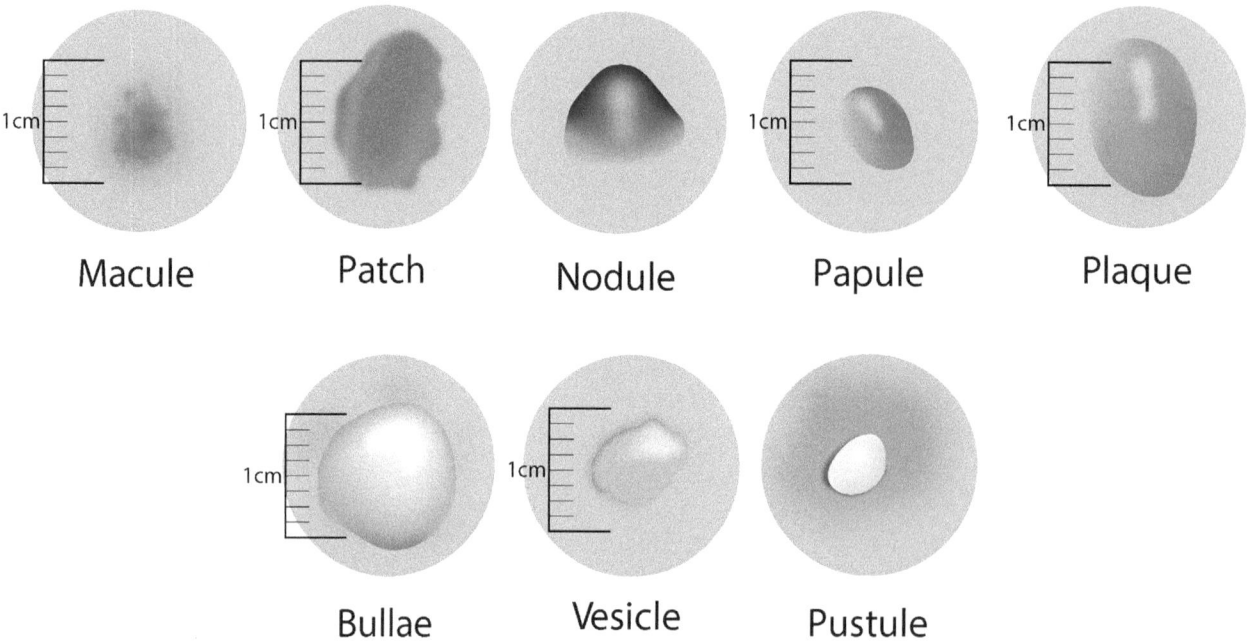

Fig. 22.4 Primary morphologies

22.2 Fundamentals of Dermatology

22.2.1 How to Approach a Skin Lesion

Dermatology is a very visual specialty, and being able to notice the details of a skin lesion is key. One good way to practice is by looking at everyday objects and observing them in detail.

When examining skin lesions, you can use a systematic approach, such as the following:

1. What is the primary morphology of the skin lesion? (Table 22.1, Fig. 22.4). The easiest way to make sure you are looking at a primary lesion is to first have the patient try and point out lesions on their body that resemble what the lesion looked like when it first appeared. See below on how to describe morphology.

Secondary morphologies

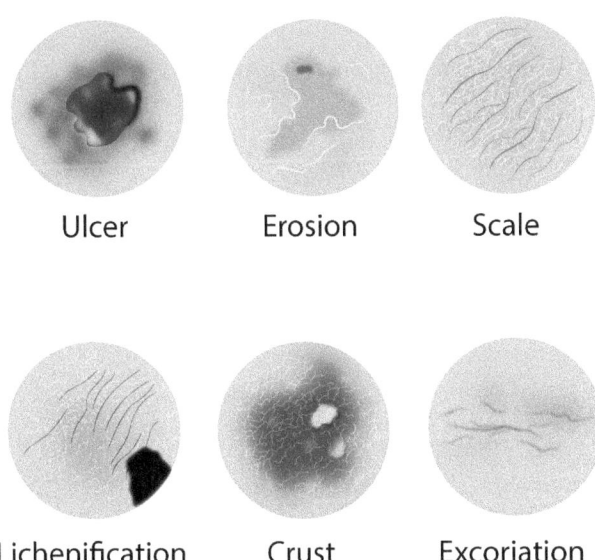

Ulcer   Erosion   Scale

Lichenification   Crust   Excoriation

◧ **Fig. 22.5**   Secondary lesions

2. Where is the lesion located? If applicable, where did the eruption start and where did it spread to?
3. Note any secondary lesions (below) as a clue to the symptoms of the lesion and how it is evolving.

Dermatologists use the term "morphology" to describe what a *primary* skin lesion looks like. Understanding the proper terms used to describe morphology is key to communicating what the skin condition looks like and establishing a differential diagnosis.

Primary skin lesions can be divided into the following categories.

Important subtypes of skin lesions are:

- Cyst: well-defined nodule filled with fluid or other debris.
- Wheal: edematous papule/plaque with erythematous borders and pale center; often transient in nature; one example is a hive.
- Telangiectasia: small dilated blood vessels that blanch on diascopy (see ▶ Sect. 22.2.5.2 "Other Clinical Exam Techniques").

Secondary lesions are changes to the primary lesion (◧ Fig. 22.5). These changes can be due to trauma, such as scratching, or evolution of the primary lesion.

- Erosion: loss of epidermis (often appears red with serous fluid); will heal without scarring
- Ulcer: loss of epidermis and part or all of the dermis (may be bleeding or have crusting; may see the ▶ Sect. 22.1.1.3); will typically scar
- Scale: flakes of stratum corneum
- Crust: dried blood, pus, or other exudates
- Oozing: active drainage present
- Excoriation: scratch marks
- Lichenification: thickening of epidermis with increased skin markings, leading to leathery appearance

Koebner phenomenon is the spreading of a skin condition to sites of trauma (e.g., when a patient scratches his or her arm and develops psoriasis there)

- Scar: replacement of normal skin with fibrosis secondary to trauma or disease process. Can oftentimes be indurated, which means that there is hardening of the skin.
- Fissure: superficial cut, typically linear
- Atrophy: thinning of skin
- Petechiae/purpura/ecchymoses: non-blanchable bleeding into skin

You may also want to describe the shape or configuration of the lesions with the below terminology:
- Nummular: coin-shaped
- Annular: ring-shaped
- Targetoid: like a target (ring-shaped with center involvement)
- Umbilicated: indentation in the center
- Retiform/reticulate: web or lace-like; usually occurs due to vasculature pathology
- Linear: in a line
- Serpiginous: wavy like a snake

Besides the shape and configuration, you should also describe the distribution of lesions.
- Grouped: multiple lesions clustered together
- Focal: in a particular area of the body
- Generalized: distributed generally throughout the body
- Extensors: on the elbows and knees
- Flexures: on the antecubital or popliteal fossa
- Intertriginous: in areas of skin folds, such as armpits or groin
- Palms and soles
- Photo-exposed areas: face, upper chest, and back (like in lupus)

Finally, you may also describe the borders of the lesion and how distinct the lesion is from the surrounding skin.
- Well-circumscribed or well-demarcated
- Poorly circumscribed or poorly demarcated

Below is a template with a mnemonic to help you put together a concise and detailed description of skin lesions (▶ Box 22.1).

Mnemonic for the components of a good description: Annie needed colorful crayons since preschool started (anatomic site, number, configuration, color, size, primary lesion, secondary lesions)

> Box 22.1   Template for Describing Skin Lesions
> Now, let's put all of what we learned together! Below is a template and example of how you can describe a skin lesion on rounds or in your notes:
> Template: Located on (anatomic site/s), there are (#) (configuration) (color) (size) (primary lesion) with associated (secondary change features)
> Example: Located on the lateral right thigh, there is one annular pink 4 cm plaque with overlying scale and excoriation marks

Let's practice! Describe the following lesions. We have included a sample description below the images for you to compare your description with.
   Sample descriptions:
1. Located on the upper chest, there are hundreds of diffusely scattered erythematous follicular-based papules and pustules with associated comedones (◉ Fig. 22.6).

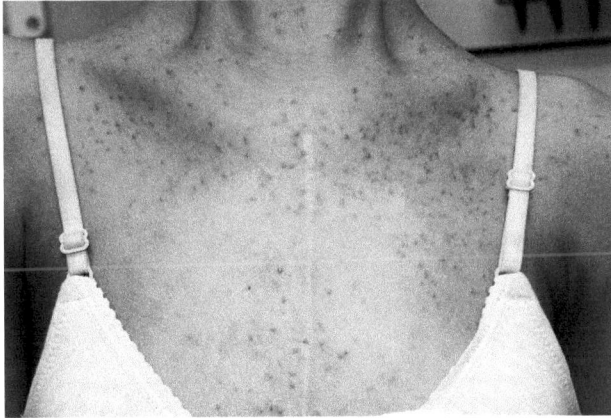

◨ **Fig. 22.6** Practice describing these lesions

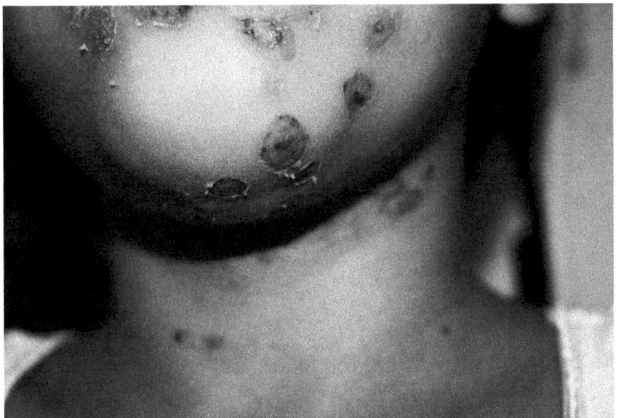

◨ **Fig. 22.7** Practice describing these lesions

2. Located on the chin and upper neck are approximately 15 erosions 1 cm in diameter, some with honey-colored crusting (◨ Fig. 22.7).
3. Located 1 cm below the left ear is a 1 cm dark brown papule with focal areas of darker pigmentation and hairs growing normally throughout (◨ Fig. 22.8).

22.2.2 **Fitzpatrick Skin Type**

The Fitzpatrick skin type is a way to classify skin based on the skin's reaction to sunlight (◨ Fig. 22.9). It is based on the amount of melanin in skin, which gives skin its color. The more melanin in skin, the darker the skin color and the quicker the skin tans and the less likely it will burn in the sun. The less melanin, the lighter the skin, the harder it is to tan, and the more likely it will burn. This is useful to document in dermatology notes to determine the patient's susceptibility to skin cancers or scarring. Lighter skin phototypes may be more susceptible to basal and squamous cell cancers, whereas darker skin phototypes may be more susceptible to post-inflammatory hyperpigmentation.

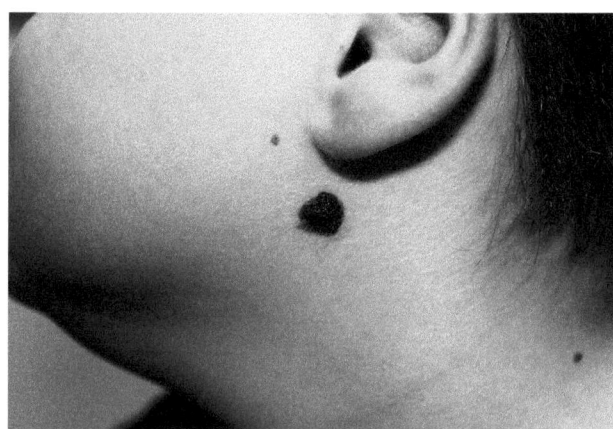

Fig. 22.8 Practice describing these lesions

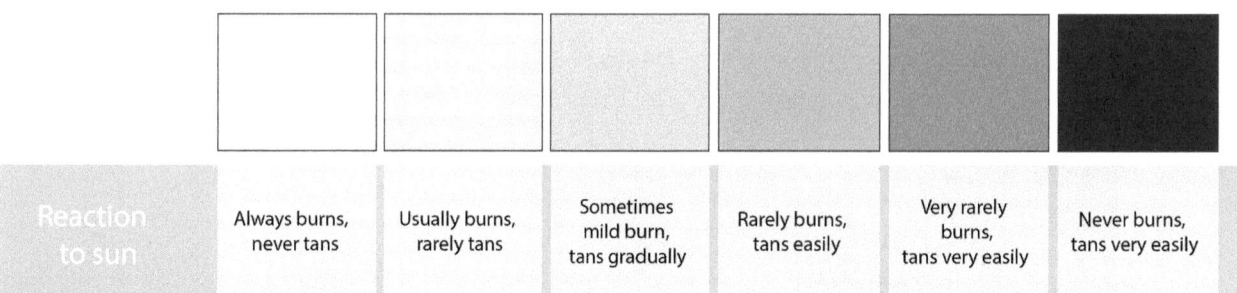

| Reaction to sun | Always burns, never tans | Usually burns, rarely tans | Sometimes mild burn, tans gradually | Rarely burns, tans easily | Very rarely burns, tans very easily | Never burns, tans very easily |

Fig. 22.9 The six Fitzpatrick skin types

Fun fact: the thinner the vehicle (excluding oil), the more it may sting because of the surfactants and emulsifiers in those vehicles. These vehicles are also less occlusive with worse percutaneous absorption, so they are not as effective for thick lesions.

To determine how much body surface area is affected, know that one patient's palm size is equal to 1% body surface area.

22.2.3 **Basics of Dermatologic Therapy**

22.2.3.1 **Topical Steroids**

Topical medications are commonly prescribed in dermatology. They are typically beneficial for treating the skin directly without generating systemic side effects. There are several vehicles in which these medications, such as corticosteroids, can come in. Below are the most common types of vehicles and when they should be used (Table 22.2).

For topical steroids, you will not only need to consider the vehicle but also the potency (strength) of each steroid type. As a medical student, it will be helpful to remember one steroid from each class (Table 22.3). Use higher (numerically low) class steroids on thicker skin, such as the back, arms, and legs, or for more severe conditions. Use lower (numerically high) class steroids on thinner skin, such as the face, eyelid, intertriginous areas (body folds), and genital areas. Two things that may change the potency of the steroid are the vehicle and the dosage: the more occlusive the vehicle, the higher the potency (e.g., ointments are more occlusive and potent than creams and lotions); the higher the dosage of steroid, the more potent the steroid (to the extent that the steroid may shift up or down a potency class). While you will not need to know off the top of your head the exact dosages of topical steroids, you can look on UpToDate or VisualDx for the correct dosage of steroid for a particular disease.

While steroids are fantastic for inflammatory lesions, prolonged use of steroids can have serious *side effects*, including skin atrophy, telangiectasias, and striae. As such, the general recommendation is to not use a topical steroid

22

□ Table 22.2 Pros and cons of various vehicles for dermatologic therapy from most to least occlusive

Vehicle	Pros	Cons
Ointment	Does not sting; occlusive; good for thick, hyperkeratotic lesions	Greasy
Cream	Good for intertriginous areas and acute exudative inflammation	May sting; less occlusive
Oil	Less sting; keratolytic (removes scale); good for scalp	Greasy
Foam	Good for scalp/hair and inflamed skin	May be expensive
Lotion	Good for hairy areas and acute exudative inflammation; easy to apply; less greasy	May sting; less occlusive
Gel	Good for scalp and hairy areas; good for acne as it can dry out pustules	May sting; less occlusive

□ Table 22.3 Steroid potency and preferred locations

Class/potency	Steroid example	Where to use
I (very high)	Clobetasol	Thicker skin such as back, arms, and legs
II (high)	Fluocinonide	
III–V (medium)	Triamcinolone, mometasone	
VI–VII (low)	Desonide, hydrocortisone	Thinner skin such as face, eyelids, genital region, and intertriginous areas (e.g., armpits)

consecutively for more than 14 days on any individual lesion (usually 2 weeks on, 2 weeks off, though can be adjusted for severity of lesion). *Use the least potent class of steroid that is effective.*

One fingertip worth of steroid = 0.5 g treats up to 2% BSA. Thus, for someone who has 2% BSA of psoriasis, if he or she needs enough steroids to apply BID × 20 days, you will need 20 g of steroid. It takes about 30 g to cover an average adult human body in one application. In general, you want to avoid under-prescribing a steroid amount. For a couple patches of psoriasis, you may choose to prescribe a 60 g tube of steroid. For a whole body rash, you may choose to prescribe a 1 lb jar.

Besides topical steroids, you may also use a wide variety of medications, depending on the underlying condition. Below are some basic principles of therapy in dermatology (□ Table 22.4). Details of the skin conditions are described in "Differential Diagnoses."

◻ **Table 22.4** Other medications you may want to consider

If you suspect	Potential treatment
Bacterial infection	Topical antibiotics or oral/IV antibiotics if the infection is severe or if the patient is immunocompromised
Fungal infection (e.g., the plaque is annular and has a scaly, active border)	Topical antifungal. Instances where topical antifungals will not work are tinea capitis and onychomycosis – you will need oral antifungals in those cases
Autoimmune skin disorder	Immunosuppressive medications, such as prednisone, rituximab, azathioprine, mycophenolate mofetil, etc.
Wounds/ulcers	Topical antimicrobial ointments, growth factors, and wound dressings (see ▶ Sect. 22.2.3.3 for more details). If very severe, patient may need to undergo surgical debridement

22.2.3.2 Cryotherapy

Cryotherapy is a procedure that uses extremely cold temperatures (in the form of liquid nitrogen) to destroy tissue. The liquid nitrogen is in a metal spray canister, and you pull the trigger to spray the affected area. Cryotherapy is often used to destroy actinic keratoses, seborrheic keratoses, and skin tags.

22.2.3.3 Wound Care

Wound care is very complex, but one basic principle is simple: if the wound is wet, make it dry; if the wound is dry, make it wet. Wounds heal more quickly when they are relatively wet, probably because of easier migration of epidermal cells and nutrients found in the wound fluid. However, if the wound is too wet, that can lead to maceration (softening of the skin due to extended exposure to moisture) and worsening of the wound.

There are several types of dressings that can be used for wounds.

1. Open dressings: gauze. Usually, you would use wet-to-moist gauze for large soft tissue defect until wound closure can be performed. Dry gauze is highly discouraged in most cases as it doesn't allow for proper moisture for the wound to heal.
2. Semi-open dressings: usually fine mesh gauze with some sort of ointment like petroleum. Examples are *Xeroform, Adaptic, and Jelonet.* These dressings are cheap and easy to apply. However, they do not maintain a moisture-rich environment for long, and if the wound is particularly exudative, then fluid can be trapped and lead to maceration. Thus, these dressings need to be changed frequently.
3. Films: permeable to gases, like water vapor, but not to protein and bacteria. Examples are *Tegaderm, Cutifilm, and Blisterfilm.* These provide the fastest healing rates, lowest infection rates, and most cost-effectiveness. Advantages are that they maintain moisture and encourage rapid reepithelization; disadvantages are that they have limited absorptive capacity and are not appropriate for heavily exudative wounds.
4. Foams: film dressings with absorbency. Examples are *Allevyn, Lyofoam, and Adhesive.* Advantages are that they are highly absorptive. They should not be used on minimally exudative wounds as they can dry out the wounds.
5. Alginates: made of natural polysaccharides found in algae. They are good for moderate to heavily exudative wounds. They are also great at hemostasis.
6. Hydrocolloids: the colloid traps exudates and creates a moist environment. Good for gentle, painless mechanical debridement. Disadvantages are malodor and possible contact dermatitis. Examples are *Duoderm and Tegasorb.*

7. Hydrogel: good for dry wounds because they can absorb or release water, depending on the hydration state of the tissue.

In addition to dressings, you can use topical therapy.
1. Antimicrobials to prevent infection
   1. Iodine, silver, honey
2. Growth factors: platelet-derived growth factors, epidermal growth factor, granulocyte-macrophage colony-stimulating factor
   1. Used for ulcers, particularly on the lower extremities
3. Chemical debridement to remove dead tissue from wounds to promote the healing process
   1. Collagenase and Santyl

22.2.4 Basics of Dermoscopy

During your dermatology rotation, you may have opportunities to examine lesions more closely using a dermatoscope – a handheld instrument that magnifies and illuminates skin lesions. While you will not be expected to be an expert on using the dermatoscope, below are some basics that will be helpful when you are handed a dermatoscope in clinic.

22.2.4.1 How to Use a Dermatoscope
Although there are many types of dermatoscopes, the basics on how to use them are the same:
- Turn on the dermatoscope light.
- Place the dermatoscope close to the skin lesion (sometimes directly on the skin, depending on the dermatoscope) (◘ Fig. 22.10).
- Adjust your body so that your eyes can look directly into the dermatoscope.

Depending on the type of dermatoscope, your eyes may need to be very close, just an inch or 2 from the lens. If you are unable to see a lesion well, continue adjusting the distance between your eyes and the lens until the lesion comes into focus.

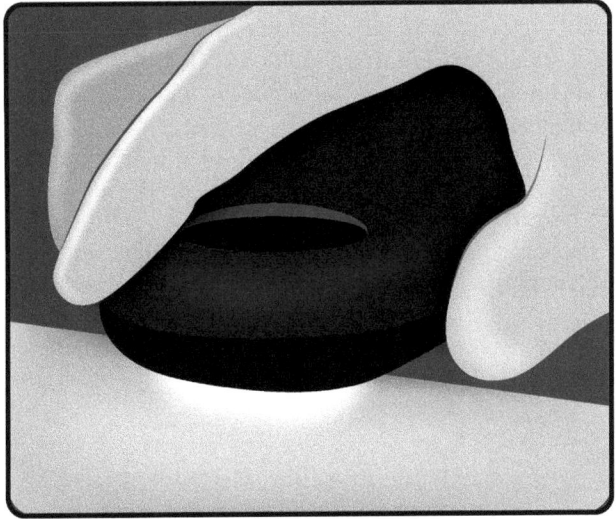

◘ **Fig. 22.10** How to use a dermatoscope

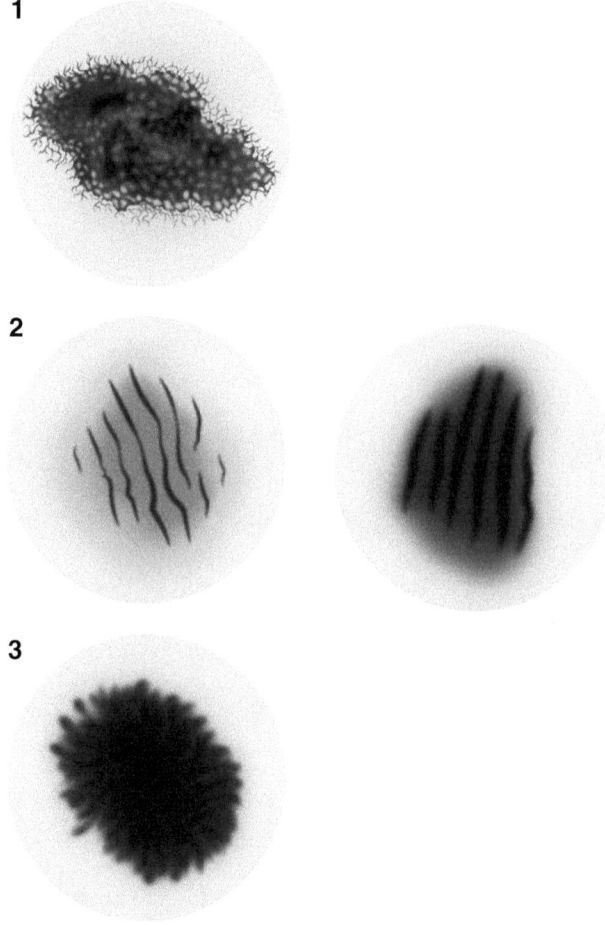

◘ Fig. 22.11 Common dermatoscopic features for pigmented lesions

22.2.4.2 **How to Describe What You See**

You can use the dermatoscope to look at any and all skin lesions, but one of the most common uses for dermatoscopes is to examine pigmented lesions. You will not need to know the nuances of looking at pigmented lesions, but here is some useful terminology to help you describe what you see (◘ Fig. 22.11).

1. *Reticular pigment with pigment globules:*
    1. Reticular pigment: a honeycomb pattern of pigment. This is usually benign if spread evenly throughout.
    2. Pigment globules: the darker pigmentation within a lesion; can be seen in both benign and malignant lesions.
2. *Parallel furrow pattern:* seen on palms and soles. If the pigment is in furrow (the valleys), then the lesion is most likely benign. If the pigment is in ridges (the raised parts), the lesion may be malignant.
3. *Pigment streaks:* streaks of pigment that spread out like sunrays. Can be seen in melanoma, a sign that the lesion is spreading outward.

22.2.5 **Other Clinical Exam Techniques**

Below are other clinical exam techniques. For invasive techniques, such as the Nikolsky sign, you will not want to perform the test by yourself. Instead, make sure a resident and/or attending agrees that this test should be performed and that they supervise you.

Nikolsky sign

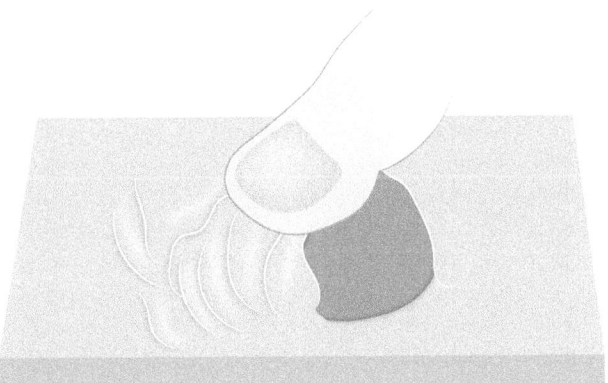

Fig. 22.12   Positive Nikolsky sign

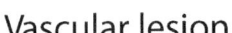
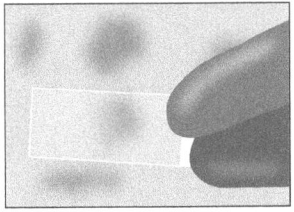

Vascular lesion

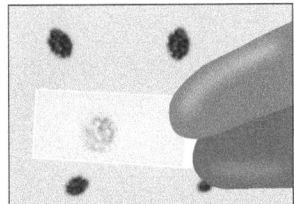

Sarcoid lesion

Fig. 22.13   Diascopy of a blanching vascular (top) and apple jelly granulomatous lesion (bottom)

22.2.5.1 Nikolsky Sign

The Nikolsky sign is relevant when you see vesicles or bullae. To perform this test, *gently* rub the top of the bullae. If the bullae shear, then you have a positive Nikolsky (Fig. 22.12). This means that the bullae are very superficial and the cleavage is above the dermal-epidermal junction. If the bullae do not shear, then you have a negative Nikolsky and the damage is in the dermis.

- Diseases with positive Nikolsky sign: Stevens-Johnson syndrome, staphylococcal scalded skin syndrome, pemphigus vulgaris
- Disease with negative Nikolsky sign: bullous pemphigoid

22.2.5.2 Diascopy

Diascopy is a test of blanchability. Use this when you have a vascular lesion or a substantive lesion suggestive of a granulomatous condition. To perform the test, press a glass slide on the lesion, and see if the lesion blanches or changes in color.

In vascular lesions, if the lesion blanches, then the lesion is a result of vasodilation (e.g., telangiectasia) (Fig. 22.13). If it doesn't blanch, then there is red blood cell extravasation (e.g., purpura) (see ▶ Sect. 22.4.12).

In granulomatous lesions, you will see an *apple jelly* color (brownish-yellow color) when you press the lesion with a glass slide (■ Fig. 22.13).

22.2.5.3 Wood's Lamp Skin Exam

A Wood's lamp is a blacklight that emits wavelengths between 320 and 450 nm (peak 365 nm). It can be used to aid in the diagnosis of many skin conditions including pigmentary disorders, skin infections, and even porphyria. It is most commonly used to evaluate patients with hypopigmented or depigmented skin lesions (see ▶ Sect. 22.4.6). To perform this exam, first turn on the Wood's lamp, and then turn off the room light (otherwise, the room will be completely dark!). Shine the lamp on the patient's skin, moving the lamp to illuminate areas of interest. In patients with loss of pigment (e.g., vitiligo), you will see a milky white or sometimes green fluorescence of the affected skin. In patients with hypopigmented skin (no loss of melanocytes), you will not see fluorescence of the skin.

22.2.6 Diagnostic Tests by Clinical Presentation

Below are a list of diagnostic tests by clinical presentation (■ Table 22.5).

■ **Table 22.5** Diagnostic tests by clinical presentation

Presentation	Test
Red and scaly lesion Concern for: fungal infection	*KOH prep:* gently scrape lesion with a #15 blade scalpel to get scales on a glass slide. Add 1–2 drops KOH which dissolves keratinocytes to visualize the fungal hyphae. Put a coverslip on. May need to heat the slide, depending on which KOH preparation you are using. Under the microscope, first scan at low power to find your cells. Then use 10× to visualize hyphae if there is a fungal infection (■ Fig. 22.14)
Grouped vesicles Concern for: HSV or VZV infection	*Nucleic acid amplification (NAAT):* this method amplifies and detects a certain sequence of the viral genome and is more sensitive than the Tzanck preparation. To perform this, you swab the base of an open vesicle and send the sample for testing. Your resident/attending will walk you through the detailed steps *Tzanck preparation:* this method is not often used anymore, but it is still helpful to understand. To perform this, use scalpel to gently scrape base of a freshly opened vesicle, and then stain with toluidine blue or Giemsa stain. Look for multinucleated giant cells using 100× magnification in suspected Herpes simplex or varicella zoster infections (■ Fig. 22.15)
Extreme pruritus +/− other household members affected Concern for: scabies	Place mineral oil on a #15 blade, the area to be scraped, and the microscope slide. Scrape the black dot at the end of a burrow (raised tracked lines that are skin-colored, signifying burrowing of a mite), and place on the mineral oil on the glass slide. Cover with a coverslip. The presence of scabies mite or eggs under the microscope at 40× confirms diagnosis of scabies (■ Fig. 22.16)
Pustules, bullae, or abscesses Concern for: infection	Culture for bacteria
Blistering Concern for: bullous pemphigoid or pemphigus vulgaris	Skin biopsy with additional biopsy for direct immunofluorescence testing to look for autoantibodies against portions of the skin

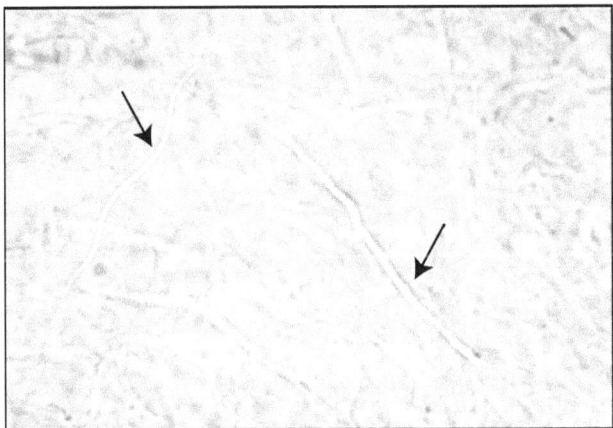

Fig. 22.14 Hyphae visualized in a KOH prep

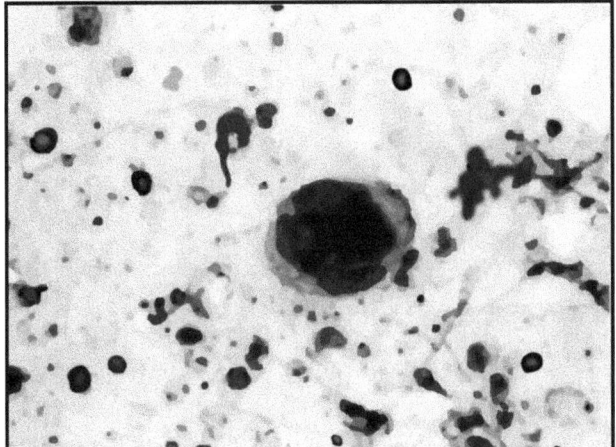

Fig. 22.15 Multinucleated giant cell visualized under microscopy

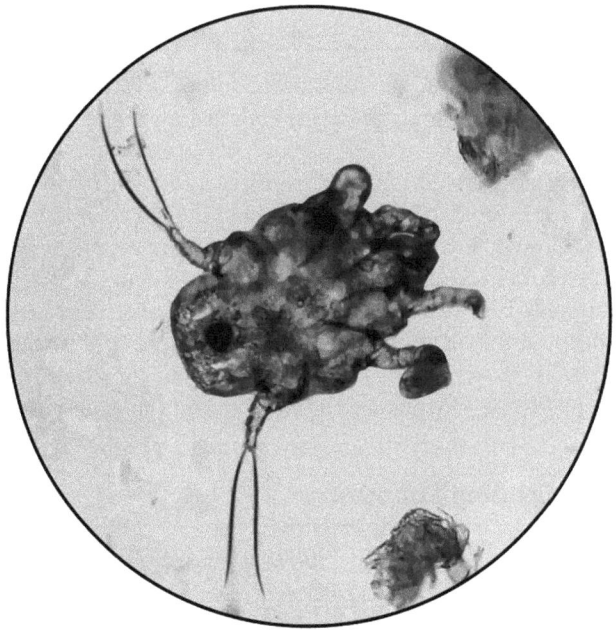

Fig. 22.16 Scabies visualized under microscopy

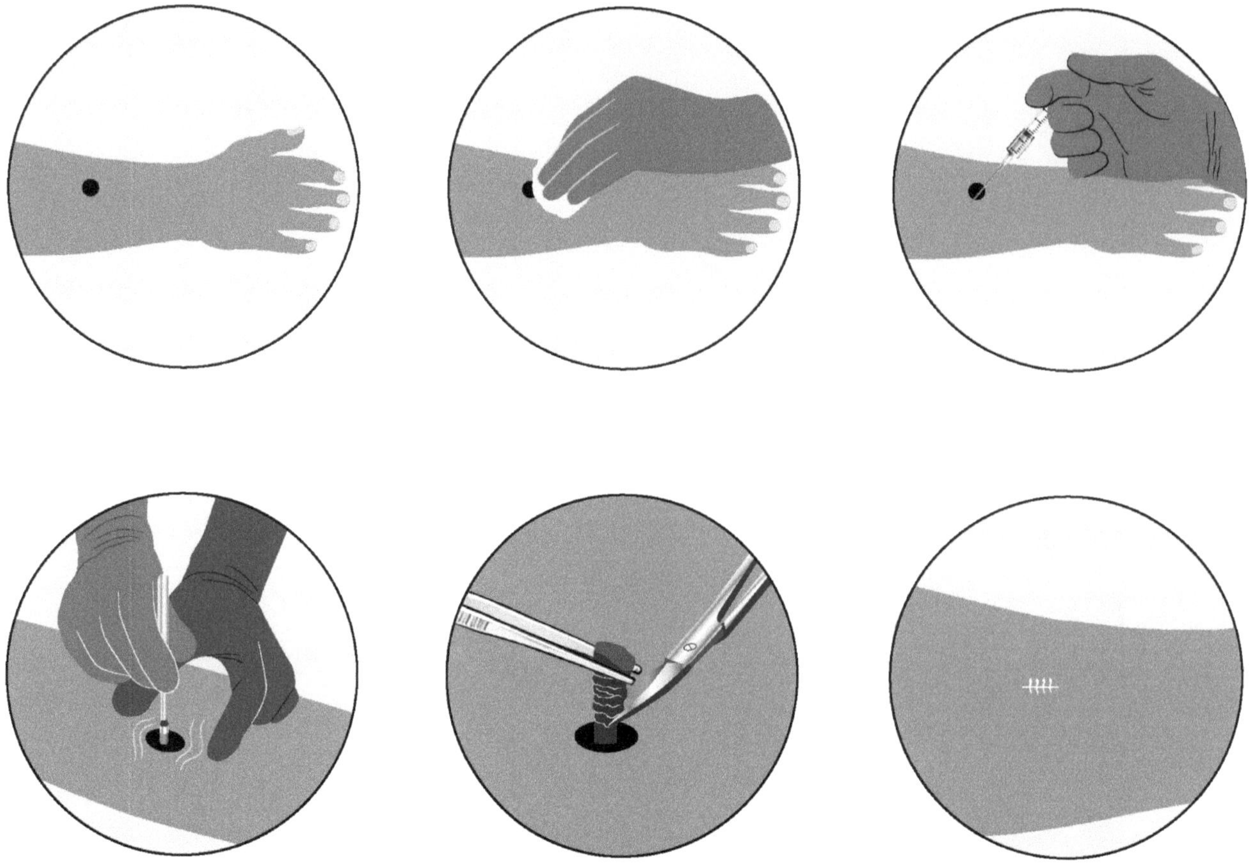

■ **Fig. 22.17** Steps of a punch biopsy (from top left to right). (1) Mark the lesion that you want to biopsy and take a photo. In general, you want to biopsy a fresh lesion. Note that for some conditions, you will want to biopsy the edge of a lesion, whereas for other conditions, you want to biopsy the center. You may look up the specifics of where to biopsy for each condition you are concerned about, and your resident/attending will walk you through this. (2) Clean the area. (3) Inject numbing medication and wait a few minutes for the area to numb. (4) Holding the biopsy tool like a pencil, twist with firm pressure to perform punch biopsy. (5) Use forceps to remove the skin tissue and cut the base with a pair of scissors. (6) Close the site using one or two simple interrupted sutures

22.2.7 Skin Biopsies

The most definitive way to diagnose a skin condition is through a skin biopsy. In general, you should sample a fresh *primary* lesion. There are two main ways to obtain a sample of the skin:
1. Punch biopsy (■ Fig. 22.17): used most commonly as you will get a full-thickness sample (epidermis, dermis, subcutaneous tissue). It is more invasive than a shave biopsy, and you will need to suture the biopsy site. However, it is very helpful in seeing how all layers of the skin are affected.
2. Shave biopsy (■ Fig. 22.18): used for rapid removal of raised lesions; it samples the deep dermis at most so you will not get subcutaneous tissue. The advantage of a shave biopsy is that it heals quickly without the need for suturing – just some Vaseline and a bandage and the patient is ready to go!

22.3 Patient Clinical Encounter

A patient encounter in dermatology follows a similar format to patient encounters in other fields in medicine, but there are a few notable differences highlighted in blue below as well as outlined in ▶ Box 22.2.
1. HPI:
   1. Location: important to know where the skin lesion is located or where a rash started and where it spread.

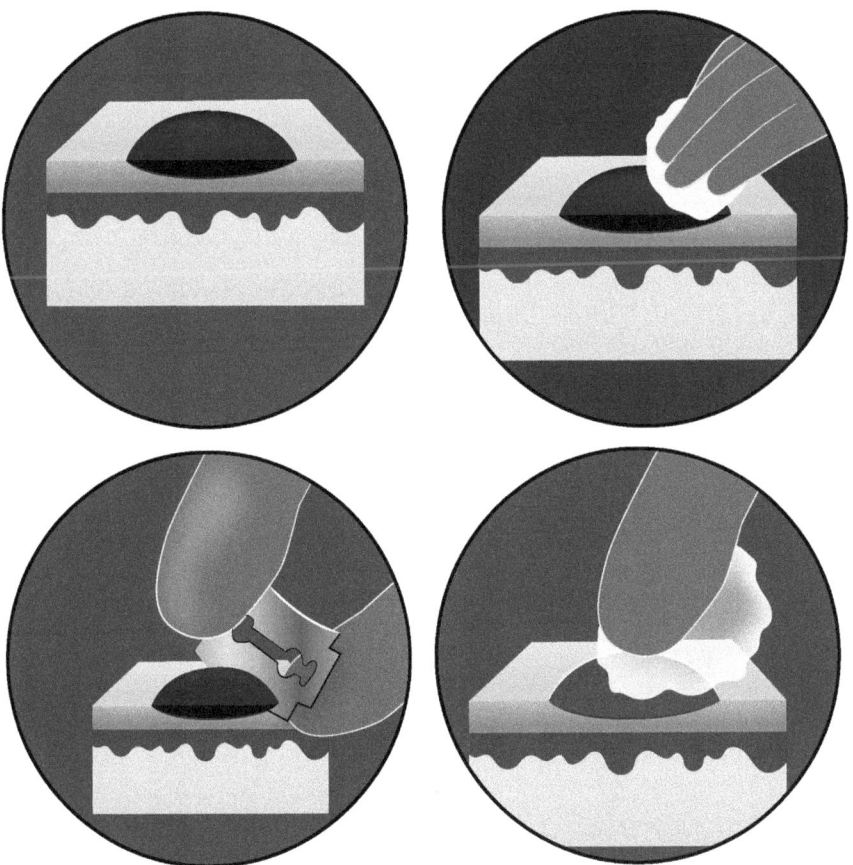

Fig. 22.18 Steps of a shave biopsy (from top left to right). (1) Mark the lesion you want to biopsy and take a photo. (2) Clean the area. (3) Fold in the sides of the shaving tool so that the blade makes a U shape. Rock the blade back and forth while applying gentle forward pressure to perform the shave biopsy. (4) Apply Vaseline and bandage

2. Duration.
3. Symptoms: itchy, painful, numb?
4. Prior treatment.
5. Previous episodes/biopsies.
6. Changes in skin lesions over time.
7. For patients who are here for a skin check, ask about four key risk factors for skin cancer: (1) history of blistering sunburns, (2) tanning bed use, (3) prolonged immunosuppression, and (4) family history of skin cancer, especially melanoma.
8. ROS: when relevant, ask for a review of systems, which could give you a clue to some big bucket diagnoses.
   1. Fevers/chills: infection or malignancy.
   2. Weight loss: malignancy.
   3. Shortness of breath: sarcoidosis, cancer metastasis.
   4. Abdominal pain: inflammatory bowel disease is associated with erythema nodosum.
   5. Back pain: cancer metastasis to bone.
   6. Joint pain: psoriasis.
2. PMH:
   1. Skin cancer.
   2. Relevant comorbidities for skin conditions are listed below in ▶ Sect. 22.4.
3. Medications – pay particular attention to immunosuppressive agents, photosensitizing agents, or common causes of drug-induced eruptions.

4. Allergies
5. Family history
    1. Anyone else in family with similar skin lesions? Important if you are suspecting an infection, infestation (e.g., scabies or lice), or an autoimmune etiology
    2. Skin cancer
6. Social history:
    1. In patients with chronic wound or skin infection, consider history of immunosuppression, either from medications or immunocompromised state such as HIV/AIDS.
    2. In patients with suspected contact dermatitis, consider exposure history (any new laundry detergent, perfumes, lotions, soaps, recent yardwork, etc.), new hobbies, or employment.
    3. Ask if the patient wears sunscreen, how often, and what SPF.
7. Physical exam: Observe if the patient looks well or ill overall. Check vitals. Then proceed with the skin inspection:
    1. Ensure adequate room lighting and that patient is situated properly for optimal lighting over the skin areas to be examined.
    2. Clean hands before and after. You may use gloves, but it may affect palpation. In patients with suspected infectious diseases, infestations, weeping lesions, or mucosal lesions, wear gloves.
    3. Start with the lesion of interest. Then look over the whole body as there may be related or unrelated (incidental) findings that are important to the patient's health.
    4. Always ask for permission when repositioning the gown and examining sensitive areas (e.g., "Is it ok if we lift up your gown to look at your abdomen?"). It is helpful to say what you are doing out loud to the patient.
    5. When doing the total body skin exam (TBSE), have a systematic way of looking over the body. One example is:
        1. With the patient sitting on the exam table, examine his or her hands first since this is the least invasive.
        2. Move up to examine the arms.
        3. Have the patient lie down on their back.
        4. Examine head to toe: scalp, face, neck, chest, abdomen, anterior surface of lower extremities, dorsum of feet.
        5. Have the patient roll onto his or her abdomen.
        6. Examine head to toe again: back of scalp, back, posterior arms, posterior legs, and soles.
    6. Palpation is useful to assess:
        1. Texture: running your fingers lightly across the lesion, how does it feel? Scaly, bumpy, no change?
        2. Consistency: pressing deeper on the lesion, do you feel fluctuance (like there is fluid in the lesion) or induration (hardening of the skin)?
        3. Tenderness: does the patient complain of pain when you gently press on the lesion?
        4. Drainage: is there fluid expressed out of the lesion to suggest an underlying collection?
    7. Make sure to check the scalp, mouth, and nails!
        1. Nails: nail pitting can be seen in psoriasis.
        2. Dilated capillary nail folds: can be seen in dermatomyositis and other connective tissue diseases (scleroderma and lupus).
        3. Scalp: scaling can be seen in psoriasis, seborrheic dermatitis, dermatomyositis, and other connective tissue diseases (scleroderma and lupus).
        4. Oral mucosa: check for blisters in blistering disease, such as bullous pemphigoid and pemphigus vulgaris.

Palpation helps reassure patients that you are not afraid to touch their skin lesions.

22

- Symptoms: do the lesions itch, burn, or hurt?
- If concerned about infectious etiology: other household members affected?
- Previous biopsies
- Previous treatments – did they work?
- New medications or exposures that could cause their skin lesions
- Risk factors for skin cancer (history of blistering sunburns, tanning bed use)
- History of skin cancer or skin conditions
- Family history of skin conditions
- Depending on attending preference, may be helpful to take a picture of the lesion for the patient's chart

22.3.1 Oral Presentations

Dermatology presentations should be short and focused. Do not list irrelevant comorbidities in the one-liner, and remember that the chief complaint should be symptoms or skin findings that the patient complains about rather than what you have observed on the physical exam. There is no need to present medications, allergies, family, or social history, unless they are directly relevant. Of course, make sure to ask the patient all of this so you can include the information in your note or answer your attending when he or she asks!

▶ Example

"Ms. S is a 60-year-old woman with a past medical history of eczema who presents with an itchy rash on her neck for the past week. The rash appeared 3 days after wearing a new necklace and has been itchy and painful. She has had similar rashes in the past. She has not used any creams or medications for her rash. She stopped wearing her new necklace 2 days ago. The rash has not blistered or had any discharge."

"Past dermatologic history is significant for eczema, which resolves with topical corticosteroids. She has not had any skin cancers, including melanoma, though she does have a history of significant sun exposure, including blistering sunburns as a child."

"She has no other relevant significant past medical history, medications, allergies, family history, or social history."

"Vitals are within normal limits, no fevers. On physical exam, the patient is well-appearing. She has widespread erythema circumferentially around her neck with fine scaling and excoriation marks. No vesicles or bullae seen. She has no similar rashes elsewhere on the body."

"Given her history and exam, I think Ms. S most likely has an allergic contact dermatitis to her new necklace. Another item on my differential is atopic dermatitis, given her history of eczema. I think we should counsel her to stop wearing the necklace and prescribe hydrocortisone 2.5% ointment BID for 14 days maximum. We can schedule a follow-up appointment in 1 month to see how her rash is doing. She has an annual full body skin exam scheduled in 4 months." ◀

22.3.2 Note-Writing

Dermatology notes are concise with detailed descriptions of the skin lesions. Attendings will structure their notes differently so you can ask for their template before you write a note. Below is a sample template that includes the key information.

Date:

Chief complaint:

Date of last clinic visit:

History of present illness: Ms. S is an 80-year-old female who presents for evaluation of the following...

Past dermatologic history (usually note as below)

- Hx of melanoma: none

- Hx of NMSC: angiosarcoma

- Any other derm hx

Review of systems

- Feels well overall; no bleeding or bruising; no fevers/chills

Past medical history

Medications

- In particular, highlight medications if you are concerned about a drug eruption (see the section on Drug Reactions for what drugs to look out for)

Allergies

Social history

Family history

- Skin cancers
- Skin conditions

Relevant results/labs

Prior skin biopsies

Physical exam

- Fitzpatrick skin type.
- A skin exam was performed including [name the body parts examined].

Insert photos taken in clinic, if applicable.

Assessment/plan

- Seborrheic dermatitis: [describe the skin lesion in detail. e.g, patchy erythema of scalp with focal scaling, consistent with seborrheic dermatitis]
    - A.   Counseled patient on etiology of seborrheic dermatitis.
    - B.   [In terms of topical steroids, be sure to state the name of the steroid, potency, vehicle, area to which apply the medication, frequency of application, and duration of application].
        - 1.   Note that for most steroids, you will not want to apply it for more than 14 days consecutively.
        - 2.   State refills if applicable.
    - C.   [State other therapies, such as "Start ketoconazole 2% shampoo"].

22.4 Differentiating the Differential

When approaching skin lesions, you can take a systematic approach that involves first identifying the primary lesion's appearance and then differentiating further with characteristics such as color, size, and texture, as well as the patient's comorbidities.

In this section, we will go over the important skin lesions you should know for clinic as well as on inpatient consults. As a student, it can be overwhelming to consider the numerous skin conditions that you may encounter, so we suggest knowing the conditions introduced at the beginning of each section really well before your rotation. Then, as you go through your rotation, you can refer to the tables of other diagnoses in each section. Bolded terminology are keywords you can use in your presentation and notes, and conditions marked with a star are those you should know about. Of note, the lists of diagnoses presented here are not comprehensive, and you should look into VisualDx or any other preferred resource for additional diagnoses and detailed information.

Diagnoses in the tables are color-coded based on whether they are:

> Malignant-purple
>
> Inflammatory-orange
>
> Infectious-green
>
> Autoimmune-blue

22.4.1 Pigmented Lesions

You will come across many pigmented lesions in dermatology clinic. These lesions are brown to black in color because of melanocytes, which live in basal cell layer (◻ Fig. 22.2). While most pigmented lesions are benign, such as age spots (solar lentigines), freckles, or moles (nevi), it is important to check for features that may be concerning for melanoma.

22.4.1.1 Melanoma

Melanoma is skin cancer of the melanocytes. The etiology is not completely understood, but UV radiation is thought to play some role. In clinic, especially during annual skin checks, you should ask patients their risk factors for developing melanoma (▶ Box 22.3).

> **Box 22.3   Risk Factors for Melanoma**
>
> - Personal or family history of melanoma
> - History of severe or blistering sunburns
> - Giant congenital nevus (>20 cm)
> - Lighter skin phototype
> - Multiple atypical nevi
> - Older age (mean age of diagnosis is 63 years of age)

Other questions to ask the patient during the history are when the lesion first appeared (benign nevi usually appear before the age of 30), changes to the lesion, and any symptoms, such as pain or itch.

A common location for melanoma in men is their back and in women is their legs. Make sure to carefully examine these locations!

752   C. Zhong

Ugly duckling sign: watch out for moles that do not look like the others (🔳 Fig. 22.19)!

When examining a pigmented lesion, look to see if the lesion is similar to or different from other lesions in the area. If it is similar to other lesions, it is more likely benign.

Characteristics of melanoma are easily remembered by the mnemonic ABCDE (🔳 Fig. 22.20).
- A: asymmetry (is one side of the lesion different than the other side?)
- B: border irregularity (is the border smooth or are there irregularities?)
- C: color variation (is the lesion one color or are there color differences within the lesion?)
- D: diameter >6 mm (is the diameter of the lesion greater than a pencil eraser?)
- E: evolution (has the lesion been changing in the past several weeks?)

Once you have examined the lesion grossly with your eye, you may use your dermatoscope to look at the pigment network and globules (see ▶ Sect. 22.2 for details). Melanoma may have pigment that radiates outward and irregular patterns of color.

There are four subtypes of melanoma:
1. Superficial spreading: fast radial growth; good prognosis if detected early
2. Lentigo maligna: in sun-damaged skin of elderly patients; considered in situ melanoma
3. Nodular: progresses quickly
4. Acral lentiginous: on palms and soles; more common in people of color
   1. Subungual: in the nail; more common in thumbnail or big toenail (see ▶ Sect. 22.4.16)

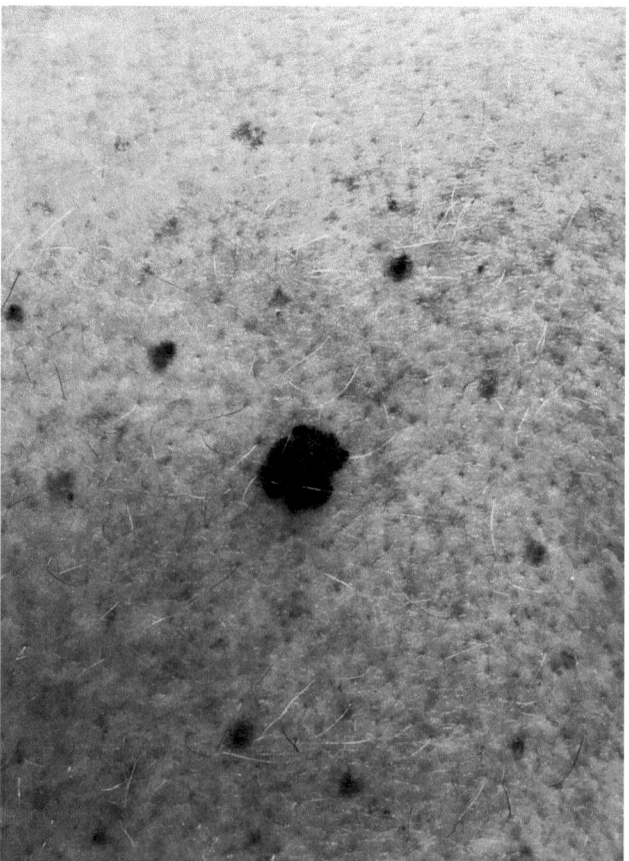

🔳 **Fig. 22.19** Melanoma. Grossly, this pigmented lesion looks very different than surrounding nevi ("the ugly duckling sign"). Furthermore, this lesion meets all of the ABCDE criteria

22

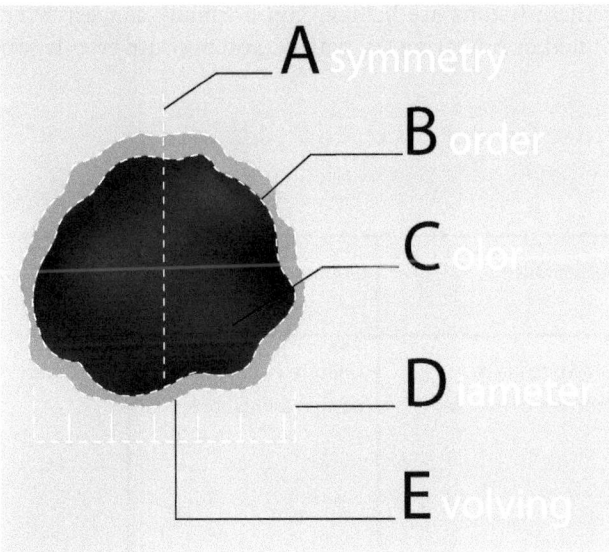

◘ Fig. 22.20 ABCDE of melanoma

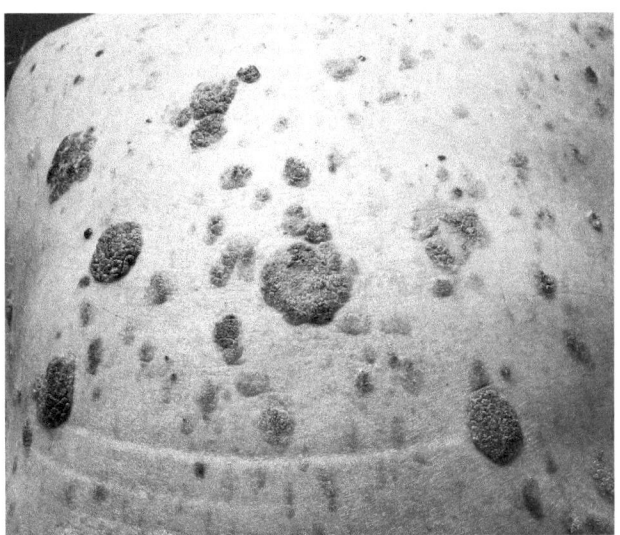

◘ Fig. 22.21 Seborrheic keratosis

If you and your attending are concerned about melanoma, your attending will choose to biopsy the lesion. It is important to sample all the way to the subcutis because one major prognostic factor is the *Breslow depth*, which refers to how deep the melanoma has invaded. The deeper the invasion, the worse the prognosis.

22.4.1.2 Seborrheic Keratosis

Seborrheic keratoses (SKs) are benign overgrowths of the epidermis that are common in older people. Because they can grow rapidly and look heterogeneous, patients may be concerned that they have skin cancer.

On exam, SKs have a waxy, stuck-on appearance (◘ Fig. 22.21). There may be little bumps on the surface, and the color may vary within the lesion. They are most commonly found on the chest and back. When you look under a dermatoscope, you will see keratin horn cysts (small cysts on the surface of the lesion).

The most common sites of melanoma metastases are the liver, lung, and brain.

Because these lesions are benign, you normally can leave them alone. If they are irritated or bothering the patient, you may use cryotherapy to remove the lesion.

22.4.1.3 Other Conditions to Consider

Condition and overview	Patient population	Appearance	Dermoscopy	Management
★ **Nevi ("mole"):** cluster of melanocytes that are benign	New ones appear within first three decades of life	Brown to black macules or papules.	Uniform pigment pattern and globules	Reassurance
Lentigo ("liver spot"): brown macules that appear with chronic sun exposure	>40 years old	Light brown macules on sun-exposed skin (face, dorsal hands, and arms) **(Fig. 22.24)**	Uniform reticular network	Encourage use of sunscreen to prevent developing new lentigines. May use cryotherapy, laser, or chemical peels to remove lentigines if bothering patient.
★ **Seborrheic keratosis (SK):** neoplasms of the epidermis that appear as one ages	> 40 years old	**"Stuck-on," waxy** brown to black papule. Has little bumps that feel rough to the touch and may have varied color within one lesion A variant of SKs are stucco keratoses. These are small white-gray SKs usually on the extremities	Keratin horn cysts	Reassurance Irritated: cryotherapy to remove the SK.
★ **Dermatofi broma:** benign skin neoplasm made of	Anyone	Firm, hyperpigmented papule that dimples inward when you squeeze it. **(Fig. 22.25)**	-	Reassurance

Dermatology

fibroblasts (what makes up scar tissue) and histiocytes (a type of white blood cell) that is well-circumscrib ed and firm		Color varies from pink to brown to black. Usually in sites of bug bites or small trauma Dimple sign: dimpling of the center when you squeeze the lesion borders		
☆ Melanoma: cancer of melanocytes	Mean age of diagnosis: 63 years	Meets the ABCDE criteria	Atypical pigment network, globules, or vascular structures	Excisional biopsy to diagnose Surgery, chemotherapy, radiation, and immunotherapy

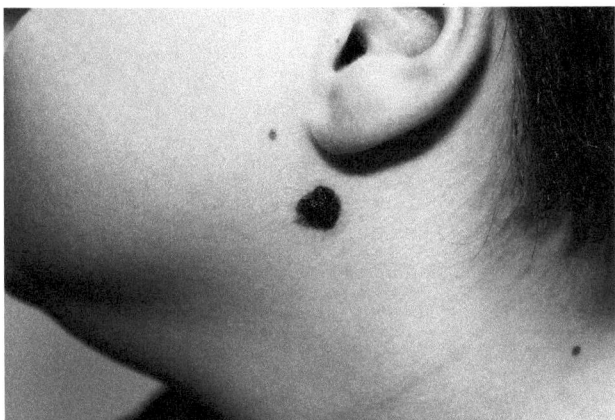

■ **Fig. 22.22** A nevus that is raised, which is called a compound nevus

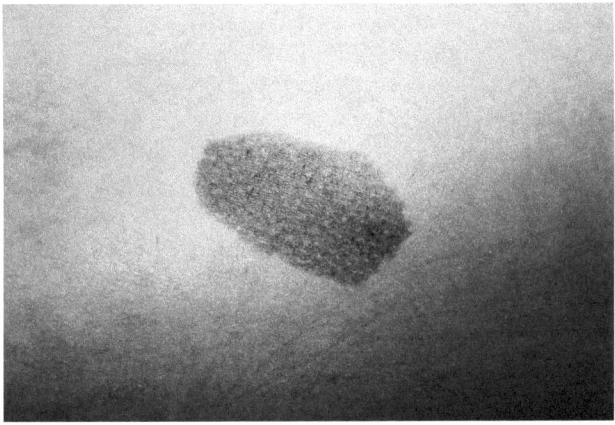

■ **Fig. 22.23** A congenital nevus

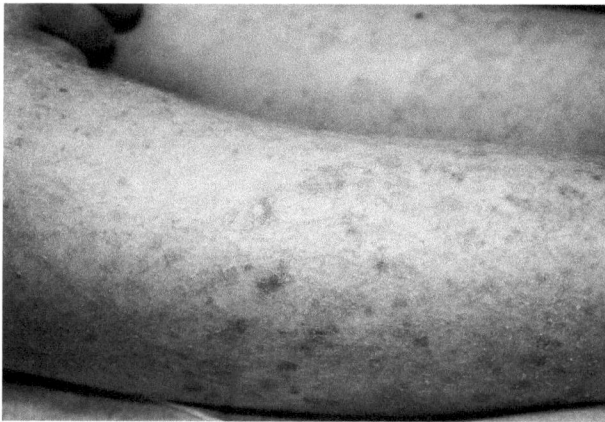

Fig. 22.24 Lentigines

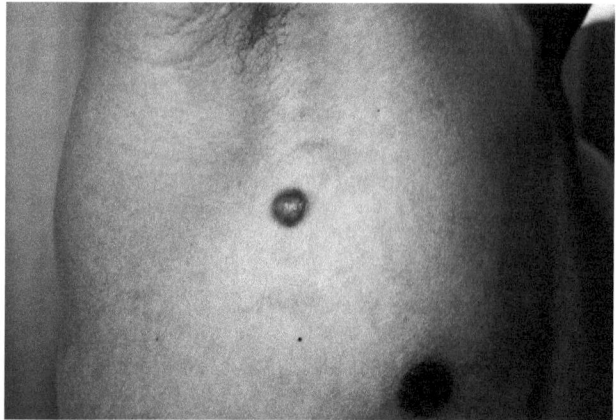

Fig. 22.25 Dermatofibroma

22.4.2 Scaly Patch

When you see a scaly red patch in a patient, there is most likely an inflammatory or infectious process (such as a fungal infection). Important questions to ask the patient are if he or she has ever had:

- A similar lesion before (suggesting a recurrent process like atopic dermatitis or psoriasis)
- A family history of these skin lesions
- Other medical conditions (e.g., atopic dermatitis occurs with asthma and allergic rhinitis, whereas dermatomyositis may occur in patients with cancer)
- Preceding illnesses (pityriasis rosea is often preceded by a viral infection)
- Previous treatments and whether or not they worked (e.g., patients who have a fungal infection will get worse with topical steroids alone)

On exam, note the distribution on the lesions (if it is localized, that suggests contact dermatitis or fungal infection, whereas if it is symmetric and diffuse, that suggests a systemic process). Also note the size of the scales (large, thick scales are more likely psoriasis) and whether or not there is an active red border (suggesting a fungal infection).

Usually, a clinical exam is enough to make the diagnosis. If not, the simplest test to determine if the scaly patch is a fungal infection is a KOH exam (see ▶ Sect. 22.2). If the diagnosis is still unclear, a skin biopsy may be helpful.

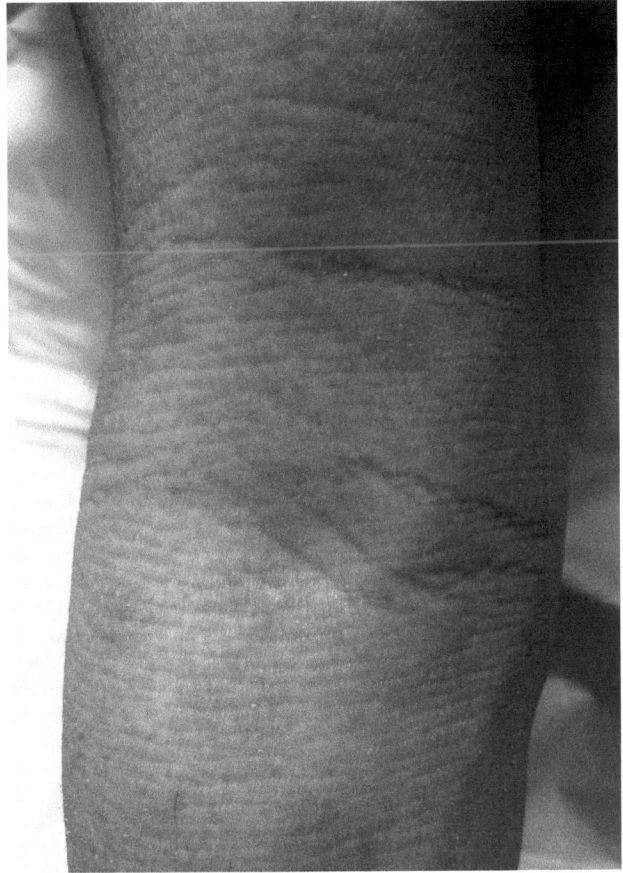

◪ Fig. 22.26   Atopic dermatitis with lichenification of the arm

22.4.2.1 **Atopic Dermatitis**

Atopic dermatitis (AD), also known as eczema, is a pruritic (itchy) chronic skin condition caused by a variety of genetic and environmental factors. *Filaggrin*, a protein that retains water in keratinocytes in the stratum granulosum, is thought to be mutated in some patients with AD (see ▶ Sects. 22.1.1 and 22.2). People with atopic dermatitis may also have asthma and allergic rhinitis; this triad of conditions is known as the *atopic triad.*

On exam, you will see erythematous scaly plaques with ill-defined borders. You can check the patient's palms to see if he or she has accentuation of skin lines (also known as *hyperlinear palms*). In adults, the flexural areas are more commonly involved (◪ Figs. 22.26 and 22.27), while in infants, the extensors are more often involved (◪ Fig. 22.28).

Topical steroids are the most common treatment for atopic dermatitis. Remember to recommend a steroid strength that is appropriate for the body area that is affected (see ▶ Sect. 22.2.3). In addition to steroids, you should remind patients to moisturize their skin, especially right after showers, and to avoid food or chemical triggers.

For some patients, the lesions may be infected. You can tell if the lesions are infected if the lesions have honey-colored crust (known as *impetiginization*) or oozing. For these patients, you should give mupirocin ointment or PO antibiotics to cover *Staph aureus* (e.g., cephalexin).

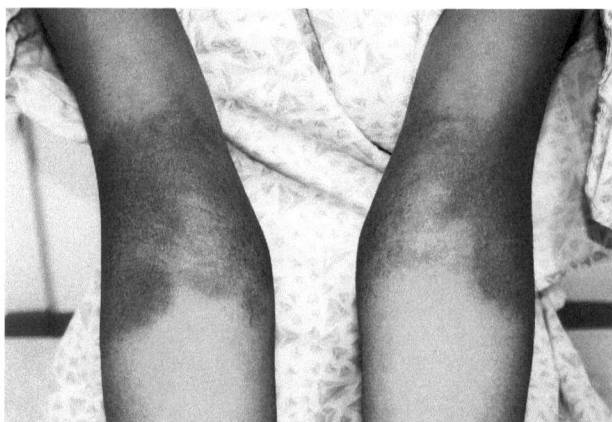

Fig. 22.27 Atopic dermatitis in darker skin tone

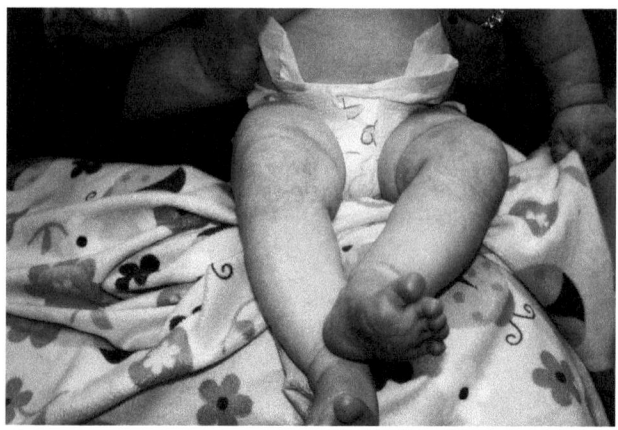

Fig. 22.28 Atopic dermatitis on the extensor surfaces of an infant

Eczema herpeticum is when the infection of eczema is due to herpes simplex virus. On exam, look for punched-out erosions. Treatment is to give acyclovir.

In patients with severe eczema who have failed topical steroids, you may suggest starting them on *dupilumab*, a monoclonal antibody against IL-4 and IL-13. These are given as injections every 2 weeks. One interesting side effect of dupilumab is conjunctivitis (pink eye).

22.4.2.2 Contact Dermatitis

Contact dermatitis is a skin reaction to an environmental trigger. Like atopic dermatitis, these rashes are scaly and red. However, unlike atopic dermatitis, these rashes tend to be geometric with defined borders because these reactions are in response to an outside exposure (□ Fig. 22.29). Contact dermatitis may also sometimes have vesicles from the inflammation (□ Fig. 22.30). With airborne exposures, swelling of the eyelids is common.

Contact dermatitis is divided into *allergic contact dermatitis* and *irritant contact dermatitis*. Allergic contact dermatitis is a delayed Type IV hypersensitivity reaction that occurs when allergens activate T cells. For this to occur, the person needs to have been exposed and sensitized to the allergen before. Because T cells are activated in this response, these rashes are usually delayed, appearing 24–48 hrs after exposure to the allergen.

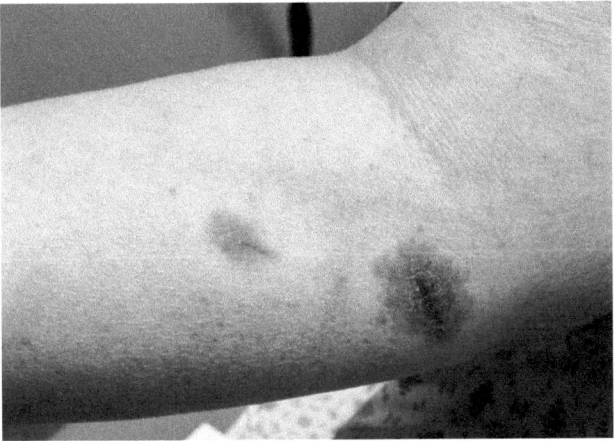

Fig. 22.29   Allergic contact dermatitis from poison ivy

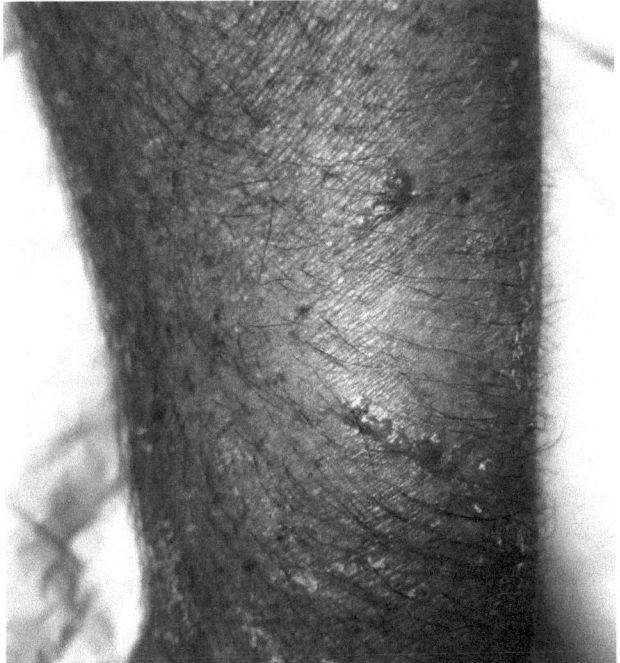

Fig. 22.30   Allergic contact dermatitis with vesicles

Irritant contact dermatitis is due to a direct toxic effect of an exposure and can appear just a few hours after exposure. Whereas pruritus is common in allergic contact dermatitis, burning and stinging are more pronounced in irritant contact dermatitis.

In patients that you suspect have a contact dermatitis, ask about the following exposures:
- Detergents
- Perfumes
- Outdoor activity, such as yardwork or hiking
- Lotions
- Jewelry
- Adhesives, such as bandages

Treatment involves avoiding the offending agent and using topical steroids to calm the inflammation. Antihistamines may be used for the itching.

22.4.2.3 Psoriasis

Psoriasis, like atopic dermatitis, is a chronic inflammatory disease. It is thought to be caused by abnormal T-cell function and keratinocyte response. Several genes have been identified that are associated with psoriasis, and in patients with these genetic variants, they may develop psoriasis after exposure to environmental triggers, such as medications or infections.

Psoriasis classically presents as well-demarcated red plaques with silver scale (❑ Fig. 22.31). Unlike atopic dermatitis which is found on the flexural surfaces in adults (antecubital fossa and popliteal fossa), psoriasis is found on the extensor surfaces (elbows and knees) (❑ Fig. 22.32).

Besides the skin, psoriasis can affect other parts of the body:
- Joints (psoriatic arthritis).
- Nails: you may see little indentations in the nail called "*nail pitting.*"

Treatment of psoriasis involves topical steroids, calcipotriene (vitamin D analog that helps with skin turnover), and topical retinoid. For patients with more severe disease or joint involvement, you can try phototherapy or a systemic immunosuppressive.

Psoriasis has been associated with cardiovascular disease, cerebrovascular accidents, metabolic syndrome, mood disorders, and hepatic disease.

If you remove a psoriatic scale, you may see pinpoint bleeding, known as the *Auspitz sign.*

Psoriasis that affects the axilla, groin, and intergluteal cleft is called inverse psoriasis.

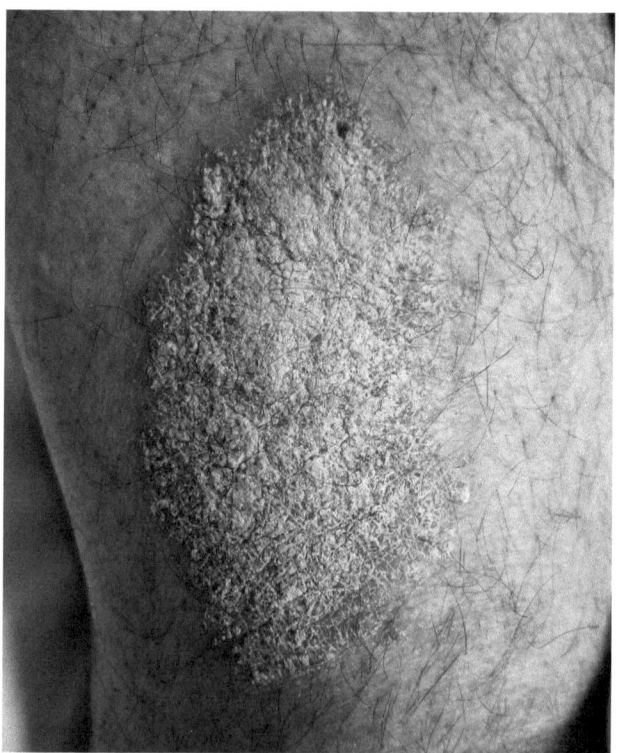

❑ **Fig. 22.31**   Psoriasis with thick silvery scale

22.4.2.4 Seborrheic Dermatitis

Seborrheic dermatitis is a common inflammatory condition that is probably due to a variety of factors, but one of the most well-known is an abnormal immune response to *Malassezia* yeast that normally lives on the skin. It can occur in children on the scalp, in which it is known as "*cradle cap*" or in adults on the scalp, which is known as "*dandruff*." Seborrheic dermatitis can also occur on the face, upper chest, and back – areas that are sebum-rich. The scales of seborrheic dermatitis are loose and greasy (◘ Fig. 22.33).

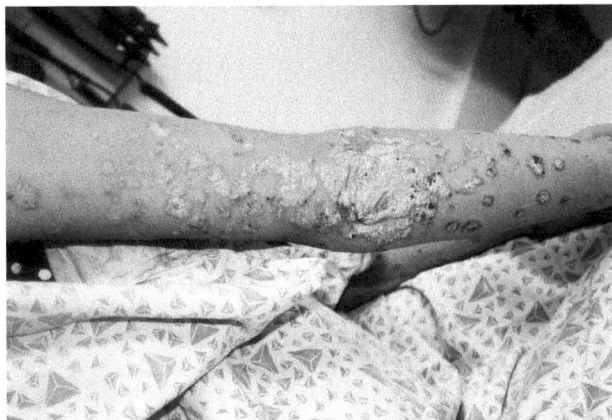

◘ **Fig. 22.32** Psoriasis over the extensor surfaces, unlike atopic dermatitis which is often on the flexural surfaces in adults

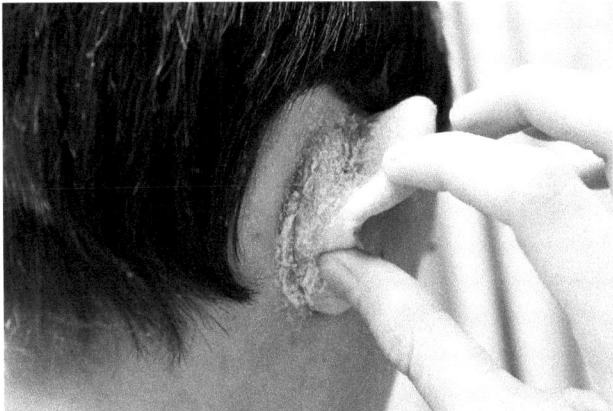

◘ **Fig. 22.33** Large, greasy yellow scales of seborrheic dermatitis behind the ear

Common treatments are over-the-counter shampoos that have salicylic acid (Neutrogena T/Sal), selenium sulfide (Selsun Blue), pyrithione zinc (Head and Shoulders), or tar (Neutrogena T/Gel). Shampoos can also be prescribed, such as ketoconazole 2%. These therapies aim at exfoliating the scalp and/or killing the *Malassezia* yeast.

In patients who have intractable itching and inflammation, a topical steroid may be helpful. If the seborrheic dermatitis is on the face, a cream is the best vehicle, and if it's on the scalp, then a solution or gel may be best.

22.4.2.5 Other Conditions to Consider

Condition and brief overview	Patient population	Appearance	Management
★ **Atopic dermatitis (AD):** also known as eczema; a chronic relapsing condition of itchy patches; may be associated with asthma and allergic rhinitis	Anyone	Scaly, erythematous papules and plaques with ill-defined borders	Flares: topical steroids Pruritus: antihistamines Remind patients to moisturize skin often and avoid triggers Severe AD: **dupilumab**, a monoclonal antibody blocking IL-4 and IL-13
★ **Psoriasis:** inflammatory disease of thick silvery scaled plaques	Anyone	Well-demarcated red plaques with silver scale, commonly on **scalp, elbows, and knees**. Psoriatic scales are much thicker and larger than in atopic dermatitis	Topical steroids Calcipotriene Topical retinoid (tazarotene) Severe disease: phototherapy or systemic treatment (methotrexate, mycophenolate mofetil, tacrolimus)

			Joint involvement: TNF-alpha inhibitors, such as infliximab and etanercept, apremilast (PDE4 inhibitor), or guselkumab (IL-23 inhibitor)
★ **Contact dermatitis:** itchy or painful skin reaction to allergens	Anyone	Erythematous scaling patches that may be in **geometric patterns** (from exposure), often with distinct borders	Avoid offending agents Topical steroids, calcineurin inhibitors, antihistamines If symptoms are persistent, may consider referring for **patch testing** to detect what the patient is allergic to
★ **Seborrheic dermatitis**: also known as **"dandruff"** if on the scalp; greasy yellow scaling in sebum-rich body areas	Anyone Association with HIV and Parkinson's disease In babies, seborrheic dermatitis is referred to as **"cradle cap"**	**Erythematous plaques with large greasy scales** in areas with many sebaceous glands, such as forehead, nasolabial fold, chin, eyebrows, scalp, chest, and back.	Topical ketoconazole; anti-dandruff shampoo (e.g., active ingredient pyrithione zinc, selenium sulfide) Flares: topical steroids
Pityriasis rosea: benign skin rash that may be triggered by a viral infection	Adolescents and young adults Possibly due to reactivation of HHV-6 and HHV-7	**Discrete salmon-colored oval, scaly plaques and patches (Fig. 22.34).** Starts with a **"herald patch"** (one larger patch, often on the trunk; **Fig. 22.35)** and then spreads in a "Christmas tree" distribution (oriented along skin cleavage line) Spares face, palms, and sole	Supportive treatment, such as topical steroids and antihistamines for itch
★ **Tinea corporis ("ringworm"):** superficial skin infection of	Athletes, people living in hot/humid conditions	**Annular scaly plaque with central clearing and active, scaly border.** Often itchy	Isolated plaque: topical antifungal (e.g., clotrimazole)

dermatophytes (fungi that live on the skin) on the trunk and extremities		Sample for KOH exam should be taken from the red scaly margin	Widespread lesions: oral antifungals (e.g., griseofulvin) Topical steroids will worsen the fungal infection!
Tinea cruris ("jock itch"): superficial skin infection of dermatophytes in the groin region	Risk factors: obesity, diabetes, men	**Erythematous plaque with sharp margins and active border;** may lack scale because of occlusion May perform KOH exam to diagnose	Drying powders and topical antifungals (e.g., terbinafine) Widespread involvement: oral antifungals
✯ **Tinea pedis** ("athlete's foot"): superficial skin infection of dermatophytes on the feet	Risk factors: athletes, older people	Multiple subtypes: 1. Interdigital: maceration with scaling and redness in between toes 2. Moccasin-type: patchy erythema and scaling of the soles in a moccasin distribution 3. Vesiculobullous: bullae or vesicles 4. Ulcerative: ulcerations and erosions of the webspace; seen in immunocompromised May perform KOH exam to definitively diagnose.	Drying powders and topical antifungals Bullous tinea pedis may be refractory, in which case you will need to treat with oral antifungals (terbinafine)
Mycosis fungoides: most common T-cell lymphoma of the skin	More common in males, older adults, and African-Americans	Progression over years 1. Patch stage: Erythematous or hypopigmented patches and plaques on **buttocks and sun-protected areas**	Topical steroids Stage 2 or beyond: systemic therapies (chemotherapy, biologics, radiation)

		2. Plaque: annular or polycyclic 3. Tumor: ulceration may be present	
Lichen planus: autoimmune inflammatory condition in which lesions are described by the 6 Ps	30-60 year olds May be associated with hepatitis C. Medications can also cause lichen planus-like eruptions	**5Ps: purple, polygonal, pruritic, planar (flat-topped), papules** **Wickham striae:** fine scaly white lines on lesions Look for oral lesions	Topical and intralesional steroids for thick lesions If the above doesn't work, then can try oral corticosteroids, methotrexate, phototherapy, and oral acitretin
★ **Dermatomyositis:** multisystem autoimmune connective tissue disease that may be associated with an internal malignancy	Children 5-14 years old and adults 45-65 years old Inflammatory myopathy that is associated with cancer!	Photodistributed rash and a diagnosis of cancer (**Fig. 22.36**). The rash may or may not be associated with muscle weakness. If it is not, the diagnosis is **amyopathic dermatomyositis** Key findings of dermatomyositis: - **Heliotrope sign:** violaceous erythema and edema of upper eyelid - **Shawl sign:** pink patch/plaque on upperback like a shawl	Check for extracutaneous findings: - Muscle: aldolase, creatine kinase, clinical muscle weakness - Cardiac: ST-T changes - Lungs: Interstitial lung disease (poor prognosis) - Malignancy For skin findings: photoprotection, topical steroids Muscle involvement: oral steroids or other immunosuppressive

		- **V-neck sign:** red telangiectatic patch on upper chest - **Gottron sign:** violaceous erythema on knees - **Gottron papules:** violaceous papules over DIP and PIP - **Holster sign:** pink scaly plaque on lateral thighs - **Mechanic's hands:** hyperkeratotic papules on lateral second digits - **Dilated capillary folds** at nailbed	medications (e.g., methotrexate, mycophenolate mofetil, azathioprine)

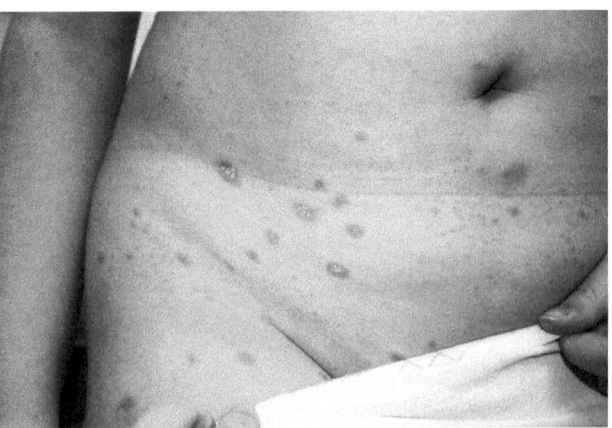

■ **Fig. 22.34** Salmon-colored circular plaques with fine collarettes of scale in pityriasis rosea

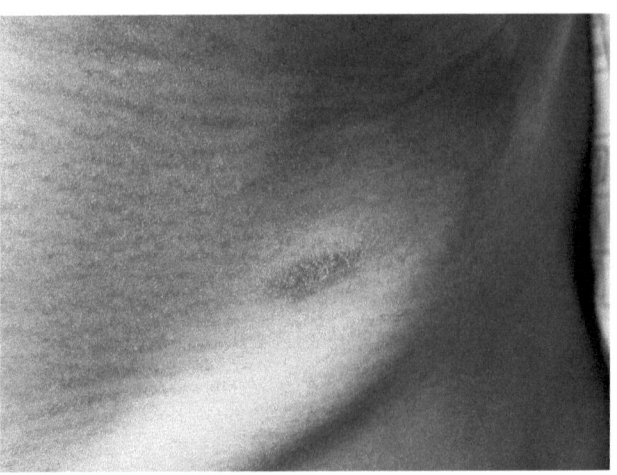

■ **Fig. 22.35** Herald patch of pityriasis rosea

22

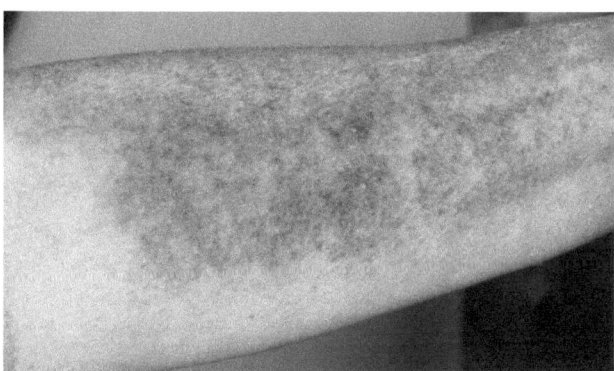

Fig. 22.36 Dermatomyositis with photodistributed rash

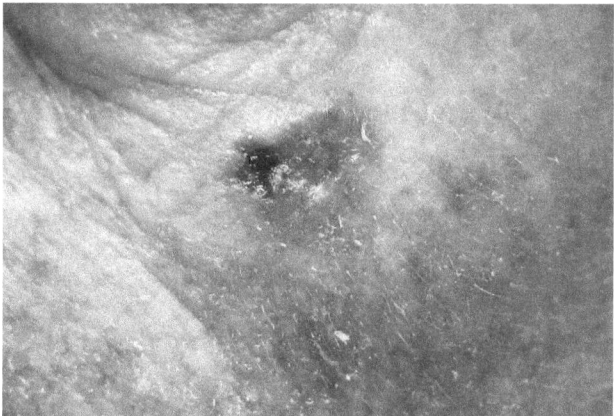

Fig. 22.37 Nodular basal cell carcinoma

22.4.3 Non-melanoma Skin Cancer and Other Discrete Scaly or Smooth Papules

Two common non-melanoma skin cancers (NMSCs) are basal cell carcinoma and squamous cell carcinoma. Both of these skin cancers are related to sun exposure and are more common in older people with lighter skin phototypes. On the body, they are often found in sun-exposed areas, such as the face, upper chest, and arms.

22.4.3.1 Basal Cell Carcinoma

Basal cell carcinoma (BCC) is the most common skin cancer. It is a neoplasm of the basal keratinocytes and generally presents as a smooth pearly papule or nodule with rolled borders and maybe some overlying telangiectasias (dilated blood vessels). On histopathology, you will see basophilic cells in nests in the dermis and subcutis. While the rates of metastases are low, as with any malignancy, it is still important to detect BCCs early.

22.4.3.2 Squamous Cell Carcinoma

Squamous cell carcinoma (SCC) is the second most common skin cancer. Like BCCs, they are related to UV exposure, but they can also be related to solid organ transplantation, human papillomavirus, immunosuppression, and chemical exposure, such as arsenic. SCCs present as hyperkeratotic, scaly papules or plaques (■ Fig. 22.38). On biopsy, you will see foci of keratinization (*keratin pearls*) with atypical keratinocytes beyond the basement membrane.

> While the nodular type is the appearance you should remember when you enter rotations, be aware that there are three types of BCC, which all present differently.
> 1. Nodular BCC: appears as *pearly papule* with telangiectasia (■ Fig. 22.37)
> 2. Superficial BCC: appears as chronic eczema
> 3. Sclerotic BCC: appears as chronic scar

> Marjolin's ulcer is an SCC that occurs on a chronic wound.

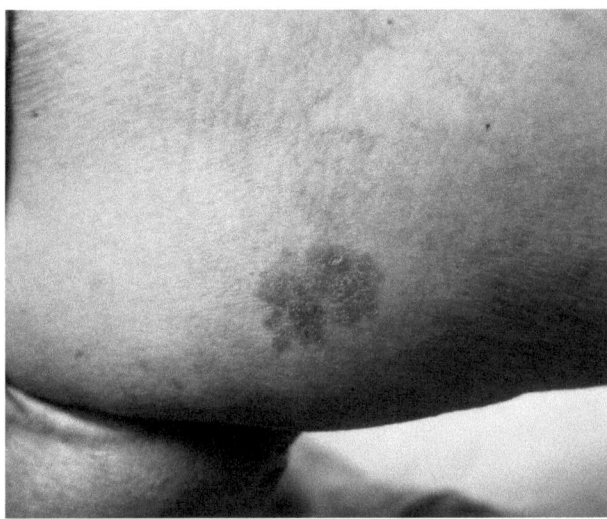

□ Fig. 22.38   Squamous cell carcinoma in situ

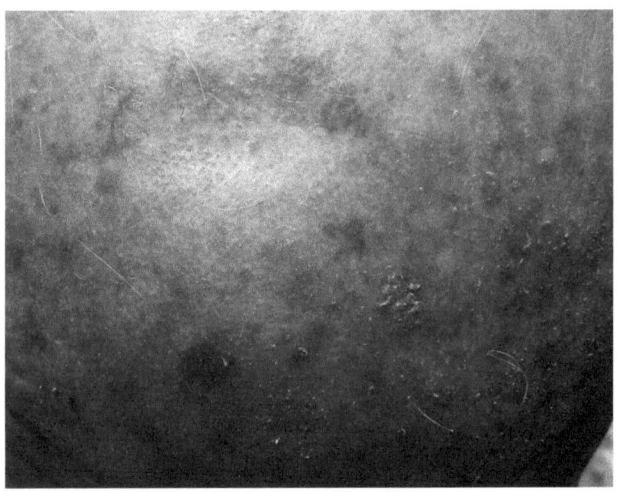

□ Fig. 22.39   Actinic keratosis of the scalp

22.4.3.3 **Actinic Keratosis**

Actinic keratoses (AKs) have the potential to evolve into SCCs, though the rate is very small with every AK having a 0.075–0.096% chance of evolving into an invasive squamous cell carcinoma. AKs appear as rough scaly papules or plaques with ill-defined borders on sun-exposed areas (□ Fig. 22.39). They may be tender and can be skin-colored, pink, or brown. Management is often cryotherapy, but for patients who have many AKs, you can do field therapy, whereby you apply topical 5-FU or imiquimod to the affected and nearby unaffected areas to prevent development of more AKs.

22.4.3.4 **Other Conditions to Consider**

In the table below, we have listed other discrete scaly or smooth papules that may look like the NMSCs we discussed. In general, important questions to ask when a patient presents with a discrete papule are: when did the papule appear and are there any changes to the lesion, bleeding or discharge, and history of skin cancer?

On exam, note where the lesion is. Warts and clavi appear more frequently on the hands and feet, whereas actinic keratoses, BCC, and SCC appear more frequently on sun-exposed areas like the arms or face. If you are concerned about cancer, you may suggest obtaining a biopsy of the lesion.

22

Condition and brief overview	Patient population	Appearance	Management
★ **Actinic keratosis:** precancerous epithelial overgrowth on sun-exposed areas	Elderly; lighter skin phototypes	Ill-defined scaly, rough papule on sun-exposed areas, such as scalp, arms, and face Some patients may have many AKs that coalesce into plaques	Cryotherapy
★ **Squamous cell carcinoma** (SCC): cancer of the squamous cell	Elderly; lighter skin phototypes	Hyperkeratotic papule or plaque on sun-exposed areas	Biopsy to confirm diagnosis Excision, electrodessication and curettage, Mohs surgery In situ disease: topical therapy such as 5-FU or imiquimod
★ **Basal cell carcinoma:** cancer of the basal keratinocyte; most common skin cancer	Elderly; lighter skin phototypes	**Pearly papule** with telangiectasia	Biopsy to confirm diagnosis Excision, electrodessication & curettage, Mohs surgery In situ disease: topical therapy such as 5-FU or imiquimod Systemic therapy: **vismodegib** (Hedgehog pathway inhibitor)
★ **Verrucae** (warts): epidermal proliferation due to HPV infection, commonly on hands and feet	Anyone, but most common in immunocompromised and children	Hyperkeratotic papule that **disturbs skin lines (Figure. 22.40)**. Has black/red dots representing **thrombosed capillaries**	Usually self-limited so may not need to treat Treatment options: salicylic acid, cryotherapy, 5-FU, imiquimod, intralesional Candida or bleomycin
Clavus (aka corn): benign epidermal thickening from repeated pressure or friction	Risk factors: elderly, those who play sports or perform repetitive actions	Well-circumscribed hyperkeratotic papule **without disturbed skin lines or thrombosed capillaries**	Reassurance. If bothering patient, can use salicylic acid creams or pare down with scalpel in clinic
Molluscum contagiosum: dimpled papules caused by **poxvirus**	Children In adults, molluscum is often in the anogenital distribution from sexual transmission	Dome-shaped papules with central **umbilication (Figure. 22.41)**	Usually self-limited. Can do curettage or cryotherapy Advise patients that these are **contagious**

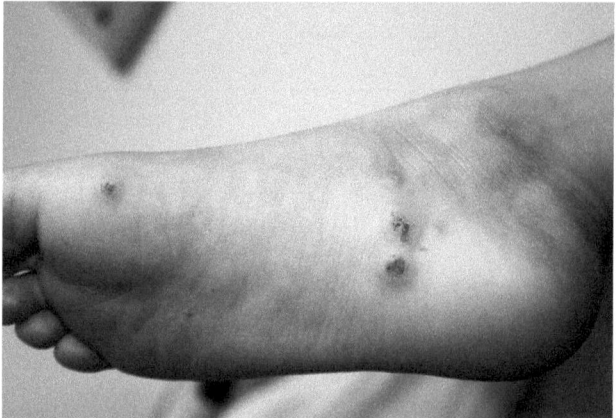

Fig. 22.40 Warts that disturb skin lines on feet

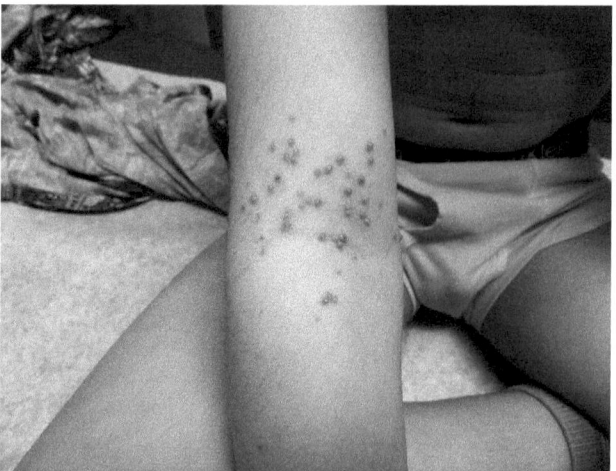

Fig. 22.41 Umbilicated papules of molluscum contagiosum

22.4.4 Follicular-Based Papules/Pustules

Papules and pustules that develop around follicles are often due to a disorder of the pilosebaceous unit (see ▶ Sect. 22.1.1 "Structure of the Skin").

22.4.4.1 Acne

A very common condition is acne vulgaris (commonly known as acne). Acne is caused by (1) plugging of the follicles from excessive keratinocytes, (2) bacterial growth, and (3) inflammation. It is common in teenagers but can also be seen in adults.

On exam, you may see erythematous, inflammatory papules, pustules, or nodules usually on the forehead, chin, or cheeks (■ Fig. 22.42). In patients with darker skin phototypes, there may be post-inflammatory hyperpigmentation, and in patients with nodular acne, there may be atrophic scarring. If you look closely at acne, you can see *comedones* which are skin pores that can be

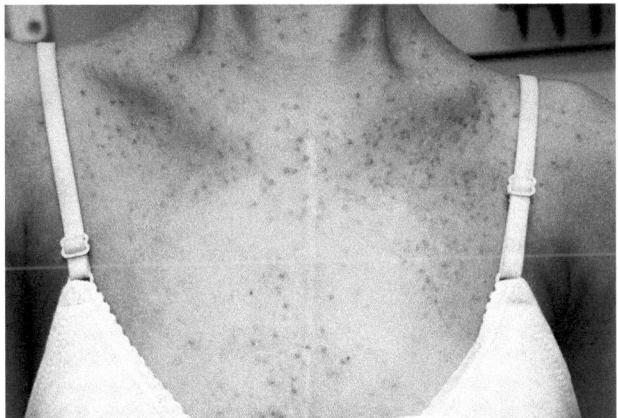

■ **Fig. 22.42**   Acne on the upper chest

either open (blackhead) or closed (whitehead). The presence of comedones is a distinguishing factor between acne and similar-appearing conditions, such as rosacea.

There are several treatments you can use for acne. To combat the plugging of follicles, you can suggest a topical retinoid (such as Adapalene), benzoyl peroxide, or salicylic acid, which are all exfoliators. To minimize bacterial growth, you can suggest a topical antibiotic, such as clindamycin. Treatment should be tailored to the severity and nature of the acne. In general:

- If the acne is predominantly comedonal without redness or inflammation → topical retinoid
- If the acne is comedonal with some pustules:
  - Mild: topical antibiotic plus a topical retinoid or benzoyl peroxide
  - Moderate: oral antibiotic and topical retinoid and topical benzoyl peroxide
  - Severe (nodular acne): oral isotretinoin
    - Oral isotretinoin (Accutane) reduces oil production and can essentially "cure" acne, though for some people, they will need to go on several courses of the medication. Isotretinoin is a teratogen so patients need to participate in iPledge, a contract that requires using two forms of contraception and monthly pregnancy tests. While on isotretinoin, patients also need to have regular blood draws.
- Women with jawline acne that worsens when she is about to have her period (also known as *hormonal acne*) → oral spironolactone

22.4.4.2 Hidradenitis Suppurativa

Hidradenitis suppurativa (HS) is a chronic condition characterized by inflammatory nodules and papules in apocrine gland-bearing regions (e.g., axilla, groin, breasts). It is often misdiagnosed and can be debilitating for the patient. The pathophysiology is thought to be from occlusion of the follicles that leads to trapping of bacteria and inflammation. HS usually occurs after puberty, and risk factors include obesity and smoking.

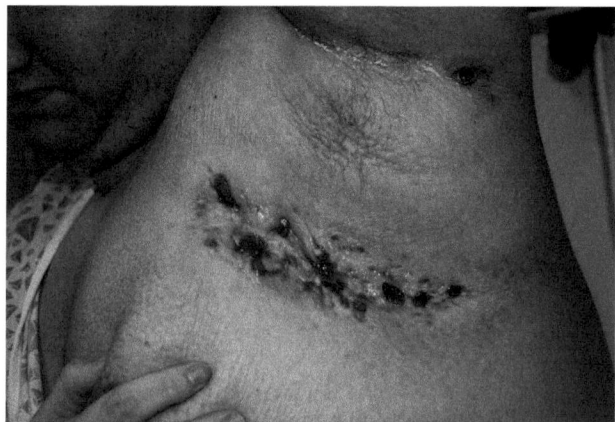

Fig. 22.43   Hidradenitis suppurativa

On exam, look for pink to brown papulonodules and abscesses, common in the axilla, groin, buttocks, breasts, and areas of friction (e.g., waistband area) (■ Fig. 22.43). You may see *double-headed comedones on a single nodule,* which is indicative of HS.

To categorize the severity of HS, you can use the *Hurley staging system*:
1. Abscesses without sinus tract or scarring
2. Recurrent abscesses with sinus tracts and scarring
3. Multiple abscesses and sinus tracts with diffuse involvement

Treatment will be multipronged:
1. Address underlying conditions: For those with metabolic syndrome, encourage weight loss, and for those who smoke, you should counsel on smoking cessation. If patient has diabetes, start medication, such as metformin.
2. Cleaning the area: Hibiclens is an antimicrobial skin cleanser that is often used in HS. Another option is bleach baths.
3. Treatment ladder for lesions themselves
   - Intralesional corticosteroid in active lesions
   - Topical clindamycin 1% BID
   - Oral doxycycline
   - Spironolactone
   - Oral clindamycin with rifampin
   - TNF-a inhibitor (adalimumab)
   - Acitretin, an oral retinoid (not great for women of childbearing age because they can't drink alcohol because that increases side effects)

22.4.4.3 Other Conditions to Consider

Condition and brief overview	Patient population	Appearance	Management
Folliculitis: inflammation of superficial hair follicle	Risk factors: shaving, obesity, friction, occlusion, diabetes, HIV	Erythematous papules and pustules centered around follicles **(Fig. 22.44)** **Furunculosis:** nodules due to deeper involvement	Avoid shaving or other triggers Topical antibiotics (mupirocin, clindamycin) Furunculosis: oral cephalexin or clindamycin (if MRSA suspected)
Milia: minute epidermoid cysts that present as small white/yellow papules	Anyone, common in newborns	White, yellow 1-2 mm papules; common on cheeks, nose, eyelids	Benign, but if patient is concerned about appearance, can extract in clinic May use tretinoin chronically to prevent recurrence
Sebaceous hyperplasia: benign hypertrophy of sebaceous glands	Older adults	Small yellow papules with **central dell**; common on forehead, nose, cheeks **(Fig. 22.45)**	Reassurance
☆ **Acne:** inflammation of pilosebaceous unit due to hormonal change	Adolescents and adults	Erythematous, inflammatory papules, pustules, or nodules. +/- postinflammatory hyperpigmentation and atrophic scarring Can distinguish from other conditions because this has **comedones**! In females, acne may be cyclical with menstruation	Topical retinoids, antibiotics, benzoyl peroxide, oral antibiotics, isotretinoin **Hormonal acne**(acne that worsens with menstruation): **spironolactone**
☆ **Hidradenitis suppurativa:** inflammation in apocrine-gland-bearing regions	Risk factors: obesity and smoking	Pink to brown papules, nodules, and abscesses, common in axilla, groin, buttocks, breasts, and areas of friction (e.g., waistband area). May see **double-headed comedones on a single nodule**	Address risk factors, careful cleaning of areas, intralesional corticosteroid, topical or oral clindamycin

Pilonidal cyst: disruption of epithelium on coccyx that leads to abscess formation	Young male adults Risk factors: obesity, hirsutism, prolonged sitting	Tender, erythematous nodule over coccyx. May have purulent drainage.	Incision and drainage followed by warm sitz baths. Antibiotics not usually indicated unless patient is immunocompromised or there is cellulitis.

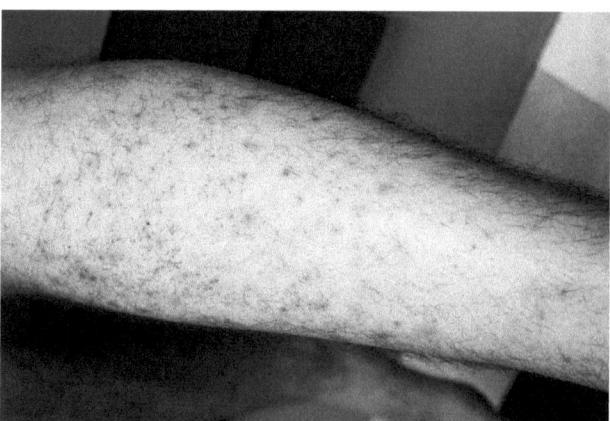

Fig. 22.44 Folliculitis

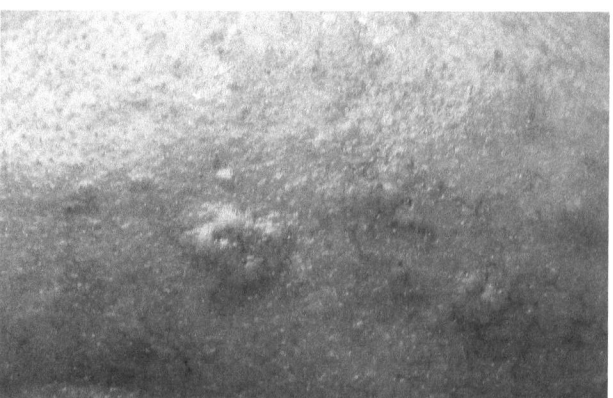

Fig. 22.45 Sebaceous hyperplasia

22.4.5 **Erythematous Cheeks**

When patients present with redness of the cheeks, there can be a variety of reasons for the redness. Some clues as to what may be going on are:

- If the redness is associated with triggers → rosacea
- Varies with the menstrual cycle → acne
- Has scaling → seborrheic dermatitis
- Worsens in the sun or associated with oral ulcers, alopecia (hair loss), or other systemic symptoms → lupus

On examination, make sure to look closely at how the redness is distributed and whether or not it involves the nasolabial folds. If the rash spares the nasolabial folds, this suggests that the rash is photodistributed because the nasolabial folds do not get as much sunlight. An example of a rash that spares the nasolabial folds is the malar rash in lupus.

22.4.5.1 **Rosacea**

Rosacea is a chronic inflammatory condition that is commonly seen in 30–50-year-olds with women presenting younger than men. The pathophysiology of the condition is not well understood, but vascular changes and immune activation in response to certain triggers are implicated. Common triggers for flushing in rosacea are:

- Spicy foods
- Chocolate
- Alcohol
- Hot foods

The typical appearance of rosacea is erythematous cheeks, maybe with telangiectasias, papules, and pustules, that spare nasolabial folds. There are four main subtypes of rosacea that may present differently:

- Erythematotelangiectatic: persistent erythema with intermittent flushing
- Papulopustular: acneiform pustules (to distinguish from acne, rosacea does not have comedones!)
- Phymatous: thickening of skin, most commonly on the nose
- Ocular: conjunctivitis, blepharitis, hyperemia

Rhinophyma is seen in phymatous rosacea, whereby there is thickening and cobblestoning of the nose skin.

Treatment for rosacea involves avoiding triggers and using topical treatments, such as metronidazole, azelaic acid, or erythromycin. For patients with more severe rosacea, you may consider oral tetracycline or metronidazole.

22.4.5.2 Other Conditions to Consider

Condition and brief overview	Patient population	Appearance	Management
Acne (see Sect. 22.4.4)	–	–	–
Seborrheic dermatitis (see Sect. 22.4.2)	–	–	–
Rosacea: facial flushing with telangiectasias and papules in response to certain triggers	30-50 year–olds Lighter skin phototypes	Erythema on cheeks that typically spares nasolabial folds	Avoid triggers Topical metronidazole, azelaic acid, or erythromycin Can also use oral tetracycline or metronidazole
★ **Systemic lupus erythematosus:** multisystem autoimmune disorder with butterfly rash that spares nasolabial fold	Women of child-bearing age; more common in African-Americans	Erythema of central face that spares nasolabial folds (**malar rash**). Unlike rosacea, this rash is not papular and not worsened with triggers for vasodilation In addition to malar rash, patient may have oral ulcers, renal disease, arthritis, serositis, and neurologic disorder Lab abnormalities may include **+ANA, +dsDNA, anti-Smith,** leukopenia, anemia, and thrombocytopenia	Hydroxychloroquine Flares: oral prednisone, azathioprine, or methotrexate, mycophenolate, cyclosporine, or rituximab

22.4.6 Lighter Skin Patches

When a patient presents with patches of skin that are lighter than other parts of their skin, you should consider the distribution of the patches, their appearance, and any preceding symptoms. Lighter skin patches may be caused by infection, inflammation, UV radiation, or an autoimmune etiology.

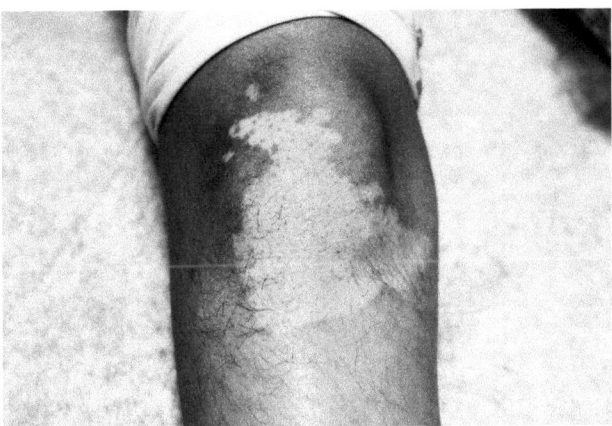

▫ Fig. 22.46   Depigmented patch of vitiligo with perifollicular repigmentation

22.4.6.1 Vitiligo

Vitiligo is a condition whereby there is complete loss of melanocytes in certain areas of the skin, either by an autoimmune response or intrinsic melanocyte defects. Patients who develop vitiligo are usually otherwise healthy, though they may have hyper- or hypothyroidism, diabetes, or Addison's disease – diseases that are all associated with an autoimmune process. Thus, you should ask patients whether or not they have these other conditions if you are suspecting vitiligo.

Vitiligo is different from other hypopigmenting conditions in that vitiligo macules and patches are *depigmented* (complete loss of melanocytes) (▫ Fig. 22.46), whereas other conditions tend to have *hypopigmented* lesions (lighter skin color, but not completely devoid of melanocytes). As a result of the complete depigmentation in vitiligo, you will see vitiligo patches "light up" (be a bright milky white) on Wood's lamp exam. A biopsy is definitive in making this diagnosis.

The goal of vitiligo treatment is to stop progression of the disease and promote repigmentation. First-line treatments involve topical corticosteroids and calcineurin inhibitors. Other treatments include phototherapy and skin grafts. Interestingly, when the skin starts to repigment, it often repigments around hair follicles. Thus, you may counsel patients on *perifollicular repigmentation* so that they are not surprised.

22.4.6.2 Other Conditions to Consider

Condition and brief overview	Patient population	Appearance	Management
★ **Tinea versicolor:** benign superficial skin fungal infection	Active individuals; more common in the summer	Scaly asymptomatic hypo– or hyperpigmented macules that coalesce into patches on the trunk and proximal extremities (**Fig. 22.47**) **Versicolor:** can be a variety of colors (pink, brown, white) **KOH exam shows spaghetti and meatball** (non-septated hyphae and spores)	Large affected areas: Anti-dandruff shampoos as body wash; ketoconazole 2% wash Limited areas: topical antifungals, such as clotrimazole cream Severe: oral fluconazole
Post-inflammatory hypopigmentation: loss of skin pigmentation after inflammation	Anyone; common in people with inflammatory skin disease, such as atopic dermatitis or seborrheic dermatitis	Hypopigmented patches **in location of previous inflammatory lesions**	Reassurance; sunscreen
Idiopathic guttate hypomelanosis: benign small hypopigmented macules on shins and forearms	More common in people with lighter skin phototypes with extensive sun exposure	**3-5 mm hypopigmented macules**symmetrically on extensor arms and legs	Reassurance; sunscreen; discourage excessive sun exposure
Pityriasis alba: hypopigmented patches in children with atopic children	Children with atopic dermatitis	**Poorly demarcated hypopigmented patches** with fine scaling (**Fig. 22.48**); usually symmetrically on cheeks. **Starts as scaly pink plaque**	Topical steroids; topical calcineurin inhibitors (tacrolimus, pimecrolimus) Moisturizers
★ **Vitiligo:** autoimmune disorder that leads to depigmentation (complete loss of melanocytes)	Anyone **Screen patients for other autoimmune diseases.** E.g., hypothyroidism, alopecia areata, Addison's disease, type 1 diabetes	**Depigmented** macules or patches. Under **Wood's lamp,** you will see milky white depigmentation Skin biopsy shows **absence of melanocytes**	Sun protection Local disease: topical steroids or calcineurin inhibitors; phototherapy Rapidly evolving disease: oral steroids Surgical option: skin grafts

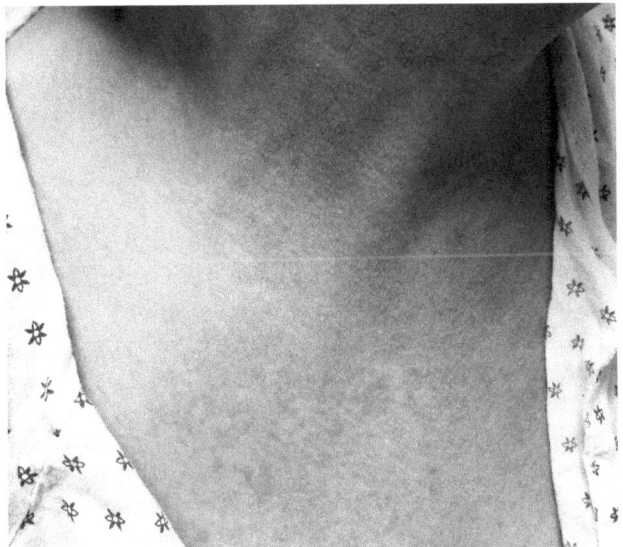

Fig. 22.47   Tinea versicolor on upper chest

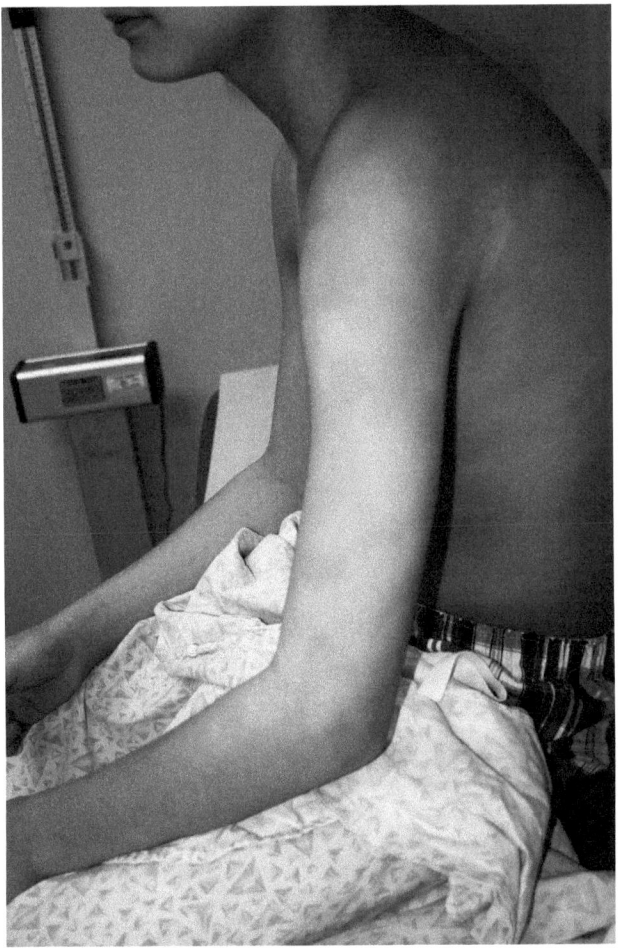

Fig. 22.48   Pityriasis alba of the arm

22.4.7 Leg Conditions

In this section, we will discuss common conditions of the lower extremities. It is important to note that most of these conditions can be seen elsewhere on the body as well.

22.4.7.1 Cellulitis

Cellulitis is an infection of the deep dermis and subcutaneous tissue (compared with *erysipelas* which is an infection of the superficial dermis and lymphatics). It can be seen in anyone, though people with diabetes or tinea pedis are particularly susceptible because those conditions lead to small cuts that are entry points for bacteria.

Patients with cellulitis may have fevers and chills. Their legs display four cardinal signs of inflammation: redness, swelling, heat, and pain. Mark the edge of the erythema, and check every 4–6 hours to see if the borders have expanded, which would indicate that your therapy is not effective. If the leg displays any crepitus (crackling when you press on it), then you should be concerned about necrotizing fasciitis which is an emergency and requires immediate surgical debridement. Other conditions to rule out are deep venous thrombosis, stasis dermatitis, and erysipelas.

In patients with cellulitis, the white blood cell count may be normal or elevated. Blood cultures are usually negative in immunocompetent patients. If the drainage is purulent, you can do a wound swab to check for MRSA. If there is no drainage, a wound swab is usually not helpful.

Treatment is dependent on the patient's immune status and MRSA risk factors. Methicillin-sensitive *Staph aureus* is the most common organism, so PO cephalexin or penicillin is usually adequate (use clindamycin if the patient has a penicillin allergy). If MRSA is suspected, you could try trimethoprim-sulfamethoxazole or doxycycline. For patients with severe cellulitis (fever, tachycardia, or leukocytosis), you may need to give IV antibiotics.

Cellulitis is usually unilateral. If both legs are red and swollen, consider other diagnoses!

22.4.7.2 Other Conditions to Consider

Condition and brief overview	Patient population	Appearance	Management
★ **Cellulitis:** infection of deep dermis and subcutaneous tissue	Risk factors: diabetes, minor skin trauma on legs, IV drug use, tinea pedis, peripheral vascular disease Most common organisms: Group A beta-hemolytic strep (*Strep pyogenes*) and Staph aureus	**Unilateral** erythema with classic signs of inflammation (redness, warmth, pain, and swelling) May have fever/chills and leukocytosis	Elevate leg Consider tissue cultures prior to starting antibiotics in immunocompromised patients! Mild infection in healthy patient: oral antibiotics (e.g., cephalexin) Severe infection or patient with comorbidities: IV antibiotics (e.g., cefazolin) MRSA risk factors(e.g., if patient is hospitalized): PO clindamycin or IV vancomycin

Erysipelas ("superficial cellulitis"): infection of superficial dermis and lymphatics	Risk factors: venous insufficiency, stasis dermatitis, and poor lymphatic drainage Most common organism: beta-hemolytic group A streptococci (*Strep pyogenes)*	**Sharply defined erythematous plaque that is very tender** Commonly on face and lower extremities Different than angioedema or contact dermatitis in that the patient has fever and elevated leukocyte count	Mild disease in healthy patient: PO penicillin IV treatment: cefazolin
Necrotizing fasciitis: deep bacterial infection that spreads rapidly and is a surgical emergency	Risk factors: recent surgery, trauma, diabetes, old age	Progresses rapidly with escalating pain and little response to antibiotics. **Pain out of proportion to visible skin changes.** May see skin necrosis, bullae, and **crepitus** (indicating gas in soft tissue). Systemic signs such as fever, tachycardia, hypotension If anogenital region is affected, it is called **Fournier gangrene**	This is a surgical emergency! Immediate debridement, IV antibiotics, and IV fluids Check labs: CBC, CRP, CPK, urea, creatinine, blood and wound cultures, X-ray of limb
Stasis dermat it is: inflammation of lower extremities due to poor circulation	Risk factors: **venous insufficiency,** obesity, congestive heart failure, varicose veins, elderly	Erythematous scaly plaque on **bilateral** lower extremities	Leg elevation, compressive therapy, topical steroids
Asteatotic dermatitis (aka eczema craquele): very dry skin on lower extremities	People with chronic xerosis (dry skin); elderly Worse in winter	**Erythematous plaque with polygonal cracked skin** that looks like "dried-up riverbed"	Minimize hot showers and soap; moisturize immediately after bathing with emollient-based creams Topical steroid to areas of erythema and pruritus
Erythema nodosum: inflammation of subcutaneous fat associated with inflammatory bowel disease	More common in females age 20-45 Associated with: pregnancy, lymphoma, infection (Streptococcal), sarcoidosis, IBD, drugs (sulfonamides and OCPs)	**Tender, erythematous deep-seated nodules on anterior shins** (could also be on buttocks and thighs); associated with fever, malaise. **Often bilateral(Fig. 22.49)** This is an inflammatory disease of the fat (panniculitis)	Treat underlying disease; elevate extremities, cool/wet compresses Supportive treatment: NSAIDs

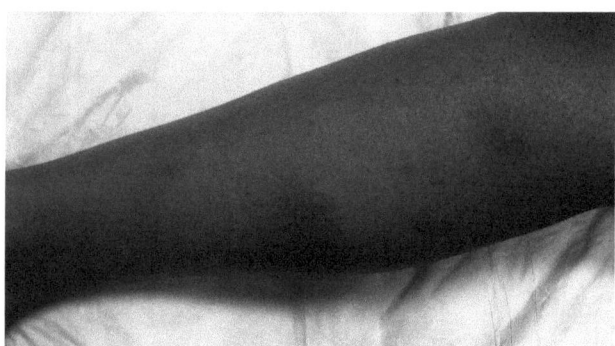

Fig. 22.49   Erythema nodosum

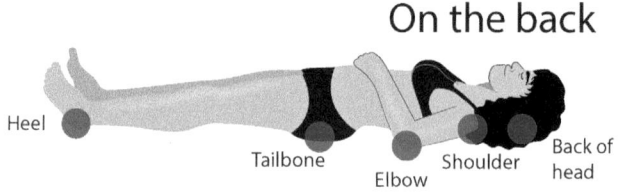

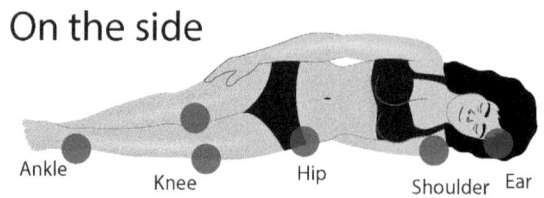

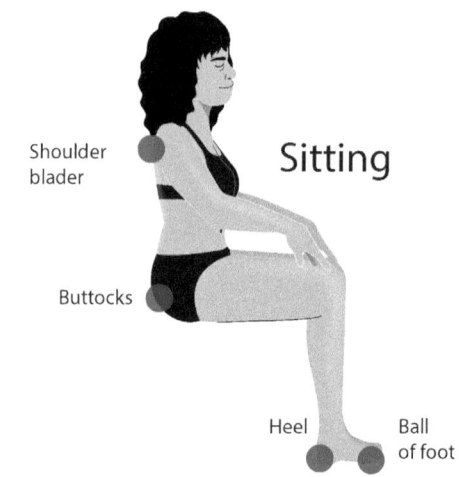

Fig. 22.50   Location of pressure points

22.4.8 Ulcers

Ulcers are when there is loss of the epidermis and part of, or all of, the dermis. You will encounter many patients with ulcers, and your team will be asked to formulate a treatment plan. In general, ulcers form because either pressure (■ Fig. 22.50) or vascular disease leads to compromised blood flow and necrosis of the skin.

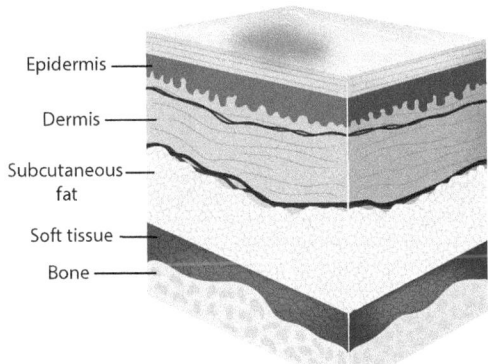

Stage I: nonblanchable
erythema on intact skin

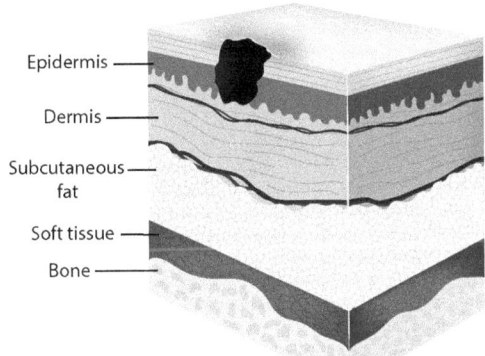

Stage II: epidermis loss leading to
shiny red underlying dermis

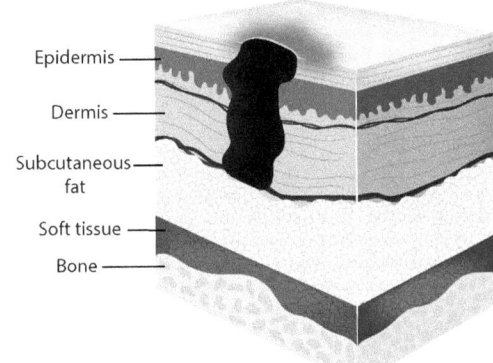

Stage III: loss of epidermis, dermis, and possibly
subcutaneous tissue that extends to the fascia

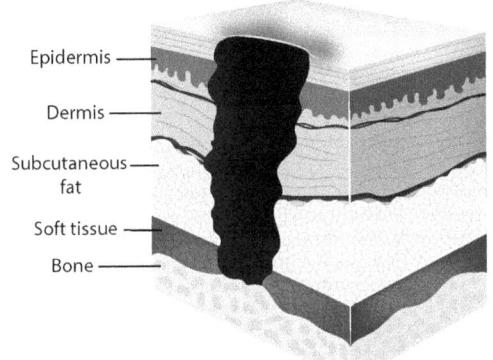

Stage IV: loss of epidermis, dermis, subcutaneous
tissue, and fascia that extends down to muscle/bone

Fig. 22.51 Four stages of ulcers

When assessing an ulcer, make sure to assess its stage (■ Fig. 22.51) and any neurovascular compromise (strength of nearby pulses and sensation around the ulcer). Complications of ulcers are soft tissue infection, osteomyelitis (infection of the bone), and squamous cell carcinoma (Marjolin's ulcer).

Wound dressings and care should be used for these patients (see ▶ Sect. 22.2). You would choose the wound dressing based on how much exudate the wound is producing, the risk for infection, and convenience for the patient to change dressings. As a medical student, you would not be asked to know the precise wound dressing, but knowing the basics of wound care will be helpful as you hear what attendings and residents choose to recommend.

22.4.8.1 Pyoderma Gangrenosum

Pyoderma gangrenosum (PG) is a rare inflammatory (but not infectious) disease that causes ulcers. It is a neutrophilic disease meaning that on skin biopsy, you will see a lot of neutrophils. However, remember that these lesions are not infectious. The exact etiology of PG is unknown, but patients with *inflammatory bowel disease*, monoclonal gammopathy of undetermined significance, granulomatosis with polyangiitis, and Behcet's disease are particularly susceptible to developing PG.

PG lesions usually start as an extremely painful pustule or papule that ruptures and develops into an ulcer with a purulent base and violaceous rolled borders (■ Fig. 22.52). It is commonly found on the hands or legs.

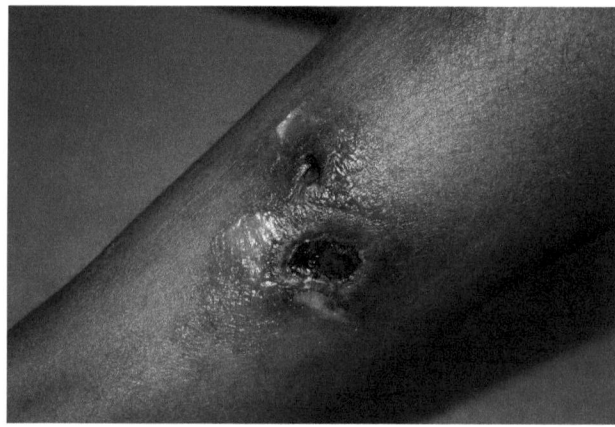

◘ Fig. 22.52 Pyoderma gangrenosum ulcer with rolled violaceous borders

Treatment involves good wound care. Do not suggest debriding the ulcer as this may increase the size of the ulcer via pathergy. You may use intralesional or topical steroids for mild disease and systemic immunomodulators for severe disease.

22.4.8.2 Other Conditions to Consider

Condition and brief overview	Patient population	Appearance	Management
Decubitus ulcers, also called pressure ulcers or bed sores	Risk factors: limited mobility, smoking, or elderly	Ulcers on pressure points, such as the tailbone, heel, or hip	Repositioning, wound care (see Sect. 22.2), infection and pain control
Leg/feet ulcers	Risk factors: diabetes, smoking, vascular disease	Ulcers on feet, usually on the soles, or distal legs	Treat underlying diabetes, wound care, infection and pain control
★ Pyoderma gangrenosum	Middle-age adults	**Extremely painful** nodule or pustule that ruptures and forms **ulcer with purulent base and violaceous rolled border**	Wound care and treat underlying condition Mild disease: topical or intralesional corticosteroids Severe disease: systemic immunomodulator, such as infliximab or adalimumab

22.4.9 Urticaria and Angioedema

Urticaria and angioedema are two types of swelling that can be associated with anaphylaxis. Urticaria is swelling of the upper dermis and looks more superficial (◘ Fig. 22.53), whereas angioedema is swelling of the lower dermis/subcu-

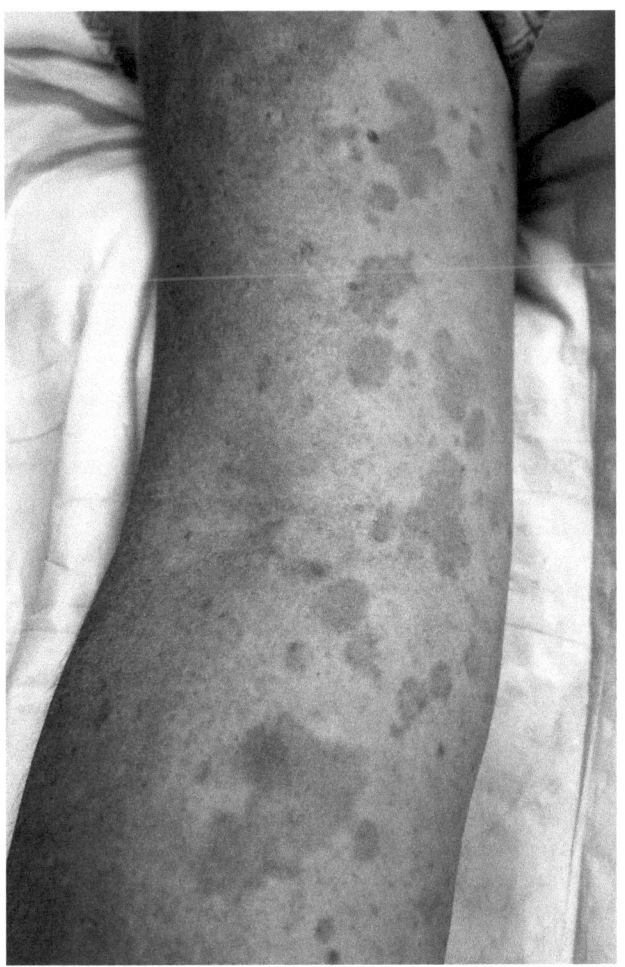

■ **Fig. 22.53**   Urticaria on arms

taneous tissue and is more raised/swollen. Urticaria tends to be itchy, whereas angioedema tends to be painful.

Both may be triggered by medications or foods or be idiopathic. Some patients may experience *chronic urticaria,* which is defined as urticaria for *more than 2 days/week for greater than 6 weeks.*

The presence of angioedema is an emergency, as it may herald imminent respiratory compromise. Thus, it is crucial to check airway, breathing, and circulation in a patient who presents with angioedema. If there are signs of anaphylaxis, epinephrine, IV fluids, and oxygen should be administered.

22.4.9.1 Table of Urticaria vs. Angioedema

Condition and brief overview	Patient population	Appearance	Management
☆ *Urticaria:* also known as hives; swelling of upper dermis	Anyone	Well-circumscribed, erythematous papules/plaques with pale center called wheals. *Individual lesions last <24 hrs. Pruritic*	Oral H1 antihistamines (cetirizine, fexofenadine, loratadine) Referral for allergy testing as needed

Condition and brief overview	Patient population	Appearance	Management
Angioedema: swelling of lower dermis and subcutaneous tissue	Anyone	*Localized swelling*, most frequently involving lips, tongue, and face. Can *last several days*. *Burning/painful*	Check airway, breathing, circulation (ABCs!) If anaphylaxis occurs, administer epinephrine, IV fluids, and oxygen

22.4.10 Blistering Diseases

Blisters (classified as *vesicles* if <1 cm and *bullae* if >1 cm) can be due to:
1. Trauma: e.g., wearing uncomfortable shoes causing physical disruption of bonds between epidermal cells.
2. Inflammation/infection: e.g., in contact dermatitis, fluid accumulates within the epidermis.
3. Autoimmune: e.g., in bullous pemphigoid, autoantibodies attack adhesion molecules in the dermoepidermal junction.
4. Genetic: e.g., in epidermolysis bullosa, there are loss of cell adhesion proteins.

For any blister, you could examine for the presence of the *Nikolsky sign* to assess whether the damage is at or above the dermal-epidermal junction (i.e., very superficial) or deeper (see ▶ Sect. 22.2).
- Diseases with positive Nikolsky sign: Stevens-Johnson syndrome, staphylococcal scalded skin syndrome, pemphigus vulgaris
- Disease with negative Nikolsky sign: bullous pemphigoid

If vesicles are localized to one particular area, the location can be a great clue for the diagnosis (◘ Table 22.6).
  Besides location, symptoms before the onset of blisters are also important.
- Pain: herpes zoster, HSV
- Itch: contact dermatitis, dyshidrotic eczema, herpes zoster
- Trauma: friction blister
- Recurrent: HSV

A common secondary feature of vesicles or bullae is *erosion* when the vesicle/bulla pops.

22.4.10.1 Pemphigus Vulgaris
Pemphigus vulgaris (PV) is an autoimmune bullous disease that affects the skin and mucosal membranes. It is caused by autoantibodies to *desmoglein 1 and 3*, proteins responsible for keratinocyte adhesion in the stratum spinosum. On biopsy, you will see *suprabasal epidermal acantholysis* (cell separation above the basal layer) leading to "*tombstoning*" whereby the basal cells look like tombstones (◘ Fig. 22.54).
  Because the split in the skin occurs in the epidermis, the blisters you see in PV are very thin and fragile. If you perform the Nikolsky sign (see ▶ Sect. 22.2), you will be able to slough off the skin (a positive Nikolsky sign). PV often affects mucosal membranes so make sure to ask if the patient has been having difficulty eating and swallowing, which can be very debilitating. Also, perform a thorough exam of the oral cavity when a patient presents with suspected PV.

▪ Table 22.6 Location of vesicles with corresponding differential diagnoses

Location	DDx
Trunk in dermatomal distribution (on one side, does not cross midline)	Herpes zoster (shingles)
Fingers	Herpetic whitlow (HSV on fingers) Contact dermatitis Dyshidrotic eczema
Eyes, mouth, nose	HSV Bullous impetigo
Genitals	HSV
Legs and arms	Contact dermatitis
Feet	Tinea pedis Contact dermatitis Dyshidrotic eczema
Diffuse	Pemphigus vulgaris Bullous pemphigoid Stevens-Johnson syndrome Varicella zoster Bullous drug eruption

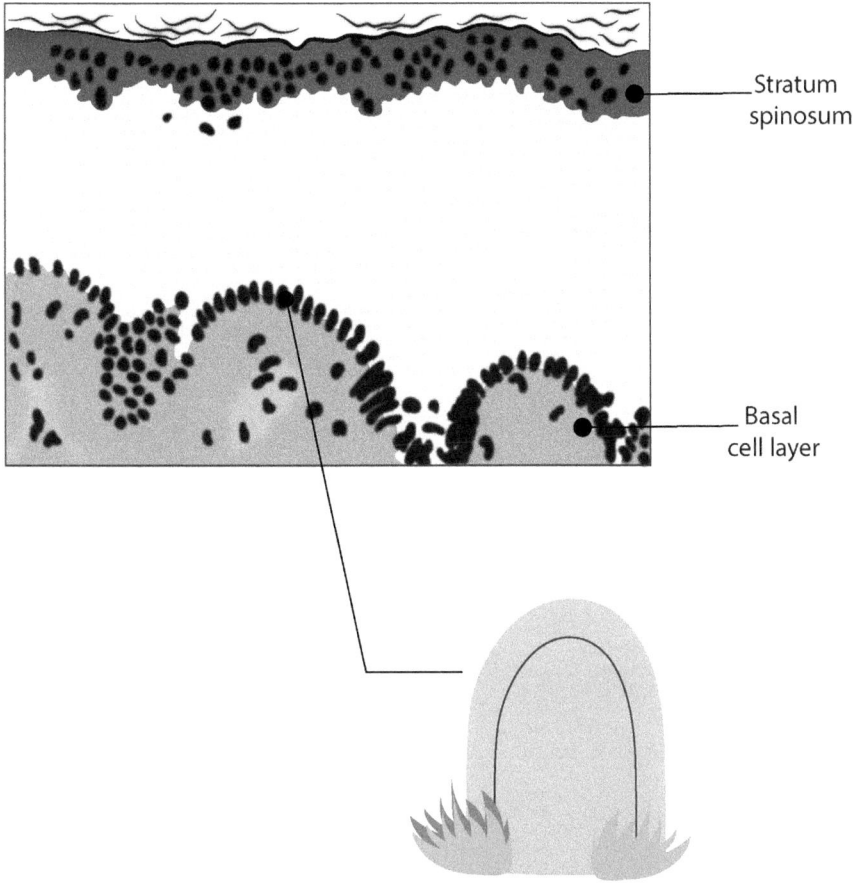

▪ Fig. 22.54 Tombstoning of the basal cell layer in pemphigus vulgaris

Rituximab works because it targets B cells that are creating the autoantibodies!

Definitive diagnosis involves taking a skin biopsy on the edge of a blister. Direct immunofluorescence will be performed on the normal-appearing skin adjacent to the lesion and will reveal IgG deposition in the epidermis if it is PV.

When a patient has confirmed PV, management will involve suppressing the immune system using prednisone and/or other immunosuppressive medications (e.g., azathioprine, rituximab).

22.4.10.2 Bullous Pemphigoid

Bullous pemphigoid (BP) is another autoimmune blistering disease caused by autoantibodies to *hemidesmosomes (proteins that attach basal cells to the basement membrane)*. Prior to the onset of the blisters, patients may complain of itching or urticaria. These lesions are more common in older individuals, so suspect this disease when an elderly patient complains of itching followed by the appearance of blisters.

Unlike pemphigus vulgaris where the split in the skin is in the epidermis, the split in bullous pemphigoid is below the epidermis. Thus, BP blisters are more tense and less fragile than those in pemphigus vulgaris (◘ Fig. 22.55). They will be *Nikolsky negative* (will not rupture when you slide you finger across them). BP can affect the oral mucosa, though it is less common and more minor than in PV.

Diagnosis for BP is similar to PV. Perform a skin biopsy on the edge of the lesion and direct or indirect immunofluorescence on the normal skin. If the diagnosis is BP, you will see IgG on the basement membrane.

In terms of treatment, for localized disease, you can use high-potency topical or intralesional steroid. For diffuse disease, use prednisone and/or other immunosuppressive medications. If you suspect that a medication was causing the BP, stop that medication.

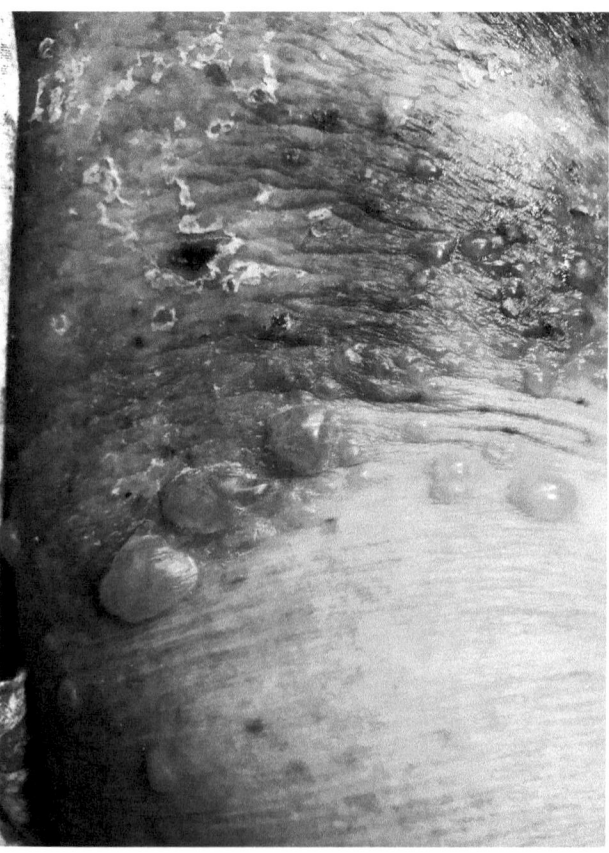

◘ **Fig. 22.55**   Bullous pemphigoid with tense blisters

22.4.10.3 Other Conditions to Consider

Condition and brief overview	Patient population	Appearance	Management
Allergic contact dermatitis (see also Sect. 22.4.2.2 under Scaly Patch)	Anyone	Vesicles in a pattern of exposure (e.g., in poison ivy, the vesicles are often in a linear streak). Vesicles appear 24-72 hrs after exposure	Topical steroids, oral antihistamines. Severe involvement may require oral steroids
★ **Herpes zoster** (shingles): reactivation of varicella zoster infection that is very painful and in a dermatomal distribution	More common in adults	**Grouped vesicles on erythematous base in a dermatomal distribution** (rarely crosses the midline) (**Fig. 22.56**) Usually **preceded by burning**; it is often very painful	Valacyclovir. Best if administered within the first 72 hrs of symptom onset to reduce length and severity of episode Complication of shingles: **postherpetic neuralgia** (residual hypersensitivity/pain in affected area even after lesions have resolved)
★ **Herpes simplex:** viral infection with characteristic grouped vesicles on erythematous base HSV 1: favors **mouth** (transmitted through direct contact) HSV2: favors **genitals** (sexually transmitted) Clinical subtypes: Herpes labialis: cold sores on mouth Herpetic whitlow: painful, distal finger Herpes gingivostomatitis: ulcers on lip and tongue Herpes genitalis: blisters/erosions in genital region	Anyone; in patients with severe/recurrent disease, consider HIV or immunosuppression	**Grouped vesicles on erythematous base; bright red borders and may present as crusts/erosions (Fig. 22.57)** **Lesions are often recurrent**	Acyclovir; initiate within first 72 hrs May also use prophylactic acyclovir in patients with >6 episodes per year

★ **Varicella zoster virus** (chickenpox): itchy skin lesions at different stages	Children	Pruritic macules and papules that start on face and spread to trunk/extremities. Turns into vesicles with erythematous base– **"dewdrops on a rose petal."** Hallmark is **lesions at different stages**	Symptomatic treatment with acetaminophen, cool compresses, calamine lotion, systemic antihistamines. Acyclovir can lessen severity if administered within first 72 hrs **Varicella vaccine** is live-attenuated and contraindicated in immunocompromised patients
Bullous impetigo: *Staph aureus* infection in children that causes blisters	Children <2 years	**Blisters with negative Nikolskysign with honey-colored crust (Fig. 22.58)** If very diffuse and severe, consider MRSA as the cause (**Staph scalded skin syndrome**)	Limited disease: topical mupirocin Systemic: PO cephalexin MRSA suspected: doxycycline
★ **Pemphigus vulgaris:** severe autoimmune disease of blisters on skin and mucous membranes like mouth	Adults	Diffuse **erosions.** Frequently involves mucous membranes **Nikolsky positive**	Prednisone and/or other immunosuppressive medications (e.g., azathioprine, rituximab)
★ **Bullous pemphigoid:** autoimmune condition that causes development of intact bullae in older individuals	Older adults	Diffuse **tense bullae** **Nikolsky negative**	Localized disease: high–potency topical steroid Widespread: prednisone +/-other immunosuppressives
Drug eruptions (see that section)	–	–	–

22

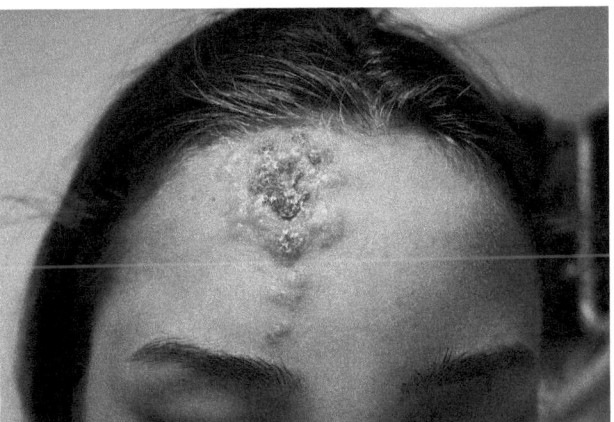

Fig. 22.56   Herpes simplex on the forehead

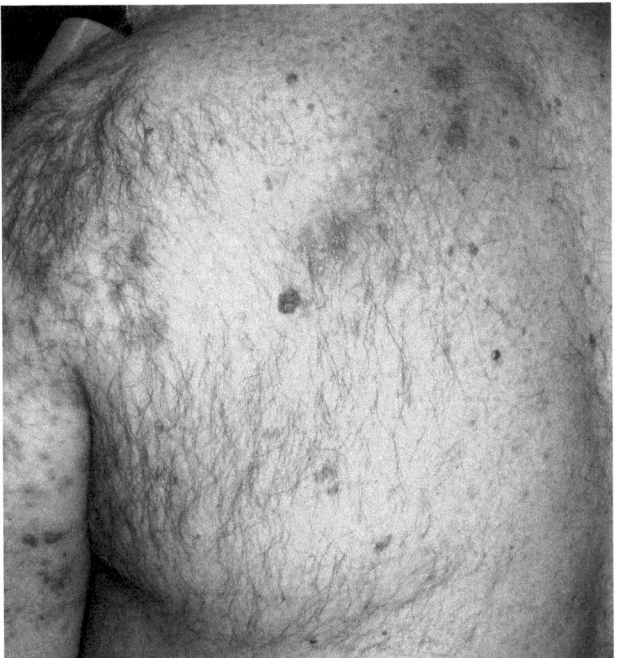

Fig. 22.57   Herpes zoster in a dermatomal distribution

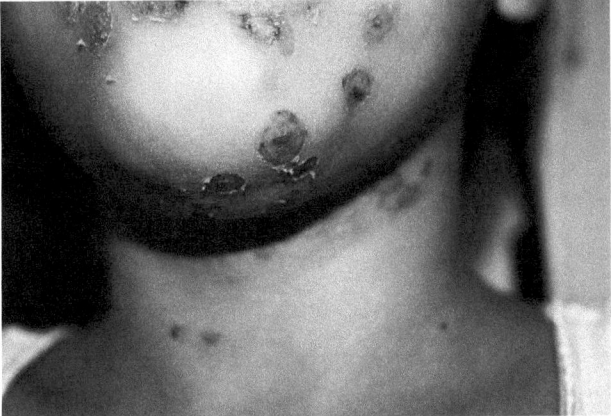

Fig. 22.58   Secondary erosions of bullae in bullous impetigo

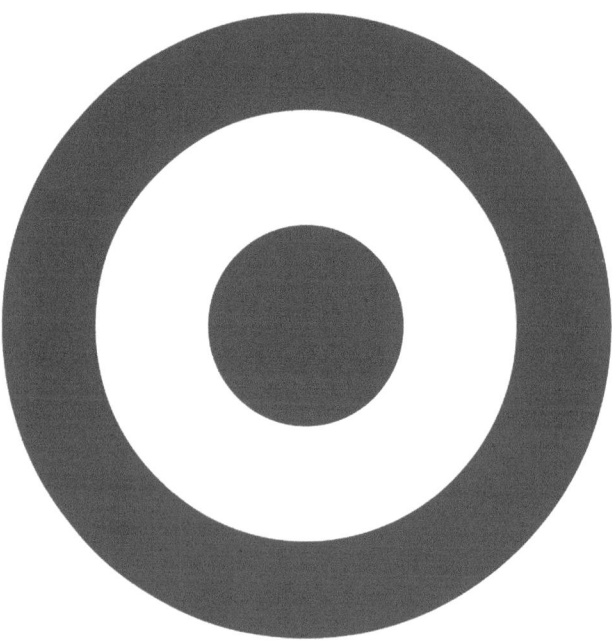

☐ **Fig. 22.59** A true "target" lesion has three zones: a dark center, pale ring around the dark center, and a peripheral ring of erythema

22.4.11 Target and Targetoid Lesions

The two main diagnoses for target or targetoid lesions are erythema multiforme and erythema migrans. The definition of "target" is that the lesion has three zones: a dark center, pale intermediate zone, and peripheral rim of erythema (☐ Fig. 22.59). Targetoid lesions look similar to target lesions, except that they do not have the exact three zones. Targetoid lesions are seen in Stevens-Johnson syndrome and toxic epidermal necrosis.

When a patient presents with target or targetoid lesions, make sure to ask about any recent infections, new medications, or tick bites. Look closely at the lesions and the distribution, which can give you a clue to the diagnosis.

22.4.11.1 Other Conditions to Consider

Condition and brief overview	Patient population	Appearance	Management
Erythema multiforme: hypersensitivity reaction with target lesions, most commonly triggered by HSV infection	Adolescents and young adults; more common in males Can be caused by infection (HSV, EBV), medications, and malignancy. It can also be idiopathic.	Classic target lesions though may appear targetoid (**Fig. 22.60**). Usually asymptomatic. **Erythema multiforme minor:** no mucosal involvement	Address the underlying cause. Symptomatic treatment with antihistamines, topical steroids, cool compresses, and wet dressings.

		Erythema multiforme major: mucosal involvement and systemic symptoms, such as fever, arthralgias, and malaise	
Erythema migrans: targetoid rash in Lyme disease	More common in the Northeast, Midwest, and West coast. Risk factors: hiking and tick bites.	A red macule at the site of tick bite that spreads outward into a target lesion. Usually asymptomatic.	Doxycycl ine. Watch out for disseminated Lyme disease, which can cause neurologic abnormalities, atrioventricular block, and myocarditis. The lesions in this case may be widespread across the body.

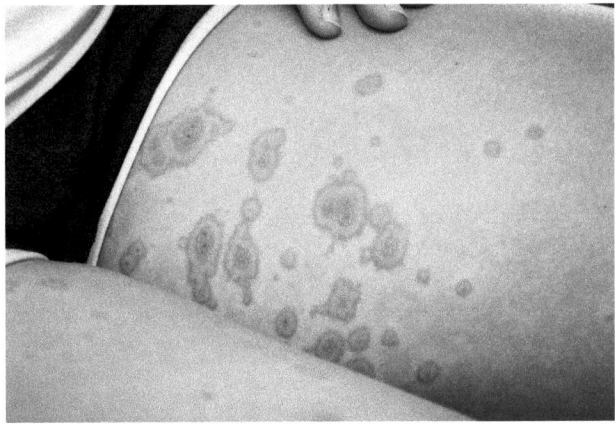

☐ **Fig. 22.60** Erythema multiforme target lesions on inner thigh

22.4.12 **Red/Violaceous Papules and Plaques**

Red/purple lesions of the skin can range from benign cherry angiomas to vasculitis. The redness in these lesions is due to blood vessels. As discussed in Fundamentals of Dermatology, you can perform a diascopy test on vascular lesions to see if the redness is due to dilated blood vessels or extravasated blood. The former will blanch on pressure (turn a paler pink when you press a slide on it), and the latter will not blanch (will remain a similar color when it is pressed) (☐ Fig. 22.61). An example of something that will blanch is a *telangiectasia*, which is a dilated small blood vessel. An example of something that will not blanch is *purpura*, a lesion due to leakage of blood from vessels.

We will focus this introductory section on purpura since it can be intimidating for medical students and is worth providing a framework for. Purpuric lesions that are smaller than 3 mm are called *petechiae*; lesions that are larger than 5 mm are called *ecchymoses*. Besides the size of the lesion, two questions you should ask when you see purpura are: is it palpable and is it retiform

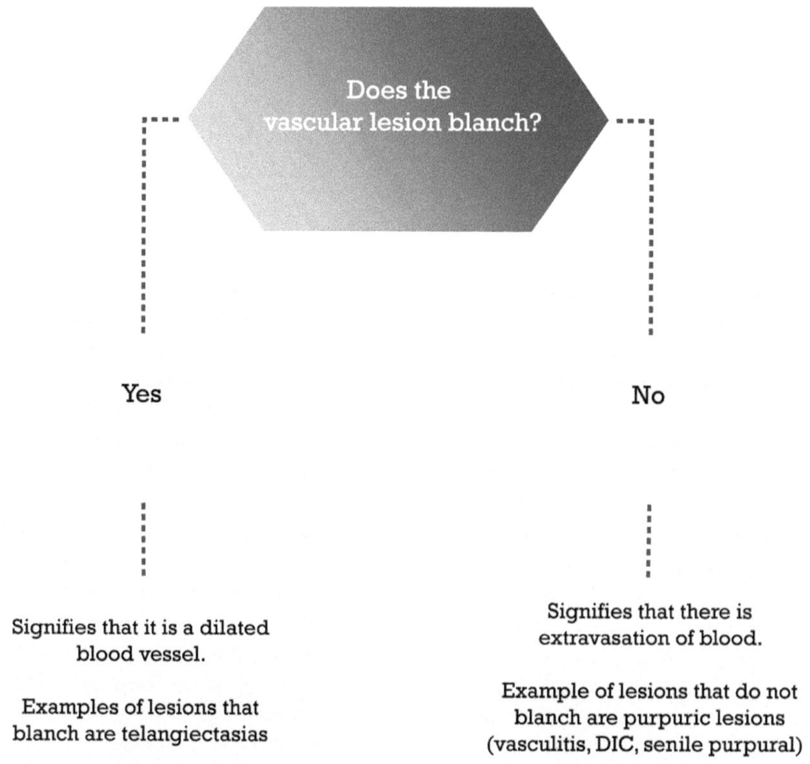

Does the vascular lesion blanch?

Yes   No

Signifies that it is a dilated   Signifies that there is
blood vessel.   extravasation of blood.

Examples of lesions that   Example of lesions that do not
blank are telangiectasias   blanch are purpuric lesions
                                          (vasculitis, DIC, senile purpural)

Fig. 22.61 Flowchart of whether the vascular lesion blanches

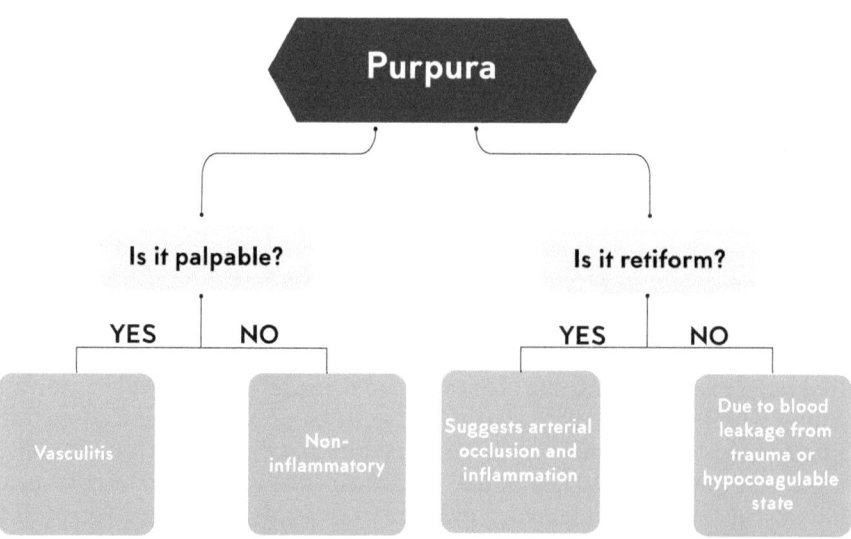

Fig. 22.62 Categorizing purpura based on whether or not it is palpable or retiform

(**Fig. 22.62**)? *Palpable* means that if you close your eyes, you can feel substance to the lesion. *Retiform* means the lesions have a netlike pattern because of vessel occlusion.

- Palpable: due to vascular inflammation (vasculitis)
  - Vasculitis, such as Henoch-Schonlein purpura, ANCA vasculitides, and polyarteritis nodosa
- Non-palpable: non-inflammatory causes, such as DIC, coagulation defects, external trauma, skin weakness, thrombocytopenia, abnormal platelet function

22.4.12.1 Other Conditions to Consider

Condition and brief overview	Patient population	Appearance	Other features	Management
☆ **Telangiectasia:** dilated superficial blood vessels also called "spider veins"	Older people with extensive sun exposure	Dilated small blood vessels (diameter approximately 1 mm) that blanch upon pressure	Blanches under diascopy	Reassurance Can use lasers to remove
☆ **Cherry angioma:** benign bright red to violaceous papule caused by proliferation of dilated venules that appear as you age	>40 year-olds	**Bright red to violaceous papule** most frequently on trunk and upper extremities. Patients may have several of these	May or may not blanch under diascopy due to how fibrotic the lesion is	Reassurance May be excised or treated with laser per patient preference
☆ **Solar/senile purpura:** atrophy of the dermis due to sun exposure that leads to easy bleeding	>60-year-olds	**Asymptomatic violaceous macules and patches on hands and extensor surfaces of the arms** usually after minor trauma	Does not blanch; not palpable; not retiform	Encourage sun avoidance and protection
Disseminated intravascular coagulation (DIC): coagulopathy in critically ill patients	Critically ill/septic patients; often associated with meningitis and meningococcemia	**Retiform purpura** symmetrically and diffusely on body, in particular on the buttocks and breasts	Does not blanch; not palpable; retiform	Patient should be managed in ICU with multidisciplinary team Treat underlying disease process, supportive measures, monitor labs

				Make sure to check: CBC: anemia with schistocytes, low platelets Fibrinogen: low D-dimer: elevated PT and PTT: variable, but over half of patients have prolonged value
Henoch-Schonlein purpura (aka IgA vasculitis): small vessel vasculitis with gastrointestinal involvement in children	Children: ages 3-15 Peaks during winter; **check for streptococcal infection, which may be a precipitating factor**	**Palpable purpura** (erythematous/violac eous macules symmetrically on legs and buttocks; occasionally on upper extremities and trunk), arthritis, abdominal pain Skin biopsy shows leukocytoclastic vasculitis; **IgA immune complex deposition in vessel walls**	Does not blanch; palpable; not retiform	Supportive treatment +/- prednisone Check a urinalysis for renal involvement
Leukocytoclastic vasculitis: small vessel vasculitis that usually erupts on lower extremities 7-10 days after trigger of medications, infections, malignancy, inflammatory bowel disease, or connective tissue disease	Anyone, though more common in adults	**Palpable purpura** of non-blanching **3-5 mm bright pink / red or violaceous, round papules (Fig. 22.63).** Older lesions may turn brown	Does not blanch; palpable; not retiform	Skin biopsy within 48 hrs of onset for highest diagnostic yield Treat underlying disease Limited with no systemic involvement: supportive treatment Ulcers or visceral involvement: prednisone and other immunosuppressives

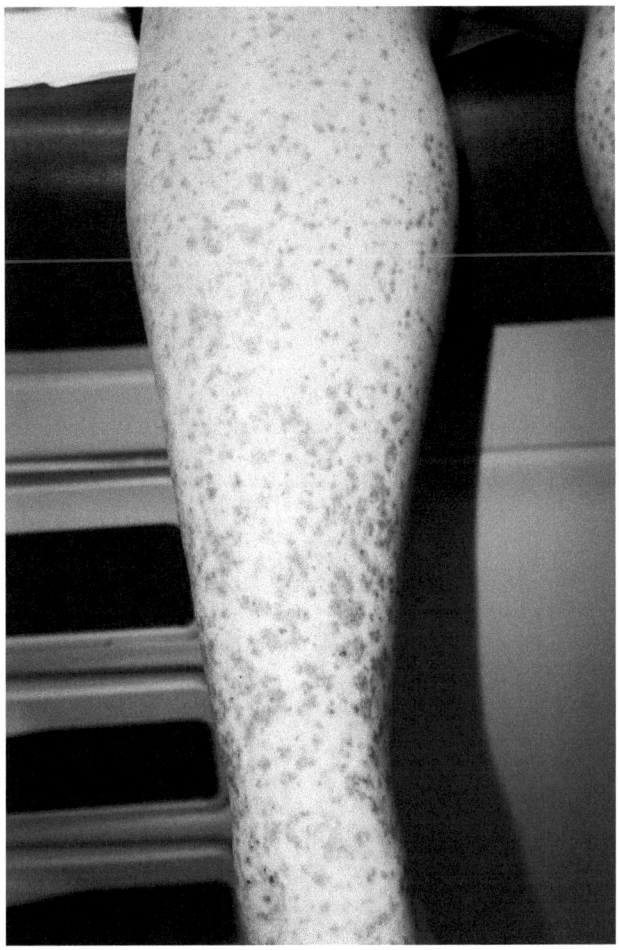

◘ Fig. 22.63   Leukocytoclastic vasculitis of the lower extremities

22.4.13 **Viral Exanthems**

A morbilliform eruption literally means "like a measles rash." These rashes are composed of erythematous macules and papules. The main differential diagnosis for morbilliform eruptions includes drug reactions and viral exanthems (exanthem = rash that appears abruptly and affects several areas of the skin). The key way to distinguish between the two is age – viral exanthems are more common in children, and drug rashes are more common in adults.

In this section, we will focus on viral exanthems, whereas in the next section, we will focus on drug eruptions. Viral syndromes that cause exanthems in children include measles, rubella, roseola infantum, erythema infectiosum, and hand-foot-mouth disease. In adults, a variety of viruses can cause a nonspecific morbilliform eruption, such as enterovirus, adenovirus, and parainfluenza virus. In all viral exanthems, the rash is usually preceded by systemic symptoms of fever, myalgia, cough, runny nose, etc. Blood tests may reveal reactive lymphocytosis, as opposed to eosinophilia which is more suggestive of a drug reaction. The best way to distinguish between different viral exanthems are the age of the patient, unique findings as outlined below, and blood test for IgG and IgM antibodies.

Measles and rubella are rare in the USA because most children are vaccinated. Ask about vaccinations to assess the risk of the child having either of these diseases!

■ Unique Findings

Koplik spots (little white spots surrounded by red inside the mouth)	Measles
Forchheimer's sign (petechial lesions in mouth)	Rubella
Rapid spread of rash from face downward in less than 24 hrs	Rubella
High fever preceding rash	Roseola infantum
Bright red cheeks	Erythema infectiosum
Rash on palms and soles	Hand-foot-mouth

22.4.13.1 Table of Important Viral Exanthems

Condition and brief overview	Patient population	Appearance	Management
★ **Nonspecific viral exanthem:** non-specific viral rash	Common causes: enterovirus, adenovirus, parainfluenza virus, rhinovirus.	Prodrome of fever, myalgia, and fatigue and then **morbilliform eruption with no unique morphology or distribution**	Self-limited to about 1 week; supportive care
Measles: caused by rubeola virus	Children	Prodrome of fever, conjunctivitis, runny nose, cough, and **Koplik spots** (tiny white spots inside of cheek). Then, erythematous macules and papules start on face and spread downward	Supportive care. **Vitamin A may help** Complications include: otitis media, pneumonia, and laryngotracheobronchitis (croup)
Rubella (German measles): caused by rubella virus	Children	Prodrome of systemic symptoms followed by pruritus pink red macules and papules that start on face and spread downward **in 24 hrs** **Forchheimer's sign:** petechial lesions on soft palate and uvula; seen in 20% of patients	Supportive care
Roseola infantum (Sixth disease) : caused by HHV-6 or HHV	Children: <5 years old	Prodrome of **high fever x 3 days** and then sudden appearance of **pink macules and papules with white halos that begin on trunk and spread to proximal extremities**	Supportive care

| Erythema infectiosum (fifth disease): caused by Parvovirus B19 | Children: 4-10 years old | Prodrome of low-grade fevers, myalgias, runny nose → **bright red cheeks** → reticular (lacelike) erythema on trunk on extremities | Supportive care

! Some infections can lead to chronic erythroid hypoplasia (severe anemia) and transient aplastic crisis in patients with sickle cell disease. In pregnant women, can cause hydrops fetalis (accumulation of fluid in fetus) and fetal death. |
| Hand-foot-mouth disease: caused by Coxsackie and entero virus | Children: <5 years | Prodrome of systemic symptoms and then **erythematous erosions like canker sores in mouth that spread to extremities, trunk, palms, and soles (bright pink macules, papules, and painful vesicles)** (Fig. 22.64). | Supportive care |

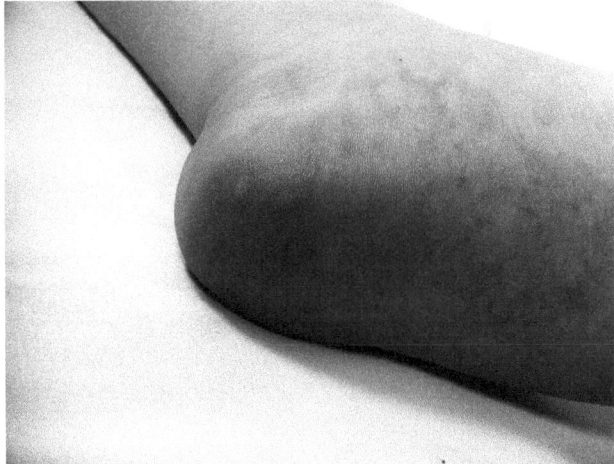

☐ **Fig. 22.64** Erythematous macules on soles in hand-foot-mouth disease

22.4.14 **Drug Reactions**

Drug reactions that look like morbilliform eruptions are called *exanthematous eruptions*. However, drug eruptions can appear a variety of ways. In general, when you are suspecting a drug reaction, ask if the patient started any new medications in the past several months.

Risk factors for drug reactions are:
- Previous drug reaction
- Recurrent drug exposure
- Comorbidities
  - Patients with EBV infection are more likely to have a drug reaction to aminopenicillins.
  - Patients with HIV are more likely to have a drug reaction to sulfonamides and other drugs.
- HLA type
  - HLA-B*1502 in Southeast Asians: associated with SJS/TEN when taking carbamazepine
  - HLA-B*5701: associated with DRESS when taking abacavir
  - HLA-B*5801 in East Asians: associated with SJS/TEN when taking allopurinol

FDA recommends screening all Southeast Asian patients for HLA-B*1502 before starting carbamazepine and all patients for HLA-B*5701 before starting abacavir.

Drug reactions can first be divided according to when they occur (◘ Fig. 22.65). If they occur less than 1 hr of taking the offending drug, they are *immediate reactions*. Immediate reactions consist of urticaria, angioedema, or anaphylaxis.

If the reaction occurs more than 6 hrs from taking the offending drug, then the patient has a *delayed reaction*. These reactions can take as long as months from initiation of the offending drug. Delayed reactions include exanthematous drug eruption, fixed drug eruption, DRESS, and SJS/TEN.

There are many drugs that can cause each of the below reactions. You will not be expected to memorize them, although it is helpful to remember some big buckets of drugs: antibiotics, anticonvulsants, HIV antivirals, NSAIDs, and gout medications. When you are suspecting a drug reaction, you can find an extensive list of causative drugs on websites like ▶ VisualDx.com.

When taking a history, there are five important things to ask:
1. Drug timeline (◘ Fig. 22.66): Day 0 is when the rash first started. Ask about any drugs that were started or discontinued up to at least 2 months before the rash started. This timeline is important because it can give you clues as to what type of drug reaction it is.
2. Previous exposure to the medication and similar reactions in the past.
3. Symptoms of the rash. If the predominant feature is pruritus, consider exanthematous drug eruption. If the predominant feature is pain, consider Stevens-Johnson syndrome (SJS)/toxic epidermal necrolysis (TEN).

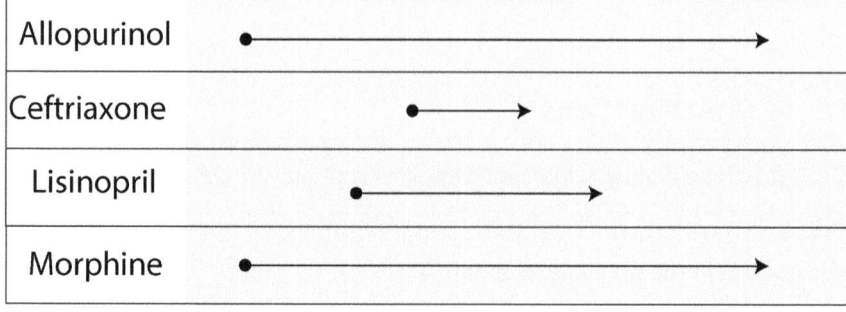

◘ **Fig. 22.65**   Common time of onset for drug eruptions

Timeline of onset

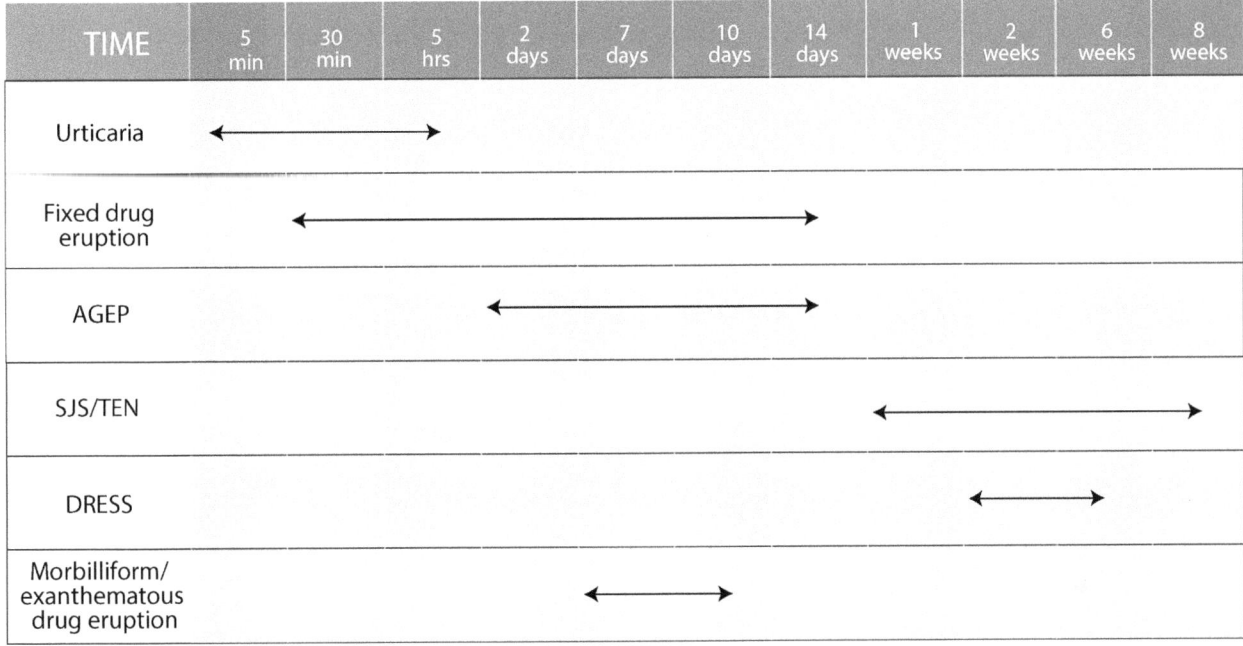

TIME	5 min	30 min	5 hrs	2 days	7 days	10 days	14 days	1 weeks	2 weeks	6 weeks	8 weeks
Urticaria	←——————→										
Fixed drug eruption		←————————————————→									
AGEP				←——————————————→							
SJS/TEN								←——————————————→			
DRESS									←————→		
Morbilliform/ exanthematous drug eruption					←————→						

◘ Fig. 22.66 Example of drug timeline

4. Mucosal involvement: if involved. Consider SJS/TEN.
5. Review of systems: important to do a thorough ROS to understand what other organ systems may be affected.
   1. Labs to consider are CBC, LFT, BUN/creatinine, and UA. In patients with elevated LFT and eosinophilia, consider DRESS.

The management of all drug reactions is to stop the offending drug. In cases in which the drug must be continued and there are no alternatives, you may continue if the patient has a mild or moderate exanthematous drug rash and treat symptomatically with close observation. Patients may require desensitization to a critical medication causing an exanthematous drug rash if there are no other treatment alternatives.

22.4.14.1 Table of Cutaneous Drug Reactions

Condition and brief overview	Patient population	Appearance	Management
Urticaria (see also ► Sect. 22.4.9)	Anyone Minutes to hours after drug exposure. Shorter when patient has had previous exposures to the drug Drugs: penicillin, other antibiotics	Erythematous, edematous papule and plaque with pale center	Discontinue offending drug

Condition and brief overview	Patient population	Appearance	Management
☆ *Exanthematous drug eruption:* morbilliform drug eruption	Anyone 7–10 days after drug exposure (can be as early as 24 hrs if patient has been exposed to drug before) Drugs: beta-lactams, anticonvulsants, dapsone, allopurinol	"Morbilliform": erythematous macules and papules that start on trunk and spread outward to extremities (◻ Fig. 22.67) May have pruritus and mild fever	Discontinue offending drug; topical steroids, oral antihistamines Will resolve through scaling/desquamation
Acute generalized exanthematous pustulosis (AGEP): pustular drug eruption	Anyone 48 hrs – 2 weeks after drug exposure Drugs: penicillins, other antibiotics, isoniazid, anticonvulsants	*Small nonfollicular pustules on erythematous plaques.* Start spreading within a few hours *High fever for up to a week is common*	Discontinue offending drug; symptomatic treatment with antipyretics and topical steroids to relieve itching
Fixed drug eruption: well-demarcated patch/plaque that recurs in same place with re-exposure to drug	Anyone 30 min to 8 hrs after drug exposure Drugs: laxatives, barbiturates, NSAIDs, sulfonamides, metronidazole, tetracycline	*Well-demarcated erythematous or violaceous round patch/ plaque that recurs when exposed to the same drug.* May evolve to become a bulla → erosion. Healing phase: violaceous with post-inflammatory hyperpigmentation Common locations: mouth, genitalia, face, acral areas	Discontinue offending drug If lesion is not eroded, can use topical steroids; if eroded, use antimicrobial ointment
☆ *Drug reaction with eosinophilia and systemic symptoms* (DRESS): multisystem disorder from hypersensitivity to a drug	Anyone 2–6 weeks after drug exposure Drugs: allopurinol, antibiotics, isoniazid, anticonvulsants, NSAIDs, abacavir	Face swelling, pharyngitis, lymph-adenopathy, eosinophilia, and elevated liver function tests Labs to check: LFT, CBC, Cr/BUN	Discontinue offending drugs If mild, use topical steroids and systemic antihistamines. Trend lab values If severe, start prednisone 1 mg/kg/day and taper over weeks

Condition and brief overview	Patient population	Appearance	Management
☆ *Stevens-Johnson syndrome*: serious skin rash from drugs that may cause sloughing of skin; it is called SJS if <10% body surface area is affected *SJS/TEN*: 10–30% body surface area *Toxic epidermal necrolysis* (TEN): >30% body surface area	Typically begins several weeks after drug initiation Drugs (SATANN): Sulfa antibiotics Allopurinol Tetracyclines Anticonvulsants NSAIDs Nevirapine	Rash preceded by fever, headache, myalgias *Erythematous irregularly shaped red to purpuric macules/ targetoid lesions that coalesce* (◧ Fig. 22.68). There may be bullae with positive Nikolsky sign. Usually *painful* (signifies necrosis) *Mucosal involvement* may precede skin involvement. Ask about pain when moving eyes!	This is a medical emergency! Stop offending drugs. Administer immunosuppressive medications, such as IVIG, cyclosporine, cyclophosphamide SCORTEN is used to assess severity and predict mortality! For patients with high body surface involvement, you should send the patient to the burn unit Complications include corneal damage, urethral or introital adhesions, bronchiectasis, sepsis

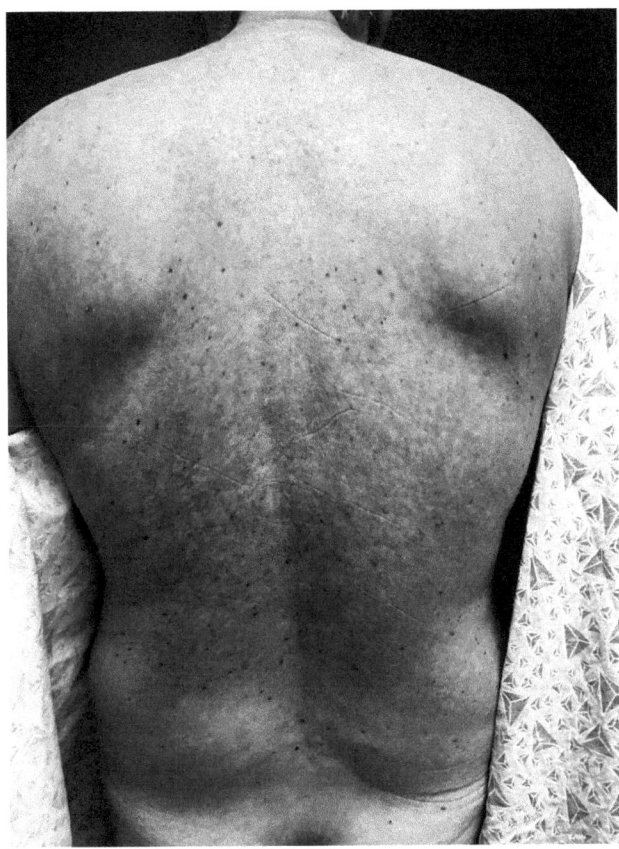

■ **Fig. 22.67** Morbilliform reaction of an exanthematous drug reaction

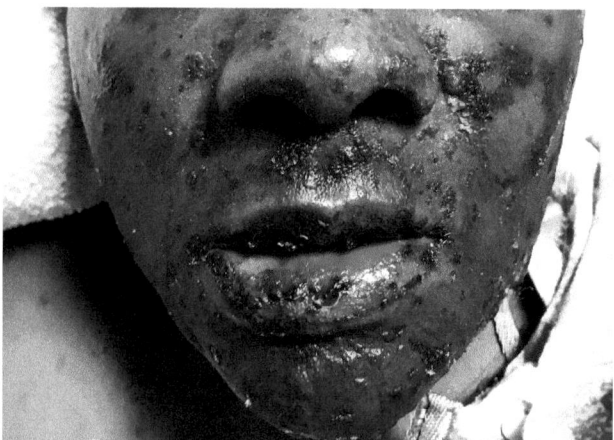

◘ Fig. 22.68   SJS of the face and lips

22.4.15 Erythroderma

Erythroderma is generalized redness or scaling of the skin that involves >80–90% body surface area. Erythroderma is not a diagnosis itself, but is a clinical manifestation of underlying disease.

Mnemonic for causes of erythroderma is REDMAN:

- R: radiation
- E: eczema/psoriasis
- D: drugs
- M: malignancy (e.g., mycosis fungoides, lymphoma)
- A: autoimmune (dermatomyositis)
- N: no cause (idiopathic)

Common symptoms include fevers, chills, malaise, and pruritus. In patients with long-standing erythroderma, patients can have diffuse alopecia, keratoderma (thickening of stratum corneum), nail dystrophy (nail plate abnormalities), and ectropion (outward turning of lower eyelids). Potential complications include sepsis, severe metabolic derangements, hypothermia, and cardiac failure.

- History: obtain thorough medication history since drugs can cause erythroderma.
- Physical exam: focus on vital signs, nails, mucosa, lymph nodes, hepatosplenomegaly
  - *Shiny, erythematous, scaling skin diffusely on the body.* May first start as a morbilliform exanthem (little red macules and papules). Progresses to patchy erythema followed by scaling and desquamation (peeling).
- Labs: CBC, BMP, LFTs.
- Repeat skin biopsies may be necessary to make a definitive diagnosis.

One unique form of erythroderma is *red man syndrome,* an IgE anaphylactic response to parenteral vancomycin. This appears 5–10 minutes after infusion of vancomycin. Patient experiences generalized burning and erythema over the body. Significant hypotension, fever, dizziness, and dyspnea may all occur. To prevent red man syndrome, administer antihistamines prior to vancomycin infusion, limit vancomycin dose to 500 mg, and administer vancomycin slowly over 2 hours.

Management of erythroderma includes:
- Discontinuing offending medications
- Evaluating for cardiac and respiratory involvement
- Addressing electrolyte imbalances
- Maintaining aggressive hydration to offset insensible fluid losses
- Applying topical steroids to affected skin two to three times daily
- Administering oral antihistamines for pruritus

22.4.16 Nail Disorders

Disorders of the nails can present a wide variety of ways. Medical terminology that describes nails usually starts with the root "onycho-." Below are some terms you should be familiar with:
- Onychodystrophy: abnormal growth and development of the nail
- Onychomycosis: fungal infection of the nail
- Onycholysis: lifting of nail from the nail bed

22.4.16.1 Onychomycosis

Onychomycosis is a fungal infection of the nail and is a common condition seen in older people. Onychomycosis causes thickened, yellow nails with onycholysis. While the infection is not life-threatening, patients can be disturbed by their nails' appearance and want their onychomycosis to be treated. For treatment, topical antifungals are not effective; instead, you should confirm that the patient has onychomycosis by performing a fungal culture, KOH, or histology, and then start the patient on oral terbinafine. While the patient is on terbinafine for 6–12 weeks, the doctor will need to monitor the patients' liver function. Despite the aggressive therapy, treatment success is only about 50%. Thus, for patients who are not bothered by their onychomycosis, it does not need to be treated.

When someone presents with onychomycosis of his or her toenails, make sure to check if he or she also has tinea pedis, as the same fungus (most common *Trichophyton rubrum*) can cause both.

22.4.16.2 Pigmentation in the Nail

Pigmentation in the nail can be caused by a variety of reasons. If the patient had traumatized his or her nail and the pigmentation is slowly moving up and out of the nail as the nail grows, then you can be fairly certain that the patient had a subungual hematoma. If the patient has a darker skin phototype and has narrow (1–2 mm in width) vertical bands of pigmentation that isn't growing or causing any symptoms, the bands may be a benign condition called longitudinal melanonychia (◘ Fig. 22.69). Longitudinal melanonychia can affect multiple nails.

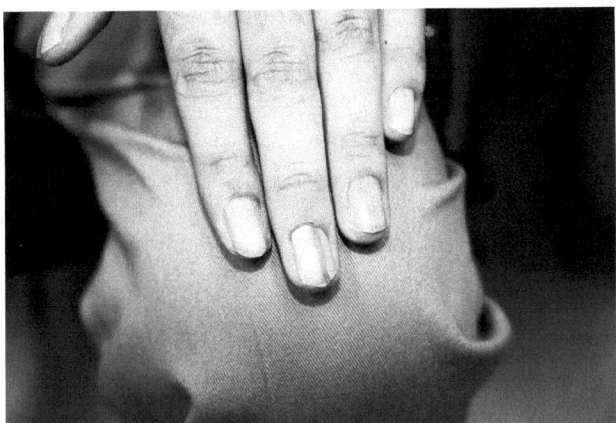

◘ **Fig. 22.69**   Longitudinal melanonychia affecting several fingernails

The most important condition to watch out for is subungual melanoma. This type of melanoma is more common in darker skin types. Unlike in longitudinal melanonychia, subungual melanoma is usually wide (3 mm in width), has blurry borders, and is most commonly on the big toe or thumb. *Hutchinson's sign*, a sign of subungual melanoma, refers to the brown-black discoloration of the nail fold where the pigmentation of the nail starts.

22.4.16.3 Other Conditions to Consider

Condition and brief overview	Patient population	Appearance	Management
★ **Onychomycosis:** fungal infection that causes thickening and yellowing of the nail	Elderly	Thickened, yellow nails with onycholysis and subungual debris	**Oral terbinafine** (though treatment success rate is only 50%). If not bothering the patient, can go without treating
Acute paronychia: infection and tenderness of skin around nails	Anyone Can be caused by trauma or medications (e.g, retinoids or epidermal growth factor receptor inhibitors)	Pain, swelling, and redness of the lateral nailfolds **(periungual) (Fig. 22.70).**	Topical antibiotics such as mupirocin Severe disease requires oral antibiotics. Consider if MRSA coverage is needed. If so, use clindamycin or doxycycline For drug-induced paronychia, may try doxycycline 100 mg BID along with topical steroids to decrease inflammation
Subungual hematoma: bleeding under the nail from trauma	Anyone History of trauma	Red, purple, or black discoloration in areas where trauma occurred. Usually does not extend across the entirety of the nail from nailbed to distal nail (like melanoma). **Will grow out as the nail grows out.**	Monitor the nail discoloration to make sure it is resolving or growing out with the nail

Subungual melanoma: melanoma under the nail	Age 50-70	Broad (>3mm) pigmented band with blurry borders on nail. More common on big toe or thumb. Consider ABCDEs of melanoma (see Sect. 22.4.1)	Shave biopsy of nail matrix If confirmed, work with medical oncologist to treat
Longitudinal melanonychia : vertical dark lines on nails that can be normal/physiologic (ethnic melanonychia) or caused by trauma, medications, or other conditions, such as psoriasis and lichen planus	>50 years old Skin phototype V-VI	Brown-black longitudinal lines on nails (usually involves several nails, unlike melanoma).	Reassurance and monitoring

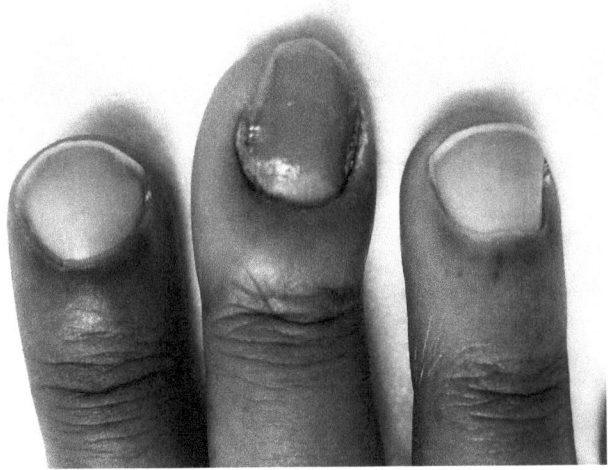

◨ **Fig. 22.70** Paronychia: swelling and inflammation around the nail

22.4.17 **Hair Loss**

Hair is a form of self-identity and for many, its loss (also called alopecia) can be extremely distressing. Alopecia can be divided into scarring (*cicatricial*) and non-scarring. *Scarring alopecia* can lead to irreversible hair loss from scalp inflammation and destruction/fibrosis of hair follicles. Because of the inflammation, there are often associated scalp symptoms, such as itching, burning, and flaking. Examples of scarring alopecia are discoid lupus erythematosus and lichen planopilaris (lichen planus of the scalp). Early diagnosis and initiation of treatment is crucial for scarring alopecias.

Non-scarring alopecia, on the other hand, is more common and not associated with any inflammation of the scalp. There are usually not any symptoms besides the hair loss itself, which can be reversible.

Key questions to ask someone who presents with hair loss include:
- Timeline, location, rate of hair loss
- Associated pain, pruritus, or burning sensations
- Stress and diet
- Medication (changes in medications, hormonal medications, etc.)
- Hair regrowth (if present, this would indicate the alopecia is not scarring)
- Tight hairstyles and use of chemical relaxers
- Family history of hair loss

On exam, look at where the hair loss is occurring and if you notice any changes to the scalp – any flaking, redness, or changes to the hair follicles? For looking at the hair follicles, you may use a dermatoscope to look more. If you see *follicular ostia* (hair follicle openings), this is suggestive of non-scarring hair loss. If you don't see ostia, this is suggestive of scarring hair loss. If scarring alopecia is suspected, a biopsy at the edge of active disease may establish diagnosis and management.

To determine underlying causes of hair loss, check the following labs:
- CBC
- TSH
- Iron, ferritin
- Zinc
- Vitamin D [25(OH)D]

22.4.17.1 Telogen Effluvium

Hair loss can occur in response to stressful events, such as pregnancy, surgery, or stress at work. This is because the stressor causes excessive shedding of resting (telogen) hairs. When this occurs, the condition is called telogen effluvium.

Telogen effluvium can affect anyone, though is most common in women 30–60 years of age. On exam, you will notice diffuse hair loss with no inflammation or scarring of the scalp. There should not be patches of complete hair loss. You can conduct a *hair pull test*, whereby you grab 10–20 hairs in your hand and pull gently. A positive test means you pull out >3–6 hairs – this may be seen in telogen effluvium.

Telogen effluvium is usually self-limited, and you can reassure the patient that the hair should grow back, though it may take 6–12 months.

22.4.17.2 Alopecia Areata

Alopecia areata is an autoimmune disorder caused by T cells destroying the hair follicle. In most cases, patients will have patches of hair loss on the scalp, eyebrows, or body hair (Fig. 22.71), but in some cases, there is complete loss of hair on the scalp, which is called *alopecia totalis*, or complete loss of hair on scalp and body, called *alopecia universalis*. Alopecia can affect anyone, though there seems to be increased incidence in those with autoimmune disease.

When the hair loss occurs, there may be scalp burning with some redness. Despite these symptoms, on exam, look for round areas of *non-scarring* hair loss. There may be *exclamation point hairs*, which are hairs that are more tapered/thinner at the base near the scalp than at the ends of the hair. There may also be pitting and ridging of the fingernails. If you have a positive hair pull test at the periphery of the hair loss patches, then that signifies that the disease is active and may continue to progress.

You may get a false-negative hair pull test if the patients washed their hair that day, so be sure to ask when they last washed their hair.

Because alopecia areata is an autoimmune disease, consider checking for other autoimmune diseases, such as hypothyroidism, vitiligo, etc.

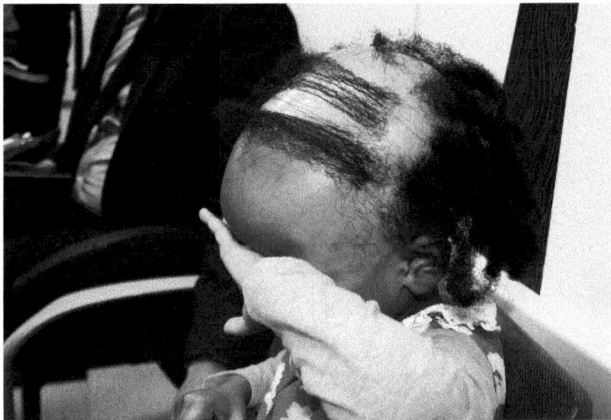

◼ **Fig. 22.71** Alopecia areata in a young child

Treatment depends on severity of the condition. In limited and mild disease, you may use topical steroids. For moderate disease, you may use intralesional steroids. For severe disease (e.g., alopecia totalis or alopecia universalis), you may consider psoralen ultraviolet A (PUVA) or systemic immunomodulators like methotrexate or tofacitinib.

22.4.17.3 Other Conditions to Consider

Condition and brief overview	Patient Population	Appearance	Management
★ **Telogen effluvium:** diffuse hair loss 6-9 months after a stressful event	More common in women	Nonscarring alopecia; **diffuse hair loss** with no associated redness or flaking	Self-limited; reassurance
★ **Androgenetic alopecia** : male pattern hair loss	More common in men	**Bitemporal recession**, hair loss at **vertex/crown of scalp (Fig. 22.72)** Will see **miniaturization of hair** in areas of hair loss Negative hair pull test except in areas of active hair loss	Minoxidil 5% foam or solution; oral finasteride 1mg Hair transplantation, platelet-rich plasma injections, or laser and light-based therapy
Traction alopecia : hair loss from wearing tight hairstyles	Women and girls, particularly of African descent because of hair features and hairstyles	Nonscarring; hair loss at anterior margins of the scalp **Fringe sign:** retained hair on frontotemporal edge	Encourage patients to stop tight hairstyles Topical minoxidil 2%; topical steroids

Tinea capitis: fungal infection of scalp leading to hair loss	Children Caused by dermatophytes and is infectious.	Scaly **annular** hair loss with possible inflamed papules or pustules (**Fig. 22.73**). **Kerion** is a severe presentation involving boggy plaque with pustules. May be associated with **neck and postauricular lymphadenopathy**.	Oral antifungals, such as griseofulvin or terbinafine. Topical treatments are not effective, but ketoconazole or selenium sulfide shampoo can be used in addition to oral therapies.
★ **Alopecia areata:** autoimmune destruction of hair follicles leading to patchy areas of complete hair loss	Anyone	Nonscarring alopecia; **patchy round areas of hair loss; exclamation point hairs** (small hairs with tapered bases) May see nail pitting and ridging	Topical and intralesional steroids. In severe cases, PUVA and immunomodulators
Lichen planopilaris: a type of scarring alopecia thought to be caused by cell-mediated immunity; it is lichen planus of the scalp	More common in lighter skin photoypes 40-60 years of age	Perifollicular fine scale around patches of alopecia. In more progressive disease, you may see loss of follicular ostia.	Topical and intralesional steroids For more aggressive disease, may try hydroxychloroquine and systemic immunomodulators

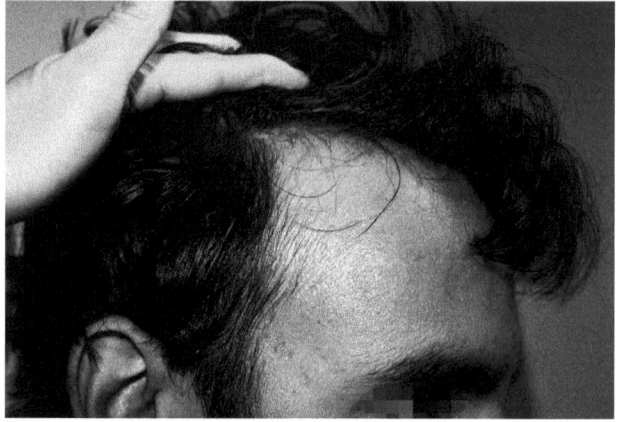

Fig. 22.72 Androgenetic alopecia with hair loss in frontotemporal regions

22

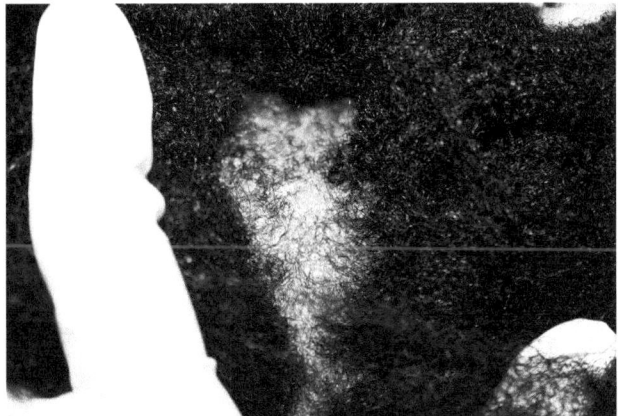

Fig. 22.73 Tinea capitis causing hair loss

Orthopaedic Surgery

Ameen Barghi

Contents

© The Author(s), under exclusive license to Springer Nature Switzerland AG 2021
S. H. Lecker, B. J. Chang (eds.), *The Ultimate Medical School Rotation Guide*,
https://doi.org/10.1007/978-3-030-63560-2_23

23.1 Introduction

Orthopaedics (ortho) is a fulfilling specialty that deals with the musculoskeletal system and all relevant structures such as bones, muscles, tendons, ligaments, nerves, and blood vessels, including all subspecialties from pediatrics to oncology. Orthopaedic surgeons ("orthopaedists, orthopods") are familiar faces to many people from all walks of life. Some children interact with ortho early on in life, perhaps for a broken arm after falling off the monkey bars or a congenital deformity of the spine or limb. Teenagers and young adults may require orthopaedic care after tearing a meniscus or an ACL while playing soccer, or after others forms of trauma. Others receive surgical care much later in life after experiencing chronic joint pain or fractures related to osteoporosis. There are multiple subspecialties within orthopaedic surgery including: arthroplasty (hip and knee replacement, "joints, recon"), foot and ankle, hand and upper extremity, musculoskeletal oncology ("onc, tumor"), sports medicine, spine, trauma, pediatrics ("peds, pedi"), and shoulder and elbow. According to the American Academy of Orthopaedic Surgeons (AAOS, one of the largest orthopaedic professional societies), more than 90% of recent graduates choose to pursue fellowship training. Among these specialties, surgeons may choose to further develop a specific area of interest or pursue multiple fellowships – for example, a hip and knee total joints fellowship, or a sports/shoulder/knee sports fellowship. This is typically seen in academic centers where such niche practices are viable.

A strong understanding of anatomy and physiology, biomechanics, and patterns of injury are critical to a medical student and resident physician's arsenal. While ortho is a surgical specialty, it is a common misconception that a majority of problems are surgically treated. Historically, a majority of problems have been treated nonoperatively, and this trend is likely to increase in the future. Furthermore, knowledge of musculoskeletal medicine is a useful skill even if one chooses a field other than orthopaedics – approximately 15% of primary care office visits are for musculoskeletal complaints.

23.2 What Is the Role of an Orthopaedic Surgeon?

23.2.1 Clinic Days

Just like any physician, an orthopaedic surgeon's primary obligation is to his/her patients. The typical orthopaedist splits their week between clinic and the operating room. The average orthopaedic surgeon performs surgeries 2–3 days a week complemented by office hours/clinics 2 days a week. While this ratio is certainly dependent on surgeon seniority, patient population, and other individual factors, it is important to realize that seeing patients during clinic is the foundation of a surgical practice. This is particularly true in some of the outpatient orthopaedic subspecialties, such as arthroplasty or sports, in which the procedures are elective (i.e., not urgent or emergent). The role of a surgeon during clinic is to apply their robust knowledge base to best determine which patients require nonoperative treatment and which patients would benefit from a surgical intervention. Perhaps just as important as knowing how to operate is when to operate. Surgeons, as they become more experienced and have a better understanding of their own technical skills and limitations, are better able to foreshadow the prognosis of a surgical procedure given a specific patient's risk profile.

Clinic days are critical for establishing rapport, developing trust, and building the patient–doctor relationship – the key to a successful musculoskeletal practice. Understanding a patient's desires and needs will set the stage for a successful surgical plan that includes both preoperative and postoperative plans. It is well-known that patients who do not adhere to postoperative physical therapy for certain procedures have worse outcomes both in the short and the long term. Therefore, it is incumbent on the orthopaedic surgeon to see the patient regularly during the postoperative rehabilitation process to ensure optimal progress to functional recovery. In addition, through a consistent dialogue with the patient, a surgeon can better understand some of the social barriers that may present as challenges to recovery and subsequent therapy.

There is a common misunderstanding among medical students that surgical specialties like orthopaedics have very short-term relationships with their patients. However, while that may be the case in some practices, that is often not true in many settings. There may be short-term appointments such as preoperative evaluations and postoperative follow-up care. These visits are very complaint-driven and typically do not last more than 15 or 20 min, unless something unexpected arises. Alternatively, chronic painful disorders such as osteoarthritis, congenital deformities and malformations of the limbs and the spine, or oncologic diseases may result in long-term relationships between patient and surgeon that can span decades or the lifetime of the patient. Therefore, understanding one's own preferences, whether they are longitudinal or shorter-term relationships with patients can help better mold a satisfying practice setting and post-residency subspecialty selection.

For those surgeons for whom operating is their passion, clinic days serve as a conduit to building their surgical caseload. It is accepted that to become well-respected in your subspecialty within orthopaedics, you must first become the best surgeon you can be and always do right by your patients. Without clinic days, that is simply impossible.

23.2.2 OR Days

The operating room (OR) is usually where medical students fall in love with orthopaedic surgery. While to the inexperienced eye, all surgical ORs may seem similar, there are a few key distinctions that make an orthopaedic OR unique. Perhaps the most eye-catching OR environment is that of a total joint replacement surgery. Students often associate these surgeries with "space suits" where members of the surgical team are donning longer protective gowns, heavier gloves, and full helmets with a shield reminiscent of a "space suit." Orthopaedic ORs are also often more spacious than other ORs – they require space for external imaging devices (i.e., "C-arm") or may have specialized airflow technologies designed to reduce infection rates.

The best way to understand what an OR day for a surgeon looks like is to first understand what it looks like for the patient. While the logistics vary between institutions, they are generally similar. Cases are scheduled in advance in designated ORs. The dates must be arranged with enough time for patients to undergo preoperative visits and medical clearance (i.e., via a primary care, anesthesia, or specialty medical visit). Surgeons typically have one or two ORs. Patients arrive several hours before their scheduled surgical time. After their admission, they are held in the preoperative unit. There, they are visited by the nursing teams, the anesthesia team, and the surgical team. The surgeon will visit the patient one more time before surgery and answer any last-minute questions and sign their operative site with a marker. Intraoperatively, surgeons interact closely with the perioperative team, which consists of nursing, scrub techs (individuals who keep instrumentation organized and ready), and anesthesiologists. In academic institutions, surgeons may be working with fellows, residents, physician's assistants, or medical students. Pure private practice settings lack medical students or residents, unless they hold academic affiliations. They do, however, work with PAs, nurses, and technicians. Corporate device representatives may also be present in the OR ("industry reps"). They may serve to answer questions regarding manufacturer details for devices or implants.

23.2.3 Emergency Department

An orthopaedic surgeon's involvement with the emergency department depends on call schedules and institutional frameworks. Call schedules are premade calendars that determine when an attending surgeon will be present to consult or take cases from the emergency room during nonbusiness hours, such as in the late evening, overnight, or on weekends. Medical students, residents, and fellows all have their own respective call schedules. For a medical student, the call schedule is designed to introduce them to orthopaedic care during off hours and which includes evaluating patients in the emergency room.

Regardless of whether your interaction with the emergency room is on call or not, emergency room orthopaedic consults are eye-opening opportunities for learning. Attending surgeons at academic institutions are not the first-line providers who receive orthopaedic consults. Either a resident, physician's assistant, or other provider interacts with the patient prior to a surgeon's interaction. Oftentimes, it is the responsibility of this person to see patients, work them up for the team, and then present them to the attending physician as the night proceeds or the following morning. Depending on the organization of the institution, surgeons will decide whether to operate on emergency room consults, admit patients into the hospital under the purview of orthopaedic surgery, or simply allow for care to continue with emergency room staff that then have discretion over the patient's complaint and subsequent discharge. The emergency room consults are managed either by a "day call" or a "night call" surgeon. Patients may be requested to follow up with outpatient orthopaedic clinics after they are referred from the emergency room.

23.2.4 Practice Settings

There are several practice settings available to orthopaedic surgeons. Practice settings may be described as occurring on a spectrum – from "academic" to "private." *Academic centers* typically take care of complex patients with multiple comorbidities who require the care of several medical and possibly surgical specialties. Some examples may include a recurring prosthetic joint infection in need of an explant and several weeks of IV antibiotics treatment, a pathological fracture secondary to metastatic renal cell carcinoma, or a patient with several comorbidities and a femur fracture. These centers are often associated with a university hospital, and they train medical students, residents, and fellows. Clinical and basic science research is heavily emphasized. Patient care is escalated from the broadest of learners (medical students) to an attending surgeon so that all trainees may maximize their learning from each patient encounter. These surgeons are often involved in medical education and enjoy teaching and research. *Academically affiliated private groups* (colloquially known as "privademic" centers) are hybrid entities, adopting some practices of both academic institutions and a pure private practice environment. They are often associated by practice location or educational interests with a university or academic institution, but function as a private practice within that setting. They may be involved in resident education and cover complex cases, but they most often are financially independent entities from the academic centers. *Private practice* settings are by far the most common practice setting for orthopaedic surgeons. According to the AAOS, while the most popular practice setting in 2014 was a "group private practice" (35%), many orthopaedic surgeons are leaving group and solo private practice settings and moving to academic and hospital centers. They are typically extremely efficient, volume-driven, and geared toward high patient satisfaction. They are rarely involved in medical education and seldom conduct high volume research. These practices are often modeled similar to a business or firm, where the partnership model determines salaries, workload, and institutional seniority. Mid-level providers or allied health professionals (i.e., physician assistants or nurse practitioners) are often key members of a private practice surgeon's team. As a medical student on a clerkship, you are more likely to rotate in academic centers, depending on your school's affiliation. Regardless of the program or institution type, all residency programs are accredited by the Accreditation Council for Graduate Medical Education (ACGME), which outlines the core competencies required of all graduating orthopaedic surgeons. These surgical residencies all produce exceptional surgeons who understand the fundamentals of orthopaedic surgery and thoughtful patient care. Therefore, selection of program type is entirely based on applicant needs and desires.

Some of the largest and most popular orthopaedic organizations are listed below and available on the AAOS website (▶ https://www5.aaos.org/CustomTemplates/Content.aspx?id=22703&ssopc=1)

Orthopaedic Organizations:
- AOA – American Orthopaedic Association
- AAOS – the American Academy of Orthopaedic Surgeons
- State Orthopaedic Societies (▶ https://www7.aaos.org/govern/state/state_societies/statesocieties.aspx)
- RJOS – Ruth Jackson Orthopaedic Society – organization devoted to supporting and promoting women in orthopaedics
- The Perry Initiative – pipeline to promote women in engineering and medicine; conduct outreach events (▶ https://perryinitiative.org)
- Nth Dimensions (▶ http://www.nthdimensions.org) – Pipeline program for promoting women and minorities in orthopaedic surgery
- J. Robert Gladden Multicultural Orthopaedic Society (▶ http://www.gladdensociety.org) – society dedicated to increasing the number of minorities in orthopaedic surgery

23.3 Useful Resources

23.3.1 Web-Based Services

23.3.1.1 Orthobullets

Located at ▶ https://www.orthobullets.com/, Orthobullets is a free online service that is an offshoot of the general medical website, Medbullets. It is an ever-growing, collaborative platform designed to provide descriptions of orthopaedic complaints, technique guides, anatomy overviews, instructional videos, multiple-choice questions for residency board review (lower yield for medical students), and more. Some Orthobullets contents – e.g., "premium" questions and videos – are available only by subscription. The free version is more than sufficient for a medical student. There is also a free Orthobullets phone app and a podcast that is useful for quick studying and learning on the go. As a student you may even catch residents reviewing Orthobullets immediately before a case or looking up a certain classification to evaluate a fracture in the ED. It is clear, concise, and well-formatted for learners in operative and nonoperative settings. It is a recognized resource in the orthopaedic community, from medical students to attendings.

Best For:

- Quick review of musculoskeletal complaints, syndromes, and orthopaedic procedures
- Bulleted reading of high yield orthopaedic topics
- Simple diagrams
- Review steps of classic orthopaedic cases
- Forum, Q bank, Practice-guiding articles

23.3.1.2   AO Surgery Reference

AO is an international, nonprofit organization for orthopaedic trauma and musculoskeletal surgery education and research. They have some of the most comprehensive educational materials and were one of the earliest organizations to describe bone healing, fracture plating, and surgical fixation. Their surgery reference website, found at ▶ https://surgeryreference.aofoundation. org/, is a well-designed user interface that provides detailed step-by-step guides with animations and graphics to describe a surgical procedure. This is often reviewed by residents and attending surgeons; therefore, reviewing it can be useful to get an overview of all of the steps of a procedure as well as some of the dangers to watch out f or and postoperative treatment regimens.

Best For:

- Detailed and one-line descriptions of steps of case, great for case prep!
- Simple diagrams
- Official organization

23.3.1.3   Digital Anatomy Atlas

While the classic Netter's Anatomy textbooks will most likely never lose their value, there is something to be said about a digital, three-dimensional anatomy atlas that is interactive and available on a mobile device. While each of these has its pros and cons, we have found that the following have been useful to medical students on their rotations, both in the clerkship as well as the advanced sub-internships and away rotations. Oftentimes, institutions will provide access to one of these, or a functionally equivalent substitute. Though certainly not required, we recommend a 3D digital atlas, as it can save time and be more memorable than a traditional Netter's atlas. It is also important to study imaging references that review ultrasound, radiographs, MRIs, and CT scans so you are prepared to interpret orthopaedic imaging (◻ Table 23.1).

23.3.2   Textbooks

23.3.2.1   Netter's Concise Orthopaedic Anatomy

This text covers in detail almost all orthopaedic anatomy relevant to a medical student clerkship or advanced rotation. It borrows many of Dr. Frank Netter's images from his original textbook. It also has several illustrations that seem to

□ Table 23.1 Pros and Cons of common digital atlases used on orthopaedic rotations

Product	Link	Primary function	Pros	Cons
IMAIOS	► https://www.imaios.com/en/e-Anatomy	Scrollable imaging atlas	Covers all anatomy MRI available Radiographs available Cartoon illustrations available Extremely detailed and accurate Used by MSK radiology residents High resolution images	Subscription service, not free
Visible body	► https://www.visiblebody.com/en-us/	Three-dimensional illustrations of the entire human body	Covers all anatomy Cartoon illustrations are excellent All anatomy is interactive ("click to read more") Has a specific focus to musculoskeletal anatomy and physiology Musculoskeletal application has movement videos and cartoons to illustrate muscle insertions and origins Images are customizable Usable on iPad, computer, iPhone 3-dimensional rendering is invaluable for intraoperative understanding of anatomy	Not free (may be available by your institution)
Stanford MSK MRI atlas	► http://xrayhead.com/	Free scrollable MRI atlas	Free Accurate labels High resolution images If you haven't had a radiology course this can be a good place to start for familiarizing yourself with ortho imaging and anatomy	Not the best user interface Does not cover all body parts
HIP AND KNEE BOO	► https://hipandkneebook.com/	Comprehensive arthroplasty resource	Excellent beginner to intermediate resource for arthroplasty and total joint history Overview on implants and hardware Kinematics and history explained Special maneuvers also included Diagrams easy to follow and understand Easy to follow text	Only useful for arthroplasty/joints

be specifically drawn for orthopaedics and musculoskeletal physicians. The drawings are crisp, clear, and exactly what you would expect from a Netter illustration. In addition to the illustrations, there is a descriptive text for every chapter that goes through major pathologies and functional classifications. The illustrations are well-organized, memorable, and useful for quick referencing. This text also illustrates many of the different fracture pattern classification systems. This is the anatomy textbook that most ortho medical students swear by and can often be found in the pocket of a student's white coat.

Best For:
- Reviewing relevant ortho anatomy
- Reading small blurbs on high-yield ortho diseases
- Visualizing classification systems of disease

23.3.2.2 Surgical Exposures in Orthopaedics: The Anatomic Approach (Hoppenfeld, Surgical Exposures in Orthopaedics)

Known as "Hoppenfeld's" in the orthopaedic vernacular, this textbook best describes surgical exposures. Explanations are detailed, but not overwhelming. Most medical students may read this to get a first-pass grasp of the anatomy and steps for relevant procedures. Explanations are accompanied by illustrations that are not the most modern, but serve their purpose well. Hoppenfeld's does a particularly good job outlining "do not miss" anatomy as well as critical portions of the surgical exposure. Additionally, Hoppenfeld's comments on virtually every exposure type you will encounter on a clerkship; it is comprehensive and well-written. It seems to be a textbook that most students start with to establish a foundation for anatomy that can be complemented with something more lighter, accessible, and concise like Orthobullets. A common approach is to read Hoppenfeld's the night before a case and to refresh your memory the morning of the case with more concise and readily available resources like Orthobullets.

If you study up on cases with Hoppenfeld's you can feel confident that you will be able to answer most of the anatomy questions your attending may ask.
Best For:
- Reviewing step-by-step surgical approaches and diagrams
- Reviewing the relevant and "critical" anatomy of a given procedure
- Studying up on the tomorrow's cases so that you can nail every anatomy question the attending asks and are prepared for what might happen next in the case

23.3.2.3 Pocket Pimped: Orthopaedic Surgery

This is a new series of books that features handy collections, organized by specialty, of high-yield questions for orthopaedic surgery as well as general surgery. It is reminiscent of the more popular text "Surgical Recall." The book is a collaboration between residents, fellows, and attendings and is essentially 1500 of the most commonly asked pimp questions. Online reviews and the student reviews we have solicited seem to be very favorable, though we do not have personal experience with this resource.
Best For:
- On-the-go Q&A when you have got downtime or are tired of reading textbooks

23.3.2.4 Other Textbooks

The following materials are by no means required. Many students do very well without ever even opening one of the below resources. However, they are provided to you to share some of the other material you will see being used by residents and surgeons on your rotations. This way, you won't feel like you are "missing out" on any resources. These resources are particularly useful when preparing for a presentation (such as a presentation at the end of a rotation). They are also nice fodder for downtime on call.

23.3.3 Surgical Technique Guides

Surgical technique guides are documents that describe the step-by-step methods for a surgical procedure. They are typically written by industry to describe the steps on how to use that company's specific device. While technique guides are typically used by residents, they can be a useful resource to get a general understanding of the steps of a procedure. To use a surgical technique guide, one must know the exact device and brand of the device being used for the procedure. This information may not be available in the electronic medical records, so you can always ask your resident the day before. Technique guides can be extremely detailed, given the depending on the number of steps in a procedure, and therefore feel overwhelming for a medical student. Nevertheless, some students find them helpful to keep up with a procedure they've never seen before, or to gain a higher-level understanding of each step of a procedure. Technique guides also provide well-illustrated images of devices that can help better orient students in the procedure. Technique guides are certainly not a mandatory resource for medical students and may even detract time from learning critical concepts like anatomy and physiology.

To find a technique guide, you can Google the name of the implant or device being used followed by "technique guide," and typically the first PDF result is the technique guide. For example, when googling "zimmer nextgen technique guide," the first link (▶ https://www.zimmerbiomet.com/content/dam/zimmer-biomet/medical-professionals/000-surgical-techniques/knee/zimmer-nexgen-lps-fixed-knee-surgical-technique.pdf) is the PDF for the Zimmer® NexGen® LPS Fixed Knee. It is 44 pages and has the 12 general steps necessary for this implant.

23.3.4 Zuckerman and Koval's (*Handbook of Fractures*)

This handbook is a pocket-sized text that is intended to function as a quick, reliable reference for everything to do with fractures in orthopaedics. It is filled with tables and illustrations describing the typical fracture patterns, classifications, treatments, complications, and more for all body parts (for adult and pediatric patient populations). You may see some students carrying this around on the wards. The text is well-written and relatively succinct (think somewhere between Orthobullets and Rockwood and Green's *Fractures in Adults*) but probably contains more than is required of a medical student. Most students seem to prefer the easily accessible, digital format of Orthobullets to this handbook for everyday utility. Nevertheless, consider keeping this text on your bedside table so after a long day you can review the epidemiology and management of a specific fracture pattern.

23.3.5 Rockwood and Green's *Fractures in Adults*, Rockwood and Wilkin's *Fractures in Children* (Three Volume Set)

This compendium is referred to as "THE go-to reference" for everything fracture-related and the "leading textbook" for orthopaedic surgeons and residents. If you pick up one of these volumes, expect to gain a full understanding of the epidemiology, history, mechanisms of action, treatment, and much more of essentially every fracture in adults and children. It is a textbook written by some of the most eminent names in orthopaedics. While it is an extremely good resource for orthopaedic residents, it is by no means required for medical students on their rotations. You may see these volumes scattered among your attendings' offices. There may be a copy in the call room next to the bed or in the resident work room. It is a good resource to read if you have downtime during a call shift or need material for a presentation at the end of the rotation. If you do have the time to read this text, it will rapidly elevate your fund of knowledge and solidify your understanding of any challenging concepts. Of note, the first two volumes are for adult pathology, while the third volume is exclusively a pediatrics text.

23.3.6   Miller's Review of Orthopaedics

This guide is specifically designed to prepare residents, fellows, and surgeons to ace their board exams (the "OITE" – Orthopaedic In-Service Training Exam). Therefore, it is filled with highly tested topics including useful images, tables, and pathology slides. It is written in an easy-to-read, bulleted format. While it is, in total, above the level of knowledge required of a medical student on rotation, it can be useful for getting a quick, advanced understanding of any one specific topic. For example, while you may not benefit from reading the entire "lower extremity" section, reviewing the "total knee arthroplasty" section may be useful preparation for a case the next day.

23.3.7   VuMedi and the Orthopaedic Video Theater (OVT) from AAOS

Surgical videos may be another useful resource for case preparation and general orthopaedic learning.

- VuMedi (▶ VuMedi.com)

This free, educational resource features thousands of videos from surgeons and manufacturers (more than 15,000 videos!). The videos can be great learning tools for students and cover a wide variety of topics related to surgical practice. For example, you can watch a video on interpreting shoulder anatomy on MRI, a presentation from a conference in 2016 on reconstructing rotator cuffs, or a video demonstrating the anterior approach to the hip for a total hip replacement. Be aware that anyone, including industry, can post videos and there may be promotional content for certain products and "sponsored" (i.e., industry paid for) content.

- JOMI (▶ jomi.com)

The Journal of Medical Insight (JOMI) offers high-quality, professionally edited, peer-reviewed surgical videos for student, resident, and surgeon education. The videos feature procedures (orthopaedic and more) from incision to wound closure. The videos include key educational content for learners including a preview of the procedure to be performed, surgeon narration, and a full-text article for a thorough understanding of the procedure. An account is not free unless your institution has a subscription. Although not quite as comprehensive as OVT or VuMedi, the videos are incredibly well-edited and detailed (you can watch at >1× speed, which is ideal, considering some videos may be over an hour).

- Orthopaedic Trauma Association (▶ OTAonline.org)

The Orthopaedic Trauma Association (OTA) curates a useful Video Library featuring educational content. There are about 250 videos in the "Procedures & Techniques" category and 450 videos in the "Annual Meetings & Conferences" category. Although we have not used this content it is free (!), features high-quality content from a reputable organization (the OTA), and offers videos that are about 10 min or less (digestible for a student).

- The Orthopaedic Video Theatre (OVT, ▶ aaos.org)

The American Academy of Orthopaedic Surgery (AAOS) presents the Orthopaedic Video Theatre (OVT). This resource offers nearly 1000 high-quality orthopaedic surgery videos, free with your AAOS membership (otherwise access is $350.00, which we consider too steep for a medical student). This resource may be a great way to watch procedures (e.g., tumor resection from a humerus or application of a spica cast) and your home institution or where you are rotating may let you use their subscription!

23.4 A Typical Day: OR

23.4.1 Introduction

Most of the information in this section applies to both general surgery and the surgical specialties. While there is a slight variation for orthopaedic surgery rotations, the information is generally the same. A layout of a typical OR is also presented in the ▶ Chap. 7 and may help you orient yourself. We recommend reviewing this content in the ▶ Chap. 7, as well.

Understanding a program's expectations of a student, whether in a clerkship or on an away rotation, is critical. Expectation-setting should definitely happen at the beginning of your rotation with the resident or intern. You should make sure to ask your intern the first day of your rotation if they can carve out 5 or 10 min of time to discuss your mutual goals during the rotation. You can assess whether it is within institutional culture to set expectations with your attending surgeon. Typically, however, a student's point person is a resident or intern. While it intuitively seems helpful, if not advantageous, to assume the appropriate culture based on prior experiences, this approach can be damaging as institutional cultures can be wildly different. For example, in some institutions it is reasonable, maybe even expected, that a medical student requests suture material from the scrub tech toward the end of the case to help close. In others, it may be perceived as presumptuous. Clarifying such expectations with your residents will help avoid many awkward misunderstandings between you and the staff. When in doubt – ask before doing!

» *The advice below is what the authors and student reviewers have seen. It is meant to be general advice – please do not be surprised if/when your rotation and experiences differ from what is described. When in doubt, ask your residents!*

The amount of time a medical student spends in the OR during a clerkship, advanced rotation, or an away rotation is institution-dependent. On some rotations, your time in the OR will be prioritized. On others, high case volume necessitates medical student involvement in managing patients on the inpatient floors or in clinic. Come with an open mind and a good attitude – you will have many, many days in the OR as a resident and surgeon.

23.4.2 General

A typical OR day starts a few hours before the first case and ends an hour or so after the last case. What time the first case starts depends on the institution, service, and surgeon. Surgeons who "run multiple rooms" will typically assign you to be with the resident in one of the rooms while they work with a physician's assistant or a fellow in another room. Typically, you are only responsible for preparing and understanding cases in your respective room. How long your day lasts is variable – trauma services have more unpredictable schedules while elective services (i.e., joints) are much more predictable and rarely change. In addition to clinical work there will be meetings such as morning rounds to discuss overnight admissions (this may be called "rounds" or "hand off," depending on the institution). In addition to discussing the night's events, there may also be an indications conference in an elective service (i.e., when and why to operate), or morbidity and mortality conferences ("M&M"), or one or more service-specific research meetings. Be aware of these and never miss the ones where you are expected to participate or are a member of that team.

23.4.2.1 A Typical Day: Morning Rounds (Fig. 23.1)
- Pre-Rounding
- Rounding
- Progress Notes
- Dressing Changes
- Morning Conference

Rounding is the activity performed almost universally across medical specialties wherein patients are evaluated first thing in the morning and their condition overnight is assessed. While it is more common on inpatient trauma services, elective services, such as joints, may also have a rounding component in the morning. How you round and when you round is dependent on your institution and the culture that has been set for medical students. Typically, the adage for medical students is, "first to arrive and last to depart." While this may be useful if you have no sense of your expectations, we recommend speaking with your residents and understanding how you would best be helpful on a team. Some may want you to come in first and "update the list" of inpatients. Some may request you attend the morning conference and not worry about rounding. Sometimes, it is disruptive to team dynamics if you arrive before

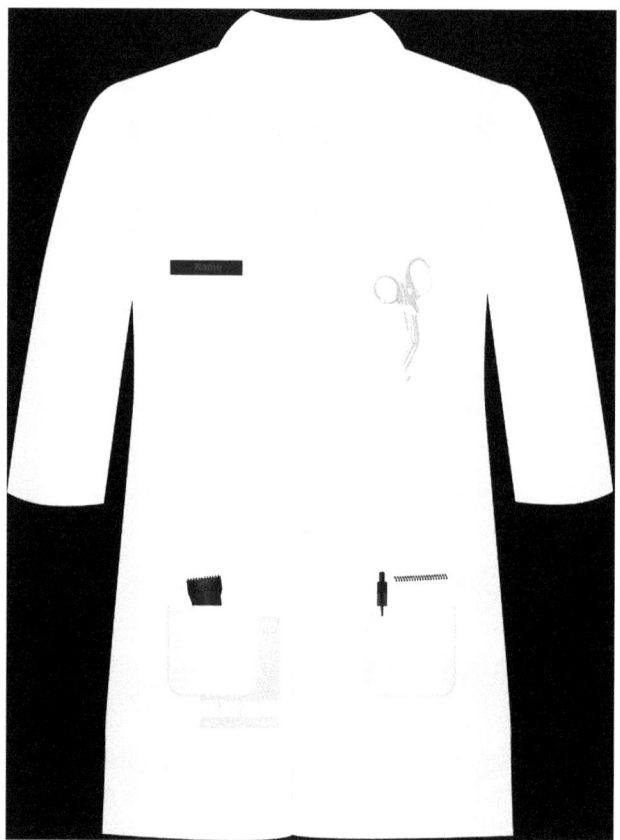

 Fig. 23.1   What's often found in the Ortho student white coat

everybody else and round "just because that's what a medical student should do." You should always double check with your resident and understand their needs and see how you best fit into their workday.

If you are arriving early to *pre-round* (i.e., round before the resident arrives), you typically are responsible for what an intern or resident would otherwise be doing: making the patient list, visiting all the patients that you have operated on the previous day, and writing the progress notes for those patients. The idea of pre-rounding is to give you a little bit of extra time so you can carry out the full obligations that an intern or resident would. You should never feel as if it is expected for you to immediately know the appropriate standards to do the above. Instead, simply speak to your resident your first day to set expectations. For example, if it is your first time printing a list on a surgical service, you may ask, "I've never printed a list before. Would you have a second to show me how you guys like your lists printed?" Even if it is not your first time, this is an appropriate question as every surgical specialty may print lists differently. You should try to master the content of the list as best as you can. If you notice any vital sign or other medical abnormalities, you can let the resident know and they will certainly appreciate it. It is also helpful to have an extra copy of the list, just in case somebody else needs it.

Since every orthopaedic subspecialty operates on different regions of the body, the *progress notes* on inpatient services will be slightly different. Understanding what kind of history and physical exam is critical for a pediatrics service is different than an arthroplasty service. An easy way to get a sense of the most important points for a specific service is to acquire the note templates that the residents used to write progress notes. These templates often have a preset history and physical exam that you can use to guide your questions for the patient. Be careful with the "copy forward" function on many EMRs! It can lead to false information being carried forward. And, although this may seem obvious, never make up exam findings or answers to questions. Honesty is always the best policy – if you didn't check distal pulses, go back and reexamine the patient or leave that part out of the note. If you *did* check the pulses but couldn't feel any and *think* there should be pulses, do not lie in the note! Say you didn't feel the pulses and then ask a resident to double check – maybe you will learn a modified approach to your physical exam, or maybe you will be the first to detect an urgent situation!

You should try to have dressing supplies ready to help with any *dressing changes*. You may even find out which patients need dressing changes by using the previous days' progress notes. Never change a dressing without confirming with your residents, as sometimes the notes are incorrect and certain dressings are laborious to reapply (and may require a visit to the OR). Having a "dressing kit" ready to go as a medical student can be very helpful. Some services even round with a "dressing cart" with all the necessary supplies. In general, it is never a bad idea to carry tape, bandages, ACE bandages, xeroform, and gauze. Also, always have your trauma shears – when rounding, in the OR, in the ED or in the clinic!

Morning conferences are an opportunity for medical students, residents, and even fellows to learn about a topic that either a colleague or an attending is presenting. Typically, medical students observe during these conferences. Again, the medical student role is variable in different institutions: in some institutions medical students simply listen and learn, in others, students are asked questions and present talks. It is ill-advised for the medical student to correct a resident, fellow, or attending. How you participate in morning conference should mostly be dictated by what you observe of the institution's culture. Are medical students encouraged to ask questions? Do medical students make presentations at morning conference at the end of their rotation? Do medical students simply sit in the back and listen? Will you be able to give an oral presentation of your patients, or does the resident present all of the patients? These are questions that you will need to figure out and act accordingly. Grand rounds, subspecialty conferences, teaching conferences, and core curricula for the residents are all opportunities for you to learn more about orthopaedics and the musculoskeletal system.

23.4.2.2   The Night/Day Before

You will benefit from speaking with your resident to confirm the surgeon's preferences the day before your OR day. Please do not arrive to the operating room ill-prepared! Do your best to be ready using the resources we mentioned above. Some questions you might ask your resident to guide your preparation include:

- What is typically the medical student role during the operation?
- What are the expectations for medical students?
- What are the surgical approaches (i.e., anterior or posterior approach to the hip) that you will be using for the day?
- Is this a primary procedure or a revision? Is it a "typical" case, or modified in any way?
- Is this a service that encourages rounding on patients that you have operated on? May I join you for rounds in the morning before hand-off?
- If it is your first day, understanding basic logistics is also important: What time and where should I show up?

The night before an OR day is best spent preparing for the next day's cases. If you have access to the electronic medical records (EMR) from home, you can read about the patient history and better understand their disease progression. If you do not have access, spending a few extra hours in the hospital will be worth a comprehensive understanding of your patients and their medical history. Expectations vary among attendings – some expect the medical student to understand surgical indications for every patient. Other surgeons may expect you to know something about the patient – e.g., what do they do for work or fun? The resident may be able to give you a tip on what to expect and when in doubt, definitely look at any orthopaedic clinic notes in the EMR. Overall, we believe that the above approach to surgical preparation leads to a deeper understanding and more durable appreciation of musculoskeletal disease and the patient experience, and therefore recommend it regardless of your attending's preference.

After reviewing the patient history, understanding the surgical approach is your next priority. This can be done independently using an anatomy atlas (such as listed in the resource section, above), using the guidance of a specific approaches textbook (i.e., Hoppenfeld's), or a more summarized resource such as Orthobullets. Below is a checklist that you can use to make sure you have covered most of what you need to prepare for a case. We will be using a total joint arthroplasty of the hip (posterior approach, the "Southern" Approach) as an example. Keep in mind, there are many different ways to prepare for a case, and every student does it differently. Find what methods work for you by trial and error. This is simply an example that we have found to be effective. Take some notes on a piece of fresh printer paper or patient list so that you aren't trying to remember all of this in your head. (A word of caution – do NOT misuse or misplace protected health information, PHI, when doing your case preparation. This applies to all rotations!).

Case Prep Checklist (■ Fig. 23.2):

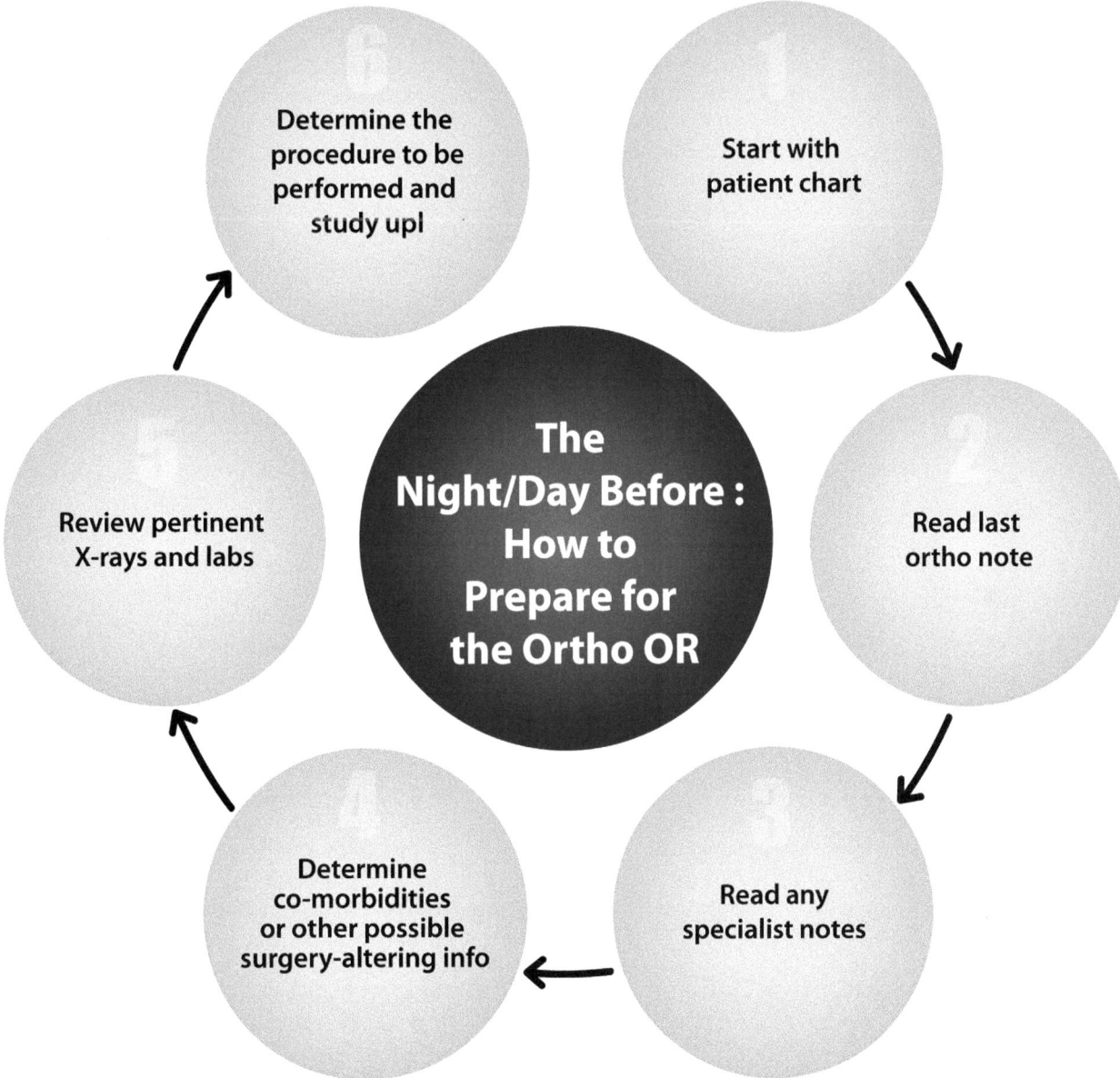

■ **Fig. 23.2** Flowchart of topics to review the night or day before a case

- Day before the case: Use the EMR or your resident to identify the approach the surgeon will be using. In this case, the posterior approach.
- Review the patient's chart:
  - Read most recent attending surgeon visit note
    - Pay specific attention to the history and physical exam (Did they fall? How long have they had hip pain? Do they have a history of osteopenia/porosis?)
  - Rad initial attending surgeon visit note
  - Search for any medical specialty notes (i.e., cardiology)
  - Search for any comorbidities (e.g., check a primary care note!)
  - Make note of their medication list (specific medications to look out for include blood thinners, insulin, and other diabetic medications, antibiotics, etc.)

- Make note of any allergies (do they have a betadine allergy? Penicillin? What about latex…for our gloves?)
- Search for any significant social determinants of health (are they homeless? Do they have a support system within their community?)
- Review most recent X-rays
- Review initial X-rays
- Review any advanced imaging (MRI, CT, etc.)
- Review any relevant labs – hemoglobin is usually important but it doesn't hurt to check the most recent INR, WBC/ "white count" or another lab that may be appropriate (e.g., ESR, CRP for an infection)
  - You may need to wait until the morning of the case to check the most up-to-date labs!
- If you have never seen this case before:
  - Read all of "Hip Posterior Approach (Moore or Southern)" section in Orthobullets
    - Are you a visual or kinesthetic learner? Some students have success with drawing out each step of the procedure in addition to reading about it
    - Remember! A thorough understanding includes knowing everything from the first skin incision to the final closing suture/staple/drain/you name it!
    - Consider the postoperative protocol, too – is the patient getting a drain? Antibiotics? Posterior hip precautions? When can they start working with physical therapy?
  - Read relevant section of Hoppenfeld's
  - Read relevant section of Netter's Concise Orthopaedic Anatomy
  - Spend time reviewing anatomy on a 3D digital atlas alongside one of the above resources
  - Watch a video on VuMedi or JOMI of the procedure
  - Read relevant sections of the "Hip and Knee book" (▶ website)
  - Tip: if you want a description of how the surgeon does this procedure review their dictation for this procedure in the EMR – the resident can probably help you find this (they usually have a smartphrase for their own note writing).
- If you've seen this case a few times:
  - Review anatomy on Orthobullets
  - Review anatomy on a 3D digital atlas
  - Review do-not-miss anatomy on Orthobullets
  - Skim "hip and knee book" (website)
- If you have seen this case several times:
  - Review anatomy on orthobullets

Also, remember that sleep is important. An extra 30 min to an hour of sleep may be more worth your time than a deep, comprehensive review of the neurovasculature of the hip.

Before the case, at your own discretion, review any essential anatomy (i.e., the anatomy emphasized in the resources listed in the prepping checklist) and go over the surgical approach. This may be as quick as scrolling through Orthobullets while walking to the hospital or waking up a little early and reviewing Hoppenfeld's. If you find yourself short on time, make sure to review the anatomy involved in the approach, specifically muscles, nerves, and blood vessels that are encountered or cut. It is wise to also meet your resident and ensure your understanding of the approach and confirm any anatomy or common pimp questions to be prepared for intraoperatively. Residents are often very open to sharing their knowledge with medical students. If you have not met the attending surgeon before, this is a good time to also introduce yourself and state your role. This way, they can better plan their case to maximize your learning opportunities as well as ensure patient safety. While involvement may be limited the first time you work with an attending, most surgeons also think of medical student involvement in terms of graduated autonomy, whereby you are given increasing responsibilities in each case as long as you demonstrate you are capable and prepared.

You should make sure that you introduce yourself to any patient for whom you will be present during their operation. It is your ethical duty as a student to be transparent about your role with patients. In our experience, patients are often very eager to have a medical student be involved in their care, specifically patients who elect to receive their care at a teaching institution. In the event that the patient does not consent to your involvement, you should be mindful and respectful of their wishes and discuss it with your resident. We do not condone medical student involvement in operations when patients do not consent, as this a violation of their informed consent and autonomy. Introducing yourself to a patient also allows you to better be involved in their care, understand the impact of the burden of disease, and establish a personal connection. You can consider examining your patient before their surgery, if this is the norm in your institution (ask your resident!). It is important to correlate the history and physical exam that *you* acquire with the surgical indications. Show initiative to review these pertinent findings with your resident or the attending.

You should always try to be present when your resident or attending speaks to your patient. Speaking with patients before an operation also gives you a perspective on what patients typically worry about before a surgery. Logistics that may seem mundane to you (i.e., how long will it be after my operation before my family member/friend can see me?) can be the most important concern to a patient. It is also very educational to hear what clinical symptoms the patient is experiencing that necessitates the surgery and go over the clinical examination with the resident for maximal learning opportunity. When speaking to a patient, be mindful to not speculate answers to questions that seem "common" or "obvious" to you. For example, you may have been with Dr. Smith last week and noticed that he removes bulky jones dressings after 3–4 days. This week, however, you are with Dr. Jones. Maybe she will do the same? Remember – even in similar procedures, perioperative care can be different. You never want to unintentionally give incorrect information about the nuances of a procedure. This only leads to confusion for the patient and surgical teams, as well as creates more work.

After you have spoken to the patient, you should go to the OR before the patient is rolled back, typically by the anesthesia team. That way, you can introduce yourself to everyone in the room: the scrub tech, the nurses, the anesthesia staff/residents, industry representatives, and anyone else. After introductions, there is often a whiteboard or equivalent where all staff members involved in a case list their names. Nurses appreciate when medical students take the initiative to "put their name on the board." This way, they can more easily enter your name in the electronic medical record as a participant in the surgery. Sometimes, you may even be asked to put your glove sizes next your name, as your gloves may be pulled for you. However, you should *never* assume that someone will pull your gloves. In fact, it is helpful for you to not only pull your gloves, but also offer to pull the gloves of the resident or any other personnel who may seem busy. Maybe even pull all the gloves you will use during the entire day in that room (i.e., 4 pairs of gloves for the 4 cases of the day). When doing this, make sure you have checked all the patients in the queue for latex allergies and pull gloves appropriately and always ask the circulator (i.e., the Nurse who is documenting and grabbing extra supplies during the case) and scrub tech in advance. A final task that may be useful, depending on institutional preference, is pulling up the patient's imaging (usually X-rays) on the computer system in the OR. Again, it is never a bad idea to check with the resident first and keep out of the way of the rest of the team.

If you have completed the above and still find yourself with ample time before a case, you may consider offering your help to the intern, if there is one on your service. Many elective services do not have a surgical intern, but rather a midlevel provider (PA, NP, etc.). You may also consider offering your help to these providers, as they often carry the brunt of the floor work on a service. They are excellent resources for learning. You should always ensure that you have "one eye on the clock," so that you do not miss the patient's rollback from the perioperative area to the operating room. Depending on the electronic medical record system, there may be an option to estimate time remaining until rollback. Alternatively, your resident may be able to give you an anecdotal estimate.

If you still have free time, refueling is wise (i.e., via snacks, a quick trip to the cafeteria, or a protein bar). While elective services have a more predictable schedule, your next chance to grab a meal or snack may be unpredictable.

23.4.2.3   During the Case

Overview:
- Room set up
- Prepping the patient
- Your role in the procedure
- Useful skills
- Final words on sterility in the OR

The highlight of the OR day, of course, is the intraoperative experience. While the rest of the day is valuable for understanding workflow, the actual operation is where students often fall in love with orthopaedics. Some attendings may prefer you watch and observe your first time with a procedure; others may want you scrubbed in right away. Every attending has their own preference for how the room is set up and how the case runs. Thus, it may be ill-advised to implement what you have learned with one surgeon to another (even in the same procedure – a hip replacement with Dr. Smith is not the same as a hip replacement with Dr. Jones). Once you have observed and feel comfortable with the room set up, you should ask for permission and then feel free to participate in the set up. Some residents may help teach you appropriate sterile technique and want to walk you through the setup. Others may give you more freedom with leading the room setup. You should always feel empowered to ask for help. *Please never feel as if asking will "look bad" or hurt your performance evaluation. In fact, the opposite is true. Not putting the patient at risk of infection or harm is your first duty as a medical professional.* As an aside, remember to silence your phone when in the OR and, if applicable, put your pager on a shelf or other designated area.

Setting up the room starts with helping roll the patient from the preoperative area to the OR. At this point, everyone in the OR will be wearing a surgical mask – don't forget yours! Also, at this time, all the materials for the case (e.g., hardware, suture, and other sterile items) will be open on the "back table" so be careful with how you're moving about the OR. After arriving in the OR, you may help move the patient from the gurney to the OR table. Never attempt a patient transfer alone as this is a danger for both the patient and yourself.

Depending on the workflow, the resident, nurse, or anesthesia will take the lead. You may also help by moving any digital monitors that are used for arthroscopy cases. Ensure you have introduced yourself to everyone, if that was not done before the patient arrived. During some services, there may be necessary equipment that the team needs – step stools, headlamps, batteries for headlamps, etc. – that you can gather before scrubbing in while the patient is getting comfortable on the table. Remember it is cold in the OR and you might make yourself useful by grabbing a couple warm blankets to make the patient comfortable. You may find the orthopaedic instrumentation set overwhelming at first. However, understanding the names and roles of all of the devices that a surgeon uses is not a high priority for you and your role. That is better saved for "on the job," experiential learning on the rotation and as a resident. You will slowly learn to pick up device names as you pay attention to what the residents and surgeons are asking of the scrub tech. After a few repetitions, you may even be comfortable asking for basic instruments yourself (after asking if this is appropriate!).

Medical student involvement in *prepping a patient* is also variable by institution. As with all things, it is most useful to learn how to clean a surgical site from a resident or nurse before attempting it yourself. This typically involves chlorhexidine sticks, betadine washes, or some combination of the two. While the setup is variable, the main components involve the type of disinfectant, the setup materials, and the cleanup materials. The setup materials are often chux pads that are placed under the body part that is to be washed. The cleanup material is blue sterile towels or simply nothing (air dry). When using the chlorhexidine sticks, be mindful that the disinfectant (orange color) is contained in a glass ampule that shatters with external grip force. Often, students shake the stick vertically, in an attempt to "soak the pad" with the orange prep. However, there have been cases where over-vigorous shaking has led to glass expelling into the pad and causing lacerations on patients. Gentle, circular movements of the wrist are sufficient. Be aware of the fire precautions and the waiting times after draping. These are universal precautions. Additional aspects of prep may include shaving the skin (there is usually an electric shaver somewhere in the room) and removing all hair with tape or special sticky pads. A hip case won't use a tourniquet, but be aware that other cases may and learning how to apply tourniquets before sterile prepping, is a useful skill for your OR team.

Once a case has started, a *medical student's role* is determined by the resident and the surgeon. Some surgeons may only allow a student to retract while others may walk a student through the entire case. The concept of "graduated autonomy" is used to describe the ever-increasing responsibilities garnered to a trainee based on their performance and preparation. In some academic institutions, medical students mostly observe and retract. At other institutions, medical students are more involved and may even function as a "first assist" (or second surgeon) in cases. The first time you are seeing a case should feel very different than the fourth or fifth time. The difference is your comfort with the steps of the procedure, anticipation of what happens next and what could go wrong, and your confidence in being involved. The first time, you are most helpful to the team if your involvement is minimal. You will probably retract or be instructed to carry out certain tasks when needed. As your repetitions with a certain case increase, you will find you can self-identify where you are most helpful and go on to anticipate need for retraction or suction. A pitfall for students is that they often simply replicate tasks they had carried out in previous cases, not taking into consideration that this case may be slightly different and that the task is now either unnecessary or actually harmful. Therefore, it is often better for the patient and the entire team if you do not assume steps in a case. Whether you feel involved or not, maintain a good attitude and remember to always ask before doing.

At some point in the case, you may find that the surgeon has gotten into a familiar rhythm with the case and may ask you about yourself. Don't be surprised if the surgeon is curious what institution you are from, what you studied in undergrad, where you grew up, what your hobbies are. These kinds of friendly questions may catch you off guard, but are commonly asked. There is also a certain culture about speaking in the OR: When is it appropriate? Should I ever ask questions? Initially, it is wise to speak when spoken to. After you have established rapport, you will find yourself becoming more comfortable with the team.

Understanding how to suture and tie surgical knots may be the most common *skill/ procedure* with which a medical student is tasked. There are many free videos online for you to practice at home. While it is by no means a requirement, we recommend investing in a cheap suture practice kit. Alternatively, your institution may have a simulation center or other facility where you can practice while on call or after hours. This way, you can comfortably practice at home as much as you would like on standardized materials. Alternatively, you can also practice on orange peels, bananas, towels, pig's feet (available at the butcher counter of some grocery stores), or grapes. Please be mindful of your sharps when practicing at home. Do not dispose of sharps in the normal recycling or trash at home. Collecting them at home in a provided sharps container (from the hospital) or, if in a pinch, an empty water bottle and disposing the water bottle in the hospital sharps bin is best practice. You can also learn how to tie knots at home using YouTube videos and some shoelaces. After you have learned on shoelaces, feel free to ask the scrub tech or circulator for some expired free hand ties or suture for a finer experience. You may even choose to do all of the above activities wearing wet gloves, for an added challenge.

Maintaining sterility is critical in all surgical environments. You will either have a tutorial at your institution on sterile technique, or be taught by one of your residents. If you have already completed your clerkships, you have learned sterility in your general surgery blocks. If not, some quick tips include:

- Move *slowly* so everybody can anticipate your movements
- Keep your arms above your waist and below the nipple line
- Do not touch your gown above your elbows
- Do not approach the field and patient until told to do so
- Remember that everything covered in blue drapes is sterile!
- Careful to watch out for the large and lumbering c-arm or mini-c!
- Respect everybody's personal space
- If in arthroplasty, inquire whether the institution considers your hood sterile or not
- If using boots, change them every time you enter and exit the operating room and wing of the hospital
- If you contaminate a field, do not be embarrassed and pretend it didn't happen. It can be detrimental to the patient and is unethical – *speak up!!*
- If need be, step back from the field so you don't contaminate anything (if your glove falls off, if you need to sneeze or vomit, etc.)

23.4.2.4 Do's and Don'ts on Orthopaedic Services

You will develop a mental checklist of some of the common pearls and pitfalls of different cases and services. This list is by no means exhaustive, but rather a starting point for you to develop your own list (◘ Table 23.2).

▣ Table 23.2 Some common Do's and Don'ts for the different orthopaedic subspecialties

Specialty	Do's	Don'ts
Arthroplasty (joints)	Anticipate retraction Read the Hip-and-Knee book (online) Try to get involved in closing, as appropriate Learn how knots are tied and tie some when closing Learn to apply staples on patient skin Respect time when cementing – this is a critical portion of the case	Touch the implants/hardware Touch your hood unless your institution considers them sterile Play with the extra cement, unless invited to do so (then make a femur or volcano!)
Hand/upper extremity	Spend time learning hand anatomy and appreciating radiography of hand, wrist, and elbow Learn arthroscopic views of shoulder/elbow Enjoy being able to sit while operating Be *gentle* when retracting nerves, vessels, muscles, etc. Avoid being in the way of the mini c-arm As applicable, be ready with a tourniquet before prepping	Expect to use micro instruments as a medical student – this includes wearing loups, using fine suture and delicate instruments, etc. Make large, rapid movements (the hand is very valuable real estate) Speak without thinking – some hand procedures do not use general anesthesia and the patient may be awake and listening!
Foot and ankle	Learn how lower extremities are positioned and help position them in the future Appreciate the anatomy and innervation of the lower extremity and foot As applicable, be ready with a tourniquet before prepping	Forget to scrub the feet really well during prepping Avoid touching toes with your sterile gloves even after prepping unless warranted
Oncology	Learn most common MSK sarcomas and cancers, their treatments, and typical prognosis (available on Orthobullets under "Pathology") Learn relevant anatomy for the specific case Expect more sensitive patient conversations	Memorize pathology/histology slides
Sports medicine	Learn the basics of arthroscopy and common ports and views (Orthobullets, Hoppenfeld's) Wear booties that go up to your knees – it can be a watery mess during arthroscopy	Smash into articular cartilage during arthroscopy Put the camera down on the drapes! The bulb is HOT and will melt the drapes and potentially harm the patient
Spine	Come prepared to stand for many hours Know neuroanatomy of spinal cord and nerve root function Consider volunteering to do skin closure – these are some of the largest incisions in surgery and excellent learning opportunities!	Suction recklessly (may be on dura or neural structures) Volunteer to retract the muscles unless you are confident in your endurance to do so
Trauma	Learn how to roll a quick and accurate splint. Be available and able to help with splints in the tauma bay, ED, or OR Learn broad anatomy Master your "anatomy review system" and resources Review basic fracture classification systems Learn your way around the ED and the wards and where to find materials you might need on call If applicable, start notes or take notes on patients to help your resident	Don't expect a "nine to five" work day Try not to get in the way of the C-arm
Pediatrics	Understand patient–parent dynamics Respect pediatric patient vulnerability Review how pedi X-rays are different than adult Skim some of the highest yield pediatric fractures (supracondylar fracture, both bone forearm)	Expect to be involved without establishing good rapport

23.4.2.5 Pimping

Pimping is one of the most feared aspects of a surgical rotation, particularly for more inexperienced medical students on the core clerkships. Pimping is a modern version of the Socratic method, whereby the teacher asks the learner questions about a specific topic, oftentimes spontaneously. The teacher may ask individual questions, or "dig deeper" and ask questions in increasing detail and difficulty until the learner no longer answers correctly. The Socratic method may be dreaded by students because it seems punitive or puts someone "on the spot." However, this is rarely the case. Most of the time, teachers simply want to determine how much a student knows on a particular topic so that they may tailor their own teaching and/or adjust the content material.

As a medical student, we hope you will begin to look forward to pimping. This may seem counterintuitive but hear us out. This is direct, one-on-one tutoring that you are receiving from experts whose time is precious and valuable. The more you read and prepare, the better you will be at answering questions and engaging in the material you are being taught. Often, attendings ask the same questions of everybody, so you may ask your resident if there's anything specific you should prepare for or read about. This way, you come to the case more prepared and therefore will benefit much more from teaching. At the end of the day, the impact of answering questions correctly on your final rotation evaluation is often overemphasized by students. Do your best to avoid dwelling on questions you got wrong or could not answer. Passing the "do I want to get a beer with you" test is often more valuable than answering surgical minutiae correctly.

Nevertheless, an adequate fund of knowledge is critical for you to benefit from the rotation and maximize your time. If there's a question you do not know the answer to, it is OK to say, "I'm not sure." Sometimes, when students are unsure of an answer, they will instead dance around the topic with what they *do* know. This strategy may be helpful because it demonstrates that your fund of knowledge is adequate but simply incomplete. At the same time, in front of a different surgeon, it may be damaging because it may be interpreted as an attempt to evade the question. Perhaps, your best strategy may be to gauge your audience and, if the situation becomes increasingly awkward, find time later in the day to ask the resident for feedback and help. Overtime, you will develop your own way of handling topics and questions you're unsure of. Some people simply stick to "I'm not sure" or "I'll look it up after the case." In the end, it is important to realize that the Socratic method is there for your learning and not meant to be a punitive social shaming experiment. If you are asked to "look something up for tomorrow," always do so. This is a great learning opportunity to read more about a topic that is clinically relevant.

When giving answers to a question, you should always make an effort to not embarrass someone else on the team who did not know the answer to the question if they were asked before you. You want to be thought of as a "team player" and must be diplomatic when explaining a topic. Remember: no one likes a "know it all."

23.4.2.6 Closing/After the Case

Closing the case is typically when most of the surgical procedure is complete and it is time to close the patient's wound layer by layer. Often, there are both deep and superficial closures. Typically, the deep closure is done by the resident or even the attending depending on case/institution. The superficial closure, however, is a task that may be offered to the medical student. While you should certainly observe and learn your first few times, it is not unreasonable to ask your resident if you can participate in the superficial closure of a wound. They will often agree, unless it is a special closure, such as a patient with extremely frail skin or a previously infected site. If you have been practicing your suturing at home, the superficial closure is your chance to shine! Embrace feedback, as it is the only way you will improve your technique. After all, a surgical residency is, in some ways, 5 years of feedback. There are different closure techniques at different institutions; different knot types are preferred. You will quickly learn what your institution prefers, and this will be most apparent when you are on the away rotation season experiencing different hospitals. After closing the skin, most wounds will need some sort of dressing – you can help with this. It is good form to hold the limb or otherwise help with dressings, as needed.

After the closure and dressings have been applied, you may help by transferring the patient onto the hospital bed from the OR table. Be mindful that certain procedures can make transfers difficult. For example, after a total hip replacement, you must be very mindful of positioning during transfer as the hip may dislocate. In a spine case, patients are prone and flipped supine. Therefore, when you are first starting, it is wise to follow the resident's lead and take instruction from the nurses and anesthesia. The anesthesiologist, holding the patient's head and sometimes the endotracheal tube, will typically lead with a countdown when moving the patient or moving the bed, so please pay attention to your colleague at the head of the bed. You will then help roll the patient to the Post Anesthesia Care Unit (PACU), after which you have completed your case. Don't forget to thank the OR team for letting you participate! While in many institutions "writing orders" is fairly repetitive and automated, you should volunteer to learn. This way, you will get a sense of the perioperative medications and nursing orders that a patient needs for their care. Writing orders is not only useful for a medical student to learn, but also can be one less burden for your already busy resident.

During some trauma rotations, you may be asked to *"roll the splint"* before or after the case. If you already know how to roll a splint, you can ask the nurse/resident if there is a designated location/table where you may lay your splint on and how they typically handle pre-rolled splints (if at all). If splints are not typically pre-rolled, working on your splinting skills can pay off, as you can quickly roll the splint immediately post-op while the patient is still on the table. Speed and accuracy are appreciated. Knowing where the plaster, Webril, and ACE bandages are is key.

23.4.2.7 In Between Cases

There is typically turnover time – i.e., time spent by specialized teams that scrub and restock the OR – in between cases. The time varies on your institution type: private groups often have much faster turnover times than academic institutions. The time between cases can be used for:
- Reviewing anatomy for the next case
- Looking up any topics that you were unsure of during the first case
- Discussing the next case with your resident
- Checking in with the intern (or whoever is doing floor work) to see if they need any extra hand
- Attending case conference, grand rounds, or academic meetings
- Grabbing a bite to eat (very important!) and a drink of water

23.4.2.8 Ending the Day

You may offer to write brief operative notes after each case. You will find that these notes are typically done immediately after the surgery. They are very short and can take less than a few minutes. Your institution may even have a simple template you can use. You may also go visit the intern or floor person and offer your help with any floor work that needs to be done. You may also be at a point in the day when you can do postoperative checks on patients that you operated on earlier in the day. Check with your resident before you visit these patients as institutional policy may vary.

After all the cases are done, it is often expected that you may leave when determined by your resident. This may seem old fashioned but is still a safe way to approach a rotation, especially if you do not yet know the team well enough to know how they will respond to you asking to depart. If you're finding yourself at a point where you are idling and have exhausted all of the ways you can be helpful to the team, consider asking your resident the classic question: "Is there anything else that you need help with?" This is a universal signal understood by all residents to mean, "is there anything else that you need help with? If not, can I go home?" Residents will often dismiss you if there is truly nothing else left to be done. There are different views on asking your resident for permission to leave, as some people swear by the "the first one to arrive last one to leave" mentality of a surgical rotation. However, we find that simply being honest and trying your best to be helpful to the team is the best policy.

23.5 A Typical Day: Clinic

Clinic days are often integrated into orthopaedic rotations. They provide a good representation of an actual orthopaedic surgeon's week. Clinic days are important for following up on patients after surgery as well as determining whether new patients need operative or nonoperative treatment of their musculoskeletal complaint. Confirm your schedule for clinic with the program coordinator or clerkship coordinator at the start of your rotation. Schedules often change last-minute and you don't want to find yourself wasting half of your day being idle or searching for a clinic.

23.5.1 The Night Before

The night before clinic is a good time to get yourself prepared to see patients the following day. If you have remote access to the electronic medical record, you should spend time reading about your patients the next day. Even without remote access, you may consider spending an hour or two in the hospital after your day ends to prepare. The patients you will see on clinic days are often not predictable. You may shadow the attending on your first day (you should try to start seeing patients on your own as soon as you feel comfortable), alternate seeing patients with the resident, or be directed into certain patient rooms based on the patient pathology. If somebody has a pathology that will serve as a useful teaching moment, the resident or attending may direct you to that room. Therefore, it is generally not possible to predict which patients you will be seeing the next day (after day 1 or 2, you will have a better sense of the workflow). As such, depending on how many patients are on the list, you may consider skimming through the histories of all of the patients by looking at their most recent clinic note, if that patient is known to that clinic. This is useful because (1) you will spend less time during clinic doing so and can therefore see more patients, and (2) you will know a little bit about patients that you have not even seen and can potentially predict a couple of teaching moments of the day. As the rotation progresses and your stamina decreases, you may find yourself wanting to skip reviewing the patient list prior to clinic. However, we strongly recommend that you stay strong and continue coming prepared. After all, the goal of the rotation is to learn as much orthopaedics as you can as well as put yourself in the mindset of being the patient's primary provider. Don't despair! Over time, as your fund of knowledge increases, you will naturally spend less time reviewing patients beforehand. Also, use your resources.

Orthobullets, or other quick reviews, can be useful immediately before seeing a patient to brush up on a topic. You may also consider reviewing some of the patient's prior visit notes to better understand what the attending you are working with considers important during the visit.

23.5.2 During Clinic

You should introduce yourself to all of the nurses and clinic staff. A clinic day should be treated similarly to an OR day. The same general principles apply:

- Introduce yourself
- Familiarize yourself with the environment
- Learn common locations for equipment such as injection kits, ACE wraps, soft braces, chux pads, suture removal kits, etc.
- Set expectations with the resident and attending
- Understand the logistics of when you should arrive and leave

Make sure you wear proper attire. Some clinics allow scrubs. Most require conservative attire for students (ties, professional blouses or shirts, no sandals or sneakers, you will be familiar with this uniform after your other clerkships). Confirm with the residents before clinic about attire. You don't want to show up in scrubs when everyone else is wearing a suit.

If it is your first day with an attending in their clinic, you should probably wait for the attending to arrive before seeing their patients. Sometimes, attendings have particular preferences about whether students should see patients independently or not. There is a careful balance between showing initiative and being disrespectful of an attending's workflow. You may consider asking the resident whether you can see patients if you have arrived early.

For a typical patient visit, you should read about their history and why they are in clinic. You can use note templates that the institution provides on the electronic medical record to start taking notes while you were reading about the history. If you are unsure what to ask during the patient encounter, you may consider printing off the note template that is used in clinic. This typically covers information that is considered critical and can guide your approach. After you have seen a patient, you will often present the patient to the attending and resident. How the oral presentation is structured is dependent on the attending's preference. Speak with your resident to understand how much detail you should present. Orthopaedic oral presentations are typically quick and to the point, lasting under 2 min. Presentations may be as short as, "Mr. Johnson is a 62 your old man who underwent ORIF of the left tibia with you two weeks ago. He is here for follow-up today and is doing well." While this is not a very descriptive oral presentation, it is not uncommon for follow-up patients. New patients will most certainly require a longer presentation that includes any key history, physical exam, and radiographic findings with an assessment and plan. We recommend reading Mehlman and Farmer's "Teaching Orthopaedics on the Run: Tell Me The Story Backward" article for a better understanding of how your oral presentations can improve to augment your learning experience. Our ► Chap. 7 has more detail on the components of an oral presentation.

When visiting a patient, you may treat this as any other medical rotation. You should go through the history and physical with a targeted approach. If you are unfamiliar with the disease, you should read about it on Orthobullets before seeing the patient so that you can maximize your interaction with the patient. Old notes can be helpful, but also may serve as a crutch – you may find yourself struggling with new patient encounters. After your visit with the patient, you should present the patient to the attending or resident and then go see the same patient with the group. Make note of any changes in the history or physical exam during the attending/resident encounter, as that will be the official record in the patient note. You may start working on your note while the attending visits the next patient with the resident (if the attending is alternating patients with the resident). Try to finish your notes as the day moves along, so you don't have to stay afterward and catch up on notes. This will also provide for higher-quality notes, since as the day progresses, patients may start blending together, and you may forget details. While it is a good goal to match the resident's speed in clinic, this is unreasonable when you first start. You should, however, get a sense of the expectation for how many patients a typical medical student sees. Of course, try to meet the expectation; it is OK to start slow and build up early on during the rotation season. The number of patients you see is often not as important as the quality of your visit. Residents and attendings would much prefer to see a well-written note and oral presentation than several sloppy visits. Of course, make sure all of your notes are "assigned" to the appropriate attending; there is usually a function to do this in the EMR.

There are often many providers who collaborate to deliver the best musculoskeletal care in the orthopaedic clinic. If you have downtime, consider spending some time with the physical therapists or hand therapists to see how patients benefit from rehabilitation. Try your hand at ultra-sounding a joint to see if you can see an effusion. There may even be opportunities to learn from the radiology teams. Keep your eyes and ears open to make the most of your clinic days.

23.6 A Typical Night: Call Nights

Whether you have call nights as part of your rotation or not will depend on your institution. "Call" is what happens in the hospital after the business day is over and before the next business day starts. You should also be aware that there are providers assigned to take care of the call responsibilities during business hours ("day call"). Medical students are typically not involved in day call as this is when clinics and elective cases are scheduled. Typically 6:00 PM to 6:00 AM is the normal call schedule for night call. The day before you were on call, you should ensure you get adequate rest for your overnight shift. If it is your first time doing an overnight or you are starting a burst of call shifts (i.e., about to start a series of call nights), then your adjustment will be more difficult. You should confirm the logistics of your call:

- What time does call start?
- Where is the call room?
- Who are you working with? (often, the resident you have been with is not the same resident that is on call)
- What is the call schedule? (i.e., q2 (every 2 days), one weeknight plus a weekend, etc.)
- What is the medical student role on call? Do you see patients in the emergency room first? Do you see them with a resident together?
- Are the electronic medical record note templates different for call nights?

The night of your call, if you were working with a resident that you haven't met before, you should start with setting expectations. You will notice that setting expectations is a recurrent theme. You may be at an institution where call is extremely busy and residents see consults throughout the night. Alternatively, your institution may have very calm call nights. Whatever the case, call nights can be a good opportunity to learn the responsibility of an orthopaedic resident on call. You may be more involved in patient care, as there are fewer learners in the hospital. If there are no consults/cases, being on call is an excellent time to bond with your residents, catch up on orthopaedic literature, and work on research projects. If you do find yourself with a chance to sleep, let your resident know so that they can wake you up if there is a consult that they are going to see. Typically, exchanging cell phone numbers is a good idea before the night gets busy.

Seeing patients in the emergency room is similar to seeing them in a clinical setting. Please refer to the above section detailing clinical visits for more details. You can expect to see and potentially participate in a lot of fracture reductions on an orthopaedic rotation. If there is a reduction pending, make sure you gather necessary equipment (see Procedure section) to assist. If you are on an extremely busy service, you should consider writing the patient notes (e.g., ED notes, admit notes, post-op checks) during any downtime you may have. This way, you can help offload some of the resident workload and ensure both of you leave on time the next morning. The following morning during rounds, you may be asked to present some patients to the incoming team. You should also assist in finishing any unfinished notes. If you go to all of the patient encounters overnight, you can help contribute to all of the notes.

23.7 Procedure Guide

Like many things, your level of involvement in procedures will vary based on institution, your preparation, and your willingness to participate. Typically, you will be supervised for most procedures and will often learn from residents, including in the emergency room or the OR. The medical student is typically most helpful as an extra set of hands when applying and removing splints, casts, and braces.

23.7.1 Supplies

Gathering supplies is a useful task for medical students. It can be helpful to understand where the supply closets are in the emergency room, as this is where the typical student will be rolling splints and applying casts. It is particularly helpful if you can visit the emergency room before your call shift and speak to a nurse and learn where the orthopaedic supplies are kept. At some institutions, there is a dedicated "ortho room" in the emergency room, and all of the supplies are centrally located in that place. It may also be nice to know where there is an industrial sink for filling up buckets for splints and disposing of sharps and other waste products. Getting a lay of the land before your call shift is extremely helpful so you can quickly pick up what you and the resident need.

23.7.2 Splint Rolling and Application

Rolling a splint is a quintessential procedure in orthopaedics for medical students. A splint requires plaster, Webril, and an ACE wrap. A splint is not a cast – which is made from fiberglass material and is more rigid (see next section). A splint is important in immobilizing and supporting fractures. While there are different types of splints that are used for different extremities and fractures, the basic concept is the same. You will also need a bucket of water to get the plaster wet and ready to take shape. In order to get the correct length for your splint, you can use Webril as a measuring tape on the extremity. Your template piece of Webril will serve to guide how long you will make your plaster and subsequent pieces of Webril. Typically, the plaster to Webril ratio is 10–13 to 5 (i.e.,for every 10–13 "slabs" of plaster, you will have 5 sheets of Webril). Each institution may have slightly different approaches to the most common splints, so you should ask the resident what the preferred way is where you are working. ◘ Figure 23.3 *illustrates some of the splints you will encounter on your rotations and their most common indications.*

A common trick when rolling plaster is to measure the first piece with your template Webril, drop the roll into an empty bucket (typically the bucket that you brought all of the materials in) and fold the plaster over itself 10 times. This will create identical sized pieces of plaster, as they are folded on top of one another. This is much faster than rolling out a piece of plaster, tearing it, rolling another piece of plaster, and repeating. Ask your resident for their tips on rolling a splint efficiently. When it is time, you will dip the plaster into your bucket of water, which will start to set the plaster.

Now, your countdown timer is ticking until the plaster will harden. You will then lay out the plaster onto a table or surface (i.e., chux) and put the Webril on top. The plaster plus Webril combination will be transferred to the patient and applied as a splint. The Webril will be touching the skin and keeping the plaster from doing so. You don't want plaster on skin. As plaster hardens, it always warm up – it is an exothermic chemical reaction. Do not use hot water (lukewarm is fine) to set your plaster – the exothermic reaction is more intense, faster, and should be avoided. Often, in order to prevent plaster from touching skin, the Webril pieces will be slightly wider than the plaster pieces.

Application of the splint requires understanding of fracture anatomy. Splints typically are associated with a certain type of molding pattern whereby different forces are distributed across the fracture to help it maintain reduction and heal in proper orientation. Therefore, you should always ask before you apply a splint and do so under supervision. After a splint is applied, it may be wrapped in ACE wrap that serves to not only keep the splint pieces together but also create a more aesthetically appealing final product for the patient. Make sure the ACE wrap is not too tight; you do not want to cause a compartment syndrome – damaged tissue needs some room to swell.

23.8 Compartment Syndrome

This is important for all medical students. Often, if a splint or wrap is too tight, a patient may complain of "throbbing pain that is not responding to medication," one of the earliest symptoms. It is helpful to elevate such extremities and, if there is concern for compartment syndrome, loosen dressings and feel the patient's skin to verify if the skin is taught. Urgent findings include numbness, tingling, and discoloration. For a more detailed medical discussion of compartment syndrome, please read the Orthobullets (if you're on an ortho rotation, this is a must-read).

23.8.1 Splint Takedown

Taking a splint may be done both in the OR (i.e., if a temporizing splint was applied in the emergency room) or in the office. While it may seem intuitive, there are a few pitfalls to watch out for. For example, sometimes you may be

Orthopaedic Surgery

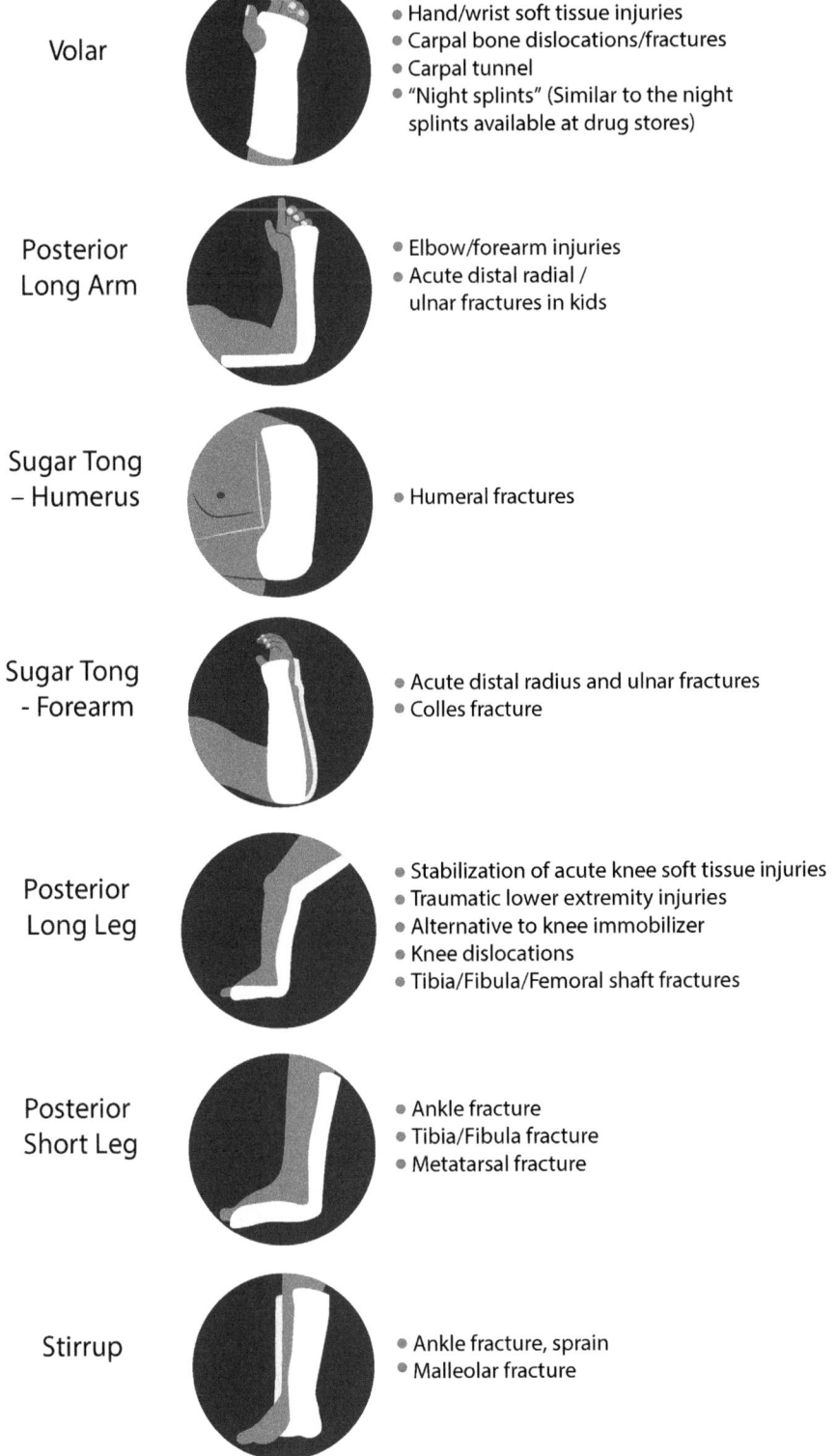

Volar
- Hand/wrist soft tissue injuries
- Carpal bone dislocations/fractures
- Carpal tunnel
- "Night splints" (Similar to the night splints available at drug stores)

Posterior Long Arm
- Elbow/forearm injuries
- Acute distal radial / ulnar fractures in kids

Sugar Tong – Humerus
- Humeral fractures

Sugar Tong - Forearm
- Acute distal radius and ulnar fractures
- Colles fracture

Posterior Long Leg
- Stabilization of acute knee soft tissue injuries
- Traumatic lower extremity injuries
- Alternative to knee immobilizer
- Knee dislocations
- Tibia/Fibula/Femoral shaft fractures

Posterior Short Leg
- Ankle fracture
- Tibia/Fibula fracture
- Metatarsal fracture

Stirrup
- Ankle fracture, sprain
- Malleolar fracture

◻ **Fig. 23.3** Common splints often seen in the Emergency Department for common fracture patterns. Based on the fracture pattern, splints may be definitive fracture management or a temporizing measure for surgery

required to take down splints applied by other providers or services. If you are not familiar with the procedure or fracture pattern, you may encounter pins or other devices hiding underneath the now-wispy Webril. Therefore, if you are not gentle or mindful of these pins, you may pull them out unintentionally causing pain, disruption of the fracture reduction, or another trip to the OR. Alternatively, there may be some type of skin graft or advanced wound closure underneath the splint that has now dried to the Webril. Any aggressive removal of the splint may also disrupt this wound. Therefore, given the almost infinite possibilities that may lie underneath a splint, it is important to understand the history of the patient and why the splint was put on in the first place before removing. This way, your removal is informed and safe.

23.8.2 Cast Application

Casts are less frequently used in the adult world than they are in the pediatric world. The basic ingredients for a cast are fiberglass cast material, a moleskin sleeve, Webril, a bucket of cold water, ± a cast saw, and ± cast spreader. Applying a cast is more difficult and tedious than a splint. Casts, if not applied properly, can result in pressure ulcers and sores on a patient skin or in malreduction.

The order of operations is: moleskin → Webril → fiberglass. The moleskin sleeve is first inserted over the extremity. Then, the extremity is very well wrapped and padded with Webril, taking particular care over joints and bony prominences (to prevent pressure ulcers). When applying the Webril, you may even tear little pieces off when you encounter curvature in the extremity to provide extra padding for bony prominences. Applying Webril appropriately may be one of the most difficult parts of cast application. Afterwards, fiberglass is dipped in cold water (which slows down the hardening process; if you opened the fiberglass before it was ready to be applied and left it out, it would quickly harden). The wet fiberglass is rolled over the Webril.

After the fiberglass has been applied, the resident will typically apply a mold onto the fracture pattern to help it set in alignment. When molding, it is best to use your wrist or palm to apply pressure, not individual fingers, as this can create a pressure point that results in an ulcer. Sometimes, casts will be "bivalved," meaning they will be cut along their medial and lateral edge to create a pressure valve of sorts. Bivalving can also result in sharp fragments along your cast, so be mindful of these shards as they may cut patient skin or you. After the cast is set, it is no longer expandable. Therefore, if there is any type of pressure buildup in the extremity, the cast forms a rigid body that can imitate compartment syndrome. Bivalving can help with creation of a pressure release in a cast and does require a cast saw.

A cast saw may seem intimidating at first. The saw has a reciprocating, not circulating, blade. This means that the blade simply moves back and forth (reciprocates) at very high speeds and does not go in circles (circulate). Therefore, the blade should not cut through soft tissues. Reciprocating blades can still be dangerous for two reasons: (1) they can develop small metallic sharp edges overtime as they blunt, which will cut through soft tissue, (2) they heat up extremely fast. Cast burns are "never events" that result from keeping a cast saw too close to skin for too long and therefore burning the patient. A nice trick to cool down your cast saw blade is to use a roll of Webril that you have dunked in cold water. You can put this roll next to your patient's extremity and every few seconds pull out the saw and press it against the cold, wet Webril. You should also never drag the cast saw along the cast – this only speeds up the heating of the blade. Rather, you should cut and raise, repeating a "dipping" motion, rather than a drag. You can also intermittently check the temperature of the blade by pushing your index finger along the side of the blade (not the actual teeth of the blade). Some institutions have cast saw protectors, which are long pieces of plastic that look like rulers. For these protectors, the plastic protector is placed underneath where you will be running the cast saw to protect the patient's skin.

23.8.3 Fracture Reduction

Your cast or splint will be useful in keeping your fracture reduced. Medical student involvement in fracture reduction varies by institutional culture as well as caseload. You should never attempt a reduction on your own. Inappropriate reductions can be extremely harmful to a patient. After you have observed several, you may ask your resident to teach you and walk you through one. The principles of fracture reduction are outside the scope of this text.

Neurosurgery

Malia McAvoy and Zack Abecaissis

Contents

24.1 Neurosurgery Mentality

Neurosurgery will be a culture shock to you. You need to approach the rotation with the mindset of entering basic training for the Marine Corps. If you are considering neurosurgery, ask yourself, are you tough? Here are some tips to help you improve your mental fitness.

- As a future neurosurgical resident, *you will be held to an extremely high standard and you must maintain a high level of responsibility.* Many of the cases you will encounter carry a high level of acuity. Treatment of neurosurgical patients requires a constant level of near obsessive vigilance.
- *Rule number one: Get things done.* Get there first and be the last to leave. Your goal in this rotation is to learn as much about neurosurgery as possible. Scrub into as many cases as possible. If you don't think you are learning anything while doing seemingly small things such as putting in a foley or turning a patient, think again.
- *Be humble yet confident.* You must entirely remove any sense of self-importance that you have. No task is too small for you to complete. Respect the hierarchy within neurosurgery.
- *Be organized.* You will need to maintain an up-to-date list and write down everything, as you will not be able to remember all of the exams and things to do for each patient. Create *checklists* and do everything *systematically.* Eventually, you will learn to triage tasks. Assume that every patient has a disaster waiting to happen and it is your job to find it.
- *Examine all patients yourself.* If you are called with any change in neurological exam, it is important to go see the patient immediately. Do not rely on others' exams of the patient.
- *Never complain.* You are not the only person who is tired. Never speak poorly about ANYONE. That includes residents from other services and other sub-interns. *You are part of a team and other people's lives depend on how well you work within that team.*
- *Be resilient.* You will screw up. It is not enough to admit wrongdoing; do it right next time.
- *Integrity above all else.* Never lie. Never make anything up. If you don't know how to do something, ask. Be the person everyone trusts to get things done.
- *Take initiative.* As a sub-intern, there are MANY things you can do to make your residents' lives easier. Set up the Mayfield before the case, balance the scope, take out the drains. Do things for your resident without them asking. You will complete tasks to help push the cases and patient care forward without any recognition.

24.2 The Neurosurgical Neuro Exam

One of the key goals of your sub-internship should be to master the Neurosurgical neuro exam. The Neurosurgical neuro exam is different than the neuro logical exam you learned while in medical school. You must tailor your exam to the answers you are trying to elicit in order to be as efficient as possible. Use ◘ Tables 24.1, 24.7, and 24.9 as references for full exams and only do the portions of the exam that are relevant to your patient (◘ Table 24.10).

High yield point #1: Never do a full neuro exam in neurosurgery. You must tailor your exam to the patient's history to save time.

Table 24.1 Neuro exam for the conscious patient

Mental status	*Step 1*: Wake the patient up. "Sleeping soundly" should never appear on the note.
	Step 2: Determine if the patient can follow commands. Use visual cues for aphasic patients.
	Step 3: If patient does not follow commands and does not display purposeful movements, determine if the patient responds to central stimuli (sternal rub or pinching neck) and document the response (i.e., localizes with L hand, opens eyes).
	Step 4: If the patient does not localize to the stimuli, determine response to peripheral stimuli by pinching the antecubital area of the knee or arm.
	Record Exam:
	  Alert, following commands (f/c)
	  Opens eyes, not f/c, purposeful
	  Not f/c, localizes to central stimuli
	  Not f/c, nonspecific movements to central stimuli, withdraws to painful stimuli

CN II	*Pupils:* Shine light and alternate into each eye, look for asymmetry. *Tell the patient, "look at my nose"* *If the patient has unilateral or bilateral dilated pupils (or is obtunded) call your senior resident immediately.* *Visual acuity: Tell the patient, "look at my nose."* Hold up 1–3 fingers in 4 quadrants of visual field to determine if patient has hemianopia or quadrantanopia. This is very important to do in pituitary patients or patients with possible stroke (PCA). Look at *fundi* (check for *papilledema*).
CN III, IV, VI	*Extraocular movements: Ask the patient to follow your thumb with their eyes without moving their head.* Move thumb in shape of an "H." Report any asymmetry or double vision.
CN V	*Facial sensation:* Lightly touch skin over forehead (V1), cheeks (V2), and chin (V3) on each side. Report any asymmetry or lack of sensation.
CN VII	Have patient close eyes tightly and smile. Report any asymmetry. Patients undergoing surgery for acoustic neuromas may have facial weakness. It is essential to report the ability of the patient to fully cover the pupil when closing eyes to prevent corneal injury.
CN VIII	Rub fingers next to the ears. Report any lack of hearing.
CN IX, X	Have patient open mouth and say "ah." Determine if palate rises symmetrically.
CN XI	Test shoulder shrug and head turning to resistance. Note any weakness against resistance.
CN XII	Have patient stick out tongue. Report any tongue deviation.

Motor exam	*Pronator drift:* Have patient hold both arms with palms facing the ceiling, elbows off the bed, and then have the patient close their eyes.
	  If patient slowly drops or pronates hand, it is a sign of contralateral UMN pathology.
	Muscle tone: test tone/rigidity of both upper and lower limbs to passive movement. Record the *Modified Ashworth scale* (Table 24.2) for each limb.
	Cervical spine:
	  Test each muscle for any patients with cervical pathology (Table 24.3)
	  To test biceps, have patient make biceps curls with both arms, support the elbow while examining each arm
	  Test interossei of hands using your own pinkies
	  Record exam with scale 0–5 using table as follows:

	Deltoid	Bicep	Tricep	Wrist flexion	Wrist extension	Inter-ossei
R						
L						

Lumbar spine:
  Test each muscle in patients with any cervical or lumbar pathology (Table 24.4)
  If patient is lying in bed, raise the leg off the bed to examine

	Hip flexion	Hip exten-sion	Leg flexion	Leg extension	Ankle flexion	Ankle extension	Ankle inversion	Ankle eversion	EHL
R									
L									

(continued)

■ Table 24.1 (continued)

Sensation	Test sensation to light touch in each dermatomal region (■ Table 24.5). Have patient close their eyes and guess which side you are touching (■ Fig. 24.1).
Deep tendon reflexes	Document reflexes according to the scale listed in ■ Table 24.6.

	Biceps	Triceps	Brachialis	Patellar	Ankle
R					
L					

UMN signs	Babinski sign (check for all spine patients) Triple flexion (check for spinal cord injury patients) Hoffman's sign (check for cervical spine pathologies)
Cerebellum	Finger-toe nose exam. Make sure the patient is fully extending to touch your finger. Finger tap: have patient tap index finger to thumb rapidly. Heel-shin Romberg sign

■ Table 24.2 Modified Ashworth scale

0	Normal tone
1	Slight "catch"
1+	Significant "catch
2	Mild, limb moves easily
3	Moderate, passive range of movement difficult
4	Severe, rigid limb

High yield point #2: Always include a Glasgow Coma Scale (GCS) score on new consults, especially traumas.

High yield point #3: GCS 8 = intubate.

High yield point #4: To determine whether a patient can follow commands use commands such as:
– "squeeze my hand"
– "wiggle your toes"
– "show 2 fingers"
– "stick out your tongue"

■ Table 24.3 Cervical spine exam

Level	Motor	Reflex	Sensory
C5	Deltoid (shoulder abduction)	Bicep tendon	Lateral upper arm
C6	Bicep (elbow flexion)	Brachioradialis	Radial forearm, thumb & index finger
C7	Triceps (elbow ext)	Triceps tendon	Middle finger (may have some C6 or C8)
C8	Finger flexion (grip)	None	Ulnar forearm, ring and little finger
T1	Interossei (finger abduction)	None	Upper medial forearm & medial arm

◨ **Table 24.4** Lumbar spine exam

Level	Motor	Reflex	Sensory
L2	Psoas (hip flexor)	None	Antero-medial thigh
L3	Quadriceps (leg extension)	None	Med thigh around knee
L4	Tibialis anterior (dorsiflex & foot inversion)	Patellar tendon	Medial foot
L5	EHL (great toe extension)	None	Dorsum foot
S1	Gastrocnemius	Achilles tendon	Lateral foot

◨ **Table 24.5** Levels of principal dermatomes

Lateral parts of upper arms	T12	Inguinal region	
Medial sides of upper arms	L1–4	Anterior and inner surfaces of lower limbs	
Thumb	L4–5, S1	Foot	
Middle finger	L4	Medial side of great toe	
Ring and little finger	S1–2, L5	Posterior and outer surfaces of lower limbs	
Nipples	S1	Lateral margin of foot and little toe	
Umbilicus	S2–4	Perineum	

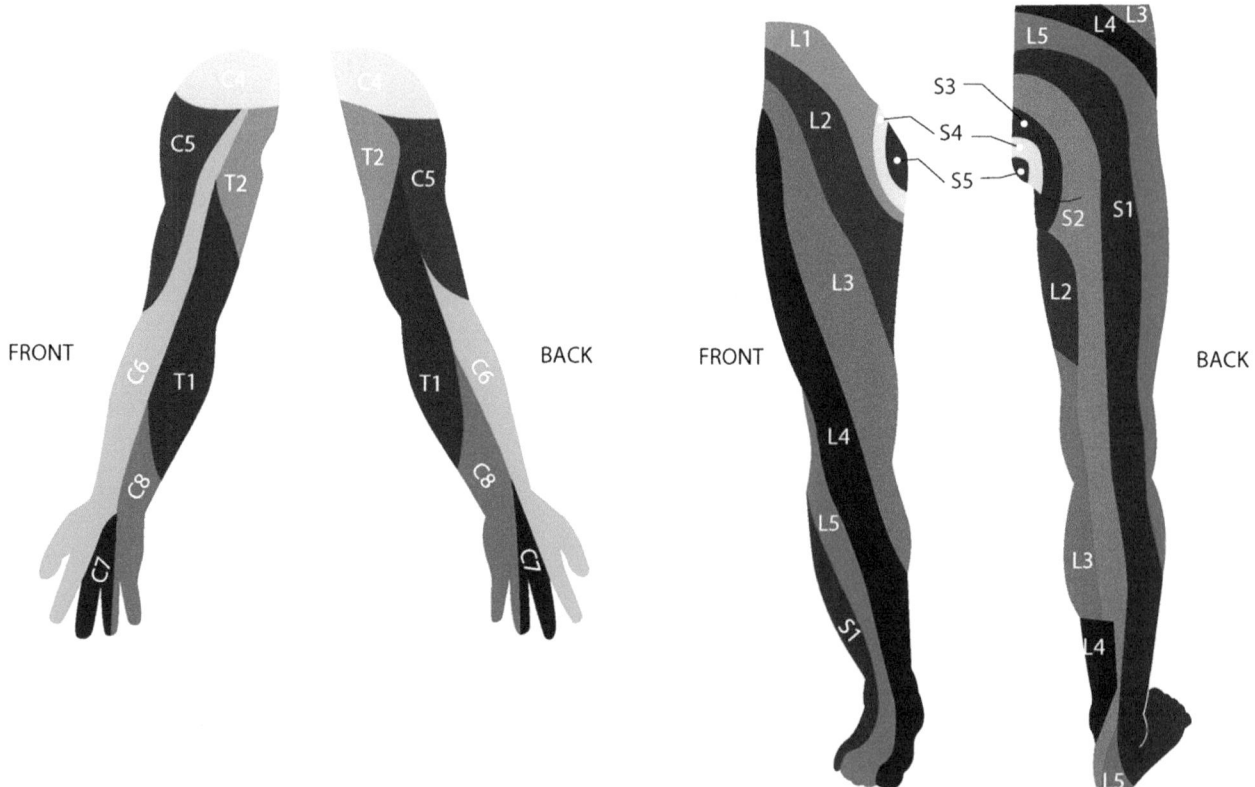

◨ **Fig. 24.1** Testing of dermatomes is part of the neurological examination looking for radiculopathy as sensation changes within a specific dermatome may help in determining the level of pathology

◘ Table 24.6 Reflexes scale

0	No response
1	Minimal response
2	Normal
3	Slightly hyper-reflexic
4	Exaggerated with clonus

◘ Table 24.7 Neuro exam for the unconscious patient

GCS	*Record as*: E: _____ V: _____ M: _____ (◘ Table 24.8) True *localizing* (AKA "purposeful movement") is defined as patient bringing arm up to site of pain *Withdrawing* is where the patient flexes at the arm to a central stimuli or flexes away from peripheral stimuli (◘ Fig. 24.2)
Respiration	"Overbreathing" the ventilator (i.e., pt is breathing at a higher rate)? *Cheyne-Stokes:* diencephalic lesions or bilateral cerebral hemisphere dysfunction
Mental status	*Record response to:* (1) voice, (2) central stimuli (trapezius pinch, sternal rub), (3) peripheral stimuli (antecubital pinch, nailbed pressure) In the NICU, you will likely hear the terms "obtunded", "stupor," and "comatose." These words can mean different things to different people and it is best to just describe what you observe.
Eyes	Observe any *spontaneous* eye movements *Windshield wiper eyes:* nonlocalizing *Ping pong eyes*: 2–5 s of side-to-side movement. Bilateral cerebral dysfunction *Ocular bobbing:* vertical deviation. See if crossing midline. Pontine lesion Test *blink to threat* Elicit *oculocephalic (doll's eyes) reflex* Test *pupil response* Look at *fundi* (check for *papilledema*)
CN V	*Corneal reflex* Use a syringe filled with sterile saline and apply drops to assess for corneal reflex Avoid testing corneal reflex using q-tip or cotton, can damage corneas
CN IX, X	*Cough reflex* Use the suction to stimulate a cough and remove excess secretions
Muscle tone	Test muscle tone and record Modified Ashworth Scale as above
DTRs	Test reflexes and record as above

☐ **Table 24.8** Glasgow coma scale

Response	Scale	Score
Eye opening response	Eyes open spontaneously	4 pts
	Eyes open to verbal command, speech or shouting	3 pts
	Eyes open to pain (not applied to face)	2 pts
	No eye opening	1 pt
Verbal response	Oriented	5 pts
	Confused conversation, but able to answer questions	4 pts
	Inappropriate response, words discernible	3 pts
	Incomprehensible sounds or speech	2 pts
	No verbal response	1 pt
Motor response	Obeys commands for movement	6 pts
	Purposeful movement to painful stimulus	5 pts
	Withdraws from pain	4 pts
	Abnormal (spastic) flexion, decorticate posture	3 pts
	Extensor (rigid) response, decerebrate posture	2 pts
	No motor response	1 pt

Minor brain injury = 13–15 pts, Moderate brain injury = 9–12 pts, Severe brain injury = 3–8 pts
GCS 8 = intubate

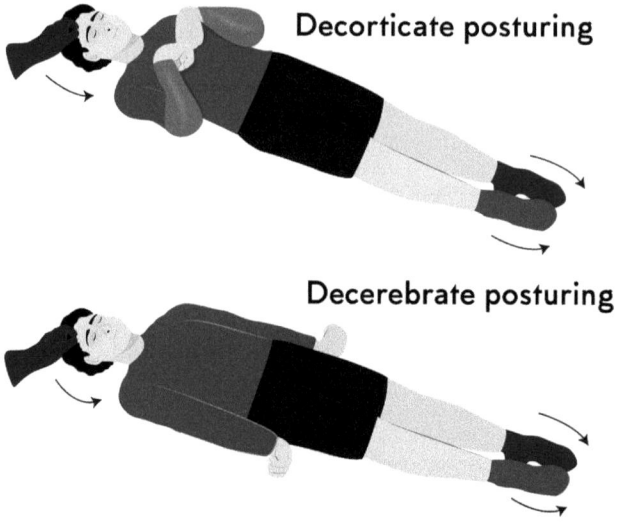

☐ **Fig. 24.2** Decerebrate posture indicates upper midbrain damage whereas decerebrate posture indicates upper pontine damage

◾ Table 24.9 Neuro exam of the neonate

Vitals	Observe for bradycardia, desats, apneic spells
Mental status	Is the infant arousable with minimal stimuli, irritable or lethargic with a weak cry?
Cranial nerves	*CN II:* blink response to light (3–4 months), pupillary light reflex *CN III, IV, VI:* observe spontaneous eye movements, ability to track objects *CN V:* test suck/swallow reflex *CN VII:* look if face is symmetric, ability to suck and cry *CN VIII:* test reaction to sharp sounds in each ear (e.g., clapping) *CN IX, X:* gag reflex *CN XI:* observe for shoulder droop
Motor exam	Observe for spontaneous movement Check tone Note any asymmetry in posture of movements Pull infant from lying to sitting and note head position Check for hypotonia by holding under axilla Check *grasp reflex* if <5 months Check limb recoil (*parachute reflex*) by extending limbs and releasing
Sensory exam	Observe grimace or withdrawal of limbs in response to pain in extremities
Head	Check *head circumference* Palpate *fontanelle*
Back	Check for sacral/coccygeal dimple or tufts of hair and asymmetry of gluteal fold

◾ Table 24.10 Tailored exam by pathologic location

Unconscious head bleed	[ ] GCS [ ] Pupils [ ] Cough reflex [ ] Corneal reflex [ ] Response to central stimulation (trap squeeze, supraorbital pressure, sternal rub) *always check to see if there is sternal/facial injuries before doing sternal rub/supraorbital pressure* [ ] Response to peripheral stimulation (pinch, fingernail pressure)
Cervical spine	[ ] Upper and lower extremity motor exam [ ] Sensation to light touch along dermatomes of all extremities [ ] Hoffman's reflex [ ] Patellar reflexes [ ] Assess for clonus [ ] Babinski
Lumbar spine	[ ] Upper and lower extremity motor exam [ ] Sensation to light touch along dermatomes of all extremities [ ] Patellar reflexes [ ] Assess for clonus [ ] Babinski [ ] Rectal exam *wait to do this with a resident present but always propose this in your plan*

Any examples of different types of masses with brain MRIs

24.3 How to Look at Images

24.3.1 Tips for Being Pimped

You will be pimped by an attending to describe what you see in an image. To be successful, you must develop a systematic approach. It may also be helpful to review the chapter on Radiology prior to your rotation.

1. Take a deep breath. Be confident.
2. If you are only given one cross section of the lesion, ask if the driver can scroll through. Don't be afraid to also ask for sagittal and coronal views. When in doubt, just *ask for more views*.
3. First, describe the *imaging modality*. For instance, say, "this is an axial section of a T1 weighted MRI with contrast."
4. Next, measure the lesion, if possible, and note the *size* of it. Can generally say "large" for lesions >5 cm.
5. If the imaging modality has contrast, describe the lesion as *enhancing or nonenhancing*. If the lesion is enhancing, describe it as *homogenously or heterogeneously enhancing*. If it is a non-contrast CT scan, describe the lesion as *hyperdense or hypodense*. If it is an MRI that is not T1 with contrast, describe the lesion as *hyperintense or hypointense*.
6. Describe any unique *components* of the lesions such as calcifications or cysts.
7. Describe the *location* of the lesion.

Finally, note any 8) *midline shift*, 9) *hydrocephalus*, or 10) *IVH*.

Examples of this approach are shown in ◘ Table 24.11.

In summary, here is what you need to hit when being pimped: (1) be confident, (2) ask for more views, (3) imaging modality, (4) size, (5) homogenously/heterogeneously enhancing or nonenhancing (if contrast) or density/intensity, (6) components, (7) location, (8) midline shift, (9) hydrocephalus, and (10) IVH.

24.3.2 How to Read a Head CT

You must look at a head CT systematically, the same way every time, so you don't miss anything. Use the mnemonic, "*Blood Can Be Very Bad*," to scroll through axial sections from bottom to top. Repeat for sagittal and coronal sections although can skip cisterns for these.

Blood   scroll through axial sections from bottom to top on blood window looking for the following:
- *EDH*: lens shaped, does not cross sutures, often low temporal
- *SDH*: crescent shaped, crosses sutures, may be bright (acute) or dark (if chronic)
- *IVH* and subsequent HCP
- *SAH*: blood in basilar cisterns (suprasellar, interpeduncular, ambient, quadrigeminal), Sylvian, or interhemispheric fissures

Cisterns (◘ Figs. 24.3 and 24.4)   keep same blood window while looking for asymmetry in the following cisterns
- *Ambient*: lateral to the midbrain
- *Interpeduncular*: between cerebral peduncles, behind chiasm
- *Prepontine*: space between clivus and pons
- *Suprasellar*: above pituitary gland

☐ **Table 24.11** Examples of describing a lesion on a brain MRI

Radiographic image of a T2 weighted MRI with a tumor in the basal ganglia. Any tumor. I can adjust the text to fit the image

"This is an axial section of a T2 weighted MRI showing a large, T2 hyperintense mass extending through the R thalamus and basal ganglia."

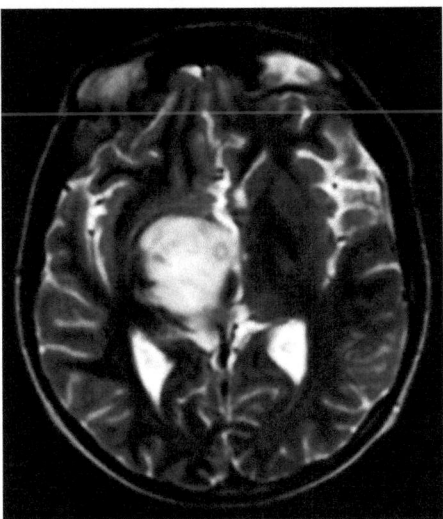

T1 weighted MRI with mass in fourth ventricle

"This is an axial section of a T1 weighted MRI without contrast showing a large, T1 hyperintense mass filling the fourth ventricle."

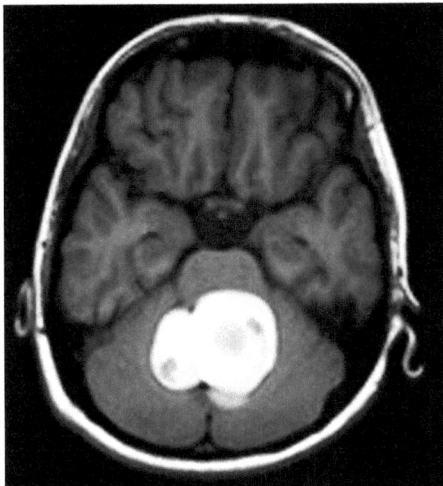

T2 weighted MRI with cystic mass in sella

"This is an axial section of a T2 weighted MRI showing a large, T2 hyperintense, cystic mass extending through the premedullary and prepontine cisterns."

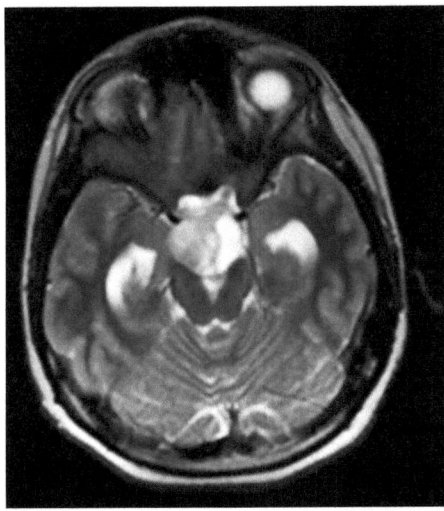

◻ **Table 24.11** (continued)

T1 weighted MRI with periventricular mass

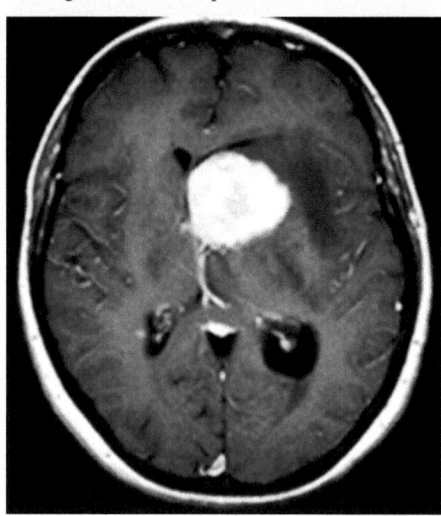

"This is an axial section of a T1 weighted MRI with contrast showing a large, homogenously enhancing periventricular mass in the L basal ganglia."

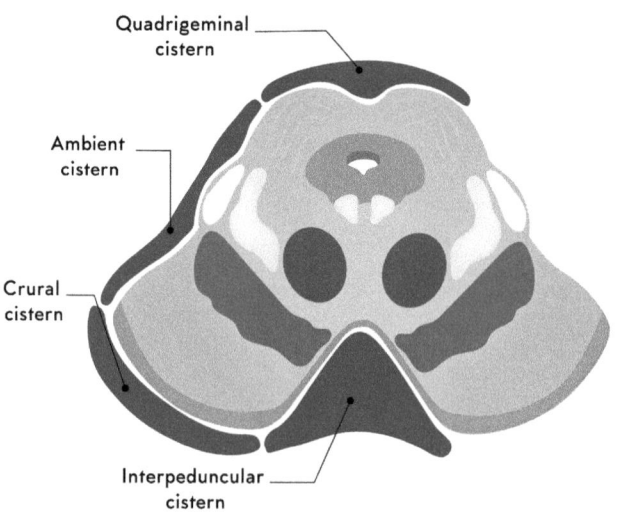

◻ **Fig. 24.3** Cisterna of the midbrain

— *Cisterna magna*: base of the skull, also look for tonsillar ectopia >5 mm = Chiari
— *Sylvian fissure*

High yield point #5: Identify the motor cortex on an axial head CT using the "omega sign" (◻ Fig. 24.6).

Brain switch to brain window (white matter: 20–30 HU, grey matter: 37–45 HU). Evaluate the following for symmetry:
— *Gray-white border*: blurred in edema, anoxic injury such as stroke (calculate ASPECTS score using MedCalc)
— *Shift*: observe interhemispheric fissure for displacement and measure (◻ Fig. 24.5)
— *Hyper or hypodensities*: look for mass or edema, stroke

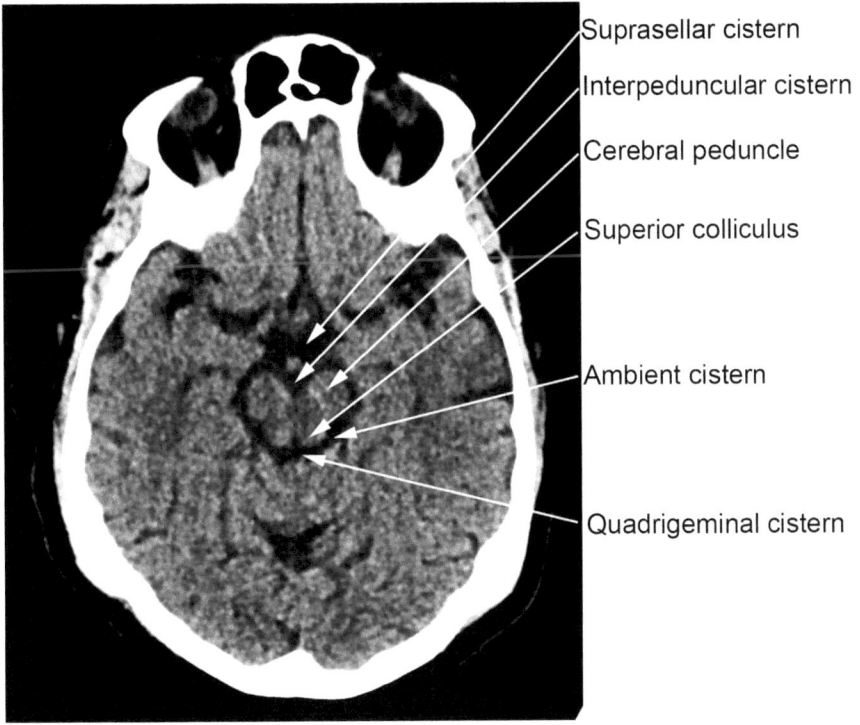

Fig. 24.4 Cisterna of the midbrain on axial sections of a non-contrast head CT

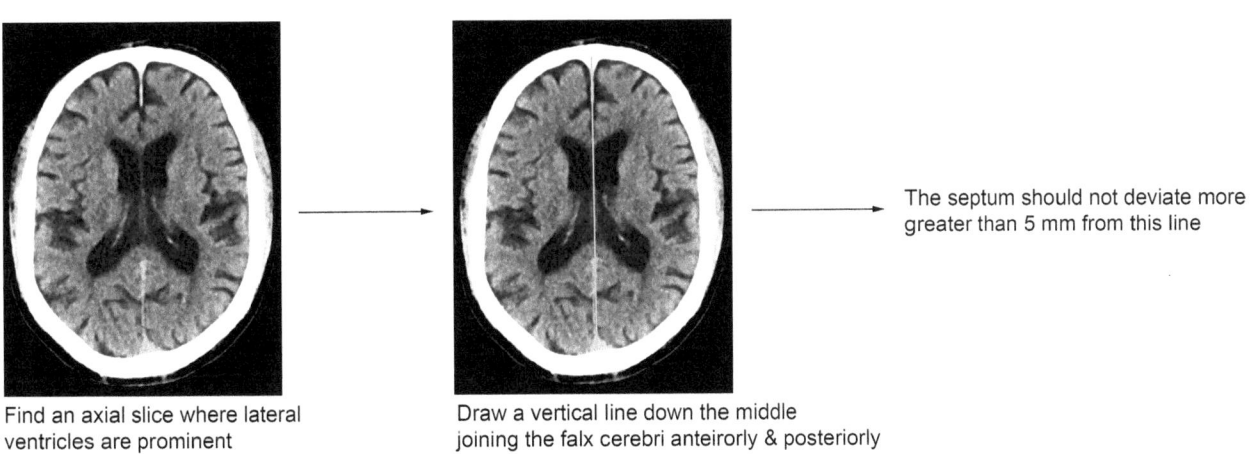

Find an axial slice where lateral ventricles are prominent

Draw a vertical line down the middle joining the falx cerebri anteirorly & posteriorly

The septum should not deviate more greater than 5 mm from this line

Fig. 24.5 How to measure midline shift. Perpendicular distance between the vertical line and the septum pellucidum should not deviate more than 5 mm

- *Pneumocephalus*: often associated with open fracture or fracture through the sinus
- *Gyri and sulci*: evaluate for effacement (loss of gyri/sulci) or atrophy (wide gyri/sulci)

Ventricles   use same window as brain. Evaluate for effacement or asymmetry of all ventricles.
- Look at all four ventricles systematically: (1) fourth ventricle, (2) third ventricle, (3) both lateral ventricles
- Look for any blood in ventricles or periventricular white matter lesions (DDx: PCNSL, infectious epididymitis, primary glial tumor, MS)

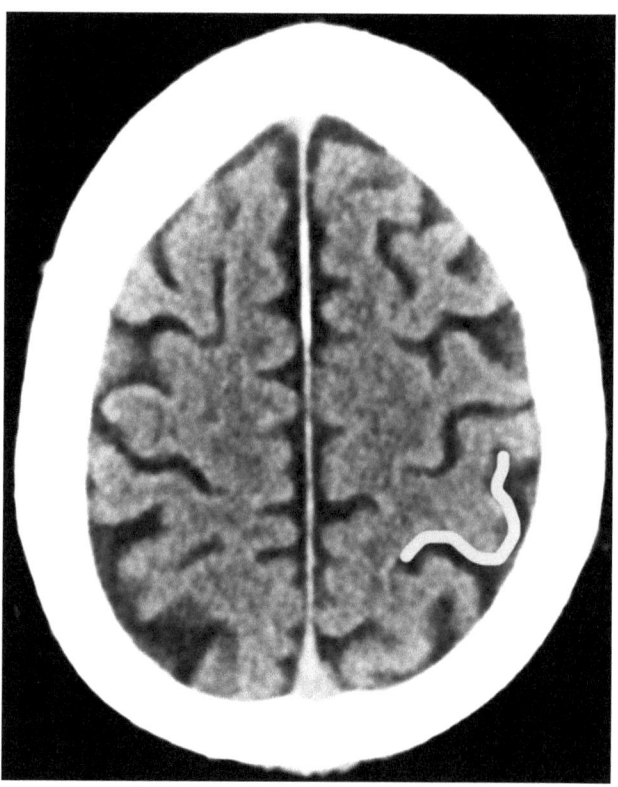

Fig. 24.6 The hand area of the motor cortex bulges out in a way that is reminiscent of the Greek letter omega

Bone   use bone window. Look for fractures, especially temporal bone, and examine sinuses and air cells looking for air/fluid levels.

24.3.3   How to Read a Head MRI

High yield point #6: The differential diagnosis for a diffusion restricting mass on a head MRI includes abscesses and cysts.

Also look through a head MRI systematically. Look at two axial sequences scrolling bottom to top at the same time as follows.

1. *T1 without contrast (left window) and T1 with contrast (right window)*: observe for
   - Any obvious masses, noting whether they are enhancing or not
   - Look for any ventricle asymmetry
2. *T2 (left window) and T2 FLAIR (right window)*: scroll through T2 looking especially in the posterior fossa for masses and T2 FLAIR for any hyperintensities
3. *DWI (left window) and ADC (right window)*: use both sequences to look for areas of acute ischemia. Cytotoxic edema from an acute stroke will appear bright on DWI and dark on ADC. Note whether a mass is diffusion restricting or not. Most tumors do not restrict diffusion, even necrotic or cystic components
4. *T1 without contrast sagittal and coronal*: scroll through these quickly to note any lesions you may have missed

Table 24.12 Images to load during rounds

Consult	Images
Spine	Axial/sagittal/coronal bone windows, cross-linked
Vascular	Initial CT, CTA, 3D recons of angio (if available)
Tumor	T1 w/out contrast, T1 w/contrast, T2, FLAIR

24.3.4 How to Present Images on Rounds

Residents are expected to present images of new consults during rounds and, as a future resident, you should learn how to do this well.
- Have images uploaded and ready to go BEFORE ROUNDS (Table 24.12). Emergent/need to crash right now → show first
- Treat this presentation like a lecture in front of the whole department → PREPARE!
- Have your list of all admissions from the night before in front of you
- Give the one liner (name, location, age, story) while showing the films
- Typically, do not show any scan that the neurosurgery team does not do anything about (chest X-rays, CT abdomen/pelvis, etc.)

High yield point #7: Pay attention to how the resident moves through the films using the imaging software when he/she presents and practice using the software before presenting.

24.4 Rounding

24.4.1 Pre-Rounding

Arrive approximately 45–60 min before the start of rounds to pre-round (or whenever your resident tells you to come). Reserve about 10 min per patient. Pre-round on all patients, even those whom you are not presenting on rounds so you have all data available in case the resident needs it. Generally, seeing and examining the patient on the floor before rounds is not required as the team examines the patients together.

High yield point #8: While pre-rounding, collect the most up-to-date drain outputs by calling or going to see the nurses of the patients you will be presenting.

Organize your rounding list   First, ask your resident how they organize their list. Here is one strategy for organizing your rounding list:
- [ ] Print a *small list* consisting of the patient's MRN, name, room number and one liner. Write a checkbox next to the room number of each patient to track which patients have been seen on rounds.
- [ ] Fold the small list "hotdog" style
- [ ] Print a *longer list* consisting of other information including 24-h vitals, drain outputs, labs, action plans.
- [ ] Staple the longer list behind the small list. Fold the small list "hotdog" style so just the names of the patients are showing. Draw lines across the page separating each patient and create small checkboxes for each patient so you can keep track of tasks to do for all patients very easily (Fig. 24.7).

High yield point #9: Create your *own* system for organizing your list. It is helpful to use a multicolor pen at first. I will write patient data (vitals, labs, drain output, etc.) in **black**, last exam in **blue** next to the patient room number so I can write new exam findings on rounds, checkboxes for rounds in **blue** and "to do" checkboxes in **red**.

Collect data   Once you have your list printed, the first thing you should do is read the most recent notes on the patient including nursing notes and consult recommendations. Then begin collecting the patient's data in the following order:

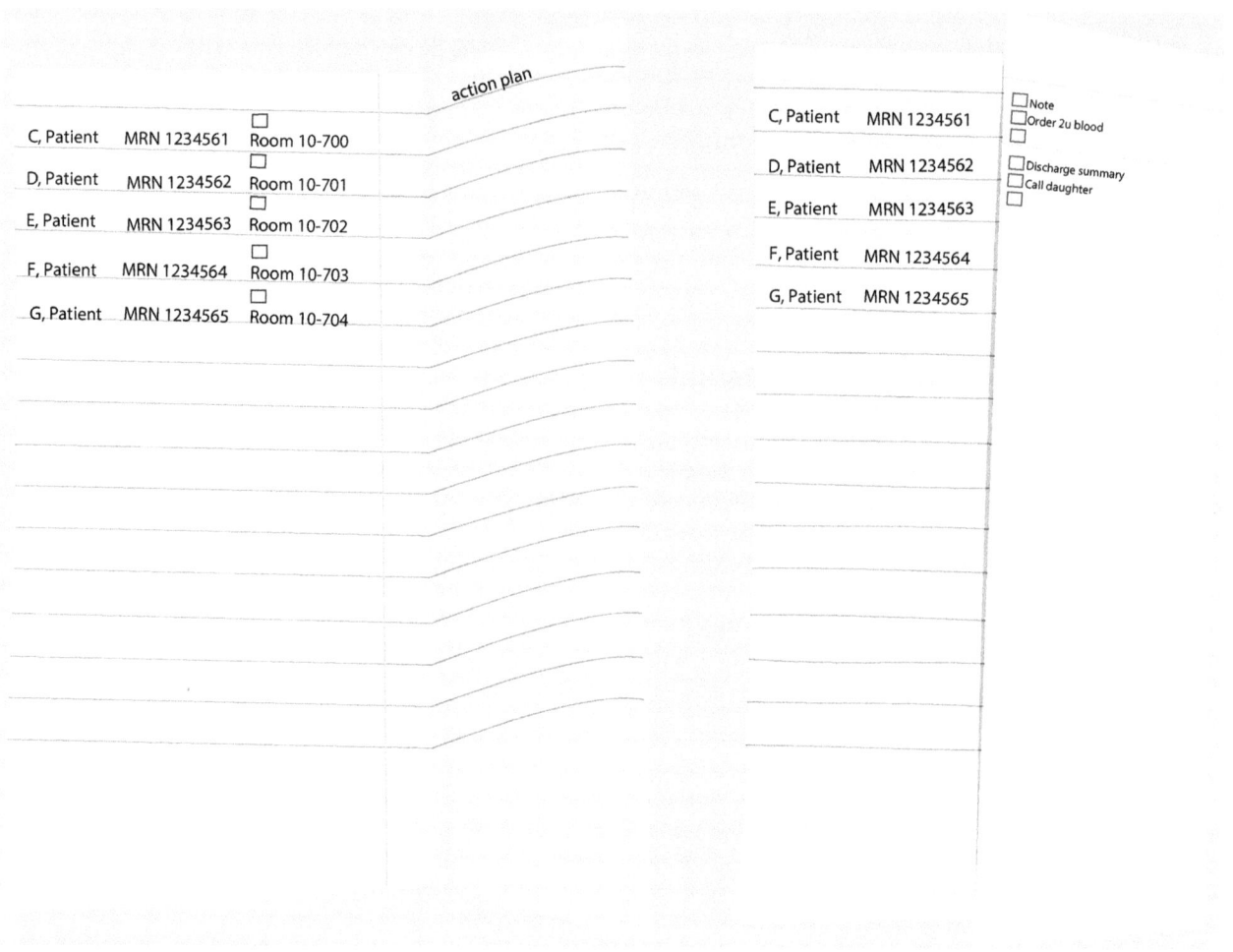

□ Fig. 24.7   Create checkboxes for tasks to do and keeping track of who you have seen on rounds

EPIC Tricks #1: Set up your list on EPIC so you can click through each tab in the same order every day as follows: *Index/Notes/Comp/I/O/ Lab Table/60 day micro/Meds/MAR/ Gluc/Blood/Handoff*
The vitals, vent settings, last ABG and 24 h ICPs are all located under the Comp (Comprehensive) flow sheet) tab.

High yield point #10: Ask your resident for note templates. Write the notes with the preliminary plans for all patients and share them with the resident. Include screenshots of scans as appropriate. Notify the resident that you shared it.

- [ ] Vitals: T, HR, BP 24 h ranges and most recent, SpO2% on _L
- [ ] Ventilation settings: Vent mode, PEEP, FiO2
- [ ] Last ABG: pH, PaCO2, PaO2
- [ ] Drips @ _
- [ ] 24 h ICPs
- [ ] Drain (EVD, subgaleal, subdural, back) outputs: 24h/12h. Get the most up-to-date drain outputs by asking the nurse directly
- [ ] Labs: Na (last 3), creatinine, WBC, Hgb/Hct, coags, gluc (last 3)
- [ ] Microbiology: CSF stains and cultures, urinalyses, urine/blood/wound cultures
- [ ] Meds: AC, abx, anti-seizure, BP meds, DVT prophylaxis, bowel regimen
- [ ] Imaging

[ ] *Make a plan:* The plan will depend somewhat on what procedure the patient had (□ Table 24.13). See the following table for things that ought to be considered for all post-ops in addition to plans specific to the procedure performed.

◘ **Table 24.13** Plans for post-ops

All	[ ] Transition to po meds
	[ ] Antibiotics (day #, when to discontinue)
	[ ] Antiemetics
	[ ] Pain control
	[ ] Imaging
	[ ] Keep vs. pull foley
	[ ] Keep vs. pull drains
	[ ] Consult recommendations
	[ ] Electrolyte repletion
	[ ] Blood products
	[ ] Fluids
	[ ] DVT prophylaxis
	[ ] PT/OT
	[ ] Wounds management: staples out?
	[ ] Discharge timeline
Crani	[ ] EVD: raise or lower or clamp
	[ ] Antiseizure meds
	[ ] BP control meds
	[ ] Steroids
	[ ] HOB elevation
	[ ] Neuro exam checks and frequency
	[ ] Speech, language pathology evaluation (stroke patients)
Spine	[ ] Brace
Pituitary	[ ] UO monitor
	[ ] Sinus precautions
	[ ] AM cortisol?
	[ ] Na checks, goals
Vascular	[ ] Nimodipine
	[ ] TCDs

◘ **Table 24.14** Dos and Don'ts of neurosurgery rounds

Do	**Don't**
For each day on rounds, try to check of as many of these as you can.	*Don't get in the way of rounds.* It is a well-oiled machine and you can very easily become a cog in the wheel if you're not paying attention.
[ ] Help lead rounds with the chief. Keep up.	Interrupt a resident during rounds
[ ] Track which patients have been seen and which patient is next on the list (use a checklist).	Answer a question directed at another resident or medical student
[ ] Lead the team to the most efficient route to see the next patient.	Just stand there in the back for rounds. You should be front and center helping.
[ ] Move overbed trays and other obstacles to allow the resident to examine the patient.	Try to outshine other medical students. You are a team.
[ ] Offer the resident gloves.	Present an ICU patient for longer than 20 s. Floor patients should be <10 s.
[ ] Turn the patient to examine spine wounds.	
[ ] Shine a light (flashlight or headlamp) on all wounds/drains.	
[ ] Shine a penlight in the patient's eyes for pupillary reflex.	

High yield point #11: Recall Rule Number One: Get things done. This is more important than your knowledge base!

High yield point #13: Have tape already ripped and on your scrubs to speed up dressing changes.

High yield point #12: Always have gloves on when seeing each patient and help the resident remove the dressings.

High yield point #14: Your patient presentation should be less than 20 s for ICU patients. Period. In fact, aim for 10 s. Practice saying the presentation before rounds.

High yield point #15: Coordinate cases with the other subinterns the night before but be aware cases often get cancelled or changed to another date. Neurosurgery requires you to be flexible!

24.4.2 On Rounds

Lead rounds   The chief will be the one directing rounds; however, you should be helping track which patients have been seen and which one is next on the list. Do not let the team miss a patient! Place checkboxes next to the names of each patient and check off each one that is seen. Know the best route to take to see the next patient and lead the team there. This will help the chief tremendously to make rounds as efficient as possible without leaving out any patients. Keep up on rounds. You should be front and center helping with rounds.

Help on rounds (◻ Table 24.14)   Always be prepared to assist in examining the patient and in wound care. This will involve moving overbed tables so the resident can have access to examine the patient, turning the patient to see spine incisions, shining a flashlight on all wounds and drains, shine a penlight in eyes for pupillary reflex, removing and replacing dressings and obtaining gloves for the residents. It may be helpful to have a headlamp around your wrist to have easy access to a bright light.

- Items to keep in your pockets
- [ ] Gloves
- [ ] Penlight
- [ ] Headlamp
- [ ] Scissors
- [ ] Marking pens (multiple)
- [ ] Staple removal kits
- [ ] Suture removal kits
- [ ] Dressing tape
- [ ] 4 × 4 dressings
- [ ] 4 × 8 dressings
- [ ] Notecards for cases
- [ ] Rounding list
- [ ] Small notebook

24.4.3 Patient Presentations (◻ Table 24.15)

24.5 OR

24.5.1 Night Before the Case

Take a look at the OR schedule and decide which case you will be going to the next day. Complete the following step-by-step process the night before the case to prepare.
1. *Atlas reading*: There are two excellent neurosurgical atlases and you should read the section pertaining to the case the night before. For a more in-depth description of these resources, please see the resource section of this chapter. The first atlas is divided into two volumes and these are called *Atlas of Neurosurgical Techniques: Spine and Peripheral Nerves* and *Atlas of Neurosurgical Techniques: Brain*. The second atlas is available for free online called *The Neurosurgical Atlas by Dr. Aaron Cohen-Gadol*. Read the Volumes section pertaining to the procedure and watch the Operative Video Cases in the Cases section.

Table 24.15 Presenting patients on rounds

ICU	Floor
Name, POD __ s/p __	Name, POD __ s/p __
O/N events: check with nurse. List any transfusions	O/N events
Vitals: Only say *notable* vitals. AF, HR, SBP, % on __ L O$_2$. If all vitals are within normal range, can say "AVSS on RA." Give 24 h range of vitals	Vitals, mostly "AVSS"
I/O: Give 24 h and 12 h outputs of drains. For EVDs, give 24 h and 12 h outputs plus ICP range, Say "foley in" (but know UO).	Relevant meds
Vent settings: Mode/RR/TV/PEEP/FiO$_2$. *ABG:* pH/PaCO$_2$/PaO$_2$	Labs: Na, WBC, Hct, plt,INR
Labs: Na (last 3), hct.	Micro
Micro: list any *notable* cultures, urinalysis, gram stains	Relevant meds
Meds: Drips (sedation/pressors/anti-HTNs), AC, abx, anti-sz, bowel reg, DVT proph	Plan
Imaging: say findings for imaging in past 24 h	
Plan	

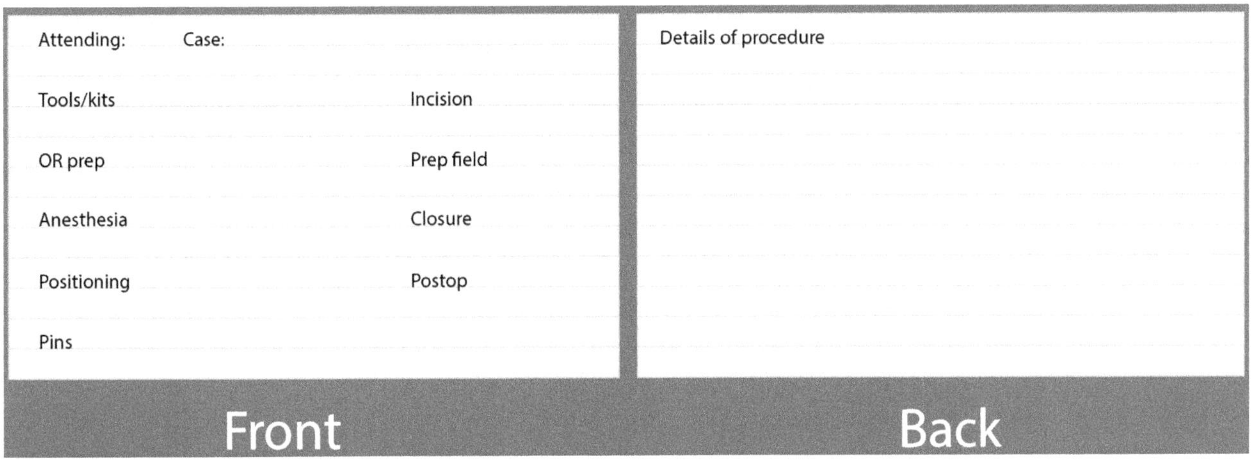

Fig. 24.8 Attending preference notecard. Make the notecard the night before the case and fill it out throughout the case. Keep all notecards together on a ring for future reference

2. *Master the anatomy*: Review the anatomy of the case by reading and taking digital notes for reference on the *Rhoton collection* (online for free for AANS members: ▶ http://rhoton.ineurodb.org/). Keep these digital notes on an application such as OneNote or EverNote that you can access on a portable device and review as you are waiting for the case to start. Also, be sure to master the *Rhoton Top 100 Surgical Anatomy Images*. I would review 10 of these images daily. As a resident, you will be expected to master every one of these 100 images and you will be tested on this knowledge during your PGY 2 year in the Neuroanatomy exam as part of board certification. Get started now. For endovascular/vascular cases, review the corresponding sections relevant to the case on ▶ neuroangio.org.
3. *Attending book and notecard:* as a resident, you will be required to set up the case according to each attending's preferences. Therefore, *you must keep meticulous notes of how each attending sets up each case*. To accomplish this, keep a stack of index cards for each attending, one index card for case, detailing the following for each case: tools/kits, OR prep, anesthesia, positioning, pins, incision, prep field, closure, post-op, and details of the procedure. Setup the *attending preference index card* (◘ Fig. 24.8).
4. *Review the patient's history* (◘ Fig. 24.9) *and imaging* (◘ Table 24.16)

CASE PREP TEMPLATE	
Attending: Resident: Procedure: OR/time	Patient name / age: MRN: DOB:
Allergies	
H&P (include prior op notes)	
Vitals	
Exam	
Labs	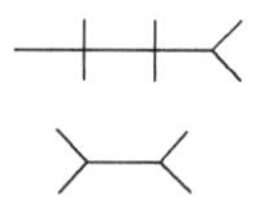 PT/PTT/INR: Micro:
Imaging	ECHO: EF
Home meds	
Case prep	☐ Neurosurgical atlas ☐ Neuroanatomy atlas (e.g.Rhoton) ☐ Video ☐ Attending book, attending preference card
OR prep	☐ Images up ☐ Crani: mayfield Spine: table ☐ Mayo Stand ☐ Navigation ☐ Consent ☐ Interval H&P ☐ Site mark, examine, spine: (1) cough, (2) fever, (3) weakness ☐ Patient chart sticker
OP note	Operative findings: Pathology: EBL: Closure, drains:
Poston plan	☐ Update handoff ☐ Postop check ☐ Postop imaging ☐ Prep D/C sum
Post case	☐ Log Case ☐ Write up attending book ☐ Re-read atlas, make notes

Fig. 24.9 Template to use for case prep. The night before the case, look up and write the patient' s H&P (including prior op notes), exam findings, imaging findings, and home meds. Also, complete the tasks in the "case prep" section. The morning of the case, write the patient's vitals and labs. Complete all tasks for prepping the OR right before the case. During the case, note the findings you will need to help write the op note and help with the post-op plan.

5. *Look up patient orders*: You will want to make a habit of checking the patient's orders and making sure everything is set for the next day so when you are a resident, this will be automatic. Make sure you understand all of the orders that were made by the resident. Check the following:
   - *A*ntibiotics: Ancef 1 g IV (if allergic, vancomycin 1 g IV) on call to OR for all surgical patients
   - *B*lood work: CBC, lytes, BUN, Cr, INR/PTT, type/screen or X-match, AM cortisol for pit patients

◻ Table 24.16 Review preoperative imaging

Any crani	[ ] Skull thickness (abnormally thin skull from chronic HCP? Previous craniotomy?) [ ] Size of frontal sinus [ ] Degree of mastoid aeration
MCA aneurysm clip	[ ] Length and morphology of M1 (lenticulostriate arteries distal to bifurcation of MCA?) [ ] Direction of aneurysm dome [ ] Develop a mental map of M2 branches (M2 trifurcation?) [ ] Presence of calcium plaques across the neck or dome of the aneurysm or within M1 (can interfere with clipping)
Bypass	[ ] Donor vessels along the scalp (e.g., superficial temporal artery or occipital artery)

- Consent for surgery/embo and blood products
  - Discuss treatment options and pros/cons
  - Describe proposed interventions (pts often concerned about cosmetics, i.e., incision location/scar, hair shaving)
  - Discuss rationale and benefits of proposed intervention
  - Discuss general risks – anesthetic, infection, bleeding
  - Discuss specific risks relevant to the procedure – neurologic/endocrine, injury/worsening associated with intervention, treatment failure, CSF leak, … coma, death
  - Discuss post-op medical risks – infection, drug rxns, DVT/PE, electrolyte disturbances
  - Consent for blood products (given only when necessary)
- Dexamethasone (10 mg IV the night and morning prior to surgery, depending on surgery)
- Everything else (EKG, CXR)
- Food (i.e., make NPO), films available
- Gang (ensure patient/family, OR aware)
- Hibiclens shampoo (time permitting, night before)

24.5.2 Before Rounds

Look up patient labs   If labs are still cooking, make a reminder in your phone with an alarm to look at the labs after rounds.
- For every patient: Na, K, creatinine, WBC, Hgb/Hct, Plts, coags
  - Plts should be >100,000 generally
- For pituitary patients, check AM cortisol level
  - Patients with low pre-op serum AM cortisol (<4 ug/dl) ought to be offered stress-dose steroid coverage peri-operatively (50 mg hydrocortisone IV every 6 h for 36 h then oral replacement)(1)

High yield point #16: Get to know Siri well. You will need constant reminders to complete tasks at certain times because you will not remember everything.

24.5.3 Before the Patient Rolls In

- [ ] Ask the CN for you to place the foley
- [ ] Pull images up for case (◻ Table 24.17)
- [ ] Set up the scope

□ Table 24.17   Pulling images for a case

Case	Images
Spine	T2 sagittal and axial CT sagittal and axial XR lateral and AP
Crani for tumor	4 × 4: head MRI axial T1p (top left) sagittal T1p (top right) coronal T1p (bottom left) axial T2 (bottom right)
Open vascular	axial CT head (left) diagnostic angio (right)
Crani for trauma	3 × 1: head CT axial (left) sagittal (middle) coronal (right)
Shunt	3 × 1: head CT axial (left) sagittal (middle): measure skull to lateral ventricle, skull to foramen of monro coronal (right): measure from skull to foramen of monro

- *Eyepieces:* Spine and open vascular cases "face to face," crani for tumor "left to right" (place assistant eyepiece on opposite side of tumor)
  - Check eyepiece setting is correct on scope: *Config → OPMI → setting*
  - Check once more to make sure eyepieces are screwed in correctly
  - Look at your thumbs side-by-side under both eyepieces
- *Light:* Test to make sure light turns on, can set to 75% intensity for beginning of the case.
- *Balance:* Before a case, all scopes must be "balanced" so it moves properly during the case. *Autobalance → Complete system auto.* Test the balance by pressing green button with right hand and let go of the scope. The scope should not move at all.

- [ ] Set up the Mayo stand
  - Set up the following items on the Mayo stand: clippers, mitts, comb, bacitracin, marking pen, xeroform, tegaderm
  - Draw up the lidocaine into the syringe for the resident
- [ ] Set up the Mayfield
  - Place pins in clamp
  - Apply betadine or bacitracin to pins (ask resident)
- [ ] Set up for patient positioning
  - Make the axillary roll
  - Make a bump for shoulder
- [ ] Set up navigation
  - Watch and ask resident how to set up navigation properly and take notes so next time you can set it up for the case.
- [ ] Roll the patient in
  - When all tasks in the OR are complete, go see the patient and help anesthesia roll the patient back to the OR.

High yield point #17: *How to make an axillary roll*
1. Roll a towel along the short side and tape the towel on the sides OR
2. Wrap a towel around a 1L bag of saline and tape

Table 24.18 Patient positioning

Position	Procedures used for
Supine	Endoscopic transnasal Pterional crani Orbitozygomatic crani Frontal crani Temporal crani Interhemispheric crani Anterior parietal crani
Modified park bench	Posterior parietal crani Occipital crani Posterior fossa and posterior skull base Craniocervical junction Pts with severe cervical stenosis or morbid obesity to avoid neck turn
Sitting	Posterior fossa

24.5.4 When the Patient Rolls In

- Before induction
- [ ] Help move the patient to the bed by standing next to the OR table on the opposite side of the bed to make sure the patient doesn't fall off the table.
- [ ] Once the patient is securely on the table, take the bed out of the room.
- [ ] Get blankets for the patient.
- [ ] Put pneumatic compression boots on the patient. Plug into the machine and turn on.

- Positioning (Table 24.18)
- *Goals of positioning*: prevention of pressure injuries, expansion of the operative corridor using gravity retraction, minimization of surgeon fatigue.
- Lesion should be the highest point in the operative field.
- Exposed surface should be parallel to the floor.
- Torso should be positioned before the head.
- Skull clamps typically used for microsurgical procedures, doughnut and horseshoe head rests used for nonmicrosurgical operations.

- Pinning a patient
- The pins should be inserted along the plane of an imaginary *head band* to provide good mechanical support avoiding thin portions of the squamous bone and the bulk of the underlying temporalis muscle (Fig. 24.10)
- Single pin should bifurcate the space between the double pins.
- Hold the side with two pins in your right hand; firmly plant these pins to the skull first. Slowly close the clamp to place the side with one pin. When both pins are firmly in place apply pressure to both sides to click the clamp in place *twice*.
- Clamping pressure should be *60–80 pounds for adults* and *30–40 pounds for pediatric patients*
  - May require more pressure during awake craniotomy (e.g., 80 pounds)
  - Integra recommends minimum 5 years of age for Mayfield clamp

High yield point #18: Help the resident with positioning and anticipate next steps. THIS is the part of the case where the sub-intern can shine!

High yield point #19: Each line that extends out of the torque knob on the Mayfield corresponds to 20 pounds, common to have three lines or 60 pounds of pressure to fixate the adult skull.

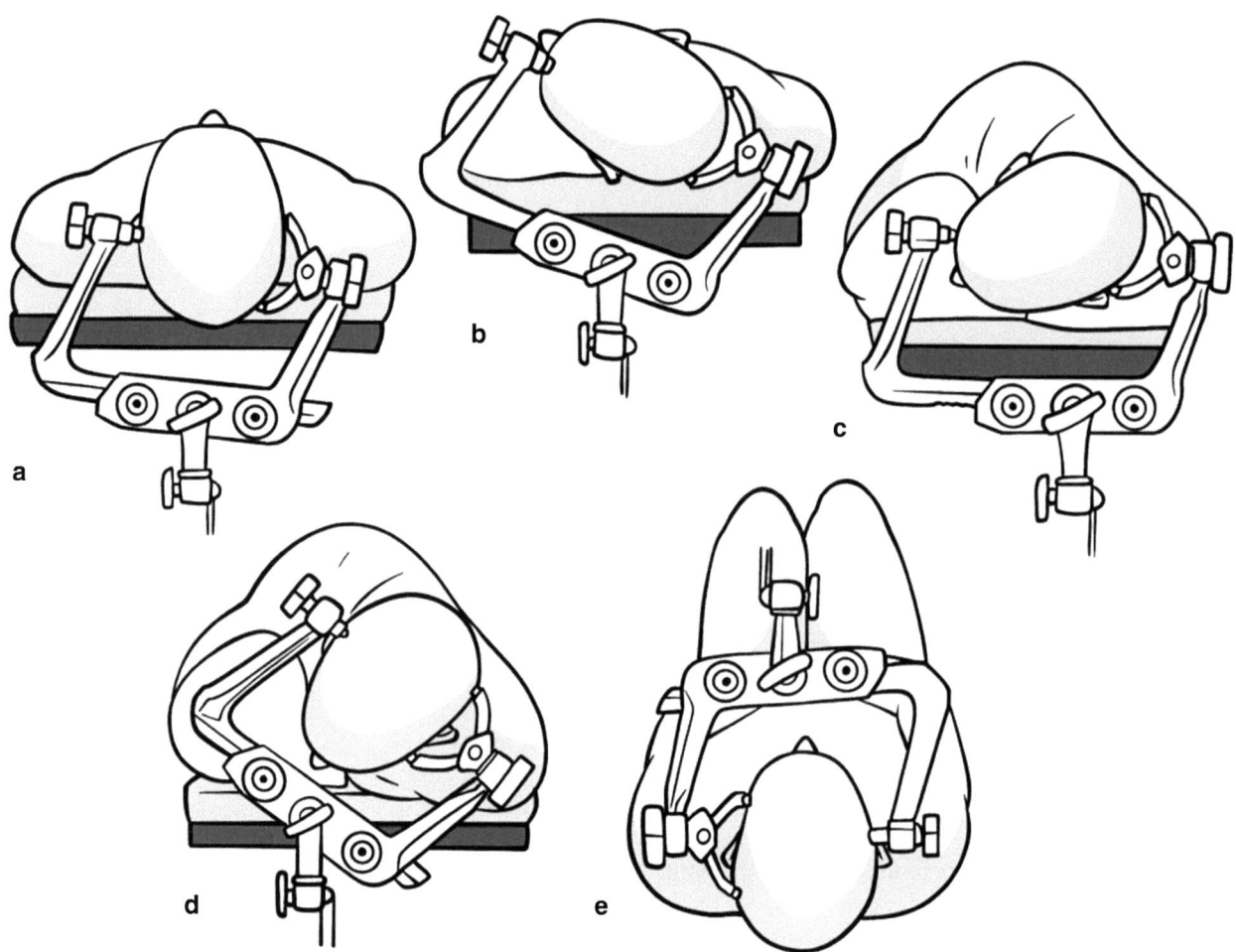

Fig. 24.10 **a** Unilateral or bilateral frontal approach. **b** Pterional craniotomy. **c** Retrosigmoid approach to cerebellopontine angle. **d** Midline suboccipital approach. **e** Midline suboccipital approach with the patient in the semi-sitting position

High yield point #20: Pins are placed well behind the planned incision.

- **Supine position**
  - Before fixation with the skull clamp, the *back of the bed should be elevated* to maintain the patient's head *10–15 degrees above the level of the heart*, aiding in venous drainage, which is compromised could lead to increased ICP and cerebral edema. The patient's legs are flexed at the knees.
  - *Pinning* (Table 24.19)
  - Head is *extended for basal lesions* (allows frontal lobes to fall away with gravity, *malar eminence becomes the highest point in the field*) and *flexed forward for posterior frontal or parietal lesions*
    - When the neck is flexed, make sure there is *at least two fingers' breadth between the mandible and the sternum to avoid airway obstruction*
      - Also try to maintain the neck in a neutral position to minimize jugular vein occlusion and maximize venous return.
  - Elevate the head above the level of the heart.
  - Keep in mind excessive flexion and rotation of the head may occlude the vertebral artery if it is very dominant on one side and causes quadriparesis.
  - In general, the closer to the midline the lesion is, the less the head is turned (30° turn), and the more lateral the lesion is, the more the head is turned (45°) (Table 24.20 and Fig. 24.11).

Table 24.19 Pin placement for craniotomies

Crani	Pin positioning
Pterional	Pins are placed well behind the planned incision. *Double pin*: contralateral superior temporal line. *Single pin*: behind the ear over the mastoid bone.
Temporal and subtemporal	Patient's head is turned contralaterally and the ipsilateral shoulder is placed on a bump. *Double pin*: positioned posteriorly, just superior to the nuchal line. One pin set adjacent to the inion and the other laterally. *Single pin*: ipsilateral supraorbital region, at least 1 cm superior to the eyebrow and lateral to the supraorbital notch. Avoid placement of this pin or slippage into the orbital region of the frontal sinus.
Frontal	All three pins should be below the cranial equator to allow the cranium to fall into the pins. Head should be turned contralateral to pathology except for the interhemispheric approach in which the patient's head should be positioned at a neutral anatomic position. *Double pin*: posterior aspect of the superior temporal line. *Single pin*: superoposteriorly to the pinna.
Parietal	All three pins rest above the ears, avoiding temporalis muscle. Be sure there is good clearance between the patient's face and the arm of the clamp, may apply padding to nose. *Single pin*: thin posterior aspect of the temporalis muscle superior to the ipsilateral ear.
Bifrontal	Pin placement can be challenging due to large incision spanning from ear to ear. Pins must be sufficiently posterior to the incision to avoid traction on the scalp, which could complicate closure. *Double pin*: rotated, one pin is posterior and superior to pinna, other pin is closer to the vertex. *Single pin*: superoposteriorly to the pinna.
Retrosigmoid	All 3 pins may be placed superior to the patient's ears. *Double pin*: parallel and just posterior to the superior temporal line. *Single pin*: above the superior temporal line just along the hairline.
Suboccipital	Pins are placed superior to the pinna bilaterally and slightly anteriorly to facilitate neck flexion. Pins should be placed at or above the superior temporal line.

Table 24.20 Degree of head turn in the supine position

Degree of head turn to contralateral side	Pathology
0°	Cranial procedures involving the *anterior or middle fossa* Approach is along the midline
30°	Lesion is unilateral *along the Sylvian fissure* Head is turned 30° contralateral to *avoid obscuration by the temporal lobe*
45°	Lesions close to the *opticocarotid cistern or the upper clival basilar artery*
60°	Greater than 45° turn, place a large roll behind the shoulder and back Lesion near the *anterior communicating artery, optic chiasm or anterior third ventricle*
70°	Lesion near the *tentorial notch or posterior temporal region*

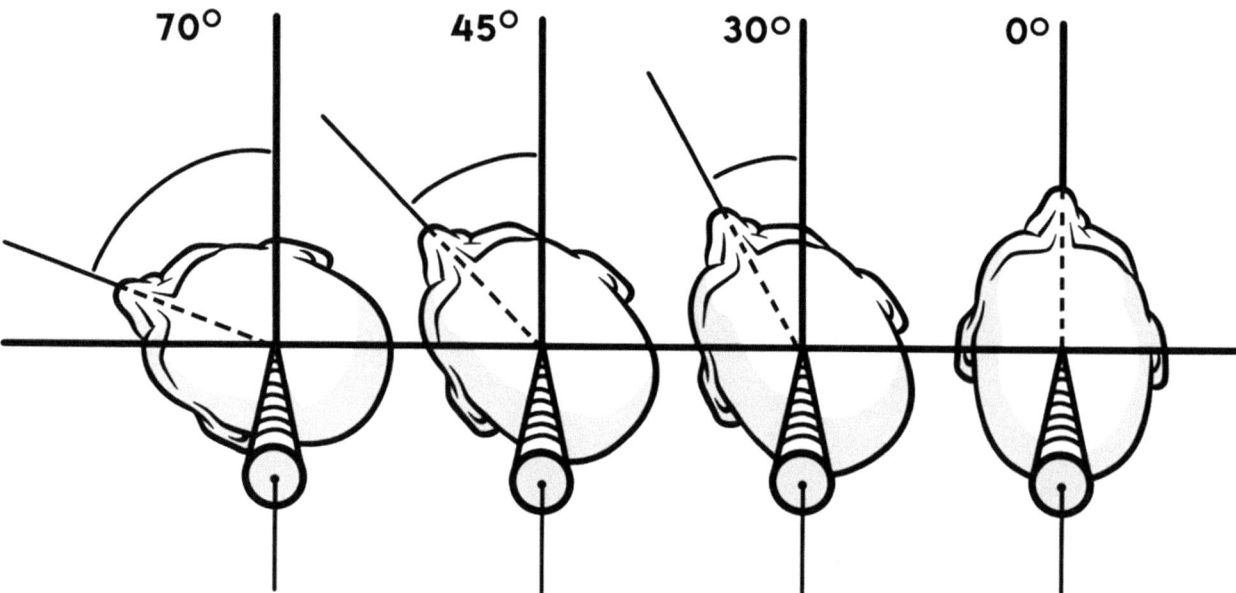

Fig. 24.11 Degree of head turn depends on how close the lesion is to the midline. The closer the lesion is to midline, the less head turn is required

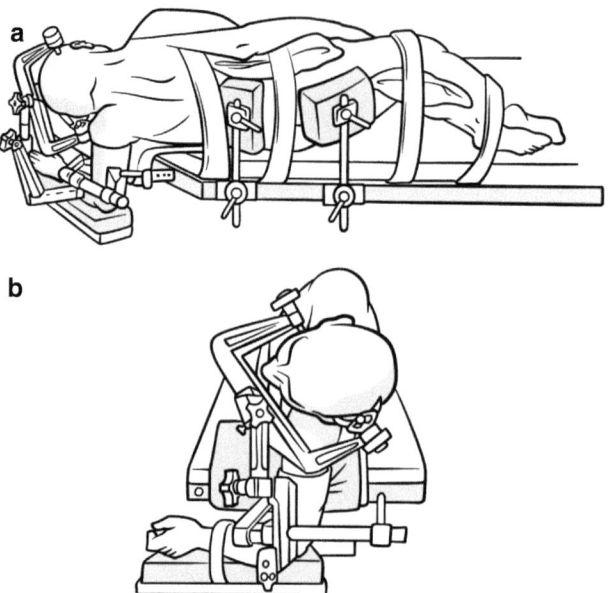

Fig. 24.12 Lateral oblique or park bench position view. **a** Lateral view. **b** Anterior view

- **Lateral Oblique or Park Bench Position (☐ Fig. 24.12)**
- Place *axillary roll* under the dependent axilla or the dependent arm may be held in a sling.
- Head and thorax elevated to about 15° to facilitate venous return.
- Upper shoulder is retracted caudally using adhesive tape to access suboccipital space. Make sure the tape is secured to the metal portion of the bed.
- Rotate patient's head 20° toward the floor and continue to adjust the turn by tilting the tape.

- **Prone and Semi-Prone Position (▣ Figs. 24.13 and 24.14)**
- ▬ Flexion and tuck of the chin is maximized without airway compromise to open the cranial–cervical junction

- **Sitting Position (▣ Fig. 24.15)**
- ▬ Gravity assists with cerebellar retraction
- ▬ Can be used for morbidly obese patients where prone or park bench position may cause cranial venous drainage and ventilation to be compromised
- ▬ Higher risk of air emboli

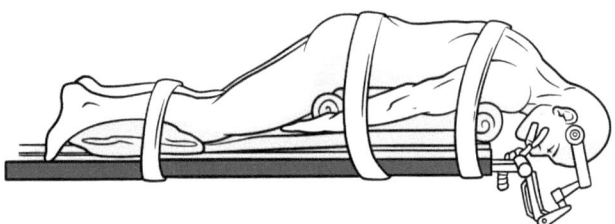

▣ **Fig. 24.13** Prone position

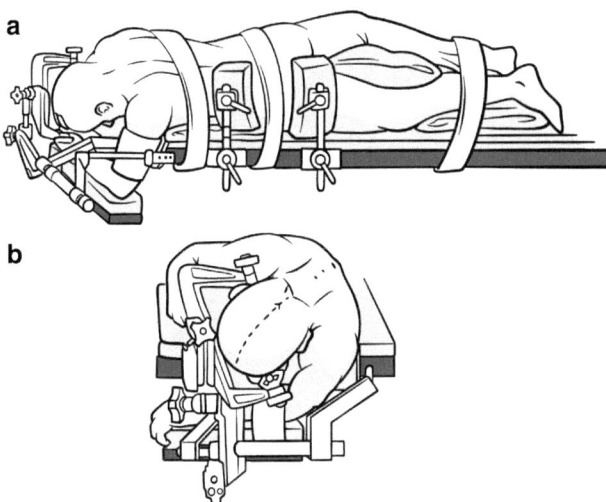

▣ **Fig. 24.14** Semi-prone position. **a** Lateral view. **b** Anterior view

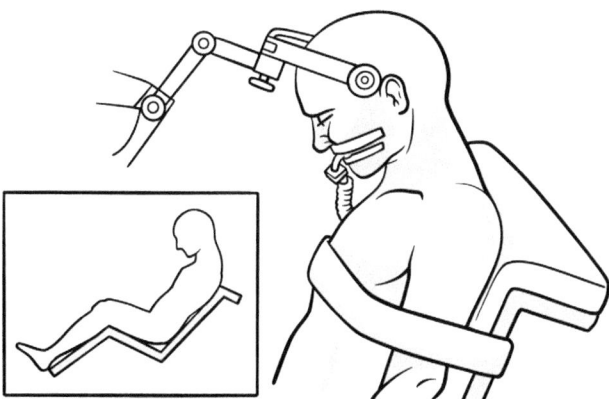

▣ **Fig. 24.15** The sitting position

High yield point #21: During the case, try to remember the following: operative findings, pathology sent, EBL, closure, and drains. This will help you help the resident to write the operative note.

24.5.5 During the Case

- Right before scrubbing, fill out your **attending preference notecard** as much as possible. After you scrub, try to remember the key findings of the procedure while you are scrubbed. See ◘ Table 24.21 for details about what you should be writing about on your notecard.

◘ Table 24.21 To do/note during a case

	All cases	Crani	Spine
Equipment	Scope in the room? Navigation in the room? Special trays available? **Note what equipment was in the OR for the case and the equipment that the resident made sure was available.**	Fiducials placed before the case? Ultrasound?	C-arm?

OR prep	Introduce to CN, ask about foley, set up foley
	Yours and resident's gloves
	Pull images up in OR
	Set up navigation
	Go introduce yourself to patient and *help push patient to OR*
	Take bed out of OR
	Help CN put boots on patient
	Put in foley after intubation (ask anesthesia if OK)
	Note everything the resident did to prep the OR for the case
		Mayo stand: clippers, mits, comb, bacitracin, marking pen, xeroform, tegaderm, draw up lidocaine into syringe
		Mayfield setup
		  Place pins
		  Apply betadine or bacitracin to pins (ask resident)
		Balance microscope (if in room)
		  "side to side" for tumor cases (eyes on opposite side of tumor), "face to face" for vascular
		Make bump
		Make axillary roll
			Mayo stand
			Balance microscope
			  Most spine cases will be "face to face"
			Adjust table
			Make bump

Anesthesia	**Note any special anesthesia considerations for the case**	Steroids? Esp. for pituitary cases Hyperosmotic agents? Anticonvulsants? Antibiotics? Blood in room? A-line? Ventricular or lumbar drainage? Intraoperative evoked potential or other special monitoring?	Antibiotics?
Positioning	How was the patient's body taped to the bed? Set up lights Where was padding placed? Lollipops? OR ergonomics	Bump used? Axillary roll used? How was the bed angled?	
Navigation	Anticipate next steps for setting up the navigation: hand the resident the chicken foot, screw in the star How were the screens set up? **Note the EXACT steps the resident took to set up the navigation**		
Incision	What does the incision look like? How large is it? What local anesthesia is used? How much?	How much hair needs to be shaved? Does attending prefer the hair to be braided?	
Field prep	How are drapes set up?	Set up bar for fishhook retractors? (i.e., Leyla bar)	
Details of procedure	Note important anatomy Key tips from attendings		

(continued)

▣ Table 24.21 (continued)

	All cases	Crani	Spine
Closure, Dressing	How was the incision closed – type of suture/staples, stitch What dressing was used?		
Post-op	Floor vs. ICU Drains? Post-op imaging? SBP range? Steroids? Antibiotics? Pain control? Hours until shower? Diet? Foley? DVT ppx? Anticipated discharge? Page NSGY when….	Neuro checks?	

24.5.6 Technical Skills

Become a sniper   Achieving great OR technical skills is akin to being a great sniper. You must master three things:
1. Position: Both you and the patient must be in the correct position before you take any actions. Make sure the bed is at the right height, rest the ulnar aspect of your hands on something sturdy; try to avoid supination of your wrists.
2. Visualization: You must see your target accurately before you take any actions. Do not lie and say you see something when you don't. Make sure you have adequate lighting and retraction.
3. Authorization: You must have the authorization from someone senior to you before you take any action. This means that a resident or attending must give you permission to do something in the OR before you do it.

24.5.7 Instruments and Proper Handling (▣ Table 24.22)

– Instruments should generally be held in a pencil grip between the thumb and index finger rather than in a pistol grip by the entire hand (▣ Fig. 24.16). The pencil grip allows the instrument to be manipulated finely by the fingers rather than by coarser movements with the wrist.

▪ Scalpel
– Proper application of the scalpel is shown in ▣ Fig. 24.17. The belly of the blade, not the tip, is used to make the incision. The blade should stay perpendicular to the skin.
  – 10 blade used for skin incisions
  – 15 blade used for making the initial dural opening. Then transition to Metzenbaum scissors to extend the initial durotomy

Table 24.22 Instruments in neurosurgery

Frazier suction	Teardrop thumb hole. By releasing, suction pressure drops precipitously, releasing the suck structures.
Fishhook retractors	Retract the scalp Used for most pterional and anterior skull base craniotomies because the force of retraction is more controlled
Weitlander retractors	Retract on flatter surfaces of the skull
Periosteal elevator	Reflect muscle and galea
Cerebellar retractors	Incisions on a curve, such as during a midline suboccipital craniotomy
Penfield dissector	#1 Penfield dissector used to remove inner table bone fragments in burr holes Dura is stripped from skull using #3 Penfield
Leksell rongeurs	Remove lateral sphenoid wing
Kerrison rongeurs	Expand burr holes

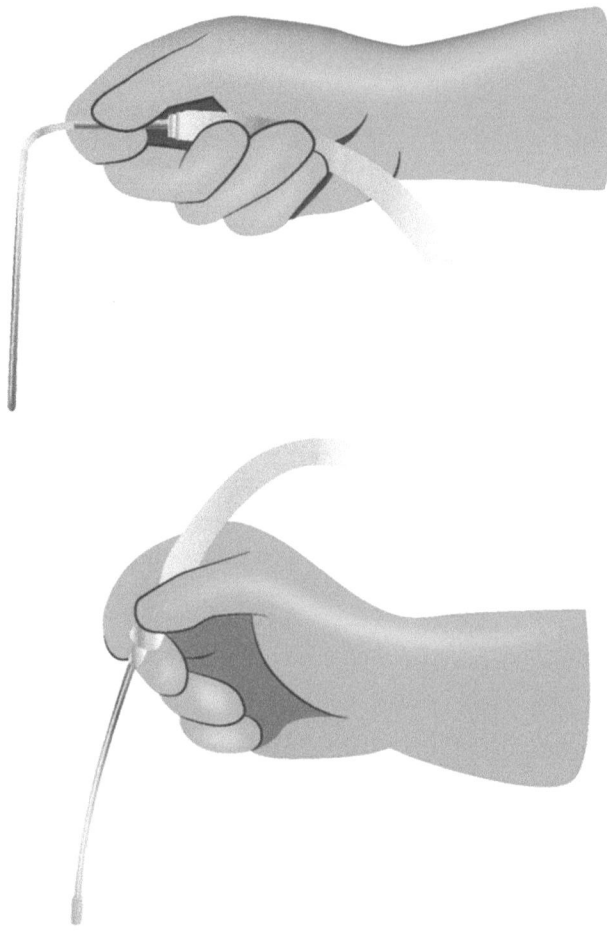

Fig. 24.16 Top: Pistol grip with the entire hand; movements of the instrument are performed using the wrist. Bottom: Pencil grip between the thumb and index finger allows for the instrument to be manipulated by the fingers

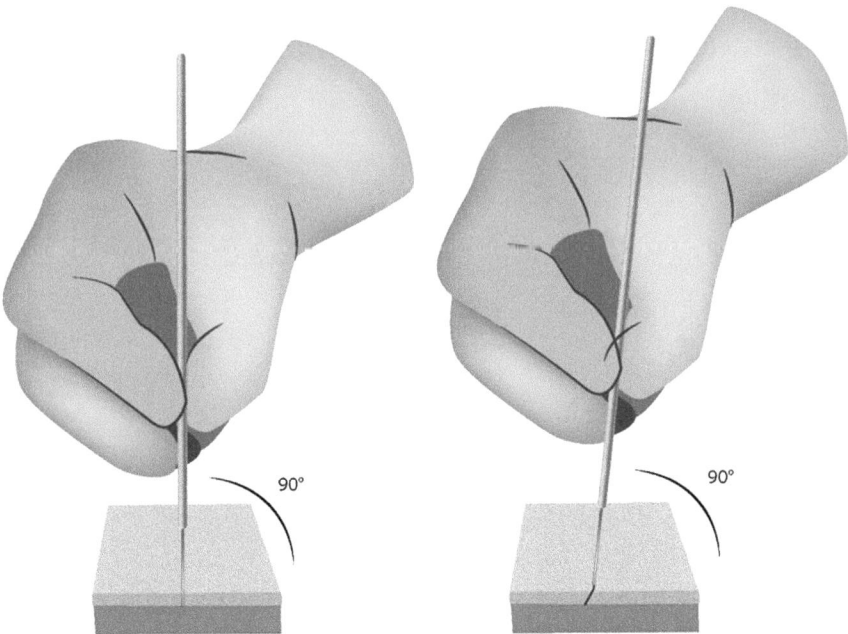

Fig. 24.17 Use the belly of the blade, perpendicular (90°) to the skin, to make the incision

- Hand drills
- *Perforator drill bit:* These drill bits have an automatic stop mechanism when the inner table is penetrated.
- *Acorn drill bit:* Controls burr holes more effectively than perforator with an acorn drill bit the most important task is to avoid plunging. The drill should be braced with one hand while the other stabilizes the drill to avoid plunging.
- *Craniotome:* Footplate ought to stay tangential to the inner surface of the skull to avoid dural tears, especially around the dural venous sinuses. The dural sinuses can embed themselves within the inner table of the skull. There is a gentle concavity that the footplate must respect to avoid massive hemorrhage (Fig. 24.18).
  - To maximize the expanse of bony exposure, the craniotomy must run along the outer edge of each burr hole (Fig. 24.19).

- Bipolar coagulation
- Allows coagulation in areas where unipolar coagulation would be hazardous such as near the CNs, brainstem, cerebellar arteries, and fourth ventricle.
- When the electrode tips touch each other, the current is short-circuited, and no coagulation occurs.
- There should be enough tension in the handle of the forceps to allow the surgeon to control the distance between the tips because no coagulation occurs if the tips are too far apart.
  - Coagulate for only 1–2 s at a time

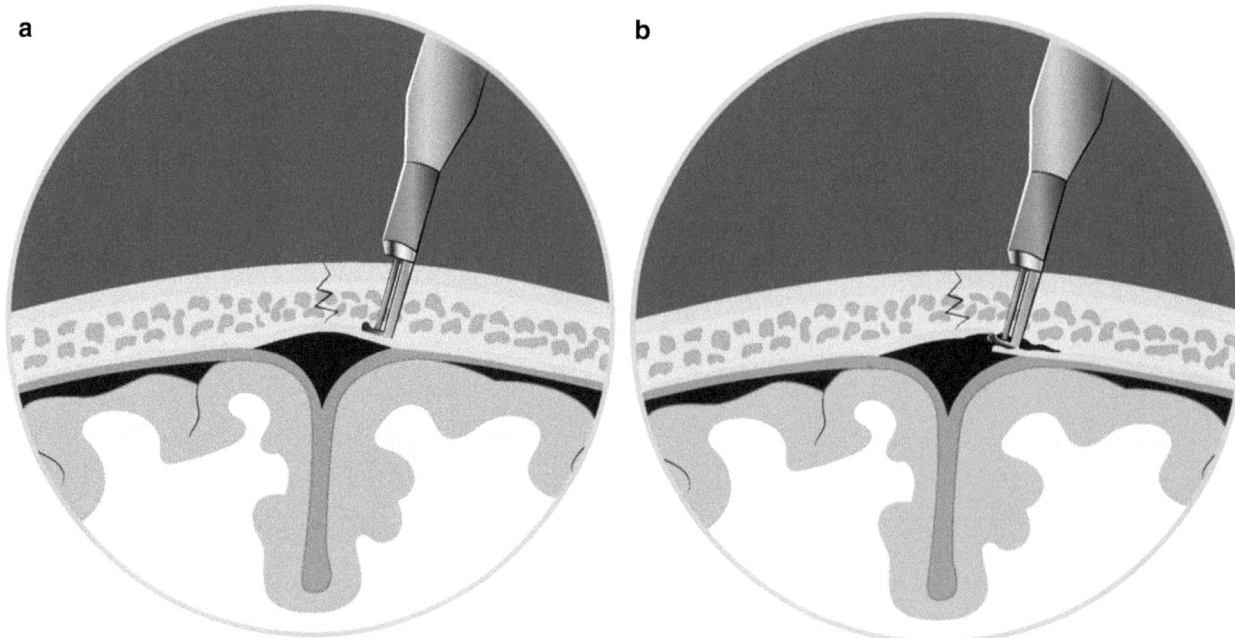

◘ Fig. 24.18 **a** Footplate of the craniotome ought to stay tangential to the inner surface of the skull to avoid dural injury as shown in **b**

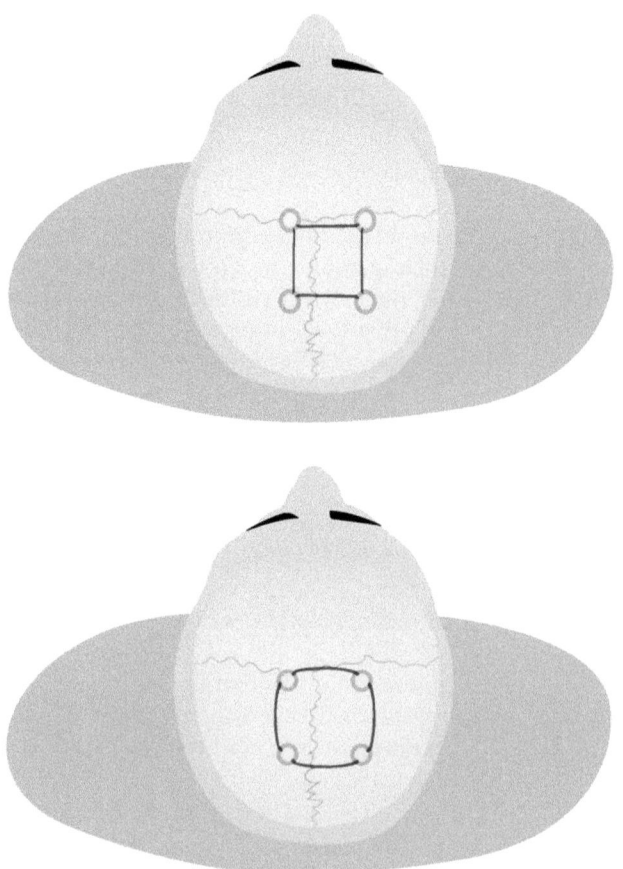

◘ Fig. 24.19 Avoid a smaller craniotomy (top image) by running the drill along the outer edge of each burr hole (bottom image)

24.5.8　Pterional Cranial Exposure

Positioning　see supine position section

- **Incision and scalp flap**
  - Mark the midline and the zygomatic root to inion line to approximate the superior sagittal sinus and transverse sinus, respectively.
  - Large "question mark" incision drawn along the sagittal midline; starting at the hairline (6 cm anterior to the coronal suture in the absence of a hairline) continue low to just above the pinna of the ear where it turns to just above the zygomatic arch.
  - Incision 1 cm off midline with bone flap 1 cm off incision (should keep out of superior sagittal sinus).
  - Flap length should be about equal to width to maintain vascular supply (◻ Table 24.23).
  - Skin incision is made with a 10 blade scalpel → control bleeding with bipolar, Frazier suction to clear operative field → apply Raney clips → muscle and galea reflected using periosteal elevator → scalp retraction using rubberbanded fishhooks attached to a Leyla bar.
  - Temporalis muscle is elevated off the temporal bone and retracted carefully to avoid injury to the *frontal branch of the facial nerve* (◻ Fig. 24.20).

High yield point #22: The frontal branch of the facial nerve courses across the zygoma in the superficial fat overlying the temporalis muscle to innervate the frontalis muscle. You will be pimped on this!

◻ **Table 24.23**　Scalp vascularization

Artery	Location	Course
STA	Anterior and middle scalp	Courses over the zygomatic root in front of the tragus Preauricular incision <0.5 cm from the tragus typically avoids the STA
OA	Posterior scalp	Exits the skull behind the mastoid along the digastric groove

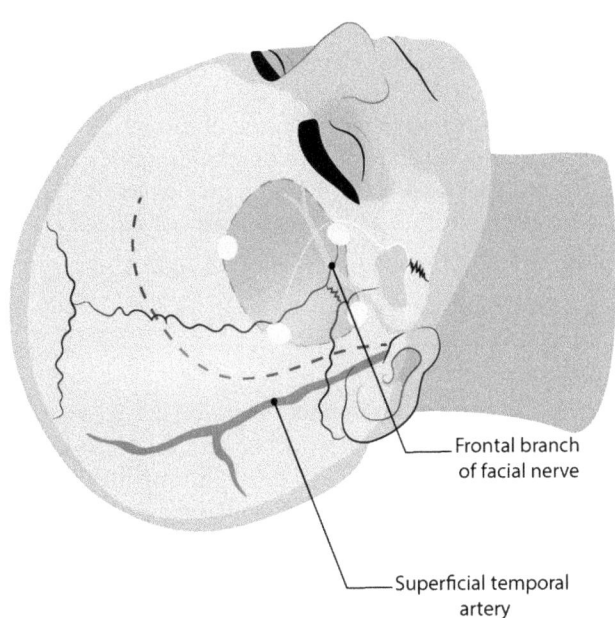

Frontal branch of facial nerve

Superficial temporal artery

◻ **Fig. 24.20**　The frontal branch of the facial nerve diverges from the main trunk below the zygomatic arch and courses across the zygoma in the superficial fat overlying the temporalis muscle

- Incisions reaching the zygoma more than 1.5 cm anterior to the tragus commonly interrupt this nerve unless the layers of the scalp in which it courses are protected.
- Both the vascular and nerve supply of the temporalis muscle course tightly in the fascial attachments of the muscle to the bone.
- Optimal preservation of the muscle's bulk is best achieved through separation of the muscle from the bone by accurate dissection using a sharp periosteal elevator.
- Reflect scalp and temporalis anteriorly. Wrap scalp and temporalis complex in a wet lap band. Held out of the way using rubber banded fishhooks to the temporalis muscle and attached to a retraction bar.

- Craniotomy and bone flap elevation
- Craniotomy should lie 2 cm from the skin incision, so the skin infection does not go through the craniotomy edge to involve the epidural or subdural space.
- Bur holes are made using either a perforator or an acorn drill bit.
  - One burr hole in the anatomic keyhole.
  - One in the squamous temporal bone.
  - An additional burr hole posteriorly at the superior temporal line may be avoided in older patients to avoid unintentional disruption of the dura.
- Once the burr holes are created, the inner table bone fragments can be removed with a bone curette or a #1 Penfield dissector.
- Dura is typically stripped from the overlying inner table using #3 Penfield.
- Use a drill with a B-1 attachment and footplate to elevate the craniotomy flap.
- When the bone flap is elevated, use oxidized cellulose rolls along the craniotomy edge to stop epidural bleeding or drill small holes around the craniotomy site and secure the dura to the bony edge using 4-0 Nurolon sutures ("tack-up sutures").

- Dural opening
- Dura is opened in a semicircular fashion with the base of the dural flap centered on the lesser sphenoid wing.
- A 15 blade scalpel can be used to make the initial dural opening and next, the Metzenbaum scissors extend the initial durotomy.
- Dural retraction involves placing 4-0 sutures along the line of the dural fold closest to the brain or skull base, not along the edges of the dural flap. An extra 2–3 mm of exposure is gained using this technique.

24.5.9   Open Posterior Lumbar Approach

- Relevant anatomy
- Fascia is extremely robust in the L5-S1 region reinforced by the aponeuroses of the latissimus dosi and posterior serratus inferior muscles.
- Lumbar paraspinous muscles are arranged into superficial and deep layers.
  - Superficial layer: erector spinae muscles (spinalis, longissimus, and iliocostalis from medial to lateral).
  - Deep layer: multifidus, rotatores, intertransversarii.

- Positioning
  - Jackson rail system is commonly used to avoid pressure on the abdomen, producing elevated pressure in the epidural venous system causing bleeding during surgery.
  - Lumbar spine is flexed widening the interlaminar space.
  - Head is typically supported on a foam headrest but in elderly patients with cervical spondylosis, use of a Mayfield facilitates neutral cervical alignment.
  - Avoid excessive abduction (>90°) or flexion of the shoulder to prevent brachial plexus injury.
  - Elbows must be appropriately padded to avoid ulnar neuropathy.
  - Knees are flexed to relax the sciatic nerve.

- Incision
  - Injected with 1% lidocaine/1:200,000 epinephrine to prevent excessive bleeding.
  - Subcutaneous tissue is retracted using a self-retaining Weritlander.
  - Scalpel is taken down to the spinous process where the lumbodorsal fascia is encountered.

- Exposure
  - Muscles are stripped from the spinous process superficial to deep.

24.5.10 Minimally Invasive (MIS) Posterior Lumbar Approach

- Case
  - *Indications for MIS approach:* compression worse in lateral recess rather than central spinal canal.
  - *Contraindications to MIS approach:* grade >1 spondolisthesis, instability of flexion-extension, significant lateral listhesis, scoliosis >30°. Congenital spinal stenosis and profound facet hypertrophy are relative contraindications owing to the narrow laminar space available for docking.

Positioning   see positioning for Open Posterior Lumbar Approach

- Incision
  - Stab incision is made at the entry point, about 1.5 cm off midline on the side of pathology.
  - Smallest dilator is inserted through the lumbodorsal fascia and paraspinal muscles.
  - Confirm spinal level is correct on fluoroscopy.

- Exposure
  - A series of progressively larger dilators is advanced onto the lamina using a muscle-splitting technique (twisting motion).
  - Another fluoroscopic image is obtained.
  - Tubular retractor is placed over the largest dilator and secured to a table-mounted holder.
  - Any paraspinal muscle obscuring the bony anatomy is resected using pituitary rongeur and monopolar cautery.

24.5.11 **Closure**

The majority of your technical skill will be tested when assisting the resident with closure.
- Practice the following closure techniques at night using a suture practice kit.
- Always use a one-handed tie in neurosurgery. Be comfortable throwing one handed ties with both hands.

■ Dura closure
- Dura is closed by 4-0 silk interrupted or running sutures.
- Avoid any tension on the dura with the needle.
- Small bits of fat or muscle may be sutured over small openings caused by shrinkage of the dura.

■ Bone flap
- Your resident may ask you to place titanium plates and screws or absorbable PGA plates and screws to attach the bone flap. When inserting screws, always use your nondominant hand to secure the bone flap. Insert screw perpendicular to the bone flap. Make sure the screws are flush with the plate.
- If there is significant bony defect from extra bone removed beyond craniotomy, bone cement or methylmethacrylate can be used to fill the defect.

High yield point #23: DO NOT DROP THE BONE FLAP. This will cost the patient another surgery.

Temporalis muscle   reattach to the superior temporal line using 2-0 absorbable sutures, muscle is stretched and kept under some tension to avoid muscle atrophy.

■ Galea closure
- Buried, interrupted, inverted stitches using 3-0 vicryl. 1 cm between stitches.
- Be sure that you are biting galea with needle. Take needle out halfway between galea and skin within subcutaneous tissue.
- Suture in parallel. Make sure your bite on one side of the incision matches directly parallel to your bite on the other side.
- Push the needle all the way through with the needle driver, hold the needle with Adson, then reload the driver by grabbing the needle from Addison so you don't have to readjust the needle. This "no-touch" technique will save you time.
- First knot should be a granny knot that allows you to adjust the tightness before securing it. When securing knot, pull the suture tight with nondominant hand, perpendicular to incision. Pull knots in the same direction as the incision.

■ Scalp closure
- Skin is approximated using either a permanent 3-0 monofilament or staples (see technical skills section for more detail about closure).
- When tying with needle driver, try to make as few movements as possible.

■ Spine closure
- *Subcutaneous closure*
    – Deep fascia closed with interrupted 0 Vicryl
    – Skin closed with buried, interrupted stitches using 3-0 Vicryl

– Similar technique to galea closure, avoid buttoning, reload the needle using a single move. Make sure the knot is TIGHT. DO NOT create an air knot. Knots are tied the same as galea closure: two granny knots then two knots to secure.

■ Secure drains
═ How a drain is secured may be resident/attending dependent, but a purse string closure will sufficiently secure the drain.
═ The first bite will be on one side of the drain, parallel to the drain but in the opposite direction. The second bite is on the other side of the drain, also parallel to the drain but in the same direction.
═ An air knot is created with four throws. Wrap around the drain once then tie with four throws. Wrap around the drain three more times. Then, tie with four throws.

24.5.12 After the Case

Finish filling out attending preference notecard.

Look at post-op admission orders read the orders the resident made for post-op admissions. Make sure you understand each order. General post-op admissions NICU orders will include the following:
═ NPO → Sips → DAT (if NPO, order GI ppx)
═ Bed rest
═ HOB 30° (depending on surgery)
═ NVS q1h
═ Foley I/O
═ CBC, lytes, BUN, Cr daily
═ IV NS +/− KCl (consider D5NS in diabetic)
═ Cefazolin 1 g IV q8h × 3 doses
═ Gravol 25–50 mg iv/po/im q4-6h prn (or other antinausea med)
═ Ondansetron 4–8 mg po/iv q8h prn
═ Neuro bowel reg protocol
═ Labetalol/hydralazine 5–10 mg iv q10 min to maintain SBP <150 (may adjust based on surgery and premorbid HTN)
═ Pre-op meds (hold anti-hyperglycemics until eating, avoid iatrogenic hypotension with BP meds)
═ Standard analgesics
  – Tylenol 1 g q4-6h prn
  – Morphine 5–10 mg sc/im q3-4h prn
  – Morphine 1–2 mg iv q1h prn
═ Decadron 4 mg iv/po q6h and then taper (e.g., 4 mg bid ×2d, 2 mg bid ×2d, 1 mg bid ×2d), depending on surgery
═ DVT ppx unless ICH/bleeding. Use heparin ppx if any AKI/CKD

24.6 Neuro ICU Essentials

To be successful in the NICU, you must master all concepts in the chapter on MICU and the Neurology chapter in addition to the following topics.

High yield point #24: Suspect DI if: (1) serum Na > 148, (2) UO > 250–300 cc/h × 3 consecutive hours OR (3) urine specific gravity < 1.003

24.6.1   Management of Post-Op Neurosurgical Patients

- Before examining the patient, review the following:
  - [ ] Recorded preoperative deficits
  - [ ] Preoperative and postoperative imaging
  - [ ] Op report
  - [ ] Write down, with checkboxes, all exam findings you will check so you don't forget when you see the patient
- In the op report, check whether there was:
  - *Frontal sinus invasion?* → check for CSF leak (e.g., watery drainage from nose – have patient sit up and lean forward; salty taste in mouth)
  - *Vascular manipulation?* → check for signs of vasospasm (e.g., focal motor deficits, speech or receptive aphasias, anomia if dominant side, increasing confusion)
  - *Peri-orbital invasion?* → check for malignant edema of the orbit. Will have decreasing vision in the affected eye, limited ROM of eye, significant pain
  - *Disturbance of pituitary stalk?* → observe for DI: check q4h Na, urine specific gravity, UOP

- Supratentorial lesions (◻ Table 24.24)
- If exam is concerning, immediately obtain a STAT CT head and look for: parenchymal hematoma (think about mass effect), pneumocephalus, epidural hematoma
- Compare with previous imaging to evaluate for any midline shift. Think about repeat imaging.

◻ **Table 24.24** Exam of post-op patients with supratentorial lesions

Lesion location	Potential deficits to monitor
Temporal	[ ] *Language*: expressive aphasia, word generation and any pauses or poverty of speech [ ] *Hearing* (temporal lobe has bilateral representation): blunted hearing due to post-op fluid in the sinuses, especially if air cells were entered or a middle fossa craniotomy [ ] *Short-term memory:* have patient remember the words, "apple, table, penny" and have the patient repeat them back at a later time. [ ] *Seizures:* especially if present preoperatively or if lesion is intraparenchymal [ ] *Visual fields:* bilateral quadrantanopsia affecting the contralateral visual field due to interruption in Meyer's loop = "pie in the sky" (◻ Fig. 24.21)
Parietal	[ ] *Motor or sensory deficits:* check pronator drift. [ ] *Apraxia:* cannot use pen or button shirt [ ] *Hemispatial neglect:* especially R parietal lesions [ ] *Gerstmann's syndrome for dominant parietal lesions:* agraphia, acalcula, finger agnosia, left-right disorientation
Occipital	[ ] *Visual field deficits:* may not be obvious to the patient. Have patient cover eyes separately and test visual fields. Anton–Babinski Syndrome (cortical blindness): patient thinks they can see but they are blind
Frontal	Typically don't cause significant deficits unless they extend posteriorly into premotor area or occur bilaterally [ ] *Motor deficits* [ ] *Loss of executive function* (poor decision making, unacceptable social responses, abulia)

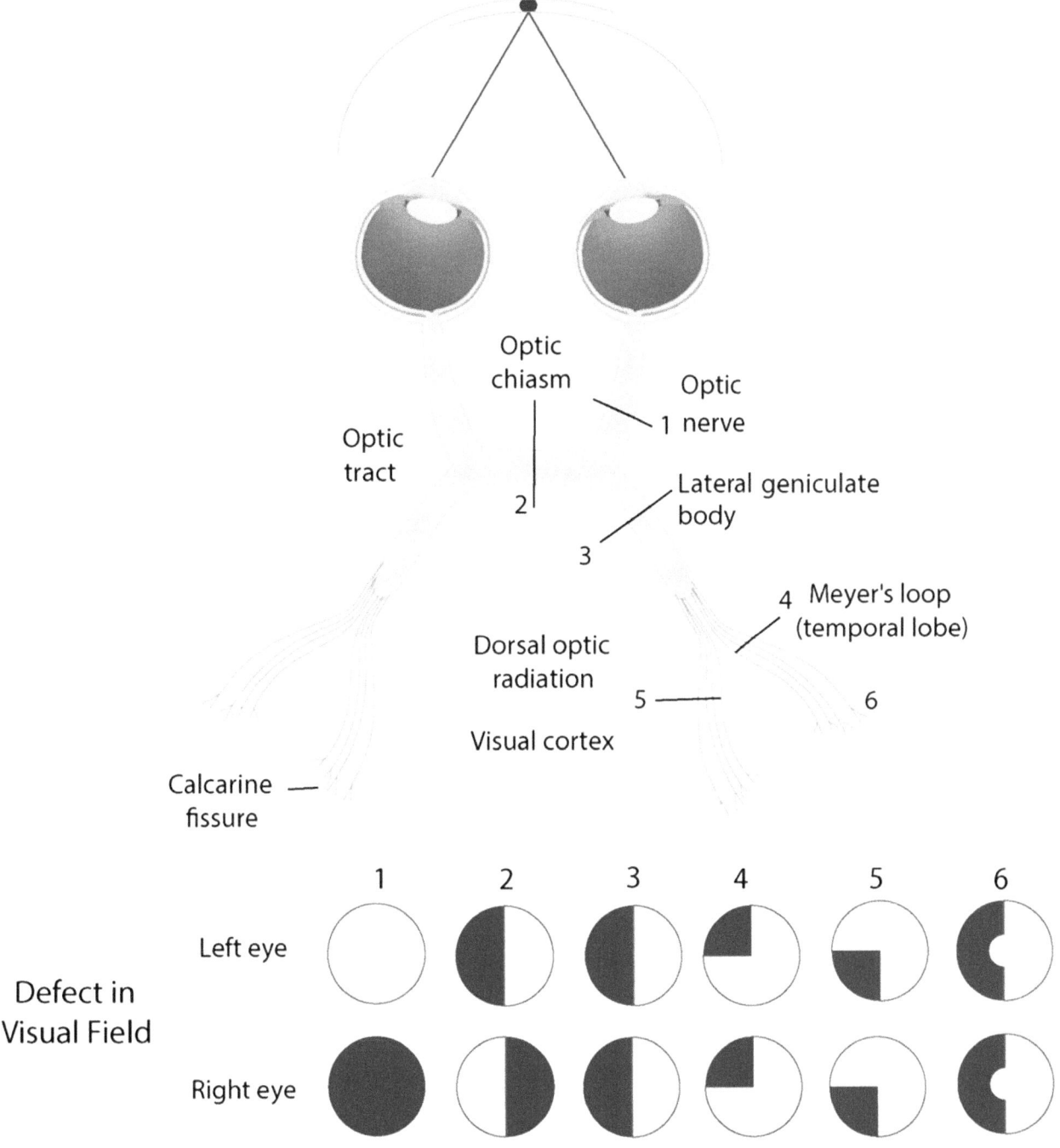

- Infratentorial lesions (□ Table 24.25)
- Important to monitor several urgent issues including *obstructive HCP, wound leakage, stroke, IPH*
- HOB usually elevated to 30°
- Obtain imaging and look for
  - Hematomas
  - Morphology of the 4th ventricle, lateral ventricles (checking for HCP)
  - Pseudomeningocele

■ **Table 24.25** Exam of post-op patients with infratentorial lesions

Lesion location	Potential deficits to monitor

Cerebellar	[ ] Check for *wound leakage* (may not occur until POD 2–5)
	[ ] *Nystagmus*
	[ ] *Coordination/balance/posture*
	  Limb ataxia (lesions of the cerebellar hemisphere)
	  Truncal ataxia (more central vermian lesions)
	[ ] *Dysmetria*
	[ ] *CN exam*
	[ ] Check for *word generation and spontaneous speech* (associated with "cerebellar mutism")

CP Angle	Focus exam on *CNs 3–12* [ ] *CN 3,4,6*: eye ROM [ ] *CN 5:* facial sensation [ ] *CN 7*: facial symmetry [ ] *CN 8*: hearing and balance [ ] *CN 9, 10*: palate, swallow [ ] *CN 11*: shoulder shrug [ ] *CN 12*: tongue midline, side to side

■ **Table 24.26** Exam of post-op patients with interventricular lesions

Lesion location	Potential deficits to monitor
Interventricular	[ ] *EVD*: is it draining [ ] *Mental status* [ ] All *CNs* (especially eyes) [ ] *Motor exam* [ ] *Drift* [ ] Look for signs of *DI* due to injury of the hypothalamus and median eminence (symptoms include excessive urine, rising Na)

- ■ Intraventricular lesions (■ Table 24.26)
- – Know which approach was performed before you examine the patient:
  - – Transcortical
    - – Burr hole made through Kocher's point and entry is made into the frontal horn of the lateral ventricle
    - – *Watch for slightly higher risk of postoperative seizures*
  - – Interhemispheric transcallosal
    - – Midline craniotomy is made and dissection down between the two hemispheres
    - – Callosotomy is made and the 3rd ventricle is entered

- ■ Skullbase approaches (■ Table 24.27)

- ■ Vascular surgeries (■ Table 24.28)
- – *Endovascular patients*
  - – Patients may have either had pressure held or a Starclose (small metallic device used to close the artery) post procedure.
    - – If pressure was held, the patient must be flat for 4 h.
    - – If Starclose was used, may mobilize the patient immediately.

◘ **Table 24.27** Exam of post-op patients with skullbase approaches

Approach	Potential deficits to monitor

Orbitozygomatic	This approach takes both the zygoma and lateral orbital wall. If modified OZ, lateral orbital wall is taken with fronto-temporal bone in one piece and zygoma is left intact.
	[ ] Check *eye ROM* since the lateral wall of the orbit is disturbed in this approach
	  Post-op patients may have difficulty with ipsilateral lateral gaze
	  Monitor for malignant edema of the orbit (increased pain, decreased vision, limited ROM)
	[ ] Check *all other CNs, including CN 1*
	[ ] Look for *CSF leak*
	[ ] Check for signs of *vasospasm*
	[ ] Check for facial asymmetry, including *frontalis palsy* (have patient raise eyebrows)

Supraorbital	This approach can be done with either a traditional pterional skin incision or via minimally invasive "eyebrow" incision [ ] *CN exam* [ ] Look for *CSF leak* [ ] Check for *frontalis palsy* (have patient raise eyebrows) [ ] Assess *eye ROM* and *visual fields*, look for *signs of malignant edema of the orbit* [ ] Check for signs of *DI* [ ] Check for signs of *vasospasm*
Far Lateral	This approach gives access to the lateral brainstem, medulla, lower CPA, lower CNs 9–12 and the lower cranio-cervical vasculature (vertebral, PICA, and lower basilar) Typically involves removal of the lateral C1 ring with mobilization of the vertebral artery [ ] Look for *CSF leak* (enlarging wound, weeping around sutures, positional headaches) [ ] *CN 9, 10*: palate, swallow [ ] *CN 11*: shoulder shrug [ ] *CN 12*: tongue midline, side to side

◘ **Table 24.28** Exam of post-op vascular patients

Case	Potential deficits to monitor
Endovascular	[ ] Look at groin site. Check for hematoma or oozing. [ ] Check DP pulses
Ruptured aneurysm	*EVD:* typically, the drain may be lowered to 10 after securing the aneurysm. If no EVD is in place, monitor for signs of HCP (decreasing mental status, increasing HA) [ ] Check *post-op CT* looking at temporal horns, 3rd ventricle, lateral ventricles for dilation [ ] Monitor for *vasospasm* Typically peaks POD 7–10 Check for any focal deficit New motor drift Evidence of cerebral salt wasting (increased urine Na, decreased serum Na, increased fractional Na excretion) Increasing confusion or agitation may be signs of early vasospasm Monitor daily transcranial doppler (TCD) [ ] *Exam:* depends on location of the aneurysm MCA – language difficulties, paresis of contralateral side ACA – weakness of contralateral leg, contralateral neglect ICA – contralateral paresis or plegia PCA – visual deficits, lower extremity weakness Vertebral/PICA – look for lateral medullary syndrome (*Wallenberg syndrome*: dysphagia, dysphonia, dysarthria, ataxia, nystagmus, loss of pain and temperature on contralateral body and Horner's)

- When Endo patients arrive to the unit: *check bilateral dorsalis pedis pulses.*
- If groin hematoma develops, apply direct pressure for 20 min, check repeat CBC
    - If hemodynamically unstable, give IVF NS bolus. Consider transfusion and order direct pressure with Femstop.
    - If puncture site continues to ooze, can order femstop but be careful to not occlude the artery. Make sure you can feel DP pulse.
    - If large hematoma or dropping HCT, get CT abd/pelvis to evaluate pseudoaneurysm or retroperitoneal hemorrhage.
    - If unexplained drop in HCT <30, without obvious hematoma, may be retroperitoneal bleed. Repeat CBC. CT abd/pelvis if continues to drop.

■ Functional neurosurgery (◘ Table 24.29)

■ Chiari cases (◘ Table 24.30)

◘ **Table 24.29**   Exam of post-op functional neurosurgery patients

Case	Potential deficits to monitor
Microvascular decompression	These patients often have post-op nausea/vomiting [ ] *CN 7:* check facial symmetry (puff cheeks and show teeth) [ ] *CN 8:* check hearing (often have decreased hearing on surgical side due to fluid in the mastoids or manipulation of nerve) [ ] *CN 9:* check for swallowing and palatal symmetry
Amygdalohippo-campectomy	[ ] *Visual fields:* check for "pie in the sky"
DBS, thalamotomy	Look for evidence of misplaced electrodes [ ] *Contralateral motor weakness* → involvement of internal capsule [ ] *Dysarthria* → usually affected in VIM DBS, electrode is near VOC
Baclofen/pain pumps	[ ] Look for evidence of *Gabaergic overdose* (vomiting, weakness, drowsiness, slowed breathing, coma)

◘ **Table 24.30**   Exam of post-op Chiari patients

Case	Potential deficits to monitor
Chiari	These patients may have significant postoperative pain due to dissection of the posterior cervical muscles Check lower cranial nerves to elicit evidence of brainstem infarction due to manipulation of vertebral artery or PICA [ ] In the *op note*, look to see whether the decompression was intradural or extradural [ ] Ensure *pain* is controlled [ ] Check for *CSF leak* around suture line if duraplasty was done [ ] *CN 9, 10:* check swallow, gag, cough and monitor for aspiration [ ] *CN 11:* shoulder shrug [ ] *CN 12:* tongue midline, side to side

- Pituitary via Transphenoidal Hypophysectomy (TSH) (◻ Table 24.31)
- If concern for DI
  - Keep foley in for 48 h
  - Check q4h Na and specific gravity for 24 h
  - Don't be fooled by post-op fluid mobilization/diuresis
  - Orders to call for concerns of DI
    - UO > 300 cc/h × 3 consecutive h
    - Serum Na > 148
    - Urine spec grav <1.003
- Treatment of DI:
  - If awake and alert, have patient drink as much free water as able
  - If unable to tolerate oral repletion due to nausea/vomiting or altered, may treat with ½ NS + 20 mEq KCl and give DDAVP if Na > 150
    - DDAVP dosing
      - DDAVP IV/SQ 1–4 mg BID
      - DDAVP PO 0.05 mg BID up to 0.6 mg BID
      - DDAVP nasal insufflation 10mcg (one puff) qhs up to 40mcg qd

- Trauma (◻ Table 24.32)
- Close monitoring of trauma post-op patients is essential to avoid secondary injury to brain tissue from hypoxia or ischemia. This is done with pressure monitors (e.g., EVD or Camino ICP monitor) or in conjunction with a Licox for the monitoring of cerebral perfusion.

- Spine patients (◻ Table 24.33)
- Always check a motor/sensory exam.
- Check for evidence of CSF leak if a durotomy was encountered (fluid near incision, positional HAs).

◻ **Table 24.31** Exam of post-op pituitary TSH patients

Case	Potential deficits to monitor

Pituitary via TSH	[ ] In the *op note*, look to see *whether the CSF was encountered*
	     Often there is a lumbar drain placed if CSF leak was seen and nasal
	     packing will likely be in place.
	 [ ] Assess *visual fields*, look for bitemporal hemianopsia.
	 [ ] Check for active *CSF leak* by having the patient lean forward and observe
	     for continuous watery drip.
	 [ ] Monitor *lumbar drain output*, drain should be placed at level of defect
	     (level of tragus), order may be written to titrate 10–15 cc/h.
	 [ ] Monitor for *DI*

◻ **Table 24.32** Exam of post-op trauma patients

Case	Potential deficits to monitor
Trauma	[ ] GCS [ ] Drain output (amount and consistency) [ ] Check for swelling out of craniotomy site [ ] Follow ICPs

Table 24.33 Exam of post-op spine patients

Case	Potential deficits to monitor
Cervical	Anterior approach – ACDF [ ] Monitor for *stridor, trachea deviation, swallowing, egophany* (say EEE), *C5 palsy* [ ] Compare *pre/post-op motor/sensory exams, DTRs* [ ] Monitor *drain output* Posterior approach – laminectomy/fusion [ ] Compare *pre/post-op motor/sensory exam, DTRs* [ ] Monitor *drain output* [ ] Check *wound for leakage* [ ] Check and arrange for *post-op imaging*
Tho-racic	Anterior [ ] Compare *pre/post-op motor/sensory exam* [ ] Check for *chest tube, check breathing* [ ] Check a *post-op CXR* to evaluate for PTX and serve as a baseline [ ] Monitor *H/H* for a minimum of 24 h to ensure no hemothorax is developing Posterior [ ] Compare *pre/post-op motor/sensory exam* [ ] Check *post-op imaging* [ ] *Drain output*
Lumbar	Anterior [ ] Compare *pre/post-op motor/sensory exam, DTRs* [ ] Monitor *drain output* [ ] Monitor *H/H* for a minimum of 24 h to ensure no occult retroperotineal bleed [ ] Check *post-op imaging* Posterior [ ] Compare *pre/post motor/sensory exam, DTRs* Check for any new post-op motor deficits, esp. foot drop, new radiculopathies. If exam is concerning, check post-op imaging. May require advanced imaging (i.e., CT) to evaluate screw position, or presence of post-op hematoma [ ] Check *drain output* [ ] If durotomy occurred, keep flat for 24 h

24.6.2 Postoperative DVT Prophylaxis (Table 24.34)

- Dose: lovenox 40 mg sc q24h or heparin 5000 units sc q12h

24.6.3 Paroxysmal Sympathetic Hyperactivity (Storming)

- Management (Table 24.35)
- Avoid triggers that provoke the paroxysms
- Mitigate excessive sympathetic outflow
- Address the effects of PSH on other organ systems

24.6.4 ICP Management

Cerebral Perfusion Pressure (CPP) = Mean Arterial Blood Pressure (MAP) – Intracranial Pressure (ICP)

◻ **Table 24.34** Post-operative DVT prophylaxis

Cranial surgery

1. Standard risk – no risk factors = SCD alone + early ambulation
2. Moderate/high risk – 1 or more risk factors = SCDs + lovenox 18–24 h post-op

Spinal Surgery elective OR spine fracture w/out SCI

1. No risk factors = early ambulation
2. Moderate risk – 1 risk factor = SCDs + early ambulation
3. High risk – multiple risk factors = SCDs + lovenox at 24–48 h

Risk factors:
Immobility (defined as not out of bed and ambulating at 12 hrs after surgery)
Cancer/malignancy
Glioma/glioblastoma
Meningioma
Neurologic motor deficit
Previous DVT/CTE
Anterior lumbar spine procedure
Advanced age (>75 years)
Known hypercoagulable state

◻ **Table 24.35** Pharmacotherapy for paroxysmal sympathetic hyperactivity

Drug class	Medications with clinical evidence	Clinical features mitigated
Opioids	Morphine, Fentanyl	HTN, allodynia, tachycardia
Anesthetics	Propofol	All features
B-blockers	Propranolol, labetalol	Tachycardia, HTN, diaphoresis? dystonia
A2-agonists	Clonidine, dexmedetomidine	HTN and tachycardia
Neuromodulators	Bromocriptine (D2 receptor)	Temperature and sweating
	Gabapentin (calcium channels)	Spasticity and allodynia
	Baclofen (GABAB receptors)	Spasticity and dystonia
Benzodiazepines	Diazepam, lorazepam, midazolam, clonazepam	Agitation, HTN, tachycardia, posturing
Sarcolemmal Ca	Dantrolene	Posturing and muscular spasms

- Optimization of CPP is what we aim to control by measuring ICP.
- The Brain Trauma Foundation Guidelines recommend *target CPP values of 60–70 mmHg* for survival and favorable outcomes.
  - Landmark study by Robertson, et al. (2) demonstrated that CPP targets >70 mmHg were associated with a higher rate of ARDS.
- ICP is considered pathologically elevated when >20 mmHg for >5–10 min.

Cerebral Blood Flow (CBF) = Cerebral Perfusion Pressure (CPP)/ Cerebrovascular Resistance (CVR)

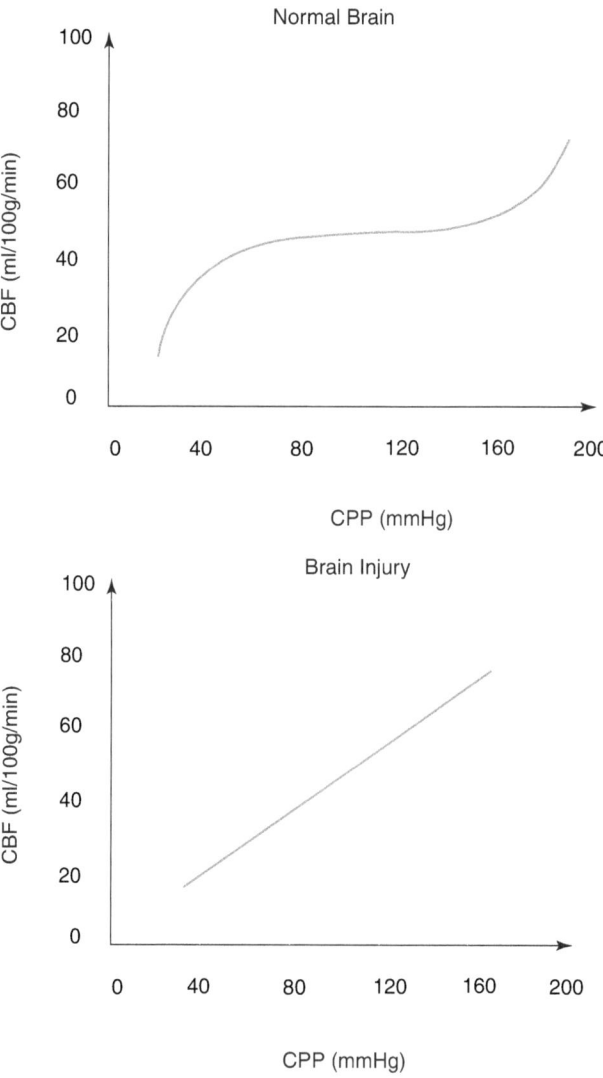

Fig. 24.22 Relationship of MAP and CBF in both normal brain and during brain injury. Local tissue ischemia causes a failure of autoregulation and CBF becomes passively dependent on CPP

- Usually CVR holds the CBF constant over a broad range of BPs. In brain injury, local tissue ischemia causes a failure of autoregulation. CBF becomes passively dependent on CPP, which can result in an inability to maintain a stable CBF over a broad range of MAPs and CPPs (■ Fig. 24.22).

- Ways to monitor ICP (■ Fig. 24.23)

- Indications for ICP monitoring (■ Table 24.36)

- When to wean the EVD
- EVD is typically placed at 10 cm H2O (higher = less drainage)
- As the acute injury resolves and the patient neurologically stabilizes, think about EVD wean
  - This is typically done by raising the EVD to 20, however can also be done more gradually
- If the exam and ICPs remain stable, can trial clamping. The EVD is clamped for 24 h and a CT scan is completed
- If CT/exam stable, discontinue EVD

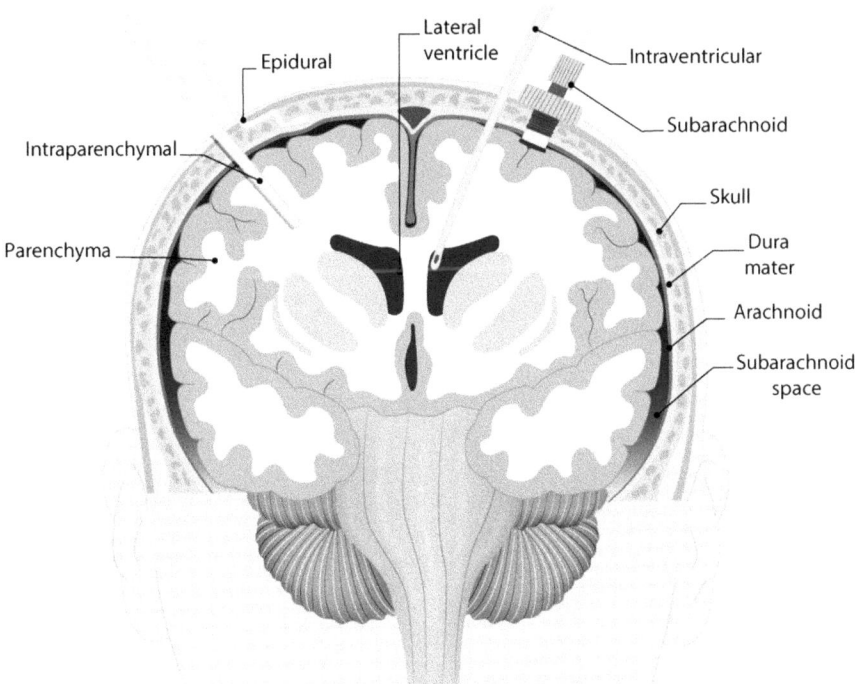

■ Table 24.36 Indications for Increasing ICP Monitoring

If TBI	If not TBI

GCS score ≤8 and CT scan showing evidence of mass effect OR normal CT plus:
  Age > 40 years
  Motor posturing
  Systolic BP <90 mmHg
	No strict management guidelines. In general, patients with conditions that would put them at high risk for developing elevated ICP should be considered for monitoring:
	  IVH, SAH
	  Evidence of shift, herniation, or effacement of basal cisterns
	  Those with signs of increased ICP (unilateral or bilaterally fixed and dilated pupil(s), decorticate or decerebrate posturing, bradycardia, hypertension, and/or respiratory depression)

■ Strategies for managing ICP prior to starting hyperosmolar therapy
 = *Fluid management*: goal euvolemia and normo- to hyperosmolar
   – *Limit all free water (enteral, 1/2NS, D5W)* but provide adequate fluids with NS or LR
 = *Stimulus management*: provide adequate sedation
 = *BP management*: goal is to minimize hypotension and HTN to maintain an adequate CPP
   – Generally, MAP >65 provides adequate CPP
 = *Positioning*: HOB 30–45° (make sure no unstable T/L spine fractures, check yourself), loosen cervical collar
 = *Fever*: aggressively manage, goal normothermia.
   – Note that hypothermia is a recommendation for refractory elevated ICP. Can use chilled saline, cooling pads, or the Arctic Sun. Relative contraindications include patients with active bleeding or infections.

  – If cooling:
    – Electrolyte panel
    – Glucose
    – CBC
    – Blood cultures at 12 h and again at 24 h
    – Watch for hypoK

- ▪ **Strategies to combat shivering**
- ▬ Apply Bair hugger
- ▬ Meds + specific dosages to specify in presentation and notes:
    – Demerol 25–50 mg/h, intermittent IVP or continuous drip
    – Propofol 10–300 mg/h
    – Buspirone 20 mg every 6 h
    – Precedex 0.1–1mcg/kg/h
- ▬ *Paralyze + sedate if severe*

- ▪ **Hyperosmolar therapy (◘ Fig. 24.24)**
- ▬ Most common treatment is 20% Mannitol, 3% hypertonic saline (HTS) or 23% HTS

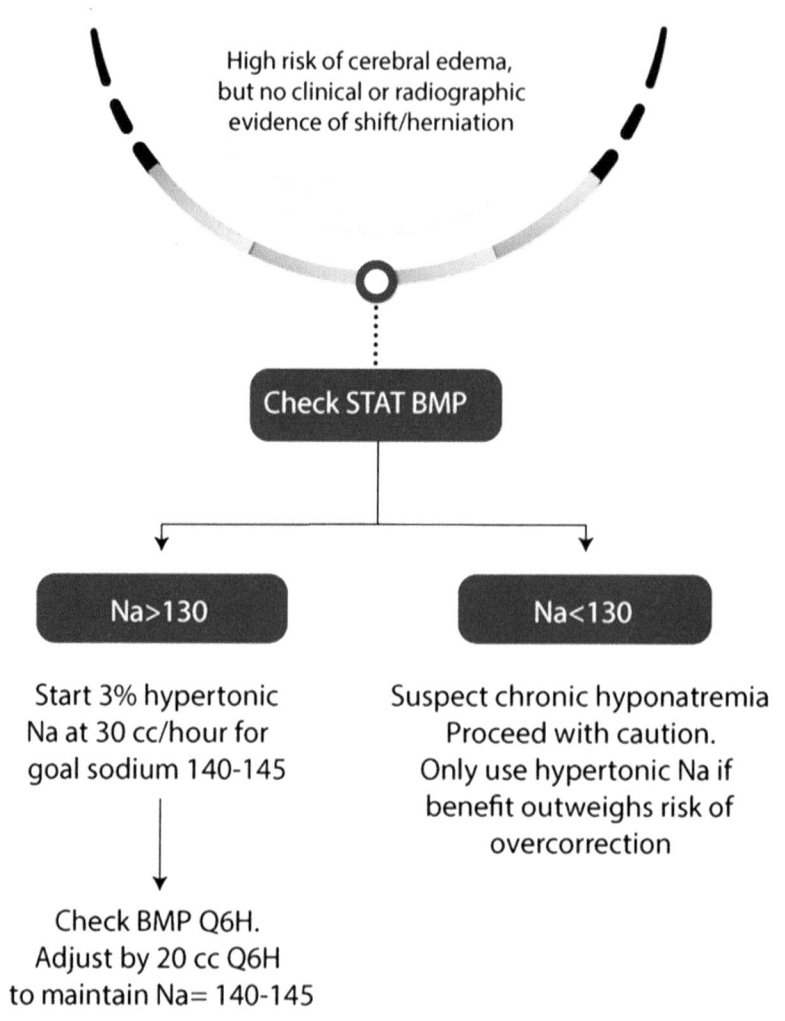

High risk of cerebral edema, but no clinical or radiographic evidence of shift/herniation

Check STAT BMP

Na>130

Na<130

Start 3% hypertonic Na at 30 cc/hour for goal sodium 140-145

Suspect chronic hyponatremia Proceed with caution. Only use hypertonic Na if benefit outweighs risk of overcorrection

Check BMP Q6H. Adjust by 20 cc Q6H to maintain Na= 140-145

◘ **Fig. 24.24** Algorithm to decide whether hyperosmolar therapy is appropriate as part of managing cerebral edema

◼ Table 24.37 Monitoring needed while on hyperosmolar therapy

For Mannitol	1. Na, Glu, BUN/Cr, Osms Q6H 2. Watch for hypotension that can lower CPP
For HyperNa	1. Na Q6H
For Both	1. Daily BMP (monitoring kidney, both can cause ATN, mannitol is more likely to do this though) 2. Daily CXR

- Mannnitol usually 0.5–1 g/kg IV (50–75 g for avg adult) followed by lasix 10–30 mg IV push
  - Watch for hypovolemia (may impair CPP)
- HTS 3% – 50 cc/h through peripheral IV
- HTS 23.4% – 30 cc (120 mEq) given over 15–20 min (2 ml/min), *centrally only*
  - *Contraindications:* serum Na > 160 mEq/l, serum osm > 320 mOsm/kg

- **Always know Na when using HTS (◼ Table 24.37)**
- Steroids were studied in the MRC CRASH trial (Lancet 2005) and demonstrated increased mortality. Thus, steroids are usually avoided UNLESS the increase in ICP is 2/2 to tumor.

- **Licox Brain Tissue Oxygen Monitoring System (◼ Fig. 24.25)**
- LICOX uses near-infared spectrum to measure the partial pressure of brain tissue oxygen ($P_{bt}O_2$) that correlates hypoxia and ischemia as a result of TBI. It aids in the decision making for management of ICP issues, i.e., when to use pressors, hyperventilation, etc. with the end goal of preventing secondary injury to brain as a result of ischemia or hypoxia. This can be used in conjunction with jugular venous O_2 ($SjvO_2$).
- It comes as a 3-lumen BOLT that measures $P_{bt}O_2$, temp, and ICP.
- *Brain oxygenation*
  - Normal is approx. 30 mmHg (when treating, keep *above 20–30 mmHg*)
  - Cerebral ischemia <15 mmHg (PbO_2 < 5 for 30 min = 50% incr. risk of death)
  - SjO_2 normal is >55% and <75%
    - <55% = cerebral hypoperfusion
    - >75% = luxury perfusion, brain death or hyperemia (high PCO_2)
- *Treatment:* keep CPP ~60 (50–70), avoid CPP >70 mmHg

- **Refractory ICP or clinical deterioration (◼ Fig. 24.26)**
- *Maximal hyperosmolar therapy (HyperNa + Mannitol) dose as follows:*
  - Start: draw labs and give Mannitol
  - 2 h later: give 23% Na
  - 3 h later (5 h from start): check labs, send as STAT
  - 1 h later (6 h from start): redose Mannitol if below hold parameters
  - Repeat bolus of 23% (if Na < 160)
- *EVD vs. craniectomy*
- Lower classes of evidence
  - Mild hypothermia – treat temperature > 37.5 °C
    - Cooling blankets 35–36 °C
    - Indomethacin 50 mg q6h, not in acute setting with bleeds

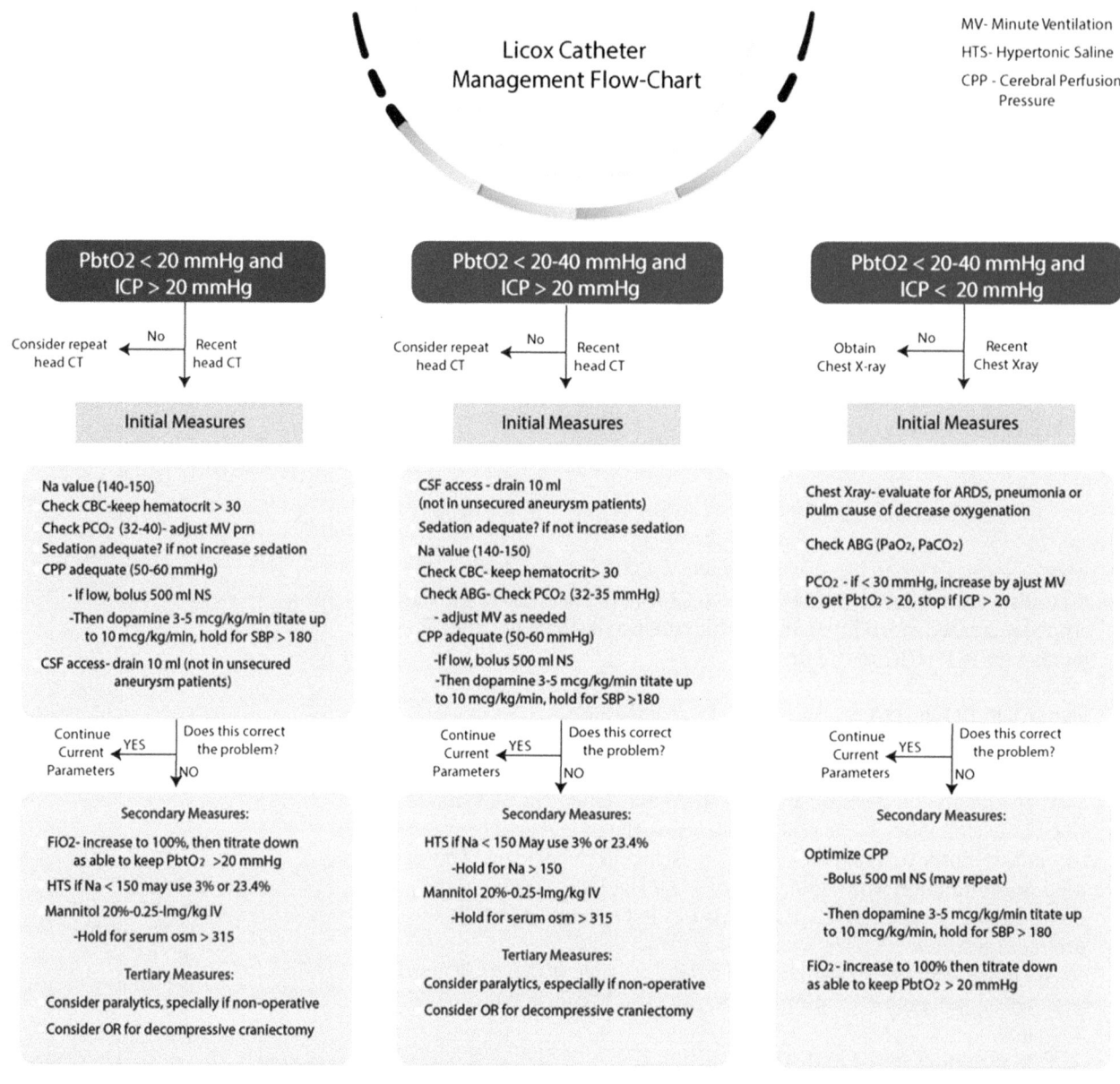

Fig. 24.25 Flow chart for management based on Licox monitoring

- Increased sedation
- Barbiturate coma
  - Pentobarbitol load 10 mg/kg over 30 min then 5 mg/kg qh for 3 h, then continue 1 mg/kg/h infiusion
  - Use continuous EEG, titrate to burst suppression
- Hyperventilation (temporary): hypocapnia-induced cerebral vasoconstriction
  - Peak impact 30 min after intervention
  - PaCO2 level 30–35 mmHg
  - *Guideline*: no prophylactic hyperventilation (PaCO2 < 35 mmHg) during the first 24 h of head injury as it can be harmful.
  - *Risks:* rebound vasodilation and ischemic injury
- Barbiturate coma to suppress brain metabolism

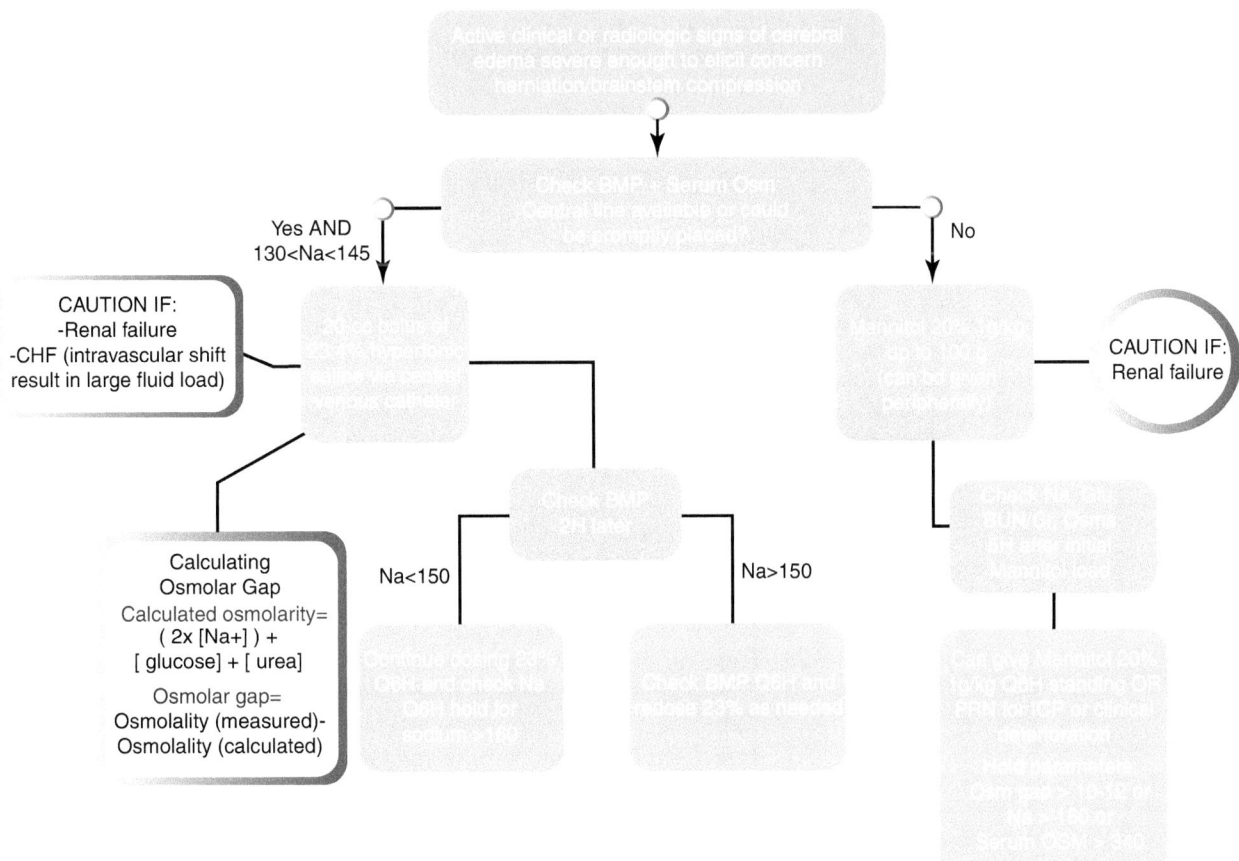

Fig. 24.26 Steps for managing cerebral edema

24.6.5 **Procedures**

- Shunt tap
- *Supplies needed:*
  - [ ] sterile gloves
  - [ ] chloraprep stick or 4 × 4s with betadine prep
  - [ ] 25 g butterfly needle with syringe
- *Procedure:*
  1. Look at the CT/MRI and the X-ray series.
  2. Determine type of shunt valve present and palpate the reservoir.
  3. Prep over the valve reservoir with a good margin.
  4. Break the seal on the syringe.
  5. Puncture the reservoir with the 25G butterfly needle, ideally at 45° angle without syringe attached.
  6. Observe for spontaneous flow into tubing, and if present, estimate an opening pressure based on how high the column of CSF rises in the tubing.
  7. Collect CSF depending on clinical scenario: about 4 cc if routine diagnostics are needed or high volume for ICP management.
  8. Send CSF for gram stain, cell count with diff, culture, protein, glucose.

- Lumbar Drain
- *Indications:*
  - Patients with CSF leaks
  - Patients with HCP

– *Contraindications*:
- Thrombocytopenia (<50,000)
- Increased ICP
  - Increased BP with widened pulse pressure
  - Papilledema
  - Change in MS until imaging studies have ruled out mass effect
- Patients receiving anticoagulant therapy
- Cutaneous infection at the site of procedure

– *Supplies needed:*
- [ ] Lumbar access kit (14G Tuohy needle, catheter, connectors)
- [ ] Lumbar drain collection system
- [ ] Four OR towels
- [ ] Chloraprep sticks ×2 or 4 × 4s with betadine prep
- [ ] Lidocaine 19% and 25G needle for injection
- [ ] Mastisol, tegaderm, metapore tape

– *Procedure:*
1. Check labs (coags, CBC).
2. Consent patient verbally
3. Position: lateral decubitus, same as for LP, 1 ft from edge of bed.
4. Prep with chloraprep or iodine prep and drape with four sterile towels.
5. Open all supplies on table in sterile fashion.
6. Numb skin, subcutaneous insertion tract and interspinous ligament well.
7. Insert Tuohy needle bevel facing laterally between spinous processes, direct needle about 10° toward umbilicus, until you pop through dura, then rotate bevel to head.
8. Have lumbar drain ready and remove stylet, if you get CSF insert LD into Tuohy needle (fenestrated, black-tipped end goes into thecal sac).
9. If you have a hard time, angle the needle more cephalad, insert as much as you can.
10. Remove needle over drain, cap the catheter (NEVER pull back on catheter – it can fracture off inside the thecal sac).
11. Mastisol all around site. Spiral drain around on mastisol and cover with tegaderm or cloth tape. Some prefer to suture down catheter along spiral tract.
12. Hook drain to collection bag. Make sure catheter is secured with tape to prevent pullout.

– *Management of LDs*
- All LDs are to drain at the level of the tragus
- Should titrate to drain 10–15 cc/h
- Avoid overdrainage as it can cause herniation.
  - If overdrainage is suspected, immediately clamp and place patient in Trendelenburg.
  - If patient is lethargic/obtunded or there is suspected herniation, slowly inject 10 cc of preservative-free NS into the LD.

■ EVD

– *Supplies needed:*
- [ ] Sterile gloves and gown
- [ ] Chloraprep sticks or betadine and 4 × 4s
- [ ] Hair trimmers
- [ ] Cranial access kit
- [ ] EVD

– *Procedure:*
1. Check labs (INR <1.3, CBC, plts 80–100 K).
2. Look at head CT. Measure distance from skull to foramen of Monroe, should be around 6.5–7 cm.
3. Consent
4. Give sedation/pain meds (0.5–2 mg versed, 1–4 mg morphine or 75 mg fentanyl for average adult), antibiotics (1 g vancomycin or ancef).
5. Position head of bed 30–45°. Tape head facing forward on the bed.
6. Placement of EVD should be specific to the pathology: if SAH, try to place on opposite side of aneurysm, or if known side of approach for surgery. If no preference, place on right side.
7. Mark out Kocher's point (10–11 cm posterior to glabella, 2.5–3 cm off midline, midpupillary line). Place EKG leads on glabella and external acoustic meatus.
8. Trim hair over location planned, leaving about 3 cm posterior for tunneling of EVD. Prep shaved area with chloraprep/iodine scrub.
9. Open cranial access kit on a stand in sterile fashion. Gown and glove, then drape with towels provided leaving midline, ipsilateral eye and ear visible.
10. Plastic drape over towels with opening placed posteriorly for tunneling.
11. Inject skin with lidocaine at your incision, down to periosteum and trocar tract.
12. Incision made to bone. Small self-retaining retractor is placed.
13. Dissect periosteum away.
14. Have nurse hold head. Affix drill bit and make hole perpendicular to skull. Feel cortical bone, then cancellous, then cortical bone. Cortical bone will pull drill in. Be careful to not plunge.
15. Carefully pierce dura (either with trocar or #11 blade). Feel that the dura has been pierced using the blunt stylet. Make sure the dura is actually pierced because passing the catheter with intact dura can cause EDH.
16. Holding EVD at 7 cm, pass the catheter perpendicular to the skull, to 6–7 cm toward ipsilateral medial canthus and tragus. Do not go deeper than 6–7 cm.
17. A pop can often be felt as the tip penetrates the ependyma; CSF flow is then confirmed.
18. Remove the stylet and advance the catheter tip for another 1 cm so the catheter tip is at the foramen of Monro.
19. Tunnel the catheter under the skin posteriorly. *Control the EVD so it does not plunge or pull out.* Use your Addison to hole up the skin and prevent the trocar from advancing too far in the scalp.
20. Cap the EVD. In SAH patients, do not let off much CSF as it increases the risk of aneurysmal rupture.
21. Close incision with nylon, purse string, and roman sandal the EVD with 3-0 nylon. Tie down at a second location with nylon (◘ Fig. 24.27).
22. Connect to collection bag and make sure you have drainage.

– *Management of EVD*
  – SAH 15–20, trauma 10 or closed

■ BOLT-Camino-Licox Placement
– *Supplies needed:*
  – [ ] Sterile gloves and gown
  – [ ] Cranial access kit
  – [ ] Camino monitor kit

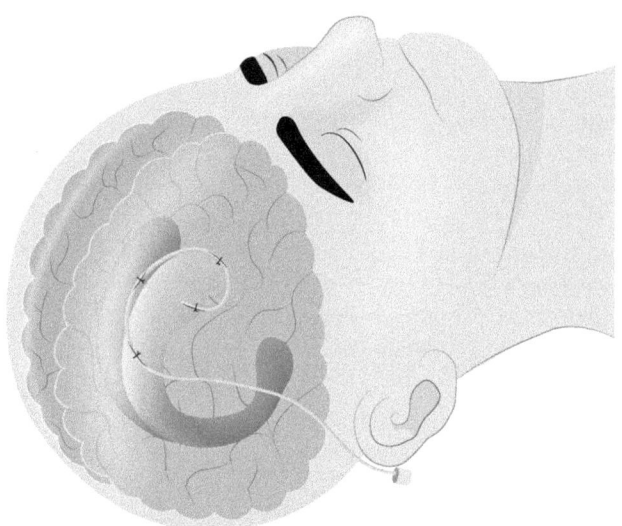

Fig. 24.27 The roman sandal technique for securing external ventricular drains (EVDs) against pullout

 - [ ] Head shaver
 - [ ] Lidocaine
 - [ ] Chloraprep or betadine prep and 4 × 4s
- *Procedure:*
    1. Look at labs (coags, CBC).
    2. Consent family if available, otherwise document as an emergency.
    3. Place monitor on the side of the pathology. If both sides or equal, place on the right side.
    4. Give sedation/pain meds (0.5–2 mg versed, 1–4 mg morphine for average adult) and local anesthetic.
    5. Mark out *Kocher's point* (10–11 cm posterior to glabella, 2.5–3 cm off midline, midpupillary line). Shave this area.
    6. Infiltrate with local anesthetic.
    7. Prep skin and surrounding area, drape with provided towels and plastic drape.
    8. Make stab incision at Kocher's point. Use provided twist drill and smaller drill bit provided with the camino system to drill until you drill through the skull. *Careful* not to pierce the dura.
    9. Screw the BOLT into the skull (make sure the stylet guide is protruding from the end of the BOLT) and tighten hand tight.
    10. Remove the guide and puncture dura with spinal needle.
    11. Connect the Camino to the monitor system and zero with provided screwdriver.
    12. Insert the Camino monitor so that the red dot is at the depth mark and tighten the retaining nut.
- Wait 1 h before reliable $P_{bt}O_2$ can be gathered.
- Must perform oxygen challenge test to ensure correct placement:
    - Turn vent to 100% O_2 for 2–5 min, if monitor is working, will see an increase in the $P_{bt}O_2$ number.
    - If no change, get CT head and troubleshoot.
    - Then turn FiO2 down and maintain goal >20 mmHg.

24.7 Consults

Here the most common consults are described including important indications for surgery, relevant RCTs and scoring systems, things to review in the chart or ask the consulting physician before seeing the patient, potential neurosurgery recommendations, and checklist for a neurosurgery admission.

- Admissions orders
- Even though you will not likely be inputting admission orders, it is important to understand what the orders will be so you can make an accurate plan and understand what you need to order when you become a resident.

- Presenting a consult to a chief

If you present a consult to a chief, follow the following steps:
1. Pull images up on a screen.
2. "Hey chief, I have a [operative vs. nonurgent] consult for you."
- Always start with whether the consult is operative so the chief is not wondering whether he/she needs to operate the whole time you are giving the story.
3. Give the one liner: "This is a XX year old M/F presenting with [symptom/mechanism of trauma] found to have [describe scan]. Exam is XX. Other injuries are XX. Labs are XX. I think we should XX."

> EPIC TRICK #2: Under "My Lists," create the following lists: "Consult Stage 1 (not seen)," "Consult Stage 2 (note)," "Consult Stage 3 (staffing)," "Cases"

24.7.1 Consult 1: Malignant Cerebral Edema ISO MCA Infarction (◻ Table 24.38)

- Diagnosis and evaluation
- *Signs of cerebral edema on CT:* low density parenchyma, decreased gray-white differentiation, effacement of the sulci and subarachnoid spaces, compressed ventricles, parenchymal herniation, vascular compression, infarction

- Management
- The DECIMAL, DESTINY and HAMLET RCTs suggest an improvement in good outcomes (mRS of 3 or less) and improvement in survival with no increase in patients with severe disability among patients who underwent hemicrani for management of malignant cerebral edema 2/2 MCA infarction.
- Should be considered within 48 h of ictus
- Patients likely to benefit from hemicrani meet all *STATE criteria* (◻ Table 24.39)
  - *May benefit from early hemicrani*: age < 82 years and meets many but not all state criteria
    - Hemicrani is offered if there is consensus among treating teams
  - *Unlikely to benefit from early hemicrani*: age > 82 years or terminal illness or signs of active herniation
- *Consenting a patient for a hemicrani:* ensure the consenting party understands the deficits the patient will likely sustain. The goal of the intervention is to preserve the patient's life, despite a probable long-term limitation in function.

□ Table 24.38 Evaluation/management of a patient with malignant cerebral edema

Steps before seeing patient	[ ] Review NCHCT [ ] Review vessel imaging [ ] Confirm received ASA/tPA [ ] Review STATE criteria [ ] Review CBC, coags [ ] Confirm type and screen sent
NSGY recs	? to OR for hemicrani ? give plts [ ] repeat 6 h imaging
Admissions checklist	Usually admitted by neurology service Confirm patient ordered for: [ ] Consider ordering: lipids, HgbA1c, Troponin [ ] Dysphagia screen [ ] Telemetry monitoring [ ] ASA (unless s/p tPA) [ ] Statin, if stroke presumed to be atherosclerotic in origin [ ] ECHO, consider if high concern for intracardiac thrombus [ ] DVT ppx (hold until 24 h NCHCT if s/p tPA) [ ] PRNs for HTN, glucose, fevers, constipation [ ] Consider fluoxetine 20 mg QD per FLAME Unless: trop elevated, h/o severe CAD, CHF, aortic dissection, hemorrhagic transformation, or s/p tPA (goal <180/105) [ ] Restart or antiHTNs in patient with BP >140/90 to target normotension once neurologically stable [ ] Treat hyperglycemia to target 140–180 Special considerations [ ] If s/p tPA: no foley, no arterial punctures at non-compressible site [ ] If s/p tPA: 24 h repeat NCHCT [ ] If severe carotid stenosis or severe non-occlusive extracranial thrombosis, consider anticoagulation [ ] If s/p tPA: BP goal <180/105 [ ] If significant edema: review STATE criteria and consider the need for hyperosmolar therapy [ ] If s/p tPA and neurological worsening: consider tPA related bleed [ ] If neurologic worsening: consider if patient has a blood pressure dependent exam

□ Table 24.39 State criteria for hemicrani ISO MCA infarction

Factor	Criteria
Score	NIHSS item 1a $\geq$ 1 or GCS $\leq$ 8 and NIHSS >15 or >20
Time	$\leq$48 h since last seen without neurological deficits
Age	18–60 years
Territory	Infarct lesion volume >150 cm^3 >50% MCA territory
Expectations	Life expectancy "reasonable" in the opinion of neuro ICU fellow

◻ **Table 24.40**   Evaluation/management of patient with ich

Steps before seeing patient	[ ] Review NCHCT [ ] Review vessel imaging [ ] Check SBP <140 [ ] Confirm reversal of a/c [ ] Review CBC, coags [ ] Confirm type and screen sent
History	[ ] Ask patient about meds, specifically blood thinners
NSGY recs	[ ] Repeat 6 h imaging [ ] BP <150–160 ? Reversal of anticoagulation ? To OR for hemicrani ? Need for conventional angiogram (young/atypical/unexplained bleed) ? Give plts ? Seizure ppx
Admissions checklist	[ ] Consider need for CTV/MRV if c/f VST [ ] Review EKG Labs to review or order [ ] Coags, CBC, BMP, LFTs, type and screen, Utox/serum tox [ ] Review glucose, aim for <185 Confirm patient ordered for [ ] Repeat 6 h scan [ ] Anti-HTN meds (nicardipine or labetalol preferred) [ ] No chemical DVT ppx for 48 h [ ] PRNs for hyperglycemia, fevers, constipation, sedation, vent [ ] PT/OT/SLP

24.7.2 Consult 2: Intracerebral Hemorrhage (ICH) (◻ Table 24.40)

■ Diagnosis and evaluation
═ Examine the patient completely so you have an accurate baseline as a reference in case the patient deteriorates
═ Determine the need for intubation, have a low threshold
═ STAT CT head, repeat in 6 h
═ Review the head CT
  – Is there a large clot that needs to be evacuated?
  – If IVH/signs of HCP, consider EVD
  – Determine if consistent with HTN bleed or other cause such as AVM, aneurysm, trauma
═ Strict BP parameters (usually <150–160)
  – Labetalol 10 mg IV q5min SBP >160
  – Nicardipine gtt if SBPs consistently high: 5–15 mg/h, start at 5mgh/h, titrate up PRN
  – Hydralazine 10 mg IV q6h (can cause reflex tachycardia)
═ Determine need for seizure prophylaxis (◻ Fig. 24.28)
═ Determine need for anticoagulation reversal
  – Decision to give patient FFP vs. NovoSeven (factor VII)/Profilnine rests on urgency of need for OR
    – In general, large clots in patients needing OR or potential OR get Factor VII/Profilnine
    – If patients are stable and clot is stable, proceed with FFP

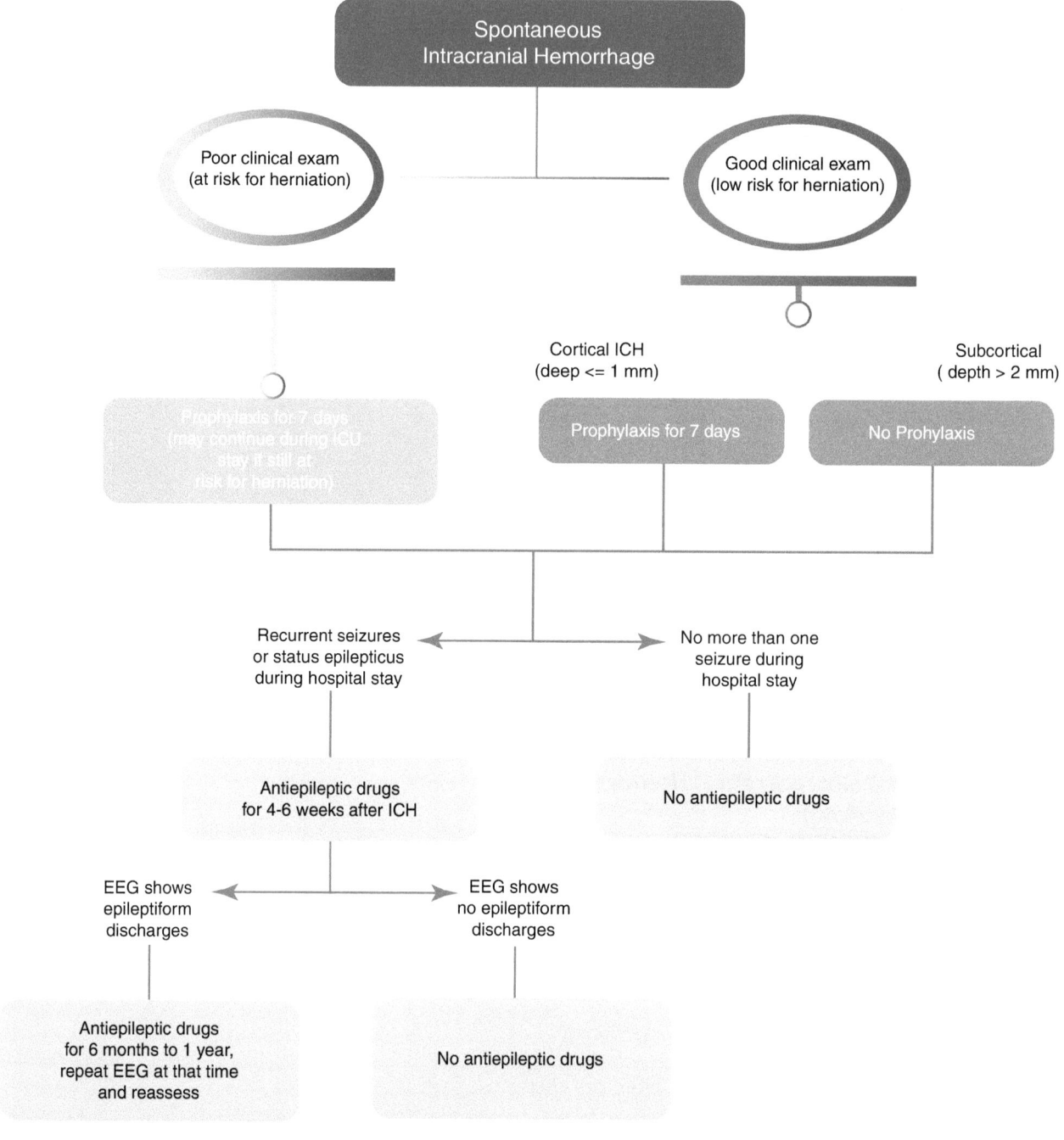

The Neurologist vol. 16:3; May 2010

Fig. 24.28 Algorithm to determine whether a patient with intracranial hemorrhage (ICH) requires seizure prophylaxis

24.7.3 Consult 3: Traumatic Brain Injury (TBI)

- Concussion
  - Most common symptom is headache. Other symptoms include nausea, dizziness, confusion, double or blurry vision.
  - Recovery from symptoms within 7 days to 6 weeks

- Neuroimaging is typically normal
- Measures of assessment include balance testing and neuropsychological testing
- Most patients will have spontaneous resolution of their symptoms with conservative measures
- 10–20% of patients will experience a protracted recovery and benefit from pharmacologic treatment, physical therapy, vestibular therapy and cognitive therapy

- Diagnosis and Evaluation of Severe TBI
- *IMPACT prognostic calculator (IPC)*
  - IPC was developed to predict 6-month outcome and mortality
  - It is based on patients in the IMPACT trial, including 8509 patients with moderate to severe TBI(3)
  - IPC includes 13 variables available at admission such as age, motor score, pupil reactivity, hypoxia, hypotension, imaging findings, blood glucose, and hemoglobin
  - The IMPACT model demonstrated a high accuracy (AUC 0.7–0.8), especially when the predicted risks of unfavorable outcomes were <80%
  - The calculator is available at: ▶ http://www.tbi-impact.org/?p=impact/calc

- Management of Severe TBI (■ Table 24.41)
- Measure ICP if GCS < 8 and head CT shows signs of increased ICP
- Position patient in full reverse Trendelenburg position (20°) and elevate the HOB an additional 10° (except in patients on spine precautions) for a total of 30° HOB elevation
- Maintain neutral neck position and avoid flexion at the hips
- Sedation general guidelines (doses given for presentations, notes):

■ **Table 24.41** Evaluation/management of patient with TBI

Steps before seeing patient	[ ] Review vessel imaging (r/o dissection)
NSGY recs	? Invasive ICP monitoring [ ] NPO, bed rest, NVS q1h [ ] PP× Keppra 500 mg BID ×7 days if no e/o seizures [ ] SBP <140, but avoid hypotension [ ] Management of elevated ICP [ ] C-collar if poly-trauma [ ] Agitation PRN so long as you can rouse the patient to examine (e.g., Nozinan 6.25–12.5 mg iv/im/po q1–2h prn) [ ] Follow up serial CT scans according to rule of 2 s (2 days, 2 weeks, 2 months post injury to look for increased mass effect). Immediate CT scan if neuro deterioration.
Admissions checklist	Usually admitted by trauma team especially if poly-trauma [ ] Consider LTM, high risk of NCSE [ ] Consider early MRI for diagnosing DAI Special considerations for trauma patients [ ] Syncope? Need telemetry and ECHO [ ] Alcohol intoxication and dependence? Consider phenobarbital, Ativan, or Precedex sedation. Thiamine, folate, MVI. Review if cirrhosis may affect medication dosing [ ] Found down? Check CK, watch for rhabdo [ ] Eval for paroxysmal sympathetic hyperactivity (storming) [ ] Fever? High risk for aspiration, low threshold for abx

- Fentanyl 25 mcg/h and titrate to optimal pain control (max 200 mcg/h)
- Titrate propofol drip to goal Richmond Agitation Sedation Scale (RASS, ► https://www.mdcalc.com/richmond-agitation-sedation-scale-rass)
- Dexmedetomidine IV drip maintenance gtt = 0.2–1.4 mcg/kg/h. Titrate q30min to achieve goal RASS
- Seizure prophylaxis
  - Keppra 500–100 g IV q12h
- Maintain normoglycemia
- VTE prophylaxis:
  - Pneumoboots
  - Pharmacologic prophylaxis 48 h after repeat CT head shows no progression of bleeding
- Nutrition
  - Feeding tube?
  - Achieve full enteral nutrition within 24–48 h of admission
- *Crash* (◘ Table 24.42)
  - Think "crash crani" AKA decompressive hemicraniectomy when:
    - Acute SDH: >1 cm thick, >5 mm MLS
    - Acute EDH: >15 mm, >5 mm MLS, volume > 30 cc or GCS <9 regardless of size
    - Bad neuro exam (e.g., unconscious and extending) in a young patient
  - If you are thinking of crashing someone:
    - [ ] Know history and exam
    - [ ] Check labs and attempt to normalize PT/PTT/INR/platelets ("coags")

High yield point #25: NOTH-ING, except polytrauma + hypotensive, should hold up a crash crani

◘ **Table 24.42** Surgical vs. medical management of TBI

	Immediate surgical intervention	Medical management
Epidural hematoma	Pts with temporal EDH, lower threshold for surgery (higher risk of herniation) Volume >30 mm^3 regardless of GCS Volume <30 mm^3 but with MLS >5 mm, clot thickness >15 mm, GCS <8, deteriorating exam, or location in low temporal regions	Pts with intact neuro exam and not meeting the surgical criteria may be observed
Acute subdural hematoma	Thickness >10 mm or MLS >5 mm, regardless of GCS score GCS <9 with aSDH 20 mmHg or fixed dilated pupil All patients with GCS <9 should get ICP monitor	
Intraparenchymal hemorrhage & contusion	IPH volume > 50 cc Progressive neuro decline, medically refractory intracranial HTN or mass effect on CT GCS 6–8 with frontal or temporal contusions >20 cc in volume with MLS >5 mm or compression of cisterns	No neurologic compromise, controllable ICPs, no significant mass effect
Posterior fossa hemorrhage	Pts with p-fossa mass effect, neuro deficit or deterioration should get decompressed urgently Mass effect = compression or obliteration of 4th ventricle or loss of cisterna If obstructive HCP, need EVD first then decompression Treatment is suboccipital craniectomy	Pts with incomplete loss of 4th ventricle, no HCP and no neuro deficit may be observed clinically
Depressed skull fracture	Open fractures depressed greater than the thickness of the cranium, involving the frontal sinus, wound contamination (i.e., open wound), gross cosmetic deformity	May defer surgery if no indications of dural penetration, no hematoma All open compound fractures should be covered with antibiotics

- [ ] Give mannitol (1 g/kg) or 23.4% via central line (UNLESS hypotensive)
- [ ] Talk to the chief about the patient ASAP – give the chief the story, exam (incl. pupils, motor), coags, medications and extent of other injuries
- Should be able to get someone down to the OR in 10 min – time is brain!

24.7.4 Consult 4: Spontaneous SAH

- Incidence of aneurysmal SAH reaches an annual rate of 6–8 per 100,000. Mortality rates as high as 45%.
- *Etiologies of spontaneous SAH*: ruptured IC aneurysm (75–89%), cerebral AVM, dural and pial AV fistula, dural venous sinus thrombosis, pretruncal/perimesencephalic nonaneurysmal SAH, cerebral artery dissection (internal carotid and vertebral arteries), rupture of an infundibulum, pituitary apoplexy, coagulation disorder (bleeding dyscrasias and thrombocytopenia), CNS vasculitis, brain tumor, spinal AVM (cervical or high thoracic).
- *Presentation:* worse HA of life, rapid onset, meningismus, LOC, nausea, vomiting, photophobia, diplopia, back pain, seizure, weakness, association with another activity (e.g., cocaine use, sexual activity).
- *Physical exam:* perform a quick but thorough neuro exam consisting of: GCS, MS, CNs, motor.
- Intubate patient if needed, have a low threshold for doing so (poor GCS, very sleepy, seizing, labored breathing, unstable BP or HR).

- Diagnosis and evaluation
- CT scan has a sensitivity of 98% for detection of SAH
- Next step is to perform CTA
  - Sensitivity of 96–99.7% and specificity of 100% for aneurysms that are 4 mm or larger
  - Tends to underestimate the size of the aneurysm
  - Can be difficult to detect small aneurysms (<4 mm), especially within the crowded Sylvian cistern
- CTA is superior to MRA for detection of aneurysm and study of aneurysm's morphology. Patients with iodine-based allergy may undergo MRI/MRA
- If CT scan is unremarkable for SAH but symptoms are still suspicious for SAH, an LP is indicated
  - When CT and CTA are unremarkable, there is a 99% chance that SAH is ruled out. 1% rate of misdiagnosis is reduced by performance of LP.
  - Xanthochromia is found within hours of ictus and remains within CSF for 3–4 days.
  - CTA is the next step. If CTA is unremarkable then angiogram is indicated.
- CTA and diagnostic angiograms play complementary roles. CTA is invaluable for detection of calcium or thrombus within the aneurysm neck and dome as well as depiction of the anatomy of the skull base.
- *Threshold for vasospasm*: diagnosed when the mean CBF velocity is >200 cm/s or a Lindegaard ratio of >6. Mean CBF >120 should be monitored carefully. Mean CBF is <120 cm/s.

Table 24.43 Hunt and hess grade

1	Asymptomatic, mild HA, slight nuchal rigidity
2	Moderate to severe HA, nuchal rigidity, no neurologic deficit other than CN palsy
3	Drowsiness, confusion, mild focal neurologic deficit
4	Stupor, moderate-severe hemiparesis or other moderate focal disability
5	Coma, decerebrate posturing

Table 24.44 Fisher scale (imaging appearance)

1	No blood detected
2	Diffuse deposition or thin layer with all vertical layers of blood (in interhemispheric fissure, insular cistern or ambient cistern) less than 1 mm thick
3	Localized clots and/or vertical layers of blood 1 mm or more in thickness
4	Intracerebral or intraventricular clots with diffuse or no subarachnoid blood

- Scoring systems (Tables 24.43 and 24.44)

- Management (Table 24.45)
- In patients with SAH, management of Airway, Breathing, and Circulation must be a priority. *GCS < 9 should be considered for intubation.*
- Decide whether the patient needs an EVD right away or can wait
  - Presence of intraventricular blood or ventriculomegaly indicate the *need for placement of EVD*
    - Laterality of EVD should not interfere with surgical approach
    - Liberal drainage of CSF is not advised because abrupt changes in intracranial and transmural pressures may lead to aneurysm rerupture. Leave drainage at 20 cm H2O prior to securing aneurysm
- If EVD can wait until the patient gets to the NICU, the following orders are made:
  - SBP <120 with IV administration of calcium channel blocker such as nicardipine or beta blocker such as labetalol
  - Keppra 500 mg q12h
  - Q1h neuro checks
  - Normalize coags
- *Imaging*: CT/CTA, diagnostic cerebral angiogram, EKG, echo
- *Labs:* CBC, BMP, ionized Ca, Mg, Phos, coags (PT, PTT, INR), blood type and screen, ABG, initial troponin level, urine drug screen
- *Consent* for EVD, angio and OR at the same time, if possible
- *Arterial and central venous catheters* must be considered. A-line is indicated for close monitoring of BP and frequent blood draws. CBC is indicated to assess volume status and determine etiology of hyponatremia
- *Statins* are likely to decrease the risk of vasospasm, delayed neurologic deficits, and mortality; they are continued *for 30 days.*
- Absence of seizure activity limits the *anticonvulsant medication* dosing to *7 days.*
- *CCBs* are administered for *21 days.*

High yield point #26: Many of the patients with SAH will require EVD. Rare exceptions will include those with low grade bleeds that are minimally symptomatic and have no evidence of hydrocephalus or those with perimesencephalic bleeds.

◻ **Table 24.45** Evaluation/management of patient with spontaneous SAH

Steps before seeing patient	[ ] Review meds. Hold/reverse anti-plts/AC [ ] Review NCHCT and vessel imaging [ ] Review EKG
History	[ ] Worse HA of life [ ] Rapid onset [ ] Meningismus [ ] LOC [ ] Nausea [ ] Vomiting [ ] Photophobia [ ] Diplopia [ ] Back pain [ ] Seizure [ ] Weakness [ ] Association with another activity (e.g., cocaine use, sexual activity)
PE	[ ] GCS [ ] Mental status [ ] CNs [ ] Motor, drift
NSGY recs	[ ] NPO [ ] Labs: CBC, BMP, ionized Ca, Mg, Phos, PT/PTT/INR, blood type and screen, ABG, initial troponin level, urine drug screen [ ] SBP <140 [ ] Four vessel angiography ? EVD if symptomatic HCP or blood casting in ventricles, drain at 15 cm H2O ? OR vs. endovascular suite pending angiography [ ] Levetiracetam 500 mg BID × 7 days (if no seizure history) [ ] Nimodipine 60 mg q4h × 21 days [ ] Statin × 30 days [ ] LTM for all Fisher 3+ or H/H4/5 patients for ischemia detection or where there is suspicion for nonconvulsive szs [ ] Daily TCDs [ ] Initial labs: CBC, BMP, ionized Ca, Mg, Phos, coags (PT, PTT, INR), blood type and screen, ABG, initial troponin level, urine drug screen [ ] EKG [ ] ECHO
Admissions checklist	See NSGY recs plus: [ ] Admit to NICU [ ] Consider arterial and central venous catheter [ ] Maintain euvolemia, normothermia, normoglycemia [ ] Aim for eunatremia. If hyponatremia determine SIADH vs. salt wasting (refer to chapter on Nephrology, for further details). AVOID free water restriction, use 3% sodium or mineralocorticoids if needed to ensure euvolemia [ ] If new neurologic decline: prompt CT/CTA, consider EVD [ ] If clinical decline and imaging suspicious for delayed cerebral ischemia initiate rescue therapies: [ ] Induce HTN, [ ] ensure euvolemia, and [ ] notify endovascular for potential directed therapy

– Optimal treatment for ruptured aneurysm is evaluated on a case- by-case basis. *Four main considerations that influence treatment options (microsurgical vs. endovascular):* (1) aneurysm morphology, (2) patient's age, medical status, presenting symptoms (e.g., HH grade), (3) preferences of the patient and family, (4) expertise of the treating surgeons/interventionalists

Table 24.46 Evaluation/management of patient with a brain tumor

Steps before seeing patient	[ ] Review imaging for MLS, reactive edema
History	[ ] Nausea [ ] Vomiting [ ] Headache [ ] Seizures [ ] Weakness [ ] Numbness [ ] Ataxia
PE	[ ] MS → intubate? [ ] Complete neuro exam
NSGY recs/admissions checklist	[ ] NPO [ ] Labs: CBC, BMP, ionized Ca, Mg, Phos, PT/PTT/INR, blood type and screen [ ] Steroids + PPI [ ] Keppra load + prophylaxis [ ] MRI spine r/o drop mets [ ] MRI brain w/navigation protocol

High yield point #27: The patient is at risk for vasospasm after SAH on days 3–14 post-injury. The critical window is 7–10 days. If any changes in daily TCDs are observed, immediately examine and obtain CT/CTA followed by angiogram.

– Regardless of treatment mode, early intervention (within 24 h of ictus) has been shown to decrease mortality rate caused by re-hemorrhage.
– May obtain angiogram on 9th posthemorrhage day to confirm exclusion of aneurysm and relief of vasospasm before transfer to floor
– Watch for rebleeding – ICPs shoot up with bradycardia and worsening of neuro exam with blood in EVD
  – If this happens, clamp EVD, CT head STAT, patient may need OR

24.7.5   Consult 5: New Brain Tumor (Table 24.46)

■ Diagnosis and Evaluation
– When the patient arrives, complete a complete neuro exam, documenting any deficits
– Assess patient's MS, need for intubation (rare)
– Look at imaging, assessing degree of MLS, mass effect and reactive edema

■ Management
– If CT shows MLS, significant mass effect or reactive edema, give bolus of 8–10 mg Decadron, continue 4 mg q6h (may be less if elderly or diabetic)
  – When ordering steroids, always order GI prophylaxis (Pepcid/Ranitidine) at the same time. ICP and steroids double the risk for ulcers.
– If significant MLS or patient is somnolent, give mannitol 25–60 g IV
– Keppra load + prophylaxis
– MRI brain w/protocol for navigation (e.g., Stealth protocol)
– *Pediatric brain tumors*: posterior fossa tumors (medulloblastoma, IPAs) often present with HA and obstructive HCP. These pts must be observed in the ICU and may require EVD.
  – If suspect medulloblastoma, obtain MRI of total spine w/wo contrast to evaluate for drop met

Table 24.47 Evaluation/management of patient with a pituitary tumor

Steps before seeing patient	
History	[] Eating and drinking habits [] Weight loss/gain [] Taste or smell changes [] Vision changes
PE	[] Visual field testing [] Signs of endocrine dysfunction (acromegaly, stria, hyperpigmentation, myxedema, proptosis, cushingoid appearance)
NSGY recs/ admissions checklist	[] Labs: TSH, FSH, LH, ACTH, prolactin with dilution, T3, T4, alpha su, estrogen, GH, IGF-1, serum cortisol

24.7.6   Consult 6: Pituitary Tumor (◘ Table 24.47)

- **Diagnosis and Evaluation**
- Thorough history including eating, drinking habits, weight loss/gain, taste or smell changes, or vision changes
- Perform a complete neuroexam, detailed visual field testing. Look for signs of endocrine dysfunction (acromegaly, stria, hyperpigmentation, myxedema, proptosis, cushingoid appearance)
- Think about apoplexy – rapid onset HA, visual disturbances, ALOC, endocrinopathies or low cortisol, hemodynamic instability
- Also evaluate for DI
- *Imaging*: MRI pituitary protocol w/wo contrast
- *Labs*: TSH, FSH, LH, ACTH, prolactin with dilution, T3, T4, alpha su, estrogen, GH, IGF-1, serum cortisol

- **Management**
- Acute treatment of apoplexy
  - 20–40 mg hydrocortisone q4hrs
  - Decadron 4q6h with 10–20 mg IV bolus ×1

24.7.7   Consult 7: Shunt Evaluation (◘ Table 24.48)

- **Diagnosis and Evaluation**
- Make sure the patient is NPO, IV, continuous pulse ox (observe for apnea, bradycardia)
- *Labs:* CBC, AED levels, electrolytes (especially if patient has been vomiting)
- *Micro:* UA
- *History*:
  - Etiology of HCP (e.g., congenital, IVH, neonatal meningitis, aqueductal stenosis, tumor)
  - At what age first shunted
  - Total number of revisions and why (e.g., failure, infection, disconnection, outgrowth)
  - Date of last revision, cause of failure, by who (surgeon's name) and where
  - Typical symptoms of failure

High yield point #28: Shunt failure can be an emergency! Do not wait on these patients if failure is suspected.

High yield point #29: If a patient says that he/she had a prior shunt revision because of infection, ask the patient whether he/she knows what the organism was. Many of these patients have been in the hospital for shunt failure multiple times and know their medical histories well.

Table 24.48 Evaluation/management of patient for shunt evaluation

Steps before seeing patient	[ ] Read op note – what type of shunt is it?
History	[ ] Nausea/vomiting [ ] Etiology of HCP [ ] Date of last revision and where [ ] Typical symptoms of failure [ ] Seizure disorder? If so, when was the last and how often [ ] Is patient having seizures now?
PE	[ ] MS [ ] CNs [ ] Fundi [ ] Incision [ ] Abdominal exam [ ] Palpate valve for refill
NSGY recs/admissions checklist	[ ] Quick brain MRI vs. head CT [ ] Shunt series ? Abdominal u/s vs. CT [ ] Labs: CBC, BMP, AED levels, ESR/CRP, [ ] UA, CXR [ ] NPO [ ] Continuous pulse ox [ ] Shunt tap ? Admit to floor for observation vs. shunt tap vs. shuntogram vs. OR for revision

– History of ventricles that do/do not dilate in setting of documented shunt failure
– Seizure disorder? If so, when was the last and how often
– Site of VP shunt
– Model of shunt
– Last known valve setting of shunt
– Why presented to ED this time and progression of symptoms over time
– Positional in nature
– Worse at a particular time of day
– ROS:
  – Fever/chills
  – Nausea/vomiting
  – Vision changes (e.g., blurry vision)
  – Sick contacts/recent travel
  – Abdominal pain
  – Diarrhea/UTI
  – Trauma history
– Medications: AC, ASA, Plavix (why and last dose), any medication changes
= *Exam*:
  – Vitals (HR, temp)
  – MS, cranial nerves, fundi (check for papilledema), incision, abdominal exam, myelo closure if MM patient
  – Have the resident show you how to palpate a valve and check if there is refill
  – Have the resident show you how to check the shunt valve setting
= *Imaging*:
  – Quick brain MRI

High yield point #30: If a shunt patient has a headache that is worse upon supine/laying down, this is suggestive of shunt underdrainage.

- Head CT (shunt protocol) if unable to obtain MRI in timely fashion or crashing patient
- Compare old and new scans for change in vent size
  - Look closely at old CT during last shunt failure – do the ventricles change in size or do they remain slit like?
- Shunt XR series:
  - Look for kinking/disconnections
  - Coiling in abdominal wall
  - Look and identify valve brand and setting
- Abdominal u/s: if suspect chronic infection to look for pseudocyst, if questionable, obtain CT
- *Labs*: CBC with differential, BMP, coags, AED levels, ESR/CRP, UA, CXR

■ Management
- If there is any evidence of increased ICP (large vents, papilledema, Cushing triad of irregular and decreased respirations, bradycardia, and HTN), patient requires an urgent shunt tap and schedule for OR stat
- Shunt tap if infection is suspected
- If after workup, failure is still suspected, admit to floor and may proceed to radionuclide shunt tap (shuntogram)

24.7.8 Consult 8: Cauda Equina (☐ Table 24.49)

■ Diagnosis and Evaluation
- Caused by large disk herniation into spinal canal causing compression of the cauda equina

☐ **Table 24.49** Evaluation/management of patient with cauda equina

History	[ ] What deficits they have [ ] Onset [ ] Progression of symptoms (how quickly it changed) [ ] Why did they come in today if they have chronic issues [ ] Pain: location, character, radiation, alleviating and worsening factors [ ] LE weakness – are they weak because of pain or poor coordination vs. true motor weakness [ ] Sensory deficits and distribution [ ] Claudication [ ] Perianal and saddle anesthesia [ ] Urinary retention [ ] Bowel/bladder incontinence
PE	[ ] Motor exam: strength exam 0–5 for all major muscle groups, make them push through paint to give maximum effort [ ] Sensory exam Reflexes: [ ] DTRs [ ] Conus [ ] Babinski [ ] Midline spine tenderness [ ] Rectal exam [ ] Post void residual
NSGY recs/ admissions checklist	[ ] STAT MRI L spine [ ] STAT PVR [ ] Labs: CBC, lytes, PTT/PT/INR ? OR for emergency laminectomy/discectomy ? Foley

- *Symptoms*: may be acute or chronic
  - *Acute*: sudden onset lower back pain, radiculopathy, progressing to LE weakness, perianal and saddle anesthesia followed by urinary retention and bowel/bladder incontinence
  - *Chronic*: recurrent back pain, gradual LBP, sensorimotor loss, bowel/bladder incontinence developing days to weeks
- *Imaging*: look for massive disk herniation into the neural canal with compression of cauda equina

- Management
- If imaging is truly concerning for cauda equina, will need emergent OR for laminectomy/discectomy

24.7.9 Consult 9: Spinal Cord Injury (SCI) (◘ Table 24.51)

- Examine the patient immediately. Determine if there are any neurologic deficits and document detailed motor/sensory exam.
- For *acute SCI < 8 h*, start:
  - *Solumedrol SCI protocol (30 mg/kg IV over 15 min, then 5.4 mg/kg/h IV for 23 h)*

- Scoring systems (◘ Table 24.50)

- Cervical SCI
- *NEXUS criteria*: patients meeting all five criteria are at low risk and don't need imaging
  - No posterior midline tenderness
  - No neurological deficits
  - Normal GCS of 15
  - No evidence of intoxication
  - No distracting pain elsewhere
- *Imaging*: trauma patients will get a CT
  - Identify type of fracture on CT:
    - Atlas (single ring fracture, Jefferson fracture), Axis (odontoid, Hangman fracture, etc.)
      - Which vertebrae? Body, pedicle, lamina, facet, TP pars?
    - Determine alignment (kyphotic, lordotic, spondylotic, jumped facets, AOD, etc.)
    - Determine mechanism (flexion/compression w/wo compression or distraction)

◘ **Table 24.50** Asia impairment scale (AIS)

A	*Complete injury:* no motor or sensory below injury level including S4–5
B	*Incomplete injury:* sensory but no motor below injury level including S4–5
C	*Incomplete:* motor preserved below injured level but major muscles are motor <3
D	*Incomplete:* motor is preserved, majority muscles motor >3
E	*Normal:* motor and sensory normal

◼ **Table 24.51** Evaluation and management of SCI

	Cervical spine injury	Thoracolumbar spine injury
Steps before seeing patient	[] Identify fractures on CT [] STAT MRI	
PE	[] Palpate and check for neck tenderness. If no tenderness check ROM. [] Motor exam [] Sensory exam [] DTRs [] Hoffman's [] Conus [] Babinski [] Bowel and bladder function [] Post void residual [] Bulbocavernosus reflex if patent is out	[] Motor exam [] Sensory exam [] DTRs [] Conus [] Babinski [] Bowel and bladder function [] Post void residual [] Bulbocavernosus reflex if patent is out
Classification	[] AO spine: upper cervical or subaxial cervical classification system	[] AO spine thoracolumbar classification system
NSGY recs	[] Solumedrol SCI protocol for acute SCI <8 h ?OR	[] Solumedrol SCI protocol for acute SCI <8 h [] Flat in bed with logroll precautions ?OR

- MRI indications: *50/50/20/neuro*
  - 50% of greater vertebral body height loss, compared to neighboring vertebral bodies
  - 50% of greater canal stenosis
  - >20° Cobb angle (measured as angle from endplate of superior vertebra to inferior endplate of inferior vertebra)
  - Neurologic deficit
  - MRI spine should be done emergently if: (1) clinical and radiographic findings don't match or (2) suspicion of a ruptured disk or epidural hematoma
- *CTA neck*: evaluate for vascular injury to vertebral arteries
  - Upper cervical fractures: occiput – C2
  - Fracture through transverse foramen (C6 and above)
  - Jumped or locket facet, unilateral or bilateral
- Report the *AO upper cervical or subaxial cervical classification*
  - AO upper cervical injuries classification categorizes based on location-specific patterns and then further subdivided according to injury type and presence of neurological injuries: ▸ https://radiopaedia.org/articles/ao-classification-of-upper-cervical-injuries?lang=us
  - AO subaxial cervical spine injury classification categorized into nine groups based on morphology of the injury. Additional features include facet joint injury and neurologic status: ▸ https://radiopaedia.org/articles/ao-classification-of-subaxial-injuries?lang=us
- Determine if this injury is urgently operative
- If locket facets → emergency → cervical traction vs. OR for reduction
  - For the neuro intact, or very mild deficits – traction starting at 10 lbs then gradually add 5–10 lbs every 10–20 min until max 5–10 lbs per level (e.g., C5/6 locked facet max of 25–50 lbs depending on the body habitus)

High yield point #31: In patients where clinical injury differs from the radiographic findings, be suspicious for traumatic disk rupture or epidural hematoma

- Get a new lateral C-spine fluoro after each time of adding weight
- If unable to reduce locket facets, set up OR for surgical reduction (NPO, labs, consent)

  — *Cervical spine clearance:*

  - Flexion/extension contraindicated in patients with acute fracture or ligamentous injury
  - Must have *negative* CT c-spine
  - No distracting injuries
  - Not intoxicated
  - If awake and alert, palpate and check for neck tenderness
    - If neck *tender*, KEEP collar in place, d/c patient and schedule follow-up in clinic for final clearance in 2 weeks
    - If neck *non-tender*, then have patient do full range of neck motions for you. If non-tender with ROM, then remove collar.
  - Clearance of comatose patients require MRI o the cervical spine (done in acute setting <72 h). Evaluate for STIR signal of the ligaments

- Thoraco-lumbar SCI
— Major types of fractures:
  - *Compression fracture*: axial loading causing compression of the anterior column (◘ Fig. 24.29). Usually stable.
  - *Burst fracture*: axial and flexion loading with fracture through anterior and middle columns, fracture through posterior wall with retropulsion of fragments and loss of vertebral body height
  - *Chance fracture* (flexion-distraction): AKA seatbelt injury. Flexion, rapid deceleration injury axially along disk space or bone (ligamentous chance and bony chance). Usually have seatbelt sign.
  - *Fracture dislocation*: flexion, rapid deceleration; usually complete disruption of ligaments with distraction and malignment between two contiguous levels.
— *Exam*
  - Quick, thorough motor and sensory exam
    - Is the injury complete or incomplete?
    - What is the level of injury based on the exam?
    - Where is the lesion on the imaging? Does it correlate with exam?

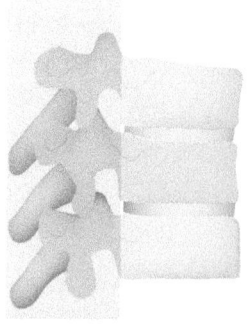 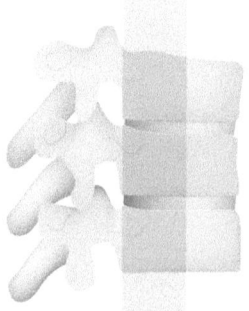 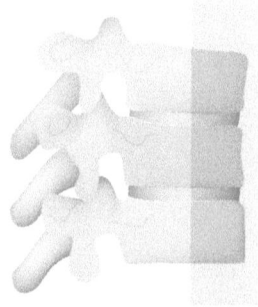

Posterior Column

Anterior Longitudinal
Ligament (ALL),
1/2 of vertebral
body and annulus

Middle Column

Posterior 1/2 of vertebral
body and annulus,
Posterior Longitudinal
Ligament (PLL)

Anterior Column

Posterior elements

◘ **Fig. 24.29**   3-column model of Denis

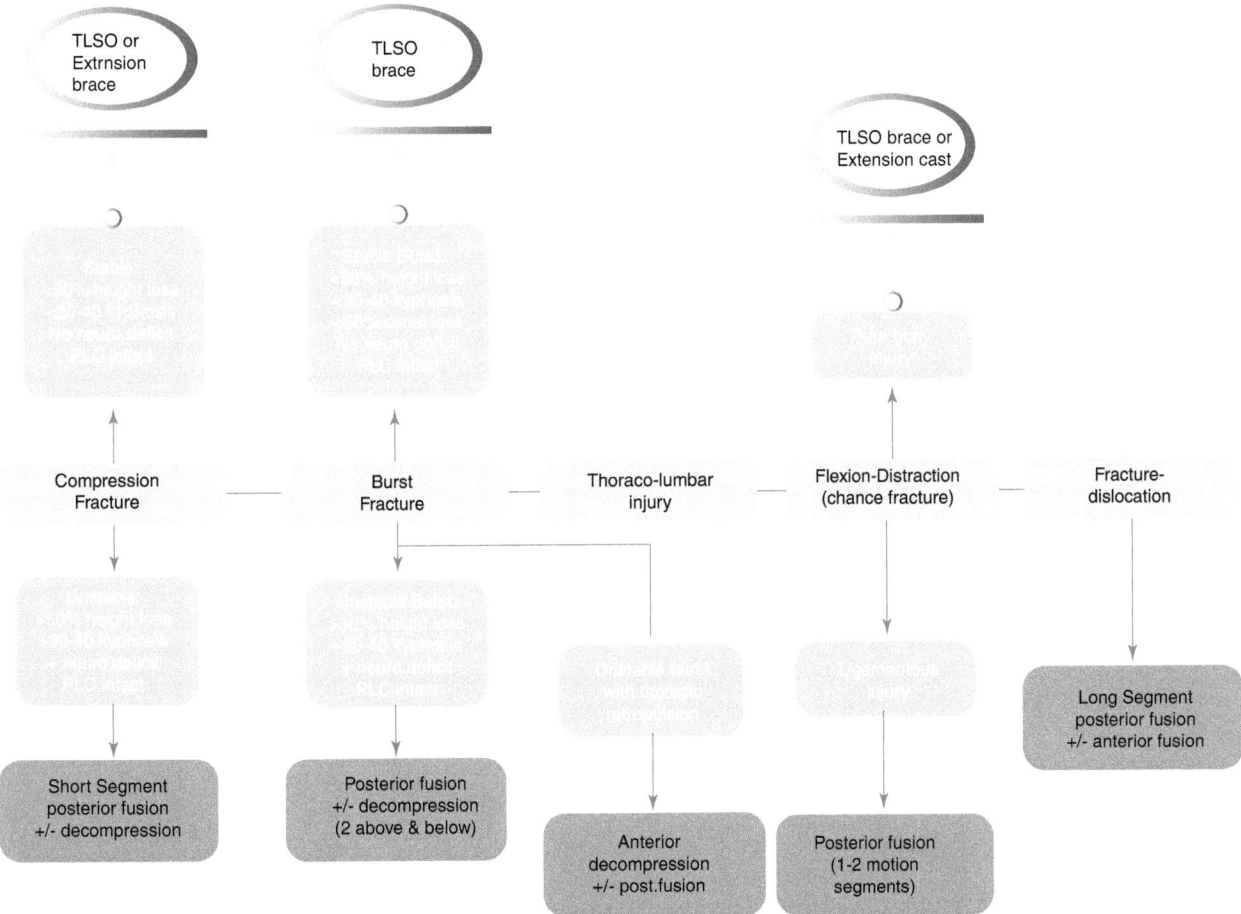

Fig. 24.30 Flow chart for fixation of thoracolumbar fractures

- Report the *AO spine thoracolumbar classification system*
  - Report the *AO spine thoracolumbar classification system* for thoracolumbar spine fractures
  - This system categorizes according to morphology of the fracture, presence of neurological signs, presence of ligamentous injuries, and comorbid conditions: ▶ https://radiopaedia.org/articles/ao-spine-classification-of-thoracolumbar-injuries?lang=us
- Order activity as flat in bed with logroll precautions
- If incomplete neurologic injury, surgical reduction is *urgent*
- If complete, less emergent but patient will likely require surgery within 24 h
- *Imaging*: trauma patients meeting NEXUS criteria will have full spine CT
  - MRI indications as above
- *Treatment* (**□** Fig. 24.30)
  - *Compression fracture:*
    - *Stable* if not meeting criteria below and posterior elements intact
      - Treat in extension brace or TLSO
    - *Unstable* compression fracture:
      - 25–30° progressive kyphosis
      - >50% loss of height or symptomatic, treat
    - Or if develop any neurologic deficits, treat
  - *Burst fracture*:
    - *Stable burst*: 2-column injury. Treat in TLSO brace
      - <50% canal compromise

– >40° kyphosis
– Posterior column intact
– Neurologically intact
– *Chance fracture*
  – Bony chance fracture through body → usually treat in TLSO or extension cast
  – Ligamentous/bony + ligamentous injury – posterior fusion
– *Fracture-Dislocation:* highly unstable, high rate of neurologic injury requiring long segment posterior fusion

High yield point #32: If bulbocavernosus reflex is negative, the patient may have spinal shock instead of complete SCI.

24.8 Essential Cases

24.8.1 Case 1: Decompressive Hemicrani ("Crash Case")

■ OR Prep

Pre-crash checklist:
- [ ] Correct patient
- [ ] Correct side
- [ ] Looked at labs, especially coags, platelets
- [ ] Consent
- [ ] Staff available/in agreement
- [ ] Appropriate imaging up: review bone fractures, air sinuses, thickness. If CTA available look for aneurysm, venous sinus asymmetry or abnormal location

■ Positioning (◘ Fig. 24.31)
- Supine, lollipops on ipsilateral side
- Bump ipsilateral shoulder
- Turn head parallel to floor
- Reverse T 15–20°

■ Pins
- May consider resting head on doughnut
- Single pin: contralateral forehead *above the frontal sinus*
- Double pins: occiput, make sure pins are securely *in bone* not in muscle

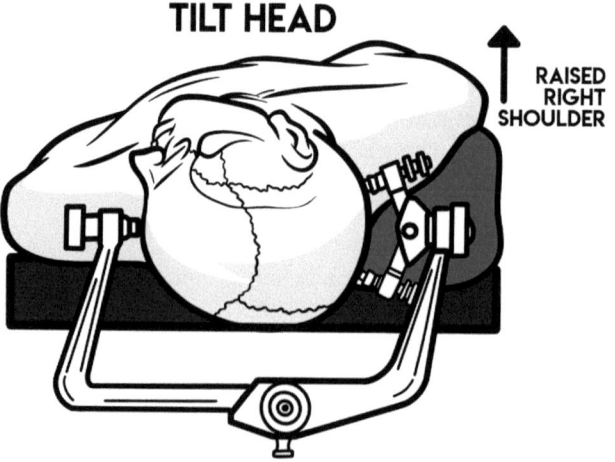

TILT HEAD

RAISED RIGHT SHOULDER

◘ **Fig. 24.31** The patient is placed supine on the operating table, secured with straps, tape, or braces and a bump is placed under the ipsilateral shoulder. The head is turned *away* from the operative site

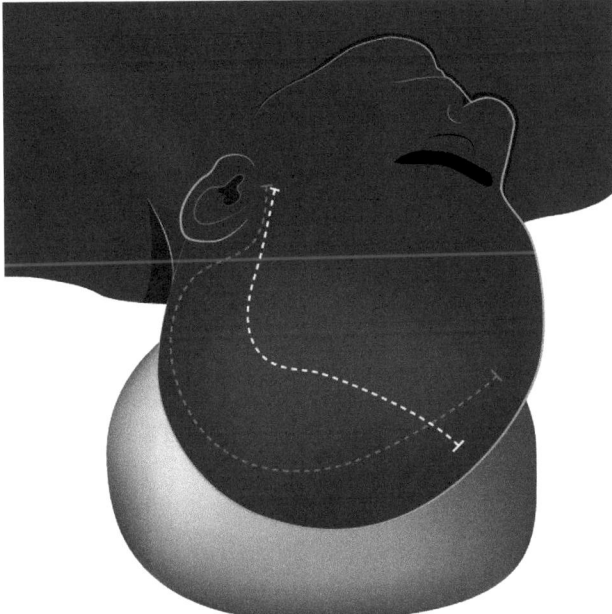

☐ **Fig. 24.32** Use a large incision for a crash crani. The purple line represents the appropriate incision. Yellow line is too small, resulting in an even smaller craniotomy

Incision planning   see Pterional cranial exposure
- Go BIG (☐ Fig. 24.32)
- Try to incorporate lacerations but avoid skin islands

■ **Field prep**
- Drape *in* midline

■ **Procedure details**
- *Skin and muscle flap:* incise to bone rostromedially sharply → incise through the galea sharply over the temporalis → use scissors to dissect over superficial temporalis fascia and incise sharply to inferior extent of the incision (try to preserve STA with the incision almost on tragus and blunt dissection around the zygoma when possible) → bovie through any remaining periosteum → apply Rainey clips generously → bovie through temporalis along incision line at root of zygoma → reflect scalp and temporalis anteriorly (dissect temporalis up with periosteal in direction of muscle striations).
- *Bone flap:* Identify the sagittal suture and stay at least 2 cm off. Place burr holes at the root of the zygoma and the keyhole *always*. Outline the craniectomy widely. Achieve hemostasis at the burr holes. Dissect dura form the bone and connect burr holes using Pennfield 3. Take bites with kerrisons at the base of the burr hole to allow better angles for dissection. Use craniotome to connect burr holes. Visualize underneath bone flap while removing to avoid tearing adhesions dura/veins. *Carefully give the bone flap to the SN. DO NOT DROP THE BONE FLAP.*
- *Decompression:* remove bone from sphenoid wing using Leksell rongeurs both inferiorly and anteriorly. Get to the floor (squamous temporal) and anterior (lesser sphenoid) limit of the middle fossa to completely decompress the temporal lobe/brainstem. *Adequate bony decompression over the lateral temporal lobe is paramount to prevent herniation.* Use bone wax to stop any bone bleeding (especially sphenoid) and plus any exposed air cells in the mastoid.

- *Dura opening:* Place dural tack up sutures circumferentially. Can be done after dural opening in cases of severe edema. The dura may be opened in a cruciate fashion with several incisions directed into the apices of the "corners" of the craniotomy to maximize exposure.
- *Hematoma evacuation:* Be gentle and use lots of irrigation. Use blunt instruments for clot removal. Just buzzing a cortical bleed with bipolar leads to more bleeding and damages brain.

- Closure
  - Dural substitute is onlayed over the dura. In a crash setting, it is not necessary to achieve a watertight closure.
  - One or two drains are typically placed along the borders of the wound and brought out through separate stab incisions to closed bulb suction.
  - Portable CT scan may be performed before leaving the OR
  - Cranioplasty usually delayed for 6 weeks

24.8.2 Case 2: MCA Aneurysm Clipping

- Relevant anatomy
  - *MCA course*: begins within the Sylvian fissure, forms a genu (right angled turn) over the limen insula, exits through the opercular cleft and terminates over the lateral convexity as superior and inferior divisions.
  - There are 4 segments of the MCA (◘ Table 24.52).
  - *MCA aneurysm locations:* The bifurcation is the most common location for MCA aneurysms, accounting for 80–82% of all MCA aneurysms. Aneurysms arising from the M1 segment account for 12–16% of all MCA aneurysms and are most often associated with other intracranial aneurysms.

- Indications for surgery (◘ Table 24.53)
  - Indications differ based on the following presentations: incidental, hemorrhagic, ischemic, mass effect

◘ Table 24.52 MCA segments

M1 sphenoidal	Begins at the terminal bifurcation of the ICA Gives rise to two branches First branch (inferiorly): *anterior temporal artery* projects along the temporal surface of the Sylvian cistern to supply parts of the temporal cortex Second branch (superiorly): *lenticulostriate arteries* divided into medial and lateral Medial: supply the lentiform nucleus, caudate and IC Lateral: supplies the basal ganglia, caudate Occlusion is associated with significant morbidity
M2 insular	Bifurcation of the MCA into superior and inferior trunks occurs at the junction of the M1 and M2 segments With a bifurcation proximal to the genu, it is possible to find lenticulostriate arteries distal to the bifurcation
M3 opercular	Originates at the insula Courses laterally along the frontoparietal operculum Terminates at the surface of the Sylvian fissure
M4 cortical	Originates at the Sylvian fissure Courses superiorly on the lateral convexity Terminates at final cortical territory

□ **Table 24.53** Indications for MCA aneurysm clipping

Incidental	Incidentally found aneurysms ought to be treated if they have an irregular morphology, recent growth or change or at high risk for rupture due to size. Based on data from the International Study of Unruptured Intracranial Aneurysms (ISUIA), MCA aneurysms have a low rate of rupture when small (less than 7 mm) of 0–1.5% over 5 years, 2.6% over 5 years between 7 and 12 mm. For aneurysms larger than 12 mm, the risk of hemorrhage jumps to 14.5% over 5 years and to a staggering 40% over 5 years for giant aneurysms (≥25 mm).
Hemor-rhage	Most common presentation of MCA aneurysm (55% of all MCA aneurysms, 34% of all intracranial aneurysms) Most ruptures are presented by SAH, up to 45% will present with an *intraparenchymal hemorrhage* MCA bifurcation aneurysms account for 87% of these ruptures, followed by 9% for proximal MCA aneurysms
Mass effect	Symptoms of mass effect: headaches, seizures, dysphagia
Ischemia	Intraluminal thrombus may lead to hemiparesis or speech impairment

- MCA aneurysms often are more effectively treated by surgical clipping than by endovascular therapy due to:
  - Relative ease of access to the MCA through the Sylvian fissure
  - Higher association with intracerebral hematoma
  - Higher rate of recanalization after embolization from the broad neck anatomy of most MCA aneurysms

Equipment microscope, brain navigation

- **OR Prep**
- [ ] Balance the scope
- [ ] Set up brain navigation
- [ ] Set up the Mayfield
- [ ] Set up the mayo
- [ ] Make bump

Anesthesia Goals of anesthesia include:
- Minimizing the risk of aneurysm rupture by keeping MAP well controlled throughout the procedure
- Provide an anesthetic environment that permits adequate brain relaxation to aid the surgeon with exposure and clipping
  - Brain relaxation is achieved by *mannitol 0.5–1 g/kg body weight* along with a *small dose of furosemide* at the time of skin incision
  - *Hyperventilation* is also commonly used to induce *mild-to-moderate hypocapnia (pCO2 30–35 torr)* further reducing intracranial pressure
    - Must also balance with hypocapnia-induced vasoconstriction to avoid cerebral ischemia
- Cerebral protection during temporary arterial occlusion
  - Requires administration of cerebral protective agent: often propofol, pentobarbitol, or etomidate to reduce ischemic complications and achieve burst suppression on EEG
- Typically accompanied by induction of a modest increase in MAP
- Prepare for induction of cardiac arrest using adenosine in case of intraoperative rupture

Positioning/Pins/Navigation/Incision planning   see Pterional Cranial Exposure

- Field prep
  - If an extracranial-intracranial bypass is being considered, the ipsilateral cervical carotid region should also be prepped and included inside the sterile drapes

- Procedure details
  - *Skin and muscle flaps:* Sufficient exposure is achieved by subperiosteal elevation of both the skin and temporalis muscle together in a standard myocutaneous flap. It is unnecessary to elevate the skin and muscle flaps separately since this procedure typically does not involve an extensive approach, such as an orbitozygomatic craniotomy.
  - *Bone exposure:* See Pterional cranial exposure for steps of bone flap. The craniotomy is completed by performing removal of the lateral sphenoid ridge using ronguers and a high-speed drill for optimal exposure of the Sylvian fissure. Exposure should provide view of the proximal and distal Sylvian fissure, inferior frontal lobe and superior temporal lobe.
    - Bony removal is taken medially to the lateral edge of the superior orbital fissure that is marked by the meningo-orbital artery
    - Inadequate removal of the sphenoid ridge will result in an obstructed view of the cranial window because of "tenting" of the dura over the residual bone
  - *Split the Sylvian fissure* (Table 24.54): Scope is brought in the field and the Sylvian fissure is opened starting medial to the Sylvian vein at the level of the pars triangularis of the inferior frontal lobe where the Sylvian fissure is typically broadest. Mobilization of the superficial Sylvian vein to the temporal side allows the fissure to be completely divided while sparing the vein. Then the surgeon must decide among three distinct approaches to

Table 24.54 Techniques for splitting the Sylvian fissure

	Technique	Advantages	Disadvantages
Distal to proximal	most common dissection of the fissure begins approximately 3cm posterior to the sphenoid wing proceeding proximally to trace the M2 segments back to the bifurcation	Allows for wide dissection of the fissure with less need for retraction. For MCA bifurcation aneurysms, allows access to more proximal M1 without exposing the aneurysm neck or dome	Obtaining proximal control before encountering the aneurysm can be difficult. Especially with the presence of a thick clot within the fissure, the early bifurcation of the dominant M2 branch can be confused with the M1 bifurcation
Proximal to distal	starts at the opticocarotid cistern and dissection continues anterograde along the ICA to the MCA bifurcation	Allows more CSF drainage to aid in brain relaxation. For this reason, may be particularly useful among patients with SAH to relax inflamed brain.	Increased need for retraction. Risk for frontal lobe or lenticulostriate artery injury.
Superior temporal gyrus	Start by making a small incision made in the superior temporal gyrus followed by subpial resection to access the MCA branches and follow them proximally to the aneurysm	Avoids dissection through a complex network of Sylvian veins within the distal fissure. Best suited when M1 segment is long. Large temporal hematoma limiting proximal access. Aneurysm is projecting inferiorly (toward the frontal lobe)	Subpial dissection leads to more tissue damage. Requires caution because the aneurysm may rupture during evacuation of the hematoma

splitting the Sylvian fissure: distal to proximal, proximal to distal and superior temporal gyrus dissections.

  - "Proximal" vs. "distal" Sylvian fissure is defined by the Sylvian point, which is the confluence of the ascending, horizontal, and posterior rami dividing the inferior frontal gyrus into the pars orbitalis, pars triangularis, and pars opercularis. The "proximal fissure" corresponds to the fissure proximal to the Sylvian point and distal to this point is the "distal fissure." Most cases need a proximal Sylvian fissure dissection.

- *Temporary clipping:* After splitting the Sylvian fissure, enough of the distal M1 must be dissected to place a temporary clip. Temporary clips have been shown to reduce the overall incidence and associated morbidity and mortality of intraoperative aneurysm rupture.

  - Curved or angled temporary clips are typically selected

- *Definitive clipping*: Definitive clipping of the aneurysm is achieved through proper clip selection (length, shape) and placement that provides complete occlusion of the aneurysm neck without compression of the parent vessel.

  - Optimal clip length 20–30% longer than the diameter of the unclipped aneurysm except in cases of multiple clips

- *Intraoperative assessment:* The gold standard for ensuring complete obliteration of the aneurysm and assessing patency of the parent and branch vessels is diagnostic angiogram. Indocyanine green (ICG) videoangiography is also often used to achieve this purpose. The fluorescent properties of ICG under near-infared light are used to provide arterial capillary and venous phases of blood flow.

Closure see Pterional Cranial Exposure.

Post-op care Standard craniotomy post-op care plus continuation of nimodipine for 21 days for all patients with ruptured aneurysms.

24.8.3 Case 3: ACDF

- **Relevant anatomy**
- *Right- vs. left-sided approach:* historically, the left side was favored because the right recurrent laryngeal nerve makes a more oblique angle after looping around the subclavian artery. Right-sided approach also puts the thoracic duct at risk; injury may cause chylothorax.
- Aberrant vasculature should be noted on preoperative imaging. Carotid artery has been shown to be medial to its typical position (lateral to the transverse foramen) in as high as 12.3% of the population.

- **Equipment**
- Scope

- **OR Prep**
- [ ] Set up the scope
- [ ] Set up the Mayfield
- [ ] Rolled towel for between the scapulae

24.8.3.1 Anesthesia
- **Positioning**
- Head is stabilized using a Mayfield.
- A rolled towel is placed between the scapulae to increase accessibility to the anterior spine.

- Incision planning
- Transverse incision

24.8.3.2 Field Prep

- Exposure
- After skin incision, the platysma can be dissected in line with the skin incision using electrocautery.
- The sternocleidomastoid, enveloped by deep cervical fascia, should be identified an d blunt dissection is carried along its anteromedial aspect.
- Finger dissection is directed medially toward the anterior cervical spine between the carotid sheath laterally and the trachea and esophagus medially.
- Omohyoid muscle may be encountered (usually at C5–6), in which case the surgeon can push the muscle either caudally or cranially.
- The prevertebral fascia can be bluntly stripped away with a Kittner to expose the medial edge of the longus colli muscles.
- Self-retaining retractor is inserted beneath the longus colli.
- Sharp dissection should halt when the vertebral body begins to slope downward to the edge of the transverse foramen.
  - Straying lateral to the longus colli muscles places the sympathetic chain at risk, leading to Horner's syndrome.
- Spinal needle may be used to confirm the proper operative levels. Placement of a needle in the adjacent disc space can lead to higher rate of degeneration, so needle may be placed in a vertebral body.

- Procedural details
- Anterior annulotomy is performed sharply with a 15-blade scalpel.
- Caspar pins are placed in the vertebral bodies cranial and caudal to the corresponding disk.
- Scope is introduced.
- Discectomy is completed with a combination of rongeurs and curettes.
- Uncinate processes are used as lateral borders of the decompression. Removing bone lateral to these structures places the vertebral arteries at risk.
- After adequate bony resection, an angled Epstein curette may then be used to detach the posterior annulus fibers, exposing the posterior longitudinal ligament (PLL) either centrally or in the foramen.

24.8.4 Case 4: Open Posterior Lumbar Laminectomy

- Procedure details
- After exposure, the spinous processes are removed at the level of decompression using a rongeur.
- Ligamentum flavum is detached from the inferior aspect of the lamina with a sharp curette.
- A Leksell rongeur can be used for the initial portion of the laminectomy.
- Removal of the lateral portions of the lamina and medial facets is performed using a series of Kerrison ronguers.
- The plane between the ligamentum flavum and the dura should be clearly identified before inserting the footplate of the instrument.
- In patients with significant stenosis, the ligamentum may be adherent to the underlying dura and associated with CSF leak.

Closure   See Spinal Closure under Technical Skills

24.8.5 Case 5: Ventriculoperitoneal Shunt Insertion

- OR Prep
- Set up navigation
- Bump underneath one shoulder
- Donut underneath head

- Anesthesia
- *Antibiotics:* Surgeon requests IV cefazolin (30 mg/kg) before making the first incision. If patient is allergic to cephalosporins, vancomycin (15 mg/kg) is used.

- Positioning
- Supine for flat and straight trajectory for tunneling the catheter.
- Head is placed on doughnut and turned opposite the site of the proximal catheter, 45–60°.
- Place bump under both shoulders to provide a straight line between the thorax, neck and retroauricular region
  - The mastoid process and clavicle should be approximately in the safe horizontal plane, facilitating safe tunneling.
- EKG leads on glabella and external acoustic meatus for palpation of landmarks.

- Field prep
- Hair is liberally clipped
- Skin scrubbed with 3% chlorhexidine solution and isopropyl alcohol before applying three sticks of Chlorhexidine
- Sterile towels and staples to position
- Antimicrobial incision drape with iodophor impregnated adhesive

- Incision
- Curvilinear incision ("hockey stick") is made on the scalp such that the incision is positioned away from the shunt hardware.
- Incision made using scalpel, deepened to level of the periosteum using monopolar cautery.

- Procedure details
- Periosteal elevator to remove periosteum from skull.
- Flap is secured back in place with a 2-0 vicryl stitch and hemostat.
- *Subgaleal pocket:* Immediately adjacent to the incision, a small subgaleal pocket is made in the plane between the periosteum and the galea within the loose areolar tissue to accommodate the shunt valve. Remaining in the subgaleal plane when creating the pocket is important to promote wound healing and reduce the risk of hardware erosion.
- *Burr hole:* See ▢ Table 24.55 for different locations of Burr holes for proximal catheter insertion. Frazier's point most commonly used for occipital VP shunt insertion. Measure 3–4 cm from midline, 6–7 cm above the inion. Use Kerrison to make the hole bigger.
- *Dura:* Bipolar the dura and sharply.
- *Insertion of ventricular catheter*
  - *Trajectory:* Insert the catheter parallel to skull base. Initially aim for the middle of the forehead. If this fails, aim for ipsilateral medial canthus.
  - *Insertion length:* The tip should be just anterior to the foramen of Monro in the frontal horn. Depth of the catheter may vary widely 4–10 cm.

☐ **Table 24.55** Proximal catheter position

	Region	Indication	Location	Trajectory	Insertion length
Kocher's point	Frontal	Common for ICP monitors	3 cm from midline, which is approximately mid-pupillary line, 1 cm anterior to coronal suture (to avoid motor strip)	Direct catheter perpendicular to surface of brain, which can be approximated by aiming in coronal plane toward medial canthus of ipsilateral eye and in AP plane toward EAM.	Advance catheter with stylet until CSF is obtained (should be <5–7 cm depth; this may be 3–4 cm with markedly dilated ventricles). Advance catheter without stylet 1 cm deeper. If CSF is not obtained until very long insertion (>8 cm), the tip is probably in a cistern (e.g., prepontine cistern), which is undesirable.
Frazier's point	Occipital-parietal	Placed prophy-lactically before p-fossa crani for emergency ventriculostomy	3–4 cm from midline, 6–7 cm above inion	Insert catheter parallel to skull base. Initially aim for middle of forehead. If this fails, aim for ipsilateral medial canthus.	The tip is just anterior to the foramen of Monro in the frontal horn. In adults, the inserted length is usually 12 cm. Use the stylet for the initial 6 cm of insertion then remove it and insert the remaining length. Keep the catheter straight during penetration of occipital parenchyma and prevent the tip from dropping into the temporal horn.
Keen's point	Posterior parietal		2.5–3 cm posterior and 2.5–3 cm superior to pinna	Pass the catheter perpendicular to the cortex in a slightly cephalic trajectory.	Will hit CSF around 5 cm
Dandy's point			2 cm from midline, 3 cm from inion		

Confidently pass catheter with stylet for 5 cm, should get CSF. Advance catheter 1 cm. Then remove stylet and insert the remaining length (usually 12 cm total). Catheters that are inserted too far may end up through the foramen of Monro and lead to functional obstruction.

- *Troubleshooting:* If CSF flow is not seen, several techniques can be sued to assess catheter position. Common mistake is to see sluggish flow and assume the catheter is correctly positioned. Lower the catheter gently or flush to remove an air lock.
- After insertion, the ventricular catheter is secured with a hemostat and attention is turned to the distal access site.

◼ *Peritoneal exposure*
- The most common exposure is a minilaparotomy with a small (2 cm) transverse incision made to the right of midline at the level of the umbilicus.
- Dissection is performed down to the level of superficial rectus fascia.

◼ *Distal catheter tunneling*
- Tunneling is the most immediately dangerous part of the procedure!
- Catheter is generally passed from the head to the abdomen.
- Most resistance is encountered in the neck.
- After the nuchal fascia is penetrated, *keep the passer above the clavicle to avoid a pneumothorax.*
- Always hold head of tunneler to avoid poking through the skin. Tunneling should not be too close to the skin to minimize future erosion.
- Avoid tunneling through breast tissue (that is "poor form").

- *Confirm distal flow.*
- Cover the distal catheter with a sterile towel once it is passed.

- **Closure**
- 1 mL (10 mg/mL) of vancomycin mixed with 2 mL (2 mg/mL) of gentamicin is injected into the shunt reservoir with a 25-gauge needle.
- Copious irrigation with bacitracin.
- Good closure of the galea is essential to prevent wound breakdown.
- Skin closure with absorbable, antibiotic impregnated Monocryl.

- **Post-op**
- Observed overnight with serial neuro exam
- Stat post-op CXR with VA or ventricular-pleural shunts
- Head CT depending on attending preferences
- Pain with NSAID or low-dose oral/IV narcotics
- Most patients discharged the day after surgery

24.9 Resources

The Neurosurgical Atlas by Aaron Cohen-Gadol, MD
- Online operative neurosurgical text that is free with registration (▶ neurosurgicalatlas.com)
- Excellent videos and text to review cases the night before

CNS Neurosurgery Survival Guide
- App-based resource
- Can also purchase a hard copy version that fits in white coat – highly recommend
- Useful to lookup as resource both before case and during consults

Neuroanatomy through Clinical Cases by Hal Blumenfield, MD, PhD
- Textbook
- Particularly useful as a beginning guide for medical students to master basic neuroanatomy
- Can review before sub-internship

Ortho bullets
- Free, online resource (▶ orthobullets.com)
- Useful to review for spine cases and consults

Greenberg
- Serves as reference to lookup protocols/management during consults
- Do not read front to back, use as a reference

The NeuroICU Board Review by Saef Izzy, David Lerner, Kiwon Lee
- Textbook
- Board-style questions, useful before neuro ICU rotation

Atlas of Neurosurgical Techniques by Laligam N. Sekhar, Richard G. Fessler
- Two operative neurosurgical textbooks – one covering cranial and other spine/peripheral nerve procedures
- Excellent review for the night before cases
- Before starting residency, useful to go through front to back

The Rhoton Collection
- Online, free for AANS members (▶ http://rhoton.ineurodb.org)
- Useful for mastering anatomy before cases
- Be sure to master The Rhoton Top 100!

Abbreviations

2/2 – Secondary
ABG – Arterial Blood Gas
ACA – Anterior cerebral artery
ACoA – Anterior communicating artery
ACP – Anterior Clinoid Process
AICA – Anterior inferior cerebellar artery
ALOC – Alert Level of Consciousness
CN – Circulating Nurse
CPP – Cerebral Perfusion Pressure
CVA – Cerebrovascular Accident
DDx – Differential diagnosis
DI – Diabetes Insipidus
DTR – Deep Tendon Reflexes
EDH – Epidural hematoma
EHL – Extensor Hallucis Longus
EVD – External Ventricular Drain
f/c – Follows commands
GCS – Glascow Coma Scale
HCP – Hydrocephalus
I/O – Ins/Outs
ICP – Intracranial Pressure
ISO – In setting of
IVH – Intraventricular hemorrhage
Levo – Levophed
MAP – Mean Arterial Pressure
MCA – Middle cerebral artery
MS – Mutliple sclerosis
OA – Occipital Artery
PCA – Posterior cerebral artery
PCNSL – Primary CNS Lymphoma
PICA – Posterior inferior cerebellar artery
Prop – Propofol
RAS – Reticular Activating System

RCT – Randomized Controlled Trials

SCA – Superior cerebellar artery

SDH – Subdural hematoma

SN – Scrub Nurse

STA – Superficial Temporal Artery

T1p – T1 weighted MRI, post-contrast

UMN – Upper Motor Neuron

UO – Urine Output

Ophthalmology

Theodore Bowe

Contents

© The Author(s), under exclusive license to Springer Nature Switzerland AG 2021
S. H. Lecker, B. J. Chang (eds.), *The Ultimate Medical School Rotation Guide*,
https://doi.org/10.1007/978-3-030-63560-2_25

25.1 Introduction

Medical students entering an ophthalmology clerkship often express the concern that they will largely be "shadowing" an attending. Medical students do not typically write notes and may not be asked to give formal presentations, leaving many students unsure of ways to stand out. However, there are many opportunities to learn, contribute, and impress. The most effective way is by being genuinely interested and well prepared (reading up on patients before clinic, knowing your preceptor's area of interest, etc.) and by asking good questions/dropping "hints" in any presentations you give that demonstrate your knowledge of ophthalmology. Most students struggle to provide a therapeutic plan for patients and end their presentation at the data gathering point. Always try to take the presentation a step further and propose a management plan.

Additionally, ophthalmology is a very visual specialty. The exam is difficult to learn and takes extensive practice to master. Avoid the temptation to confirm to your resident or attending that you see a finding that you cannot! Being honest with yourself and asking when you need help visualizing a finding will help your skills grow immeasurably. This chapter will be full of content review, so you can demonstrate your knowledge, in addition to offering high-yield tips and clinical pearls to help you shine as an excellent medical student on your ophthalmology rotation. Additionally, consider shadowing an ophthalmologist before your rotation if possible to increase your familiarity with the slit lamp, an elegant instrument used for most exams that takes practice to master! Consider checking out ▶ https://eyeguru.org/essentials/slit-lamp-tips/ for high-yield tips on using the slit lamp.

The first section of this chapter serves as a review of high-yield abbreviations, anatomy, investigative tools, and a discussion of keys to the history, exam, and presentation. This is followed by content review, clinical pearls, and information to make you stand out, organized by subspecialty to allow for targeted review.

25.2 High-Yield Abbreviations

As a field, ophthalmology relies heavily on abbreviations. Here is a list of some of the more frequently used abbreviations to help you make sense of EMR notes you read!

AC – Anterior chamber
APD – Afferent pupillary defect
DFE – Dilated fundus exam
IOL – Intraocular lens
IOP – Intraocular pressure
OD – Right eye
OCT – Optical coherence tomography
OS – Left eye
OU – Both eyes
PH – Pinhole
PVD – Posterior vitreous detachment

RD – Retinal detachment

SLE – Slit lamp exam

VA – Visual acuity

VF – Visual field

Consult   ▶ https://www.aao.org/young-ophthalmologists/yo-info/article/learning-lingo-ophthalmic-abbreviations for a more comprehensive list!

25.3 High-Yield Anatomy

It is vital to understand basic ocular and orbital anatomy in order to grasp disease processes and to think through differential diagnoses. There is great variability in the depth and quality with which ocular anatomy is taught in medical school, so consider reviewing this section for both the content review and for the clinical pearls mixed in. Practice and contextualize this section with helpful interactive Ophthalmic Figures from the American Academy of Ophthalmology found at ▶ https://www.aao.org/interactive-figures.

25.3.1 Eyelids

Eyelids are composed of skin, muscle, and a cartilaginous tarsal plate (◻ Fig. 25.1). Within the tarsal plate lie lipid-producing meibomian glands which contribute oils to the tear film. Meibomian glands can become clogged and cause eye irritation and a burning sensation from meibomian gland

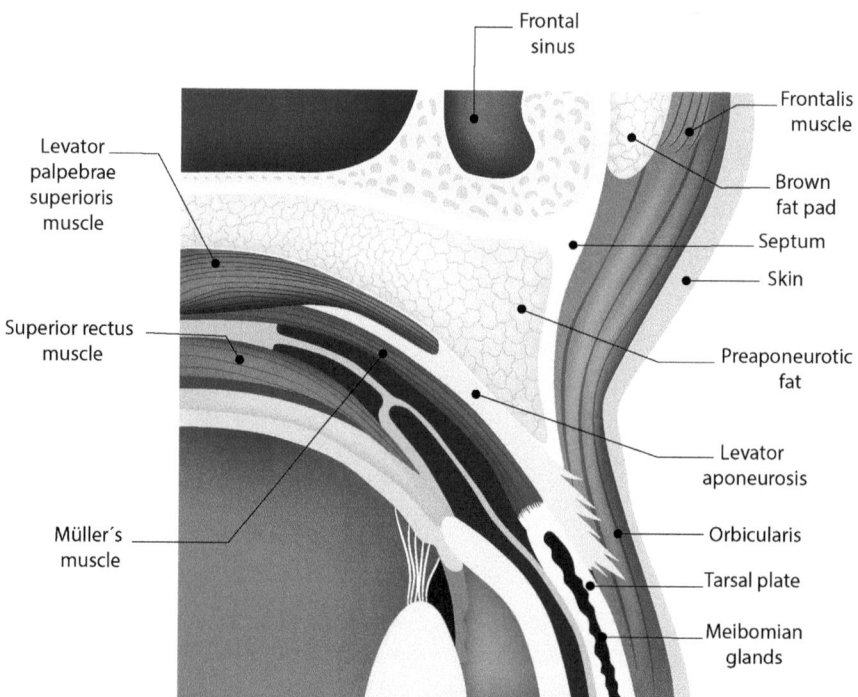

◻ **Fig. 25.1** Diagram of eyelid and orbital anatomy

dysfunction (MGD). Eye lashes grow from hair follicles with sebaceous glands. These glands can become infected resulting in pimple-like styes or inflamed in a more chronic condition of the eyelid with characteristic scaling, redness, and crusting known as blepharitis. Tears are produced in the accessory tear glands located in the eyelids and conjunctiva. The lacrimal gland contributes reflexive tears. The medial aspects of the upper and lower lids have small puncta for tear drainage into the canalicula and the nose. The eyelid is opened by the levator palpebrae (controlled by CN III) and closed by the orbicularis oculi (controlled by CN VII).

25.3.2 EOMs and Cranial Nerves

The globe is moved by six extraocular muscles, controlled by three cranial nerves. There are four recti (superior, inferior, lateral, and medial) and two obliques (superior and inferior). The lateral rectus is controlled by CNVI, the superior oblique by CNIV, and the rest by CNIII. *Memory Aid* (said like a chemical formula): $LR_6SO_4R_3$ (R = rest of them)

The four recti mostly pull in their directions. The obliques act to move the eyes up/down and to intort/extort the eye, depending on the direction of gaze. The superior oblique inserts via the trochlea (so it can be thought of as originating at the trochlea in regard to its actions) (◻ Fig. 25.2). Its effect is intorsion and depression of the eye. The inferior oblique is responsible for extortion and elevation of the eye.

The cavernous sinus sits behind the eyes, and the third, fourth, sixth, and the V1 and V2 divisions of the fifth cranial nerve run through it. This can be relevant in the ED when a patient shows up with limited extraocular movement (EOM) and sensory deficits that don't map to a single nerve. Cavernous sinus thrombosis can present with severe headache, diplopia, ptosis, and paresthesias in the V1 and V2 distributions.

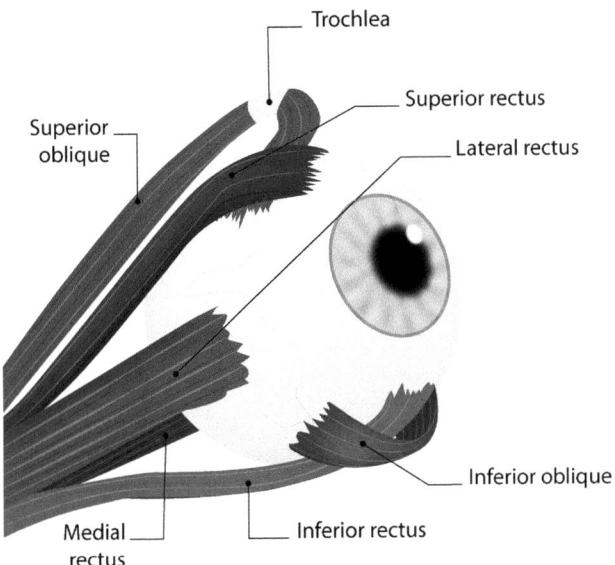

◻ **Fig. 25.2** Diagram of extraocular muscles

25.3.3 Globe

The globe ("eye ball") is surrounded by an outer wall of white collagenous tissue called the sclera. This layer is continuous with the optic nerve sheath posteriorly and the clear cornea anteriorly. The sclera is 0.3 mm thick in most places and is thinnest at the muscle insertions (0.1 mm) (upon blunt force trauma it is most likely to rupture there, at the equatorial pole behind the insertions of the recti muscles).

The globe is separated into three chambers; anterior, posterior, and vitreous (☐ Fig. 25.3). The anterior and posterior chambers are separated by the colored, muscular iris. They are both filled with nutrient-rich aqueous humor. The posterior chamber is separated from the vitreous cavity by the clear lens and its supporting zonules. The vitreous cavity makes up the largest volume and is filled with a gel-like collagenous material called vitreous humor.

25.3.4 Conjunctiva/Sclera

The conjunctiva is the clear "skin" of the eye that overlies the white, tough sclera. Between the conjunctiva and sclera, there is another connective tissue layer called *Tenon's capsule*. The conjunctiva can become inflamed in conjunctivitis, secondary to bacterial, viral, allergic, or chemical etiologies. The sclera can become inflamed in scleritis or episcleritis from rheumatological, infectious, or idiopathic processes. The conjunctiva terminates at the limbus, which is the outer edge of the cornea.

25.3.5 Cornea

The cornea is the clear "window" of the eye. It provides ~66% of the eye's refractive (light-bending/focusing) power, with the lens providing the remaining ~33%. There are five layers of the cornea: epithelium (very well innervated and with excellent regenerative capacity – which explains why a corneal abrasion is so painful but heals so quickly), Bowman's layer, stroma (90% of the cornea's thickness), Descemet's membrane (which can become visibly folded when the cornea is edematous), and endothelium (this *single-cell thick* layer is

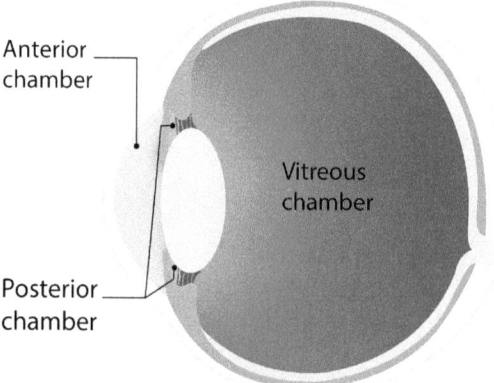

☐ **Fig. 25.3** The three chambers

vital for keeping the cornea dehydrated and clear). *Memory aid:* **B**owman is a**B**ove, **D**escemet is **D**eep. The cornea becomes cloudy when it is edematous and swollen with aqueous humor. It is the job of the endothelial cells to pump this fluid out of the cornea. The endothelial cells can die or undergo damage in several ways (commonly from trauma during surgery or endothelial corneal dystrophies). Sometimes, cataract surgery may be followed by corneal edema due to the high ultrasound energy usage damaging these cells (resolved by better phacoemulsification machines and the use of shock-absorbing viscoelastic material).

Corneal transplants are often needed to restore sight to patients with corneal scarring, corneal edema, or those who with advanced corneal dystrophies. The transplants can be full thickness (penetrating keratoplasty, "PK") or partial thickness (Descemet stripping endothelial keratoplasty, "DSEK," or Descemet membrane endothelial keratoplasty, "DMEK").

At the edge of the cornea internally lies the angle where the cornea and the iris meet. This area requires a special lens called a gonioscope to visualize. The gonioscope is necessary because the location is otherwise invisible due to total-internal reflection – a concept you might recall from physics. This angle is where the aqueous humor leaves the eye, via the trabecular meshwork and Schlemm's canal. Obstruction of this angle limiting aqueous outflow causes angle-closure glaucoma.

25.3.6 Uvea

The uvea is composed of three, contiguous structures: the iris, the ciliary body, and the choroid. The iris is the muscular "aperture" of the eye, contracting and relaxing due to light stimulation, neuroendocrine signals, or during accommodation. The ciliary body lies out of sight, behind the iris. It produces the aqueous humor that fills the posterior and anterior chambers and is the attachment point for the zonules – string-like structures which hold the lens capsule in place and play a role in changing the lens's shape during accommodation. The uveal structures can become inflamed, in a condition called uveitis, secondary to many etiologies discussed later.

25.3.7 Lens

The lens is a proteinaceous, clear, light-focusing structure of the eye that lies behind the iris. It has three layers: the capsule (a thin bag), the cortex, and the harder, central nucleus. It can be helpful to picture this as a peanut M&M. Cataracts, or clouding of the lens, can occur in various locations and are named for where they occur. The lens is suspended by the zonules, behind the iris, and provides ~33% of the eye's refractive power (◘ Figs. 25.4 and 25.5). When the ciliary body contracts (moving inward with the contracting iris), the bungee cord-like zonules release tension on the lens capsule (their origin, the ciliary body, and their insertion, the lens capsule move closer together). This allows the lens to "round out" and increase in refractive power. This is part of the mechanism in accommodation.

When we age, our lens becomes less flexible and isn't able to change shape when the zonules release tension. Therefore, we are unable to change our focusing power to see near objects, a condition called presbyopia – requiring older folks (or anyone with an intraocular lens implant, which has a fixed focal length) to use reading glasses in order to properly focus on near objects.

T. Bowe

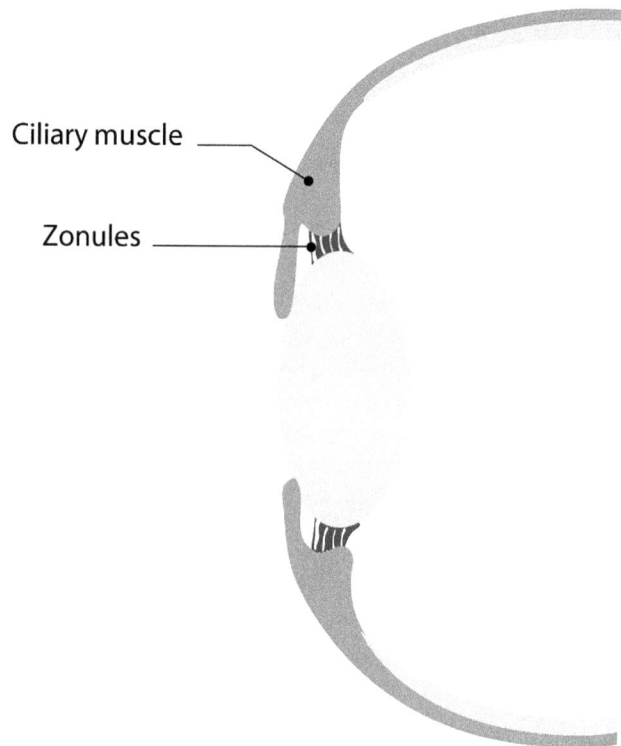

Fig. 25.4 The suspensory zonules and the ciliary muscle

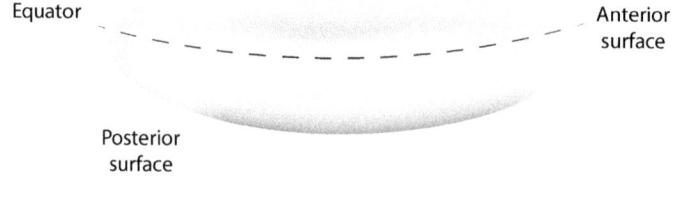

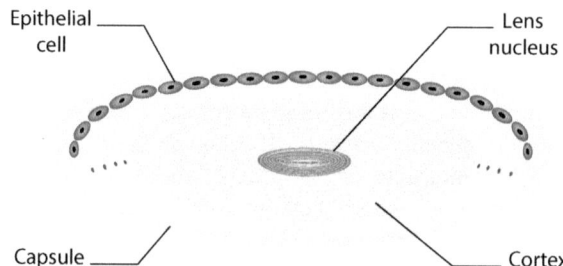

Fig. 25.5 Cross-sectional diagram of the lens

25.3.8 Vitreous

The vitreous cavity is filled with the jellylike vitreous humor. As we age, the vitreous can liquefy and collapse on itself, causing "floaters" in the patient's field of vision. When the edge of the vitreous separates from the retinal surface, it is called a posterior vitreous detachment (PVD). This usually happens acutely during middle age, and patients may see flashing lights and new floaters. The vitreous is attached relatively securely on the optic disc, and when the vitreous pops off the optic disc during formation of the PVD, you can sometimes see the ring of collagen where the vitreous edge was previously attached to the optic disc, called the *Weiss ring*. In the course of PVD formation, the vitreous can pull on the retina to cause a retinal tear and subsequent retinal detachment. The differential diagnosis for the chief complaint "floaters" will be discussed in depth later. In other disease processes with neovascularization, blood vessels can grow from the retina into the vitreous resulting in traction and increased likelihood of retinal detachment or vitreous hemorrhage.

Surgical removal of the vitreous (vitrectomy – see ◘ Fig. 25.34 in "Retina") is a common surgery performed by vitreoretinal surgeons for a variety of indications including retinal detachment and vitreous hemorrhage.

25.3.9 Retina

The retina lines the inside of the globe and is the neurosensory layer of the eye. The macula is the area of highest-resolution visual acuity and is densely packed with both rods and cones. It sends information to the brain via ganglion cells, which come together and exit the eye via the optic nerve. The retina is nourished by two blood supplies. The inner 2/3 of the retina (closest to the vitreous) gets its blood supply from the retinal vasculature, branching from the central retinal artery, which enters the eye within the optic nerve. The blood supply of the outer retina and macula (including the photoreceptors – light-sensitive rods and color-sensitive cones) comes from the underlying choroid (supplied by the long and short posterior ciliary arteries). When the neurosensory retina detaches due to a pathologic process, it is separated from the retinal pigment epithelium. *While the retinal vasculature continues to supply the inner retinal layers, the photoreceptors are damaged if not reattached in time.*

25.3.10 Optic Nerve/Disc

The optic nerve, central retinal artery, and central retinal vein enter the eye at the optic disc. There is a natural cup slightly off center of the optic disc. The vessels exit the disc on the nasal aspect and the macula is temporal to the optic disk (knowing this allows you to deduce which eye is depicted in an unlabeled fundus photo). The "cup-to-disc ratio" (◘ Fig. 25.6) is monitored for glaucoma patients as increases in this ratio are predictive of worsening disease. Examination of the optic disc also focuses on the sharpness of the disc edges (sharp? evidence of papilledema?) and the color of the disc (pallorous? hyperemic?).

25.3.11 Orbit

There are seven bones that make up the orbit: the frontal, zygoma, maxilla, sphenoid, ethmoid, lacrimal, and palatine. The maxilla is the most clinically relevant. It makes up the medial aspect of orbital floor, which can fracture in traumatic injury. If it does, the fracture can create a "trap door" that opens (especially common in kids), entrapping a portion of the orbital tissue and/or the inferior rectus, thereby restricting EOM (remember – this may also cause injury to CN V2, leading to numbness above the upper lip). This is evaluated

Small   Mid   Large

Rim of Nerve Tissue

Central Cup

Blood Vessels

C/D: 0.3   C/D: 0.5   C/D: 0.8

◻ **Fig. 25.6** Depiction of various cup to disc ratios

by clinical exam and CT scan and can require surgical intervention to avoid death of the muscle and to reestablish free movement of the eye. Large fractures are also repaired to prevent the eye from having a sunken in appearance and associated double vision.

25.4 History, Exam, and Presentation

As in most fields of medicine, obtaining a good history of the presenting complaint is essential to providing optimal care for the patient. Consider using a mnemonic you are comfortable with and likely employed in the past in order to be thorough (e.g., *OPQRST* – onset, provocation/palliation, quality, radiation, severity, timing). All of these questions can lead to insights that steer you towards or away from a particular etiology. If this is a new patient, be sure to take a gathered past medical/surgical/ocular/family/meds/allergies/social history (e.g., "have you ever had an eye surgery/needed to see an ophthalmologist/ taken any medicines for your eyes/had any trauma to your eyes, any eye diseases in the family, anyone blind/low vision/take drops, are you on any meds/ drops, allergic to anything, what do you do for work – if relevant – do you use appropriate eye protection). If the patient says yes to any of these, be sure to gather more information. For instance, if the patient says they remember a grandmother being blind, ask if they know why. If not, see if you can tease out the etiology with questions about timing (was she always blind or only in later life? Gradually developed worse vision or sudden onset? Was it fixed with an operation? The answers to these questions might point to a wide variety of etiologies such as glaucoma, numerous childhood blindness etiologies, retinal detachment, or cataracts).

Consider checking out ▶ https://timroot.com/history-and-physical-of-the-eye-video for a high-yield video review of this topic.

For the review of systems, consider asking patients about the following concerning signs or symptoms:

- New-onset vision loss (permanent or transient episodes), flashes of lights, or floaters
- Eye pain or redness
- Change in visual acuity
- Diplopia (double vision) or ophthalmoplegia (weakness or paralysis of one or more extraocular muscles)
- Metamorphopsia (distortion of straight lines that can be a sign of macular pathology)
- Proptosis (eye bulging)
- Nystagmus
- Headaches, scalp tenderness

When evaluating a patient in the clinic or the emergency room, after taking a history, gather the "vitals of the eye": vision, pressure, and pupils. If the visual acuity is decreased, see if looking through a pinhole improves it (improvement with pinhole points to a refractive problem). Test confrontational visual fields and extraocular movements. For most patients you would then move on to the slit lamp exam. This exam should be performed in the same order every time: external structures, lids and lacrimation, conjunctiva and sclera, cornea, anterior chamber, iris, lens, vitreous, retina (abbreviated: EXT, L/L, C/S, K, A/C, iris, lens, Vit).

25.4.1 External Structures

A holistic external exam is the first step. Here you are looking for evidence of proptosis (extrusion of the eyes), ptosis (drooping of the eyelids), discoloration/bruising of the surrounding skin, or any other abnormalities. If you have concern for infection (e.g., conjunctivitis, cellulitis) assess preauricular, mandibular, and mental lymph nodes.

25.4.2 Lids and Lacrimation

Inspection of the lid position and lid margin can shed light on common etiologies that bring patients to the ophthalmologist. Diffuse edema or erythema could point to an allergic etiology or infection. Localized swelling could point to a stye or chalazion. Blepharitis can be diagnosed by visualizing "scruff" around the base of the hair follicles of the eyelid margin, as well as by eyelid margin telangiectasias and thickening. By pressing on the eyelid margin with a Q-tip, you can evaluate for clogged meibomian glands – if the lipid-rich secretions do not flow out freely, this may be a sign of meibomian gland dysfunction.

25.4.3 Conjunctiva and Sclera

Conjunctivitis is often apparent on exam. The four main causes of conjunctivitis are bacterial, viral, allergic, or chemical. A "Differentiating the Differential" box later in this chapter will discuss the exam findings of conjunctivitis due to each of these etiologies. Scleritis or episcleritis is distinguished by red, injected vessels deep to the relatively clear conjunctiva.

25.4.4 Cornea

Examining the cornea is best approached with a thin beam of light angled obliquely at the cornea to allow for greater depth perception. Corneal ulcers appear as whitish patches on the surface, although more advanced cases may penetrate deeper into the cornea. If a fluorescein dye is applied to the ocular surface and the light source is switched to blue, defects in the epithelium will become much more apparent at the slit lamp. If the cornea is edematous, the cornea will look swollen and cloudy. Another characteristic finding of corneal edema is folding of the Descemet's membrane, referred to as Descemet's folds (◘ Fig. 25.7).

25.4.5 Anterior Chamber

The anterior chamber is also best examined with the light at an angle. It can contain many findings based on the pathology, including red blood cells (hyphema) or white blood cells (hypopyon). While there can be layering of these cells in the anterior chamber inferiorly, an appreciable layer of WBCs or RBCs may not be seen if there is insufficient quantity of cells or if the patient hasn't kept their head still (effectively "shaking up the snow globe"); cells may still be seen floating in the anterior chamber. The beam length should be shortened and positioned obliquely to the eye to appreciate cells floating in the AC. The cells will be seen as white or red specs floating between the entrance of the beam (on the cornea) and the back of the beam (on the iris). This is analogous to looking up in a movie theater and seeing dust floating in the light coming from the projector. The phrase "cell & flare" has a specific meaning as an ophthalmology exam finding. "Cell" refers to inflammatory cells, while "flare" refers to the foggy appearance of protein that has leaked from inflamed vessels (◘ Fig. 25.8).

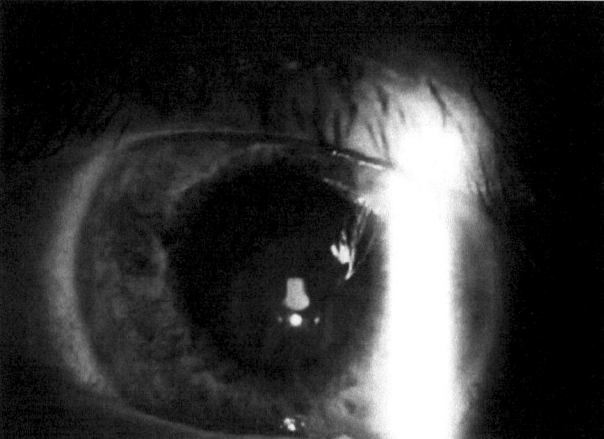

◘ **Fig. 25.7** Anterior segment photograph of corneal edema with notable Descemet's folds. (From "A Review of Corneal Endothelitis and Endotheliopathy: Differential Diagnosis, Evaluation, and Treatment" PMID: 30859513)

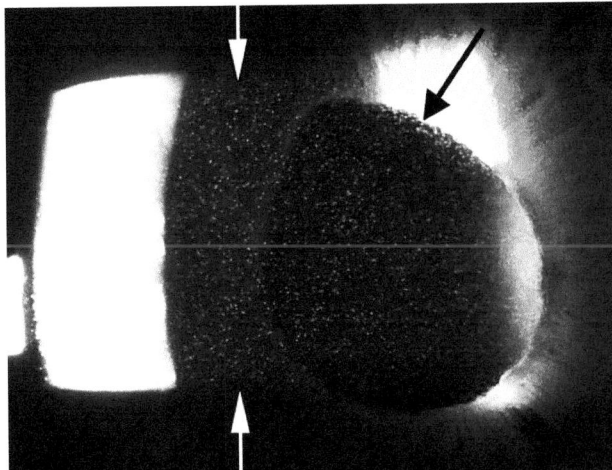

■ **Fig. 25.8** "Cell and flare" seen in the anterior chamber of an eye with acute iritis. Between the white arrows is hazy aqueous fluid and suspended white cells. (From "The Columbia Guide to Basic Elements of Eye Care pp 27-36" ISBN: 978-3-030-10885-4)

25.4.6 Iris

Patients with diseases that increase VEGF production (like diabetic retinopathy and retinal vein occlusions) may have neovascularization of the iris (NVI) and/or neovascularization of the angle (NVA). NVA is a risk factor for glaucoma as a result of vessels growing into the trabecular meshwork causing decreased drainage of aqueous humor. This type of glaucoma is called neovascular glaucoma.

25.4.7 Lens

The lens is typically evaluated for cataract or occasionally for positioning (displaced down and in homocystinuria or up and out in Marfan syndrome). Cataracts are named for what portion of the lens they occur in (nuclear sclerotic, cortical, or posterior subcapsular). Advanced nuclear sclerosis appears as a yellowish browning ("brunescence") of the lens. Cortical cataracts appear as a spoke pattern when light is directed perpendicularly at the cataract. Posterior subcapsular cataracts can appear as grains of sand or a sheetlike opacity at the back of the capsule (see ▶ Sect. 25.7 subsection for photos).

25.4.8 Vitreous

Vitreous can be clouded by red blood cells from a vitreous hemorrhage or more rarely white blood cells from an infection of the eye (endophthalmitis) or inflammation (posterior uveitis). As mentioned previously, posterior vitreous detachments (PVDs) can be visualized as gray, congealed strands of vitreous humor, and the most easily seen form is the Weiss ring. Pathologic states can cause friable blood vessels to grow off of the retina into the vitreous, and these can also be visualized during the exam.

25.4.9 Retina

The retina is the final portion of the slit lamp exam. It requires the use of a handheld lens (e.g., a 90-diopter lens) in addition to the slit lamp. Four areas of the retina should be visualized and examined for pathology at the slit lamp. First is the *optic disc*. As mentioned previously the cup-to-disc ratio should be estimated and the symmetry or lack thereof between fellow eyes should be noted. Make sure there is no papilledema (swelling of the optic disc), or disc pallor (white coloration of the disc indicating axonal death). Then the *macula*, the area responsible for central vision, should be examined for edema, hemorrhage, drusen (yellow dots seen in age-related macular degeneration – ◻ Fig. 25.9), or other abnormalities. *Vessels* should be examined for signs of pathology; examples of these that will be discussed later in this chapter include arteriovenous nicking, flame hemorrhages, cotton-wool spots from diabetes and hypertension, etc. (◻ Fig. 25.10). Finally, the *periphery* should be examined for evidence of degeneration, tears, or other abnormalities. Many ophthalmologists use the indirect ophthalmoscope for the peripheral retinal exam, and this requires a larger lens such as the 20D lens (check out this link for some great tips – ▸ https://eyeguru.org/essentials/indirect-ophthalmoscope-tips/). The retina exam is technically challenging, but keep practicing, and remember to line up all the elements of the exam: there should be a straight line between your eye, lens, and the patient's eye.

An epiretinal membrane is a clear fibrous membrane that can develop on the surface of the retina. While usually innocuous, it can contract and cause traction on the retinal surface with subsequent distortion of vision because the retina needs to be perfectly smooth. An epiretinal membrane can be visualized on fundus exam and confirmed with optical coherence tomography (OCT) (refer to ◻ Fig. 25.28 in ▸ Sect. 25.12 subsection of this chapter). These membranes can be peeled off during retinal surgery. OCT is essential in diagnosing many macular diseases, including age-related macular

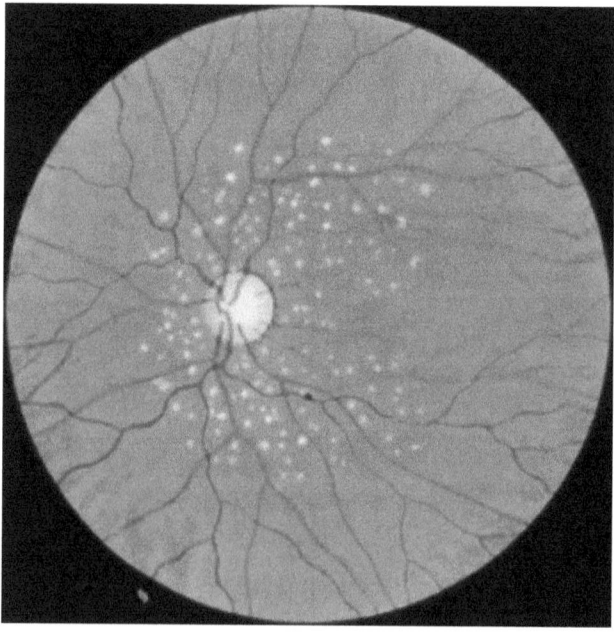

◻ **Fig. 25.9** Drusen in an eye with an unrelated macular disorder. (From "OCT in the Management of Diabetic Macular Edema")

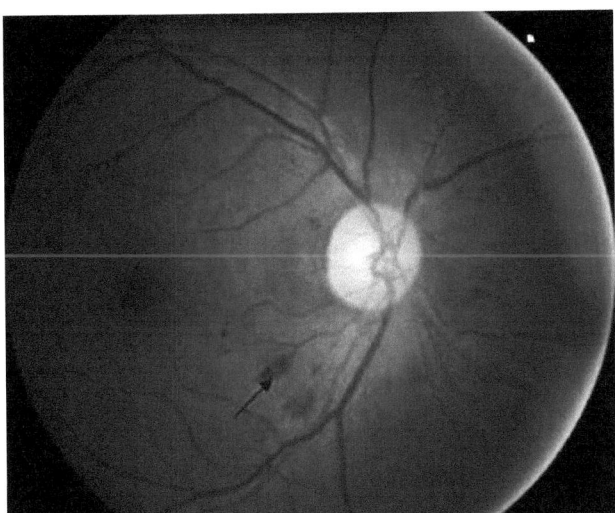

◨ **Fig. 25.10** Arteriovenous nicking, flame-hemorrhage (arrow), and dot blot hemorrhages in an eye with moderate retinopathy. (From "How does hypertension affect your eyes?" PMID: 21509040)

degeneration, diabetic macular edema, macular hole, and many others. It would be useful to study what a normal OCT looks like, and some common macular disorders (See "High-Yield Investigative Tools" for a description, resources, and images).

As mentioned previously, ophthalmology is a very visual specialty. During an exam, you might see something strange that you don't have the vocabulary to describe precisely. Don't be afraid to be candid about what you see (or what you don't see!). As long as you are honest and trying to improve with every exam, most attendings will view your attempts favorably.

When presenting your first patient, it is important to ask for expectations as they will vary from attending to attending. It would be very unusual for them to request a medicine-style, exhaustive presentation. Short presentations with only pertinent details are most often requested. These can be challenging as deciding what is pertinent can be difficult for a beginner. In many sections of this chapter, we have included sample presentations for common patient complaints that might be useful to review. Generally, they follow the template of who (with relevant info), new patient or established, their problem/the history, what is currently being done for the problem, what the status of the problem is by your history and exam, and what you think next steps should be. Remaining concise is key, but there is often an opportunity to add a sentence in the next steps section to demonstrate your knowledge and depth of your thinking about the patient's problem.

25.5 High-Yield Investigative Tools and Resources for In-Depth Orientation

- *Hertel exophthalmometer* – a tool used to measure the axial positions of the eyes, useful for evaluating for proptosis. Getting these measurements is often referred to as getting "Hertels."
- *Corneal topography* (◨ Fig. 25.11) – a graphical display of the curvature and thickness of the cornea used to evaluate for many corneal diseases discussed later. Check out ▶ https://eyeguru.org/essentials/corneal-topography/.

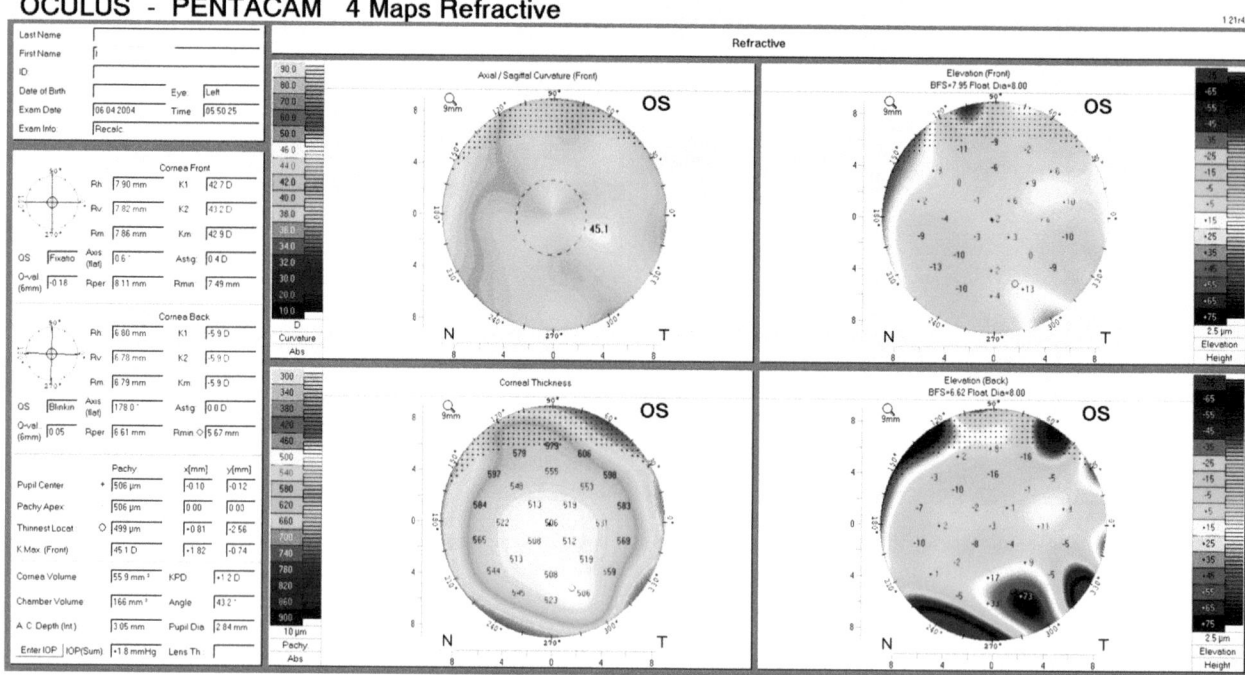

■ **Fig. 25.11** A readout of a Pentacam topography of a patient with mild keratoconus. (From Advanced Surface Ablation in Mild (Fruste) Keratoconus: A Case Report" PMID: 32323165)

- *Slit lamp* – as mentioned before, practice, practice, practice. Consult ► https://eyeguru.org/essentials/slit-lamp-tips/ for some tips and orientation.

- *Indirect ophthalmoscope* – as mentioned before, this tool allows for a much better view of the retina than can be obtained by direct ophthalmoscopy. An excellent resource to review before attempting this difficult-to-master skill can be found at ► https://eyeguru.org/essentials/indirect-ophthalmoscope-tips.

- *Optical coherence tomography (OCT)* (■ Fig. 25.12) - is a commonly employed technique to get in vivo, cross-sectional images of the pre-retinal vitreous, the layers of the retina, and the choroid. It can be thought of to be similar to an ultrasound (and findings are described in the same manner – hyper-/hypo-*reflective*). Check out ► https://eyeguru.org/essentials/interpreting-octs/.

- *Fluorescein angiography* (■ Fig. 25.13) – an imaging technique that uses an injectable dye that fluoresces when illuminated by blue light which allows for detailed investigations into the structure and function of the retinal vessels (the dye cannot permeate through intact, healthy endothelial cells, which allows for excellent visualization of defects!) Consult ► https://eyeguru.org/essentials/fluorescein-angiography/ for a detailed review.

- *Visual fields* (■ Fig. 25.14) – a visual field analysis is vital in the evaluation and monitoring of a number of diseases, particularly of glaucoma and neuro-ophthalmological complaints. Consult ► https://eyeguru.org/essentials/visual-fields for a detailed review.

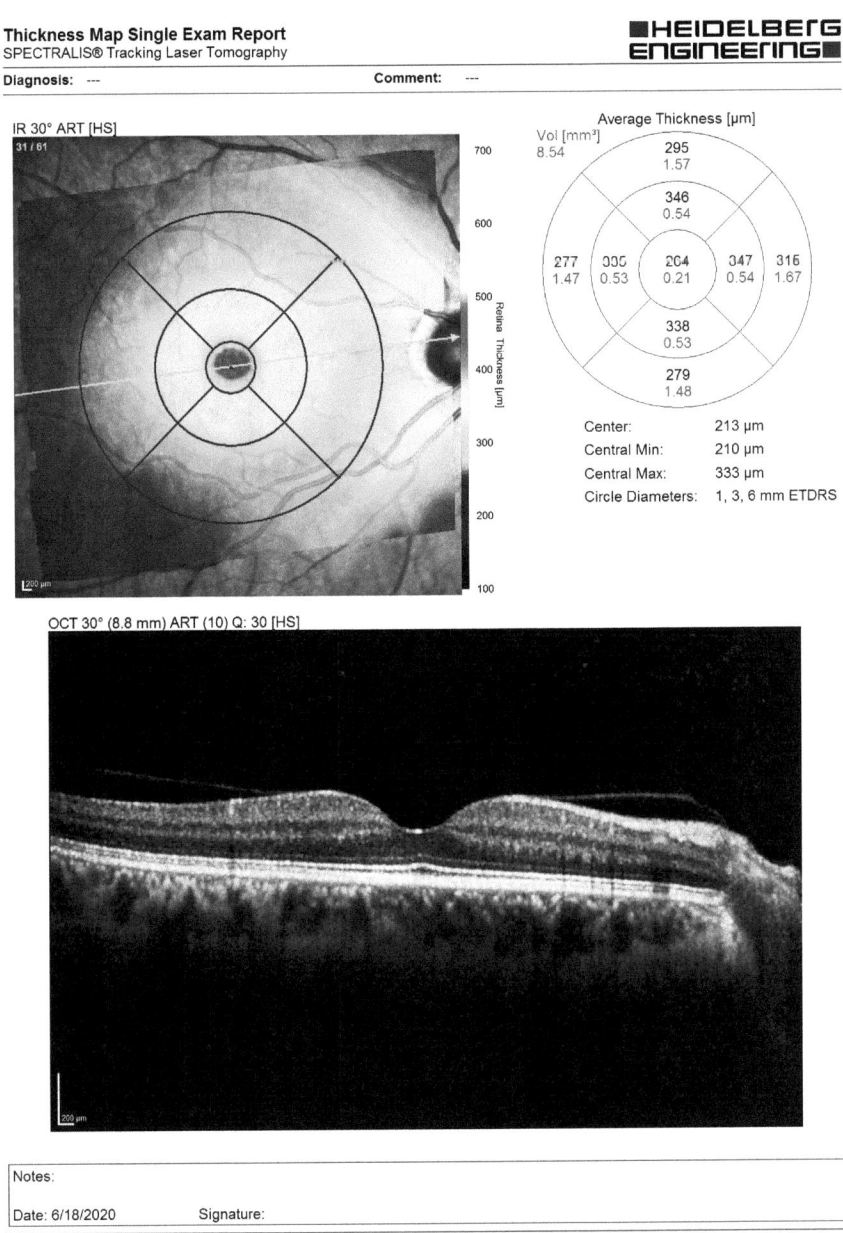

Thickness Map Single Exam Report
SPECTRALIS® Tracking Laser Tomography

HEIDELBErG ENGINEErING

Diagnosis: ---   Comment: ---

IR 30° ART [HS]
31 / 61

Average Thickness [µm]
Vol [mm³]
8.54

295
1.57

346
0.54

277 / 335 / 264 / 347 / 316
1.47 / 0.53 / 0.21 / 0.54 / 1.67

338
0.53

279
1.48

Center: 213 µm
Central Min: 210 µm
Central Max: 333 µm
Circle Diameters: 1, 3, 6 mm ETDRS

OCT 30° (8.8 mm) ART (10) Q: 30 [HS]

Notes:

Date: 6/18/2020   Signature:

Software Version: 6.12.4   www.HeidelbergEngineering.com   Thickness Map Single Exam Report

Fig. 25.12 A readout of an unremarkable Heidelberg OCT. (Contributed by Dr. Ankoor Shah, Assistant Professor of Ophthalmology, Harvard Medical School)

25.5.1 Conditions by Subspecialty

For the remainder of the chapter, we will delve into content review of common conditions and high-yield tips, pimp questions, trials, and resources to excel on your rotation. It is structured by subspecialty, so be sure to review at minimum the ones that pertain to the attendings that you will be working with! In order, we will cover cornea and refractive, cataract and lens, glaucoma, pediatric ophthalmology, trauma, neuro-ophthalmology, retina, infection and inflammation, and oculoplastics.

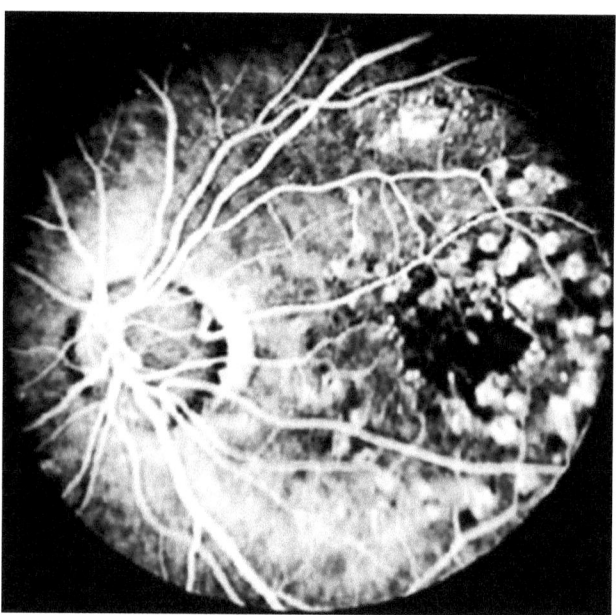

Fig. 25.13 Fluorescein angiogram demonstrating significant macular microaneurysms and areas of leakage in a patient with diabetic retinopathy. (From Oral fluorescein angiography with the scanning laser ophthalmoscope in diabetic retinopathy: a case-controlled comparison with intravenous fluorescein angiography" PMID: 15184968)

25.6 Cornea and Refractive

Comprehensive ophthalmology clinics will include a variety of corneal pathology. We will cover the bread and butter cornea conditions you might run into and their medical and surgical treatments. While it is less likely you will run into many refractive surgery cases during your rotation, we will also mention the different mechanisms of refractive surgery and their pros and cons.

The cornea is a sensitive tissue that relies on many cell types to function optimally. The cornea is the most densely innervated tissue in the body. The epithelial layer contains many nerve endings, making abrasions particularly painful. Blink reflexes and eyelid closing ability must remain intact in order to avoid corneal damage from exposure. The cornea's refractive potential and comfort relies on lacrimation and meibomian gland secretions. The single-cell thick endothelial layer must pump fluid out of the cornea to keep it clear and non-edematous.

A very common diagnosis made in the clinic is that of *dry eye*. Dry eye can cause visual distortions, monocular double vision, discomfort, or pain. The etiology of dry eye for most people is either due to insufficient tear production or a problem with the quality of the tears. The tear film consists of three layers (inner to outer: mucous, aqueous, lipid). Mucous layer helps tears adhere to the eye. The lipid layer (produced by meibomian glands) keeps the tear film from rapidly evaporating. An unstable tear film can be evaluated with a tear break up time (TBUT) test. On slit lamp exam you might see punctate corneal erosions or conjunctival surface irregularities. Patients are advised to practice good lid hygiene (scrub with baby shampoo, frequent warm compresses, etc.) and may use lubricating drops, but compliance is often inadequate. Other options include prescription drops or a punctal plug insertion (keeps tears from draining too fast). In severe cases, doctors may prescribe serum tears, which are made of the patient's own blood serum.

CENTRAL 24-2 THRESHOLD TEST

FIXATION MONITOR: BLIND SPOT
FIXATION TARGET: CENTRAL
FIXATION LOSSES: 0/15
FALSE POS ERRORS: 10 %
FALSE NEG ERRORS: 13 %
TEST DURATION: 07:13

FOVEA: OFF

STIMULUS: III, WHITE
BACKGROUND: 31.5 ASB
STRATEGY: SITA-STANDARD

PUPIL DIAMETER:
VISUAL ACUITY:
RX: +2.50 DS   DC X

DATE: 19-01-2018
TIME: 08:53
AGE: 77

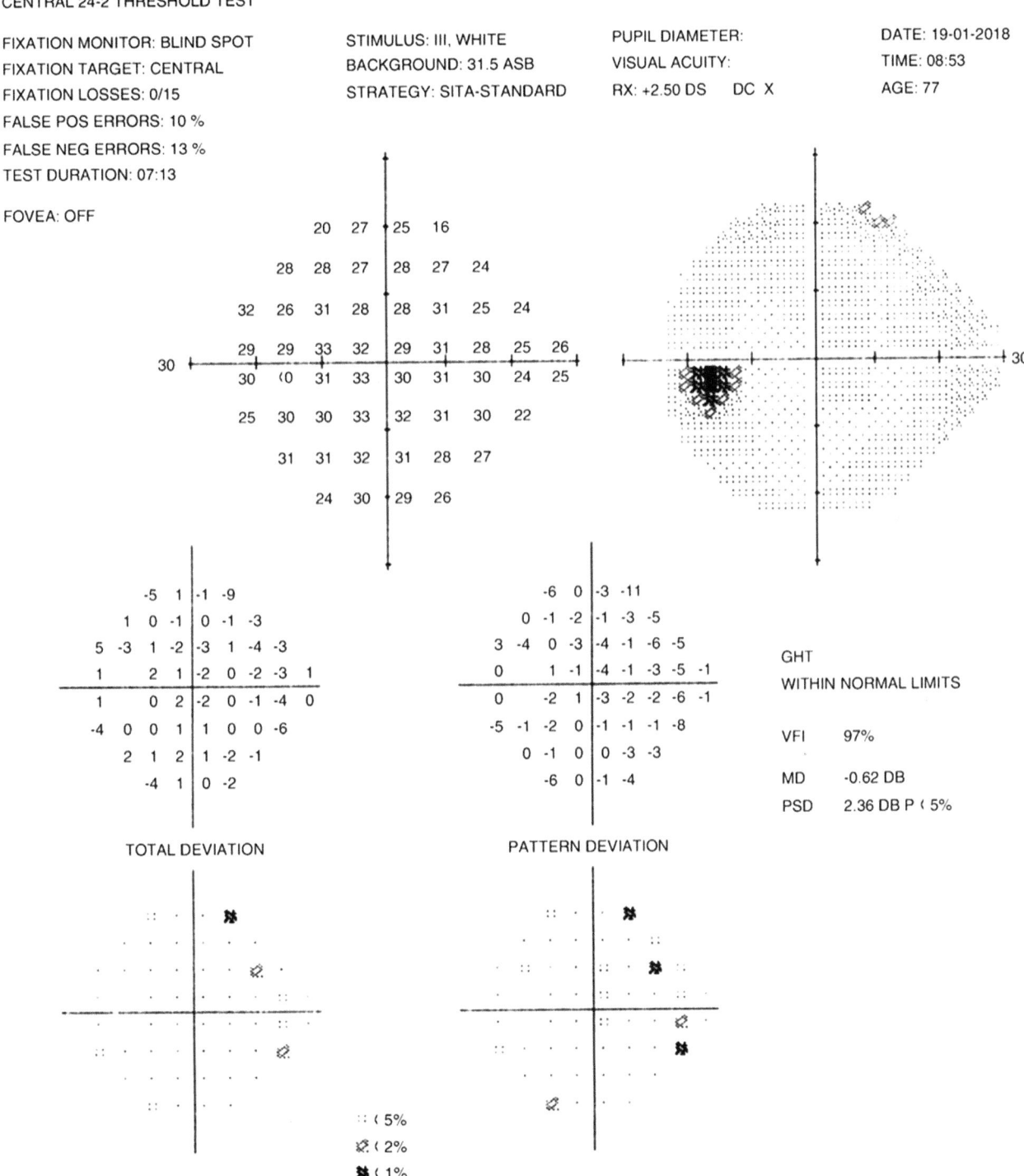

GHT
WITHIN NORMAL LIMITS

VFI   97%

MD   -0.62 DB
PSD   2.36 DB P (5%

TOTAL DEVIATION

PATTERN DEVIATION

:: (5%
⊘ (2%
✻ (1%
■ (0.5%

Fig. 25.14 A readout of an unremarkable Humphrey Visual Field. (From "Optical Coherence Tomography in Non-Glaucomatous Optic Neuropathies from Optical Coherence Tomography in Glaucoma" **ISBN: 978-3-319-94904-8**)

Astigmatism is football-shaped (as opposed to spherical) curvature of the cornea (or less commonly of the lens). This characteristic in the corneal shape leads to imprecise focusing of light rays onto the retina, leading to decreased visual acuity and/or blurred vision. It can be quantified in the clinic and corrected with numerous interventions including eyeglasses, contact lenses, or laser-assisted corneal surgery.

Pinguecula and pterygia (◻ Fig. 25.15) are benign growths of conjunctival tissue thought to be caused by a combination of dry eyes and exposure to the elements (UV light, dust, wind, etc.). They are commonly referred to as "surfer's eye" for this reason. Pinguecula are growths that appear as mounded up conjunctiva at the limbus (the intersection of the sclera and the cornea). They are rarely surgically removed and are instead managed with lubricating drops as needed for irritation. Sometimes, if they become inflamed, steroid eye drops are used. Pterygia are classically wedge-shaped, vascularized conjunctival growths that extend from the conjunctiva and cross the limbus onto the cornea. They are often surgically managed when symptomatic.

When should I bring a pterygium to the OR? Pterygia are removed when they begin to interfere with vision, or if there is a concern that they soon will because of their extension toward the visual axis. It is also reasonable to perform the surgery for cosmetic function or for symptoms including pain, foreign body sensation, or irritation.

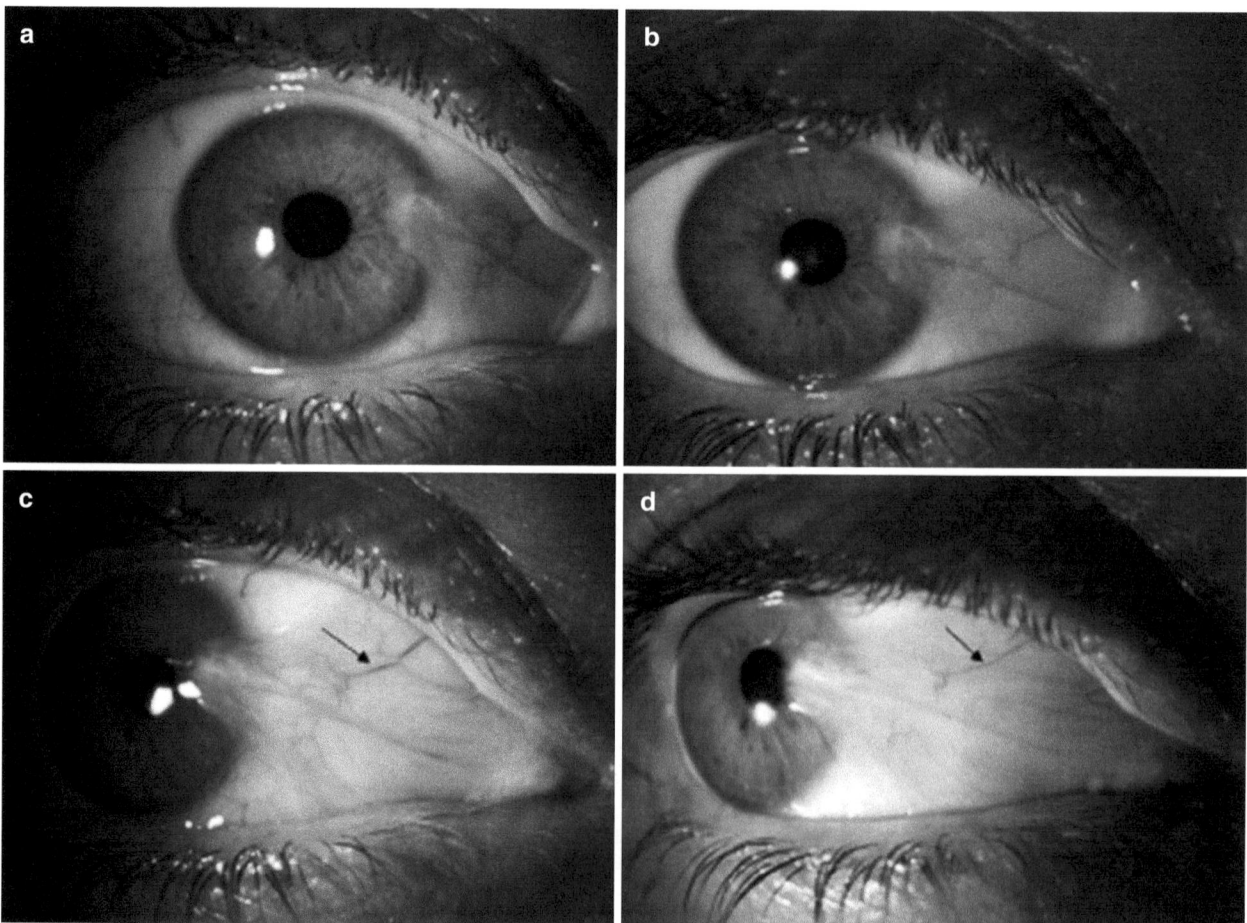

◻ **Fig. 25.15   a–d** A pterygium with notable vascularity (arrow). (From "Management of primary pterygium with intra-lesional injection of 5 fluorouracil and bevacizumab (Avastin)" PMID: 31217579)

Eyelids play a major role in maintaining the ocular surface environment. If they cannot perform their protective function, *exposure keratopathy* can develop. This can present with pain, although advanced cases might not have pain if the nerves in the cornea are destroyed. On slit lamp examination, corneal erosions can be seen, particularly with fluorescein applied to the ocular surface and using blue light. Depending on the severity and the expected length of the exposure (brief vs indefinitely), treatment options range from lubricating ointments and drops to amniotic membrane transplants to suturing the eyelids together with a procedure called a tarsorrhaphy.

Keratoconus is a progressive corneal thinning disease that is invariably bilateral, although it can develop at significantly different rates between the fellow eyes. It causes thinning and outward bulging of the cornea which manifests as optical aberrations that are impossible to correct with glasses. Keratoconus progression may also be associated with eye rubbing. The corneal curvature is assessed with corneal topography (refer to ▢ Fig. 25.11). Treatments for keratoconus include conservative management with hard contacts (e.g., rigid gas-permeable lenses), corneal crosslinking (which slows down progression), and eventually corneal transplant if necessary. You might hear about an artificial cornea, a keratoprosthesis (KPro), but this is used very rarely, and only for eyes not amenable to standard corneal transplant.

More about corneal crosslinking? This new technique is employed in patients with documented worsening of their keratoconus. The procedure involves dropping riboflavin (vitamin B12) onto the cornea while the eye is irradiated with UVA light for a period of ~30 min. While it can often halt progression of keratoconus, it is contraindicated in patients with severe corneal scarring or opacification, history of poor wound healing, severe dry eye, or severe autoimmune disorders.

Fuchs' endothelial corneal dystrophy is a disorder of the endothelial cells that are required to pump fluid out of the cornea. These cells degenerate, and this leads to corneal edema. Corneal edema manifests on exam as corneal thickening and cloudiness, and in severe cases with visible folds of the Descemet's membrane. Fuchs' patients also have guttae on exam, which are punctate, collagenous outpouchings of Descemet's membrane in areas of absent endothelium. It can be treated with dehydrating (hyperosmotic) eye drops or with surgical interventions. The two most common surgical interventions are procedures to replace the corneal endothelium with donor endothelium (DSEK or DMEK).

Corneal abrasions and ulcers are common complaints that bring patients to ophthalmologists. Abrasions of the cornea can be very painful and if they become infected can cause ulcerations. Ulcers can also be caused by viruses such as HSV, VZV, or adenovirus. They can easily be seen at the slit lamp under blue light with fluorescein applied to the cornea. HSV corneal ulcers have a very pathognomonic "dendritic" appearance (▢ Fig. 25.16). The ophthalmologist may decide to culture or to treat empirically based on the appearance of the ulcer. It is vital to stop an abrasion from becoming an ulcer and/or to stop ulcers from progressing to perforations or endophthalmitis. Antibiotic drops are the primary treatment for ulcers (not systemic because remember – the cornea is *avascular*, so systemic would only make sense if there was concern for scleral expansion of the infection or perforation). Pressure-patching the eye can provide pain relief for an abrasion, but this should be done with frequent checks to ensure an ulcer is not developing under the patch! Additionally, contact lens wearers should discontinue their use and should be treated with fortified antibiotic drops as they are at higher risk for infection with more resilient

25

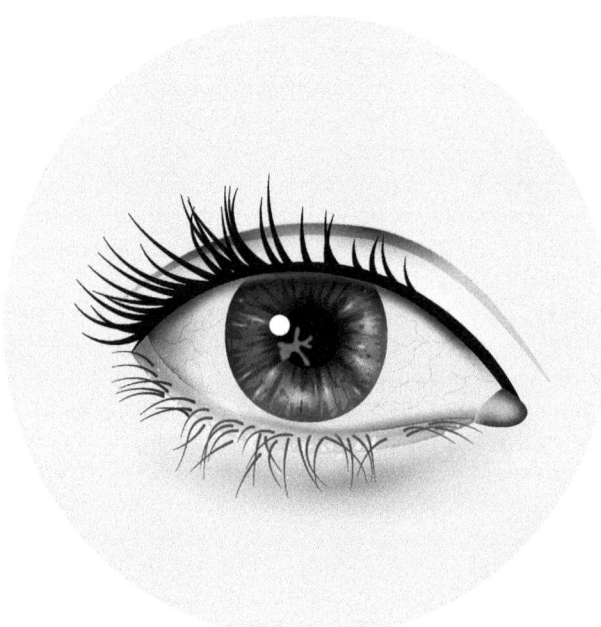

Fig. 25.16 Drawing of the classic, dendritic appearance of an HSV corneal ulcer examined with fluorescein at the slit lamp

bacteria (commonly *Pseudomonas aeruginosa*). Over the long term, ulcers can leave a scar on the cornea, which appears as a whitish patch that may affect vision depending on its location.

25.6.1   DtDx: Corneal Abrasion vs Corneal Ulcer

A corneal abrasion vs a corneal ulcer can be thought of to be analogous to a skin scrape vs an infected laceration. This analogy can be useful when you are considering which diagnosis is accurate. The patient with the abrasion will complain of pain and photophobia as their most prominent symptoms (remember, the corneal epithelium is densely innervated). Patients with ulcers might have a visible bacterial infiltrate or discharge/pus-like material coalescing at the area of the epithelial defect. On slit lamp exam, you might appreciate a depth to the whiteness.

Refractive surgery changes the light-bending power of the eye by altering the shape of the cornea to correct for myopia (nearsightedness) or hyperopia (farsightedness). The most common surgeries to do this are LASIK and PRK (◘ Fig. 25.17). These are all surgeries that use a laser to change the shape of the cornea, and they vary in the methods by which they access the portion of the cornea they reshape. At the end of the day, understand that patients may ask about these procedures, that many would be able to derive significant benefit from them, and that while the risks change based on the patient factors (contraindicated in extremely thin corneas and keratoconus), all carry some degree of risk (the most common complication is dry eye).

■   Sample Presentation
Mr. D is a 24-year-old man who presents for evaluation of right eye pain after getting "poked in the eye" while playing basketball last night. He endorses for-

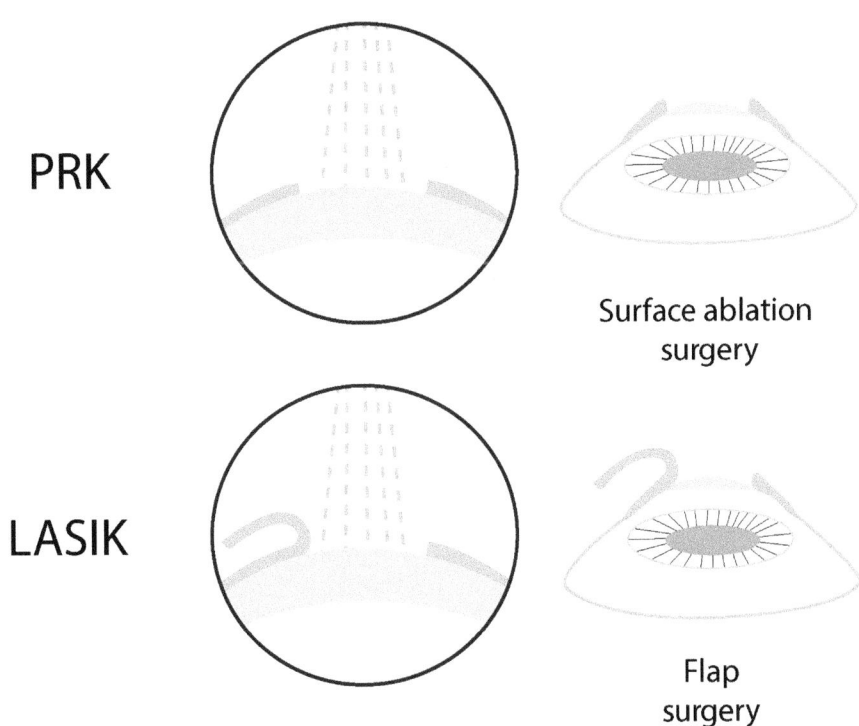

PRK

Surface ablation
surgery

LASIK

Flap
surgery

Fig. 25.17 Depiction of PRK vs LASIK

eign body sensation, increased tearing, and stinging, and constant, 4/10 pain in the right eye. On exam, his VA is 20/20 and pupils are equally round and reactive to light. His right eye is Seidel negative and I see no evidence of a foreign body. There is a small abrasion on the periphery of the cornea which stains with fluorescein. There is no appreciable discharge. I would recommend him to use lubricating drops and ointments for comfort, along with an antibiotic drop for 1 week due to the mechanism of injury. I would also counsel him to call if his symptoms worsen rather than improve over the next few days, or if he experiences any "red flag symptoms" such as severe eye pain, nausea/vomiting, new worsening of his vision, or new double vision.

25.6.2 High-Yield Trials

SCUT (2006) (Steroids for Corneal Ulcers Trial)
- *Is there a benefit to steroids drops in addition to abx drops in the treatment of bacterial corneal ulcers?*
  - No difference in visual outcomes between the steroid + abx and placebo + abx (except better vision in steroid group for subgroup with central ulcers and subgroup with count fingers vision or worse). No safety issues either, so sometimes used for inflammation in corneal ulcers even outside of those subgroups

CDS (2013) (Corneal Donor Study)
- *Does the age of the donated cornea matter for visual outcomes?*
  - No difference at 10 years between corneas from 12–65-year-old donors and 66–75-year-old donors. However, when analyzed as a continuous variable, older < younger at 5 years ($p < 0.001$)

25.6.3 Procedures for Further Review

- DMEK vs DSEK
- PRK vs LASIK vs LASEK vs SMILE

25.7 Cataract and Lens

Cataract is opacification of the lens. They can occur due to numerous etiologies and are named based on the layer of the lens that they opacify. We will discuss commonly seen etiologies of cataracts and their presentation, how to help the patient decide when to proceed with surgery, which surgical options are best, and lastly, the steps of cataract surgery – the most common operation performed in the USA.

Age-related cataracts (nuclear sclerotic cataracts) (◻ Fig. 25.18) are the most common type and could be considered to be the natural consequence of exposure to light for many years rather than a pathologic state. They typically present as decreased visual acuity or increased glare. On exam they appear as a yellowish-brown ("brunescent") opacification of the lens nucleus. A good question to get at the progression of a cataract is asking about the difficulty of night driving. A test done by technicians before the ophthalmologist sees the patient, called a brightness acuity test (BAT), gives an objective measure of this. On examination, direct the slit lamp beam obliquely at the eye and focus on the lens to appreciate the cataract. A decision to proceed to surgical removal of the clouded lens and replacement with an intraocular lens (IOL) is subjective and should be made with the patient after a discussion of the risks and benefits. The decision to pursue cataract surgery greatly rests on the degree to which the cataract is impacting the patient's functional status and quality of life. When working up the patient, it is also crucial to assess the patient's visual potential (e.g., does the patient have concomitant vision-limiting retinal pathology?) in order to appropriately counsel the patient regarding the degree of vision improvement they can expect and properly discuss the risk/benefit of the operation.

Cortical cataracts (◻ Fig. 25.19) develop in the cortex of the lens. On exam they can appear as spoke-shaped opacifications, particularly when the slit lamp light source is directed perpendicularly to the lens.

Posterior subcapsular cataracts (◻ Fig. 25.20) develop at the back of the lens capsule. They appear as small, punctate opacifications on the posterior capsule, reminiscent of scattered grains of sand. Over time, they can present as a confluent sheet on the posterior capsule. Because of their posterior position on the visual axis, they can have a substantial effect on vision. They are often

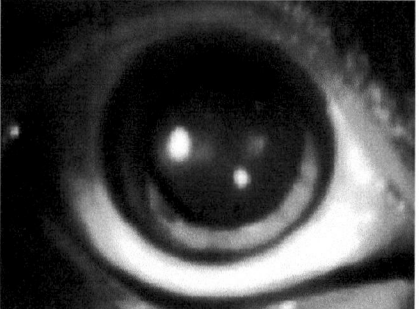

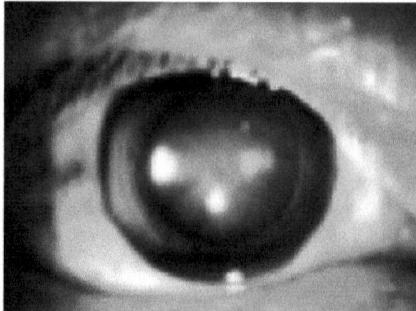

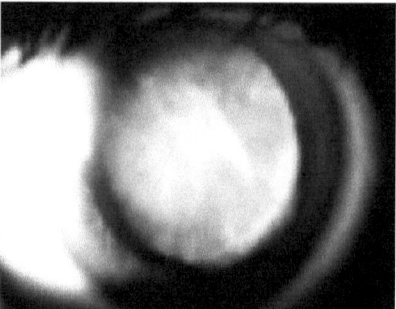

◻ **Fig. 25.18** Mild (left), moderate (middle), and advanced (right) nuclear sclerotic cataract. (From "Cataract" in Nature Reviews Disease Primer PMID: 27188414)

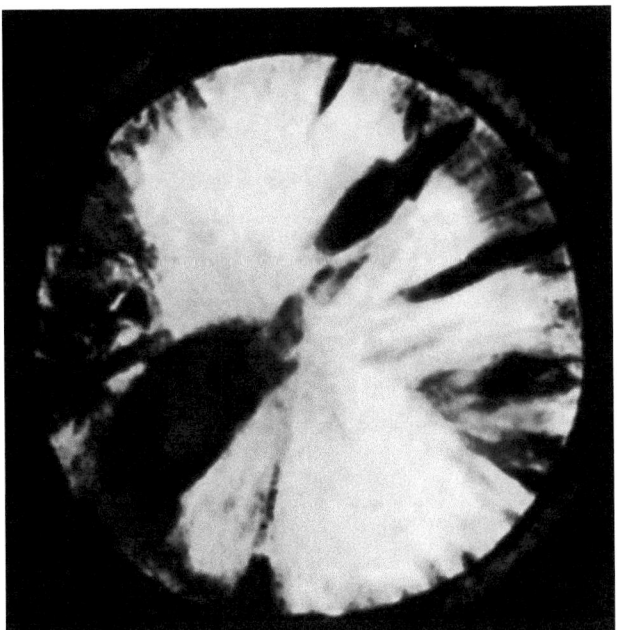

◘ Fig. 25.19 Cortical cataract. (From "The morphology of cataract and visual performance." PMID: 8325426)

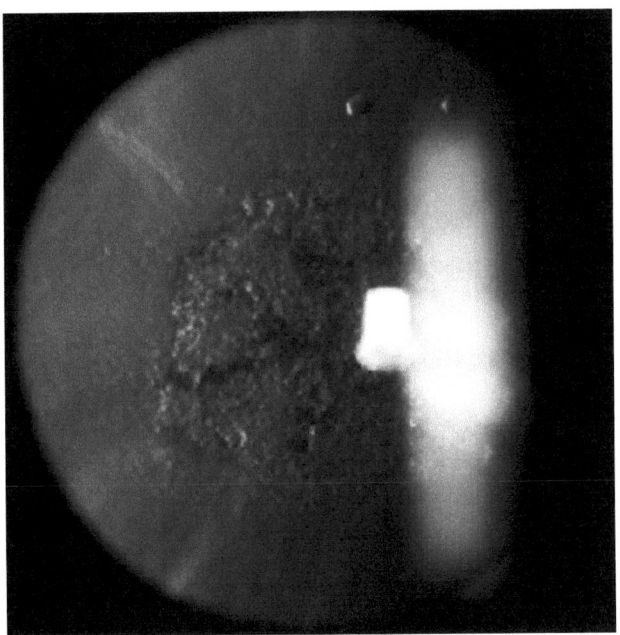

◘ Fig. 25.20 Posterior subcapsular cataract. (From "Morphology of Pediatric Cataract" ISBN: 978-981-13-6938-4)

associated with diabetes, steroid use, ocular inflammation, or previous ocular surgery.

Posterior capsule opacification (PCO) can develop months to years after cataract removal. They form as a result of lens epithelial cell migration over the posterior capsule. When it is visually significant, it can be removed using an in-clinic laser procedure called a YAG capsulotomy (◘ Fig. 25.21) which creates a hole in the posterior capsule removing the opacification from the visual axis.

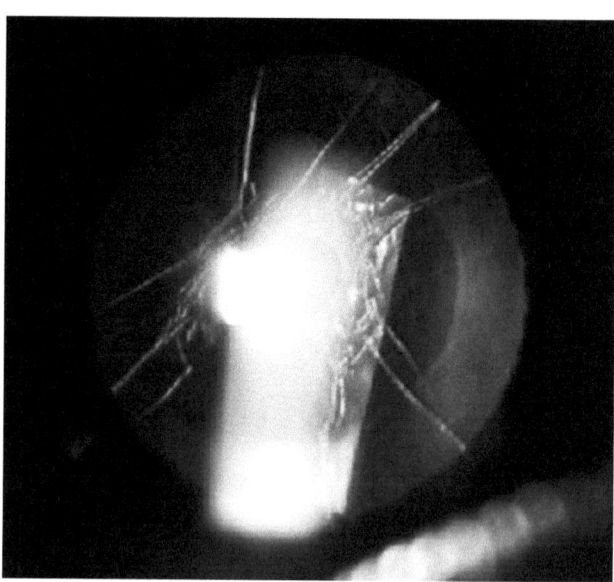

□ **Fig. 25.21**   Posterior capsule 3 months after YAG capsulotomy. (From "Spontaneous closure of Nd:YAG posterior capsulotomy in capsular blockage syndrome" PMID: 15877087)

Traumatic cataracts occur following trauma to the eye. Pathophysiologically, the lens capsule bursts from the force of the trauma, fluid enters the capsule, and the lens becomes edematous and subsequently opacifies.

Congenital cataracts most commonly occur due to metabolic disease or pre-/perinatal infections. These must be removed early in life to prevent the development of amblyopia (discussed further in ▶ Sect. 25.9 subsection).

25.7.1   Grading of Nuclear Sclerotic Cataracts in Clinic

This is based on the appearance of the nucleus of the lens
- NS tr or 1+ = evidence of cataract on exam but nucleus is still clearer than the anterior/posterior portions of the lens
- NS 2+ = nucleus is equal to the anterior/posterior portions of the lens
- NS 3+ = nucleus is denser than the anterior/posterior portions of the lens
- NS 4+ = nucleus is completely yellow/brown (brunescent)

■ Sample Presentation

Mr. S is a 79-year-old man here for his yearly exam. He reports his vision has worsened over the past few months with difficulty reading small print and dealing with glare of oncoming headlights while driving at night. His best corrected visual acuity is 20/80. He BATs to 20/100. On exam his bilateral nuclear sclerotic cataracts are dense and brunescent, thus I would grade them as 4+. They are affecting his activities of daily living, so I would recommend removal and IOL placement. He has no significant comorbidities that keep him from lying flat or staying still, so topical anesthesia should be appropriate, and he has never had ocular surgeries or taken Flomax, so the surgery should be fairly standard.

A note on the *types of IOLs*. There are two main options other than a basic intraocular lens that you may come across. The first is a Toric lens for patients with regular astigmatism. This lens has to be positioned correctly in the eye in order to counteract the astigmatism. The second is called a multifocal lens.

Pearl: Sometimes a patient will come to clinic reporting that they no longer need their reading glasses. They are pleasantly surprised! However, this may actually be a sign that their cataract is progressing. This presentation is referred to as the "Second Sight Phenomenon." It occurs because a developing cataract makes the lens rounder (making the patient more myopic), and thus reducing the need for reading glasses (which refract light rays to focus on the macula).

Pearl: Eyes that cannot properly dilate make cataract surgery more difficult. One common cause of floppy iris syndrome (over-relaxation of the iris) that should be screened for prior to undergoing cataract surgery is use of tamsulosin (you'll likely hear ophthalmologists refer to it by its trade name, Flomax), which is commonly prescribed to relieve symptoms of benign prostatic hyperplasia.

This lens provides different focal points, allowing for patients to function without reading glasses (which patients with basic IOLs will invariably require).

■ **Step by Step of Cataract Surgery**

A bare bone explanation of the most commonly performed surgery is worthwhile. Notably, there are many variations. See "Topics for Further Review" for an excellent resource to review cataract surgery in further depth! The basics are:

1. Dilate the pupil and anesthetize the eye with topical anesthesia and provide some intravenous sedation.
2. Incise the cornea (paracentesis) in two places.
3. Fill the anterior chamber with viscoelastic material, which cushions the sensitive endothelium of the cornea from the high energy phacoemulsification machine.
4. Drag a curved needle (cystitome) across the anterior capsule and then use forceps to peel and create the capsulorhexis (hole through which the lens can be accessed).
5. Hydrodissection – inject balanced salt solution (BSS) just under the capsule to cleave cortex from capsule. Rotate lens to ensure that it is freed from the underlying cortex.
6. Use the phacoemulsification handpiece to chop up and remove the lens from the capsule, without damaging the posterior capsule.
7. Cortical aspiration – grab and peel the cortex off the capsule.
8. Fill capsular bag with viscoelastic.
9. Inject the IOL into the capsule and position it properly.
10. Remove the viscoelastic material.
11. Close the corneal wounds by hydrating them. This swelling of the cornea causes temporary local opacification and closure of the small incisions.

Consenting patients in clinic can be an excellent way to stand out! Therefore, know that the (rare) complications of cataract surgery include the usual complications of any surgery (bleeding, inflammation, infection) and the ophthalmological specific (high IOP requiring medical or surgical treatment, corneal edema and haziness, retinal detachment leading to the requirement for another surgery (or even possibly blindness), or dislocation of the IOL requiring re-operation).

25.7.2 Topics for Further Review

- To optimally prepare for your time in the operating room, I would highly encourage you to use on of the many available resources to review cataract surgery in depth. A favorite resource can be found at ▶ http://cataractcourse.com/. I would strongly recommend going through this course before your rotation! It is very high yield!
- YAG capsulotomy for treatment of PCO.

25.8 Glaucoma

Glaucoma = optic nerve damage. It is a complex and multifactorial disease that is highly prevalent in older populations. The chronic version is referred to as a "silent thief of sight," as vision loss is slowly progressive and classically

25

Pearl: ISNT rule
(◻ Fig. 25.22) – in normal eyes, the thickness of the rim of the optic disc is I (inferior) > S (superior) > N (nasal) > T (temporal). This often deviates in glaucomatous eyes.

Pearl: Dilation of the pupil
(thickening of the iris muscle) causes a narrowing of the angle and this can precipitate an episode of acute angle closure glaucoma. Clinically, this dilation could be precipitated by being in the dark or dilating medications/drops. Many people are born with narrow angles (especially far-sighted people with smaller eyes and people of Asian ancestry) and are at higher risk of angle closure.

moves from the peripheral vision in towards central vision, so patients do not often recognize their vision loss until it is severe.

Glaucoma is strongly associated with increased intraocular pressure (IOP), but the cause of the vision loss is theorized to be due to a number of factors that are poorly understood. Some theories include mechanical, vascular, and biochemical factors. It is monitored with Humphrey visual field testing, IOP, OCT, and fundus examinations with particular attention paid to the optic nerve. The nerve is examined for the "cup-to-disc ratio" as well as the orientation of the cup within the overall disc.

While the pathophysiologic basis of glaucoma is poorly understood, the basis for increased IOP can often be determined and requires an understanding of aqueous humor production, flow through, and egress from the eye.

Aqueous humor is produced by the ciliary body in the posterior chamber. It flows anteriorly through the pupil where it nourishes the cornea. It exits through the trabecular meshwork, which is located in the anterior chamber at the angle where the cornea meets the iris, into the canal of Schlemm and out of the eye.

Glaucoma can present as acute with a closed angle, or more commonly chronically with an open angle. The angle refers to the outflow tract through which the aqueous humor flows through (which can be evaluated by gonioscopy, as discussed previously) on its way through the trabecular meshwork and out of the eye. *Acute, closed angle glaucoma* is an emergency. It most commonly occurs when the lens plasters against the back of the iris, preventing any flow of aqueous humor into the anterior chamber and out of the eye (this is called pupillary block). The pressure gradient across the iris causes it to bend anteriorly and close the angle. On presentation, the patient will be nauseated, and the eye will be red, injected, and painful (and even hard to the touch if you were to palpate over the lids) (◻ Fig. 25.23). Normal intraocular pressure range is roughly 8–22 mmHg and in acute glaucoma it is often 30 mmHg or greater. Irreversible vision loss can occur within hours so a "throw the kitchen sink at it" approach to treatment is taken, with any intervention that might decrease pressure employed. (See below in "Options for Management" – effectively *the*

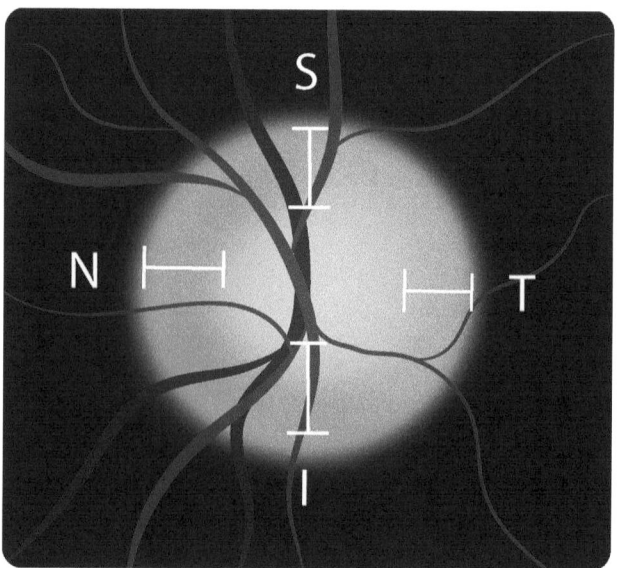

◻ **Fig. 25.22** ISNT rule in a non-glaucomatous eye

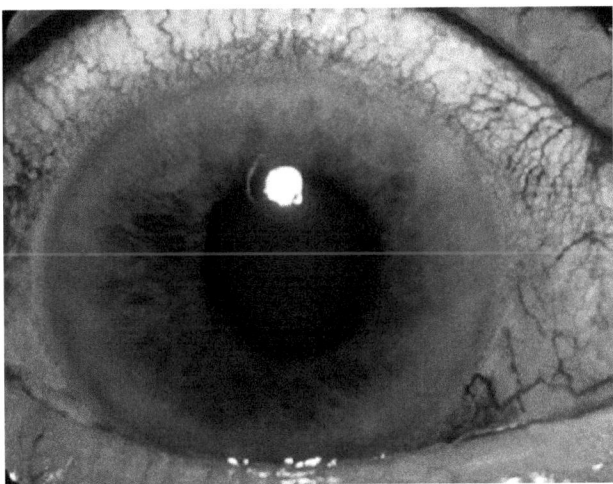

Fig. 25.23 External photo of acute angle-closure glaucoma. (From "Acute Angle-Closure Glaucoma" ISBN:978–3–319-78,944-6)

goal is to immediately lower IOP in order to reduce corneal edema, relieve iris ischemic changes, prevent future episodes, and prevent permanent visual loss. Pain and nausea should also be addressed in the acute setting.)

Primary open angle glaucoma (POAG) risk factors include age, family history, African-America race, and thin corneas. These patients are typically picked up by screening at yearly eye exams. Visual fields and nerve fiber layer OCT are used to evaluate if there are any sequelae of their elevated IOP (referred to as ocular hypertension until there are functional or structural deficits). Medical and/or surgical treatments (discussed below) are initiated with a goal of lowering IOP.

■ **Sample Presentation**

Ms. M is a 57-year-old woman with a history of glaucoma s/p bilateral trabeculectomy in 2016 who presents for a 6 mo follow-up visit. She has no new visual complaints and reports good compliance with her drop regimen. Her pressures are 15 OD 14 OS and her VA is 20/25 OU, stable from last visits. Her visual fields and OCT are unchanged from her last visit. The visual field testing demonstrates a classic superior arcuate defect (see topics for further review – "Classic Scotomas"). No notable findings on slit lamp exam, beyond her 1+ nsc OU that are not affecting her daily life. On gonioscopy, her angle is open to scleral spur OU. Since her pressures are stable on her current drop regimen and she has no complaints or disease progression, I would recommend that her current regimen be continued, and we see her for follow-up in 6 months.

There are a few other etiologies worth mentioning that can lead to decreased outflow of aqueous humor. One is *neovascular glaucoma*, which is crowding of the angle by new vessels which grow secondary to a VEGF stimulus (often from an ischemic process like diabetes). *Pigment dispersion syndrome* can also decrease outflow and is caused by the zonules rubbing against the back of the iris. Small particles of pigment rub off and flow forward to eventually clog the trabecular meshwork. Similarly, *pseudoexfoliation syndrome* is a systemic disease that results in clogging of the trabecular meshwork. A coarse material is deposited on the anterior lens capsule. When the iris dilates and contracts over this material, pigment is "shaved off" the iris and flows forward with the aqueous humor to clog the trabecular meshwork.

25.8.1 Options for Management

- *Medical*
  - Many eyedrops! Know them, their MOA, and their side effect profiles!
    - Prostaglandins like *latanoprost* (SEs: stinging of eye, darkening of the eyelids, eyelashes, and/or iris) increase outflow of aqueous humor
    - Beta blockers like *timolol* (SEs: systemic effects of beta blockers like difficulty breathing, bradycardia, hypotension, or fatigue), alpha-agonists like *brimonidine* (SEs: arrhythmia, HTN, dry mouth), and carbonic anhydrase inhibitors like *dorzolamide* (SEs: frequent urination) reduce the production of aqueous humor
    - Cholinergic agents like *pilocarpine* (SEs: blurred vision, miosis, headache/eye ache) increase the outflow of fluid from the eye (these are not often prescribed for glaucoma anymore because of their frequent dosing schedule and their side effects)
  - Don't forget! For acute angle closure glaucoma, give something for pain and an antiemetic in addition to pressure-lowering drops +/− surgery!
- *Surgical*
  - Laser iridotomy – laser creates hole in iris allowing flow between the posterior and anterior chambers to avoid a pressure gradient between them. Trabeculectomy surgeries – small hole in the sclera surgically created allowing for aqueous humor to flow into a "bleb" under the conjunctiva.
  - Tube shunt surgeries – flexible tube implanted into the anterior chamber allowing for outflow of aqueous humor into device implanted beneath the conjunctiva
  - Minimally invasive glaucoma surgery (MIGS) - Less "major" operations than traditional trabs/tubes with fewer complications. This group of procedures, united under the "MIGS" umbrella, work by using tiny incisions and equipment. While they are safer than traditional glaucoma operations, there may be some tradeoff between safety and magnitude of effect. MIGS procedures include mini versions of trabeculectomies, trabecular bypass operations, suprachoroidal shunt operations, or milder versions of laser iridotomies.

25.8.2 High-Yield Trials

- EMGT (2002) (Early Manifest Glaucoma Trial)
  - *Should we treat early POAG? YES!* – this is the first trial to show there is benefit to early IOP reduction in open-angle glaucoma patients
- OHTS (2002) (Ocular Hypertension Treatment Study)
  - *Should you treat elevated IOP (24–32) if there is no evidence of glaucomatous damage on exam or visual fields?* Definitely consider it – treating these patients decreases incidence of glaucoma within the next 5 years by ~50% (from 9.5% to 4.4%). However, be cognizant of side effects and realize that patients with OHT and few risk factors might be best off delaying treatment.
- TVT (2012) (Tube vs Trabeculectomy Study)
  - *Should tubes be reserved for higher-risk eyes? Not necessarily,* tubes had a higher long-term success rate and had fewer short-term complications. However, trabeculectomy had less use of adjunctive pressure-lowering therapy at 2 years.
- UKGTS (2013) (Latanoprost vs. Placebo for Open-Angle Glaucoma)
  - *Is there a benefit in terms of VF preservation in starting patients on IOP controlling therapy immediately upon diagnosis of POAG? Yes*

25.8.3 Visual Field Findings in Glaucoma

A scotoma is defined as a blind or low vision spot in an otherwise normal visual field. As mentioned earlier in the chapter, visual field testing evaluates for scotomas. As taught in medical school, the classic visual field deterioration in glaucoma moves from the periphery towards the center. However, there are many nuances to this. While beyond the scope of this chapter, consider using online resources (including those listed below) to learn about classic scotoma patterns in different stages of disease.

Learning how to *monitor patients, set IOP goals, and develop appropriate, evidence-based treatment plans* to reach those goals can make you stand out in your plans. Consider the below topics worthwhile to review to really stand out on a glaucoma rotation!

25.8.4 Topics for Further Review

- A quick read about glaucoma visual field testing with classic scotomas shown (Visual Field Testing for Glaucoma – a practical guide PMID: 23520423
- The Iowa Glaucoma Curriculum, found at ▶ http://curriculum. iowaglaucoma.org/, is an invaluable resource for students (or residents) who want an increased depth of understanding, although is an investment of your time to complete!
  - *Key tip:* glaucoma is a field with many trials! Consider visiting ▶ https:// www.aao.org/eyenet/article/landmark-glaucoma-studies-key-findings-treatment-1 for many more relevant trials to review.
- Specifics about various MIGS procedures (indications, contraindications, expected IOP lowering, etc.)
- Ahmed vs. Baerveldt shunts (differences and the pros/cons)
- How to set a targeted IOP goal per patient, and the pros/cons of doing so (▶ https://glaucomatoday.com/articles/2018-nov-dec/target-iop-to-set-or-not-to-set)

25.9 Pediatric Ophthalmology

Children present to the ophthalmologist for many reasons, ranging from refractive error to neurological issues or life-threatening conditions. As you might imagine, examining a child in clinic can be very difficult and requires a skillful and patient pediatric ophthalmologist and often the help of the child's caregiver.

Subconjunctival hemorrhage is an alarming presentation of a benign condition. It occurs when a blood vessel under the conjunctiva bursts. A small volume of blood can create an impressively red eye. This can occur in any age but is common in children. The impetus for the bursting vessel is some increase in pressure, typically a Valsalva (coughing, vomiting, etc.). It will typically self-resolve in a week and only requires reassurance!

Epiphora, or excessive tearing, commonly occurs unilaterally or bilaterally in children due to poorly developed or clogged nasolacrimal ducts. If the history and exam suggest this is the case and it is sufficiently bothersome, parents are asked to monitor the symptoms and provide supportive care. Most cases resolve without further intervention by 1 year. When it continues and is bothersome, a surgical intervention that can resolve the problem is a probing and removal of obstruction of the nasolacrimal duct. Another common cause of epiphora is dry eye. When the eyes are dry, they sting and reflexively cause tearing.

Amblyopia is decreased vision in an eye because of disuse during the critical time of visual pathway development, childhood. Normally, the two eyes "compete" to develop visual pathways to the cortex. If one is hampered by refractive error, cataract, ptosis, strabismus, or any other process, the affected eye will "give up" (the brain will suppress the bad eye and favor the normal eye) and the necessary neural pathways will not develop. This loss will never be able to be repaired and the patient may have issues ranging from loss of binocularity to complete blindness in one eye. Therefore, to avoid these complications, early visual impediments (such as congenital cataracts) must be treated quickly.

▪ Examining the Evidence

Penalizing (via patching or atropine drops) the "good" eye to allow for the development of visual pathways associated with the "bad" eye is an important treatment to avoid poor visual outcomes. Counterintuitively, longer periods of patching do not necessarily lead to better outcomes. Severe amblyopia is treated with 6 hours of patching each day, but there is no further improvement beyond that length. Moderate amblyopia is treated with 2 hours of patching each day, with no further improvement beyond that length. Patching can be uncomfortable for children and difficult for their parents. This difficulty can lead to poor compliance and permanent visual dysfunction, so these findings that "more isn't necessarily better" were warmly welcomed when published by the Pediatric Eye Disease Research Group (PEDIG)!

A common presenting complaint to the pediatric ophthalmologist is *strabismus*, or "misaligned eyes." In order to evaluate the alignment of the eyes, the pediatric ophthalmologist uses fixation targets and a variety of tests. If you are in the position to evaluate the degree of misalignment, first use the light reflex to evaluate for pseudostrabismus – the appearance of strabismus because of prominent epicanthal folds. If there is a true misalignment, it is important to document whether the misalignment is always equal or if it is different in different directions of gaze (comitant or incomitant) and whether the nondominant eye is directed medially or laterally (eso or exo). Finally, consider whether

Pearl: The spiral of Tillaux is an anatomical rule an attending might ask you about prior to strabismus surgery. It describes the distance from the limbus to the various rectus muscle insertions (◻ Fig. 25.24).

◻ **Fig. 25.24** Spiral of Tillaux rule depicting the length from the various recti muscles to the limbus

the misalignment is always there (−tropia) or only there under conditions of stress/during the cover-uncover test (−phoria). For example, a misalignment that is always there, is equal in all directions of gaze, and has the nondominant eye directed inwards would be a comitant esotropia. Treatment can range from prescribing glasses with corrective prisms to intermittent patching/blurring eye drops (penalizing the good eye so the other eye's visual pathways develop) to strabismus surgery.

Leukocoria, aka "white pupil," is a common reason for referral from a pediatrician. This is screened for because if it is caused by retinoblastoma, it could be the first sign of a life-threatening illness. Other causes of white pupil include cataract or severe retinal detachment, both of which may also require surgical treatment to prevent vision loss.

25.9.1 Differentiating the Differential: Leukocoria

Leukocoria can be caused by numerous life-threatening or sight-threatening processes. While a professionally done exam is the key differentiator here, targeted questions and a rudimentary exam can get you closer to the diagnosis. Is there a family history of retinoblastoma? If so this increases the likelihood of that being the cause. Was there a history of trauma that might suggest a rhegmatogenous retinal detachment? Is the child healthy and meeting milestones? If not, this might suggest a cataract secondary to a metabolic disorder. How was the pregnancy and perinatal period? A history of maternal infection could hint at congenital cataract and a very premature birth could suggest a retinal detachment secondary to retinopathy of prematurity.

- ■ Sample Presentation

Sam is a 2-week-old term-born boy who was referred by his pediatrician due to lack of red reflex in the right eye. His prenatal and birth course were unremarkable, he has not had any trauma, and he has not required any medical interventions. There is no family history of retinoblastoma. Exam was limited due to fussiness, but I appreciated a decreased red-reflex in the right eye. The most worrisome diagnosis on my differential is retinoblastoma, but it would be rare to present this early without + FH. Since he was born term and has had an uncomplicated clinical course, I think retinal detachment from retinopathy of prematurity is unlikely and a metabolic disorder causing congenital is less likely. While I am unsure of the origin of the cataract, I think a cataract is the most likely cause the of the leukocoria. It should usually be removed expediently as pediatric cataracts are highly amblyogenic.

25.9.2 High-Yield Trials

- ═ Cryo-ROP (Multicenter Trial of Cryotherapy for Retinopathy of Prematurity)
  - – While cryotherapy was supplanted by better methods of peripheral ablation (photocoagulation), this study convincingly demonstrated and standardized the need to treat and screen for retinopathy of prematurity.
- ═ ETROP (Early Treatment for Retinopathy of Prematurity)
  - – *Does treating high-risk, pre-threshold (Topics for Further Review) ROP with laser improve retinal structural function compared to waiting to treat until threshold disease develops?* **Yes** – treat early for better results at age 2.

- PEDIG (2002) (Pediatric Eye Disease Investigative Group)
    - *Is patching or atropine penalization more effective for preventing amblyopia in young (age 3–7) children?* They are roughly equivalent for patients with *moderate* amblyopia.
- IATS (2010) (Infant Aphakia Treatment Study)
    - *Should we implant an IOL into children before the age of 6mo with unilateral cataracts (which must be removed to prevent the development of amblyopia) or correct them with an extraocular lens (contact or glasses)?* Likely *leave them aphakic* for the time being if they are below the age of 6 months. Below this age there are no improved visual outcomes in the IOL group and a higher incidence of complications.

25.9.3 Topics for Further Review

- How to perform cover/uncover tests, prism evaluations of angle of misalignment, and other topics. Many resources for orthoptists may be helpful here and some skill or knowledge in this area could make you stand out.
- Retinopathy of prematurity – screening criteria, treatments, disease classifications.

25.10 Trauma

Trauma to the eye and orbit is incredibly common, particularly in younger people and in males. Projectiles of all sorts, airbags, fists, chemicals, and virtually everything else you can think of is capable of causing ocular trauma. There are many potentially significant sequelae of ocular trauma.

One of the most concerning potential outcomes of a trauma is an *open-globe injury*. This means that the cornea or sclera have been completely perforated and is a true surgical emergency. While some open-globe injuries are apparent by visual inspection, the Seidel test is a way to evaluate for one at the slit lamp (◘ Fig. 25.25). Suspected open-globe injuries should be covered with an eye-shield and taken to the OR for further evaluation. It is essential that pressure not be applied to the eye which could extrude ocular contents (no need to check pressure!). Many patients get a CT scan (Is there a retained

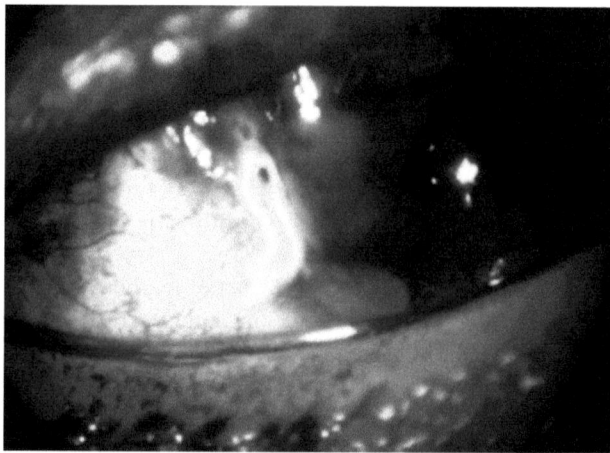

◘ **Fig. 25.25** A positive Seidel test; an anterior chamber leak evidenced by disruption of the green fluorescein by a flow of aqueous humor. (From "The Columbia Guide to Basic Elements of Eye Care" pp 91 ISBN: 978-3-030-10885-4)

foreign body? What is the lens position?). Prophylactic systemic antibiotics are given in addition to topical antibiotics, topical corticosteroids, and strong cycloplegia (such as atropine, cyclopentolate, etc.). Patients are followed closely to evaluate for healing and potential complications from the initial injury or the operation (such as orbital fracture, orbital hemorrhage, orbital compartment syndrome, posttraumatic endophthalmitis, etc.).

A trauma can cause the orbital floor (composed of the maxillary bone) to fracture. This fracture can open like a trap door, allowing the inferior rectus and/or surrounding tissue to slip in and become entrapped. This entrapment can lead to restriction of eye elevation, bradycardia (oculocardiac reflex), and eventual muscle necrosis. Consider you might also see numbness above the lip (due to CNV2 entrapment and subsequent dysfunction). While this finding does not commonly occur, it is often asked about! The best way to evaluate for this is by CT scan, and surgical correction might be necessary. While CT is the terminal method of evaluation, if extraocular movements are full, the likelihood of entrapment is very low.

Eyes are vulnerable to *foreign bodies*. Foreign bodies can present with excessive tearing, pain, "foreign body sensation" (which can also be a buzz-word for dry eye), and red eye. Mechanism of injury can clue you in to potential foreign body ("metal on metal" = grinding or hammering). Foreign bodies on the cornea or conjunctiva can be removed at the slit lamp. Others might require surgical exploration in the OR, particularly if an open-globe injury is suspected. Performing a dilated retina exam is essential, checking for a shallow anterior chamber. CT of the orbits may be needed.

Chemical injuries can be extremely severe. A known exposure is typical. The key for patients is irrigate, irrigate, irrigate! In the ED, we use a device called a Morgan lens to continuously irrigate the eye. Children can have difficulty tolerating this and might need to be restrained. Irrigation continues until normalization of ocular surface pH. Findings can include a hazy cornea, inflamed conjunctiva. Be sure to evert the eyelids to remove residual chemical.

Traumatic iritis, hyphema, and angle recession are all complications that can occur from ocular trauma. Post-traumatic surgical intervention is often necessary to avoid complications. If eye pressure is elevated, emergent glaucoma surgery is needed. Urgent retinal surgery can be required if a retinal tear or detachment is noted.

Traumatic iritis refers to iris irritation secondary to trauma. It can result in a sluggishly reactive pupil and anisocoria (pupil diameters differing by 0.4 mm) and light sensitivity. Cells may be seen floating (refer to ◼ Fig. 25.8) in the anterior chamber. Treat with a topical steroid to decrease inflammation and a cycloplegic to dilate the pupil (so that the inflamed iris doesn't spasm with light exposure and cause pain). An added benefit of dilating the inflamed iris is that it helps prevent it from sticking to the lens posteriorly and causing "posterior synechiae."

A layered *hyphema* (blood in the anterior chamber) might be visualized by the naked eye or at the slit lamp. Be sure to monitor pressure (blood can clog the trabecular meshwork and increase IOP). Initially, patients should maintain head elevation of at least 45 degrees to allow the hyphema to settle inferiorly. Pressure-lowering drops can help and a paracentesis at the slit lamp may be required to lower the pressure and through which an "anterior chamber washout" can be performed. Elevated pressure in the setting of a hyphema can stain the inner cornea with blood which can affect vision and take years to improve. Monitoring for "rebleed" (rupture or breakdown of the fibrinous clot and subsequent accumulation of additional blood in the anterior chamber) is key. The window of time in which rebleeding is highest is 3–5 days (when the clot naturally retracts), so be sure to follow the patient daily in this window and continue to monitor the IOP and size of the clot. To understand hyphema grading, refer to ◻ Fig. 25.26.

Angle recession occurs secondary to trauma when the ciliary body muscles tear. Angle recession is evaluated for via gonioscopy (an exam technique previously described in "High-Yield Anatomy" section of this chapter) with the characteristic finding of "ciliary body band widening." Angle recession is reported in degrees or clock-hours (e.g., if 75% of the angle shows recession on exam, this would be reported as either "Angle recession from 12 o'clock to 9 o'clock" or "270 degrees of angle recession"). It is relevant because subsequent scarring of the trabecular meshwork can lead to elevated pressure and increased risk of glaucoma.

■ Sample Presentation

Mr. H is a 22-year-old male in the ED following a bar fight 3 hours ago. He was punched in the right eye and is complaining of decreased VA and photosensitivity. He is unable to fully open the eye. VA is 20/40 and pressure is 14 OD. He is Seidel negative. On exam, ecchymosis and edema surrounds the right orbit, without crepitus. The upward gaze of the right eye is significantly restricted. There is 4+ cell and a 2 mm layered hyphema in the AC. The right pupil is 1 mm more dilated than the left in low light and is sluggishly reactive to light. I think this patient has a closed-globe injury OD, an orbital floor fracture, traumatic hyphema, and

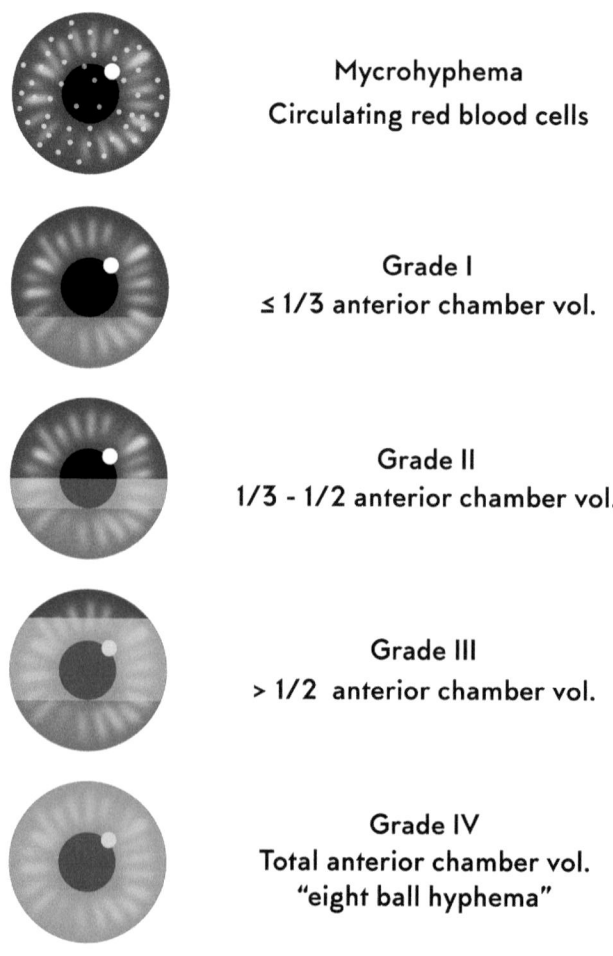

Mycrohyphema
Circulating red blood cells

Grade I
≤ 1/3 anterior chamber vol.

Grade II
1/3 - 1/2 anterior chamber vol.

Grade III
> 1/2 anterior chamber vol.

Grade IV
Total anterior chamber vol.
"eight ball hyphema"

◻ **Fig. 25.26** Grading of hyphema

*traumatic iritis. I think we should obtain a CT scan to assess for an orbital frac-
ture, steroids to decrease inflammation, and cycloplegic drops to decrease photosensitivity and to prevent rebleeding of the hyphema.*

25.10.1   Topics for Further Review

- Seidel test – key in identifying globe ruptures (▶ https://timroot.com/
  corneal-laceration-thats-seidel-positive-video/).
- For patients undergoing repair of a globe rupture with other injuries, how
  to consider whether to do multiple procedures at the time or presentation vs
  whether to stage them.
- Anesthesia concerns for traumatic optic injuries.
- How to consider scheduling follow up after traumatic ocular injuries.

25.11 Neuro-ophthalmology

Neuro-ophthalmology is a field that operates at the nexus of neurology and
ophthalmology. Neuro-ophthalmologists treat a wide variety of diseases from
those that are fairly benign to those that are imminently life threatening.

CN palsies bring many patients to the office. Here, we will discuss various
findings and etiologies of CNIII, CNIV, and CNVI palsies. Palsies may merit
ordering an MRI to rule out dangerous causes.

The *oculomotor nerve (CNIII)* innervates all extraocular muscles with the
exception of the lateral rectus (innervated by the abducens nerve, CNVI) and
the superior oblique (innervated by the trochlear nerve, CNIV). CNIII also
innervates the levator palpebrae, which elevates the eyelid. Therefore, when the
third cranial nerve is knocked out, the unopposed action of CNIV and CNVI
lead to an eye that is "down and out." There is usually ptosis as well.
Additionally, parasympathetic "pupil constrictors" run with CNIII, which
leads to dilation if they are compromised. The most common causes of CNIII
palsy are microvascular insult (due to a process like diabetes), compression of
the nerve, or trauma. In "Clinical Pearl" box, we outline how the status of the
pupil can give important hints as to the etiology.

25.11.1   Differentiating the Differential: Cause of a Third
              Nerve Palsy

When a patient arrives with a classic "down-and-out" eye and ptosis, the diagnosis of a third nerve palsy is clear. However, differentiating between the causes
is key; compression of CNIII from an enlarging aneurysm can cause this presentation, as can microvascular insult secondary to a process like diabetes.
Luckily, by understanding the anatomy of the oculomotor nerve, you can use
the pupil's status to determine which is the most likely cause. The parasympathetic nerve fibers that constrict the pupil run on the outside of the nerve and
thus are vulnerable when the nerve is externally compressed (e.g., by an enlarging aneurysm). Conversely, the small vessels affected by diabetes run within the
nerve where fibers provide motor output to extraocular muscles (i.e., vascular
disease tends to cause "down-and-out gaze" and ptosis). Therefore, if the eye
is down and out and the pupil is dilated ("blown"), you should be concerned
for a compressive etiology (e.g., aneurysm or mass lesion). If the eye is down
and out and the pupil is unaffected, it is more likely due to microvascular

insult. Third nerve palsies can be true life-threatening emergencies, so make sure you let your team know if you suspect it at any point.

CNIV trochlear nerve palsy presents with subtle findings (e.g., vertical double vision) as the only dysfunction is of the superior oblique muscle. Knocking this muscle out leads to an upward deviation and torsional changes in the affected eye. Patients tend to compensate for these changes by tilting their head, which can be a telltale sign! CNIV is particularly vulnerable to trauma as it runs all the way from the back of the brain stem. It can also be affected by microvascular insult or mass effect. Additionally, many patients have a congenitally poorly functioning trochlear nerve. Its function can continue to deteriorate during life and eventually present as a "decompensated congenital trochlear nerve palsy."

CN VI Abducens nerve is responsible for abduction of the eye via the lateral rectus. It manifests as horizontal double vision and is easily appreciable on exam, as the affected eye will not be capable of abducting beyond the midline. The most common cause of palsy is microvascular disease. It can also be caused by trauma, mass lesions, or high intracranial pressure (e.g., pseudotumor cerebri) due to its long anatomical course.

■ Sample Presentation

Mrs. T is a 65-year-old woman with DM (last A1c 12.7) who presents with new diplopia in right gaze. She first noted it upon awakening 2 days ago and saw that her right eye "wasn't moving right." She denies trauma, headache, N/V, or other visual disturbances. Her vision is 20/25 OU, pressure 15 OD 16 OS. Exam is notable for decreased EOMs. Her right eye cannot abduct beyond midline. I think she has an abducens nerve palsy due to microvascular disease and that we should counsel her about controlling her blood glucose and blood pressure, and the expected gradual recovery of her abducens nerve function.

Double vision (diplopia) is a common presenting complaint. The first question to narrow the differential should always be whether the double vision is monocular or binocular. Monocular double vision is not a neuro-ophthalmological problem. Rather, it is most commonly due to problems with anterior eye structures (e.g., astigmatism, dry eye, or cataracts, etc.). Binocular diplopia has a broad differential.

Binocular diplopia is due to the eyes not working together. This could be secondary to nerve dysfunction, muscular dysfunction, or neuromuscular junction dysfunction. Good medical history taking can often go a long way toward narrowing your differential. For instance, has the patient had a recent stroke? Any symptoms of myasthenia gravis (trouble swallowing, weakness)? Any new medications or dose changes? Any history of phorias? History of thyroid disease? CNS lesions? The appropriate next steps in the workup are dependent on the findings in the history and exam but may include neurological imaging. Treatment options depend on the underlying etiology. Unlike with children, for adults there is no risk of amblyopia. However, diplopia can often cause quite a bit of discomfort and limit activities of daily living, so patients are often highly motivated to receive interventions quickly.

Adult strabismus surgery aims to align the eyes in the neutral gaze position so that there is no double vision at rest. This is done by resecting portions of eye muscles to tighten them or by moving muscle insertions posteriorly (recession) to loosen them. The amount of resection or recession is determined by measurements of eye deviation taken in clinic.

Optic neuritis is inflammation of the optic nerve associated with rapid deterioration of vision followed by steady recovery. It is most commonly associated with multiple sclerosis but can be associated with infection. Not all patients with MS experience optic neuritis and conversely not all patients who have optic neuritis will have MS. The most common symptom is unilateral color vision changes that can be associated with pain. It typically is episodic, with episodes lasting on the order of weeks. Findings may include relative afferent pupillary defect and optic nerve edema. Treatment depends on the underlying etiology, but steroids are often central.

Anterior ischemic optic neuropathy refers to ischemia of the optic nerve. There are two etiologies of this condition: arteritic (AAION) and non-arteritic (NAION). Arteritic is the result of giant cell arteritis (GCA). Recall that GCA is a vasculitis that affects older adults and presents with headaches, fever, fatigue, jaw claudication, and vision loss. It must be treated quickly with high dose steroids, even before confirming the diagnosis with a temporal artery biopsy. Non-arteritic is due to compromise of the posterior ciliary vessels and leads to compartment-syndrome-like swelling of the optic nerve head.

25.11.2 DtDx: NAION vs AAION

To differentiate between AAION and NAION, history and exam are key. Recall the association between AAION and GCA – ask about symptoms associated with GCA like fatigue, fever, jaw claudication, and temporal pain. On exam, the appearance of the optic disc in NAION is typically hyperemic, whereas in AAION it is typically "pale with chalky-white edema." NAION classically causes sudden, painless, unilateral vision loss or blurred vision, and the visual changes may be limited to a portion of the visual field, classically to the inferior (from "sectoral optic disc swelling"). AAION can cause blurred vision, diplopia, or sudden complete vision loss unilaterally. Remember that GCA is one of the few diagnoses that can kill a patient presenting to the ophthalmology clinic, so it is a diagnosis that cannot be missed. ESR and CRP levels should be checked. Patients with GCA are treated with prolonged course of steroids.

Pseudotumor cerebri (aka Idiopathic Intracranial Hypertension (IIH)) is a condition caused by elevation of intracranial pressure. As its name ("false brain tumor") suggests, it presents with many symptoms characteristically thought of to be associated with brain tumors. Patients are typically overweight women in the 20s–40s, some of whom are on medications that are associated with this condition such as retinols, oral contraceptives, or tetracyclines. They present with headaches, visual disturbances (often short episodes of blindness after changing position rapidly, e.g., standing up after tying shoes), and pulsatile tinnitus. On exam, papilledema (Fig. 25.27) can be prominent. A more definitive diagnosis is made with a spinal tap that measures high opening pressure. The first recommended treatment is typically weight loss. This leads to resolution of symptoms for many patients. MRI and neurologist workup may be warranted. Concurrently, diuretics such as carbonic anhydrase inhibitors are started. If these interventions are successful, VP shunt placement may be recommended.

25.11.3 High-Yield Trials

- IONDT (1998) Ischemic Optic Neuropathy Decompression Trial
  - *Should you perform surgery to decompress the optic nerve head for NAION? Pathophysiology is like compartment syndrome so maybe a "fasciotomy" makes sense here? NO!* Not effective, may be harmful, many patients spontaneously resolve.

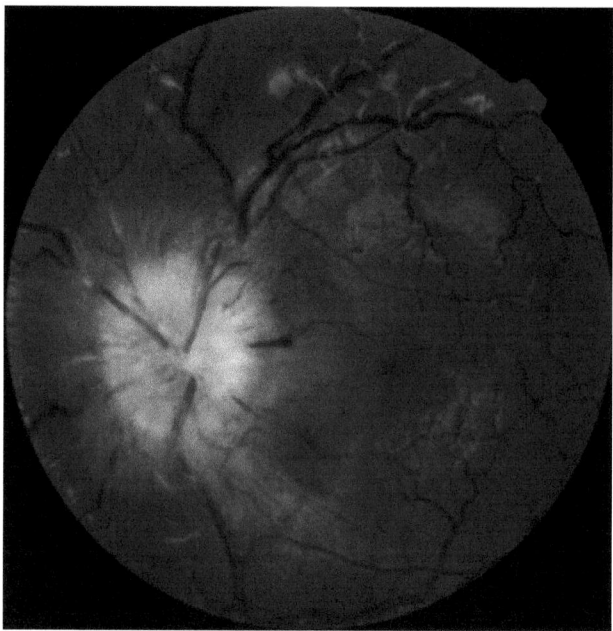

◘ Fig. 25.27 Papilledema in a 13-year-old boy who complained of 3 weeks of headaches and 1 week of double vision – diagnosed with pseudotumor cerebri. (Contributed by Dr. Eric Gaier, Assistant Professor of Ophthalmology, Harvard Medical School)

- ONTT (2013) Optic Neuritis Treatment Trial
  - *Should you give PO steroids to a patient with optic neuritis? No!* – PO steroids resulted in increased rate of recurrence. However, you should consider giving IV steroids as they accelerate rate of VF recovery (w/o improving the long-term visual outcome).
- IIHTD (2014) Idiopathic Intracranial Hypertension Treatment Trial
  - *Is acetazolamide beneficial in addition to a low-sodium diet and weight loss in the treatment of IIH? Yes* – patients who received acetazolamide achieved modest improvement on visual field tests.

25.11.4 Topics for Further Review

- The extensive differential diagnosis of papilledema (often organized by unilateral vs bilateral)

25.12 Retina

Medical students often find visualizing the retina at the slit lamp or with the indirect ophthalmoscope to be difficult. It is certainly a skill that develops with practice. This can be discouraging at the beginning but continue practicing at every opportunity and be sure to review content before, so you can know what to look for and make the most out of your time in retina clinic and ORs.

Age-related macular degeneration (AMD) is an incredibly common condition affecting over 15 million North Americans. It most commonly presents as blurry central vision, or a distortion of straight lines, called metamorphopsia. Patients are often given a grid with a dot in the center (called an Amsler grid) to monitor for progression of the symptoms. AMD is subcategorized into dry macular degeneration and wet macular degeneration. Dry is less severe and is monitored with little treatment available besides smoking cessation, green vegetables, and vitamins. Antioxidants can prevent or slow progression from dry to wet (AREDS vitamins – discussed in ▶ Sect. 25.12.2). Wet macular degeneration is characterized by choroidal neovascularization and macular edema. It can lead to rapid deterioration of visual acuity. The retinal exam of dry macular degeneration is characterized by numerous drusen (small collections of yellowish lipid deposits in Bruch's membrane deep in the retina) (refer to ◧ Fig. 25.9 earlier in the chapter). Bruch's membrane is a basement membrane that separates the retinal pigment epithelium (RPE) and the deeper choroidal vasculature. Drusen collect in Bruch's membrane and prevents the exchange of oxygen and nutrients leading to increased VEGF production and atrophy of the macula. Wet macular degeneration is characterized by hemorrhage and edema. Wet AMD can be treated with a regimen of anti-VEGF injections to decrease the neovascularization and associated edema.

Diabetic eye disease is another disease of abnormal vessel proliferation. Hyperglycemia leads to hyalinization of the endothelium of retinal vessels. These vessels form microaneurysms and can burst and create areas of ischemia, leading to the characteristic retinal findings of dot-blot hemorrhages and cotton-wool spots (fluffy gray-white lesions of microinfarction) (refer to ◧ Fig. 25.10 earlier in the chapter). There are two broad classifications of diabetic retinopathy: non-proliferative diabetic retinopathy (NPDR) and proliferative diabetic retinopathy (PDR). PDR is the more advanced form, where the ischemic state of the eye results in retinal neovascularization, which can cause vision loss from macular edema (leaky vessels), vitreous hemorrhage, tractional retinal detachments (from contracting neovascular membranes), acute glaucoma (neovascularization of the iris or angle), and higher rates of PSC cataracts. The most common cause of vision loss is diabetic macular edema (DME), which can be seen in either NPDR or PDR (◧ Fig. 25.28). DME is usually treated with anti-VEGF injections but focal laser treatments and steroids are options as well. PDR is treated with either or both anti-VEGF injection and panretinal photocoagulation (◧ Fig. 25.29).

Retinal detachment refers to a separation between the sensorineural retina and the underlying retinal pigment epithelium (and choroidal blood supply) (◧ Fig. 25.30). Without surgical intervention retinal detachments lead to ischemia and cell death. Retinal detachments are categorized into three groups based on their mechanism: tractional (TRD), rhegmatogenous (RRD), and exudative (ERD). TRDs are caused when traction from a membrane pulls the retina off its base. This is often either from neovascular diseases such as diabetic

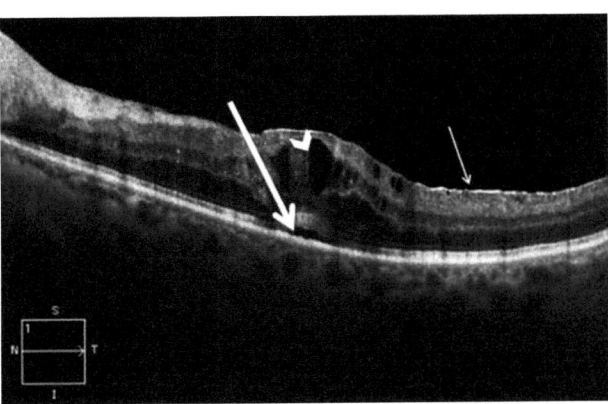

◧ **Fig. 25.28** OCT of diabetic macular edema with epiretinal membrane (arrow), cystic changes (arrowhead) and subretinal fluid (large arrow). (From "OCT in the Management of Diabetic Macular Edema")

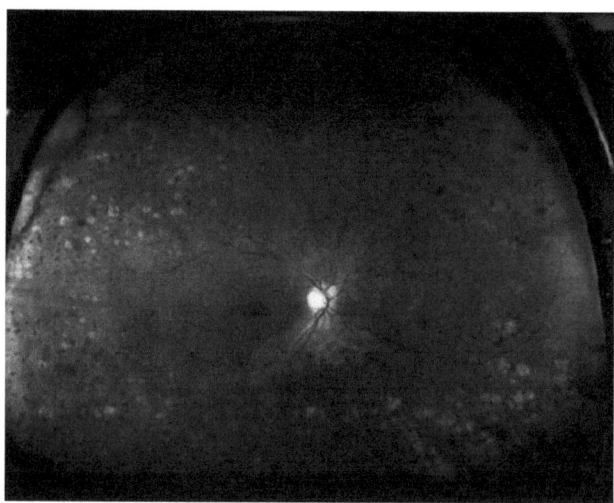

□ Fig. 25.29 Ultrawide field photograph demonstrating an eye that has undergone panretinal photocoagulation (PRP). (From "Vitreoretinal Disorders" pp 71–89 **ISBN:** 978–981–10-8544-4)

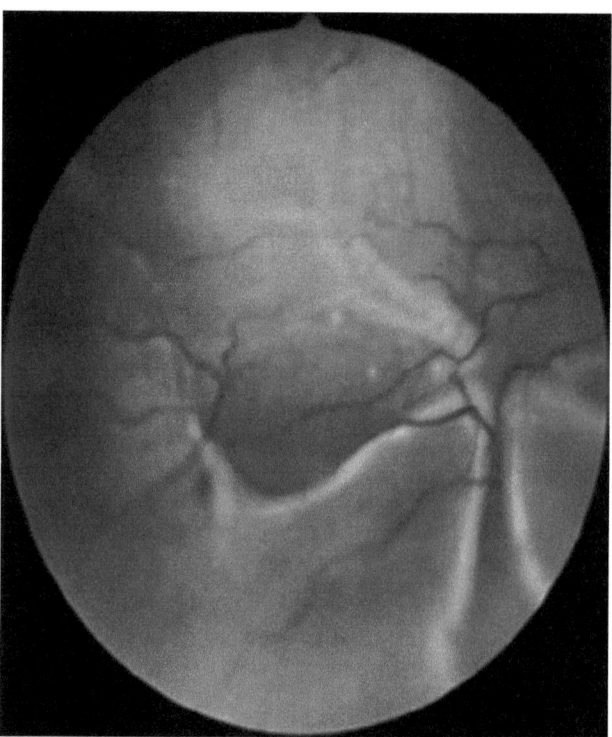

□ Fig. 25.30 Fundus photo depicting a rhegmatogenous retinal detachment with early proliferative virtreoretinopathy. (From "Hypopyon, conjunctival injection and purulent discharge associated with postoperative endophthalmitis." PMID: **18356929**)

retinopathy or retinopathy of prematurity or from scar tissue that forms in the setting of RRD, called proliferative vitreoretinopathy. RRD refers to retinal detachment caused by a full-thickness break in the retina, most commonly in the setting of PVD formation. RRDs are the most common cause of retinal detachment. ERDs are the least common type and refer to the buildup of fluid under the retina that pushes it off of its nourishing base. This could occur secondary to tumors, vascular diseases, inflammation (uveitis), and even some medications (such as chemotherapy agents – MEK inhibitors). Treatments for retinal detachment all aim to reestablish contact between the retina and RPE. The specific modality depends on the underlying cause (Topics for Further Review). Among the options are vitrectomy, scleral buckling, and pneumatic retinopexy.

What determines the urgency of the intervention? The status of the macula! If the macula remains attached ("mac-on") for RRDs, the surgery is usually urgent, as the central vision is preserved, and it is vital to prevent the detachment from spreading and affecting the macula. If the macula is already detached ("mac-off"), the surgery should still be performed promptly within several days usually, but it is not an emergency.

Pearl: A specific slit lamp finding you might observe in the anterior vitreous of a patient with a retinal tear is depicted with the buzzword "tobacco dust" (aka Shafer's sign – ◘ Fig. 25.31), which is small amounts of pigmented cells suspended in the vitreous.

25.12.1 DtDx: Floaters

Most patients will endorse floaters if you ask. It is important to get at whether they have increased in number recently. For patients who reply yes or who bring this up unprompted, consider posterior vitreous detachment, retinal tears/detachments, or debris floating in the vitreous (e.g., RBCs from a vitreous hemorrhage or WBCs from uveitis). PVDs and RDs must be differentiated by a thorough retinal exam, although patients with an RD will often report hundreds of floaters and perhaps a visual field deficit as compared to a handful of floaters and no visual field deficit with a PVD. Vitreous hemorrhage might manifest as a dark reddish tint or a "dark cloud" obscuring vision along with those floaters, and commonly occurs in patients with a known history of diabetic retinopathy. Uveitis or endophthalmitis can present with new floaters in the context of pain or photophobia.

There are some systemic medicines you might have heard about in medical school that have retinal side effects. The most common one that you'll see in ophthalmology clinic is patients with lupus or rheumatoid arthritis on hydroxychloroquine (aka Plaquenil). It can cause central vision loss and damage to the RPE called "*bulls-eye maculopathy,*" and if this develops the medication is recommended to be stopped, because the vision loss is permanent and can keep progressing. This finding presents on fundus exam as a darkening ring around the macula. There are other causes of bulls-eye maculopathy, such as retinal degenerations. Below is a sample presentation of one of these visits.

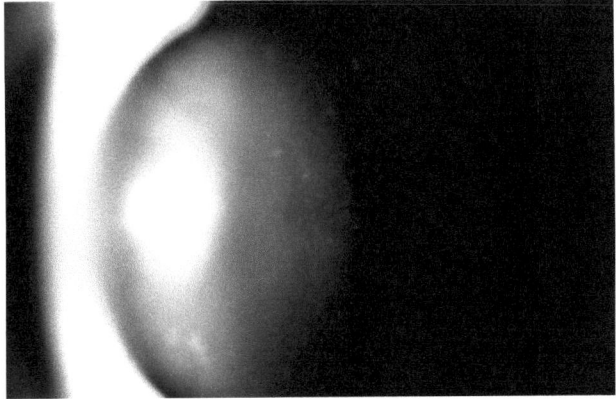

◘ **Fig. 25.31**   Depiction of a positive Shafer sign – pigment granules in the anterior vitreous. (From "Posterior Vitreous Detachment from Vitreoretinal Surgery" ISBN: 978-3-540-37581-4)

■ **Sample Presentation**

Ms. Z is a 64-year-old woman with lupus on hydroxychloroquine for the last 5 years, here for her 6-month screening. She has had no changes in her dose regimen and reports no new visual symptoms. On exam, she has 1+ nuclear sclerotic cataracts bilaterally. I did not appreciate any signs of retinal toxicity, particularly RPE changes around the macula. The OCT and visual field testing were normal. Therefore, I would plan to have her continue her current medication regimen, discuss with her the expected progression of her cataract over the next few years, and see her back for a follow-up in 6 months.

Central retinal vein occlusion (CRVO) (◘ Fig. 25.32) is caused by reduced outflow of the retinal vein, via compression or a clot. This causes fluid and blood to leak from the vein. A CRVO can be thought of as a "DVT of the eye." Patients classically complain of blurry or distorted vision, which may be intermittent. The often-striking fundus exam reveals prominent flame hemorrhages and cotton-wool spots (refer to ◘ Fig. 25.10 from earlier in the chapter). CRVO can be differentiated into "ischemic CRVO" and "nonischemic CRVO" based on the degree of the non-perfusion of the retina. Fluorescein angiography is a useful tool to differentiate between these subtypes. Risk factors for CRVO overlap with those for DVT (atherosclerosis, hypertension, diabetes, etc.). The prognosis of CRVO is often poor due to associations with neovascular glaucoma and retinal detachment. These complications are due to elevated VEGF; therefore treatment with anti-VEGF injections (bevacizumab, ranibizumab, aflibercept) is often indicated.

Central retinal artery occlusion (CRAO) (◘ Fig. 25.33) most commonly results from an embolic event but can also occur secondary to local arteriosclerotic changes. It can be thought of as a "stroke of the eye." Patients classically complain of acute, nonpainful, monocular vision loss. On fundus examination, the ischemic retina swells and loses its transparency, which results in a broadly whiter retina. However, as this swelling occurs particularly in layers of the retina (Topics for Further Review) that are not found in the fovea, the normal color of the choroid remains visible there, leading to the classic finding of a *cherry-red spot*. The risks factors for CRAO overlap with those for embolic and thrombotic stroke *[ipsilateral carotid artery atherosclerosis, cardiogenic*

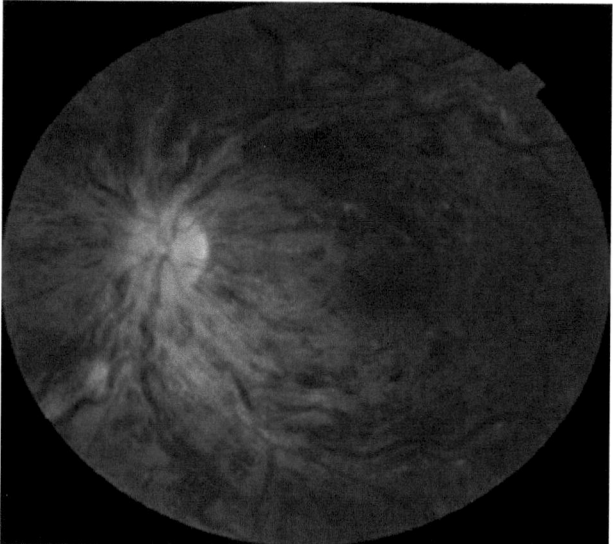

◘ **Fig. 25.32**   CRVO. (From "How does hypertension affect your eyes?" PMID: 21509040)

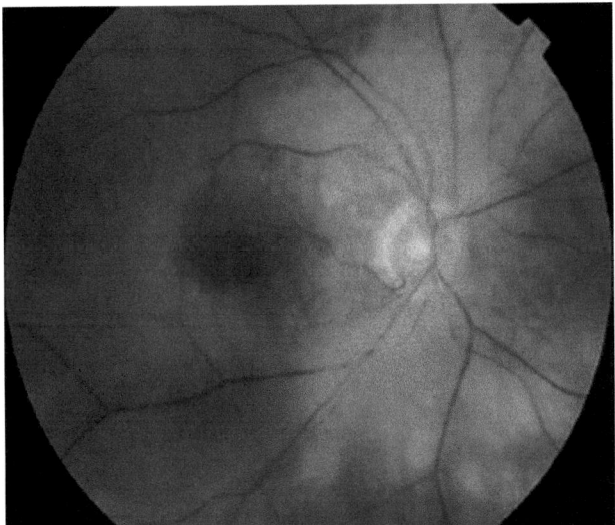

◘ **Fig. 25.33** CRAO. (From "A review of central retinal artery occlusion: clinical presentation and management" PMID: 23470793)

embolism, carotid artery dissection, diabetes/vascular disease, hypercoagulable states (especially malignancy), and sickle cell disease]. Therefore, it is easy to remember that *systemic evaluation is vital!* Patients require imaging of the carotid arteries, followed by an echo and atrial fibrillation evaluation if the carotid examination is unremarkable. Treatment is aimed at maximizing visual recovery. Goals for treatment include dislodging the clot and moving it further down the vasculature (via ocular massage and hyperbaric oxygen therapy) and managing IOP (via drops or surgery) as necessary.

25.12.2 High-Yield Trials

- DRS (1975) (Diabetic Retinopathy Study)
  - *Does photocoagulation help prevent severe visual loss from proliferative diabetic retinopathy? YES!* – subjects randomized to photocoagulation had 60% reduced risk of blindness at 2 years and the trial was ended early.
- ETDRS (1989) (Early Treatment of Diabetic Retinopathy Study)
  - *Is there a benefit to focal macular laser in the treatment of diabetic macular edema? Yes.*
  - *Does scatter laser PRP reduce the risk of vision loss? Yes.*
    - *When should it be initiated? It can be delayed until the development of severe non-proliferative or early proliferative stage retinopathy.*
- BVOS (1984) (Branch Vein Occlusion Study)
  - *For patients with macular edema and VA of 20/40 or worse secondary to BRVO, is macular grid laser photocoagulation beneficial? Yes* – although wait 3 months to allow for resolution of macular edema. If macular edema persists, use fluorescein angiography to evaluate the extent of the ischemia. If macula is still perfused and there is no fovea hemorrhage, proceed with laser grid photocoagulation.
- CVOS (1995) (Central Vein Occlusion Study)
  - *For non-perfused CRVO, is immediate prophylactic PRP beneficial? No.*
  - *For patients with macular edema and VA of 20/50 or worse secondary to CRVO, is macular grid laser photocoagulation beneficial? No.*

- Prophylactic PRP also doesn't prevent iris or angle neovascularization after CRVO. PRP should only be performed after CRVO when active neovascular disease is apparent.
= SCORE (2009) (Standard Care vs. Corticosteroid for Retina Vein Occlusion)
  - *Is there benefit to intravitreal corticosteroid injection for patients with CRVO (since CVOS showed observation is equivalent to laser)? – Yes!*
= EVS (1999) (Endophthalmitis Vitrectomy Study)
  - *Is there any benefit to vitrectomy vs a "tap and inject" for patients with endophthalmitis?* Not for patients with a VA of hand motion or better. Some benefit of immediate vitrectomy for patients with light perception VA or worse.
= AREDS (1 and 2)
  - *Is there a vitamin/antioxidant combination that can reduce the likelihood of progression to advanced age-related macular degeneration for patients at high risk of progression?* Yes – subjects given AREDS vitamins received a 34% reduction of risk of progression to advanced AMD.
= MARINA and ANCHOR (2006)
  - *Does ranibizumab (Lucentis) prevent vision loss in patients with AMD and central neovascularization?* Yes, and it actually improved visual acuity in this group, which was the first-time visual acuity improved in wet AMD.
= CATT (2011) (Comparison of Age-Related Macular Degeneration Treatments Trials)
  - *Is there an advantage to using either bevacizumab or ranibizumab in AMD? No –* there was statistical equivalence between visual outcomes of the two treatments at 2 years
= DRCR Protocol I (2010) (Diabetic Retinopathy Clinical Research)
  - *For patients with diabetic macular edema, ranibizumab + laser vs laser alone vs laser + triamcinolone? Ranibizumab + Laser*
= DRCR Protocol S (2015) (Diabetic Retinopathy Clinical Research)
  - *Is ranibizumab an effective alternative to PRP for the treatment of PDR? - Yes*
= DRCR Protocol T (2016) (Diabetic Retinopathy Clinical Research)
  - *For patients with diabetic macular edema, bevacizumab (Avastin) vs ranibizumab (Lucentis) vs aflibercept (Eylea)?* VA improved in all three treatment arms over 2 years. In eyes with presenting VA of 20/50 or worse, aflibercept had superior visual outcomes until 2 years.

25.12.3   Surgical Techniques and Topics for Further Review

= Vitrectomy (■ Fig. 25.34)
= Scleral buckles (■ Fig. 25.34)
= Pneumatic retinopexy
= Cryopexy
= Techniques of laser photocoagulation
= Extraretinal membrane peeling all of the layers and cell types of the retina

25.13 Infection and Inflammation

Infections and inflammation of the eye are a common complaint that brings patients to the ophthalmologist. Infections can vary in severity from minor eyelid inflammation to sight and life-threatening infections of the eye and

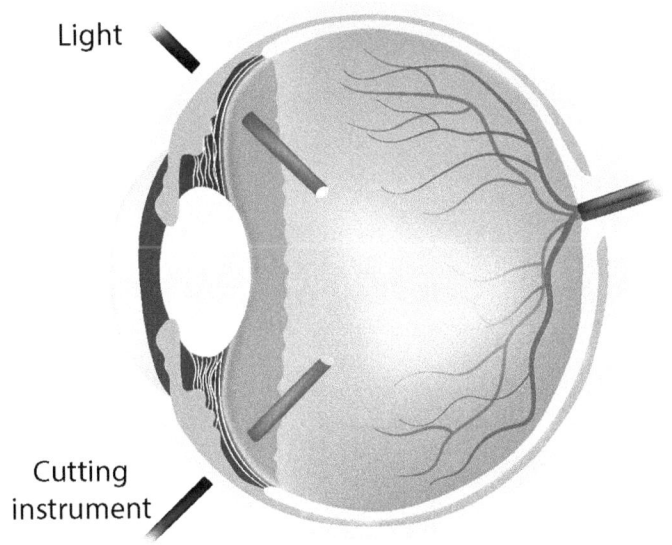

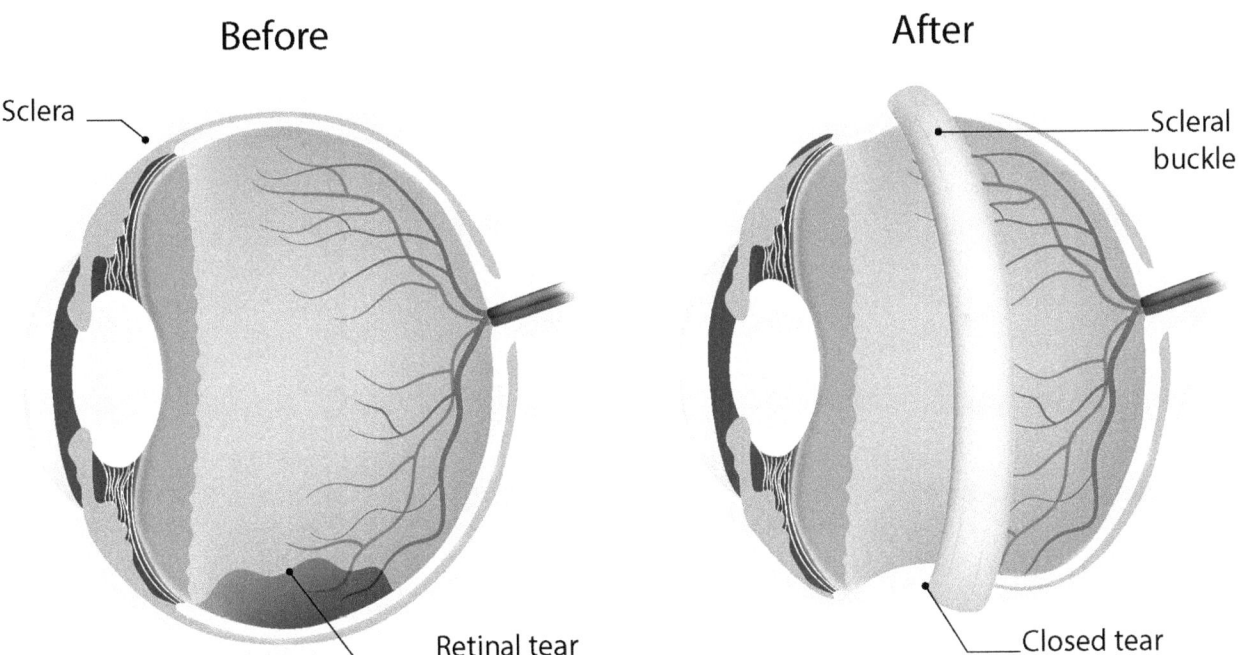

□ Fig. 25.34 Diagram of a vitrectomy and a scleral buckle placed to help treat a retinal detachment

surrounding structures. Inflammation can be secondary to infection or to rheumatologic/autoimmune processes.

Blepharitis is inflammation of the eyelid. It is a very prevalent problem, particularly among the elderly. It presents with symptoms of eyelid irritation, itching, dry eye, tearing, visible discharge, and "scruff" around the bases of eyelashes. The eyelids can also be thickened with eyelid margin telangiectasias. Applying pressure on the eyelid while visualizing the meibomian gland ducts can indicate a diagnosis of meibomian gland dysfunction if pus like material is expressed rather than clear fluid. These findings can be appreciated with a slit lamp examination. Blepharitis can be treated with "good lid hygiene." This includes warm compresses, lid massage, and occasional scrubbing of the lids with baby soap.

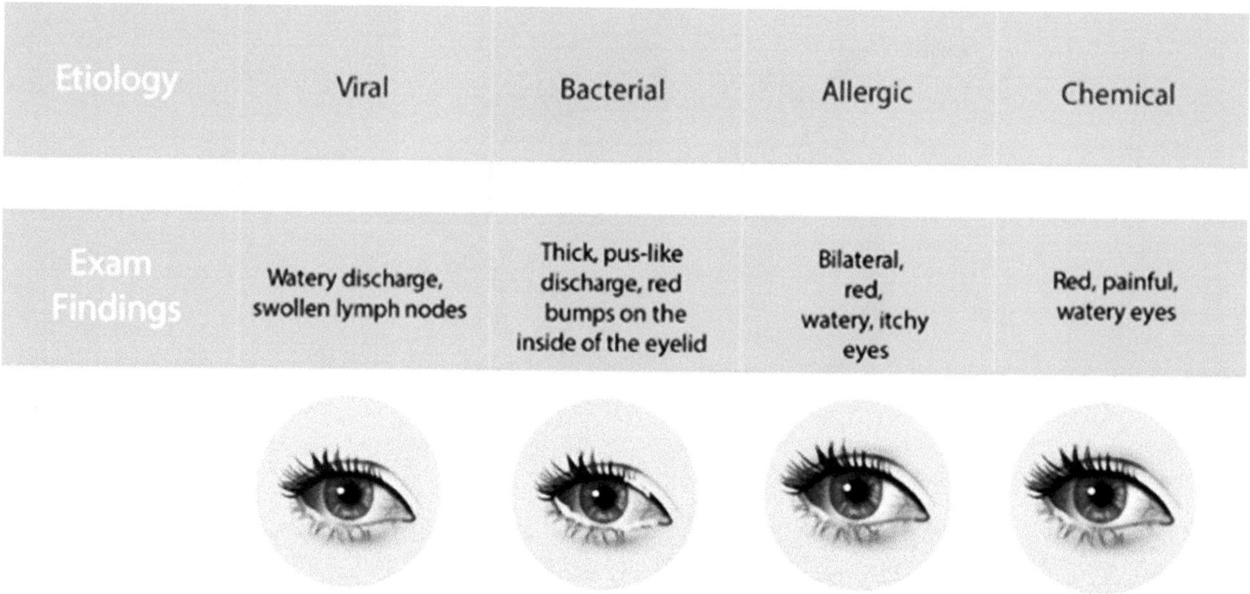

25

Etiology	Viral	Bacterial	Allergic	Chemical
Exam Findings	Watery discharge, swollen lymph nodes	Thick, pus-like discharge, red bumps on the inside of the eyelid	Bilateral, red, watery, itchy eyes	Red, painful, watery eyes

Fig. 25.35 Differentiating the differential – conjunctivitis

Conjunctivitis is inflammation of the conjunctiva. It can be subcategorized as bacterial, viral, allergic, or chemical (□ Fig. 25.35). Although the specific etiologies have different presentations (discussed in the following ▶ Sect. 25.13.1), all present with redness and discharge from the affected eye. Patients might also complain of discomfort or foreign body sensation. It is vital to ask patients whether they wear contacts, as if so, they should immediately stop wearing them as they can increase the severity of conjunctivitis and predispose to infection with more robust pathogens (particularly *Pseudomonas*). Treatment varies by etiology, but for bacterial should include antibiotic drops.

■ **Sample Presentation**

Mrs. L is a 39-year-old day care teacher who presents with 2 days of conjunctival redness and watery discharge. She reports that some children in her class had similar symptoms last week. She denies visual complaints or a history of seasonal allergies. She does not wear contact lenses. On exam she has copious watery discharge bilaterally and swollen pre-auricular lymph nodes. I think she has viral conjunctivitis and therefore should be advised to follow best hygiene practices and stay away from the day care until she is asymptomatic. She should be counseled to call if the symptoms worsen or fail to improve with time that would increase the likelihood that this may be bacterial conjunctivitis.

Uveitis refers to inflammation of the uvea (reminder: iris, ciliary body, and choroid). Uveitis is classified according to the affected structure. Anterior uveitis (iritis or iridocyclitis), intermediate uveitis (cyclitis), posterior uveitis (choroiditis, retinitis, vitritis) and panuveitis (both anterior and posterior involvement) are common terms you may hear used. It can be due to infection/inflammation of these structures or secondary to rheumatologic diseases (like sarcoidosis, IBD, lupus, ankylosing spondylitis). It can present as eye pain, eye redness, floaters, photophobia, or blurry vision. On exam, secondary evidence of the inflammation can be prominent, particularly white blood cells in the anterior chamber, either floating or layering into a hypopyon. Keratic precipitates (KPs) are WBCs that have adhered to the corneal endothelium and appear as tiny white spots on the back surface of the cornea (□ Fig. 25.36).

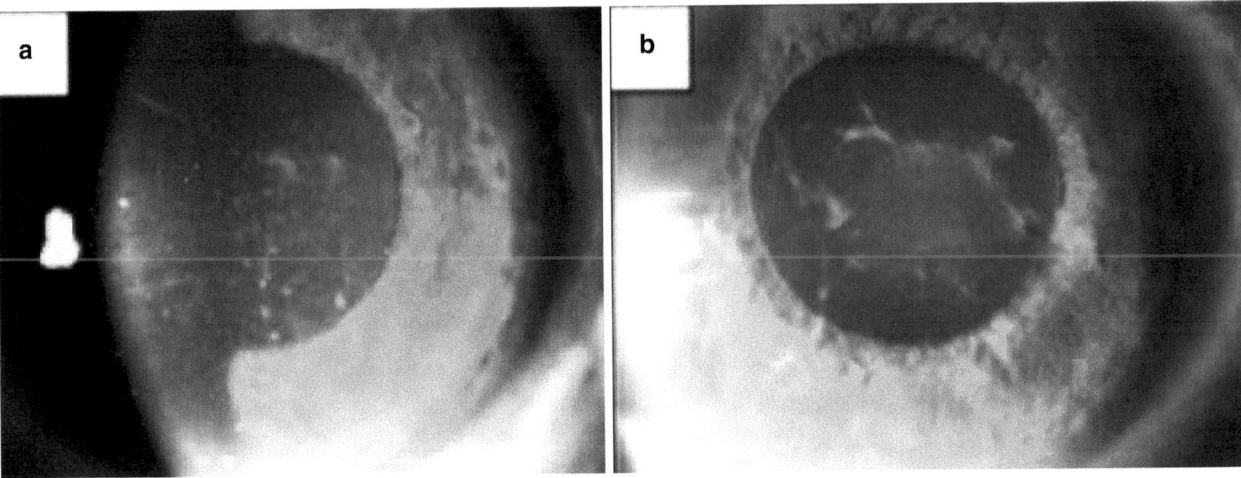

■ **Fig. 25.36   a, b** Keratic precipitates in a patient with endogenous endopthalmitis. (From *"Propionibacterium acnes* endogenous endophthalmitis presenting with bilateral scleritis and uveitis" PMID: 19648894)

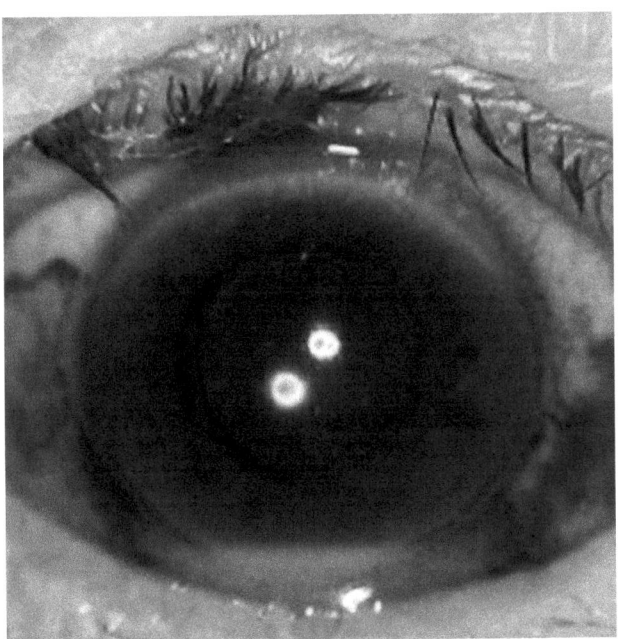

■ **Fig. 25.37**   An external photograph of an eye with hypopyon, conjunctival injection and purulent discharge secondary to postoperative endophthalmitis. (From "Postoperative endophthalmitis: optimal management and the role and timing of vitrectomy surgery" PMID: 18356929)

Ciliary flush (conjunctival injection around the limbus) is common in anterior uveitis. Signs of iritis can be found in the form of posterior synechia (iris that has adhered to the anterior lens). Treatment is based on the etiology but can include anti-inflammatory medications or eye injections, oral steroids, or various prescription eye drops (see "Options for Management of Uveitis")

Endophthalmitis is infection within the globe (■ Fig. 25.37). The biggest risk factor is recent eye surgery (exogenous endophthalmitis), but it can be endogenous endophthalmitis secondary to infection in another part of the body (like endocarditis). Endophthalmitis typically presents with a consistent history and quickly progressively increasing pain and visual dysfunction. On exam, the eye can be injected and painful with white blood cells seen in the anterior chamber and the vitreous cavity. It is evaluated and often treated with a "tap and inject." This procedure is the removal of a small amount of vitreous humor for diagnostic purposes followed by the injection of antibiotics. Close follow-up is needed, as this is a vision threatening condition that may require surgical intervention and could result in losing the eye altogether.

Soft tissue infections of the structures surrounding the eye are common. You may be called to evaluate a patient with a clear cellulitis around the eye. The primary team or emergency department will want your input as to whether the infection is preseptal cellulitis or orbital cellulitis, as they have different prognosis and require vastly different treatment regimens. The difference between these conditions is whether the infection is entirely superficial to the septum, which is connective tissue between the tarsal plate of the eyelid and the orbital rim, or whether it tracks back into the orbit.

25.13.1   DtDx: Preseptal vs Orbital Cellulitis

Both will present with redness of the skin around the orbit, swelling, and pain to palpation. However, if the infection tracts back into the orbit, it may affect the function of other orbital structures. Therefore, patients might have pain with eye movement, proptosis, decreased vision or decreased color vision (a consequence of pressure/irritation of the optic nerve), or diminished/absent function of structures that run through the cavernous sinus (CN III, IV, VI, and the V1 and V2 distributions of CNV). Treatment for preseptal cellulitis may be limited to oral antibiotics and treatment for orbital cellulitis is more aggressive, often including intravenous antibiotics and possibly surgical debridement.

25.13.2   Options for Management of Uveitis

- *Medical*
  - Eyedrops
    - Steroids, such as prednisolone, which decrease ocular inflammation
    - Cycloplegics, such as cyclopentolate, which prevent contraction of the ciliary muscle (and thus accommodation – causing blurry vision) and subsequent pain, and also prevent posterior synechiae
  - Injections (sub-Tenon, peribulbar, or intravitreal)
    - Steroids such as *triamcinolone*
  - Systemic
    - Steroids such as oral *glucocorticoids*
    - Antimetabolites such as *methotrexate*
    - Biologics such as the anti-TNF-alpha medication *infliximab*
- *Surgical*
  - Surgical correction of secondary complications such as cataract and epiretinal membranes may become necessary. Surgical implantation of fluocinolone implants (Retisert) provides local control.

25.13.3   High-Yield Trials

- MUST (2011) (Multicenter Uveitis Steroid Treatment)

> – *Is it better to treat active uveitis with systemic treatment (oral steroids +/– immunosuppressive meds) or an intraocular steroid implant?* Both treatments improve visual acuity. Neither is obviously superior. Consider the individual patient as both treatments have side effects.

25.13.4   Topics for Further Review

- Scleritis
- Episcleritis
- Rheumatologic causes of uveitis and their evaluation

25.14 Oculoplastics

Oculoplastics is a diverse subspecialty of ophthalmology. Many patients present due to lumps on the eyelid. While skin cancers and benign skin growths should always remain on the differential, often you will see them after a referral and as a student you can determine whether they are a stye or a chalazion. A *stye* is effectively a pimple of the eye: an infection of a hair follicle or sebaceous gland. It is painful to touch, and you may need to evert the eyelid to see it. A *chalazion* is a granulomatous reaction around built-up lipid secretions from a blocked meibomian gland that is generally non-tender. It can grow to significant size. Styes often self-resolve. Some chalazions can be reduced by good lid hygiene to unblock the meibomian glands and allow material to flow out, but some require steroid injection or surgical excision.

Malposition of the eyelids either turning outward (*ectropion*) or inward (*entropion*) can result from scarring, muscle weakness, or other, diverse disease processes. Ectropion is associated with laxity of the lower eyelid allowing the eyelid to pull away from the globe which can cause dry eye. Entropion can cause corneal irritation via eyelashes scraping the cornea with each blink that can result in abrasion and scarring. Both types of malposition can cause exposure keratitis if they prevent a full closure of the eyelids. Mild cases can be treated with artificial tears, rewetting ointments (ectropion), or eyelash removal (entropion). Surgical treatment is often necessary – rotating the eyelid skin accordingly into its proper position.

Ptosis is defined as drooping or falling of the upper eyelid or brow. It can be congenital, due to CNIII or sympathetic chain damage, traumatic injury, or neuromuscular disease (e.g., myasthenia gravis). Depending on the severity, it can be vision limiting. If a reversible etiology is suspected, it might be reasonable to delay surgical repair. Otherwise, for functional or cosmetic reasons, surgical repair to tighten the eyelid retractor is warranted.

Ocular malignancies can be primary or secondary (metastatic). The most common primary ocular malignancy is ocular melanoma (◻ Fig. 25.38). Periocular malignancies such as squamous cell carcinoma, basal cell carcinoma, or melanoma may first be detected at the slit lamp (refer to the dermatology chapter of this textbook for a refresher on these). While uncommon, cancers can metastasize to the eye (most commonly from lung and breast primary malignancies) (◻ Fig. 25.39).

Thyroid eye disease (TED) is an indication for a visit to an oculoplastic physician. The most common manifestation of thyroid eye disease is dry eye (from decreased tear production). It can progress to severe pain and visual field disturbances. TED can cause the eye muscles to swell and expand resulting in protruding eyes (proptosis), upper eyelid retraction, and diplopia. This disease

Pearl: Hering's Law refers to an interesting phenomenon seen following unilateral ptosis repair. If one eyelid is ptotic and surgically is lifted, often the fellow eyelid becomes ptotic. This is because the two levator palpabrae muscles are equally innervated. The surgically repaired one no longer requires as much force to remain elevated, so the force transmitted to the fellow eyelid also decreases and ptosis results. This law must be considered during surgical planning and while counseling patients before surgery.

Pearl: The most impactful thing a patient with thyroid eye disease can do to prevent worsening of their disease is to avoid smoking!

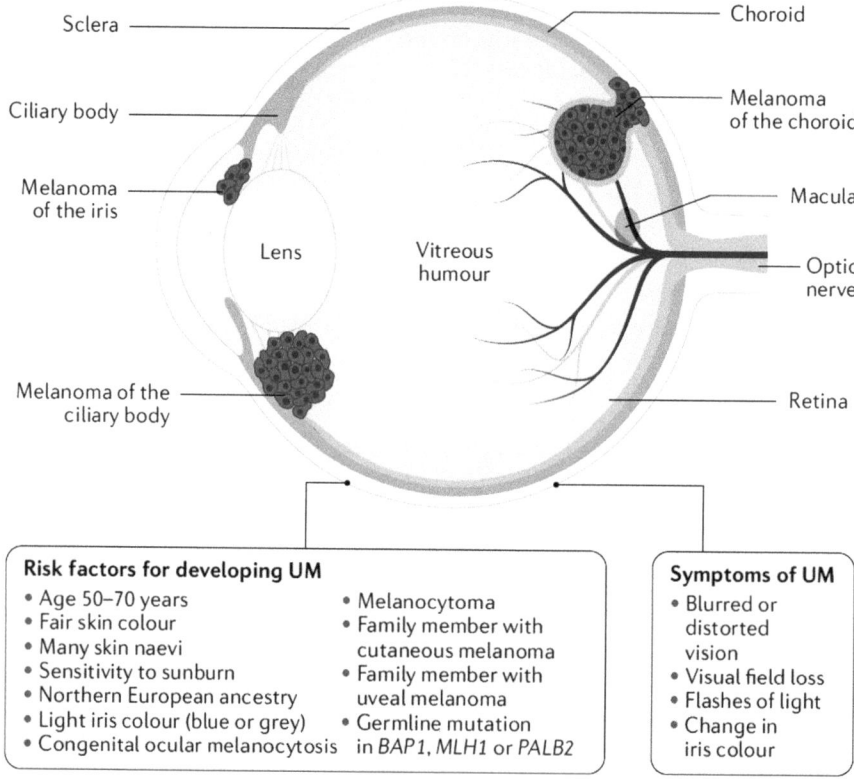

Sclera

Choroid

Ciliary body

Melanoma
of the choroid

Melanoma
of the iris

Macula

Lens

Vitreous
humour

Optic
nerve

Melanoma of the
ciliary body

Retina

Risk factors for developing UM
- Age 50–70 years
- Fair skin colour
- Many skin naevi
- Sensitivity to sunburn
- Northern European ancestry
- Light iris colour (blue or grey)
- Congenital ocular melanocytosis

- Melanocytoma
- Family member with
  cutaneous melanoma
- Family member with
  uveal melanoma
- Germline mutation
  in *BAP1*, *MLH1* or *PALB2*

Symptoms of UM
- Blurred or
  distorted
  vision
- Visual field loss
- Flashes of light
- Change in
  iris colour

◘ **Fig. 25.38** A thorough depiction of uveal melanoma: locations, risk factors, and symptoms. (From Jager MJ, Shields CL, Cebulla CM, et al. Uveal melanoma. *Nat Rev Dis Primers* 6:24; 2020)

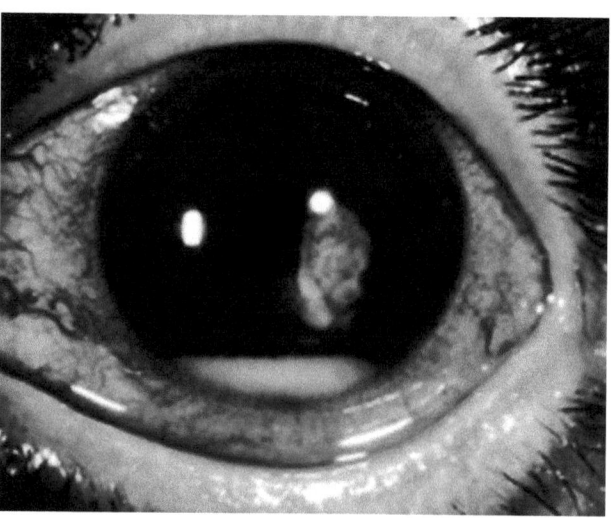

◘ **Fig. 25.39** An external photograph of an eye with a metastatic tumor and a tumor-related hypopyon. (From "Postoperative endophthalmitis: optimal management and the role and timing of vitrectomy surgery" PMID: 18356929)

typically affects hyperthyroid patients but can afflict hypothyroid or euthyroid patients as well. Management is begun with symptomatic treatment/conservative management, artificial tears and lubrication, and topical steroids, but oral/ injectable steroids may become necessary for symptom control. There are many surgical techniques for TED (Topics for Further Review), most commonly *orbital decompression surgery* (which involves the removal of bones +/− orbital fat), but also strabismus surgery, eyelid surgery, and cosmetic surgery.

■ **Sample Presentation**

Mrs. Y is a hemiparetic 83-year-old woman s/p ischemic stroke in 2016 and w/ IOL OU placed in 2008. She was referred due to her PCP noticing her eyes were not completely closing and her complaints of eye pain. She comes complaining of foreign body sensation and decreased visual acuity. On exam, left upper lid is ptotic and her left lower lid presents with significant ectropion. Her tear film breakup time is abnormal, and she has numerous small corneal erosions. I think she is developing exposure keratopathy due to her facial paralysis. She has never tried lubricating drops or any other treatment. I would suggest we try a strict regimen of lubricating ointments and drops and see her back in 2 weeks. If there is no improvement, we could consider eyelid surgery to reduce her ectropion, or a partial tarsorrhaphy.

25.14.1 Surgical Techniques for Further Review

— Consider reviewing the basic techniques involved in correcting the following pathologies:
  - Entropion and ectropion
  - Ptosis
  - TED surgeries and their pros/cons

Supplementary Information

© The Author(s), under exclusive license to Springer Nature Switzerland AG 2021
S. H. Lecker, B. J. Chang (eds.), *The Ultimate Medical School Rotation Guide*,
https://doi.org/10.1007/978-3-030-63560-2

Index

Index

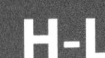